End-of-Life Care

A Practical Guide

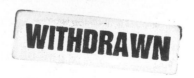

NORTHEAST COMMUNITY COLLEGE LIBRARY

Notice

Medicine is an ever-changing science. As new research and clinical experience broaden our knowledge, changes in treatment and drug therapy are required. The authors and the publisher of this work have checked with sources believed to be reliable in their efforts to provide information that is complete and generally in accord with the standards accepted at the time of publication. However, in view of the possibility of human error or changes in medical sciences, neither the authors nor the publisher nor any other party who has been involved in the preparation or publication of this work warrants that the information contained herein is in every respect accurate or complete, and they disclaim all responsibility for any errors or omissions or for the results obtained from use of the information contained in this work. Readers are encouraged to confirm the information contained herein with other sources. For example and in particular, readers are advised to check the product information sheet included in the package of each drug they plan to administer to be certain that the information contained in this work is accurate and that changes have not been made in the recommended dose or in the contraindications for administration. This recommendation is of particular importance in connection with new or infrequently used drugs.

WITHDRAWN

End-of-Life Care

A Practical Guide

Second Edition

EDITORS

Barry M. Kinzbrunner, MD

Executive Vice President and Chief Medical Officer
VITAS Innovative Hospice Care, Miami, Florida
Voluntary Assistant Professor of Medicine
Herbert Wertheim College of Medicine
Florida International University, Miami, Florida
Voluntary Assistant Professor of Medicine
Miller School of Medicine
University of Miami, Miami, Florida

Joel S. Policzer, MD

Senior Vice President–National Medical Director
VITAS Innovative Hospice Care, Miami, Florida
Voluntary Assistant Professor of Family Medicine
University of Miami Miller School of Medicine, Miami, Florida
Associate Clinical Professor of Medicine
Nova Southeastern University College of Osteopathic Medicine
Fort Lauderdale, Florida
Voluntary Assistant Professor of Medicine
Herbert Wertheim College of Medicine
Florida International University, Miami, Florida

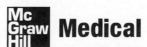

Medical

New York   Chicago   San Francisco   Lisbon   London   Madrid   Mexico City   Milan
New Delhi   San Juan   Seoul   Singapore   Sydney   Toronto

362.175
E565e

The McGraw·Hill Companies

End-of-Life Care: A Practical Guide, Second Edition

Copyright © 2011 by the McGraw-Hill Companies, Inc. All rights reserved. Printed in the United States of America. Except as permitted under the United States Copyright Act of 1976, no part of this publication may be reproduced or distributed in any form or by any means, or stored in a database or retrieval system, without the prior written permission of the publisher.

Previous edition published as *20 Common Problems in End-of-Life Care*, copyright © 2002 by the McGraw-Hill Companies.

2 3 4 5 6 7 8 9 0 DOC/DOC 14 13 12 11

ISBN 978-0-07-154527-3
MHID 0-07-154527-1

This book was set in Times Roman by Aptara®, Inc.
The editors were James F. Shanahan and Peter J. Boyle.
The production supervisor was Sherri Souffrance.
Project management was provided by Baljinder Kaur, Aptara, Inc.
The designer was Eve Siegel.
The cover design was by Barsoom Design; photo: Dennis Welsh/Getty Images.
RR Donnelley was printer and binder.

This book is printed on acid-free paper.

Library of Congress Cataloging-in-Publication Data

End of life care : a practical guide / editors, Barry M. Kinzbrunner, Joel S. Policzer. – 2nd ed.
   p. ; cm.
  Rev. ed. of: 20 common problems in end-of-life care / editors, Barry M. Kinzbrunner,
Neal J. Weinreb, Joel S. Policzer. c2002.
   Includes bibliographical references and index.
   ISBN-13: 978-0-07-154527-3 (alk. paper)
   ISBN-10: 0-07-154527-1 (alk. paper)
   1. Terminal care.   2. Terminally ill–Care.   3. Hospice care.   I. Kinzbrunner, Barry M.
II. Policzer, Joel S.   III. 20 common problems in end-of-life care.
   [DNLM: 1. Terminal Care–methods.   2. Advance Directives.   3. Palliative Care–methods.
4. Palliative Care–psychology.   5. Terminal Care–psychology.   WB 310]
   R726.8.A15 2011
   362.1'75–dc22   2010041766

McGraw-Hill books are available at special quantity discounts to use as premiums and sales promotions, or for use in corporate training programs. To contact a representative please e-mail us at bulksales@mcgraw-hill.com.

*This book is dedicated to my wife Anita and our children,
their wives, and their children (our grandchildren):
Bryan & Shira, and Zev
Eric & Suri, Avi, Eli, and Shimshon
Seth & Rebecca
Your love and devotion continue to be an inspiration and
make everything worthwhile.*
—BMK—

*I dedicate this work to:
—the memory of my beloved grandfather, Jakob Policzer,
who was the first to show me dying with grace and dignity
—my wife Madeleine, my best friend and my support,
who makes it all possible
—my children Gabe & Lia; Jacob, and Seth,
who are what life is all about*
—JSP—

In Memoriam
*We note with sadness the passing of two contributors to this work:
Judith Ann Macurda, MD, and Jeffrey K. Behrens, MD.
As skilled physicians, they were dedicated to their patients and to the
practice of hospice medicine. We were privileged to have had
Judy and Jeff as friends and colleagues.*

Contents

SECTION FIVE
Specific Populations   589

SECTION SIX
Diversity   715

Contributors

Andrea M. Adkins, RN-BC
Internal Consultant, PIS
VITAS Innovative Hospice Care
Miami, Florida
Chapter 11

Forrest O. Beaty, MD
Medical Director
VITAS Innovative Hospice Care
Walnut Creek, California
Chapter 28

Jeffrey M. Behrens, MD, CMD†
Medical Director
VITAS Innovative Hospice Care—Palm Beach
West Palm Beach, Florida
Chapter 30

Yolanda Castillo, RN
Director, Special Needs Program
Coventry Health Care
Miami, Florida
Chapter 31

Michael Clark, PharmD
Former Director of Pharmacy
VITAS Innovative Hospice Care
Miami, Florida

Richard Fife, MDiv, Dmin
President
Foundation for End of Life Care
Fort Lauderdale, Florida

Robin Fiorelli, LCSW
Sr. Director Bereavement and Volunteer
    Services
VITAS Innovative Hospice Care
Miami, Florida

---

†Deceased.

Tara C. Friedman, MD
Associate National Medical Director
VITAS Palliative Care Solutions
Senior Medical Director
VITAS Innovative Hospice Care
Blue Bell, Pennsylvania
Chapter 6

Domingo Gomez, MD
Hospice Physiciain (Retired)
VITAS Innovative Hospice Care
Miramar, Florida
Chapters 11, 22

Michele Grant Ervin, MD
Medical Director
VITAS Innovative Hospice Care
Washington, DC
Chapter 31

Jeffrey M. Kagan, MD
Hospice Physician
VITAS Innovative Hospice Care
Hartford, Connecticut
Assistant Clinical Professor of Medicine
University of Connecticut School of Medicine
Farmington, Connecticut
Senior Physician, Hospital of Central Connecticut
Newington, Connecticut
Chapter 29

Barry M. Kinzbrunner, MD
Executive Vice President and Chief Medical Officer
VITAS Innovative Hospice Care
Miami, Florida
Voluntary Assistant Professor of Medicine
Herbert Wertheim College of Medicine
Florida International University, Miami, Florida
Voluntary Assistant Professor of Medicine
Miller School of Medicine
University of Miami, Miami, Florida
Chapters 1–4, 8–10, 12, 13, 15, 18, 20, 22, 24, 29, 31, 32

Rabbi Bryan Kinzbrunner
Campus Chaplain
Oscar and Ella Wilf Campus for Senior Living
Martin and Edith Stein Hospice
Somerset, New Jersey

Judith Ann Haythorne Macurda, MD, MPH†
Medical Director
VITAS Innovative Hospice Care
Orange, California
Chapter 26

Tina Maluso-Bolton, MSN, NP, APRN-BC
Southern California Kaiser Permanente
    Medical Group
Regional Bone Marrow Transplant Program
Duarte, California
Chapters 9, 10

Gaurav Mathur, MD
Medical Director
VITAS Innovative Hospice Care
Mount Laurel, New Jersey
Chapter 19

Elizabeth A. McKinnis, DO
Private Practice
Greenville, Texas

Sarah E. McKinnon, MA
Senior Director, Education and Organizational
    Development
VITAS Innovative Hospice Care
Miami, Florida
Chapter 14

Lynn Ann Meister, MD
Director, Pediatric Hospice and Palliative Care
Pediatric Hematologist/Oncologist Joe DiMaggio
    Children's Hospital
Hollywood, Florida
Chapter 26

Melanie P. Merriman, PhD, MBA
Touchstone Consulting
North Bay Village, Florida
Chapter 5

Teresita Mesa, RN
Patient Care Administrator
VITAS Innovative Hospice Care
Miami, Florida
Chapter 31

Jeanne Micklich Ash, RN, BSN
Internal Compliance Advocate
VITAS Innovative Hospice Care
Miami, Florida

Bob Miller, MDiv
Senior Vice President for Clinical Development and Bioethics
VITAS Innovative Hospice Care
Miami, Florida
Chapter 14

Freddie J. Negron, MD
Senior Medical Director
VITAS Innovative Hospice Care
Miami-Dade Program
Miami, Florida
Chapters 7, 21, 31

Vincent D. Nguyen, MD
Medical Director
Geriatrics and Palliative Care Services
Monarch Health Care
Irvine, California
Chapters 3, 12

Joel S. Policzer, MD
Senior Vice President–National Medical Director
VITAS Innovative Hospice Care
Miami, Florida
Voluntary Assistant Professor of Family Medicine
University of Miami Miller School of Medicine
Miami, Florida
Associate Clinical Professor of Medicine
Nova Southeastern University College of Osteopathic
    Medicine
Fort Lauderdale, Florida
Voluntary Assistant Professor of Medicine
Herbert Wertheim College of Medicine
Florida International University, Miami, Florida
Chapters 3, 4, 11, 21, 23, 28

Sara Roby
Chaplain/Bereavement Counselor/Psychoanalyst
VITAS Innovative Hospice Care
West Palm Beach, Florida
Chapter 32

Syd Saxena, MD
Division of Palliative Care
VA Medical Center–Cincinnati
Associate Professor of Medicine
University of Cincinnati
Cincinnati, Ohio
Chapter 32

Bruce Schlecter, MD
Senior Medical Director
VITAS Innovative Hospice Care
Covina, California
Chapters 9, 10

Richard A. Shapiro, MD
Hospice Physician
VITAS Innovative Hospice Care
Lincolnwood, Illinois
Chapter 23

Lyra Sihra, MD
Assistant Professor of Clinical Medicine
Weill Cornell Medical College
Methodist Hospital
Houston, Texas
Chapter 24

James M. Sinclair, MD
Medical Director
VITAS Innovative Hospice Care–San Diego
Medical Director, Stevens Division
Scripps Cancer Center
Partner, Pacific Oncology and Hematology
San Diego, California
Chapter 19

Alen Voskanian, MD
Associate Physician Diplomate
UCLA David Geffen School of Medicine
Los Angeles, California
Medical Director
VITAS Innovative Hospice Care
Torrance, California
Chapter 25

Neal J. Weinreb, MD
Voluntary Associate Professor of Medicine
Miller School of Medicine
University of Miami
Miami, FL
Chapters 3, 6, 18, 19, 23

Michael Wohlfeiler, MD
Piperato & Assoc, LLC
Medical Director for Special Immunology Services,
    Mercy Hospital
Chair, Medical Care Sub-committee, Miami/Dade
    HIV/AIDS Partnership
Miami, Florida
Chapter 25

James B. Wright, DO
Associate National Medical Director
VITAS Innovative Hospice Care
Dallas, Texas
Chapters 1, 2, 10, 13

Preface

It is with great pride that we bring you *End-of-Life Care: A Practical Guide*, the second edition of the book previously titled *20 Common Problems in End-of-Life Care*.

With the many advances that have occurred in the field of hospice and palliative medicine since the first edition was published in 2002, we know that you will find the additions and updates in this edition to be timely, useful, and, in some instances, thought provoking. With the recognition by the American Board of Medical Specialties in 2008 of Hospice and Palliative Medicine as a medical subspecialty, as well as with established certification in the field of nursing, we also believe that you will find the self-assessment questions at the end of each chapter a valuable resource.

We thank you for your interest in this book and trust that you will find it useful as you endeavor to care for terminally ill patients and their families.

We would like to take this opportunity to thank all the chapter authors who devoted the time and energy necessary to contribute to this book, as well as Cecilia Amigo Haggerty for her assistance in preparing the final manuscripts and figures. We also want to give special thanks to James Shanahan, editor-in-chief of internal medicine for the Medical Publishing Division of McGraw-Hill, for his patience and support throughout this project.

Barry M. Kinzbrunner, MD
Joel S. Policzer, MD

Introduction

"No problem is more distressing than that presented by the patient with an incurable disease, particularly when premature death is inevitable.... The physician also must be prepared to deal with guilt feelings on the part of the family when a member becomes gravely or hopelessly ill."

These statements can be found in the introductory chapter of *Harrison's Principles of Internal Medicine*, circa 1980, in the opening paragraphs of a section on "incurability and death." Clearly, the goal of this section in what many consider to be the bible of internal medicine is to assist medical students, physicians-in-training, and internal medicine physicians in better understanding how to approach the care of patients who are terminally ill. And therein lies the challenge.

On the surface, these statements would seem perfectly reasonable. After all, facing an incurable or terminal illness is certainly distressing. The question is, though, distressing for whom? A careful reading reveals that the subject of the distress is not the person who is dying; rather, it is the individual "presented by the patient with an incurable disease," namely the physician.

Should the physician be distressed? Certainly, taking care of a patient when that patient is near the end of life is a formidable task, and the physician should be empathetic to the patient's distress, as well as that of family members. However, the physician's professional obligation to the patient and family requires that distress be avoided in favor of providing support, guidance, and continued hope during this most difficult and challenging time. It is this obligation, especially as it relates to providing continued hope, that raises additional issues with the statement above. For how can a physician give a patient and the family hope when the patient is thought to be "hopelessly ill"?

The above analysis is not meant to suggest that either the authors of these statements or physicians in general focus more on their own distress than on that of seriously ill patients and their families or intentionally view their patients as hopeless, even in the face of a terminal illness. Far from it! However, the statements do suggest that these feelings are subtly woven into the attitudes that physicians carry with them when caring for patients who are nearing the end of life.

With this in mind, the goals of *End-of-Life Care: A Practical Guide* remain to assist physicians and other clinicians in overcoming their "distress" and in providing the patients they care for who are near the end of life with hope in the face of apparent "hopelessness." To help accomplish these goals, the book is divided into six major sections that logically walk clinicians through the perceived complexities of providing patients and their families with quality end-of-life care.

SECTION ONE: PREPARING PATIENTS FOR END-OF-LIFE CARE

The opening section, Preparing Patients for End-of-Life Care, attempts to answer some of the fundamental questions related to the "who, what, and where" of care at the end of life. The first issue, who needs to receive this care, is addressed in Chapter 1, which discusses the various clinical guidelines and criteria that, when combined with the physician's clinical judgment, will assist the clinician in identifying patients who require end-of-life care. Chapter 2 then follows with a discussion of how and where this care can be obtained, starting with a detailed examination of the Medicare Hospice Benefit, followed by examination of the expanding palliative care options that are available in various communities to extend the benefits of end-of-life care to patients and families earlier in the course of advanced illness.

Once the patients and the type of care they need have been identified, clinicians must then confront the challenge of sharing this information with the patients and their families. Communication techniques to assist clinicians in accomplishing the formidable task of "breaking bad news" are discussed in Chapter 3. A new section added to this chapter presents professionals with guidance on how to have conversations with patients and families directed at goals of care and decision making.

Chapter 4 provides an overview of how end-of-life care interdisciplinary teams function to care for terminally ill patients, with emphasis on the multiple roles that physicians play in working with these teams. Chapter 5 examines the various ways that outcomes and quality of life can be measured, giving the clinician confidence that the providers of patient end-of-life services are doing what they say they will, improving the quality of care and life of the patients and families they serve.

SECTION TWO: MANAGEMENT OF SYMPTOMS

Having solved the logistical problems of getting patients cared for near the end of life, the clinicians' next task is to meet the physical, emotional, and spiritual needs of their patients and families.

To accomplish this, Section Two discusses the management of many of the common symptoms experienced by patients who are nearing the end of their lives.

It is fitting that the management of pain is addressed first (Chapter 6), as the challenges associated with controlling pain near the end of life have been and continue to be for many the raison d'être of hospice and palliative care. Following the discussion on pain management, Chapters 7 through 9 review the management of respiratory, gastrointestinal, and neurologic symptoms that cause challenges for the terminally ill. Because of the difficulties clinicians often face in the management of delirium, depression, and anxiety when life is coming to a close, a separate chapter (Chapter 10) is devoted to these specific symptoms.

Chapter 11 examines disorders that affect the skin and mucous membranes, with an emphasis on wound care, which often plagues patients near the end of life, especially those with advanced nonmalignant terminal illnesses, who make up an ever-increasing number of patients cared for by hospice and palliative care providers. The uniqueness of the dying experience is addressed in Chapter 12, which examines the challenges that clinicians face when managing symptoms of patients who are in their last days of life, while Chapter 13 completes the look at physical symptoms by addressing a variety of other end-of-life symptoms that were not previously discussed.

Although physicians tend to focus on the physical symptoms experienced by patients who are approaching life's end, it is important that these clinicians have a significant understanding of the psychosocial and spiritual concerns that patients, and often their loved ones, experience during their last weeks and months of life. Chapter 14 provides an overview of these symptoms in a somewhat unique way, by looking at these issues as opportunities by which these patients, with the help of the clinicians caring for them, can grow and progress even as life draws to a close. Chapter 15 examines the specific role that physicians need to play in providing spiritual support to the patients and families under their care, while

Chapter 16 discusses various techniques for performing psychosocial and spiritual assessments.

One of the cardinal principles of end-of-life care is that the patient and family together represent the unit of care; and that care, therefore, does not end when the patient takes his or her final breath. How those whom the patient has left behind deal with their loss is every bit as important a part of hospice and palliative care as is the management of pain during the final period of life of the patient. Therefore, Chapter 17 addresses the subject of bereavement care and the role that clinicians may play in recognizing the signs and symptoms of and providing appropriate interventions for both normal and abnormal grief reactions.

SECTION THREE: DIAGNOSTIC AND INVASIVE INTERVENTIONS

In the first edition of this book, the topic of diagnostic and invasive interventions was confined to a single chapter as part of the section on ethical dilemmas. However, as hospice and palliative care have evolved over the past decade to reach out to more patients with a wide variety of different needs, it has become increasingly clear that a host of diagnostic and invasive interventions has a role to play in providing appropriate end-of-life care. Hence, in the second edition, an entire section is devoted to this subject, leading off in Chapter 18 with a discussion of the principles clinicians should utilize to consider when various diagnostic and invasive procedures might be indicated. Indications for a number of specific diagnostic studies related primarily to potentially reversible mental status changes and the evaluation of pain are next explored. The chapter concludes with a review of the end-of-life indications for a number of invasive procedures, including orthopedic, surgical, and endoscopic interventions; the management of effusions, antibiotics, and transfusions; and the use of hematopoietic growth factors.

Although now consisting of less than half of all patients cared for by hospice programs, cancer patients still remain a significant proportion of patients receiving end-of-life care. With new chemotherapeutic medications and new radiation oncology techniques being developed on a regular basis, Chapter 19 explores the appropriate utilization of these interventions as part and parcel of quality palliative care. Chapter 20 evaluates the role of invasive cardiac interventions in the management of patients with advanced congestive heart failure and other forms of end-stage heart disease who are nearing the end of life. The first part of Chapter 21 looks at the palliative indications for invasive respiratory interventions, while the second part discusses the proper techniques for discontinuing mechanical ventilation when patients or health-care surrogates have made this choice, which has in many settings become the responsibility of hospice and palliative care providers.

SECTION FOUR: ETHICAL DILEMMAS

There are four major principles that comprise medical ethics: autonomy, beneficence, nonmaleficence, and justice, which are defined in the following table. As end-of-life care has evolved over the last several decades, medical ethics has had an ever-increasing influence in assisting clinicians, as well as patients and their families, in making many of the difficult decisions during this challenging final period of life. Therefore, Section Four of this book examines some of the ethical dilemmas that clinicians and the patients and families they care for face when life is approaching its end.

First and foremost in addressing medical ethical issues at the end of life is the need to respect a patient's autonomy by having advanced knowledge of the care that a patient would or would not want to receive if those desires could not

TABLE 1. Cardinal Principles of Medical Ethics

PRINCIPLE	DEFINITION
Autonomy	Self-determination by choosing among available treatment options
Beneficence	Taking action for the patient's benefit
Nonmaleficence	Avoiding harm
Justice	
Social	Doing what is good for the society as a whole
Distributive	Allocating limited resources appropriately

SOURCE: Lo B: Ethical issues in clinical medicine. In: Isselbacher KJ, Braunwald E, Wilson JD, et al, eds. *Harrison's Principles of Internal Medicine*, 13th ed. New York, McGraw-Hill, 1994.

be expressed. Hence, Chapter 22 examines the issues (both ethical and legal), around advance directives, as well as the appropriateness of providing cardiopulmonary resuscitation to patients who are near the end of life from both the medical and ethical perspectives.

Chapter 23 presents a discussion of what is probably the most difficult ethical dilemma facing clinicians today, the role, if any, of physician-assisted suicide (PAS) and euthanasia. While recognizing that this book has an editorial bias against these practices, this chapter has attempted to present both sides of this debate, which today rages throughout organized medical societies across the globe, so that the reader can form his or her own opinions. This is especially important in view of the fact that PAS is now legal in three U.S. states, with other states planning on considering the issue in the next several years, and that some form of PAS or euthanasia is permitted in several other countries.

As patients near the end of life, their desire to ingest food and fluid often diminishes voluntarily, or they may become physically unable to eat and drink. Physicians and family members often become concerned that these patients who do not eat or drink are succumbing to malnutrition or dehydration, rather than to the natural processes associated with dying. These concerns often lead to the decision to provide the patient with food and fluid by artificial means, even at the expense of increased patient discomfort. To address these concerns, Chapter 24 discusses the medical and

ethical issues that surround the provision of hydration and nutritional support for terminally ill patients.

SECTION FIVE: SPECIAL POPULATIONS

No book on end-of-life care would be complete without discussing some of the special needs that certain groups of patients have when life is almost at an end. Chapter 25 examines the special needs of patients with acquired immunodeficiency syndrome (AIDS), who may suffer from more complex physical symptoms secondary to opportunistic infections and may have more challenging psychosocial problems due to their younger average age and, for many, alternative lifestyles.

Two chapters are devoted to the special needs of terminally ill pediatric patients. Chapter 26 explores the management of physical symptoms, with special attention being paid to the evaluation of pain and other complaints based on age and developmental level, and the need for adjusting pharmacologic interventions based on the different metabolic needs of children as opposed to adults. Chapter 27 then discusses the challenges of working with grieving parents and siblings. Despite the emotional difficulty that many health care providers experience when acknowledging that children may need end-of-life care, these children, as well as their siblings and parents, need this support just as much as the elderly, when the acceptance that life is approaching its end is somewhat more palatable.

Sometimes, it becomes apparent during the course of an acute illness that, despite receiving care in an intensive-care setting, the patient is not going to recover. At other times, the realization that a chronic illness is life limiting does not occur until the patient suffers from an acute exacerbation of that illness and presents to the hospital emergency room. In these, and other similar scenarios, patients and families are put into the difficult and uncomfortable positions of having to make end-of-life decisions while being cared for in an ICU or ED setting. Chapter 28 looks at the how hospice and palliative care can provide patient and family support even in these acute care environments.

As the population has aged, it has become increasingly clear that the elderly have specific needs. Therefore, the last two chapters in this section examine issues related to the care of the elderly population. As many elderly patients are now cared for in institutions prior to the end of life, Chapter 29 discusses how hospice and palliative care can be provided safely and effectively in long-term care facilities, with the end-of-life care provider working in partnership with the facility staff to ensure that patients receive quality care. As elderly patients are on many medications and undergo various metabolic changes as life approaches its end, Chapter 30 explores how these factors affect the management of pain in the geriatric population.

SECTION SIX: DIVERSITY

Over the last decade or so, the United States has clearly evolved into a multicultural society. Perhaps nowhere is cultural diversity more apparent then when addressing issues related to end-of-life care. Individual patients and families from different ethnic, cultural, and religious groups all have differences in how they want things done when life is nearing its end, including, for example, how they want to be communicated with, how they cope with the knowledge of having a life-limiting illness, and how the deceased is to be treated when death has finally arrived.

Chapter 31 discusses the techniques needed to perform a culturally competent assessment, so that professional caregivers learn from each patient and family their specific ethnic, cultural, and/or religious needs. This chapter then explores the end-of-life needs specific to some of the larger ethnic and cultural groups in the United States today: African Americans, Hispanic Americans, and Asian Americans. Chapter 32 explores the end-of-life customs and rituals unique to several religious groups in the United States: Jewish, Muslim, Buddhist, and Hindu.

Both chapters are meant to give readers a cursory overview of some of the more important customs of each group. However, readers must be cautioned that one should never generalize and assume that patients that belong to any specific group will always follow the customs of the group. One must always remember that there is no set approach to delivering culturally competent care. The goal is to respect the wishes of and learn from each patient and family under our care how to meet their unique needs.

Whether you are a clinician in training or have been in practice for 20 years, whether you provide primary care or practice a subspecialty, whether you are in the community setting or in academic medicine, you will, at least from time to time, need to deal with the distress and the feelings of hopelessness expressed by your patients who are near the end of life. Therefore, you should find the material outlined above and contained in *End-of-Life Care: A Practical Guide* of great utility. By understanding the principles of hospice and palliative care, clinicians can look to those who provide end-of-life care as patient-care partners, assisting them in providing their patients and families with the care that they need in a positive atmosphere of hope. As stated by Dame Cicely Saunders, considered the "mother" of hospice and end-of-life care and, having been trained as a doctor, nurse, and social worker, an interdisciplinary team all rolled into one:

> You matter because you are you, and you matter until the last moment of your life. We will do all we can, not only to help you die peacefully, but also to live until you die.

BIBLIOGRAPHY

Isselbacher KJ, Braunwald E, Wilson JD, et al: The practice of medicine. In: Isselbacher KJ, Braunwald E, Wilson JD, et al, eds. *Harrison's Principles of Internal Medicine*, 9th ed. New York, McGraw-Hill, 1980, 13th ed. New York, McGraw-Hill, 1994, Chapter 1.

Kinzbrunner BM: The terminally ill patient. In: Abeloff MD, Armitage JO, Lichter AS, Niederhuber JE, eds. *Clinical Oncology*, 2nd ed. New York, Churchill Livingstone, 2000, p. 597.

Lo B: Ethical issues in clinical medicine. In: Isselbacher KJ, Braunwald E, Wilson JD, et al, eds. *Harrison's Principles of Internal Medicine*, 13th ed. New York, McGraw-Hill, 1994.

Stoddard S: *The Hospice Movement: A Better Way of Caring for the Dying*, revised ed. New York, Vintage, 1991.

Preparing Patients for End-of-Life Care

SECTION ONE

Predicting Prognosis: How to Decide When End-of-Life Care Is Needed

James B. Wright and Barry M. Kinzbrunner

INTRODUCTION

One of the major problems that physicians must address as they plan care for their patients at the end of life is to determine when, based upon a prediction of the patient's prognosis, such care should be initiated. The ability of the physician to make a reasonable estimate of how long a patient is likely to live is critical whether one is considering referral to a hospice program (which, as discussed in Chapter 2, requires the physician to certify that the patient has a prognosis of 6 months or less) or to an alternative end-of-life care program if the patient's prognosis is somewhat longer.

PROGNOSTIC ACCURACY

Studies assessing the ability of physicians to accurately predict prognosis have reported varying results, making it difficult to draw any conclusions. For example, a 1972 study suggested that physicians and other caregivers were overly optimistic when asked to predict patient survival, whereas the Study to Understand Prognoses and Preferences for Outcomes and Risks of Treatment (SUPPORT) reported that physicians tend to be pessimistic when predicting patient prognosis near the end of life. Interestingly, and in sharp contrast to both of these studies, review of SUPPORT data also suggests that for certain subgroups of patients, physician accuracy in predicting patient prognosis may actually be quite good. In one published report, 85% of patients who were identified by their physicians as having an 85% probability of dying during the next 6 months (which would be the group of patients most likely in need of hospice and end-of-life care) actually died during that period. In a second report specifically devoted to patients with cancer diagnoses, the SUPPORT investigators drew the conclusion that "physicians estimated prognosis quite accurately."

In 2000, Christakis et al, using methodology similar to the 1972 study cited earlier, confirmed that physicians and other caregivers were overly optimistic when asked to predict patient survival in patients referred for hospice care, while, in 2003, Glare reported that physicians' predictions of terminal prognosis in cancer patients were highly correlated with actual survival.

Hospice data does little to shed light on the accuracy of physicians in predicting survival. A study based on 1990 Medicare claims data reported that more than 85% of patients admitted to hospices during a 3-month period died within 6 months, indicating that physicians were fairly accurate in predicting the prognosis of this group of individuals. On the other hand, these same patients had a median survival of only 36 days. The short median survival demonstrated in this study can be explained, at least in part, by the fact that, with so much uncertainty in the medical literature surrounding this subject of predicting prognosis, physicians are understandably reluctant to consider hospice or other end-of-life care services for their patients until death is certain. That this has continued to be a significant challenge is best illustrated by hospice length of stay data reported yearly by the National Hospice and Palliative Care Organization (NHPCO), which shows that since 1995, average hospice length of stay has been in the range of slightly less than 2 months, while the median length of stay has actually fallen from the 36 days reported earlier to a range of 22–29 days.

GUIDELINES

To assist physicians in predicting prognosis near the end of life, the development of guidelines has been suggested. These guidelines would aid physicians in identifying when patients are likely in need of hospice or other end-of-life care services. Such guidelines, both formal and informal, can be found in the medical literature, and information about them will be presented in this chapter. It should be noted that these guidelines were developed primarily for identification of patients who have a prognosis of 6 months or less, which is required for eligibility for the Medicare/Medicaid Hospice Benefit (see Chapter 2). While this may be perceived as a limiting factor in the utility of guidelines, the continued uncertainty surrounding the prediction of prognosis at the end of life suggests that the guidelines may have applicability for determining patient need for end-of-life care programs outside the confines of the Medicare Hospice Benefit as well.

Guidelines for predicting patient prognosis near the end of life are not intended to be used in a dogmatic fashion and should not be converted into a scored checklist with some magic number of items required to consider a patient ready for hospice or palliative care. When the guidelines recommend the use of objective studies, such as pulmonary functions, diagnostic x-rays, or laboratory tests, for example, these studies should not be used to rule in or rule out a patient's need for end-of-life care. Specifically, patients should not be compelled to undergo testing to qualify for hospice or palliative care, nor should they be barred from receiving such care, if clinically indicated, because they choose to avoid further such testing. What is recommended is that these guidelines and associated tests be used in a thoughtful fashion, with each specific criterion representing a piece of information that should be evaluated in the context of a patient's clinical condition and clinical course at the time of assessment. When the assessment is completed, the information obtained should be combined with other clinical and psychosocial information, making the decision to recommend that a patient receive end-of-life care one of CLINICAL JUDGMENT, based on the needs of that specific patient.

GENERAL GUIDELINES

When the concept of hospice first began to take hold in Great Britain, Canada, and the United States, there was an implicit understanding that the primary intent was to care for terminally ill patients who have cancer. Cancer patients, after all, tend to show a steady decline in health as the illness progresses, making the ability to predict when a patient's life is nearing its end seemingly straightforward. However, as the decade of the 1980s came to a close, it became clear that patients with nonmalignant end-stage conditions, such as congestive heart failure, chronic lung disease, and dementia, would also benefit from end-of-life care as well. A major reason for the inclusion of patients with nonmalignant diagnoses was that physicians and others working in hospice and palliative care observed that patients who were terminally ill, regardless of the primary diagnosis, had convergence of their symptoms and treatment approaches as the time of death became closer. For example, the shortness of breath experienced by a patient who is dying of a malignancy with lung involvement is much the same as the dyspnea of a patient who has severe chronic obstructive pulmonary disease (COPD). The approach to therapy in these patients will, likewise, be similar.

The concept of similarity in presentation also extends itself to the determination of when patients require end-of-life care. Whether patients are dying of a neoplastic process, or of a long-standing nonmalignant illness, there are some characteristics shared by all patients that can be expressed in a set of General Guidelines for Determining Prognosis, as set forth in Table 1–1, and discussed in detail below.

CLINICAL PROGRESSION OF DISEASE

Crucial to determining prognosis is the demonstration that the patient's primary disease process is progressing over time. In essence, we must ask ourselves what has changed such that we now believe that this individual has a progressive and terminal disease process. There are a number of sources of important information that can help the clinician recognize when the patient's condition is worsening. As an illness progresses, patients may find themselves more frequently in

TABLE 1–1. General Criteria
Clinical Progression of Disease
Multiple hospitalizations, emergency department visits, or increased utilization of other health care services
Serial physician assessments, laboratory, or x-ray studies consistent with progressive illness
Changes in minimal data set (MDS) for patients in long-term care facilities
Progressive deterioration of the patient while receiving home health care
Declining Functional Status as Defined by:
For patients with malignant diseases:
Karnofsky performance status (KPS) ≤ 50 or ECOG ≥ 3
KPS ≤ 60 or ECOG ≥ 2 with symptoms
Decline in KPS of at least 20 units in 2–3 mo
For patients with nonmalignant diseases:
Dependence in at least 3/6 activities of daily living
KPS or palliative performance scale (PPS) score ≤ 50
Declining Nutritional Status as Defined by:
Unintentional weight loss ≥ 10% of normal body weight and/or BMI < 22 kg/m^2
Intangible Factors
Patient's personal goals, approach to his/her disease, treatment
Burden of investigation and treatment vs. potential gain for the patient

need of health care services, causing them to spend increasing amounts of time in hospitals, emergency departments, or the physician's office. Serial office visits demonstrating persistent or increasing symptoms such as fatigue or weight loss may be a marker of progressive illness. Abnormal physical findings and diagnostic studies including blood work and x-rays that show progressive abnormalities in blood gases, liver functions, elevated tumor markers, renal function, or cardiac ejection fraction (to name a few examples) also may be indicative of advancing disease and point to the need to consider the patient for end-of-life care. For patients living in long-term care facilities, deterioration in parameters measured serially as part of the Minimal Data Set (MDS), especially those related to functional status, provide important clues to the clinician regarding changes in the patient's condition. Another important source of information is the home health care nurse, who, while visiting the patient on a regular basis at home, may note that patients have reached a point in their illness when home health nursing visits alone will no longer suffice.

DECLINING PERFORMANCE STATUS

Palliative Performance Status (PPS) and Related Measures

It was recognized during the earliest phases of cancer chemotherapy development that patients with an impaired functional status would have a poorer prognosis and would not respond as well to chemotherapy as patients with the same malignancy that had better functional status. This led to development of measures of functional status, such as The Karnofsky Performance Status Index (KPS), designed in the late 1940s as an adjunctive tool to evaluate the activity levels of patients with cancer who were participating in cancer chemotherapy trials.

The KPS, assessing ambulation, self-care ability, activity level, and evidence of disease, is delineated in Table 1–2. Studies have demonstrated that there is a rapid fall in KPS of at least 20 to 30 units during the last 2 to 3 months of life and that the median survival of patients with advanced cancer was found to correlate with the KPS rating. It was also demonstrated that patients with active symptoms, including dyspnea, anorexia, weight loss, dry mouth, and difficulty swallowing, have shorter survivals than patients with the same KPS rating who are not symptomatic.

TABLE 1–2. Measures of Performance Status: KPS and ECOG		
KPS	**KPS SPECIFIC CRITERIA**	**ECOG**
100	Normal, no complaints or evidence of disease	0
90	Able to carry on normal activity, minor disease symptoms	
80	Normal activity with effort, some disease symptoms	1
70	Cares for self; unable to do normal activity or work	
60	Requires occasional assistance, able to care for most needs	2
50	Requires considerable assistance and frequent medical care	
40	Disabled, requires special care and assistance	3
30	Severely disabled, death not imminent	
20	Very ill, active care and attention required continuously	4
10	Moribund	
0	Death	

Source: Adapted from MacDonald N: Principles governing the use of cancer chemotherapy in palliative medicine. In: Doyle D, Hanks GWC, MacDonald N, eds. *Oxford Textbook of Palliative Medicine*. Oxford: Oxford University Press, 1993, p. 105.

In the field of oncology, other less complex measures of performance have been developed by such organizations as the Eastern Cooperative Oncology Group (ECOG) and the World Health Organization (WHO). These scales were designed to simplify the rated levels of patient functional status from the 0 to 100 scale of the KPS to a 0 to 4 scale. Since many clinicians are more comfortable with ECOG and WHO scales and the studies involving performance status as a marker involve the KPS, the ECOG scale is superimposed on the KPS in Table 1–2 for comparison purposes.

One of the limitations of the KPS and the other measures discussed earlier is that they are primar-ily designed as indicators of performance status for patients with malignant disease. To help overcome some of these limitations, a modification of the KPS, called the Palliative Performance Scale (PPS), was developed in the mid-1990s and is presented in Table 1–3. In addition to the activities already measured in the KPS, the PPS assesses the patient characteristics of food/fluid intake and level of consciousness. The utility of the PPS as an indicator of prognosis has been demonstrated by several studies as well as a recently published meta-analysis of those studies. However, in all but one of the studies cited in the meta-analysis, patients were already being cared for in either a hospice or palliative care program, meaning that they had already been determined to be terminally ill. Therefore, although one can conclude that the PPS may be useful in helping the clinician predict the remaining lifespan of patients already determined to have a limited life expectancy, the utility of the PPS in determining patient survival in the larger population of chronically and seriously ill patients remains to be determined.

Despite these limitations, based on clinical experience combined with the studies cited earlier, it is generally accepted that a KPS or PPS score of less than or equal to 50, or an ECOG score of 2 or higher is predictive that the patient may have a prognosis of 6 months or less. However, a score greater than 50 does not necessarily indicate a prognosis of more than 6 months. Due consideration should be given to individuals that may initially have higher functionality score but also have unfavorable prognostic disease states. For example, a patient with stage IV untreatable carcinoma that still functions at KPS or PPS score of 60 should not be excluded from consideration for hospice care.

Activities of Daily Living

The most common method of assessing the functional status of patients with diagnoses other than cancer is by the evaluation of what are called the Activities of Daily Living (ADL). The original six

TABLE 1–3. Palliative Performance Scale (PPS)

PPS RATING	AMBULATION	SELF-CARE	INTAKE	LOC	ACTIVITY	EVIDENCE OF DISEASE
100	Full	Full	Normal	Full	Normal	No evidence of disease
90	Full	Full	Normal	Full	Normal	Some evidence of disease
80	Full	Full	Normal or reduced	Full	Normal with effort	Some evidence of disease
70	Reduced	Full	Normal or reduced	Full	Unable to do normal work	Some evidence of disease
60	Reduced	Occasional assistance	Normal or reduced	Full or confusion	Unable to do hobby or housework	Significant disease
50	Mainly Sit/Lie	Considerable assistance	Normal or reduced	Full or confusion	Unable to do any work	Extensive disease
40	Mainly in Bed	Complete assistance	Normal or reduced	Full, drowsy, or confusion	Unable to do any work	Extensive disease
30	Bed Confined	Total Care	Reduced	Full, drowsy, or confusion	Unable to do any work	Extensive disease
20	Bed Confined	Total Care	Minimal sips	Full, drowsy, or confusion	Unable to do any work	Extensive disease
10	Bed Confined	Total Care	Mouth care only	Drowsy or coma	Unable to do any work	Extensive disease
0	Death					

Source: Modified from Anderson F, Downing GM, Hill J, et al: Palliative performance scale (PPS): A new tool. *J Palliat Care* 12(1):5, 1996.

activities as described by Katz in the 1960s were bathing, dressing, toileting, transfer, continence, and feeding. A patient's ability to perform each of these activities, with modifications from Katz's original work, continue to be measured routinely in hospitals as well as in long-term care facilities as part of the Minimal Data Set (MDS).

The evaluation of ADLs on a serial basis has been found to be an important indicator of patient prognosis. In a group of elderly patients receiving residential care in Great Britain, patients who had significant ADL deficits had a median survival of 6-months, with a 2-year mortality of 80%. In a study evaluating various factors as predictors of prognosis in hospitalized elderly patients, regression analysis showed that ADL deficits were the most important predictor of 6-month mortality, outranking diagnosis, mental status, and even whether or not the patient required intensive care. Comparison of ADL deficits with KPS ratings has shown that patients with a KPS score of 50 typically have dependence in at least three of the six ADL.

DECLINING NUTRITIONAL STATUS

Another key indicator of poor prognosis is a decline in a patient's nutritional status. This is best expressed as an *unintentional* weight loss of 10% of normal body weight over a period of approximately 6 months, with the loss of weight usually due to the patient's life limiting condition. Reversible causes of weight loss, such as depression and metabolic disturbances (i.e., diabetes, thyroid disease, etc.), should be excluded prior to assuming that the weight loss is due to the terminal illness and a true indicator of the patient's prognosis. (It should be remembered that terminally ill patients may still have reversible causes of weight loss.) For terminally ill patients with reversible cause of weight loss, weight loss will be less helpful in determining prognosis. Also consider whether or not the patient is consuming normal amounts of calories. Rapid and progressive

weight loss in the face of normal caloric intake without cause other than the terminal disease is suggestive of advancing terminal illness.

Corroborating evidence that a less than or equal to 10% weight loss is associated with a poor prognosis can be found in a key study published in 1994 that examined the predictability of weight loss in a group of patients living in a long-term care facility. Approximately 62% of 53 elderly patients who had unintentionally lost less than or equal to 10% body weight during a 6-month period died in the next 6 months, while only 9% of 190 patients who had not lost weight died during the same time period. In patients with advanced cancer, weight loss has been shown to negatively effect median survival regardless of the primary site of the neoplasm.

Body mass index (BMI) is another useful way to evaluate a patient's nutritional status near the end of life. BMI is a reflection of body weight in relationship to height, and therefore, might give a truer picture of the patient's nutritional status than body weight alone. The formula for BMI is:

$$\text{BMI in kg/m}^2 = \frac{703^* \times \text{Weight in lbs}}{(\text{Height in inches})^2}$$

*The factor 703 converts lbs/in^2 into kg/m^2

A recent study demonstrated that BMI values less than 22 kg/m^2 correlated with dependence in activities of daily living as well as with increased mortality rates in elderly patients. It has also been reported that in seriously ill hospitalized patients, those with BMI's less than 20 kg/m^2 had the highest risk of mortality in the 6 months following hospitalization.

Anthropomorphic measures such as triceps skin fold thickness may be useful indicators of poor nutritional status for patients who are unable to be weighed, and are used by some hospice providers as surrogate measures of weight loss. Studies correlating these measures with patient survival have not been published to date.

Low serum albumins levels have been found to have prognostic significance as well. However, the utility of serum albumin in determining patient prognosis is limited, due to the fact that there are nonterminal medical conditions, such as nephrotic syndrome, alcoholic liver disease, and others, associated with low serum albumin levels.

INTANGIBLE FACTORS

With the current emphasis of the ethical value of autonomy in health care decision making, it is critical to consider the desires of the patient or family when thinking about referring a patient to a hospice or palliative care program near the end of life. In fact, some might consider these factors relatively more important in determining the need of a patient for end-of-life care than the more objective criteria more commonly used to determine prognosis and the need for hospice care.

The physician should consider the potential benefits versus potential burdens of disease evaluation and treatment when discussing therapeutic options with a patient or family. The physician should work with each patient/family to set realistic and achievable goals, based on the wishes of the patient/family. By approaching patients with advanced illness in this fashion, clinicians, as well as patients and families, will have a better sense of when end-of-life care is the most appropriate therapeutic option for the patient/family. The option of palliative and/or hospice care is at least as important as aggressive disease modification options in patients with advanced illness.

DETERMINING PROGNOSIS IN PATIENTS WITH MALIGNANT DISEASES

In spite of the common signs and symptoms that patients demonstrate near the end of life,

there are significant enough differences between various illnesses that disease-specific guidelines are necessary to assist the clinicians in determining when patients require end-of-life care. For patients with cancer, interest in developing such guidelines has not been particularly great, as there is a sense that physicians who care for cancer patients have a fairly good sense of when a patient is terminally ill. As already noted, the SUPPORT study suggested that physicians predict prognosis of patients with cancer with a relatively high degree of accuracy. That physicians are comfortable referring cancer patients for end-of-life care would also seem to be supported by data from the National Hospice Organization (NHO), which stated that in 1995, 50% of patients dying of cancer received hospice care prior to death.

A closer look at the data, however, suggests that all is not as it seems. In its position paper entitled "Care at the End of Life," the American Society of Clinical Oncology stated that "hospice is a widely available and excellent model for managing of end-of-life care and should be better utilized." That cancer patients are utilizing hospice services is borne out be recent data, which shows that 60% to 65% of dying cancer patients access hospice services prior to death. Whether hospice care is being "better utilized" by cancer patients, however, remains open to question, as reported by Tanis and Kinzbrunner, who examined data from over 60,000 patients admitted to a large hospice from 2000 to 2006 with diagnoses of prostate, colorectal, breast, lung, or pancreatic cancer. This data showed that the average length of stay (ALOS) remained remarkably stable over the seven years reviewed, but the 40.6 days ALOS for just five malignancies was still relatively brief at just below 6 weeks.

In light of the data noted in the introduction of this chapter that found that oncologist were generally accurate in predicting terminal prognosis in their cancer patients, one is forced to ask the following: Is a less than 6 weeks length of stay an acceptable time on a hospice service for known terminal cancer patients? Or, as seems more likely, is one forced to conclude that while the majority of patients with terminal malignancies are receiving end-of-life care, most are receiving it so late in their clinical course that the full benefits of such services cannot possibly be realized? Therefore, guidelines that would help oncologists and other physicians caring for cancer patients direct those patients to a hospice or palliative care program earlier would seem to be most beneficial.

Guidelines to help clinicians specifically identify when patients with malignant disease are in need of end-of-life care must take several factors into account. These factors include the stage of disease, the natural history of the illness, and the potential responsiveness of the specific malignancy to the multiple modalities of antineoplastic therapy available today. Because of the evolving nature of the oncology field in terms of disease-specific treatments, it is generally prudent for all patients with a cancer diagnosis, with the exception of those with far advanced disease who are very near death, to undergo an oncology evaluation prior to admission to a hospice service, especially if the malignancy is one that has a reasonable likelihood of responding to antineoplastic therapy.

Stage of disease as a prognostic factor is fairly straightforward. Cancer patients who require hospice or palliative care generally suffer from advanced disease, which is defined as metastatic spread of the malignancy from the primary site to other areas of the body or massive tumor growth at the primary site.

To define the prognostic factors of natural history and responsiveness to antineoplastic therapies is much more complex, as there is a wide spectrum of variation in these factors between different neoplasms as well as between subtypes of the same malignant illness. To address this, a classification system of common neoplastic diseases has been proposed, dividing the malignancies into five categories based upon their natural history and responsiveness to treatment in patients with advanced (stage IV) disease. This classification system will be presented below, with the cancers in each category being listed in tabular form, and with a short discussion of the characteristics that neoplasms within each category share. More detailed descriptions of specific neoplasms and their applicable therapies are beyond the scope of this chapter, and the interested reader is referred to any up-to-date oncology text for further information. In addition, the reader should be aware that as new treatment modalities are defined, this classification is subject to modification based upon evidence-based changes in the various cancer therapies.

CATEGORY I

The malignancies in category I are listed in Table 1–4. These diseases represent some of the greatest successes in medical oncology, curable in the majority of patient, even when they present with

---

TABLE 1–4. Category I: Treatable, High or Moderate Expectation of Cure

MALIGNANCIES	CHARACTERISTICS
Testicular carcinoma	Stage IV
Choriocarcinoma and trophoblastic malignancy	Cure potential high to moderate
Childhood acute lymphoblastic leukemia	End-of-life care indicated when there is disease
Other pediatric malignancies	progression after extensive antineoplastic
Acute promyelocytic leukemia	therapy
Hodgkin's disease	

SOURCE: Adapted from Kinzbrunner BM: The terminally ill patient. In: Abeloff MD, Armitage JO, Lichter AS, Niederhuber JE, eds. *Clinical Oncology.* New York: Churchill Livingstone, 1st ed, 1995, p. 409; 2nd ed, 2000, p. 597.

TABLE 1–5. Category II: Treatable, High Probability of Complete Remission, Low Probability of Cure

MALIGNANCY	CHARACTERISTICS
Ovarian carcinoma	Stage IV
Adult acute myeloblastic leukemia and acute lymphoblastic leukemia	Cure potential low
	Remission potential high to moderate
Intermediate and high-grade non-Hodgkin's lymphoma	Antineoplastic therapy in stage IV disease improves quality and length of life
Small cell (oat cell) bronchogenic carcinoma	End-of-life care indicated when there is disease progression following first- or second-line therapy (depending upon the illness)

SOURCE: Adapted from Kinzbrunner BM: The terminally ill patient. In: Abeloff MD, Armitage JO, Lichter AS, Niederhuber JE, eds. *Clinical Oncology*. New York: Churchill Livingstone, 1st ed, 1995, p. 409; 2nd ed, 2000, p. 597.

advanced metastatic disease. Treatment of these illnesses, even when far advanced at the time of patient presentation, should be strongly encouraged. The only exception to this might be the elderly patient with multiple comorbid conditions that would preclude intensive therapy. Patients who require end-of-life care with one of these illnesses will generally have a lengthy medical history inclusive of extensive antineoplastic therapy and will be suffering from advanced metastatic disease that is now resistant to further disease-directed treatment.

CATEGORY II

The category II malignancies listed in Table 1–5 share the characteristic of being relatively sensitive to antineoplastic therapy, with complete remission rates, even in the face of stage IV disease, of 60% or higher. Although many of the patients who attain a complete remission relapse within 1 to 2 years of treatment, approximately 20% of patients remain without evidence of disease on a long-term basis and, thus, could possibly be considered cured. With the potential for cure, or of substantial improvement in both quality of life and length of life even if cure is not

ultimately achieved, treatment in most circumstances should be encouraged (providing that therapy is not contraindicated by comorbid medical conditions). For patients who do not achieve a complete remission from first-line antineoplastic therapy, or who develop recurrent cancer following a complete remission, there may be benefits to second-line therapy, especially in ovarian carcinoma, the acute types of leukemia, and the aggressive lymphomas. In general, however, cure is not possible once the illness has recurred. End-of-life care may be appropriate for patients with one of these malignancies when there is evidence of progressive metastatic disease following first- or second-line therapy (depending upon the illness).

CATEGORY III

The malignancies in this category, listed in Table 1–6, present the most challenges in deciding when end-of-life care is necessary. For patients who develop one of these diseases, while cure is generally not an option once the illness has spread beyond the confines of the primary site, there are numerous effective antineoplastic treatment options available. Hormonal agents such as

TABLE 1–6. Category III: Treatable, Incurable when Metastatic, Favorable Prognosis	
MALIGNANCY	**CHARACTERISTICS**
Prostate carcinoma	Stage IV
Breast carcinoma	Incurable
Chronic lymphocytic leukemia	Remission potential high to moderate
Chronic myelocytic leukemia and the myeloproliferative disorders	Indolent course with a long prognosis
	Antineoplastic therapy may be relatively side effect
Low-grade non-Hodgkin's lymphoma	free (i.e., oral hormonal therapy)
Multiple myeloma and the immunoproliferative disorders	End-of-life care indicated when there is evidence of disease progression after one or multiple regimens
Myelodysplastic syndromes	(dependent upon specific disease) of standard
Thyroid carcinoma (except anaplastic)	antineoplastic therapy

SOURCE: Adapted from Kinzbrunner BM: The terminally ill patient. In: Abeloff MD, Armitage JO, Lichter AS, Niederhuber JE, eds. *Clinical Oncology*. New York: Churchill Livingstone, 1st ed, 1995, p. 409; 2nd ed, 2000, p. 597.

tamoxifen in breast cancer and luprolide in prostate cancer, and oral chemotherapeutic agents such as chlorambucil and alkeran in the hematological malignancies listed in Table 1–6 are efficacious, easily administered to patients, and are generally well tolerated, even by the elderly and infirm. Some clinicians would even advocate not treating stage IV patients until symptoms occur, as there is no strong evidence that treatment in the absence of symptoms improves survival. The life expectancy of patients with these illnesses is generally measured in years and varies based upon the specific disease.

Therefore, end-of-life care for patients with one of the malignancies in this category is indicated in the face of disease progression only after the patient has been treated with at least one or more often with several different antineoplastic therapeutic regimens (dependent upon the specific diagnosis), and the malignancy has become resistant to further antineoplastic therapy.

CATEGORY IV

The malignancies in category IV, listed in Table 1–7, consist of the majority of adult solid tu-

mors. However one chooses to interpret the current state of the art in the treatment of these cancers, the sobering facts are that once these diseases have metastasized, they are incurable. In addition, while some patients who suffer from a malignancy in this category will benefit from systemic antineoplastic therapy, for the less than 50% of patients who do have a response to treatment, that response is generally short-lived and has little effect on long-term survival.

It is proposed that for these patients, end-of-life care be considered not when available treatment has been exhausted, but as a therapeutic option, focusing on symptom control and quality of life rather than on disease control. Viewing hospice and palliative care as a therapeutic option is not meant to exclude antineoplastic treatments. Rather, this approach is meant to reframe end-of-life care in a more positive light. By allowing patients (and their physicians) to view hospice and palliative care as a treatment choice, hope of symptom control and quality of life can replace the perception that end-of-life care should be reserved only for those patients for whom there is no longer effective antineoplastic treatment available.

TABLE 1–7. Category IV: Treatable in a Minority of Patients with Metastatic Disease, Less Favorable Prognosis

MALIGNANCY	CHARACTERISTICS
Bladder carcinoma	Stage IV
Primary brain tumors	Incurable
Glioblastoma	Responses to therapy in less than 50% of patients
Grade III Astrocytoma	Short prognosis even after response to first-line
Gynecological malignancies other than ovary	chemotherapy.
Colorectal carcinoma	End-of-life care should be presented as a therapeutic
Nonsmall cell bronchogenic carcinoma	option to patients alongside second-line
Squamous cell carcinoma	chemotherapy and for patients with poor
Adenomcarcinoma	performance status (KPS $\leq$ 50 or ECOG $\leq$ 2),
Large cell carcinoma	alongside first-line chemotherapy.
Brochioalveolar carcinoma	
Head and neck carcinomas	
Esophageal carcinoma	
Gastric carcinoma	
Pancreatic carcinoma	
Soft tissue sarcomas	

SOURCE: Adapted from Kinzbrunner BM: The terminally ill patient. In: Abeloff MD, Armitage JO, Lichter AS, Niederhuber JE, eds. *Clinical Oncology*. New York: Churchill Livingstone, 1st ed, 1995, p. 409; 2nd ed, 2000, p. 597.

CATEGORY V

The illnesses listed in Table 1–8 are among the most frustrating to oncologists. Standard antineoplastic therapy for patients with advanced stages of these malignancies are ineffective in virtually all patients treated. Some of these patients, especially those that are relatively young and have good performance status, may be interested in and should be considered for investigational

TABLE 1–8. Category V: Generally Unresponsive to Standard Therapy

MALIGNANCY	CHARACTERISTICS
Renal cell carcinoma	Stage IV
Malignant melanoma	Incurable
Hepatobiliary and gall bladder carcinoma	Generally unresponsive to standard therapy
Adrenal carcinoma	Patients who qualify may consider investigational therapy
AIDS-associated high-grade lymphoma	End-of-life care may be the treatment of choice for this
	group of patients, unless they qualify for and desire
	investigational therapy

SOURCE: Adapted from Kinzbrunner BM: The terminally ill patient. In: Abeloff MD, Armitage JO, Lichter AS, Niederhuber JE, eds. *Clinical Oncology*. New York: Churchill Livingstone, 1st ed, 1995, p. 409; 2nd ed, 2000, p. 597.

treatment. However, for the vast majority of these patients having one of these neoplasms, end-of-life care should be considered as a treatment option at the time metastatic disease is identified. Some would even suggest that hospice and palliative care would be the treatment of choice in this group of individuals.

GUIDELINES FOR DETERMINING PROGNOSIS IN PATIENTS WITH NONMALIGNANT DIAGNOSES

Although hospice and palliative care originated with the cancer model, it became apparent toward the end of the 1980s that patients with diagnoses other than cancer had special end-of-life needs that could be met by the interdisciplinary care that hospices provide. Elderly patients with relatively common chronic debilitating illness such as chronic obstructive pulmonary disease, congestive heart failure, and Alzheimer's disease, as well as younger patients with AIDS, began to find their way onto hospice programs in ever increasing numbers. As hospice programs began caring for these patients, it became clear that the clinical course of these patients differed from their counterparts with malignant disease. For cancer patients generally had a progressive downhill course, whereas patients with nonmalignant diagnoses were observed to have much more variable disease progression, with periods of severe symptoms intermingled with periods of relative stability.

The variable clinical course of patients with nonmalignant disease was, not surprisingly, perceived as a major challenge in predicting when these patients would require hospice or palliative care. Detailed analysis of 1990 Medicare claims data cited earlier showed that of the 15% of patients surviving on hospice programs more than 6 months, the majority had noncancer diagnoses.

While, as already noted, the SUPPORT study demonstrated that physicians did a good job predicting the prognosis of patients with malignant disease, the same could not be said for the ability of physicians to estimate when patients with illnesses other than cancer were likely to die.

The heightened degree of uncertainty in predicting when patients with nonmalignant diseases require end-of-life care mandated the development of clinical guidelines in this area. Articles attempting to delineate such guidelines began to appear in the medical literature toward the end of the 1980s and into the 1990s. Crystallizing the information contained in these and other articles led, in 1995, to the development by the National Hospice and Palliative Care Organization (NHPCO) of "Medical Guidelines for the Determining Prognosis in Selected Noncancer Diseases." The document included "General Guidelines," which in large part form the basis of the General Guidelines discussed earlier, and specific guidelines for determining when patients with heart disease, lung disease, and dementia would be in need of end-of-life care. A second edition of this document published in 1996 added other noncancer illnesses, including stroke and coma, renal disease, liver disease, amyotrophic lateral sclerosis, and HIV. That these guidelines have been successful in increasing hospice access for patients with nonmalignant terminal diagnoses is shown by the continued rise in the number and percentage of patients with these illnesses receiving hospice care since the mid-1990s through 2007, best illustrated by the fact that of the 1.3 million individuals who received hospice services in 2006, almost 56% (728,000) were admitted with a terminal diagnosis other than cancer.

The criteria for determining when patients with the various nonmalignant diseases require end-of-life care will be reviewed. As with the earlier discussion of malignant disease, a list of the disease-specific criteria will be presented in tabular form, accompanied by a short discussion of the criteria, with corroboration from the medical literature where appropriate.

END-STAGE LUNG DISEASE

Knowing when patients with COPD, pulmonary fibrosis, or other forms of end-stage lung disease require end-of-life and hospice care can be exceedingly challenging.

This is because the clinical course of patients with advanced pulmonary disease usually consists of periods of relatively stable disease punctuated by episodic acute decline. It is clear, however, that as time progresses, the acute episodes become more frequent and the periods of stability become the exception rather than the rule. At such a time in the course of illness of a patient with advanced pulmonary disease, interventions by a hospice or palliative care interdisciplinary team can be invaluable. Guidelines that help determine when it is time to consider end-of-life care for patients with COPD and other forms of end stage pulmonary disease are listed in Table 1–9 and are described below.

Disabling Dyspnea

Studies in the pulmonary literature have identified many factors that affect the mortality of patients with COPD, with the most important being age, postbronchodilator FEV-1, total lung capacity, maximal work capacity of the patient, and resting heart rate. Age and resting heart rate (Table 1–9) are both easy to measure and correlate directly with patient mortality, while decreases in total lung capacity, maximal work capacity, and postbronchodilator FEV-1 are associated with a poor prognosis. Specific measures of total lung capacity and maximal work capacity that specifically predict a poor prognosis have not been reported. However, it has been demonstrated that postbronchodilator FEV-1 values consistently less than 30% predicted are associated with the highest mortality rate in COPD patients.

As stated in the introduction to the general guidelines, it is not appropriate to force patients to undergo objective testing in order to ensure that they receive needed care at the end-of-life care. Therefore, it was necessary to translate

TABLE 1–9. Criteria for Hospice Care in End-Stage Lung Disease

Disabling Dyspnea Defined by the Following:

Dyspnea at rest or with minimal exertion

Dyspnea poorly responsive or unresponsive to bronchodilator therapy

Dyspnea results in other debilitating symptoms such as decreased functional activity, fatigue, and cough

FEV-1 < 30% predicted postbronchodilator, if available

Progression in Pulmonary Disease as Manifested By:

Multiple hospitalizations, emergency department visits, or physician's office visits.

Cor pulmonale

Other Indicators of Poor Prognosis

Body weight ≤ 90% of ideal body weight, or ≥ 10% loss of weight

Resting tachycardia > 100/min

Abnormal blood gases, if available
  $pO_2 \leq 55$ mm Hg or o_2 saturation ≤ 88%
  $pCO_2 \geq 50$ mm Hg

Continuous oxygen therapy

SOURCE: Stuart B, Connor S, Kinzbrunner BM, et al: *Medical Guidelines for Determining Prognosis in Selected Non-Cancer Diseases.* Arlington: National Hospice Organization, 1st ed, 1995; 2nd ed, 1996.

these specific objective parameters into more easily accessible clinical terms. Hence, a poor total lung capacity may be represented by the criteria of disabling dyspnea at rest or with minimal exertion, a postbronchodilator FEV-1 of less than 30% predicted reflects unresponsiveness or poor responsiveness to bronchodilators, and a highly impaired maximal work capacity may be manifested by decreased functional activity and fatigue. The importance of the clinical interpretation of these objective parameters in assessing patient prognosis is underscored by a study that demonstrated that patients with higher degrees of subjective dyspnea, regardless of pulmonary function studies, had significantly shorter survival times than patients who were less symptomatic.

Progression in Pulmonary Disease

Progression of disease is an important parameter of poor prognosis. This may be manifested objectively, as it has been demonstrated that persistent and significant decreases in FEV-1 measured serially over several years portends a poor prognosis.

On a clinical level, the progression of disease can be manifested in several ways. As patients with COPD worsen, they generally develop more frequent episodes of acute bronchitis and pneumonia, requiring more attention from health care providers. Therefore, as already mentioned in the general criteria, an increase in the frequency of physician's office visits, emergency department trips, and hospital admissions is highly indicative that the patient's illness is progressing and that end-of-life care interventions may be beneficial.

Progressive dyspnea and the poor responsiveness of the patient to bronchodilators often results in the development of steroid dependence. In addition, the maximization of a patient's respiratory medication with progressive diminishing of a symptomatic response provides further evidence of disease progression.

A decreasing functional status is another important parameter that indicates advancing lung disease. The finding that patients are becoming or have become largely confined to their place of residence or to one room within their place of residence may be a strong indicator of functional decline.

Cor Pulmonale

The development of pulmonary hypertension resulting in failure of the right side of the heart, termed cor pulmonale, is associated with increased mortality in patients with COPD. Studies have shown that 50% of patients with COPD and cor pulmonale succumb to their illness in 1 to 3 years and that patients with cor pulmonale and COPD are 50% more likely to die in a

$2^1/_2$-year period than COPD patients without cor pulmonale.

Other Indicators of Poor Prognosis

There are several other important characteristics of patients with advanced pulmonary disease that may be predictive of a poor prognosis. Patients with COPD who weigh less than 90% of ideal body weight have a shorter overall survival than patients with similar levels of pulmonary function impairment whose weight either is at or exceeds ideal body weight. The presence of a resting tachycardia >100/minute is another important sign that the patient's COPD may be at an end stage and the measurement of pO_2, oxygen saturation, and pCO_2 may be helpful as well. Generally, patients with a poor prognosis have pO_2 levels of 55 mm Hg or less and/or oxygen saturation as measured by pulse oximetry of 88% or less. It is also generally accepted that patients who chronically have pCO_2 levels greater than 50 mm Hg have a poor prognosis, although patients with primarily emphysematous disease may have a poor prognosis in the absence of hypercapnea (see below).

Patients with advanced COPD often require continuous or long-term oxygen therapy. Patients on continuous oxygen therapy who are unable to elevate their pO_2 above 65 mm Hg despite the oxygen therapy have a poor prognosis. Other clinical indicators of a poor prognosis in this group of patients include patients with severe bronchial obstruction, increasing age, and the presence of chest wall abnormalities. Finally, as already mentioned, patients who require continuous oxygen therapy and have normal or low pCO_2 levels have the highest mortality among this group of patients.

END-STAGE CARDIAC DISEASE

Disabling Dyspnea, Fatigue, or Chest Pain

In general, disabling heart disease can be classified by the patient's functionality and related symptoms. New York Heart Association (NYHA) class III individuals, who have up to a 45% yearly mortality rate based on data reported by Pantilat and Steimle in JAMA in 2004, are comfortable at rest, but with minimal exertion, they will have symptoms of fatigue, angina, dyspnea, or palpations. NYHA class IV individuals, with yearly mortality rates up to 50%, will have the aforementioned symptoms at rest and their discomfort will increase with exertion. The principles for determining when patients with end-stage cardiac disease require end-of-life care, found in Table 1–10, are actually similar to those for determining prognosis of patients with advanced pulmonary disease. In other words, these are patients who have symptoms of either congestive heart failure or unstable angina pectoris at rest can be classified as being in NYHA class IV.

In addition, these patients are so severely ill that either they no longer respond to optimal medical management, including diuretics and vasodilators, or they can no longer tolerate the medications due to intolerable side effects such as hypotension and renal failure.

For patients with end-stage congestive heart failure, corroborating objective evidence of a terminal prognosis would be an ejection fraction of 20% or less, based upon a study that demonstrated that such patients had a median survival of 12 weeks and a 75% mortality at 6 months. However, as already noted, clinical evidence of persistent disease far outweighs the importance of ejection fraction, as demonstrated in a study showing that the presence of clinical congestive heart failure was a more sensitive predictor of mortality than the numerical value for ejection fraction.

TABLE 1–10. Criteria for Hospice Care in End-Stage Cardiac Disease

Disabling Dyspnea or Chest Pain as Defined by

Dyspnea or chest pain with rest or minimal exertion (NYHA class IV)

Ejection fraction ≤ 20%, if available

Persistent symptoms despite optimal medical management with vasodilators and diuretics or

Inability to tolerate optimal medical management due to hypotension and/or renal failure

Other Comorbid Condition Associated with a Poor Prognosis

Symptomatic arrhythmias resistant to antiarrhythmic therapy

History of cardiac arrest and resuscitation

History of syncope, regardless of etiology

Cardiogenic brain embolism

Concomitant HIV disease

SOURCE: Stuart B, Connor S, Kinzbrunner BM, et al: *Medical Guidelines for Determining Prognosis in Selected Non-Cancer Diseases.* Arlington: National Hospice Organization, 1st ed. 1995; 2nd ed. 1996.

Other Comorbid Conditions Associated with a Poor Prognosis

Patients with end-stage cardiac disease that either suffer from or have experienced one or more of the comorbid conditions listed in Table 1–10 are likely candidates for a hospice or palliative care program. Other comorbid factors that have been identified as having negative effects on the survival of patients with advanced cardiac disease include renal failure, COPD, CVA, liver failure, cancer, dementia, symptomatic arrhythmias, smoking, diabetes, hypertension, elevated cholesterol, coronary artery disease, and age > 75 years. In 2003, a number of these factors were combined with blood pressure and several laboratory parameters to develop a prognostic model that was able to predict risk of 30 day and 1-year mortality in a cohort of patients hospitalized for acute congestive heart failure.

Recognizing the importance of ensuring that patients with end-stage heart disease have the opportunity to receive appropriate hospice and palliative care, the American College of Cardiology and the American Heart Association developed and published clinical criteria for patients having end-stage heart diseases in 2004. In a manner similar to the guidelines discussed earlier, the two organizations established that patients with end-stage heart diseases would suffer from one of a broad spectrum of diseases with severely abnormal hearts and symptoms of fatigue, angina, or shortness of breath (NYHA class III and IV) that occurs with or without congestion and often with normal ejection fractions. Such individuals have become refractory to medical management and do not choose or are not eligible for advanced specialized treatments.

END-STAGE NEUROLOGICAL DISEASES

For the purpose of determining patient prognosis near the end of life, end-stage neurological diseases have been divided into three major subgroups: Alzheimer's disease and other dementias, cerebrovascular disease, and amyotrophic lateral sclerosis (ALS) and related motor neuron disorders.

Alzheimer's Disease and Other Dementias

PATIENT HAS A COGNITIVE DISORDER CONSISTENT WITH FAST 7   Guidelines for determining when patients with Alzheimer's and other dementias require end-of-life care can be found in Table 1–11. Recognition that patients with Alzheimer's disease and other dementias required hospice or palliative care services near the end of life was first recognized in the 1980s. It was proposed that patients be stratified into one of five levels of care based upon the stage of patient's illness, and the wishes of the patient and family regarding future care. The various levels of care proposed represented points on a continuum, with levels 4 and 5, and perhaps at times level 3, all being consistent with needing some degree of hospice and palliative care. The challenge for the clinician caring for such patients was predicting when a patient's

TABLE 1–11. Criteria for Hospice Care in End-Stage Alzheimer's Disease and Other Dementias

Patient has a Cognitive Disorder Consistent with FAST 7, as Manifested by

Inability to ambulate without assistance

Inability to speak or communicate meaningfully with speech limited to approximately a half-dozen or fewer intelligible or different words

Loss of ADL functions including bathing and dressing (stage 6)

Incontinence of bowel and bladder (stage 6)

Patient has had One or More of the Following Comorbid Conditions in the Last 3–6 mo:

Aspiration pneumonia

Pyelonephritis or upper urinary tract infection

Septicemia

Decubitus ulcers: usually multiple and stages III or IV

Fever, recurrent after antibiotics

An altered nutritional status as manifested by

    Difficulty swallowing or refusal to eat such that sufficient fluid or caloric intake cannot be maintained and the patient refuses artificial nutritional support

    OR

    If the patient is receiving artificial nutritional support (NG or G tube or parenteral hyperalimentation), there must be evidence of an impaired nutritional status as defined in the general guidelines ($\geq$10% loss of body weight)

SOURCE: Stuart B, Connor S, Kinzbrunner BM, et al: *Medical Guidelines for Determining Prognosis in Selected Non-Cancer Diseases.* Arlington: National Hospice Organization, 1st ed, 1995; 2nd ed, 1996.

dementia was severe enough to warrant a shift in the philosophy of care to that of palliation.

The Functional Assessment Staging Classification (FAST) was published by Reisberg in 1986. This classification of Alzheimer's dementia defines seven stages, paralleling normal human development in reverse, with a spectrum ranging from patients with no perceptible mental status changes (stage 1) to patients who are so severely demented that they lose their ability to ambulate, speak, sit up, and even smile (stage 7). It was believed that patients who exhibited the characteristics defined as FAST stage 7-C, the loss of ambulatory ability in a patient who was unable to communicate meaningfully and who required assistance in all activities of daily living, was a good candidate for hospice services. These criteria were formally adopted by the NHPCO in 1995, and are listed in Table 1–11.

It should be emphasized that inability to ambulate without assistance appears to be the key functional deficit that identifies patients who are in need of end-of-life care. Inability to ambulate should not be confused with a bed-bound status and includes patients who can be lifted into and sit in a chair with support, or who can even walk short distances with support from caregivers. The other important criteria are those that define stages 7-A and 7-B, namely loss of intelligible speech and meaningful communication. However, it should be noted that some patients do not progress consecutively through the substages of stage 7, and may on occasion lose the ability to ambulate prior to the loss of their communication skills. These patients should still be considered eligible for hospice or palliative care services, although, as discussed later, their prognosis is somewhat more variable than patients who progress in an orderly manner through the stage 7 sub-stages. It also should be noted that predominately vascular dementias tend to have nonorderly stage 7 progression depending upon the portion of the brain most affected and that individuals can have multiple etiologies for their dementias so that their symptoms and progression of disease can be quite variable.

PATIENT HAS HAD ONE OR MORE COMORBID CONDITIONS IN THE LAST 3–6 MONTHS It is well known from clinical experience that patients with advanced dementia, even those far advanced enough to qualify as FAST 7-C, may live for many months or even years. What usually determines mortality in this group of patients is the presence of one or more comorbid conditions or inter-current illnesses, especially those related to the loss of functional status, infection, decubitus ulcers, or related to a deteriorating nutritional status.

Comorbid diagnosis, such as arthritis and other chronic conditions of aging, which would generally not stand alone as indicative of end-stage disease, can significantly impair the dementia patient's health and functionality. Diagnoses such as cardiovascular disease, COPD and restrictive lung diseases, CVA, diabetes, renal insufficiency, and malignancies when present, even if not end-stage, could well impact the prognosis of dementias and should also be considered when evaluating patient prognosis.

Patients with advanced dementias are highly susceptible to a number of infectious illnesses. Aspiration pneumonia, due to either the difficulty in swallowing or the presence of a feeding tube (either NG or gastrostomy) is a common problem, and is associated with an increase in patient mortality at six months. These patients are also more likely to develop recurrent upper urinary tract infections and episodes of septicemia requiring antibiotic therapy on an intermittent but recurring basis. Such recurrent febrile episodes in this population is not only associated with an increased mortality rate, but also studies have shown that the mortality is unaffected by the decision to treat such patients with antibiotics. On the basis of this and follow-up studies, it has been suggested that, since patients have been shown to be more comfortable and less distressed when not treated with antibiotics, they may be avoided at times in this group of patients.

Decubitus ulcers are another significant comorbid factor in this group of patients. Studies have shown that 50% of patients admitted to nursing homes with multiple stage III and or stage IV decubiti and 38% of patients who develop such decubiti within 3 months of nursing home admission die within 1 year.

An altered nutritional status is a significant comorbid condition in this group of patients as well. Patients who lose the ability to eat secondary to dementias or other neurological conditions have a higher mortality whether or not they receive nutritional support via artificial means. Patients may elect, based either upon advance directives or the instructions of durable powers of attorney, not to receive artificial nutritional support. As a consequence they have an increased mortality rate either secondary to the inability to sustain themselves due to deficient caloric intake or to the increased risk of aspiration pneumonia if oral feedings were to be continued. For patients who have elected artificial nutritional support, studies have demonstrated increased morbidity and increased mortality as well, especially if they continue to lose weight following initiation of the feedings. (For a full discussion of this topic, see Chapter 24.) Therefore, patients with advanced dementia who are losing weight and either do not elect artificial nutritional support or are losing weight in spite of artificial nutritional support are likely candidates for end-of-life care. (The reader should be reminded that these comorbid factors are not mutually exclusive. For example, patients who are being artificially fed and are maintaining weight may be eligible for hospice and palliative care if they suffer from frequent infections or multiple decubiti.)

PROGNOSTIC ACCURACY OF DEMENTIA GUIDELINES A study designed to test the accuracy of the guidelines for determining the prognosis of patients with end-stage dementia was published in 1997. This study validated the importance of comorbid factors, especially related to nutritional status, in determining prognosis in these patients. The sub-group of patients who presented with classical FAST 7-C or beyond had a median survival of significantly less than 6 months whether or not they received traditional medical interventions for acute illnesses (i.e., antibiotics for febrile

episodes). Patients who were more cognitively intact than stage 7-C had a median survival of almost 2 years. A third sub-group of patients identified in this study, and alluded to above, were patients who did not progress consecutively through the sub-stages of stage 7, losing, for example, the ability to ambulate prior to the loss of their communication skills. Interestingly, these patients succumbed to their illness in a median time of less than 6 months if they did not receive traditional medical interventions for acute illnesses, while they survived a median of almost 15 months if they did receive such interventions. Therefore, in addition to confirming the importance of stage 7-C and the presence of comorbid conditions in determining the need for end-of-life care in patients with Alzheimer's disease and other dementias, the study suggests that patients who exhibit some, but not all, characteristics of stage 7-C might be appropriate for hospice and palliative care, especially if they elect comfort measures rather than traditional medical interventions for comorbid conditions or intercurrent illnesses.

A recent alternative to the guidelines presented earlier was reported by Mitchell et al in JAMA in 2004. Taking advantage of the requirement in long-term care facilities to collect quarterly data as part of the MDS (see General Guidelines section), it was determined that there were a number of factors, including, but not limited to, advanced age, presence of cancer or congestive heart failure, shortness of breath, oxygen dependence, and bedfast status, that were associated with an increased risk of 6-month mortality in residents with advanced dementia. On the basis of the weighted importance of these factors, a scoring system was developed. Patients who had the highest scores (≥ 12) had a 70% 6-month mortality, while patients with scores of 9 to 11 had a 57% chance of dying within 6 months. The authors conclude that their model for predicting 6-month mortality is more accurate than the currently existing prognostic guidelines for dementia patients (which are the guidelines presented earlier). Although the authors' conclusion is scientifically correct, the lack of any clinical judgment inherent in this prognostic model creates the challenge of potentially denying many advanced dementia patients who are eligible for hospice care from accessing those services, and severely limits their practical utility.

Cerebrovascular Disease

Guidelines for determining when patients with advanced cerebrovascular disease require end-of-life care are listed in Table 1–12. There have

been two distinct categories of patients identified: those who have recently suffered a severe acute neurological event, and those who are experiencing the debility and aftereffects of chronic cerebrovascular disease.

ACUTE CEREBROVASCULAR DISEASE AND COMA
In considering the question of when a patient who has just experienced an acute cerebrovascular event, or has become comatose due to another cause, might need hospice or palliative care, it is

---

TABLE 1–12. Criteria for Hospice Care in Cerebrovascular Disease

Acute Cerebrovascular Disease and Coma

Patient has one of the following conditions for at least 3 days duration:
  Coma
  Persistent vegetative state
  Severe obtundation accompanied by myoclonus
  Post anoxic stroke
Other factors associated with a high risk of mortality after 3 days (ref. Hamel JAMA, 1995)
  Abnormal brain stem response
  Absent verbal response
  Absent withdrawal response to pain
  Serum creatinine $\geq$ 1.5 mg/dL
  Age $\geq$ 70 yrs

Chronic Cerebrovascular Disease, Coma, and Persistent Vegetative State (PVS)

Post stroke or multiinfarct dementia consistent with FAST 7, if patient not comatose or in PVS
Patient has had one or more of the following comorbid conditions in the last 3–6 mo:
  Aspiration pneumonia
  Pyelonephritis or upper urinary tract infection
  Septicemia
  Decubitus ulcers: usually multiple and stages III or IV
  Fever, recurrent after antibiotics
  An altered nutritional status as manifested by
    Difficulty swallowing or refusal to eat such that sufficient fluid or caloric intake cannot be maintained
      and the patient refuses artificial nutritional support
    OR
    If the patient is receiving artificial nutritional support (NG or G tube or parenteral hyperalimentation),
      there must be evidence of an impaired nutritional status as defined in the general guidelines ($\geq$ 10%
      loss of body weight)

SOURCE: Stuart B, Connor S, Kinzbrunner BM, et al: *Medical Guidelines for Determining Prognosis in Selected Non-Cancer Diseases.* Arlington: National Hospice Organization, 1st ed, 1995; 2nd ed, 1996.

important to first allow such patients some time for recovery. It is well known that patients who appear moribund or comatose during the first few hours or first day following an acute neurological insult may often, with proper support and rehabilitation, go on to a meaningful recovery. On the basis of a report from the SUPPORT investigators, it would appear that patients who suffered from acute cerebrovascular attacks or became comatose from other causes (i.e., cardiac arrest) had a high mortality rate if they did not show signs of recovering neurological function within 3 days of the acute insult. Persistent neurological deficits that were associated with the highest risk of mortality after day 3 included a decerebrate response to external stimuli, an absent verbal response, and an absent withdrawal response to pain. Older patients (age $\geq$ 70 years) and patients with renal function impairment (serum creatinine $\geq$ 1.5 mg/dL) were also associated with a poor prognosis. In fact, patients who exhibited four of the five factors after day 3 had a 97% probability of succumbing to their illnesses within 2 months.

CHRONIC CEREBROVASCULAR DISEASE For patients with chronic cerebrovascular disease, long-standing coma, or persistent vegetative state (PVS), criteria that assist in determining that end-of-life care is necessary closely resemble those for dementia, as outlined in Table 1–12. Patients who are not in coma or in a PVS will usually have signs of multi-infarct dementia, with deficits in functional activity that closely resemble FAST 7. For all patients, comorbid conditions and intercurrent illnesses, such as advanced heart or lung disease, diabetes mellitus renal failure, recent infections, decubiti, or a deteriorating nutritional status, to name a few, in other words, the same criteria described for patients with long-standing terminal dementia, would serve as additional indicators for a poor prognosis.

Amyotrophic Lateral Sclerosis and Other Forms of Motor Neuron Disease

Predicting the prognosis of patients with amyotrophic lateral sclerosis (ALS) (also known as Lou Gehrig disease) and other forms of motor neuron disease may be very challenging. Patients tend to be younger and, with nutritional or ventilatory support, can live for extended periods of time, measured in years, even in the face of severe neurological dysfunction. In today's high-tech society, patients who can do little more than blink their eyelids communicate and lead productive lives with computer aids and other technological supports.

Despite these great scientific advances, however, there are patients with ALS who, as their neurological condition deteriorates, would not choose to become dependent on feeding tubes, ventilators, or computers. For these patients, end-of-life care would become a serious option, especially when the ability of such patients to either swallow or breathe independently becomes significantly impaired.

Clinical characteristics of ALS make the timing of decisions regarding end-of-life care somewhat difficult. It has been shown that, although ALS does progress over time, the rate of neurological deterioration varies markedly from patient to patient. In addition, the location of the first muscles involved has not been shown to correlate with survival.

What seems to correlate most with short survival of patients with ALS is the development of what is described as "rapid progression," which, as outlined in Table 1–13, is basically defined as the development of severe neurological disability within a 12-month period. In addition to "rapid progression," patients who have a limited prognosis and are in need of hospice or palliative care generally will have either a critically impaired ventilatory status, significant nutritional impairment, or other life-threatening complications that bear a striking resemblance to the comorbid conditions and intercurrent illnesses that are compatible with poor prognosis of patients with dementias and cerebrovascular disease.

In general, debilitating neurological diseases other than ALS such as progressive supranuclear palsy, Lewy body dementia, Parkinson disease, and MS can be evaluated for hospice appropriate

TABLE 1–13. Criteria for Hospice Care in Amyotrophic Lateral Sclerosis (ALS) and Other Motor Neuron Diseases

Rapid Progression of ALS

Development of severe neurological disability over a 12-mo period. Examples would include
  Progression from independent ambulation to wheelchair or bed bound
  Progression from normal to barely intelligible or unintelligible speech
  Progression from normal to blenderized diet
  Progression from independence in most or all ADLs to needing major assistance in all ADLs

Critically Impaired Ventilatory Capacity

Vital capacity < 30% predicted
Significant dyspnea at rest
Supplemental oxygen needed at rest
Refusal by patient of intubation, tracheostomy, other forms of mechanical ventilatory support
Note: If patient is already on some form of ventilatory support, they may still be appropriate for hospice or
  palliative care management if they exhibit one or more comorbid conditions as delineated in the following
  text.

Critical Nutritional Impairment

Difficulty swallowing or refusal to eat such that sufficient fluid or caloric intake cannot be maintained and
  the patient refuses artificial nutritional support
OR
If the patient is receiving artificial nutritional support, the patient should be experiencing continued weight
  loss despite the feedings.

Comorbid Conditions

Aspiration pneumonia
Pyelonephritis or upper urinary tract infection
Septicemia
Decubitus ulcers: usually multiple and stages III or IV
Fever, recurrent after antibiotics

SOURCE: Stuart B, Connor S, Kinzbrunner BM, et al: *Medical Guidelines for Determining Prognosis in Selected Non-Cancer Diseases.* Arlington: National Hospice Organization, 1st ed, 1995; 2nd ed, 1996.

status using the general guidelines and in part the above three diagnostic features of impaired ventilatory status, impaired nutritional state, and the other life-threatening complications. When appropriate and where applicable, features used in the dementia guidelines, such as Functional Assessment Staging, may be useful but are not required for determining appropriateness. As always, clinical judgment is required.

END-STAGE AIDS

Access to endof-life care for patients having HIV infection and AIDS has been variable throughout the years since the syndrome was first described in the early 1980s. During the decade of the 1980s, due in part to the relative youth of the majority of patients infected with HIV virus, it was unusual to see patients with AIDS in hospice programs except during the last week or two of life. As a better understanding of AIDS was acquired, markers for poor prognosis became available. Hospices, sensing the fact that patients with AIDS tended to avoid end-of-life care because of their relative youth, developed end-of-life care programs that deemphasized the terminal nature of the illness, while giving such patients the same compassionate interdisciplinary care that patients with more traditional advanced illnesses were receiving. These two factors led to increasing numbers of patients with AIDS accessing hospice and palliative care programs for significantly longer periods of time prior to death.

As we enter the new century, the nature of HIV infection and AIDS has shifted once again. The development of new antiretroviral agents, specifically the protease inhibitors, and the ability to better control opportunistic infections, has shifted AIDS from a terminal illness to a chronic one. Patients are now living for years, as contrasted to several years ago when they would have only survived months. This has significantly decreased the number of patients that use hospice and other palliative care services, albeit for the right reasons. Nevertheless, there are patients with advanced AIDS who still require end-of-life care; hence, the need to have guidelines available to determine when this is necessary.

The guidelines for determining when patients with AIDS require end-of-life care can be found in Table 1–14. Unlike most of the other illnesses discussed earlier, where laboratory studies are helpful but not required, measurements of CD4+ count and HIV RNA (viral load) are crucial to determining when patients with AIDS require end-of-life care. Patients with CD4+ counts below 25 cell/mcL, especially during periods free of acute illness, or with persistent HIV RNA levels of greater than 100,000 copies are likely to have a prognosis of less than 6 months. Conversely, patients with CD4+ counts > 50 cell/mcL clearly have a prognosis much longer than 6 months unless they have a non-HIV illness that is life-threatening or terminal. Patients who have viral loads of more than 100,000 may be candidates

for end-of-life care only if they elect to forego antiretroviral therapy, other forms of prophylactic therapy, have a declining functional status, and suffer from an HIV-related illness or exhibit one or more poor prognostic factors as listed in Table 1–14.

There are a number of life-limiting infections and malignancies associated with HIV infection that may dictate a need for a palliative plan of care. These illnesses, as well as their approximate prognoses, are delineated in Table 1–14. Other factors that predict for a poor prognosis in patients with AIDS include low serum albumin, advancing age, persistent diarrhea, and concomitant heart disease.

Patient lack of compliance with antiviral regimens often impacts disease progression along with comorbid viral infections such as hepatitis B and C. Patients presenting with low CD4 counts and high viral loads that have never been treated with antiviral therapy should be evaluated for such care prior to hospice being offered.

END-STAGE RENAL DISEASE

Criteria indicating terminal prognosis for patients with end-stage renal disease can be found in Table 1–15. Patients with chronic renal failure who should be considered for end-of-life care include those who are candidates for hemodialysis, peritoneal dialysis, or renal transplant and choose not to be dialyzed or receive a transplant. Another subset of patients with renal failure that might benefit from hospice and palliative care would be those who have been undergoing dialysis and either decide to stop or become too ill to tolerate dialysis any longer. Patients who are still being dialyzed, but are considering stopping due to a perceived poor quality of life, pose an interesting dilemma for hospice programs. Clearly, these patients would benefit from the additional psychosocial and spiritual support that a hospice can provide while considering their options. In general, such patients are not admitted to a hospice program until they make the decision to stop

TABLE 1–14. Criteria for Hospice Care in Acquired Immunodeficiency Syndrome (AIDS)

CD4+ Count < 25 cells/mcL in Periods Free of Acute Illness
OR

HIV RNA (Viral Load) > 100,000 Copies on a Persistent Basis

HIV RNA (Viral Load) < 100,000 Copies in the Presence of
Patient refusal to receive antiretroviral or prophylactic medications
Declining functional status
One or more "other factors" listed in below

HIV-Related Opportunistic Illnesses

Disease	Prognosis
CNS lymphoma	2.5 mo
Progressive multifocal leukoencephalopathy	4 mo
Cryptosporidiosis	5 mo
AIDS wasting syndrome (loss of 1/3 lean body mass)	<6 mo
MAC bacteremia, untreated	<6 mo
Visceral Kaposi's sarcoma, unresponsive to treatment	50% 6 mo mortality
Renal failure, refuses dialysis	<6 mo
Advanced AIDS dementia complex	6 mo
Toxoplasmosis	6 mo

Other Factors Associated with a Poor Prognosis for Patients with AIDS
Chronic persistent diarrhea for 1 yr
Persistent serum albumin < 2.5 gm/dL
Concomitant substance abuse
Age > 50
Decision to forego antiretroviral therapy, chemotherapy, and prophylactic drug therapy related to HIV
   disease and related illnesses
Congestive heart failure, symptomatic at rest

SOURCE: Stuart B, Connor S, Kinzbrunner BM, et al: *Medical Guidelines for Determining Prognosis in Selected Non-Cancer Diseases.* Arlington: National Hospice Organization, 1st ed, 1995; 2nd ed, 1996.

dialysis. However, some hospices are currently evaluating the feasibility of admitting such patients and providing limited dialysis while giving them the time and support to make appropriate choices.

Laboratory criteria compatible with end stage renal failure are compatible with values established by CMS (form #2728) and include a creatinine clearance less than 10 cc/minute (<15 cc/min in patients with diabetes) and a serum creatinine greater than 8.0 mg/dL (>6.0 mg/dL in patients with diabetes). One must be careful not to use blood urea nitrogen (BUN) levels to determine whether a patient meets guidelines for end-

stage renal disease, as BUN levels can be elevated due to prerenal azotemia from volume depletion.

As patients develop progressive renal failure and their prognosis worsens, various symptoms of uremia occur. The onset of such symptoms may assist the clinician in determining the appropriate time to institute end-of-life care in a patient with borderline renal failure who is not a candidate for dialysis or transplant. These symptoms are listed in Table 1–15.

The development of acute renal failure may be associated with a poor prognosis, especially when it occurs in relationship to acute illness. Conditions that, when accompanied by acute renal

TABLE 1–15. Criteria for Hospice Care in End-Stage Renal Disease

Patient meets criteria for dialysis and/or renal transplant and refuses
Patient with renal failure on dialysis who choose to discontinue dialysis

Laboratory Criteria

Creatinine clearance < 10 cc/min (<15 cc/min with diabetes)
Serum creatinine > 8.0 mg/dL (>6.0 mg/dL with diabetes)

Signs and Symptoms of Progressive Uremia

Confusion and obtundation
Intractable nausea and emesis
Generalized pruritis
Restlessness
Oliguria: Urine output < 400 cc/24 h
Intractable hyperkalemia: Serum potassium > 7.0, not responsive to medical management
Pericarditis
Intractable fluid overload
Hepatorenal syndrome

Acute Renal Failure: Comorbid Illnesses Associated with a Poor Prognosis

Mechanical ventilation	Malignancy
Chronic lung disease	Advanced cardiac disease
Advanced liver disease	Sepsis
Immunosuppression/AIDS	Serum albumin < 3.5 g/dL
Cachexia	Platelet count < 25,000
Age > 75 yr	Disseminated intravascular coagulation (DIC)
Gastrointestinal bleeding	

SOURCE: Stuart B, Connor S, Kinzbrunner BM, et al: *Medical Guidelines for Determining Prognosis in Selected Non-Cancer Diseases.* Arlington: National Hospice Organization, 1st ed, 1995; 2nd ed, 1996.

failure, tend to predict early patient mortality are listed in Table 1–15 as well.

END-STAGE LIVER DISEASE

The guidelines for patients having hepatic failure due to nonmalignant causes may be found in Table 1–16. In essence, patients with liver disease requiring hospice or palliative care are those who suffer from persistent symptoms of hepatic failure, such as ascites, hepatic encephalopathy, or recurrent variceal bleeding, despite adequate medical management. They generally have multiple liver function abnormalities, with the most sensitive laboratory indicators of severe hepatic impairment being a prothrombin time that is at least 5 seconds over control, and a serum albumin less that 2.5 g/dL.

OTHER NONMALIGNANT TERMINAL DISEASE

Patients having advanced illnesses other than the ones described earlier will sometimes also need end-of-life care. These patients should be assessed for end-of-life care on an individual basis. In many instances, the guidelines for the various illnesses discussed earlier can be applied to other patients. As noted in the ALS section,

TABLE 1–16. Criteria for Hospice Care in End-Stage Liver Disease

Progressive Symptoms not Responsive to Medical Management or Patient Noncompliance, Including

Ascites, refractory to sodium restriction and diuretics, especially with associated spontaneous bacterial peritonitis

Hepatic encephalopathy refractory to protein restriction and lactulose or neomycin

Recurrent variceal bleed despite therapeutic interventions

Hepatorenal syndrome

Laboratory Indicators of End Stage Liver Disease

Protime $\geq$ 5 s more than control

Serum albumin $\leq$ 2.5 g/dL

Other Factors Associated with a Poor Prognosis in Patients with End-Stage Liver Disease

Progressive malnutrition

Muscle wasting with reduced strength and endurance

Continued active ethanol intake (> 80 g ethanol per day)

Hepatocellular carcinoma

HbsAg positivity

Source: Stuart B, Connor S, Kinzbrunner BM, et al: *Medical Guidelines for Determining Prognosis in Selected Non-Cancer Diseases.* Arlington: National Hospice Organization, 1st ed, 1995; 2nd ed, 1996.

for other advanced neurological illnesses, such as Parkinson disease, functional status deterioration, weight loss, and comorbid conditions such as defined in the criteria for end-stage Alzheimer's disease may be helpful determinants for directing patients with these conditions to hospice or palliative care programs.

DEBILITY, UNSPECIFIED OR ADULT "FAILURE TO THRIVE"

There are elderly patients who appear to be approaching the end of life for which a definitive terminal illness is not evident. These patients usually suffer from multiple medical illnesses or may be experiencing multiple comorbid conditions or progressive disabilities, such as declining functional status or weight loss. The combination of multiple chronic illnesses and a declining condition often prompt the patient, family, or attending physician to realize that the patient's clinical situation is irreversible, and a hospice or palliative treatment plan is sought.

Attempts to develop a standard diagnostic nomenclature for this group of patients have been challenging. One diagnostic term that would accurately characterize this group of patients is adult "failure to thrive." In fact, this term has been appearing with increasing regularity in the geriatric literature since the 1970s. However, when attempts were made to admit patients with this diagnosis to hospice programs in the 1980s, the fiscal intermediaries refused to reimburse services provided for such patients due to the fact that they perceived "failure to thrive" as a pediatric diagnosis, inappropriate for use in adult patients.

An alternative diagnosis was sought, and found in Section 16 of the ICD-9 code book, "Symptoms, signs, and ill-defined conditions" (780–799). In the subsection "Ill-defined and unknown causes of morbidity and mortality" (797–799) is code 799.3, "Debility, unspecified," which by its nature would characterize elderly, debilitated patients who are ill (morbidity) and have a high risk of dying (mortality).

A study published in 1996 reported on a retrospective analysis of 53 hospice patient charts that was performed in an attempt to identify the characteristics of patients admitted for terminal care with the diagnosis "Debility, unspecified." The study demonstrated that these patients had severe functional deficits and a variety of comorbid medical illnesses most commonly involving the central nervous system or the cardio-respiratory systems, but did not meet any of the illness-specific criteria that would determine a specific diagnosable terminal illness. These patients had a median survival on the hospice program of less than 3 weeks and average survival of approximately 2 months.

TABLE 1–17. Criteria for Hospice Care in Debility, Unspecified or Adult Failure to Thrive

Patient Meets General Criteria as Outlined in Table 1–1

Declining functional status

Declining nutritional status especially BMI < 22 kg/m²

Multiple hospitalizations over the last several months

Patient has One or More Comorbid Medical Conditions Including, but not Limited to

Heart disease	COPD
Dementia	Diabetes mellitus
Cerebrovascular disease	Sepsis and/or
Multiple decubiti	frequent infections

Patient does not meet guidelines for a terminal prognosis based on any one of the comorbid illnesses from which they suffer

And/or

It is unclear which comorbid condition is most likely to result in death.

Patient or family may have chosen not to pursue further evaluation of an undiagnosed medical condition or acute care treatment of one or more comorbid medical conditions due to advanced age or overall deterioration of patient health

On the basis of this study, it is clear that patients without a specific terminal diagnosis do constitute a population of terminally ill patients and should have access to end-of-life care. Criteria for considering patients for hospice or palliative care services when a definitive terminal diagnosis is not apparent are presented in Table 1–17. In some respect, these patients represent a population of elderly individuals who meet the general criteria for a terminal prognosis such as severe functional impairment and weight loss (see Table 1–1), but do not meet any of the illness-specific criteria defined earlier. They generally suffer from one, or more often, multiple comorbid conditions, and it is unclear which condition will prove

to be fatal. In some cases, the patient or family will elect not to pursue aggressive medical evaluation or treatment due to either the patient's advanced age or overall deteriorating medical condition.

It should be noted that, due to the increasing body of geriatric literature on the subject of "adult failure to thrive" during the early and mid-1990s, the diagnosis of "adult failure to thrive" was formally recognized and incorporated into the ICD-9 code manual (783.7) and is also recognized alongside "Debility, unspecified" as a legitimate terminal diagnosis for the patients described earlier. Whether the diagnosis of "Debility, unspecified" or a similar diagnosis, such as adult "Failure to thrive" is utilized is unimportant. What is critical is for the clinician to recognize that elderly patients with multiple medical illnesses or showing signs of rapid decline and either refuse medical evaluation or are found to have irreversible conditions should be given the opportunity to receive appropriate end-of-life care.

CONCLUSION

Although it would seem that the ability of clinicians to accurately predict when patients have a prognosis of 6 months or less seems quite daunting, it can, in reality, be broken down into just a few simple principles. When confronted with patients having a chronic and life-limiting illness, the physician should primarily rely on his or her clinical judgment in thinking about whether the illness is in its final phases. To assist their clinical judgment, the factors outlined in the "General Guidelines," including signs of disease progression, increased use of health care services, decreasing performance status, and unintentional weight loss should be considered. Disease-specific criteria should also be looked for based on the patient's primary diagnosis, and various associated concurrent illnesses and comorbid conditions should be factored in as well. Most importantly, the patient's own goals and specific wishes regarding his or her illness and how he or she wishes to be treated should be thought about. If all these factors are considered, the ability of clinicians to predict patient prognosis should be reasonably sound.

Perhaps, putting this another way is for the clinician to ask him or herself a single question, one that is often attributed to Dr. Joanne Lynn, a pioneer in end-of-life care in the US: "Would I be surprised if this patient were to die in the next six months?" If the answer to the question is "No, I would not be surprised," then it is likely that the patient will succumb to his or her illness in a period of 6 months or so, and consideration of the patient for end-of-life care planning and hospice or palliative care should begin.

BIBLIOGRAPHY

Aida A, Miyamoto K, Nakano T, et al: Dyspnea grade as a prognostic factor in patients with chronic obstructive pulmonary disease. *Nihon Kyobu Shikkan Gakkai Zasshi* 32(1):9, 1994.

Alexander HR, Norton JA: Pathophysiology of cancer cachexia, In: Doyle D, Hanks GWC, MacDonald N, eds. *Oxford Textbook of Palliative Medicine.* Oxford, Oxford University Press, 1993, p. 316.

American Society of Clinical Oncology Task Force on Cancer Care at the End of Life: Cancer care during the last phase of life. *J Clin Oncol* 16:1986, 1998.

Anderson F, Downing GM, Hill J, et al: Palliative Performance Scale (PPS): A new tool. *J Palliat Care* 12(1):5, 1996.

Anthonisen NR: Prognosis in chronic obstructive pulmonary disease. Results from multi-center clinical trials. *Am Rev Respir Dis* 140:S95, 1989.

Arkes HR, Dawson NV, Speroff T, et al: The covariance decomposition of the probability score and its use in evaluating prognostic estimates. *Med Decis Making* 15:120, 1995.

Brandeis GH, Morris JN, Nash DJ, Lipsitz LA: The epidemiology and natural history of pressure ulcers in elderly nursing home patients. *J Am Med Assoc* 264:2905, 1990.

Campbell-Taylor I, Fisher RH: The clinical case against tube feeding in palliative care of the elderly. *J Am Geriatr Soc* 35:1100, 1987.

Christakis NA: Predicting patient survival before and after hospice enrollment. *Hosp J* 13:71, 1998.

Christiakis NA, Escarce JJ: Survival of medicare patients after enrollment on a hospice program. *N Engl J Med* 335:172, 1996.

Chistakis NA, Lamont EB: Extent and determinants of error in physicians' prognoses in terminally ill patients: prospective cohort study. *BMJ* 320:269, 2000.

Ciocon JO, Silverstone FA, Graver LM, Foley CJ: Tube feeding in elderly patients. Indications, benefits, and complications. *Arch Intern Med* 148:429, 1988.

Clark LP, Dion DM, Barker WH: Taking to bed. Rapid functional decline in an independently mobile older population living in an intermediate-care facility. *J Am Geriatr Soc* 38:967, 1990.

Cohen LM, Ruthazer R, Moss AH, Germain MJ: Predicting six-month mortality for patients who are on maintenance hemodialysis. *Clin J Am Soc Nephrol* 5(1):72, 2010.

Corti M, Guralnik JM, Salive ME, Sorkin JD: Serum albumin level and physical disability as predictors of mortality in older persons. *J Am Med Assoc* 272:1036, 1994.

Cowcher K, Hanks GW: Long-term management of respiratory symptoms in advanced cancer. *J Pain Symptom Manage* 5:320, 1990.

Dewys WD, Begg C, Lavin PT, et al: Prognostic effect of weight loss prior to chemotherapy in cancer patients. *Am J Med* 69:491, 1980.

Donaldson LJ, Clayton DG, Clarke M: The elderly in residential care: Mortality in relation to functional capacity. *J Epidemiol Community Health* 34:96, 1980.

Downing M, Lau F, Lesperance M, et al: Meta-analysis of survival prediction with Palliative Performance Scale. *J Palliat Care* 23(4):245, 2007.

Dubois P, Jamart J, Machiels J, et al: Prognosis of severely hypoxemic patients receiving long-term oxygen therapy. *Chest* 105:469, 1994.

Fabiszewski KJ, Volicer B, Volicer L: Effect of antibiotic treatments on outcome of fevers in institutionalized alzheimer's patients. *J Am Med Assoc* 263:3168, 1990.

Galanos AN, Pieper CF, Kussin PS, et al: Relationship of body mass index to subsequent mortality among seriously ill hospitalized patients. *Crit Care Med* 25:1962, 1997.

Glare P: A systematic review of physician's predictions in terminally ill cancer patients. *BMJ* 327(7408):195, 2003.

Hamel MB, Goldman L, Teno J, et al: Identification of comatose patients at high risk for death or severe disability. *J Am Med Assoc* 273:1842, 1995.

Harrold J, Rickerson E, Carroll JT, et al: Is the palliative performance scale a useful predictor of mortality in a heterogeneous hospice population? *J Palliat Med* 8(3):503, 2005.

Head B, Ritchie CS, Smoot TM: Prognostication in hospice care: Can the palliative performance scale help? *J Palliat Med* 8(3):492, 2005.

Hurley AC, Volicer B, Mahoney MA, Volicer L: Palliative fever management in Alzheimer's patients: Quality plus fiscal responsibility. *Adv Nurs Sci* 16(1):21, 1993.

Hurley AC, Volicer BJ, Volicer L: Effect of fever management strategy on the progression of dementia of the Alzheimer's type. *Alzheimer Dis Assoc Disord* 10(1):5, 1996.

Karnofsky SA, Abelmann WH, Craver LF, Burchenal JH: The use of nitrogen mustard in the palliative treatment of carcinoma. *Cancer* 1:634, 1948.

Katz S, Ford AB, Moskowitz RW, et al: Studies of illness in the aged, the index of ADL: A standardized measure of biological and psychosocial function. *J Am Med Assoc* 185:914, 1963.

Kawakami Y: Prognostic factors in COPD: The importance of pulmonary hemodynamic variables. *Pract Cardiol* 11(9):124, 1985.

Keating NL, Herrinton LJ, Zalavsky AM, et al: Variations in hospice use among cancer patients. *J Natl Cancer Inst* 98:1053, 2006.

Kinzbrunner BM: Non-malignant terminal diseases: Criteria for hospice admission. *Hosp Update* 3:3, 1993.

Kinzbrunner BM: Hospice: what to do when anti-cancer therapy is no longer appropriate, effective, or desired. *Semin Oncol* 21:792, 1994.

Kinzbrunner BM: The terminally ill patient. In: Abeloff MD, Armitage JO, Lichter AS, Niederhuber JE, eds. *Clinical Oncology*. New York, Churchill Livingstone, 1st ed., 1995: p. 409; 2nd ed., 2000: p. 597.

Kinzbrunner BM: Hospice: 15 years and beyond in the care of the dying. *J Palliat Med* 1:127, 1998.

Kinzbrunner BM: Utilization of hospice services by terminally ill cancer patients. *Proc ASCO* 18: 2226, 1999.

Kinzbrunner BM, Tanis D: Average length of stay in hospice for five types of cancer. *J Clin Oncol* 25(18S):17038, 2007.

Kinzbrunner BM, Weinreb NJ, Merriman MP: Debility unspecified: A terminal diagnosis. *Am J Hosp Palliat Care* 13(6):1039, 1996.

Knaus WA, Harrell FE, Lynn J, et al: The SUPPORT prognostic model. Objective estimates of survival for seriously ill hospitalized patients. *Ann Intern Med* 122:191, 1995.

Landi F, Zuccala G, Gambassi G, et al: Body mass index and mortality among older people living in the community. *J Am Geriatr Soc* 47:1072, 1999.

Lau F, Downing GM, Lesperance M, et al: Use of palliative performance scale in end-of-life prognostication. *J Palliat Med* 9(5):1066, 2006.

Lee DS, Austin PC, Rouleau JL, et al: Predicting mortality among patients hospitalized for heart failure: derivation and validation of a clinical model. *J Am Med Assoc* 290:2581, 2003.

Likoff MJ, Chandler SL, Kay HR: Clinical determinants of mortality in chronic congestive heart failure secondary to idiopathic dilated or to ischemic cardiomyopathy. *Am J Cardiol* 59:634, 1987.

Luchins DJ, Hanrahan P, Murphy K: Criteria for enrolling dementia patients in hospice. *J Am Geriatr Soc* 45:1054, 1997.

Lynn J, Harrell F, Cohn F, et al: Prognoses of seriously ill hospitalized patients on the days before death: Implications for patient care and public policy. *New Horiz* 5:56, 1997.

Lynn J, Teno JM, Harrell FE: Accurate prognostications of death. Opportunities and challneges for clinicians. *West J Med* 163:250, 1995.

MacDonald N: Principles governing the use of cancer chemotherapy in palliative medicine, In: Doyle D, Hanks GWC, MacDonald N, eds. *Oxford Textbook of Palliative Medicine*. Oxford, Oxford University Press, 1993, p. 105.

Marantz PR, Tobin JN, Wasserthell-Smoller S, et al: Prognosis in ischemic heart disease. Can you tell as much at the bedside as in the nuclear laboratory? *Arch Intern Med* 152:2433, 1992.

MedPac (Medicare Payment Advisory Commission): Medicare Beneficiaries' Access to Hospice: Report to Congress. May, 2002.

Mitchell SL, Kiely DK, Hamel MB, et al: Estimating prognosis for nursing home residents with advanced dementia. *J Am Med Assoc* 291:2734, 2004.

Mor V, Laliberte L, Morris JN, et al: The Karnofsky performance status scale. An examination of its reliability and validity in a research setting. *Cancer* 53:2002, 1984.

Morita T, Tsunoda J, Inoue S, Chihara S: Validity of the palliative performance scale from a survival perspective. *J Pain Symptom Manage* 18(1):2, 1999.

Murden RA, Ainslie NK: Recent weight loss is related to short-term mortality in nursing homes. *J Gen Int Med* 9:648, 1994.

Narain B, Rubenstein LZ, Wieland GD, et al: Predictors of immediate and 6-month outcomes in hospitalized elderly patients. The importance of functional status. *J Am Geriatri Soc* 36:775, 1988.

National Hospice Organization: *Hospice Fact Sheet*. Alexandria, VA, 1997.

National Hospice and Palliative Care Organization: *Hospice Fact Sheet*. Alexandria, VA, 2007.

Olajide O, Hansen L, Usher BM, et al: Validation of the palliative performance scale in the acute tertiary care hospital setting. *J Palliat Med* 10(1):111, 2007.

Pantilat S, Steimle A: Palliative care for patients with heart failure. *J Am Med Assoc* 291:2476, 2004.

Parkes CM: Accuracy in predictions of survival in later stages of cancer. *BMJ* 2:29, 1972.

Postma DS, Burema J, Gimeno F, et al: Prognosis in severe chronic obstructive pulmonary disease. *Am Rev Resp Dis* 119:357, 1979.

Reisberg B: Dementia: A systematic way to identifying reversible causes. *Geriatrics* 41(4):30, 1986.

Reuben DB, Mor V, Hiris J: Clinical symptoms and length of survival in patients with terminal cancer. *Arch Intern Med* 148:1586, 1988.

Rosenthal MA, Gebski VJ, Kefford RF, Stuart-Harris RC: Prediction of life-expectancy in hospice patients: Identification of novel prognostic factors. *Palliative Med* 7:199, 1993.

Rudman D, Mattson DE, Nagraj HS, et al: Antecedents of death in men of a veteran's administration nursing home. *J Am Geriatr Soc* 35:496, 1987.

Sarkisian CA, Lachs MS: "Failure to thrive" in older adults. *Ann Intern Med* 124:1072, 1996.

Stuart B, Connor S, Kinzbrunner BM, et al: Medical *Guidelines for Determining Prognosis in Selected Non-Cancer Diseases*. Arlington, National Hospice and Palliative Care Organization, 1st ed. 1995; 2nd ed. 1996.

Stuart SP, Tiley EH, Boland JP: Feeding gastrostomy. A critical review of its indications and mortality rates. *South Med J* 86:169, 1993.

SUPPORT Principal Investigators: A controlled trial to improve care for seriously ill hospitalized patients. The study to understand prognoses and preferences for outcomes and risks of treatment. *J Am Med Assoc* 274:1591, 1995.

Vaccaro J, Patrick H, Haywood S, et al: Predicting prognosis in outpatients with advanced COPD. *Resp Care* 41(10):946, 1996.

Virik K, Glare P. Validation of the palliative performance scale for inpatients admitted to a palliative care unit in Sydney, Austrailia. *J Pain Symptom Manage* 23(6):455, 2002.

Volicer BJ, Hurley A, Fabiszewski KJ, et al: Predicting short-term survival for patients with advanced alzheimer's disease. *J Am Geriatr Soc* 41:535, 1993.

Volicer L, Rheaume Y, Brown J, et al: Hospice approach to the treatment of advanced dementia of the Alzheimer type. *J Am Med Assoc* 256:2210, 1985.

Von Gunten CF, Twaddle ML: Terminal care for non-cancer patients. *Clin Geriatr Med* 12(2):349, 1996.

Weeks JC, Cook EF, O'Day SJ, et al: Relationship between cancer patients' predictions of prognosis and their treatment preferences. *J Am Med Assoc* 279:1709, 1998.

Wilson DO, Rogers RM, Wright EC, Anthonisen NR: Body weight in chronic obstructive pulmonary disease. The National Institute of Health intermittent positive-pressure breathing trial. *Am Rev Respir Dis* 139:1435, 1989.

Yates JW, Chalmer B, McKegney FP: Evaluation of patients with advanced cancer using the Karnofsky performance status. *Cancer* 45:2220, 1980.

SELF-ASSESSMENT QUESTIONS

1. When evaluating a patient with a chronic, life-limiting illness to determine whether he or she has a prognosis of 6 months or less for the purpose of initiating end-of-life care planning, which of the following statements is true?

   A. Unexplained weight loss and a decrease in performance status are required in order to determine patient prognosis.

   B. Patients must meet all disease-specific guidelines for their specific disease in order to use that disease as the terminal diagnosis.

   C. Objective studies, such as pulmonary function tests, elevated marker studies, and MRI results are required before end-of-life care planning can begin.

   D. Clinical judgment combined with the general and disease-specific guidelines as additional factors to consider are the ultimate determinants of prognosis.

   E. Patients' goals regarding how they want their disease treated are not an important factor when determining patient prognosis and possible referral for hospice or palliative care.

2. Regarding the Karnofsky Performance Status (KPS), all of the following statements are true EXCEPT

   A. The KPS was designed in the late 1940s as an adjunctive tool to evaluate the activity levels of cancer patients participating in cancer chemotherapy trials.

   B. The KPS measures the severity of active patient symptoms in addition to measuring patient activity levels.

   C. Studies have demonstrated that there is a rapid fall in KPS of at least 20 to 30 units during the last 2 to 3 months of life.

   D. Patients with active symptoms have shorter survivals than patients with the same KPS rating who are not symptomatic.

3. When evaluating patients for a prognosis of 6 months or less, all of the following would be useful in helping make that determination EXCEPT

   A. For patients in long-term care facilities, serial measures on the minimal data set (MDS) that demonstrate a significant functional decline over the last year.

   B. Serial physical examinations that show increasing hepatomegaly in a patient with lung cancer and liver metastases.

   C. Weight loss of 15% secondary to aggressive diuresis in a patient with advanced congestive heart failure.

   D. A report from the home health nurse that the patient has deteriorated significantly in the last 2 weeks and has not recovered from his last chemotherapy treatment.

   E. A patient with advanced COPD has visited the emergency department six times in the last month with progressive shortness of breath.

4. The Palliative Performance Scale (PPS) was developed as a modification of the KPS for measuring functional status in patients receiving hospice and palliative care. Which of the following statements regarding the PPS is true?

   A. It is primarily intended for use in noncancer patients, while the KPS continues to be used for cancer patients.

   B. A patient with a PPS score of 60 clearly has a prognosis greater than 6 months and is not eligible for hospice services.

   C. Studies have clearly demonstrated that there is a correlation between PPS score and patient survival in the general patient population.

   D. PPS assesses a patient's food and fluid intake and level of consciousness in addition to the patient activity levels.

5. When considering whether patients with various forms of cancer have a prognosis of 6 months or less, which of the following pieces of information are important?

   A. The natural history of the primary cancer.
   B. The presence of metastatic disease.
   C. The availability of effective antineoplastic therapy.
   D. The patient's goals of care.
   E. All of the above.

6. Progressive decline in COPD is indicated by all of the following EXCEPT

   A. Increased frequency of visits to the emergency department or physician's office.
   B. The use of liquid morphine to control symptoms of shortness of breath.
   C. Loss of $\geq 10\%$ lean body mass.
   D. The comorbid condition of cor pulmonale.
   E. An O_2 saturation of 88% or less on room air.

7. You are caring for a patient with known advanced congestive heart failure. Recently, because of the development of hypotension and renal insufficiency, his vasodilator dosage had to be decreased by 50%. He is mostly confined to bed and chair due to dyspnea, which at times also plagues him at rest. He has significant edema. His last chest x-ray 6 months ago showed cardiomegaly and congestive changes, and his last ejection fraction, also 6 months ago was 25%. He is not interested in a heart transplant. You are considering referring him for hospice. Which of the following regarding his potential hospice referral is true?

   A. He needs to have a new ejection fraction, which must be 20% or less, in order to be admitted to hospice.
   B. He will not be accepted by hospice unless he is on a maximum dose of vasodilator.
   C. He needs to have a current chest x-ray showing progressive cardiomegaly and

congestive changes in order to be admitted to hospice.
   D. On the basis of his current clinical status, he is appropriate for hospice and should be accepted for admission.
   E. He should be convinced to accept a heart transplant and be placed on a waiting list, even if he continues to refuse.

8. A 93-year-old demented female is referred for hospice care. She lives in an assisted living environment and requires help to ambulate. Her speech is greatly reduced to a few minimal words. She is incontinent and has difficulty bathing and dressing. The family needs help with her care. She is appropriate for hospice if

   A. She has lost 5% of her lean body weight over the last year and the family does not want her to have a feeding tube.
   B. She has been hospitalized for two episodes of urosepsis in the last 3 months, and the family does not want her hospitalized again.
   C. She has a stage I decubitus that has developed on her left heel due to her lack of ambulation.
   D. She has a history of heart disease and diabetes, both currently controlled with oral medications.
   E. She has no other significant symptoms, and is appropriate for hospice in her current condition.

9. A 45-year-old ALS patient has had rapidly progressive disease since his diagnosis 6 months ago. He is on a ventilator intermittently. He recently had a gastric tube placed because of his difficulty with swallowing. He also started a new medication Riluzole, which is used to slow the progression of his disease. Is he appropriate for admission to a hospice program?

   A. Yes, if he agrees to discontinue the ventilator.

B. Yes, if he agrees to stop the Riluzole.

C. No, he has an undetermined life span due to his medication and treatments.

D. He is appropriate if he also requires the use of a wheelchair or is bed-bound.

E. He is appropriate for hospice care even with intermittent ventilatory support, the Riluzole, and G-tube feedings.

10. You are asked to evaluate a 75-year-old gentleman who has had "heart problems" in the past. He occasionally has chest pain upon exertion. He cannot recall the last time he saw a physician, but he laughs when he recalls the physician telling him to stop his smoking because he already has emphysema. Since then he has a been chain smoker, coughs uncontrollably at times, and sometimes he coughs up small amounts of blood. His wife reports that he is very weak now and has loss a lot of weight over the last 9 months, although he never weighed himself. On physical exam, he is tall, appears cachectic, and has temporal and interosseous muscle wasting. His shirt is very loose, and his belt is over-tightened in order to hold his pants up. He refuses to be weighed. He has decreased breath sounds throughout on lung exam and has a slightly enlarged liver. He refuses any blood tests, x-rays, or other diagnostic studies, and says just wants to go home and die. Does he qualify for hospice care?

A. No, he must be compelled to have appropriate laboratory and diagnostic studies.

B. No, even if he refuses testing, he must first be treated for depression before considering hospice referral.

C. No, because he does not have an established terminal diagnosis.

D. Yes, but the diagnosis of "Debility, unspecified" cannot be used without a BMI being documented.

E. Yes, and a diagnosis of "Debility, unspecified" can be used since his actual diagnosis cannot be determined.

How to Assist Patients and Families in Accessing End-of-Life Care

James B. Wright and Barry M. Kinzbrunner

INTRODUCTION

As the end of life approaches, patients, and the families who care for them, have many needs. Patients require expert management of pain and other physical symptoms. Patients and their families have a wide variety of emotional, social, and spiritual needs, and they also face significant financial and bureaucratic burdens.

The responsibility for ensuring that patients and families receive the treatments and services they need at the end of life fall in large part to the clinician responsible for the patient's care. Unfortunately, medical school and postgraduate medical education on pain and symptom management, and end-of-life care in general, is limited, leaving many physicians without the expertise needed to provide the necessary supportive care. Even when physicians are comfortable managing the physical ailments of their terminally ill patients, most physicians lack both the expertise and time commitment required to provide for the nonphysical needs of the patient and family.

Fortunately, however, help is available from the almost 4,500 hospice programs caring for terminally ill patients in virtually all parts of the United States, and from the ever-increasing number of institutional and home-based nonhospice end-of-life care providers. With the ever-growing availability of end-of-life care, the major dilemma facing physicians is not finding assistance for their terminally ill patients. Rather, the challenge is how to best determine what type and provider of end-of-life care is best for their patients.

To aid physicians in deciding whether a patient should be referred to a hospice program or to a nonhospice provider of palliative care at the end of life is the focus of this chapter. Hospice in the United States as defined by the Medicare Hospice Benefit will be reviewed, followed by a discussion of alternative end-of-life care programs that have been and are being developed. Issues that physi-cians should consider when choosing an appropriate end-of-life care program for the terminally ill patients and families under their care are then discussed.

HOSPICE IN THE UNITED STATES AND THE MEDICARE HOSPICE BENEFIT

HISTORY

Historically, hospice had its origins in the middle ages. Derived from the Latin term *hospes*, meaning host or guest, hospices served as way stations for travelers between Europe, Africa, and the Middle East. One can speculate that the association between hospices and the care of the sick and dying may have come from the fact that during the Crusades, wounded soldiers would often stop at hospices on the way home, and many would not survive their injuries.

The modern concept of hospice as an interdisciplinary approach for providing comprehensive care to patients near the end of life had its origins in Great Britain during the 1960s. Dame Cicely Saunders, using the vast health care experience she had gained as a physician, nurse, and social worker (a modern hospice team rolled into one), established the first hospice facilities in London, England, initially at St. Joseph's Hospice, and then at St. Christopher's Hospice. Drawing on the British experience, hospices began to develop in Canada in the 1960s and in the United States during the 1970s. However, unlike the British model of hospice that revolved around providing care in designated inpatient facilities, the North American hospice model developed with an emphasis on providing services to patients in the home environment, with inpatient care reserved for patients with specific needs that could not be managed at home.

As the hospice movement grew in the United States, specific funding was sought, leading to the establishment of the Medicare Hospice Benefit (MHB) as part of the Tax Equity and Fiscal Responsibility Act (TEFRA) of 1982. The benefit defined a patient's eligibility for hospice services based on life expectancy, the services that the hospice was to provide, and established reimbursement rates for these services on a per diem basis. This hospice benefit has continued to the present with only minor modifications over the years, and its provisions have formed the basis of the hospice model of end-of-life care in the United States. The MHB has also served as a model for the provision and reimbursement of end-of-life care services to patients receiving Medicaid, and for increasing numbers of managed care and private insurance medical plans.

THE PROVISIONS OF THE MHB

PATIENT ELIGIBILITY

The basic features of the MHB are listed in Table 2–1. For a patient to receive the MHB, the patient must be entitled to Medicare Part A benefits and must be certified as terminally ill: defined by the Medicare hospice regulations as having "a medical prognosis that his or her life expectancy is six months or less if the illness runs its normal course." At the time of referral and admission to the hospice program, the patient must be certified as terminally ill based on the clinical judgment of two physicians; the patient's attending physician and the hospice medical director or the physician member of the hospice interdisciplinary team. A discussion of clinical characteristics that help identify patients who meet this requirement is the subject of Chapter 1. The hospice benefit has two defined periods of 90 days, covering a total of 180 days or 6 months of care. For patients who unexpectedly survive beyond 6 months after

TABLE 2–1. Basic Features of the Medicare Hospice Benefit

The patient must be terminally ill
    Life expectancy of 6 mo or less if the illness runs its normal course
    Certified by two physicians
        Attending physician
        Hospice Medical Director
The hospice benefit is a Part A Medicare Benefit
    It replaces all other Part A and Part B Medicare Benefits except:
        Professional services of the attending physician
        All services for illnesses unrelated to the terminal illness
The benefit is divided into distinct periods.
    Two benefit periods of 90 d each followed by:
    Unlimited number of benefit periods of 60 d each
    Prior to the start of any new benefit period patients require recertification of their terminal prognosis by the Hospice Medical Director.
A patient can choose to revoke the Medicare Hospice Benefit at any time, leaving the hospice program. Regular Medicare benefits are immediately restored (without any waiting period).
Reimbursement is on a per diem basis (fixed daily rate) for a defined group of services (see Table 2–2), and for four levels of care:
    Routine home care
    Continuous home care
    General inpatient care
    Respite inpatient care
No more than 20% of a hospice's days of care may be at the General inpatient level of care.
An annual payment cap is placed on each hospice program based on the number of patients enrolled.

services begin (as discussed in Chapter 1, predicting prognosis is not an exact science), the MHB provides for continued hospice services past the 6-month point with coverage divided into 60-day benefit periods. Prior to the beginning of the second 90-day period within the first 180 days, and any subsequent 60-day period, the hospice medical director or the physician member of the hospice interdisciplinary team is required to recertify, in his or her clinical judgment, that the patient continues to have a terminal illness with a "a medical prognosis that his or her life expectancy is six months or less if the illness runs its normal course."

Patients who are no longer certifiable as terminally ill are discharged from the hospice program with an extended prognosis, and their regular Medicare benefits are immediately restored. Patients may, at any time, voluntarily choose to revoke the hospice benefit and leave the hospice program. Such patients, similar to those discharged with an extended prognosis, have their regular Medicare benefits immediately reinstated.

TABLE 2–2. Hospice Services Included in Per Diem Reimbursement
Nursing services
Medical direction and physician participation in the development of the plan of care
Medical social services
Counseling services
Pastoral or spiritual counseling
Bereavement counseling: provided to the family for up to 1 year following the death of the patient
Dietary counseling
Other counseling by qualified professionals as required
Home health aide services
Homemaker services
Drugs and biologicals
Durable medical equipment
Other medical supplies
Laboratory and diagnostic studies for care related to the terminal illness
Physical therapy, occupational therapy, and speech therapy if indicated

REIMBURSEMENT AND COVERED SERVICES

Reimbursement for care rendered to patients covered by the MHB is made to hospice programs on a per diem basis. Hospices receive a fixed sum per day per patient to provide whatever services are required to care for the patient. There are four distinct payment rates, based on the patient's level of care (see Levels of Hospice Care section).

Hospices are responsible to cover all services that are needed to care for "the terminal illness as well as related conditions." A list of these services is given in Table 2–2. The care and treatment of conditions "unrelated" to the terminal illness are not covered by the MHB and are not responsibility of the hospice. In such circumstances, patients have access to regular Medicare Part A and Part B benefits. In addition to the hands-on care provided by the various members of the hospice interdisciplinary team, hospices provide all medications, durable medical equipment, and medical supplies that are required by the patient, relieving patients and families of significant financial burdens. Therapeutic modalities less commonly associated with hospice care, such as chemotherapy, radiation therapy, and transfusion of blood products, are also covered when indicated for the treatment of symptoms related to the terminal illness (see Chapters 18 and 19 for further discussion).

A unique service provided by hospice programs is bereavement counseling, offered by the hospice to surviving family members for at least 1 year following the death of the patient. Hospices provide this service despite the fact that there is no additional reimbursement for bereavement services after the patient has died (see Chapter 17 for further discussion).

An important exception to the per diem reimbursement program is related to physician services. Included in the per diem are such physician activities as administrative medical direction and physician participation in the development and modification of each patient's individualized plan of care. Professional physician services, including visits made by either hospice physicians or consultant physicians under contract to the hospice, are paid for by the hospice. However, these activities may be billed for and are reimbursed by Medicare Part A on a fee-for-service basis. Visits made to a patient by an attending physician are not considered hospice services, and are reimbursed as usual by Medicare Part B, unless the physician is also under contract with the hospice (in which case the hospice would pay the physician and bill Part A as already described). (A more detailed discussion of this issue can be found in Chapter 4.)

LEVELS OF HOSPICE CARE

As previously stated, as hospice care evolved in the United States, it was, by intention, designed to deliver the comprehensive services required to care for patients at the end of life in the most familiar and comfortable environment possible, the patient's own home. However, it was recognized that there were times when the patient's clinical condition required care that was beyond the scope of services defined by the basic MHB. An additional concern was that, because the MHB is a Part A Medicare benefit (which covers all inpatient services, as contrasted with Medicare Part B, which primarily covers outpatient and physician services), patients who elect to receive hospice services no longer had hospitalization coverage under Medicare Part A. To address these issues, the MHB provides for alternative levels of care, reimbursed at different per diem rates, which reflect the intensity of services provided by the hospice to meet the needs of the patient. There are four distinct levels of care: routine home care, continuous home care, general inpatient care, and inpatient respite care.

Routine Home Care

Routine home care is the basic hospice care provided by the hospice in the patient's home. It incorporates the services outlined in Table 2–2 and discussed earlier. For patients who live in a long-term care facility (LTCF; i.e., a nursing home), the facility is considered their home for the purpose of the MHB, and the care received is considered routine home care (see Hospice Care in Long-Term Care section).

Continuous Home Care

Continuous home care may be indicated for patients who develop acute medical or psychosocial symptoms in the home environment while receiving routine home care, or who elect to remain at home, and require more intensive, often round the clock, care and support than can be provided under the routine home level of care. Clinical indications for continuous care are listed in Table 2–3. The care provided to the patient must be primarily (more than 50%) nursing, and must be for a minimum of 8 hours a day (not necessarily consecutively) to a maximum of 24 hours a day. Rather than a daily per diem, reimbursement for continuous care is based on an hourly rate with 15 minute increments.

General Inpatient Hospice Care

During the course of a terminal illness, some patients will experience symptoms that cannot be effectively managed even under a continuous home care level of care. Other patients, when faced with severe symptoms, will not be comfortable remaining in the home environment. For these patients, an inpatient hospice environment is indicated. However, as noted earlier, patients who elect the MHB no longer have Medicare Part A benefits to cover hospitalization. Therefore, the MHB requires that all hospices provide

TABLE 2–3. Clinical Indicators for Continuous Care and General Inpatient Hospice Care

Uncontrolled pain

Sudden onset or new manifestation of pain

   Ongoing pain management, regardless of route of administration or type of analgesia:

      When modalities used under a routine home care plan of care have proven unsuccessful

      When frequent adjustments in the dose of analgesia require constant monitoring and evaluation

      Alternative modalities of pain control that cannot be managed under a routine home care plan of care

Intractable nausea, emesis, or other major gastrointestinal symptoms

Respiratory distress

Severe decubiti or other skin lesions/wounds

Any other physical symptom defined by the interdisciplinary team that cannot be managed under a routine home care plan of care

Psychosocial problems and uncontrolled symptoms that can create significant psychosocial pathology in the patient or family

   Behavioral or cognitive abnormalities that do not appear to have neurologic or organic etiology

   Severe depression or anxiety, or both, dictating increased supervision (continuous care) or a change in environment (inpatient care)

Acute breakdown or disruption in family dynamics, preventing family members from functioning as adequate caregivers for reasons that can either be physical or emotional.

patient's access to general inpatient hospice care for the management of pain and other symptoms (both physical and psychosocial), which cannot be managed in the home environment. Clinical criteria for general inpatient care parallel those for continuous care as outlined in Table 2–3.

Hospices provide general inpatient care in a variety of venues. Free-standing hospice inpatient units are dedicated facilities owned and operated by the hospice. Inpatient hospice units may also occupy a wing in a hospital or a LTCF, usually leased by the host facility to the hospice and operated either by the hospice or jointly by both organizations. Some hospices have entered into contractual agreements with local hospitals or LTCFs to provide inpatient beds on an individual patient basis. In hospitals, these beds are most commonly located either on the general medical/surgical floor or the oncology floor, whereas in the LTCF, such patients should be cared on the skilled nursing floor. Table 2–4 reviews some of the advantages and disadvantages that hospice programs must weigh when considering the various locations in which general hospice inpatient care can be provided in their communities.

Differences in the quality of hospice inpatient care provided in the various venues have never been formally evaluated. However, anecdotal experience suggests that dedicated hospice inpatient units, whether free-standing or in a hospital or LTCF, have significant advantages over contract beds. In the former, patient care is provided by hospice-employed and trained personnel in a home-like atmosphere and is consistent with palliative care standards. In the latter, patients receive most of their care from hospital or facility staff in an acute care or skilled care setting, with the care being only supplemented by hospice personnel. Therefore, the environment and the care provided to hospice patients in contract beds are much less in keeping with the goals of hospice and palliative care than when care is provided in a hospice inpatient unit or free-standing facility.

TABLE 2–4. Comparison of Locations for Hospice General Inpatient Care

LOCATION	ADVANTAGES	DISADVANTAGES

Free-standing facility	Owned, operated by hospice
	Hospice-trained staff
	Community identity and visibility
	Home-like environment
		Need to provide ancillary
		  support services
		Cost of operation
		Limitation of location may
		  negatively affect patient or
		  physician access

Inpatient unit in hospital or
  LTCF leased by hospice
	Hospice-trained staff
	Community identity and visibility
	Home-like environment
	Partnership with other community
	  health care providers
	Avoids duplication of ancillary
	  support services
		Limitation of location may
		  negatively affect patient or
		  physician access (but less
		  than free-standing facility)
		Perception as a nursing home if
		  located in LTCF

Contract bed in hospital or
  LTCF
	Partnership with many community
	  health care providers
	Greater patient, physician
	  accessibility
		Hospital staff not as familiar with
		  hospice and palliative care
		  principles
		Acute care or LTCF environment

Respite Care

The fourth defined level of care under the MHB is respite inpatient care. This level of care is indicated when patients do not meet the requirements for the general inpatient level of care, but are placed in an inpatient environment to allow caregiver family members needed respite from the day-to-day care they are providing to the patient at home. Respite care is limited to 5 consecutive days at any time.

Determining the Level of Care

When patients are admitted to a hospice program, they may be admitted to any of the four levels of care, based on their needs at the time of initial assessment. Once on the hospice program, patients may be transferred from one level of care to another within the program. For example, if a patient on a routine home care level of care experiences uncontrolled pain requiring more intensive management than can be provided in the home setting, they could be transferred, rather than admitted, to a general inpatient level of care. Once the pain is brought under control, the patient would be transferred, rather than discharged, back to a routine home care level of care.

LIMITATIONS ON REIMBURSEMENT TO HOSPICES

To ensure the proper use of hospice services and to prevent excessive costs, certain safeguards have been built into the MHB. A global cap on payment, limiting the average reimbursement that a hospice can receive per patient admitted during a year, was established to ensure that hospice costs would not exceed what Medicare would otherwise spend on health care for a patient during the last 6 months of life. The cap amount is based on a figure equivalent to 95% of the average Medicare expenditures per patient during the last 6 months of life and is adjusted annually to account for inflation and hospice rate increases.

To determine whether a hospice program has exceeded the global cap, total Medicare reimbursement for services provided (which includes per diem payments for the various levels of care as well as physician services billed outside the per diem) is divided by the number of individual beneficiaries admitted to the hospice during the year. If the calculated amount exceeds the global cap amount, then the hospice's reimbursement for that year is limited to the global cap amount multiplied by the number of patients admitted during the year.

In addition to the global cap, a second reimbursement limitation was placed on hospice services provided at a general inpatient care level of care. As previously discussed, when hospice was established in the United States, the goal was that it should be home based, rather than centered around an institution. To encourage Medicare certified hospices to provide care primarily in the home, the Medicare benefit limited reimbursement for the general inpatient level of care to no more than 20% of its total days of care.

By instituting these caps on reimbursement, the use of higher levels of care, the numbers of long-stay patients, the use of physician services billed outside the per diem and ultimately, cost can be controlled without denying care to any specific patient that needs care.

HOSPICE AND LONG-TERM CARE

In the early years following the passage of the MHB, it was recognized that there was a group of patients who were in need of end-of-life care but could not receive it, because they were considered ineligible for the hospice benefit. These were patients who were residents of LTCF and primarily receiving custodial care (as opposed to those patients receiving skilled nursing care under Medicare Part A, who were, and continue to be, ineligible for the MHB, which is a mutually exclusive Part A benefit). Legislation subsequently

modified the hospice benefit, allowing patients residing in a LTCF to receive hospice services, with the LTCF being considered as the patient's home for purpose of the hospice benefit. Reimbursement for hospice services provided to patients living in LTCFs is the same as the reimbursement provided for those patients living in their own homes, with one exception. For patients who are receiving Medicaid benefits for custodial nursing home care and are receiving hospice care under the MHB, the hospice program is reimbursed at a "unified rate," consisting of 95% of the sum of the Medicaid nursing home room and board rate and the hospice home care per diem rate. The hospice is then responsible to pay the LTCF for the patient's room and board.

Hospices must have contractual agreements with each LTCF in which they care for patients, whereas the hospice maintains the professional management responsibility for facility patients enrolled on the hospice program. To ensure that patients' needs are appropriately met and are consistent with a palliative plan of care, hospices and LTCFs are mandated to develop "coordinated plans of care" for the patients that are jointly served by the two health care organizations.

The hospice experience in serving patients residing in LTCFs has been positive. Terminally ill patients require a complexity of care that staffing levels in LTCFs are not designed to provide. Hospice programs provide such patients with supplementary nursing and nursing aide support that assist the LTCF staff in ensuring that patients receive the necessary palliative symptom management, optimal skin care, nutritional assistance, and psychosocial and spiritual support. Hospice social workers and chaplains provide support to family members of LTCF patients, who often have strong feelings of guilt about having placed a loved one in long-term care, especially when death is near. LTCF staff, considered members of the patient's extended family, greatly benefit from the psychosocial and bereavement support that a hospice program provides. (The topic of Hospice and Long-Term Care is discussed in more detail in Chapter 29.)

HOSPICE COVERAGE UNDER MANAGED CARE AND OTHER HEALTH CARE PLANS

Medicare patients who are terminally ill and are being cared for by a managed care organization (MCO) can receive hospice services covered by the MHB, under what is termed a "Medicare carve-out." Rather than mandate that the MCO provide hospice services as part of its covered services, under the provisions of the "carve-out" the hospice is reimbursed directly by Medicare at the standard per diem rates for services provided to the patient. The MCO, however, is reimbursed at a reduced rate, as it is still responsible to provide health care to the patient for conditions unrelated to the terminal illness.

For terminally ill patients who are not covered by the Medicare program, hospice is also becoming increasingly accessible. State Medicaid programs in most states have hospice benefits that parallel the Medicare benefit. MCO's and private health insurance plans are covering hospice services with increasing frequency as well, with most commercial plans also following the Medicare model, albeit frequently with lifetime dollar limits on benefits. Plans may vary significantly from carrier to carrier. Some plans, in an effort to be "cost-effective" have asked hospice providers to "unbundle" their services, allowing the plan, for example, to purchase only nursing and home health aide care for patients (see How to Choose section for further discussion of "unbundling").

ALTERNATIVE END-OF-LIFE CARE PROGRAMS

Based on the description above, hospice, as defined by the MHB, would appear to be an excellent program, providing comprehensive end-of-life care services to patients who are terminally ill. And it is! Statistics show that the growth of hospice programs that really began in the 1990s has continued to accelerate, more than doubling from the more than 500,000 terminally ill patients served in 1997 to upward of 1.3 million served in 2006.

Although the approximately 900,000 who died under hospice care in 2006 account for only 36% of the individuals who died that year, this number has also almost doubled from 1997. This is truly a remarkable growth rate for the industry; however, the downside is that there has been little or no improvement in the length of stay. The average length of stay is in the 60 to 70-day range, which is about what it was in the mid-1990s. Even more sobering is the median length of stay, which has continued to hover at approximately 3 weeks. The reality is that although more patients are receiving hospice services now than ever before, the increase represents a proportionally larger number of very short-stay patients who are not being given the opportunity to access hospice care for the 6-month period that they are entitled to.

Physician discomfort with predicting that a patient has 6 months or less to live (see Chapter 1), lack of open communication between patients, families, and physicians regarding end-of-life care issues (see Chapter 3), new and more aggressive disease management and treatment options, and the lack of inpatient relationships between hospices and hospitals have been cited among the reasons that hospice remains underutilized by terminally ill patients and families. Although increasing physician and patient education and growing numbers of relationships between hospitals and hospices are helping to make hospice care more accessible, the recognition that patients and families require more comprehensive services at the end of life has led to the development of a growing number of alternate nonhospice "palliative care programs" throughout the United States. These alternative programs, either hospital based or home care based, are described

TABLE 2–5. Comparison of Hospice and Alternative Palliative Care Services

	HOSPICE	PALLIATIVE CARE
Eligibility	Prognosis of ≤ 6 months	None required Determined by program.

Professional Services	Interdisciplinary team
	    Physician
	    Nurse
	    Social worker
	    Pastoral counselor
	    Certified nursing assistants
	    Others as needed
		Inter- or multidisciplinary team
		    Physician
		    Nurse
		    Social worker
		    Others as needed

Other services	Medications DME Bereavement care Others (see Table 2–2)	No required services. Services provided are determined by program.

Location of services	Comprehensive
	Home care
	LTCF
	Inpatient
		Based on program
		Some comprehensive
		Some inpatient only
		Some LTC based
		Some requiring networking between
		    hospital and hospice or home-
		    based home health programs.

Funding	Medicare Hospice Benefit Most state Medicaid programs Many HMOs and commercial insurers Charity (not for profit hospices)	Traditional hospital coverage Traditional home care coverage Support from hospitals and hospice partner organizations Grants Charity

below. Some key features of these programs are listed in Table 2–5, and compared with those provided by hospice programs under the MHB.

EVOLUTION OF PALLIATIVE CARE

Historically, the "palliative care movement" originated in Great Britain. Hospice being primarily done in inpatient facilities were not reaching patients who had palliative care needs in hospitals or homes. This led to the development of hospital-based consulting services and eventually a palliative medicine specialty. Home care services, a traditional component of the health care system, became the primary provider of palliative care in the home setting.

In contrast, in the United States, the growth and development of hospice programs has primarily been as outpatient services. Perhaps as a consequence, approximately 65% of Americans were dying in hospitals with no access to hospice services at all or for only a few days prior to death. In 1995, a major multi-institutional research initiative, the "Study to Understand Prognoses and Preferences for Outcomes and Risks of Treatment (SUPPORT)" was undertaken to evaluate ways to "improve end-of-life decision making and reduce the frequency of a mechanically supported, painful, and prolonged process of dying."

Phase 1 identified seriously ill patients with estimated 6-month morality rates of 50% (hospice-eligible population?) and found serious "shortcomings" in the areas of patient/family communications with physicians, physician knowledge of patient's wishes regarding cardiopulmonary resuscitation (CPR), the number of days spent in an intensive-care unit (ICU) prior to death, and pain control.

In phase II, specific interventions included patient-specific information for the physician on improving communication, the need for ICU care, pain control, the probability of survival for 6 months, and the outcomes of CPR. In addition, groups of nurses were trained to serve as conduits for improved communications among patients, families, physicians, and hospital staff. Unfortunately, these interventions were largely unsuccessful in improving outcomes. Obviously, except for the fraction of patients accessing hospice services, the care of patients near the end of life was severely lacking and in need of improvement.

The results of the SUPPORT study and the continued underutilization of hospice services were the key factors that led to the 1997 Institute of Medicine (IOM) study on Care at the End of Life. Recommendations from the study included improving patient access to end-of-life care; relaxing regulatory barriers that impede the proper treatment of pain and suffering; the creation of research initiatives in end-of-life care; and the elevation of palliative care to a medical specialty status or at least an area of expertise within the practice of medicine. As a result of the efforts of many organizations supporting both hospice and palliative care, today, there is a recognized medical specialty board in hospice and palliative medicine.

HOSPITAL-BASED PALLIATIVE CARE PROGRAMS

Despite the increasing use of hospice services, the majority of patients, more than 50% at the beginning of the twenty-first century, continue to die in the hospital. These patients often require pain and symptom control, coordination of care among multiple providers, and assistance in transitioning between various health care settings. It is also likely that the hospital is the first place where patients are forced to confront the reality of the fact that their illnesses may be terminal, and they require a great deal of support to make appropriate decisions regarding their care. In addition, the cost of hospital inpatient care in the last year of life continues to increase significantly. For these reasons, as well as to create opportunities to train health care professionals about end-of-life care, hospital-based palliative care programs have and continue to be developed.

Patient eligibility for palliative care services, which has been a major impetus for the evolution of these programs, is, by design, less limited than required for the MHB. Although patients cared for by palliative care programs are generally expected to have life-limiting illnesses, most programs do not place a time limit on patients' life expectancies, and therefore, increasing numbers of patients with chronic, incurable, debilitating illnesses with indeterminate life expectancies are receiving care from these providers.

The typical hospital-based palliative care service consist of a multidisciplinary consultation team that includes, at a minimum, a physician, a nurse, and a social worker, who work in conjunction with each patient's attending physician, physician consultants, and other members of the primary care team. In academic institutions with teaching programs, palliative medicine fellows, residents from various services such as internal medicine, family practice, and pediatrics, and advanced trainees and students from the other health care disciplines may all participate as members of the palliative care team. Other health care professionals that would be involved in the care of the patient on an as-needed basis would include a pastoral counselor and consultants from various services in the hospital, including nutritional, physical and occupational therapy, psychiatry, and pharmacy. In addition to the consultation team, some hospitals will also have an identifiable palliative care unit, which may be operated solely by the hospital, or at times, operate in partnership with a hospice program and serve the additional role of a hospice inpatient unit. Most hospital-based palliative care programs provide outpatient services by working with one or more affiliated home health agencies that have palliative care expertise as well as local hospice programs (see below for further discussion of home-based palliative care).

Referrals of patients to these programs are usually initiated with palliative care consultations provided by the palliative medicine consultant in conjunction with the palliative care nurse and other team members as patients' needs are identified. Patients may be cared for either in the acute care wards they occupy at the time of consultation, or, if available, in specially designated palliative care units developed by the institution. These units, similar to their hospice counterparts, are decorated in a more home-like fashion than an acute care hospital ward, and are staffed with personnel that have special training in palliative care. Although hospital-based palliative care services are most commonly associated with existing oncology services, the recognition that patients suffering from advanced nonmalignant illnesses also require palliative care has led to the expansion of palliative care to virtually all services in the hospital. In fact, one of the most unique roles taken on by palliative care consult services has been to work with patients, families, and staff in ICUs to assist with pain and symptom management as well as in advanced care planning when it becomes clear that acutely ill patients, often ventilator dependent, are not going to recover. The involvement of the palliative care team in these very difficult situations has helped facili-

tate communication between the patient's family and the ICU staff, leading to more appropriate decision making and a smooth transition from the ICU to palliative or hospice care when indicated.

The greatest challenge facing these new palliative care services is, not surprisingly, funding. At present, there is no specific funding for palliative care services. Palliative care programs rely on traditional acute care reimbursement from the regular diagnosis-related group (DRG) system and through standard physician current procedural terminology (CPT) code billing. Now that hospice and palliative medicine have been recognized as a subspecialty, an effort to obtain specific funding for palliative care services by the Centers for Medicare and Medicaid Services (CMS) will certainly be sought. Until such reimbursement is possible, to prevent denial of payment due to perceived duplication of physician services, palliative medicine physicians use a symptom-based ICD-9 diagnosis code. What has allowed these programs to evolve and offer the comprehensive services required is additional funding provided by grants from organizations such as the Robert Wood Johnson Foundation and the Soros Foundation, which are currently focusing research efforts on increasing the access to and improving the quality of end-of-life care for terminally ill patients and families.

Published studies have demonstrated that inpatient palliative care services have improved the management of pain, dyspnea, and other common symptoms experienced by hospitalized patients with advanced life-limiting illnesses. In terms of cost-effectiveness, it has been shown that the presence of palliative care services in hospitals can reduce costs significantly, with at least one study showing a greater than 50% reduction in the cost of an inpatient day of care, due to a number of factors, including reduction in the number of very costly ICU days (and substituting much less expensive palliative care inpatient days), reduction in the use of unnecessary and expensive futile medical interventions, and, when the inpatient palliative care program is coordinated with a hospice or home palliative care program (see discussion below), a reduction in total inpatient days. On the other hand, with the lack of defined reimbursement for palliative care, independent palliative care units have tended to run at a financial loss. However, the net effect on hospitals' bottom lines appears to be positive. The overall success of hospital-based palliative care programs can be further shown by the growing number of hospitals that wish to join the 17% of community hospitals and 20% of academic teaching hospitals that already have such programs in place.

HOME-BASED PALLIATIVE CARE

The desire to reach patients sooner in the course of terminal illness has prompted some hospice providers to create home-based palliative care programs. Such "prehospice" or "bridge" programs are designed to provide hospice-like services to patients who do not meet hospice eligibility requirements, are not yet ready to accept the implications of hospice regarding their prognosis, or are receiving life-prolonging therapy that is not consistent with a hospice's plan of care. The "prehospice" program parallels the hospice regarding the interdisciplinary approach to care. If the "prehospice" and hospice programs are part of the same agency, continuity of care, at least in theory, may be enhanced as the same team members may care for patients from the time of admission to death, regardless of whether they are on the prehospice or the hospice.

Prehospice programs are funded primarily from basic home health benefits that provide reimbursement for skilled nursing care to a patient who is confined to the home. These restrictions place limits on the patient, who cannot receive services if they go out of the house, and on the agency, which must provide nonreimbursed services if they are to be true to the interdisciplinary nature of palliative care. Additional revenue is obtained through the billing of physician home visits. Supplementary funding from outside or-

ganizations also has been helpful in making these programs a reality.

The experience with palliative home care programs has been mixed so far. Although one program has closed due to insufficient funding, another has been very successful, demonstrating not only improved palliative care for patients in the outpatient and inpatient settings, but also increases in actual hospice referral and length of stay. In a published study comparing patients receiving classical hospice care with those receiving care from a prehospice "bridge" program established by the same hospice, the median time that "prehospice" patients were cared for was significantly longer than those receiving classical hospice (52 vs. 20 days), and twice the percentage of patients received care for at least 6 months (13% vs. 6%). However, the study failed to examine why patients who chose the "bridge" program made the choice they did, and did not provide data on how many patients "crossed the bridge" to the hospice program prior to death.

There have also been palliative home care programs associated with Medicare MCOs. The goal of these programs is to allow elderly patient with debilitating diseases to remain in their homes and receive care from physicians and nurses via house calls and telephonic communications. Patients may choose to participate after being recommended for the program by their primary physicians. One of the key features that make these programs attractive is that patients are not discouraged or prevented from accessing the hospital or receiving other forms of conventional care. The concept rather is to allow patients to make informed choices regarding the nature of their debilitating illnesses and to avoid unnecessary hospitalizations. The success of such ventures is yet to be determined. Home care physicians involved in the care of patients in these programs need to be diligent in documenting patient-informed decisions and to evaluate for appropriateness of referrals to the acute care medical system as well as to hospice, to fully evaluate the success of these programs.

PALLIATIVE CARE IN OTHER SETTINGS

Palliative care programs are also developing in other venues. Increasingly, hospices and nonhospice palliative care programs are providing services in LTCFs and adult living facilities (ALFs). (Provision of hospice care in a long-term care setting is discussed further in Chapter 29.) In addition, an increasing number of disease-specific programs have evolved, attempting to meet the specific needs of patients with advanced and terminal cancer, HIV, dementia, and renal disease. Finally, there are hospice and palliative care providers who, in an attempt to reach out to the diverse ethnic, racial, and religious groups in the United States, have developed special end-of-life care programs designed to meet the specific needs of these populations.

HOW TO CHOOSE AN END-OF-LIFE CARE PROVIDER

With a better understanding of the various end-of-life care options available to terminally ill patients, the physician is faced with the challenge of helping patients and families determine which palliative care provider will best serve their needs. This challenge is compounded by the fact that in most medium- and large-sized communities several hospice programs are likely to be available, and more and more hospitals and home health agencies are beginning to offer end-of-life care and palliative care programs outside the MHB.

To assist patients and families in accessing the end-of-life care services they need, the physician needs to determine what services are most important to the patient and family being treated, and compare these to the services that the various end-of-life care providers in the community have to offer. Although patient/family needs are, to some extent unique, there are some basic services that, based on a survey of physicians, were

TABLE 2–6. Important Features for an End-of-Life Care Program

Demonstrated effective pain management, with written guidelines and protocols
Interdisciplinary care from a team of professionals trained in end-of-life care, including:
Physician
Registered nurse
Certified nursing assistant
Social worker
Chaplain
Ability to treat the patient in the home, a LTCF, or an inpatient setting
Involvement of the attending physician, with satisfactory communication and support
Family counseling provided by skilled professionals on issues related to death and dying during the patient's illness and the bereavement period that follows

deemed to be important for all patients who are in need of palliative care. These services are listed in Table 2–6, and are discussed below.

DEMONSTRATED EFFECTIVE PAIN AND SYMPTOM MANAGEMENT, WITH WRITTEN GUIDELINES AND PROTOCOLS

A quality end-of-life care provider, whether a hospice or a palliative care program, should be able to demonstrate that patients under its care have pain and other symptoms effectively managed. The provider should have pain management guidelines or protocols that are comparable with the standards set in the medical literature, and the nurses and physicians who work for the hospice or palliative care provider should endorse and use those guidelines. The provider should also be able to demonstrate, through outcomes management and performance improvement activities, that those patients under its care actually have pain and other symptoms well controlled.

ABILITY TO TREAT THE PATIENT IN THE HOME, A LTCF, OR AN INPATIENT SETTING

End-of-life care providers should be able to serve, or at least coordinate service, for patients in whatever setting is required to care for them. Medicare certified hospices are, in general, best equipped to do this, as the MHB requires that patient care be provided not only in the home environment (which may also be a LTCF), but in an inpatient setting as well. Most hospices also have relationships with multiple LTCFs in their communities, allowing terminally patients who live in that environment to obtain palliative care.

Coordination of services may not be as simple, however, for the nonhospice providers of palliative care who are not affiliated with a hospice. Inpatient palliative care programs, by design, are centered on services provided in the hospital setting, making it imperative that hospital-based palliative care programs have working relationships with hospices or home-based palliative care programs to ensure that patients who leave the inpatient setting receive appropriate end-of-life care. Likewise, home care programs that provide palliative care should have inpatient partners to provide appropriate end-of-life care to patients who require hospitalization. Home-based palliative programs are also limited in that they may not serve patients living in LTCFs.

The location of inpatient services is another factor that can be of great importance in choosing an end-of-life care provider. As delineated in Table 2–4, hospice inpatient care can be delivered in a number of settings, each of which has advantages and disadvantages. For most patients, families, and clinicians, the preferred sites of hospice or nonhospice palliative inpatient care would be either a free-standing inpatient facility or a designated inpatient unit within a hos-

pital. For some patients and families, as well as their physicians, however, geographic constraints may create challenges in using these facilities and units, which are limited in number. Under such circumstances, flexibility is required. Hospices, for example, could make contract beds available in almost all hospitals in the community, whereas inpatient palliative care programs could provide consultation services in hospitals other than the ones in which they are based. Accommodations such as these will allow patients and families the convenience of more familiar surroundings closer to home, and allow physicians to follow their patients at a time when they are most needed.

INVOLVEMENT OF THE ATTENDING PHYSICIAN, WITH SATISFACTORY COMMUNICATION AND SUPPORT

The attending physician is generally recognized as being the most knowledgeable physician regarding any patient's medical condition. In recognition of this important relationship, the MHB provides for attending physician reimbursement through normal Part B channels, as opposed to via a contract with the hospice, and considers the attending physician an integral member of the hospice interdisciplinary team. Therefore, whether the patient is receiving end-of-life care from a hospice or from a nonhospice end-of-life care provider, communication between that provider and the attending physician is paramount to the successful care of the terminally ill patient and family (for a more thorough discussion of the role of the attending physician, see Chapter 4).

The members of the interdisciplinary team must be able to communicate in an appropriate professional manner with the attending physician. Active involvement of the hospice or palliative care medical director in patient care and physician communications provides the attending physician with consultation, advice, and expertise in the areas of pain and symptom control.

The ability of the hospice staff to provide the attending physician with accurate information about a patient's condition, in a succinct and professional manner, allows for prompt and appropriate interventions. Coupled with the confidence that attending physicians will develop in the end-of-life care program when the staff communicates accurately and profession, this ultimately results in improved patient care.

FAMILY COUNSELING

One of the features that makes end-of-life care unique is the fact that the patient and family together make up the unit of care. Therefore, it is vital that the hospice or palliative care program has adequate family support services. For Medicare-certified hospice programs, family counseling responsibilities are generally shared by psychologists, social workers, clergy, and others. The same professionals will usually serve this function for nonhospice palliative care programs as well. Physicians should be aware of the qualifications of these professionals employed by their hospice or palliative care provider of choice and should also be certain that the number of social workers and chaplains are adequate to meet patient and family needs.

In hospice and palliative care, support to the family does not cease at the time of patient death. Bereavement services are another integral component of a quality end-of-life care program. Under the MHB, bereavement support to surviving family members is mandated and considered part of the per diem reimbursement rate that the hospice receives while the patient is alive and under its care. Whether the patient is cared for on the hospice for 1 day, 1 week, 1 month, or 1 year, the hospice must provide bereavement support for at least 1 year following the death of the patient. As there is no traditional health care reimbursement for bereavement support, nonhospice palliative care programs must use outside funding sources to provide family counseling after patient death.

The importance of quality bereavement care should not be underestimated. Studies have been published suggesting that appropriate bereavement support improves the health of surviving family members, as demonstrated by a decrease in use health care resources and reduced absenteeism from work (for a full discussion on bereavement services in end-of-life care, see Chapter 17).

INTERDISCIPLINARY CARE FROM A TEAM OF PROFESSIONALS TRAINED IN END-OF-LIFE CARE

The provision of end-of-life care demands a professional expertise that requires special training and experience. Therefore, a quality end-of-life care program will be one that has a majority of full-time trained staff in each of the key disciplines: nursing, medicine, social work, and pastoral counseling. It should be noted that the hospice benefit allows the option of contracting for these services under certain circumstances, and many end-of-life care providers (both hospice and nonhospice) have found that contracting for certain services is more cost-effective than hiring and training staff. However, for most patient care needs, it is important to select hospice and palliative care services that employ trained professionals.

Full-time and properly trained end-of-life care staff is apt to be more responsive to patient and family needs than contracted staff, extending from prompt and efficient admission to the hospice or palliative care program to a sense of urgency when a patient is experiencing an uncontrolled symptom. Committed staff will also be more sensitive to the needs of patients and families on weekends, holidays, and other emotionally challenging times. None of this meant to question the clinical expertise of staff from a contracted agency. However, one would have to wonder whether such staff, if usually functioning in an acute care and curative environment, would be as sensitive to the unique needs of terminally ill patients and families as properly trained,

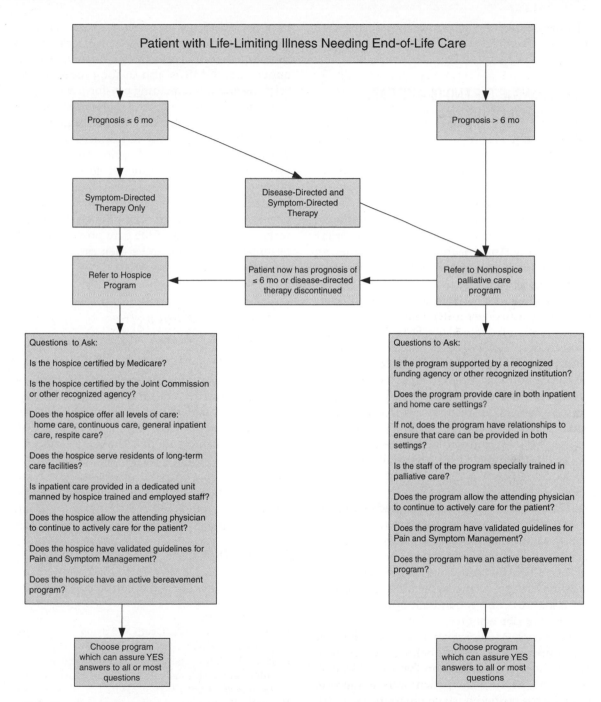

Figure 2–1. Algorithm for choosing the proper end-of-life provider.

full-time members of a hospice or palliative care interdisciplinary team.

DETERMINING IF THE END-OF-LIFE CARE PROVIDER MEETS THE NEEDS OF PATIENTS AND FAMILIES

With proper elucidation of the services that patients and families require as already described, it is incumbent upon the clinician to determine whether the end-of-life care organization of choice provides those services at an appropriate level of quality. An algorithm to assist the clinician in choosing the proper end-of-life care provider is provided in Figure 2–1.

Although it might be thought that all end-of-life care providers offer similar services at similar levels of quality, the facts are that, until recently, there has been little in the way of standardization in the field of hospice and palliative care. Eighty percent of hospices operating in the United States are Medicare certified, meaning that 20% of hospices are not. In addition, nonhospice palliative care providers are not certified by Medicare under hospice standards, and they are not compelled by regulation to provide the scope of services that a Medicare-certified hospice is obligated to offer. Therefore, although the services provided by a noncertified end-of-life care provider may appear similar to those of hospice programs that are certified, it would be prudent for a referring physician to consider whether a noncertified hospice or nonhospice palliative care program at least meets the Medicare hospice standards. It is also incumbent upon the physician to consider whether a Medicare patient referred to a non-Medicare certified end-of-life care program will incur out-of-pocket expenses, such as the cost of oral medication that would be covered by the MHB if the patient were enrolled in a Medicare-certified hospice program.

Although the Medicare benefit dictates what services must be provided, it does not adequately address the standards that define quality end-of-

life care. CMS has just issued revised Hospice Conditions of Participation, which contain very robust quality and performance-improvement requirements. CMS is also in the process of developing and implementing pay-for-performance programs for hospitals and physicians, and, if successful, it is likely that these programs will eventually find their way to hospices. For a full discussion of quality in hospice and palliative care, see Chapter 5. Suffice it so say that the quality and performance improvement program of any hospice or palliative care provider should be a strong consideration by physicians who are seeking the best end-of-life care provider for the terminally ill patients under their care.

CONCLUSIONS

It is clear from the information given above that choosing the appropriate end-of-life care provider for a patient and family can be a daunting task. With improved knowledge of the services that are available and that should be expected from an end-of-life care provider, and of the MHB and other forms of end-of-life care reimbursement this task will, hopefully, be a little less complex.

BIBLIOGRAPHY

ASCO Task Force on Cancer Care at the End of Life: Cancer care during the last phase of life. *J Clin Oncol* 16:1986, 1998.

Barrett DK, Heller KS: Death and dying the black experience. *J Palliat Med* 5(5):793-799, 2002.

Bascom PB: A hospital based comfort care team: consultation for seriously ill and dying patients. *Am J Hosp Palliat Care* 14(2):57, 1997.

Bayer R, Feldman E: Hospice under the Medicare wing. *Hastings Cent Rep* 12:5, 1992.

Beresford L: Does hospice have a role in palliative care? Hospice Manager's Monogr 3(4):1, 1998.

Beresford L, Byock I, Twohig JS: *Financial Implications of Promoting Excellence in End-of-Life Care*. Missoula, Robert Wood Johnson Foundation, 2002.

Billings JA: Massachusetts General Hospital palliative care service. In: *Pioneer Programs in Palliative Care: Nine Case Studies*. Robert Wood Johnson Foundation & Millbank Memorial Fund; 2000. http://www.milbank.org/pppc/0011pppc.html#foreword. Accessed July 7, 2010.

Billings JA: What is palliative care? *J Palliat Med* 1(1):73, 1998.

Billings JA, Block S: Palliative care in undergraduate medical education. Status report and review. *JAMA* 278:733, 1997.

Billings JA, Block SD, Finn JW, et al: Initial voluntary program standards for fellowship training in palliative medicine. *J Palliat Med* 5(1):23-33, 2002.

Capello CF, Meier DE, Cassel CK: Payment code for hospital-based palliative care: Help or hindrance? *J Palliat Med* 1(2):155-163, 1998.

Cassel CK, Vladeck BC: Sounding board. ICD-9 code for palliative or terminal care. *N Engl J Med* 335:1232, 1996.

Casarett D, Abrahm JL: Patients with cancer referred to a hospice versus a bridge program: Patient characteristics, needs for care, and survival. *J Clin Oncol* 19:2057-2063, 2001.

Center to Advance Palliative Care (CAPC): The case for hospital-based palliative care; 2009. http://www.capc.org/support-from-capc/capc_publications/making-the-case.pdf. Accessed July 7, 2010.

Center to Advance Palliative Care (CAPC): Making the case for ICU palliative care integration. A presentation of the IPAL-ICU project; 2010. http://www.capc.org/ipal-icu/monographs-and-publications/ipal-icu-making-the-case-for-icu-palliative-care-integration.pdf. Accessed July 7, 2010.

Christakis NA, Escarce JJ: Survival of Medicare patients after enrollment on a hospice program. *N Engl J Med* 335:172, 1996.

Coluzzi PH, Grant M, Doroshow JH, et al: Survey of the provision of supportive care services at National Cancer Institute-designated cancer centers. *J Clin Oncol* 13:756, 1995.

Comprehensive Accreditation Manual for Home Care 1997–1998: Chicago, Joint Commission on Accreditation of Healthcare Organizations, 1996.

Coor CA, Coor DM, eds: *Hospice Care, Principles and Practice*. New York, Springer, 1983.

Criteria for inpatient care. Policy 5:22. In: *Vitas Policy Manual*. Miami, Vitas Healthcare Corporation, 1993.

DeCourtney CA, Jones K, Merriman MP, et al: Establishing a culturally sensitive palliative care program in rural Alaska native American communities. *J Palliat Med* 6(3):501-510, 2003.

Editorial Board: New diagnosis code will track palliative care in hospitals. *Network News* 5:1, 1996.

Elyasam AF, Swint K, Roach P, et al: Palliative care inpatient service (PCIS) in a comprehensive cancer center: Clinical and financial outcomes [abstract]. Proc ASCO 2099, 522, 2003.

Evans LK, Yurkow J, Siegler EL: The CARE program: A nurse-managed collaborative outpatient program to improve function of frail older people. *J Am Geriatr Soc* 43:1160, 1995.

Ferrell BR, Virant R, Grant M: Improving end of life care education in home care. *J Palliat Med* 1(1):11, 1998.

Finn JW, Pienta KJ, Parzuchowski J, Worden F: Palliative care project: Bridging active treatment and hospice for terminal cancer patients. Proc ASCO, 1452, 2002.

42 Code of Federal Regulations, Part 418, Medicare Hospice Regulations, 1993.

Grantmakers Concerned with Care at the End of Life: *Paying for Care at the End of Life: Implications for Individuals and Families, Health Care Providers, and Society*. New York, NY, Grantmakers Concerned with Care at the End of Life, 1998.

Hanson LC, Tulsky JA, Danis M: Can clinical interventions change care at the end of life: *Ann Intern Med* 126:381, 1997.

Hospice Fact Sheet. National Hospice Organization, 1997.

Institute of Medicine End of Life Care Committee: *Approaching Death: Improving Care at the End of Life*. Washington DC, National Academy Press, 1997.

JervisMark Associates, Inc.: *Evaluation of Market for Hospice Care, Inc*. Miami, Vitas Healthcare Corporation, 1992.

Kinzbrunner BM: The terminally ill patient. In: Abeloff MD, Armitage JO, Lichter AS, Niederhuber JE, eds. *Clinical Oncology*. New York, Churchill Livingstone, 1st ed. 1995:409; 2nd ed. 2000: 597.

Kinzbrunner BM: Hospice: 15 years and beyond in the care of the dying. *J Palliat Med* 1:127, 1998.

Kinzbrunner BM: Palliative care perspectives. In: Kuebler KK, Davis MP, Moore CD, eds. *Palliative*

Practices: An Interdisciplinary Approach. St. Louis, Elsevier, Mosby, 2005, p. 3.

Knaus WA, Harrell FE, Lynn J, et al: The SUPPORT prognostic model. Objective estimates of survival for seriously ill hospitalized patients. *Ann Intern Med* 122:191-203, 1995.

Lamm M, Kinzbrunner BM: *Jewish Hospice Manual for End-of-Life Care in Hospice and at Home.* Miami and New York, Vitas Healthcare Corporation and National Institute for Jewish Hospice, 2003.

Lynch-Schuster J: Palliative care programs help perople with CHF/COPD stay home and stay healthy. ABCD Exchange 1(2):1, 1997.

Lynn J: Editorial. Caring at the end of our lives. *N Engl J Med* 335:201, 1996.

Lynn J: An 88 year old woman facing the end of life. *JAMA* 277:1633, 1997.

Mahoney JJ: Correspondance. A new diagnosis related group for palliative care. *N Engl J Med* 336:1029, 1997.

McKeen E, Billings JA: Reimbursement for physician services under the Medicare benefit. Hospice Update, December 1991.

Meier D, Morrison S, Cassel CK: Improving palliative care. *Ann Intern Med* 127:225-230, 1997.

Miller FG, Fins JJ: Sounding Board. A proposal to restructure hospital care for dying patients. *N Engl J Med* 334:1740, 1996.

Miller SC, Gozalo P, Mor V: Hospice enrollment and hospitalization of dying nursing home patients. *Am J Med* 111:38-44, 2001.

NHPCO Facts and Figures: Hospice Care in America. National Hospice and Pallaitive Care Organization, 2007.

O'Neill J, Marconi K: Underserved populations, resource-poor settings, and HIV: Innovative palliative care projects. *J Palliat Med* 6(3):457-459, 2003.

Palmetto Government Benefit Administrators: Medicare Advisory Hospice 97–11, Hospice provisions enacted by the balanced budget act (BBA) of 1997. September, 1997.

Payne R, Payne TR, Heller KS: The Harlem palliative care experience. *J Palliat Med* 5(5):781-792, 2002.

Petrisek AC, Mor V: Hospice in nursing homes: a facility level analysis of the distribution of hospice beneficiaries. *Gerontologist* 39:279-290, 1999.

Pitorak EF, Armour MB, Sivec HD: Project safe conduct integrates palliative care goals into compre-hensive cancer care. *J Palliat Med* 6(4):645-655, 2003.

Policzer JS: Hospice and Hispanics: Strategic issues in providing hospice care to an Hispanic population. AAHPM Session Abstract. *J Palliat Med* 5(1):209, 2002.

Poppel DM, Cohen LM, Germain MJ: The renal palliative care initiative. *J Palliat Med* 6 (2):321-328, 2003.

Rhymes J: Hospice care in America. *JAMA* 264:369, 1990.

Santa-Emma PH, Roach R, Gill MA, et al: Development and implementation of an inpatient acute palliative care service. *J Palliat Med* 5(1):93-100, 2002.

Schapiro R, Byock I, Parker S, Twohig JS: *Living and Dying Well with Cancer: Successfully Integrating Palliative Care into Cancer Treatment.* Missoula, Robert Wood Johnson Foundation, 2003.

Selwyn PA, Rivard M, Kappell D, et al: Palliative care for AIDS at a large urban teaching hospital: Program description and preliminary outcomes. *J Palliat Med* 6(3):461-474, 2003.

Shega JW, Levin A, Hougham GW, et al: Palliative excellence in Alzheimer care efforts (PEACE): A program description. *J Palliat Med* 6(2):315-320, 2003.

Smith DH, Granbois JA: The American way of hospice. *Hastings Cent Rep* 11:8, 1992.

Smith TJ. We can reduce the cost of in-hospital end-of-life care. *Oncology* XXV(11):4-6, 2003.

Stoddard S: The hospice movement. *A Better Way of Caring for the Dying (Revised).* New York, Vintage, 1991.

Support Principle Investigators: A controlled trial to improve care for seriously ill hospitalized patients. *JAMA* 274:1591, 1995.

Swinford S: Presentation: Successful strategies for hospice-hospital partners in palliative care. Presented at: Making the most of the Medical Director's position. A conference for Hospice administrators. The Carolina Center for Hospice and End of Life Care. August 25, 2003.

Tierney J, Wilson D: Hospice care versus home health care: Regulatory distinctions and program intent. *Am J Hosp Palliat Care* 11(2):14, 1994.

US Department of HHS: *Medicare: Hospice Manual.* Springfield, US Department of Commerce, 1992.

US Department of HHS: *Medicare: Hospice Manual,* Section 230.1 E (revised). Springfield, US Department of Commerce 1992.

US Department of HHS: *Medicare: Hospice Manual*, Section 306.1 (revised). Springfield, US Department of Commerce, 1993.

Von Gunten CF, Neely KJ, Martinez J: Hospice and palliative care: Program needs and academic issues. *Oncology* 10(7):1070, 1996.

Von Gunten CF, Ferris FD, Kirschner C, Emmanuel LL: Coding and reimbursement mechanisms for physician services in hospice and palliative care. *J Palliat Med* 3(2):157-164, 2000.

Walsh D: The Medicare Hospice Benefit: A critique from palliative medicine. *J Palliat Med* 1(2):147, 1998.

Weissman DE: Palliative medicine education at the Medical College of Wisconsin. *Wis Med J* 94:505, 1995.

Welch HG, Wennberg DE, Welch WP: The use of medicare home health care services. *N Engl J Med* 335:324, 1996.

Wilson SA, Daley BJ: Attachment/Detachment: Forces influencing care of the dying in Long-Term care. *J Palliat Med* 1(1):21, 1998.

SELF-ASSESSMENT QUESTIONS

1. Dame Cicely Saunders was the founder of the modern concept of hospice. Many consider her an interdisciplinary team (IDT) all rolled into one, as she was a degreed professional in three of the four major IDT disciplines. The only professional qualification that she did not have was that of a:

   A. Physician
   B. Nurse
   C. Chaplain
   D. Social Worker

2. Basic features of the hospice care under the MHB include all of the following EXCEPT:

   A. The patient must be terminally ill, with a life expectancy of 6 months or less if the illness runs its normal course.
   B. The patient's terminal prognosis must be certified by the Hospice Medical Director and the patient's attending physician
   C. The benefit is divided into two 90-day periods and an unlimited number of 60-day periods, as long as the patient remains terminally ill
   D. The patient continues to have full Medicare Part A and B coverage in addition to hospice coverage when electing the hospice benefit.

3. Covered services under the MHB include each of the following EXCEPT:

   A. Professional services provided by the patient's designated attending physician.
   B. Professional services provided by the hospice medical director or physician.
   C. Professional services provided by a consultant physician for a service related to the patient's terminal diagnosis.
   D. Chemotherapy if the patient has a cancer diagnosis and the chemotherapy is part of the plan of care
   E. Bereavement services for up to 1 year following the patient death.

4. Which of the following would be an indication to change a patient's level of care under the MHB from routine home care to either general inpatient care or continuous home care?

   A. The family member who is primary caregiver needs to go to an out of town wedding over the weekend.
   B. A patient has developed an increase in pain that requires a one-time adjustment of analgesic dose for better pain control.
   C. A patient has developed an increase in pain that requires frequent dose adjustments and constant monitoring.
   D. A patient with increased custodial needs at home who is awaiting an available bed in a nursing home.

5. When a patient living in a LTCF receives hospice services under the MHB, all of the following are true, EXCEPT:

   A. The LTCF is considered the patients home, and the basic care provided is the same as routine home care.
   B. Patients receiving skilled care in the LTCF under Medicare Part A can also receive care under the MHB for the same diagnosis.
   C. The room and board coverage for the patient is paid for by the family, Medicaid, or private insurance.
   D. The hospice and the LTCF require a "coordinated plan of care" to ensure that patients are properly served by both providers.
   E. The hospice is the provider primarily responsible for the professional management of the patient living in a LTCF.

6. Documented barriers to hospice access include all of the following, EXCEPT:

   A. Lack of hospice growth, limiting the number of patients that may be cared for in most US cities.

B. Physician discomfort with predicting that a patient has 6 months or less to live

C. A lack of open communication between patients, families, and physicians regarding end-of-life care issues.

D. New and more aggressive disease management and treatment options

E. The lack of inpatient relationships between hospices and hospitals

7. Which of the following features do hospices and nonhospice palliative care programs share?

A. They can only provide care to patients with a prognosis of 6 months or less.

B. They both provide care that is funded through a federally mandated benefit.

C. Informed consent must be given by patients to receive care from both providers.

D. Both provide care via a team of trained professionals including physicians, nurses, and social workers.

E. Both provide a standardized array of services to all patients.

8. All of the following regarding hospital-based palliative care programs are true, EXCEPT:

A. They have been shown to decrease the cost of an average hospital inpatient day.

B. They can provide consultative services on the medical and surgical wards, but not in the ICU or other critical care areas.

C. The management of pain and other symptoms experienced by hospitalized patients with advanced life-limiting illnesses has improved.

D. Despite the fact that many programs run at a financial loss, the net result to the hospital is usually a financial plus.

E. There is a reduction in the use of unnecessary futile medical interventions.

9. Which of the following was reported in a published study comparing patients receiving classical hospice care with those receiving care from a prehospice "bridge" program established by the same hospice?

A. Almost 50% of the patients who received care under the "bridge" program received care for at least 6 months.

B. More than 33% of the patients admitted to the "bridge" program eventually "crossed the bridge" to the hospice program prior to death.

C. The median time that "bridge" patients were cared for was more than twice as long as those on traditional hospice.

D. The main reason why patients opted for the "bridge" program was so they could still receive chemotherapy.

10. All of the following are important features to look for when determining the best end-of-life care provider for one's patients, EXCEPT:

A. Demonstrated effective pain and symptom management, with written guidelines and protocols

B. Interdisciplinary care from a team of professionals trained in end-of-life care.

C. Ability to treat the patient in the home, a LTCF, or an inpatient setting

D. Requirement that the patient's medical care by managed by the end-of-life care physician instead of the attending physician.

E. Family counseling provided by skilled professionals during the patient's illness and the bereavement period that follows.

Communicating with Patients and Families

Barry M. Kinzbrunner, Vincent D. Nguyen,
Neal J. Weinreb, and Joel S. Policzer

PART 1
HOW TO INFORM THE PATIENT: CONVEYING BAD NEWS

Barry M. Kinzbrunner,
Vincent D. Nguyen,
Neal J. Weinreb

The practice of medicine is science applied to the art of caring. To be truly competent, physicians must demonstrate an ability to listen, a willingness to acknowledge a patient's fears and concerns, an aptitude to empathize and to explain, a capability to assess and marshal social support, and a commitment to never abandon hope for the betterment of a patient's life. Nowhere are these skills needed more than when called upon to provide patients and families with "bad news."

Bad news has been defined as "any information that adversely alters one's expectations for the future" (Back et al., 2005), or "news that results in a cognitive, behavioral, or emotional deficit in the person receiving the news that persists for some time" (Ptacek and Eberhardt, 1996). In the context of end-of-life care, "bad news" conversations may include discussions regarding the discovery of a progressive, life-limiting illness, the lack of or failure of currently available therapies to control that illness, estimated prognosis, the need for hospice services, and a host of other related topics.

Conveying bad news is one of the most difficult, and all too frequent, responsibilities for a physician in clinical practice. This task is stressful, even when the focus of decision making is on curative or life-prolonging therapeutic options. How much more unpleasant the experience, and greater the level of discomfort, when the message to be given is the worst news a patient and loved ones can get: the disease process is incurable, life-prolonging treatment will most likely be ineffective, and the end of the patient's life is near. It is tempting for the physician to evade, or even to totally deny the issue, especially because physicians receive little if any formal training or effective mentoring in how to discuss end-of-life issues with patients and their families. Furthermore, the push for ever-increasing physician productivity in managed care settings has introduced constraints that do not favor the time-intensive efforts that are required to address these issues with clarity, sensitivity, and compassion. Nevertheless, the substantial attention that physician communication is attracting in the medical literature, in the lay press, and in the media, tells us that there is no excuse for physicians and other health care professionals to continue to neglect this crucial clinical skill.

Although the last several years have seen a marked increase in the number of articles in the medical literature examining the issue of how to communicate bad news to patients and families, increasing our understanding of what patients and families may want and need during this process, the medical evidence supporting the currently accepted techniques remains weak at best. Nevertheless, there are a number of articles, books, and computer software programs that are available to assist practicing clinicians in improving and perfecting their communication skills. In addition, an increasing number of medical schools and house officer training programs are including these methods in their curricula, to equip the next generation of clinicians for the tasks ahead of them. Nonetheless, although methodology can provide useful tools, and knowledge of principles of medical ethics is an important framework, successful communication is ultimately not a technological *tour de force*. Rather, it depends on motivation, dedication, and a hearty helping of common sense and decency. This chapter will highlight some of the major barriers to conveying bad news, particularly in the context of end-of-life care, and will provide some practical guidance on how to do it effectively. It is hoped that the suggestions offered here, when adapted to each unique clinical situation, will increase physician confidence in the ability to communicate, and will enhance the physician–patient relationship.

CHALLENGES WITH CONVEYING BAD NEWS

Why is this task so difficult? Consider the following scenario, quoted from a newspaper article by Jane E. Brody entitled "Bad News Well Delivered: A Prescription for Doctors":

> Breathing difficulties prompted Frank to return to the hospital days before he was to receive his next chemotherapy treatment for lung cancer. When Frank asked if he'd be getting his treatment as scheduled, a doctor neither he nor his family had ever seen before replied bluntly: "We can't give you another treatment. It would kill you." To Frank, who knew his life depended on the drugs, those 10 words were a death sentence, delivered in the cruelest possible fashion. Frank's shaken family members were left on their own to try in vain to rekindle some slim hope for his survival.

The author correctly notes the inadequacies of the above communication process. However, she misses the main point. Identifying with the patient's unrealistic expectations of the chemotherapy regimen, she finds it hard to accept that which seems medically evident. Frank's prospects for survival are not merely slim, but virtually nil, yet she criticizes the physician for giving the patient what he perceived as a "death sentence." What she failed to recognize was that the physician should not, as she suggested, focused his discussion with the patient on preserving a modicum of false hope for survival. Rather, the physician should have concentrated on helping the patient and family confront an end-of-life situation realistically, with assurance that care would be continued or even intensified with a concentration on palliation of symptoms and optimization of all dimensions of the quality of remaining life.

The denial displayed by this highly informed and well-intentioned columnist demonstrates one of the reasons why breaking bad news, particularly as related to end-of-life care, is so challenging.

CHALLENGES FOR PATIENTS

As pointed out by Dr. Robert Buckman in "How to Break Bad News," we live in a society that values the young, the healthy, and the wealthy. Those that do not belong to this group, such as the elderly, the sick, and the poor are often "marginalized" outside the mainstream of society. Patients with debilitating or terminal diseases are frequently left isolated from family and friends who themselves need to cope with the personal implications of these conditions. Therefore, it is natural that people are uncomfortable with the idea of being told that they are suffering from a life-limiting illness. They find it difficult to deal emotionally with impending losses, such as loss of control, the loss of identity as a normal, healthy person, the loss of relationships and roles, and ultimately, the loss of life itself (see Table 3–1). Serious illness is frequently perceived by patients as eroding their lifestyle, limiting choices, eliminating opportunities that healthier people enjoy, and threatening their physical and mental well-being.

Nevertheless, the literature suggests that, at least at some level, patients and families want to be informed regarding the nature of their illness, even if the news is "bad." A 2007 review article evaluating more than 150 studies and articles on patient/caregiver communication preferences found that patients and caregivers desired significant amounts of information regarding the illness, possible future symptoms and their management, life expectancy, and clinical treatment options. Of interest is that the reviewers noted that as the illness progressed patient and caregiver information needs tended to diverge, with caregivers wanting more information whereas patients wanted to be less well informed

TABLE 3–1. Implications of Life-Threatening Illness—The Patient's Perspective

TYPE OF LOSS	EXAMPLE
Loss of control	"My body has betrayed me."
Loss of identity as a normal, healthy person	"I am no longer the person I used to be."
Loss of relationships and roles	"I am afraid of losing everybody and everything."
Loss of life	

(Parker et al., 2007). Another review article published later the same year corroborates these findings, but notes that patients often do not express to the clinicians caring for them their desire to know detailed information about their illness. This study also points out that although patients and caregivers want to be informed, the majority desire to hear this information delivered in as positive a manner as possible. In addition, studies suggest that patient preferences regarding the extent of information provided to family members vary considerably. Although many patients want family members involved and present when receiving bad news, some patients do not want family members present or involved at all, whereas others would prefer the bad news be delivered to the family members, trusting the judgment of family members to tell them what they need to know (Barclay et al., 2007).

CHALLENGES FOR PHYSICIANS

For physicians, having to deliver bad news may cause great distress as well (see Table 3–2). Physicians may experience a sense of professional inadequacy for having "failed" the patient, and these feelings may be compounded by a sense of ineptness in performing such tasks, particularly when they have not been properly trained to do so. Bad news usually elicits strong reactions from the recipient that may sometimes be expressed with histrionics or even graphic physical behavior. Physicians may be intimidated or be "put off" even by a potential patient outburst, especially when they are poorly prepared to defuse such emotional or physical reactions. To further complicate matters, even nonhostile but nevertheless strong adaptive reactions by the patient may cause physicians to express their own emotions (i.e., anger, panic, sadness that may lead to tears). Although debatable, this is often perceived as weak and unprofessional behavior. However, keeping in mind that the patient is the one with the disease, why is it wrong for physicians to share in their pain and distress, provided that they can simultaneously retain professional objectivity?

Physicians are trained not to inflict pain without offering anesthesia or sedation. Bad news certainly causes pain to the person receiving it. Unfortunately, when presenting bad news, there is no place for anesthetics or sedatives. The physician must deliver it while the patient is awake,

TABLE 3–2. Implications of Delivering Bad News—The Physician's Reactions

Feelings of ineptness in performing such tasks
Feelings of inadequacies in dealing with the emotions involved
Feelings of intimidation by being blamed for the patient's illness
Feelings of professional impotence for "failing" the patient

alert, and mentally competent to understand the situation, which only magnifies the degree of physician discomfort.

Besides distaste for inflicting pain, physicians also fear being blamed for delivering bad news. Commonly, the bearer of bad tidings is inappropriately perceived as the cause of the circumstance. Anger that is misdirected at the physician should be directed at the underlying disease process or at "the slings of outrageous fortune." Nevertheless, after a good outcome, the physician usually is happy to take the credit! Thus, when things go wrong, even when out of one's control, it should be anticipated that there might be an element of unspoken or even overt hostility. The physician must be prepared to deal with this in a way that promotes the patient's best interests.

Physicians have been trained to believe that there is an effective treatment for every illness, a pill for every ill, and an ideal solution for every problem. The concept of therapeutic impotence is difficult to accept because every judgment is constantly scrutinized. One is always asking whether there is something else that could have been done, some additional test or procedure that could have been performed, or some drug(s) that could have been tried. It often feels professionally degrading to have to say: "I don't have an answer." Remember, however, that although this blow to a physician's ego may be troubling, what the physician feels pales in comparison to what the patient, faced with his or her own mortality, must endure.

HOW TO BREAK BAD NEWS WELL

An aphorism in the Book of Proverbs states: "There are those that speak like the piercing of a sword; but the tongue of the wise heals." Breaking bad news may be difficult, but it can be and should be done.

As part of the physician's duty and responsibility to the patient, being able to convey bad news in an appropriate fashion is a basic skill comparable to history taking or physical examination. The latter tools are essential to reaching a correct diagnosis and initiating treatment. Similarly, when the task of conveying bad news is done with honesty and compassion, enhanced trust strengthens the patient–physician relationship and increases the likelihood that the patient will choose an appropriate treatment approach. Conversely, bad news delivered badly can cause needless emotional pain and lead to a loss of confidence in the physician's recommendations and plan of treatment.

Not only does it benefit patients when physician are capable of conveying bad news properly, but also it is in the best interest of the physician to have these skills finely tuned. A patient rightfully expects to be spoken to in a caring and professional manner. A physician is unlikely to have a successful community practice if he is cold, impersonal, and insensitive. In addition, more malpractice litigation results from poor communication rather than from actual medical negligence. Finally, developing these skills and appropriately applying them enhances professional satisfaction in a job well done.

Delivering bad news successfully requires the physician to adequately prepare for this encounter, to relay the message in a clear and concise manner that the listener(s) can understand, and to take time tending to the patient's physical and emotional needs. Bad news will forever change the patient's reality, whether the illness is life-threatening or life-altering. Thus, it is important to note that the way the news is presented sets the tone for the patient, the family, and the physician for the entire illness experience together.

THE SPIKES PROTOCOL

"S P I K E S" is an acronym used by Dr. Buckman and his colleagues to represent a six-step protocol

TABLE 3–3. "SPIKES"—Six Practical Considerations in Delivering Bad News

	STEP	CHARACTERISTICS
S	Setting	Prepare in advance
		Face-to-face visit
		Choose a private or quiet environment
		Family/loved one/confidante
		Provide an interpreter, if necessary
P	Perception	Ask the patient what he or she knows or perceives
I	Invitation	Seek the patient's invitation to break news
		Ask how much the patient wants to know
		Listen and be present
K	Knowledge	Share information clearly and directly
		Avoid "medical jargon" and technical language
		Do not give too much information at one time
		Listen to the patient's responses
		Frequently repeat and summarize points
E	Empathy	Observe how the patient reacts
		Listen to the patient's emotions
		Allow pauses for reflection and for the patient to verbalize feelings or ask questions
		Respond by identifying and validating patient's emotions
S	Summation	Summarize the delivered news
		Review the patient's treatment options
		Schedule follow-up visits

for breaking bad news. It stands for *Setting, Perception, Invitation, Knowledge, Empathy,* and *Summation.* These steps are summarized in Table 3–3 and are discussed below.

Setting

Preparation is the essential concept in this step. Review medical notes and laboratory results beforehand. Based on how well you know the patient, think about how much the patient might want to know or not want to know, how much information the patient might be able to absorb during the meeting, and how the patient is likely to react. Although things do not always go as planned, the more prepared you are for the meet-

ing with the patient, and the more knowledgeable you are about the patient's case, the more you will feel in control. The patient and family will have greater assurance that your assessment and recommendations are based on forethought and total knowledge of the case. The more that you know about the patient's family and cultural and religious background, the better you will be able to help that patient. There are significant cultural differences that influence what and how much a patient wishes to know. In an ever increasingly multicultural society, we must be aware of and respect these varying attitudes.

Breaking bad news is done best in a face-to-face encounter. There is a great sense of rapport and humanness conveyed by a live presence that is lost in a telephone call. (It must be pointed out that although it is preferable to break bad news in person, giving patients good news over the phone is a common practice. Although there is nothing overtly wrong with that, one does run the very real and significant risk of telling a patient that the news is bad simply by requesting that this time, unlike on past occasions, you want to discuss the news face to face rather than over the phone.) If, due to distance or other circumstance, it is impossible to meet face to face, then make a point of mentioning to the patient/family that you are sorry that a personal meeting was not feasible.

Unless it is absolutely unavoidable, meetings about bad news should be done in private. A noisy public setting does not allow the parties to fully pay attention to what is being discussed, and, at worst, may be embarrassing or even insulting. Therefore, choose a quiet place and minimize any distractions.

Always try to make the patient feel at ease. If at the bedside, close the door or draw the curtain in a nonprivate room to maintain a sense of privacy. Sit comfortably and relatively close to the patient, so that you can be at or near the patient's eye level. This is a sign to the patient that you would like to engage in a nonpatronizing conversation and has been perceived in one study as a sign of compassion. In your office, pull up a chair, and try to sit on the same side of the desk rather than opposite the patient. Maintain a comfortable distance, but close enough that a holding a hand, touching an arm, or offering a facial tissue can be easily accomplished. Be conscious that your body language conveys your interest and dedication to the task at hand. Avoid interruptions as much as possible. If at all possible, turn off your cell-phone or pager and divert all incoming telephone calls. Apologize for even the briefest interruption.

At the time you set up the appointment with the patient to discuss the situation, it is important to ask the patient whether he or she would like family members or significant others present. As discussed above, there is significant variability regarding the level to which patients want family involvement, and the patient's wishes must be re-spected. If the discussion will be taking place in an in-patient setting, and the patient wants family members present, this may require a postponement of the conversation from morning rounds to a time later in the day when family can be at the hospital to be with their loved one.

If family is present, use them as a resource. Studies have shown that strong family and social bonds alleviate sickness and enhance patient cooperation with medical treatments. Furthermore, many patients, on hearing bad news, tune the physician out, and may not understand or remember what was actually said or discussed. In fact, if a patient informs you that he or she wants to speak with you alone, urge that he or she comes with at least one person who can be trusted, as the patient will likely require emotional and psychosocial support from this relative or friend. Remember, however, that the bad news may be as upsetting for the loved one as it is for the patient. Be sure that you introduce yourself and anyone else who may be present.

If the patient does not speak English, and you are not fluent in the patient's language, try not to use a family member or friend as an interpreter, as it is possible that this well-meaning loved one will not accurately translate information that he or she feels is detrimental to the patient. Rather, find a professional interpreter, if available, and ask the interpreter to translate, as accurately as possible, the thought as well as the verbiage.

Perception

Before divulging the bad news, it is wise to find out what the patient suspects or already knows. The responses from the patient will serve as a guide, particularly when the patient is prompted with open-ended questions to which the replies are usually more revealing than simple yes or no answers. The patient's level of comprehension and the vocabulary used will further set the stage for what the physician should say.

For example, if we go back to the scenario with which the chapter was opened, perhaps a better answer from the physician would have been:

"Frank, before I can answer your question about the chemotherapy, let me ask you a question. Where do you think things stand with your illness?"

Depending on the answer, the physician might follow up with a question about Frank's worsening dyspnea in terms of the extent to which it is worrisome to the patient, its importance, and implications. By doing so, the physician would develop a better idea as to whether Frank suspects or understands that he likely has a disease that has progressed despite chemotherapy, and whether he has made the connection between his worsening shortness of breath and the refractoriness of his lung cancer. Of course, if the worsening dyspnea is related to a reversible, intercurrent infection rather than to progressive disease, an immediate direct answer that chemotherapy could be resumed when the infection is resolved would be appropriate. Nevertheless, even in that circumstance, this is a propitious moment to attempt to learn what Frank understands about his disease process and course to date. In this way, the physician shows the patient that he is interested in his perceptions and input.

Invitation

In this step, the physician finds out how much the patient wants to know about his condition, and seeks the patient's invitation to break the news. How much the patient wishes to know will depend on a number of variables, including the patient's personality, religious beliefs, ethnicity, culture, age, or education level. Although at this stage many patients most likely have at least some idea that good news is unlikely, some patients still prefer not to actually hear the bad news themselves. In some cultures, there is the belief that relating bad news actually hastens or guarantees the event. Thus, before disclosure, the physician should always offer the patient a true choice, and exhibit the sensitivity to ask.

"Frank, I have looked at your chest x-rays a few minutes ago. Would you like to talk about the results?"

Depending on his response, the physician can probe further.

"It sounds as if you don't wish to talk about it. Are you afraid that the results might not be good? Would you prefer that I discuss the results with your wife?"

If the patient does not want to know or does not wish to hear the full details at that moment, the physician must not cut off all lines of communication.

"I sense that you are uncomfortable at this moment. Is there anything that I can do for you, Frank? If you prefer, let's reschedule our meeting later today or tomorrow morning."

Being sensitive to the patient's desire for realism and to his readiness for acceptance is crucial at this moment because you are about to deliver news that may confirm his worst fears. Denial is quite common at this stage. Some patients consciously or unconsciously regularly utilize denial as an adaptive technique to buffer themselves from distress, whereas others merely need to buy time to acclimatize themselves to their worsening condition.

Most often, the patient will wish to continue the discussion, at which time the physician should proceed by foreshadowing the bad news in simple language. Gauge the patient's reaction and be careful not to give the patient more information than he is ready to hear because he may not be prepared for all of the details at this time.

"Frank, I'm sorry to have to tell you that the x-ray doesn't look good. I'm afraid that the cancer has begun to grow again."

After stating the bad news, it's a good idea to stop talking and to listen. Silence at this time may be uncomfortable or even unbearable for the physician. However, a pause from speaking is essential to allow the patient to collect his thoughts and for you to watch his or her reaction. Observe the impact on the patient of the news you have conveyed. Various reactions by the patient are possible: from rage to withdrawal, from screaming to silence, from crying to anger. These first reactions can reveal a significant insight into the patient's personality. With the passage of time, it will become clear whether the patient's responses are adaptive or maladaptive. Accepted and even useful defense mechanisms for dealing with bad news include limited denial, anger (either abstract or directed at the disease), crying, fear, and sometimes, humor. Oftentimes, patients will engage the physician in a type of bargaining or channel their energy toward a realistic future goal such as a key holiday or family event. On the other hand, morbid guilt; pathological denial often associated with inappropriate behavior; anger directed at caregivers, family, or physicians; profound despair; overtly manipulative behavior; and unrealistic hope associated with "the impossible quest" are maladaptive responses that may sometimes require professional intervention. Some of these problems may be anticipated on the basis of the patient's initial reaction to the bad news.

Listening allows the physician to learn and understand what the illness means to the patient. The patient may often give clues or express what matters most to him or her. Empathy, like attentive listening, requires patience, which is a virtue that requires practice. Unfortunately, patience is rarely an inherent physician character trait and is seldom taught. However, patience and empathy promote trust. Only with the establishment of a trusting relationship will the physician be granted access to the patient's deeper feelings, values, and ideas.

Knowledge and Empathy

When imparting the bad news and the more detailed information that naturally follows, one must be careful to share this knowledge in a thoughtful manner. One must speak slowly and clearly. It is important to avoid medical jargon and highly technical language, and make sure that you explain things using terms that the patient and family can understand. Avoid giving too much information at once, as this will "overload" the patient and family, reducing the chances that

they are absorbing what you are saying to them. Another method used to help ensure that patients and families comprehend what is being said is to repeat and summarize points frequently.

Empathy is defined by Coulehan and Block (1988) as

"...a type of understanding. It is not an emotional state of feeling sorry for someone. Nor is it the same virtue as compassion. Although compassion may well be your motivation for developing empathy with patients, empathy is not compassion. In medical interviewing, being empathetic means listening to the total communication—words, feelings, and gestures—and letting patients know that you truly comprehend what they are saying. The empathetic physician is also the scientific physician because "understanding is at the core of objectivity.""

The two steps of knowledge and empathy occur consecutively as the physician follows a statement of fact (knowledge) with a response to the patient's reaction (empathy). Empathetic behavior requires you to identify the emotion that the patient is experiencing as well as the origin of that emotion. It also requires you to respond in a kind way that tells the patient that you understand him.

"Frank, I feel that I must have knocked you over with this report. You certainly have every reason to be upset, sad, and angry. I appreciate that not knowing exactly what the future holds in store is frightening, and I share your concern."

Remaining silent after an empathetic remark, perhaps by counting slowly and silently to 10 before saying anything else, is often recommended by numerous authors. This pause allows time for reflection by both the patient and the physician. The patient can use the time to absorb the feeling of being understood, while the pause permits the physician to consider how and what the patient is thinking and feeling. For the physician, it is critical to avoid the temptation to fill the void created by the pause and continue the conversation to fix the situation or to assuage the patient. It is hard to overcome the urge to quickly turn to a treatment plan so as to divert the patient from the painful news just delivered. Eventually, an appropriate action plan will need to be proposed and agreed to by the patient/family, but, at this point, it is premature.

The manner of breaking bad news is not a "one size fits all" approach. Truthfulness is important, but even the truth sometimes needs to be tailored to match individual patient needs. Sometimes, it may be wise to temper the burden of complete knowledge. However, if due to poor understanding about the diagnosis, the prognosis, or the therapeutic options, the patient may make a poor choice about proposed interventions, the physician is medically, legally, and ethically obligated to give patients or their designated surrogates sufficient information to make appropriate informed choices.

A patient's feelings of hopelessness can further exacerbate sickness and deterioration and even lead to a premature death. Even near the end of life, hope may be preserved in various ways. Studies reveal that few patients abandon hope for a cure, even when highly improbable. Other patients find hope by exercising control of their choices and ensuring that they will not suffer a lingering death complicated by prolonged tube feedings, ventilator support, or cardiopulmonary resuscitation. Even in the case of a terminal illness, a physician's offer of hope, when presented as a commitment to ensure a comfortable, peaceful, and dignified dying experience, free of pain and suffering, is not a deception.

In the era of managed care, some physicians may believe that they do not have sufficient time for empathetic communication. However, research has shown that an up front "investment" in good communication ultimately saves enormous amounts of time—time the patient will otherwise spend asking repetitive questions. Empathetic communication is one of the few panaceas in medicine. It predictably generates improved patient and physician satisfaction, fewer malpractice suits, better patient adherence to therapy, and improved clinical outcomes including the often-sought "good death."

Summation

The last task in the six-step SPIKES protocol requires the physician to summarize the delivered news and review the potential treatment options. These may include combinations of therapeutics such as chemotherapy, radiation therapy, surgery, or experimental treatment for malignant illnesses. When faced with a noncurable disease for which definitive disease-directed treatment options are lacking or futile, physicians should offer symptom-directed therapeutic options such as hospice or palliative care to assist in the palliation of symptoms, to focus on the relief of total suffering, and to help ensure that the lives of their patients end with comfort and dignity. Offering no treatment is NOT an option! Pay attention to identifying caregivers, ensuring proper living arrangements, and establishing contact with support groups or community agencies.

The patient and family need to leave the meeting with a clear understanding of what has happened to date and what is planned for the future. End by inviting future questions, scheduling follow-up visits, and planning an agenda for the next meeting. When the patient concludes this session with you, he or she should leave with assurance as to your continued availability and with a clear understanding of a mutually acceptable plan of care open to future revision as needed. He or she should also end the visit with the knowledge that his or her wishes will be respected and with reasonable hope that, even if there is no cure or chance of remission of his or her illness, pain and suffering, and other potential symptoms, will be alleviated.

CONCLUSION

Breaking bad news can be a grueling mental and emotional experience. It is easy to do it poorly because of haste, anxiety, guilt, or insensitivity.

Although desiring in principle to be supportive to patients and families, many physicians, aware of their own discomfort and lack of ease during such emotionally charged patient encounters, deliver a rapid-paced, fact-filled monologue without stopping to elicit any response from the listener. Delivering bad news in a rushed, thoughtless, uncaring manner can cause unnecessary harm to patients and to their families and can often make the bad news worse. Studies clearly demonstrate that the way bad news is communicated leaves an indelible, long-lasting impression on patients and their loved ones.

The suggestions and ideas offered in this chapter can help clinicians convey bad news more effectively and compassionately. The manner in which bad news is delivered can have a major effect on your patient's attitude and compliance. It also reflects on your image as a caring and empathetic clinician. The ability to communicate well is not inborn. It is a learned behavior. With practice, this skill can be artfully polished and become one of the most important elements of the care that you render.

In the final analysis, think how you would wish to be treated if you (as will inevitably occur) were the patient. You would hope that your experience would match that of Dr. Deborah Young Bradshaw (1999):

> I recognized that what had happened in that examination room was simply an act of love. Love in any relationship, including that between physician and patient, requires the courage to risk revealing oneself unedited, the willingness to notice and to listen, the willingness to surrender one's own ease or comfort, the willingness to share the suffering of another, and the courage to risk and accept gentle confrontation. In this way, any loving relationship can heal. Any relationship hoping to heal without love falls short.
>
> That day, I learned what it is to be in need and to be taken care of. That day, I felt healing hands upon me and was left breathless with new awareness of the awesome gift and profound responsibility I had been given as a physician.

PART 2
GOALS OF CARE AND DECISION-MAKING CONVERSATIONS

Joel S. Policzer

Patients and families have myriad decisions to make during the course of an illness. These decisions increase in frequency and complexity as the illness becomes critical or life-threatening and they are especially important when the illness has become life limiting. Often times, patients and families fall into the situation of "decision overload" where they perceive themselves to be floundering in a system that asks for decision after decision yet offers them little, if any, guidance.

A necessary role for any health care provider is to be the guide that the patient and family require to help negotiate through this decision-making process and to assist them in deciding which therapeutic options to pursue. Not only is this good patient care, it additionally leads to the patient receiving the care that he or she desires and to better satisfaction with the care, even if the patient has died.

Medical decisions should not be made as isolated events. Rather, decisions need to fit within the context of what is actually occurring medically to the patient, where the patient finds himself or herself in the trajectory of illness and how this fits into what the patient sees as his or her best option, in other words, the person's goals of care.

For example, the decision to repair a hip fracture should not be made simply because the femur is broken. If the fracture occurred in an otherwise healthy 25-year-old man who fell off a ladder while repairing roof tiles, the decision to surgically repair the hip is nearly automatic. The man is seen as having years of life before him, and clearly would want to return to normal activity and his usual life as quickly as possible. However, if the patient is a 95-year-old woman, bed-confined in a long-term care facility, who also has diabetes, hypertension, osteoporosis, and dementia, and whose fragile femur breaks while being rolled over in bed during a bath, there needs to be a careful discussion as to what the optimal care should be. Can the patient be kept comfortable and pain free without surgery? Is surgery even an option since the patient is nonambulatory and will not be able to cooperate with rehabilitation therapy? Given her multiple medical problems, would she be able to tolerate anesthesia, and so on? In this setting, the decision to operate should not be automatic. Rather, the physician and the patient's family need to discuss the situation carefully, and consider all therapeutic options, both surgical and nonsurgical, based upon multiple factors including the goals of care that the patient had expressed in the past.

In this part of the chapter we will review what constitutes goal-oriented decision making and decision making based on outcomes, barriers to decision making, and how to have the goals of care conversation with specific focus on the physician's role in this process.

GOAL-ORIENTED DECISION MAKING

Clinicians make diagnostic and therapeutic decisions for various reasons. A biopsy, scan, or procedure may be done simply because it can be, the so-called "Mt Everest Syndrome" (based on the statement attributed to Sir Edmund Hillary that he climbed Everest "because it was there"). Scans and laboratory tests may be ordered to evaluate and to correct every abnormality in the hope that this will improve the patient's outcome, or diagnostic tests are ordered to prove that no stones were left unturned in the attempt to minimize liability based on the perceived litigious nature of society.

However, the best decisions are based on the goal of providing optimal medical care. Therefore, the issue truly becomes how to define *optimal care* in the context of the patient's age; functional status; the comorbidities and secondary illnesses; care needs including medical, psychosocial, and spiritual; and the overall trajectory of the patient's illness.

GOAL SETTING

The questions that must be considered in reaching a decision for medical intervention are these: Whose goals are being considered? Are the goals achievable? Are the goals beneficial to the patient? And how are the results of the intervention going to be measured?

Whose Goals are Being Considered?

The primary goal-setter certainly should be the patient whenever possible. If the patient does not have the capacity to make decisions for his or her own care, then the patient-appointed surrogate or health care proxy will be involved in these decisions. The process should always be patient centered: the discussion should start with "what does the patient want or what would the patient want?" Although what the patient wants may not always be the final result, it should always be the beginning of any conversation.

There will be times when the goals of the patient and the family may be in conflict. For example, a woman exhausted by years of breast cancer treatment may have made peace with her impending death whereas her children, who dread losing their mother, urge her to continue to "fight on." In other situations, family members may be in conflict with each other, as in the case of the son who has been the father's primary caregiver and understands the need to withdraw interventions, whereas the daughter, who has not been involved in his care, may insist on continuing treatment to assuage her own guilt. In these situations the physician needs to keep the discussion patient centered, either empowering the patient to speak for him or herself or, if the patient is unable to participate in the discussion, reframing the conversation in terms of "if your mother were sitting here and able to speak for herself, what would she say?" If the physician is unable to successfully guide these conversations away from the conflicts and bring resolution, then it is useful to ask a social worker or chaplain for assistance.

It also needs to be recognized that physicians and health care providers often bring their own goals to the encounter. Our health care system has the imperative to "do something" as its default position; therefore, the physician may urge continuation of treatment for no other reason than this. In addition, as the medical training of physicians has been based on achieving positive outcomes for patients, the patient who is deteriorating or dying represents a situation that is neither comfortable nor intuitive for the physician. For many, in fact, the dying patient has come to be seen as a personal failure. Physicians need to continually be aware of these issues and make certain that the recommendations they make are always in the best interest of the patient.

Are the Goals Achievable?

The ability to actually achieve the goals defined by the patient or surrogate decision maker has to be a part of the conversation and has to be clearly addressed. The patient with cancer of the pancreas who wants to regain the 60 pounds that she lost may well not be able to have this happen. The man with obstructive lung disease severe enough to confine him to a chair may not be able to start walking on a treadmill to "regain strength." The man with multiple myeloma involving most of his bones may not be able to achieve full pain relief and be fully alert. The discussion in each of these situations has to be centered on what the patients want, factoring in what can be achieved completely, partially, or not at all.

Are the Goals Beneficial?

Another important element in the decision-making conversation is how the desired goals of care and any potential interventions that are being considered to achieve those goals will actually be of benefit in meeting or achieving those goals. If a patient suffers from anemia and desires to receive transfusions to avoid the symptoms of anemia and, despite having a hemoglobin level of 7.0 g/dL, has no signs of symptoms of anemia, such as headache, shortness of breath, or chest pain, how will a transfusion be of benefit and meet the goals of care? Whenever any intervention is considered, the benefits and the burdens of the intervention must be discussed fully and honestly in the context of its ability to achieve the patient's stated goals of care to allow optimal decisions to be made.

How are Results Measured?

Once a physician and patient determine a plan of action designed to achieve the agreed upon goals of care, they need to establish a time frame to allow the plan to work and at what point they will begin to measure the outcomes that will be used to determine the success of the plan. No intervention should be considered "ongoing" or "endless," as this can lead to the continuation of treatment that is not effective, or even harmful. The agreed upon time frame needs to be a reasonable one, and the parameters of success or failure must also be accepted by all parties involved. Stated in other terms, how long will the trial of therapy be, how will we know that it is working, and what will tell us that it is not working? For example, if intravenous or subcutaneous hydration is started on a dehydrated, lethargic patient with the goal of trying to make him or her more alert so that he or she can speak with his or her family, it is reasonable to offer a 24- to 48-hour trial of fluid infusion. After the requisite time frame has passed and if the patient, despite now being well hydrated, remains in the same state of lethargy, then it is reasonable to discontinue the hydration as it did not achieve the stated goal of care, and, in addition, if it were to be continued, there is the potential for the harmful complication of fluid overload.

BARRIERS TO EFFECTIVE GOAL SETTING

PATIENT AND FAMILY BARRIERS

It is not often easy or comfortable for patients and families to make their needs and wishes known to their physicians. In the patient–physician relationship, the power is heavily tilted toward the physician; this sometimes can be perceived as coercive. Patients wish to be thought of as "good patients" and therefore are often unwilling to contradict what the physician is saying, even when their goals of care may not be completely in synch with the physician. They may not wish to upset a good therapeutic relationship or are afraid that if they refuse the physician's recommendation, the physician will not want to care for them anymore. If the illness is critical, the physician is usually perceived as the person who is "keeping the patient alive," and patients will not want to jeopardize any chance for a successful outcome. It takes patients with strong empowerment to be willing to express themselves so that their needs will be taken into account. In addition, patients may be embarrassed by aspects of their illnesses or their lack of understanding of the issues, and this, as well as the fear of possible death, often prevents an open discussion that will center the decision-making on patients' goals of care.

PHYSICIAN BARRIERS

In addition to the already stated sense of failure that many physicians feel threatened by when fac-
ing the potential deterioration and death of patients they care for, physicians are reluctant to discuss goals of care with patients for several other reasons. These conversations need to be open and frank, and many physicians are concerned that the information they will be forced to convey will have significant negative effects on patients. At times, the discussion can lead to conflict and confrontation, which the physician would prefer to avoid. In addition, they may be concerned that such conversations can lead to medicolegal difficulties, especially if they are perceived as not having offered or done "everything possible."

Physicians are often not well trained in communication skills, leading to their discomfort with these difficult conversations and their fear of causing distress to their patients. A phrase that commonly used is "There is nothing more to do." It is difficult to underestimate the damage that using this short phrase causes. It creates mistrust between physician and patients and deflects the real conversation that needs to happen. It is a statement that implies abandonment; if there is nothing more that the physician can do, the relationship has ended. Most importantly, it is simply not true; there is always something that can be done. A more appropriate way to reframe this might be to say: "I wish there were more I could do to cure your illness, but let's focus on what we can do."

Discussions of the possibility of death do not always cause these patients distress. In fact, patients often welcome the open discussion of what the realities of their lives are. Regarding the issue of "taking away hope," hope is the frame within which patients construct their futures, and redirecting this from hope for a cure to hope that pain will be relieved and hope that a certain legacy will live on can be very beneficial.

HEALTH CARE SYSTEM BARRIERS

Our health care system also erects barriers to effective communication. Conversations regarding end-of-life decisions are not considered to be routine in our system and therefore are not seen as being an important part of care. As the system becomes more fragmented, with many providers involved with any individual patient, a key question is which provider has the ultimate responsibility of holding this discussion, especially if no one provider has had a long-standing relationship with the patient or family. There is decreased contact time for each encounter between physicians and patients so the opportunities for these conversations to occur are less. And finally, our health care system has a default position of "doing something," so there is little imperative to have conversations regarding the limiting or withdrawing of interventions.

HAVING THE GOALS OF CARE CONVERSATION

We all know that words matter and that physicians and health care providers have enormous impact on patients and families by what they say and how they say it. Communicating effectively to help guide patients through the process of making health care decisions is a skill that all clinicians need to acquire. Fortunately, the acquisition of this skill set is not difficult and there are formats to follow for these conversations.

STEPS TO FOLLOW IN THE CONVERSATION

The steps in having these conversations are very similar to those of other important conversations, such as "Breaking Bad News," which is discussed in Part 1 of this chapter.

First, determine who needs to be present for this conversation. The patient should be asked who he or she depends on to make decisions and should wait until the person or persons are available. If the patient lacks capacity, the important

stakeholders in the patient's care should all be present. On the health care side, there will need to be preparation to determine whether only clinical staff should attend, or whether there is the anticipation of conflict requiring the presence of an experienced social worker or chaplain.

Second, make certain the setting is correct. There needs to be privacy for all concerned, with adequate seating, writing materials, and tissues. All electronics should be turned off to avoid distraction; the physician needs to silence his or hers as well, making certain that the family knows it is off, to communicate that this conversation is so important that no interruptions will occur.

Third, the clinician has to determine the agenda so that there is a plan of what information has to be given to the patient and family and a guide for what decisions will need to be made or addressed.

Fourth, the conversation starts by determining what the patient and family know about the current clinical status of the patient and proceeds from there.

Fifth, at the conclusion of the decision-making, follow-up is planned so that everyone is clear on the plans to follow, who will do what, and when.

CONTENTS OF THE CONVERSATION

The heart of the conversation itself needs always to be patient centered; this is about this individual patient, his or her needs, and how best to serve him or her. And the needs are not only medical or clinical, the psychosocial and spiritual needs must also be addressed.

The conversation proceeds with a series of open-ended questions. Suggested questions that the clinician may use at various times during the conversation can be found in Table 3–4. The clinician should actively listen for the answer and then ask follow-up questions using the patient's own words, which communicates that what the patient said was heard. The questions should be designed to encourage the patient to talk and steer the conversation toward the practical issues that need to

TABLE 3–4. Suggested Open-Ended Questions for Goals of Care and Decision-Making Conversations

TOPIC	SUGGESTED QUESTIONS
Encourage patient to talk	"How is treatment going for you?" · "What can you tell me about the history of your illness?" "Tell me what you know about the treatment you have received and what can be done for your illness now?"
Address very practical issues	"What problems is this illness causing for you?" "What has been explained to you about how these problems can be controlled?" "Are there things about the later stages of your illness that you would like to discuss?" "Are there people who need to know what is going on?"
Assist the patient in taking control	"How are you coping with your illness?" "What, if anything, are you worried about or afraid of?" "What are your most important hopes, and your most important fears?"
Acknowledge emotions Validate feelings	"This must be very difficult for you." "It is very common for someone in your situation to have a hard time with these decisions." "Of course, talking about this makes you sad. That is normal."
Guide conversation toward goals of care and decision-making issues	"Given the severity of your illness, what is most important for you now?" "How do you think about balancing the quality of your life with the length of your life in your treatment?" "Have you thought about what you would want, and not want, for your treatment if you can't speak for yourself?" "Given what you have said, in thinking about the treatments that you could have, how would you want your treatment to be now?"
Establish a sense of what is important to the patient	"What makes life worth living for you?" "What is your quality of life now, and what can I do?" "If you are unable to speak for yourself, who is best able to speak for you?" "If you were to die sooner rather than later, what would be left undone and how can I help to make these happen?"
Concentrate on never taking hope away and reframing hope in what is possible	"Have you thought about what might happen if things don't go the way you want?" "What plans have you made to help prepare you in that case, and how can I help?" "If we can't make cure/remission/improvement happen, what other goals can we work toward?"

be addressed. They should also give the patient the license to take control of the situation.

If, during this time, the patient begins to talk about the fear of death or becomes emotional, *do not* change the subject or ignore this. Continue

to be present for the patient and ask questions that will assist in exploring what is clearly an issue of importance to him or her. Acknowledge the emotion and validate the patient's feelings. If the patient truly is expressing existential questions and raises concerns regarding the meaning of his or her life, make certain that the patient knows that this is very important to you and that you will facilitate a meeting with a chaplain. On the other hand, if the concerns center on control of physical symptoms, make certain that the patient knows that you will work with him or her to control them and that your goal is ultimately the patient's comfort.

As the conversation moves forward, the clinician should guide the conversation toward establishing the goals of care and addressing the decisions that need to be made based on those goals. Establish a sense of what is important to the patient so that you will be able to understand the patient's wishes, allowing you to be able to counsel the patient now and, when he or she can no longer make these decisions, the surrogate decision makers. Finally, concentrate on never taking hope away and reframing hope into what is possible.

CONCLUSION

It is important to remember that *goals of care and decision-making conversations* are not isolated events, but occur on multiple occasions throughout the course of a patient's illness. The goals and decisions made by patients or their surrogates may evolve and change as the clinical circumstances of the patients change during the course of the illness. By developing the necessary communication skills, physicians and other health care professionals who care for patients near the end of life and their families can do their utmost to ensure that patients receive both the care that they want and that they need, allow patients and families to be comfortable with the decisions that they make, and maintain a sense of hope, even in the face of a terminal illness. Helping the patient and family manage their hopes and their resources in a realistic way may well leave the family in the best situation after their loss.

BIBLIOGRAPHY

Annunziata MA: Ethics of relationship. From communication to conversation. *Ann N Y Acad Sci* 809:400-410, 1997.

Annunziata MA, Foladore S, Magri MD, et al: Does the information level of cancer patients correlate with quality of life? A prospective study [in English]. *Tumori* 84:619-623, 1998.

Back AL, Arnold RL, Baile WF, et al: Approaching difficult communication tasks in oncology. *CA Cancer J Clin* 55:164-177, 2005.

Barclay JS, Blackhall LJ, Tulsky JA: Communication strategies and cultural issues in the delivery of bad news. *J Palliat Med* 10:958-977, 2007.

Bradshaw DY. A visit to the doctor. *Ann Intern Med* 131:627-628, 1999.

Brody J: Personal health: Bad news. *New York Times.* August 24, 1999, Health and Fitness.

Buckman R. *How to Break Bad News: A Guide for Health Care Professionals.* Baltimore, MD, The Johns Hopkins University Press, 1992, pp. 65-171.

Chochinov HM: Dignity-conserving care—A new model for palliative care. *JAMA* 287(17):2253-2260, 2002.

Fallowfield LJ, Jenkins VA, Beveridge HA: Truth may hurt but deceit hurts more: Communication in palliative care. *Palliat Med* 16:297-303, 2001.

Fried TR, Bradley EH, O'Leary J: Prognosis communication in serious illness: Perceptions of older patients, caregivers, and clinicians. *J Am Geriatr Soc* 51:1398-1403, 2003.

Friedrichsen M, Milberg A: Concerns about losing control when breaking bad news to terminally ill patients with cancer: Physician's perspective. *J Palliat Med* 9:673-682, 2006.

Landro L: Patient-physician communication: An emerging partnership. *Oncologist* 4:55-58, 1999.

Lintz KC, Penson RT, Cassem N, et al: A staff dialogue on aggressive palliative treatment demanded by a terminally ill patient: Psychological issues faced by patients, their families, and caregivers. *Oncologist* 4:70-76, 1999.

Lo B, Snyder L, Sox HC: Care at the end of life: Guiding practice where there are no easy answers. *Ann Intern Med* 130:772-774, 1999.

Mouton C, Teno JM, Mor V, Piette J: Communication of preferences for care among human immunodeficiency virus-infected patients. Barriers to informed decisions? *Arch Fam Med* 6:342-347, 1997.

Nowak TV: The ritual. *Ann Intern Med* 130:1025-1026, 1999

Pantilat SZ: Communicating with seriously ill patients: Better words to say. *JAMA* 301(12):1279-1281. 2009.

Parker SM, Clayton JM, Hancock K, et al: A systematic review of prognostic/end-of-life communication with adults in the advanced stages of a life-limiting illness: Patient/caregiver preferences for the content, style, and timing of information. *J Pain Symptom Manage* 34:81-93, 2007.

Petrasch S, Bauer M, Reinacher-Schick A, et al: Assessment of satisfaction with the communication process during consultation of cancer patients with potentially curable disease, cancer patients on palliative care, and HIV-positive patients [in English]. *Wien Med Wochenschr* 148:491-495, 1998.

Poulson J: Bitter pills to swallow. *N Engl J Med* 338: 1844-1846, 1998.

Ptacek JT, Eberhardt TL: Breaking bad news. A review of the literature. *JAMA* 276:496-502, 1996.

Quill TE, Townsend P: Bad news: Delivery, dialogue, and dilemmas. *Arch Intern Med* 151:463-468, 1991.

Strasser F, Palmer JL, Willey J, et al: Impact of physician sitting versus standing during inpatient oncology consultations: Patients' preference and perception of compassion and duration. A randomized control trial. *J Pain Symptom Manage* 29:489-497, 2005.

Suchman AL, Markakis K, Beckman HB, Frankel R: A model of empathetic communication in the medical interview. *JAMA* 277:678-682, 1997.

Tulsky JA: Beyond advance directives: Importance of communication skills at the end of life. *JAMA* 294(3):359-365, 2005.

SELF-ASSESSMENT QUESTIONS

1. Studies documenting patient/caregiver communication preferences have demonstrated each of the following, EXCEPT

   A. Patients and caregivers desire significant information about the nature of the illness and patient life expectancy.
   B. Patient and caregivers information needs diverge over time, with patients wanting less and caregivers wanting more information.
   C. Although patients desire information, they often do not express this desire to the clinicians caring for them.
   D. Patients and caregivers want to be informed in a frank and open fashion.
   E. Patient preferences regarding family involvement is very variable.

2. All of the following are challenges that impede the ability of physicians to deliver bad news to patients and families, EXCEPT

   A. Physicians often do not have the time it takes to discuss the situation adequately.
   B. Physicians are intimidated by the thought of being blamed for the patient's illness.
   C. Physicians are well trained to communicate bad news to patients and families.
   D. Physicians develop a sense of inadequacy as they believe that they have "failed" the patient.
   E. Physicians are uncomfortable dealing with both their emotions and those of the patients.

3. Dr. X is making morning rounds and comes to see Mrs. Y, who has just been diagnosed with metastatic breast carcinoma. Mrs. Y is in a semiprivate room, so when Dr. X enters, he draws the curtain, says "Good morning" and then pulls over a chair and sits near the head of the bed. He holds Mrs. Y's wrist with his hand as if he is taking her pulse and says, "I want to discuss the results of your tests with you now. Have you given any thought to what they might have shown?" What step in preparing for this meeting did Dr. X omit?

   A. Arranging for family presence.
   B. Arranging for privacy.
   C. Sitting at eye level
   D. Holding the patient's hand
   E. Eliciting the perception of the patient

4. When imparting knowledge to patients and families about the illness, all of the following are important to follow, EXCEPT

   A. Speak slowly and clearly to aid patients and families in understanding what you are trying to tell them.
   B. Use medical jargon and technical language so that the patient and family will have confidence in your medical expertise.
   C. Avoid giving too much information at once so as not to "overload" the patient and family.
   D. Summarize and repeat information to ensure that patients and families comprehend what you are saying.
   E. Listen to the patient's responses to ensure that they are capturing the information you are providing.

5. During the summation phase of the discussion, which of the following statements would be LEAST appropriate for the physician to say to the patient and family?

   A. "I am sorry there is no treatment we can offer you. It is time for you to go to hospice."
   B. "Let's schedule an appointment after 1 week so that you can ask me any questions you have about what we discussed today."
   C. "We have agreed that we are going to use a new form of chemotherapy to try and treat your cancer."
   D. "We have agreed that we are going to focus our energies on treating your symptoms and improving your quality of life."

NORTHEAST COMMUNITY COLLEGE LIBRARY

E. "From what you have said, I understand that your daughter will be coming to live with you and take care of you."

6. All of the following statements regarding the participation of family members in a meeting to "break bad news" are true, EXCEPT

   A. Family members often remember things that were said if the patient "tunes out" the conversation.
   B. Always ask patients if they want family members present prior to discussing "bad news."
   C. If patients prefer meeting alone, try and urge them to bring along at least one other person for support.
   D. If a hospitalized patient wants his or her family present, it is important to postpone the discussion until the family can be present.
   E. If the patient does not speak or understand English, a family member should be used as an interpreter.

7. All of the following regarding medical decision making are true EXCEPT

   A. They are made based on the best treatment options available.
   B. They are made within the context of the patient's life trajectory.
   C. They are made to make certain that the patient has had every treatment available.
   D. They are made in concert with the patient's wishes.
   E. They are made on the basis of the patient's ability to tolerate the burden of treatment.

8. In considering the process of developing goals of care, all of the following are true EXCEPT

   A. If a patient and family have different goals, those of the patient are more important to follow.
   B. Decision-making surrogates should always make end-of-life decisions, even for patients with capacity, because of the distressing nature of these conversations.
   C. Physicians bring their own goals into the decision-making process.
   D. Goals should be discussed in terms of what is possible and what is not possible to achieve.
   E. An appropriate goal is one that is beneficial for the patient.

9. All of the following are barriers to effective goal setting conversations EXCEPT

   A. Physicians who avoid goal setting conversations because of their own discomfort
   B. Patients who go alongwith any of their physicians' recommendations to avoid "upsetting" them
   C. Families who encourage the patient to "fight on"
   D. Multiple physicians being involved in the patient's care
   E. Patients who confront their physicians to express their needs

10. Which of the following is true regarding goals of care conversations?

    A. When a patient begins to cry the conversation should be stopped and rescheduled.
    B. A time limit should be decided on and kept to.
    C. Only medical issues should be discussed.
    D. The patient should have people present for support and to assist in decision making.
    E. The physician should make recommendations and encourage the patient to follow them

CHAPTER

4

How to Work with the
Interdisciplinary Team

Barry M. Kinzbrunner and Joel S. Policzer

INTRODUCTION

American society has become more aware of the need to adequately provide for the needs of people at the end of life, and to this end, there has been significant growth of hospices in the system. There are now estimated to be more than 4,500 hospices in the United States and most communities have one, if not many. In addition, there are an ever expanding number of both inpatient- and outpatient-based palliative care programs. Therefore, it will be common for a practicing physician to have contact with a number of end-of-life care providers when caring for patients during the final stage of life.

American physicians tend not to be comfortable with the care of dying patients, as the necessary skills are often not taught, or if taught, de-emphasized, during medical education and training. Rather, physician training primarily revolves around the care of the living and the battle against disease. Disability and death are perceived as failures of medical care, and often failure of the physician. Although there are increasing efforts being made throughout the United States to expose medical students and resident physicians to hospice and palliative care, such training remains far from ideal and, in most cases, is only poorly integrated into the medical educational experience. In addition, the widely held attitude that death is equivalent to failure, the medico-legal climate that holds that death is suspect and may be due to physician error, and the view that hospice care is best reserved for those who are actively dying all serve to delay physician acceptance of the roles of hospice and palliative care as facilitating the end-of-life care of the patients they care for.

In caring for patients at the end of life, addressing physical symptoms alone is not sufficient to achieve adequate comfort. Patients require comprehensive care from professionals who recognize and can help with the psychological and spiritual causes of distress. From the recognition that quality end-of-life care comes from the coordinated efforts of individuals from various disciplines, the Medicare Hospice Benefit has mandated that certified hospice programs meet patient and family needs by providing care via an interdisciplinary (ID) team. The importance of the ID team approach to care is further underscored by the fact that it has been adopted by many nonhospice palliative care programs.

The ID team consists of, at the minimum, a registered nurse (RN), a physician, a social worker, and a chaplain. Other professionals often added to the team include home health aides, homemakers, pharmacists, and volunteers. With the patient at the center of the team, as well as the family, and attending physician, who are considered core members of the team, it is the responsibility of the entire ID team to develop and implement a comprehensive plan of care. With multiple disciplines offering insight into patient-identified problems from different viewpoints, individualized and innovative solutions to these problems will lead to more successful patient care outcomes.

The team approach to end-of-life care is unique among health care services offered in the United States. For physicians caring for terminally ill patients, therefore, it is important to understand how the ID team functions, how each member contributes to the whole, and how they, as physicians, may effectively participate with the team to optimize care for their patients at the end of life.

THE PHYSICIAN'S ROLE IN HOSPICE AND END-OF-LIFE CARE

The physician who works with hospices and other end-of-life care programs will need to learn how to function as do members of a team. This team approach is somewhat foreign to most physicians, who have been trained to work independently and autonomously, as well as be "the captain of the ship," holding ultimate responsibility for the outcome of care provided. This traditional view, that the physician knows best, directly challenges the basic tenet of hospice and palliative care— that the patient is the center of the team's focus and that the patient knows best.

There are distinct roles that a physician can play when caring for patients enrolled in an end-of-life care program. These roles are most clearly defined by the Medicare Hospice Benefit and the hospice approach to care. Therefore, the hospice model will be used as the template for much of this discussion. However, with the increasing of evolution of nonhospice palliative care consultation services in hospitals, long-term care (LTC) facilities, and even in the home setting, and with the formal recognition of the specialty of hospice

and palliative medicine by the American Board of Medical Specialties, the role of the palliative care consultant as an independent provider of end-of-life care outside of hospice will be examined as well.

Physician's roles can be segregated as either being outside end-of-life care organizations or inside the organizations. Physicians may interact with hospices and palliative care providers as attending physicians, long-term care medical directors, managed care medical directors, or consulting physicians. Physicians providing end-of-life care may function within hospice programs as hospice medical directors or as hospice team physicians or outside of hospice in the role of palliative care consultant. Table 4–1 lists each role with a brief description of the role and is followed by a more detailed discussion of each.

TABLE 4–1. Physician Roles in Hospice Care

PHYSICIAN ROLE	DEFINITION
Attending physician	The physician who is identified by the patient as having the most significant role in the determination of that patient's medical care.
Long-term care medical director	The physician who is responsible to oversee the medical care provided to all patients residing at all care levels in the facility.
Managed care medical director	The physician employed by a managed care organization who is responsible to oversee the medical care provided to patients on the plan.
Consulting physician	A physician contracted by the hospice to provide a specific medical service to a patient that cannot be provided by the attending physician or the hospice medical director.
Hospice medical director	A physician who is either employed or contracted by the hospice and is primarily responsible for the oversight of the medical care rendered to patients cared for by the hospice.
Hospice team physician	A physician who is either employed or contracted by the hospice and is responsible for providing hands-on medical care to patients cared for by the hospice.
Palliative medicine consultant	A physician who may be employed by a hospital, LTCF, managed care agency, or hospice, or who may be in an independent practice, and provides palliative medicine consultations to patients, generally at the request of the patient's attending physician.

TABLE 4–2. Role of the Attending Physician

Hospice responsibilities	Key member of the interdisciplinary team
	Certifies that the patient has a limited life expectancy
	Discusses need for end-of-life care with patient and family
	Actively participates in the care of the patient on the hospice program
	Professional services are reimbursable under Medicare Part B
	Office, home, and long-term care facility visits
	Care planning (30–60 min per month)
Request palliative medicine consults	Patients who have uncontrolled pain and symptom management
	Assist patients with advance care planning
	Assist in determining patient prognosis and potential hospice eligibility

ATTENDING PHYSICIAN

By Federal regulation, the attending physician is a physician of medicine or osteopathy who "is identified by the individual, at the time he or she elects to receive hospice care, as having the most significant role in the determination of the individual's medical care." The continued involvement and participation of this physician as a member of the ID team in all phases of a patient's care at the end of life is vital.

The upper part of Table 4–2 summarizes the responsibilities of the attending physician in relationship to a hospice program. The first obligation of the attending physician is to determine that a patient is entering into the final stage of life. While the argument is often made that no one knows exactly when any given person will die, guidelines published by the National Hospice and Palliative Care Organization as well as other reputable sources can be helpful to the physician in assessing patient prognosis. Combining these guidelines with sound clinical judgment, physicians can better identify when patients are approaching the end of life and in need of hospice and palliative care. (See Chapter 1 for a detailed discussion of this topic.)

The next step for the attending physician is to communicate the need for end-of-life care to patients and caregivers. This is never an easy task, and there are many tools available to the physician to illustrate how this type of information is best communicated. (See Chapter 3 for a detailed discussion of this topic.) The goal is to have patients understand where in their illness they find themselves and what forms of treatment have been used and are available. As a patient's disease-directed treatment options become more limited, the options of hospice and palliative care becomes of more value. If making the underlying disease better cannot relieve symptoms, then symptom-relief via expert palliative and hospice care is of real benefit. With appropriate counseling, it is possible to have the majority of end-of-life patients accept hospice-type care early in the course of their terminal phase, not just prior to the moment of death. At the point at which the patient and caregiver have agreed to a referral to a hospice, the attending physician refers the patient to an appropriate hospice agency and certifies that the patient has a limited life-span, expected to be less than 6 months if the disease follows its natural course.

Once the patient is admitted to the hospice program, the attending physician should be directly involved in all medical decision making and working together with the hospice medical director or team physician, as well as the other members of the ID team. The attending physician is likely to know the patient better than the hospice care-givers, and be aware of the patient's goals, preferences for treatment, and how the patient perceives the reality that his or her life is ending.

While, ideally, all attending physicians would continue to work closely with the hospice ID team, this is sometimes not the case. Some physicians are uncomfortable caring for patients near the end of life, either for personal reasons, or, more often, due to lack of formal training and expertise in palliative care. Fortunately, with the expertise of the hospice personnel, and with an open attitude of cooperation and willingness to learn, the physicians that do not have a background in palliative medicine can become comfortable and proficient in the care of their end-of-life patients. This serves not only their patients, but will add to the physician's own personal sense of accomplishment.

As a member of the ID team, the attending physician will be kept informed of a patient's course of illness, verbally by various members of the hospice ID team, and less often, in writing. The attending physician may attend the hospice ID team meeting, if not in person, then by conference call, and directly participate in the care planning of common patients. Medication orders and orders to change a patient's hospice level of care are usually provided to the hospice nurse by the attending physician, unless the attending physician is either unavailable or has asked that the hospice medical director or team physician accept that responsibility.

In recognition of the fact that the attending physician is a fully active and vital member of the hospice ID team, the Medicare Hospice Benefit has made special provisions to ensure that attending physicians are compensated for their continued care and support to patients and families at the end of life. Under the Medicare Hospice Benefit, the hospice is responsible to provide all healthcare services related to the terminal illness for patients under its care. (See Chapter 2 for a more detailed discussion of the Medicare Hospice Benefit.) However, the patient's attending physician may also receive Medicare reimbursement for professional services provided to patients via normal Medicare Part B reimbursement means. This allows the attending physician to be compensated for visiting patients either at their places of residence (home or LTC facility), inpatient hospice, or in the physician's office. Medicare also provides reimbursement to attending physicians for care planning services, so that physicians may be compensated for their active participation in care for their patients who are receiving hospice care near the end of life.

The lower portion of Table 4–2 lists some of the indications for which an attending physician may opt to call a palliative care consultant, rather than interact directly with a hospice provider. An attending physician, for example, may be unsure as to whether or not a patient is hospice appropriate and will ask the consultant to render an opinion regarding the patient's prognosis and potential hospice eligibility. Recognizing the difficulty that physicians sometimes have discussing advance care planning issues with patients, the attending physician may ask for a palliative medicine consult in order to have a more highly trained physician initiate the difficult discussion. Some patients are not interested in a hospice option, and in such situations, a palliative medicine consultant can offer the patient some of the needed care that a hospice can provide until if and when the patient may be more comfortable considering hospice care. Finally, some patients are clearly not eligible for hospice care and suffer from significant pain or other uncontrolled symptoms that require a palliative care expert to help manage. The option of calling a palliative medicine specialist in consultation provides attending physicians with the ability to ensure that all their patients, whether they are eligible or interested in hospice care or not, will be able to benefit from receiving appropriate care at the end of life.

LTC FACILITY MEDICAL DIRECTOR

One of the goals of end-of-life care is to allow patients to be cared for at home, if that is their wish. Home is defined as where the patient lives

TABLE 4–3. Role of the Long-Term Care Medical Director

Serve as attending physician
Collaborate with hospice medical director
   Coordination of patient care planning
   Development of treatment guidelines
   Education of LTC and hospice staff
Oversight of patient care in LTC facility
   Identify patients who may need end-of-life
     care
   Ensure hospice patients are receiving
     appropriate end-of-life care
Oversee palliative care consult service if one
   exists

and does not need to be a house or apartment. As patients weaken and are not able to receive adequate care in a private residence, some become residents of LTC facilities (i.e., adult living facilities and nursing homes). The LTC facility becomes the patient's place of residence or home, and care is rendered there.

The LTC facility medical director is the physician primarily charged with overseeing the medical care provided to all patients residing in the facility. In relationship to a hospice program, the LTC facility medical director interacts in a number of ways, summarized in Table 4–3.

First, in many LTC facilities, the medical director will have primary care responsibilities for some or all of the patients living in the home, and, for those patients receiving hospice services, the medical director will function as the attending physician. (See Table 4–2 and the earlier discussion.)

Second, as the overseer of the medical care provided to patients in the LTC facility, the medical director is responsible for making certain that patients receive the care that they need, including hospice and palliative care when appropriate. For patients near the end of life who are enrolled in a hospice program, the LTC facility medical direc-

tor can accomplish this by collaborating directly with the hospice medical director(s) from hospice organization(s) with which the LTC facility holds contracts. Joint activities between the respective medical directors may include ensuring that there are coordinated plans of care for common patients, developing palliative care treatment guidelines that meet patient needs while meeting safety, efficacy, and regulatory standards of both organizations, and educating LTC facility and hospice staff on how to better serve patients who are near the end of life.

Interaction between the respective medical directors may also occur when there is a conflict between the hospice plan of care and the LTC facilities plan of care. With both physicians properly communicating about the nature of the potential conflict, a solution that meets the needs of the patient and family, and both the LTC and the hospice, is more likely to be developed.

The LTC facility medical director may also provide needed oversight for patients being cared for by other facility attending physicians. The medical director can assist in identifying facility patients who might need hospice or palliative care, as well as verify that the care rendered meets both the needs of the patient and family, and the safety, efficacy, and regulatory needs of the LTC facility and the hospice.

Finally, if the LTC facility has opted to establish a palliative care consult service within the facility, the LTC facility medical director will be charged with oversight responsibility for the service, ensuring that all end-of-life patients living in the facility receive optimum palliative care.

MANAGED CARE MEDICAL DIRECTOR

The managed care medical director is a physician employed by a managed care organization whose primary responsibility is to oversee the medical care provided to patients who receive insurance benefits from the plan. Unlike the LTC facility medical director, a managed care medical

TABLE 4–4. The Role of the Managed Care Medical Director

Collaborate with hospice medical director
  Coordination of case management and
    patient care planning
  Development of treatment guidelines
  Education of managed care case managers
    and hospice staffs
Oversight of patient care
  Identify patients who may need end-of-life
    care
  Ensure hospice patients are receiving
    appropriate end-of-life care
  Determine relationship of interventions to
    terminal illness
Palliative care consult service
  "Champion" the service within the
    organization
  Collaborate with outside palliative care
    consult service provider
  Develop and implement internal palliative
    care consult service
  Oversee palliative care consult service

director rarely, if ever, carries a significant patient care role. Hence, in their interaction with hospice programs, it is much less common for the managed care medical director to function as an attending physician to a hospice patient.

Interactions between hospices and managed care medical directors are primarily administrative in nature. Examples of these interactions are listed in Table 4–4.

Much like the LTC medical director, the managed care medical director should work with his or her hospice counterpart to ensure that hospice guidelines and treatment protocols meet the standards of the managed care organization. Educating the staff is also crucial, and for the managed care medical director, this means assisting the hospice in communicating with managed care case managers and attending physicians regarding identification of patients who need end-of-life

care and disseminating palliative care treatment guidelines.

The managed care medical director must also work with the hospice medical director to ensure that patients are cared for in a comprehensive fashion. For Medicare patients cared for by a managed care organization this can be a challenge. Medicare regulations have determined that when a Medicare patient enrolls on a hospice program, Medicare will reimburse the hospice for services related to the terminal illness, just as for a fee-for-service Medicare patient, adjusting reimbursement to the managed care organization to reflect its responsibility for care that is unrelated to the terminal illness. This may create conflict between the hospice and the managed care organization around whether a particular patient need is the responsibility of the hospice program or the managed care organization. It is the responsibility of the managed care medical director, together with the hospice medical director, to determine which organization should be required to provide the particular service, based upon its relationship to the terminal illness.

For commercially insured patients, the most common arrangement between hospices and managed care organizations is a per diem contract that mirrors the Medicare Hospice Benefit. Here, the hospice provides the clinical service under contract with (and with payment from) the managed care organization; under such circumstances the managed care medical director and the hospice medical director need to work together to ensure that common patients receive appropriate services and appropriate levels of care.

Managed care organizations have become increasingly interested in providing palliative care services to patients with chronic and life-limiting illnesses, as studies have shown that quality of care improves with reduced costs of care when palliative care consultations are offered. The managed care medical director has a key role to play in the development of these services within the managed care organization. The medical director often must be "champion" of these services, convincing the nonclinical members of the management team of the importance of palliative care. He or she is often the first point of contact with a palliative care organization that might be offering these services, or, when the managed care organization is developing its own palliative care program, they may be charged with its development and initial leadership. The managed care medical director will generally remain responsible for the implementation and oversight of the palliative care services and for following the outcome measures that determine that the services remain of high quality and cost effective to the organization. Finally, it often falls upon the managed care medical director, working with the organization's nurse case managers, to encourage primary physicians to utilize the service when patients needing the service are identified.

CONSULTING PHYSICIAN

The role of the consulting physician may at first glance seem unnecessary for patients who are nearing the end of life. Principles of palliative care, after all, suggest that invasive therapies should be avoided, or, at the very least, kept to a minimum. To best meet patient needs, however, there will be occasions when invasive therapies will be the best approach to providing patient comfort. (A full discussion of invasive treatments that may be necessary for patients near the end of life can be found in Chapters 18–21.) On occasion, expert advice about a patient's condition will be required, which is outside the expertise of both the attending physician and the hospice medical director. In either of these circumstances, consulting physicians may be required.

Examples of the services that consulting physicians provide to terminally ill patients can be found in Table 4–5. What is important when considering whether or not a patient requires care from a consulting physician is to evaluate the need for the consultation in the face of the patient's current condition, the symptom or symptoms being treated, and the chances of a successful outcome.

TABLE 4–5. The Role of Consulting Physicians

CONSULTANT	EXAMPLE OF INDICATION
Orthopedics	Pathological fracture
Urologist	Suprapubic stent placement
Pulmonologist	Therapeutic thoracentesis
Radiologist	Biliary stent placement
Gastroenterologist	PEG tube placement

For patients being cared by hospice programs under the Medicare Hospice Benefit, consulting physician services are to be provided by the hospice program. Therefore, the hospice must have a contract with the consulting physician for the physician to provide services to a patient, and the hospice is responsible to compensate the physician directly. It may also bill the hospice Medicare Part A intermediary and be reimbursed for the professional services of the consultant.

HOSPICE MEDICAL DIRECTOR

The Medicare Hospice Benefit requires a certified hospice to have a medical director who is primarily responsible to oversee the medical care rendered to patients cared for by the hospice. The various responsibilities of the hospice medical director are outlined in Table 4–6 and discussed below.

Ensure that Patients Receive Quality Medical Care in Consonance with Principles of Palliative Care

The hospice medical director is responsible to ensure that patients receive care that is both necessary and appropriate. This responsibility begins by ensuring that patients who are receiving hospice services are in need of hospice services. This is accomplished by either directly certifying (together with the attending physician) that the patients have life-limiting illnesses with a predicted

TABLE 4–6. Roles of the Hospice Medical Director
Ensure that patients receive quality medical care in consonance with principles of palliative care
Ensure patients who receive care are terminally ill
Development of treatment guidelines, protocols, and standards
Participate in interdisciplinary team care planning conferences
Provide expert advice to attending physicians, hospice physicians, and hospice staff
Assume administrative and management roles within the hospice
Supervise hospice team physicians
Pharmacy utilization management
Strategic and business planning
Survey and regulatory compliance
Assist in education and training of hospice staff
Engage in community professional education and liaison activities
Develop medical education and palliative care research programs

certifying or recertifying physician, or of ensuring that the hospice physicians who are certifying and recertifying patients are composing notes that accurately support the patient's prognosis and hospice eligibility.

Once the patient is admitted to the hospice program, the hospice medical director must make certain that care being rendered to patients meets hospice and palliative care standards. This is accomplished in a variety of ways, including the development of treatment guidelines, protocols, and standards, and participation in hospice care planning meetings. The establishment of measureable outcomes and participation in hospice quality improvement functions and audits is a vehicle by which the medical director can monitor how well treatment guidelines, protocols, and standards, as well as other aspects of the quality of the patient care are being provided. This importance of measureable outcomes has recently been highlighted by the establishment in the new Hospice Conditions of Participation of the "Quality Assessment and Performance Improvement" (QAPI) program, which requires hospices to develop and track measures that are indicative of quality palliative care outcomes, to develop quality improvement projects based on these measures, and have these projects result in demonstrable improvement in those outcomes. Medical directors must play a key role in the QAPI process in their hospices in order for this to be a success.

Ensuring that patients receive treatment consistent with palliative care principles also entails frequent interaction with attending physicians, especially when there is uncertainty surrounding a patient's diagnosis or prognosis or when there is a question regarding the optimal care to be rendered. In these circumstances, the hospice medical director can function as an expert consultant, providing the patient's attending physician with advice regarding, for example, optimal approaches to relieve a patient's pain, or whether the patient is eligible for hospice services. Because of lack of understanding by many physicians regarding the principles of hospice and

survival of 6 months or less, or, if the patient is certified by another hospice physician, providing oversight to make certain that the hospice physician is exercising proper judgment. (See Chapter 1 for a discussion of guidelines that help determine patient prognosis.) If a patient's prognosis requires re-evaluation, it is the hospice medical director's responsibility to ensure that the hospice physician assesses the patient properly. (See Chapter 2 for further discussion of the Medicare Hospice Benefit.) In addition, CMS has recently added the requirement that a narrative note supporting a patient's hospice eligibility be written or dictated by the physician who certified or recertified the patient as terminally ill. The medical director, therefore, will have the additional responsibility of composing the note if s/he is the palliative care, disagreements between attending physicians and hospice medical directors sometimes occur. Although this should be expected in the normal course of patient care, the relationship between the hospice medical director and attending physician should be viewed as cooperative, with the best interests of the patient always being paramount.

In addition to serving as a palliative care expert for attending physicians, hospice medical directors may function in a similar capacity for hospice team physicians and other hospice staff. Being available to provide expertise to hospice nurses and physicians can go a long way to making sure patients receive optimum care in a timely and efficient manner.

Assume Administrative and Management Roles Within the Hospice

The hospice medical director should be the medical leader of the hospice program. Working together with other clinical and administrative leaders, the medical director should play a major role in all facets of the operation of the hospice program.

Supervision of hospice team physicians is an important medical director function. The hospice medical director provides medical leadership to hospice physicians, assisting them in appropriately participating in the ID team environment. Hospice medical directors ensure that the other hospice physicians are, for example, actively involved in the team care planning conferences. They encourage the hospice physician to follow hospice treatment guidelines and protocols, making certain that appropriate palliative care interventions are being provided to patients and families. They review hospice physicians' prognosis certification and recertification decisions and the accompanying required documentation to ensure that patients receiving hospice services are, and remain eligible for, the hospice benefit.

As palliative care has become more complex, and as resources have become less available, the appropriate use of pharmaceutical products has become a major challenge for many hospices. By understanding the efficacy of various interventions available for patients near the end of life, the medical director can, by the development of formularies and ongoing utilization monitoring, assist hospice physicians and management in providing appropriate palliative interventions in a cost-effective manner.

As the medical leader of the hospice program, the hospice medical director should be actively involved in all aspects of the hospice's strategic and business planning efforts. This includes setting goals and objectives for all aspects of the hospice operation, specifically involving areas in which the medical director is directly involved, such as quality improvement and pharmacy utilization.

Another important task for the medical director is participation in survey and regulatory compliance activities. Understanding the hospice regulations and conditions of participation will allow the medical director to respond to surveyor concerns about aspects of the care provided to patients and families. Increasing regulatory scrutiny regarding patient eligibility for hospice services has led CMS fiscal intermediaries to develop "Local Coverage Determinations" (LCDs) (formally called "Local Medical Review Policies," LMRPs) that better define patient eligibility criteria for hospice services. When reimbursement of hospice services to a patient is retrospectively denied, it is the medical director, with first-hand knowledge of the patient's clinical course, who will be in the best position to successfully argue with the fiscal intermediary as to why the patient was, in fact, eligible for hospice services.

Assist in Education and Training of Hospice Staff

The medical director needs to be actively involved in educating and training hospice staff members, including physicians, nurses, and other staff members as well. Palliative care treatment guidelines, pharmacy utilization management issues, and new developments in palliative care are among the key topics that the medical director must continually bring to the attention of interested staff to maintain high standards of patient care.

Engage in Community Professional Education and Liaison Activities

Education of hospice staff is not enough. The hospice medical director should be viewed as an end-of-life care expert in the community, providing education to health care providers throughout the hospice program's service area. Medical conferences and grand rounds programs are an effective approach to reaching physician colleagues, as are one-on-one or small group meetings. In-service presentations at hospitals and long-term care facilities are other educational activities in which the hospice medical director may participate.

Develop Medical Education and Palliative Care Research Programs

As palliative medicine evolves as a specialty, medical education and research will become increasingly important. Hospices are an excellent resource to assist medical schools and residency programs, as they have a ready source of patients for students or residents, and palliative care experts for trainees to learn from. Leading the effort for the hospice program should be the medical director, working directly with his or her academic colleagues to ensure that the training experience is a meaningful one.

Regarding research, the hospice program provides the highest concentration of patients to enroll in trials to study the effectiveness of end-of-life interventions. Observational and retrospective analysis and reporting of effective palliative care protocols are also valuable in helping improve care for patients near the end of life.

HOSPICE TEAM PHYSICIAN

The hospice physician is considered a core member of the ID team, alongside the nurse, social worker, and chaplain. In smaller hospices, the hospice medical director may also fill this role, while in larger hospices, multiple hospice physicians in addition to the medical director are usu-

TABLE 4–7. Roles of the Hospice Team Physician
Patient certification and recertification of terminal prognosis
Patient home visits and inpatient visits
Medical interventions to treat patient symptoms
Resource as expert in palliative care to other members of interdisciplinary team
Liaison with attending physicians on the current status of their patients
Staff education and support at interdisciplinary team meetings

ally required. The physician fulfills many important roles that are necessary for the proper care of the patient, outlined in Table 4–7 and discussed below. (The hospice physician may at times, also serve as a patient's attending physician.)

As the physician from the hospice primarily responsible for direct patient care, the hospice physician's responsibilities begin at the time of patient admission, by certifying, together with the patient's attending physician, that the patient has a prognosis of 6 months or less, and, based on the new CMS requirement already mentioned, documenting in a short narrative the medical information that supports the certification. (See Chapter 1 for a discussion of guidelines that help determine patient prognosis.) The goal of certification, of course, is to make certain that patients receive hospice services at an appropriate time in their illness and life.

Once on the hospice program, the Medicare Hospice Benefit periodically requires that the patient's prognosis be re-evaluated. (See Chapter 2 for further discussion of the Medicare Hospice Benefit.) These reviews, commonly termed "recertification," are meant to assess whether, due to changes in a patient's clinical condition, the patient continues to have a prognosis of 6 months or less and remain eligible for hospice services. In addition to a review of the patient's clinical course, the process includes input from other members of the ID team, a discussion with the patient's attending physician, and, on occasion, one or more diagnostic studies that may be helpful in, for example, documenting progression of a malignancy that may otherwise not be apparent on clinical examination. If the patient still has a prognosis of 6 months or less, the physician "recertifies" the patient and documents the clinical information used to make that decision in a narrative note. If a patient's medical condition has improved and the patient no longer meets the hospice eligibility criteria, the hospice physician will not recertify the patient as terminally ill. The hospice physician will work with the ID team, including the patient, family, and attending physician, to provide appropriate planning prior to discharging the patient from the hospice and back to the care of the attending physician.

While hospice visits at home are typically from nurses, home health aides, social workers, or chaplains, physician visits to patients in their homes can also be invaluable. These visits provide patients, who often are too ill to leave the house and visit their attending physicians in the office, with a sense of belonging and connection and also assure them that a physician genuinely cares about them. By visiting the patient, the hospice physician can medically assess the patient and provide direct information to assist the team in planning care. The team physician, after making a home visit, can communicate with the attending physician to make palliative care recommendations, thereby providing patients with better symptom control. In addition, patients are comforted in the knowledge that their attending physicians have up-to-date and professionally derived information about their current status.

In addition to the direct benefits to the patient provided by the physician visit, once the physician has seen the patient, ongoing care planning is more efficient, since the physician now has a live reference to associate with the verbal information shared by other team members. Follow-up physician visits are often indicated if patients develop acute problems or as deterioration and death approach. When continuous home care

(see Chapter 2 for discussion) is indicated, a periodic physician visit can provide invaluable assistance in helping control patient symptoms.

For patients that are receiving inpatient hospice care, a physician visit should occur on a daily basis. Just as in the traditional acute care hospital setting, these patients are typically very ill, too ill to remain at home. The need for daily care is mandated by the need to assure better control of the clinical symptoms. When the patient's attending physician elects to supervise patient care in the inpatient setting, the hospice physician may fill the role of an expert consultant, providing palliative care expertise if necessary. However, if the attending physician does not or cannot follow the patient, the hospice physician will provide the care.

The hospice physician serves as a palliative care expert, assisting the attending physician when the patient is at home as well as when the patient is on an inpatient hospice unit. While attending physicians are encouraged to remain actively involved in the care of their patients, when this is not feasible or not desired, or when the attending physician is not available, the hospice team physician becomes primarily responsible for medical decision making. Hospice team physician are well equipped to fill this role, as they are very knowledgeable about all the patients on their team from discussions held at the team care planning conferences and, in many cases, from having visited the patients at home. When hospice team physicians directly intervene, it is important that they communicate with the attending physicians to ensure continuity of care. Hospice physicians should also communicate with attending physicians whenever patients have changes in status or when a change in patient prognosis prompts the consideration of patient discharge from the hospice program.

The hospice physician, much like the hospice medical director, functions as an educator as well. During the ID team conference, ample opportunities for the hospice physician to teach staff present themselves. As an educational forum, team conference is particularly valuable, as it allows the physician to associate specific subjects with real examples—that is, the patients and families being cared for by the team.

PALLIATIVE MEDICINE CONSULTANT

With the recognition that palliative medicine, whether practiced in the hospice setting or independent of hospice, provides high-quality, cost-effective care, and with the establishment of Hospice and Palliative Medicine as a medical subspecialty by the American Board of Medical Specialists, physicians, in partnership with a hospital, LTCF, or hospice, or sometime independently, are now providing consultative services in palliative medicine to patients who require them. The major indications for palliative medicine consults are listed in Table 4–8.

When patients experience difficulty to control pain, dyspnea, or other distressing physical symptoms, primary physicians or even specialists who require expert assistance can call the palliative medicine expert in consultation. Such consults should not be limited to patients who have life-limiting illnesses, but could be offered to patients having a chronic disease with either a short- or long-term prognosis or to those experiencing a curable acute medical problem. Palliative medicine consultants can also assist primary physicians in evaluating patient prognosis and determining whether patients might be eligible for the Medicare Hospice Benefit.

Conversations that revolve around establishing goals of care when patients have chronic or life-limiting illnesses, much as those that involve the breaking of bad news (discussed in Chapter 3), are extremely difficult and many primary physicians are uncomfortable having these discussions with patients and families. In such circumstances, rather than try and accomplish this daunting task alone, the primary physician can seek the assistance of the palliative medicine consultant. Consults of this nature often lead to the establishment of goals of care that patients, families, and physicians can agree upon, and may result in the creation of advance medical directives, such as living wills and durable health care powers of attorney (see Chapter 22). In a similar vein, when patients or health care surrogates are confronted with the challenging decisions to accept or decline hospice services or to continue or withdraw life sustaining interventions such as mechanical ventilators and feeding tubes, the palliative medicine consultant can often be the guiding force that helps the patients or surrogates work through the process. Finally, as palliative medicine consultants have expertise in the arenas of psychosocial and spiritual care, and often bring along with them an ID team of experts similar to hospice (see discussion below), these consults can also help meet the psychosocial and spiritual needs of patients and families.

TABLE 4–8. Indications for Palliative Medicine Consultations

- Management of pain or other distressing symptoms
- Assessment of prognosis and hospice eligibility
- Goals of care discussions
- Consideration of utilization or withdrawal of life-sustaining interventions
- Patient and family support (with other members of the ID team)

STRUCTURE OF THE ID TEAM

The overwhelming majority of physicians practicing today were trained in some variation of the teaching hospital model of care, with its emphasis on vertical integration of the staff, as illustrated in Figure 4–1.

At the top of the ladder was the physician, the captain of the ship, in charge of managing

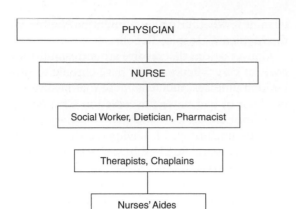

Figure 4–1. Traditional hierarchical structure of the health care team.

the patient care. Just below the physician, but very clearly subordinate, were the nurses, who were traditionally viewed as providing care ordered by the physician, usually without independent thought, question, or challenge. Below the nurses in this health care hierarchy were various ancillary personnel, including social workers, dieticians, physical and occupational therapists, pharmacists, and others whose job it was to ensure that patient care was provided smoothly and efficiently. Supporting this structure were those considered less skilled, such as nurses aides, porters, and dietary workers.

This hierarchical structure has evolved to some degree in traditional hospital and medical practices, but physician continues to be the primary driver of health care for patients and families. However, in the hospice model of care, this structure has been vastly altered. As illustrated in Figure 4–2, the hierarchical structure with the physician at the top has been replaced by the ID team, which has the patient and family as the unit of care at its center. All care providers, from the physician to the nurse to the home health aide, are all on an equal level, with the goal being for each

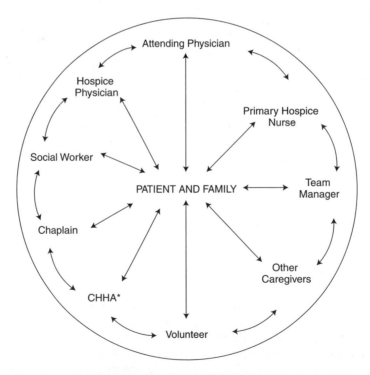

Figure 4–2. Structure of hospice interdisciplinary team.
*CHHA, certified home health aide.

care provider to use their special skills and expertise to provide expert end-of-life care as needed and directed by the patient and family.

As one reflects on the model of "suffering" or "total pain" that has been well accepted as a major dynamic in care at the end of life, the purpose of the ID team becomes clear. It is only by combining the expertise of professionals from multiple disciplines, working together collegially, and focusing on meeting the patient needs as determined by the patient and family that the outcomes of end-of-life care can be successful. To paraphrase Orwell, "All are equal, but *none are more equal* than others."

ROLES OF THE MEMBERS OF THE ID TEAM

As a member of the ID team, it is important for physicians to not only understand their role, but to understand the role of the other members of the team as well. What follows, therefore, is an overview of the role of each individual that participates in providing end-of-life care to patients as members of the ID team.

NURSE

Nurses play two distinct roles in the care of the hospice patient: management and patient care. Any group of individual acting in concert to perform a task need a leader to make certain that the job is done correctly and efficiently. The ID team is no exception. While many of the health care professionals who participate on the ID team would be capable of leading the team, that task has traditionally fallen to a registered nurse (RN), usually called the team manager or patient care coordinator. These nurse managers have multiple tasks not directly related to hands-on patient care, but related to ensuring that the professionals on the team do their jobs in an efficient and coordinated fashion.

Among the tasks of the team manager are to assign patients to the primary care nurses and make sure that all the nurses on the team have a reasonable number of patients to care for. The team manager makes certain that scheduling of visits by all disciplines is appropriate to meet patient needs and they facilitate the team care planning conferences, often referred to simply as team meetings, during which time the care plans of patients are reviewed and updated. The team manager functions as the primary supervisor of all ID team members (including the physician), resolving conflicts, ensuring that all team members perform their tasks properly and efficiently, and being responsible for the allocation of resources.

Nurses also play a major role in the hands-on care of patients and families. In most hospice programs, each patient is assigned an RN as a primary nurse, who is responsible for case management and primary patient care. At the time of hospice admission, it is the primary nurse that assesses the patient to develop, together with other ID team members, individualized care plans for patients. This nurse visits the patient on a regular basis (generally, 1–3 times per week based on patient need) to evaluate the effectiveness of the plan of care and to coordinate any changes or additions if indicated. If changes in the care plan require a physician's order, it is the primary nurse that is responsible to contact either the attending physician or hospice physician, explain what is occurring, and, often, suggest possible palliative interventions to the physician. The nurse is the primary educational resource for the patient and family, reviewing all medications, teaching the patient and family how to properly administer the medications, and monitoring to ensure appropriate medication use. The nurse will also instruct families on other aspects of care, such as wounds and decubiti care, and on how to avoid these and other problems if the patient is at further risk. The great emphasis on teaching caregivers is due to the fact that hospice programs are not meant to provide 24-hour hands-on care, but to assist the family caregivers in providing much of the basic custodial support that patients require near the end of life.

When providing hands-on care to patients, hospices often employ licensed practical nurses (LPN) or licensed vocational nurses (LVN) in addition to RNs. As the scope of practice of LPNs and LVNs are limited (i.e., medications and treatments can only be administered under the guidance and supervision of a RN), they cannot function as a substitute for the RN primary nurse. Rather, they serve to supplement the care rendered by the primary nurse, ensuring that patients receive the level of skilled nursing care that they require to manage the complex challenges they face as life nears its end.

RN primary nurses also function as case managers, overseeing patient care, interacting with family, aides, physicians, and other members of the ID team to provide optimal care. They need to know their patients in-depth, have the skills to recognize how specific patient illnesses affect the course of care, possess knowledge of the physical, psychosocial, and spiritual realities at the end of life, and be proactive in making certain that needs and potential complications of the patients under their care are anticipated and treated.

SOCIAL WORKER

The role of the social worker is varied and diverse, as there are few aspects of the patients' care in which a social worker does not become involved. Every patient that is admitted to a hospice or non-hospice palliative care program needs a psychosocial evaluation to assess the nonphysical needs of the patient and family, and this evaluation is typically performed by a social worker. (See Chapter 16 for a discussion on the psychosocial assessment.) Social workers may provide patients and families with assistance accessing community services such as Meals-on Wheels, or facilitating application for Medicaid, if the patient is eligible, to obtain LTC facility room and board coverage. Social workers may work more directly with patients and families as well to provide counseling

and support throughout the course of the terminal illness, help patients and families better cope with their current situation, and explain to patients and families what options are open to them. Social workers provide psychological support as patients' lives are drawing to a close, and often support families by attending a patient's deaths. Following a patient's death, the social worker assists the chaplain in providing grief and bereavement support to families of patients who have passed on. (See Chapter 17 for a discussion of bereavement services.)

Finally, social workers provide counseling and support to the other members of the ID team as well as to other caregivers, such as the staff of LTC facilities who work with the hospice program.

CHAPLAIN

Pastoral care has always been viewed as a core hospice service. Even though society currently has a secular orientation and many patients are not actively practicing any religion, imminent death often leads even nonreligious people to search for meaning or for a greater involvement in spiritual or religious matters. While it would be ideal to receive pastoral care from one's own minister, rabbi, or priest, the majority of Americans are unaffiliated with formal religious institutions and, therefore, are not able to directly access this vital function.

Fortunately, hospices are able to offer pastoral care, and do so by employing clergy of various religious affiliations. This allows for the multiple variations in religious practice in society to be represented, so that most specific patient requests can be met. The focus of pastoral end-of-life care is spiritual and not formally religious; hence, the individuals are seen as "generic" chaplains, rather than as members of a particular religious group, sect, or order. For chaplains working for a hospice, this means having the flexibility to serve the spiritual needs of patients that may not be of their own religious faith in a way that is nonjudgmental and without attempting to proselytize. At times, therefore, a priest may be asked to counsel Jewish patients, while a rabbi may serve Methodist patients, and so on. In recognition of patient autonomy, on the other hand, if a patient requests a chaplain of a particular faith, the hospice has the obligation to attempt to fulfill the request and not try to force the "generic" chaplain on the patient.

Chaplains initiate their work by performing a "spiritual assessment" to learn about the specific spiritual outlook and needs of each patient and family. (See Chapter 16 for a discussion on the spiritual assessment.) As there is often overlap between the role of the chaplain and the psychosocial counseling aspects of the social worker, chaplains often assist the social worker by providing additional support in the psychosocial realm, which may include anything from the performance of the psychosocial assessment to the provision of psychosocial counseling. The chaplain generally has the responsibility to coordinate grief and bereavement programs that are provided by the hospice, including one-on-one counseling, support groups, and memorial services. (See Chapter 17 for a discussion of Bereavement services.)

CERTIFIED HOME HEALTH AIDE

Often perceived as "just" a maid or cleaning lady, the certified home health aide (CHHA) performs a core function on the ID team and has been described as a "Saint from God." Unlike nurses' aides who work in hospitals and LTC facilities and must function under the direct supervision of an RN, hospice CHHAs possess a higher level of skill, receive ongoing training, and, hence, although supervised and given their specific assignments by the primary nurse, are able to function in a patient's home independent of the RN's presence.

Patients who are near the end of life often present complicated and challenging personal hygiene needs that may overwhelm families. It takes the expertise of a trained CHHA to safely see patients into a shower, bathe them in bed if they cannot walk, clean them when they have been incontinent, or give them gentle touch when others may be afraid of physical contact. In view of the intimate relationship between the patient and the CHHA, strong bonds often form. The CHHA, therefore, may be the member of the ID team who best knows what the patient truly needs and may provide the most valuable input as the ID team plans care for the patient. It is not uncommon for the family to offer their greatest thanks to the CHHA after the patient's death, and conversely, the CHHAs may experience a great deal of grief after the death of a patient in their charge for a long time.

VOLUNTEERS

Volunteers, in many respects, were the backbone of the early hospice movement. Before the creation of the Medicare Hospice Benefit, most hospice care was provided by volunteers. In keeping with that spirit, the Medicare Hospice Benefit requires that volunteers provide services to hospice programs equivalent in hours to 5% of all patient care hours. Volunteer services are appreciated by patients and families, the hospice programs they serve, and by the volunteers themselves.

By visiting with patients, volunteers can provide patients with additional human contact, especially when the patients are home-bound. They allow the patients to be distracted from the realities of their illness and to feel "normal" again. Volunteers can also provide caregivers needed respite time. As most patients cannot be left alone, volunteers can stay with a patient while the caregiver can take of personal needs, family needs, or just take a needed break to refresh and recharge. For patients who are able to get out of the house, volunteers can participate by taking patients out for rides to the mall, and for other "nonmedical" experiences.

Volunteers may also work administratively in the hospice program office. Activities from filing of records and reports, to stuffing envelopes, to making phone calls can help lighten the clerical burden of hospice personnel and allow them to focus on more direct patient care activities. Whether hospice volunteers work directly with patients or in an administrative capacity, they are usually motivated individuals, often with a prior personal hospice experience, who derive personal satisfaction from sharing of themselves with others.

A special volunteer for patients near the end of life is the "pet therapist." This is a domesticated animal, most often a dog, that has been carefully evaluated and trained to function in a healthcare environment, such as a LTC facility or a hospice in-patient unit. The animals have to be placid, not afraid of strangers, nor startle with the sudden noises that come from wheelchairs, trays, and other similar devices. It has been shown that animals bring a sense of calm to patients and caregivers and can often serve to defuse crisis situations. The gentle stroking of an animal's fur is a tactile experience that often brings back pleasant childhood memories. The right animal can be a very useful member of the team.

ANCILLARY MEMBERS OF THE ID TEAM

Pharmacist

The pharmacy consultant provides periodic review of the medications that patients on the hospice program are receiving. Often times, patients are receiving multiple medications for their various symptoms, some of which will interact with one another. The pharmacist can advise clinicians on potential drug–drug interactions, suggest alternative therapeutic approaches to difficult symptom management problems, and educate the staff on the latest medications and therapies available for use.

Nurse Practitioner

As the role of nurse practitioners (NPs) has increased throughout the health care delivery system, they have also increased their involvement in hospice and palliative care. As part of the Medicare Prescription Drug Improvement and Mod-

ernization Act of 2003, the definition of "attending physician" under the Medicare Hospice Benefit was modified to include NPs, meaning that NPs who maintained their own practice could now function and bill as an attending physician. NPs, however, were prohibited from certifying the patient's terminal prognosis at the time of hospice admission and from establishing the plan of care, both of which remain under the province of physicians only. NPs serving as specialty consultants in hospitals and LTCFs in areas such as wound care often provide consultations to hospice and palliative care patients who have problems in their specific areas of expertise. Most recently, NPs have been working as palliative care consultants alongside their physician counterparts in hospitals, LTCFs, and in patients' homes. While some hospices employ NPs, it must be noted that hospices may not bill for NP services that can be performed by an RN, nor can they bill for NP services that are being provided under the supervision of the hospice medical director or physician in the traditional NP role as a physician extender.

Others

Dieticians can be helpful in advising patients and families on the various alternatives that might assist in optimizing caloric intake for patients. Physical therapists and occupational therapists may assist hospice staff in figuring out ways of maximizing patient function, while wound specialists may provide alternative approaches to difficult-to-heal wounds. Alternative therapies such as massage therapy, therapeutic touch, and aromatherapy are being used with increasing frequency, and hospices will often engage the assistance of practitioners in these areas as well.

CONCLUSION

As was stated at the outset, the role of the physician as a member of an end-of-life care ID team is not the traditional one that physicians are accustomed to. Physicians must view themselves as a team player, which requires a greater level of cooperation and interaction with other health care professionals than is seen in other aspects of the physician's professional life. It requires a change of vision, from that of being "right," to accepting that death will occur and that what is "correct" is that which optimizes the quality of the patient's life rather than prolonging life. It requires regular discussions with the other professional members of the ID team, with physicians caring for patients, and with physicians in management roles.

Physicians have to be prepared to have their actions questioned and be able to justify how what they propose for the patient is not only accepted medical practice, but is necessary and beneficial. At times, they may have to deal with being told "No, this is not best for the patient nor what the patient wants. Therefore, it will not happen."

The relationship between the various physicians and other members of the ID team need not be confrontational. The field of hospice and palliative medicine is still relatively new and there is still a divergence between what the average physician in practice understands regarding the care of the dying and what the palliative medicine physicians or other health care professionals in the field know. Physicians who are open to cooperation and primarily concerned about the welfare of the patients under their care will see working with hospice and palliative care providers as a way of improving their knowledge and skill in caring for terminally ill patients, while providing their patients with optimal care at the end of life.

BIBLIOGRAPHY

Brumley RD, Enguidanos S, Cherin DA: Effectiveness of home-based palliative care programs for end-of-life. *J Pall Med* 6:715-724, 2003.

Centers for Medicare and Medicaid Services (CMS), HHS: *[CMS–3844–F], RIN 0938–AH27, Medicare and Medicaid Programs: Hospice Conditions of Participation, Final Rule*. Federal Register, Vol. 73, No. 109, Thursday, June 5, 2008, Rules and Regulations.

Centers for Medicare and Medicaid Services (CMS), HHS: Change to the Physician Certification and Recertification Process, §418.22. In: *[CMS-1420-F], RIN 0938-AP45 Medicare Program; Hospice Wage Index for Fiscal Year 2010, Final Rule*. FR Doc. 2009-18553 Filed 07/30/2009 at 4:15 pm; Publication Date: 08/06/2009, pp. 82-93.

Certified home health aide job description, policy 9:16. In: *Vitas Policy Manual*. Miami, Vitas Healthcare, 2006.

Chaplain job description, policy 9:18. In: *Vitas Policy Manual*. Miami, Vitas Healthcare, 2004.

Cummings I: The interdisciplinary team. In: Doyle D, Hanks GWC, MacDonald N, eds. *Oxford Textbook of Palliative Medicine*, 2nd ed. Oxford, Oxford University Press, 1998, pp. 19-30.

Gade G, Venohr I, Conner D, et al: Impact of an inpatient palliative care team: A randomized control trial. *J Pall Med* 11:180-190, 2008.

Home care team physician job description, policy 9:13. In: *Vitas Policy Manual*. Miami, Vitas Healthcare, 2004.

Hoy T: Hospice chaplaincy in the caregiving team. In: Corr CA, Coor DM, eds. *Hospice Care, Principles and Practice*. New York, Springer, 1983, p. 177.

Kinzbrunner BM: *Medical director model: Large corporate hospice*. Glenview, American Academy of Hospice and Palliative Medicine, 2004.

Kinzbrunner BM: The role of the physician in hospice. *Hosp J* 12(2):49, 1997.

Kurtz ME: The dual role dilemma. In: Curry W, ed. *New Leadership in Health Care Management: The Physician Executive*. Tampa, Lithocolor, 1988, p. 66.

Medical Director job description, policy 9:04. In: *Vitas Policy Manual*. Miami, Vitas Healthcare, 2004.

Medicare hospice regulations. In: *42 Code of Federal Regulations*, Part 418, 1993.

Miller SC, Teno JM, Mor V: Hospice and palliative care in nursing homes. *Clin Geriatr Med* 20:717-754, 2004.

National Hospice and Palliative Care Organization: Billing for nurse practitioner services. http://www.nhpco.org/files/public/billing_for_np_services.pdf. Accessed August 18, 2009.

Penrod JD, Deb P, Luhrs C, et al: Cost and utilization outcomes of patients receiving hospital-based palliative care consultation. *J Pall Med* 9:855-860, 2006.

Portenoy RK: Practical aspects of pain control in the patient with cancer. *CA Cancer J Clin* 38:327-352, 1988.

Social worker job description, policy 9:19A. In: *Vitas Policy Manual*. Miami, Vitas Healthcare, 2005.

Storey P: What is the role of the hospice physician? *Am J Hosp Palliat Care* 10(6):2, 1993.

Taylor DH, Ostermann J, van Houtven CH, et al: What length of hospice use maximizes reduction in medical expenditures near death in the US Medicare program? *Soc Sci Med* 65:1466-1478, 2007.

Team manager job description, policy 9:10. In: *Vitas Policy Manual*, Miami, Vitas Healthcare, 2008.

Vitas consultant pharmacist job description, policy 9:29. In: *Vitas Policy Manual*, Miami, Vitas Healthcare, 2004.

Vitas nurse, LPN/LVN job description, policy 9:14. In: *Vitas Policy Manual*, Miami, Vitas Healthcare, 2007.

Vitas nurse, RN job description, policy 9:14. In: *Vitas Policy Manual*, Miami, Vitas Healthcare, 2006.

Weissman DE, Meier DE, Spragens LH: Center to advance palliative care, palliative care consultation service metrics: Consensus recommendations. *J Pallit Med* 11:1294-1298, 2008.

SELF-ASSESSMENT QUESTIONS

1. Which of the following is the physician who is identified by the patient as having the most significant role in the determination of the patient's medical care?

   A. Attending physician
   B. Long-term care medical director
   C. Hospice team physician
   D. Managed care medical director
   E. Palliative medicine consultant

2. Which of the following activities is NOT part of the roles and responsibilities of the attending physician when caring for a patient on a hospice program?

   A. A member of the hospice interdisciplinary team
   B. Discusses need for end-of-life care with patient and family
   C. Certifies patient prognosis at the time of hospice admission
   D. Recertifies patient prognosis after the patient has been in hospice 90 days
   E. Visits are reimbursable under Medicare Part B

3. Which of the following hospice-related activities of a long-term care facility medial director would NOT be done in collaboration with the hospice medical director?

   A. Coordination of hospice patient care planning
   B. Education of LTCF and hospice staffs
   C. Development of hospice treatment guidelines for the facility
   D. Conflict resolution between the hospice and the facility
   E. Initial identification of patients who may need end-of-life care

4. All of the following are part of the roles and responsibilities of the hospice medical director EXCEPT

   A. Supervise hospice team physicians
   B. Document in a narrative why all hospice admissions are eligible for services
   C. Provide expert consultation to attending physicians, other hospice physicians, and hospice staff
   D. Participate in the strategic and business planning of the hospice
   E. Participate in issues related to regulatory compliance and surveys

5. All of the following are part of the roles and responsibilities of the hospice team physician EXCEPT

   A. Patient certification and recertification of terminal prognosis
   B. Assuming the overall medical care of all hospice patients on the team
   C. Participation in the interdisciplinary team meeting
   D. Patient home visits
   E. Staff education and support

6. Which of the individuals listed below is considered to be at the center of the hospice interdisciplinary team?

   A. RN team manager
   B. Primary nurse
   C. Attending physician
   D. Patient and family
   E. Hospice medical director

7. All of the following regarding nurses working for a hospice program are true EXCEPT

   A. LVNs may serve as primary nurses
   B. RNs may serve as team managers or primary nurses
   C. Team managers are the primary supervisor of all members of the ID team
   D. Primary nurses also function as case managers
   E. LVNs may provide primary patient care at the bedside

8. All of the following statements regarding the roles and responsibilities of social workers and chaplains on the hospice ID team are true EXCEPT

    A. Social workers may assist patients in accessing community services such as meals on wheels.

    B. Chaplains may assist the social worker by providing psychosocial counseling in some situations.

    C. Chaplains should help all patients ask God for forgiveness prior to the end of life.

    D. Social workers assist chaplains in providing bereavement support to family members.

    E. Social workers and chaplains provide staff support.

9. All of the following statements regarding CHHAs on the hospice ID team are true EXCEPT

    A. CHHAs may work in a patient's home independent of the supervising RN's presence.

    B. CHHAs are trained to manage the complicated personal hygiene needs of dying patients.

    C. Of all ID team members, families often offer their greatest thanks to CHHAs

    D. CHHAs often experience significant grief after the death of a patient in their charge for a long time.

    E. As CHHAs deliver personal care, their input at team meeting is not as valuable as the primary nurse.

10. All of the following statements regarding the interactions of nurse practitioners in hospice and palliative care are true EXCEPT

    A. Nurse practitioners may serve as palliative care consultants.

    B. Nurse practitioners serving as attending physicians may certify that a patient is terminally ill under the Medicare Hospice Benefit.

    C. Hospices may not bill for nurse practitioner visits when they serve as physician extenders under the supervision of the hospice medical director.

    D. Nurse practitioners can provide wound care consultations for hospice and palliative care patients.

    E. Hospice may not bill for nurse practitioner services that can be performed by an RN.

CHAPTER

5

Measuring Outcomes and Quality of Life

Melanie P. Merriman

INTRODUCTION

Quality in healthcare is determined both by what is done (or not done) by caregivers and by the results or outcomes of interventions for patients and families. According to the Institute of Medicine, healthcare quality can be defined as "the degree to which healthcare services for individuals and populations increase the likelihood of desired health outcomes and are consistent with current professional knowledge" (IOM, 2001, *Crossing the Quality Chasm*).

If outcomes focus on what happened for the patient and family, then what outcomes are important in end-of-life care? Terminally ill patients, by definition, cannot be "cured," but even a patient with no expectation or desire for prolonged survival can be "healed" in several ways. These patients can experience symptom relief, enhanced quality of life, shared decision-making, emotional and spiritual support, and continuity of care; their families can experience relief of anxiety and improved coping skills, among other outcomes.

This chapter discusses outcome measurement, including assessment of quality of life, for end-of-life care. Hospices and palliative care programs (both hospital-based and outpatient) are the primary settings of care for terminally ill patients and their families. These providers are, therefore, the most likely to use outcome measures for end-of-life care. However, individual healthcare practitioners who care for patients through the end of life should also consider how desired outcomes change when a patient is terminally ill, and clinicians may want to measure outcomes in order to improve the quality of care for these patients. In addition, individual practitioners who refer to hospice or other palliative care providers need a good understanding of desired outcomes and their measurement in order to judge the quality of care offered by different agencies.

The collection of quality measurement data serves many synergistic purposes. For individual patients and clinicians, outcome measurement provides information concerning effectiveness and quality of care. Did the patient benefit from the treatment provided? Is more or different treatment advisable? In a research context, outcomes data contribute to the evidence base for best practice by revealing which treatments are the most efficacious, safe, and cost-efficient. From the payor and consumer viewpoints, quality data also can be used for accountability. When providers document outcomes, consumers can compare providers on the basis of both quality and price, and providers become accountable for offering efficient and effective care.

OUTCOMES MEASUREMENT CHALLENGES AND OPPORTUNITIES

WHAT TO MEASURE

While end-of-life care is subject to the same internal (quality improvement, evidence-base development) and external (accountability) forces that drive quality assessment in other healthcare settings, measurement of outcomes near the end of life offers some unique challenges. Typically, healthcare outcomes are measured in the context of an episode of illness or an episode of treatment from which the patient will emerge changed by the healthcare encounter. Often, health status (defined and measured in a variety of ways) is evaluated prior to the healthcare encounter or encounters, during treatment (such as chemotherapy), and then after an episode is over (following hospital discharge or the completion of outpatient or rehabilitative care). But patients being cared for the near the end of life do not emerge from this episode of care and, during the episode, their physical and functional status will decline inexorably. Hence, "typical" measures rarely provide meaningful data for end-of-life care.

DETERMINING THE POPULATION FOR MEASUREMENT

A significant challenge in measuring the outcomes of end-of-life care is defining the population of the patients to whom the measures should be applied. Although certain diagnoses are clearly life limiting, the prospective identification of those who are in the last months of life can be difficult. Joan Teno, MD, and colleagues have referred to this as the denominator problem. While much has been written about the complexities involved in determining prognosis, particularly for noncancer patients, the fact is that hospices have a good record of admitting patients with 6 months or less to live, suggesting that accurate criteria exist to identify this population. Attempts to formalize the criteria in clinical guidelines have led to specifications that are too exclusive and leave behind many patients who are in the last months of life, largely because relevant criteria such as the psychosocial, emotional, and spiritual contexts of care are not included.

Joanne Lynn, MD, of the Center to Improve Care of the Dying, has suggested that healthcare providers, particularly physicians, think of end-of-life care as applicable to patients "who are sick enough that you would not be surprised if they died in the next several months to a year." Providers should consider measuring end-of-life care outcomes and quality of life for any patient that fits this description. At any point in time, the data can be analyzed retrospectively for patients who were in fact in the dying phase, without having to be sure exactly how close they were to dying prospectively.

For the purpose of measuring outcomes and quality of life, it seems wise to cast a wide net for prospective measurement, and then conduct data analysis and reporting on only that portion of those measured who actually died within a defined period (1, 3, 6, or 12 months) prior to the analysis date. Even though we are interested in measures that are crafted to evaluate end-of-life care, there would seem to be little downside in applying these measures to a slightly larger population, some of whom may not die, especially since many of the measures reflect excellence in outcomes even for patients who are not dying.

WHEN TO ASSESS OUTCOMES

Because patients cannot complete measures of end-of-life care following completion of care, data collection for some outcome measures must be conducted during the treatment phase. Fortunately, ongoing measurement has advantages that outweigh the burdens of continuous data collection. Elements appropriate for measurement during the course of care are those that are most meaningful when they are patient-reported. These include adverse events, pain and symptom relief, preferences and conformance to preferences, quality of life, and patient experience of care. These elements can and should be measured through a repetitive assessment process, and collection of this data also permits the analysis of intermediate outcomes that allow the provider to document and improve outcomes for individuals.

In the same way that regular measurement of vital signs provides an indicator of the patient's overall clinical condition and drives choice of interventions, measurement of symptom relief, preferences (goals), quality of life, and patient experience of care provides an indicator of the success of end-of-life care and guides adjustment in the care plan. Some providers are, in fact, implementing pain measurement as a fifth vital sign (Fig. 5–1) and tracking patient reported pain severity on a graph similar to that used for blood pressure. Data that is used daily to inform the care of individuals can be aggregated monthly or quarterly to determine overall success with end-of-life care. New Medicare regulations for hospices (see next section) require collection of data elements during routine assessment that can be used to measure outcomes for the individual patients and, when aggregated, for the specified patient groups.

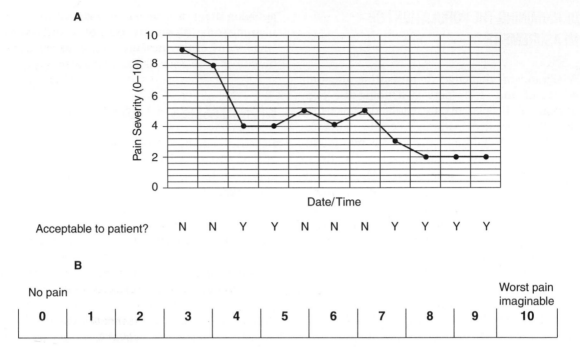

Figure 5–1. Pain as the fifth vital sign. **A**. An example of how pain might be recorded in the patient chart as a fifth vital sign. Like other vital signs, patient-reported pain severity is elicited at least daily and the date and time are recorded along with the pain severity on a specified scale. In addition, the patient may be asked whether the current pain severity is acceptable. This answer is recorded beneath the date and time using **Y** for yes and **N** for no. **B**. An example of one pain severity scale. This one uses a 0–10 scale; others use a 0–5 scale. Other scales are available from the Agency for Healthcare Policy and Research, the American Pain Society, and the medical literature.

The overall experience of end-of-life care is often assessed after the death using a questionnaire addressed to family members or close friends who have first-hand experience of the end-of-life care provided. Although in some ways, this represents "surrogate reporting" and has inherent flaws, family or close friends are often involved in end-of-life care as nonprofessional caregivers. Notably, hospice care philosophy defines the "patient and family" as the unit of care. Studies have shown that involved family members can be accurate reporters about the overall end-of-life care experience.

MEDICARE REQUIREMENTS AND OPPORTUNITIES FOR END-OF-LIFE CARE OUTCOME MEASUREMENT

In 2008, The Centers for Medicare and Medicaid Services (CMS) issued new conditions of participation for hospice providers that included key provisions for quality assessment and performance improvement. As of December 2, 2008, Medicare-certified hospice agencies are required to collect data elements during routine patient assessment and care planning that can be used to assess outcomes for individual patients. They are further required to aggregate those data elements and use the information to track and trend outcomes of care for the entire population served. Importantly, CMS did not identify required measures, instead, leaving it to each hospice to identify the measures most useful to them in their quest for optimum performance and outcomes. These requirements encourage ongoing development of outcome measures uniquely suited to assess end-of-life care; many of the measures being developed can be used in any care setting, not just in hospices.

CMS has also provided an opportunity for individual physicians to report on delivery of end-of-life care through the Physician Quality Reporting Initiative (PQRI). Professionals who successfully report on a designated set of quality measures for a specified percentage of Medicare patients served are eligible for an incentive payment of 1.5% of total allowable charges for covered services payable during the reporting period. ("Successful reporting" is determined by the number of measures on which a physician reports, and the percentage of patients who meet the measure criteria.) Among the quality measures is one aimed to increase discussions and decisions about advance care planning: *"Percentage of patients aged 65 years and older who have an advance care plan or surrogate decision maker documented in the medical record or documentation in the medical record that an advance care plan was discussed but the patient did not wish or was not able to name a surrogate decision maker or provide an advance care plan in the medical record." (2009 PQRI Measures List,* downloaded 12/6/08, http://www.cms.hhs.gov/PQRI/15_measurescodes.asp)

OUTCOME MEASUREMENT DOMAINS FOR END-OF-LIFE CARE

In the same way that time can be defined as that which is measured by the clock, quality end-of-life care will in part be defined by the ways that it is measured. Meaningful outcomes must be based on what patients and families value and on desired goals of care for patients with terminal illnesses. The challenge has been to define a group of measures that address the range of issues—physical, psychosocial, psychological/emotional, spiritual, and practical—faced by patients and families at the end of life, as well as the opportunities that are available to those who are living at end of life.

FRAMEWORKS FOR DEFINING AND MEASURING QUALITY OF CARE AT THE END OF LIFE

Following the publication in late 1995 of the SUPPORT Study, which revealed shortcomings in the outcomes of end-of-life care in major medical centers, various healthcare associations, national forums, researchers, and prayer groups began developing frameworks for quality in palliative and end-of-life care. In 1997, The American Society of Geriatrics drafted *Suggested Domains for Measuring Quality at the End of Life.* Also in 1997, The National Hospice and Palliative Care (NHPCO) published *A pathway for patients and families facing terminal disease* in which they defined three important "end-result outcomes" for terminally ill patients and their families: safe and comfortable dying, self-determined life closure, and effective grieving.

In 2004, the National Consensus Project for Quality Palliative Care (NCP) (www.nationalconsensusproject.com) published *Clinical Practice Guidelines for Quality Palliative Care* in which the authors identified eight domains of quality for palliative and end-of-life care: structure and processes of care; physical aspects of care; psychological and psychiatric aspects of care; cultural aspects of care; social aspects of care; spiritual, religious, and existential aspects of care; care of the imminently dying; and ethical and legal aspects of care. In 2006, the NCP domains were "adopted" by the National Quality Forum

(NQF) (www.natioanlqualityforum.org) in their publication *A National Framework and Preferred Practices for Palliative and Hospice Care Quality.*

OUTCOME MEASUREMENT INITIATIVES IN PALLIATIVE CARE

Recognizing the critical need to define measures that capture the care processes and unique outcomes that characterize end-of-life care, several organizations have convened groups of providers and other experts to develop measurement tools and processes for outcome measurement.

Toolkit of Instruments to Measure End-of-Life Care (TIME)

Beginning in 1996, Joan Teno, MD, and colleagues convened several conferences to design and develop a *Toolkit of Instruments to Measure End-of-Life Care* (TIME). TIME conference participants reviewed critical domains for measurement and existing measurement tools. The key products in the "toolkit" are validated and cognitively tested interview instruments, de-

signed for interviewing terminally patients, and families of patients who have died about their experiences. The scoring protocol supports quality assessment of both processes and outcomes of end-of-life care.

National Hospice Workgroup and National Hospice and Palliative Care Association

Beginning in 1998, the National Hospice Work Group (NHWG) and the National Hospice and Palliative Care (NHPCO) Outcomes Taskforce developed and pilot-tested several indicators of quality care at the end of life based on the end-result outcomes identified in *Pathways for Patients and Families Facing Terminal Illness.* Four measures, described in Table 5–1, were defined and tested. These measures are used in many hospices and other end-of-life care settings.

The PEACE Project

In preparation for hospice regulations published in 2008, CMS contracted with the Carolinas Center for Medical Excellence to develop a list of recommended quality measures for hospices.

TABLE 5–1. National Hospice Work Group/National Hospice Organization Proposed Outcome Measures

END-RESULT OUTCOME	INDICATOR	HOW IT IS ASSESSED
Comfortable dying	Percentage of patients who report that pain was brought to a comfortable level within 48 h of start of care	Patient self-report at start of care and 72 h later
Safe dying	Percentage of families who report confidence in their ability to care for the patient safely at home	Self-report by family members on a questionnaire administered 1–3 mo after death
Self-determined life closure	Percentage of patients for whom preferences regarding hospitalization and CPR are met	Patient/legal representative report of preferences and chart review to determine adherence
Effective grieving	Percentage of families who report that they were helped to cope with changes following the loss of a loved one	Self-report by family members on a questionnaire administered 1–3 mo after death

The Carolinas Center named the initiative the "PEACE Project" for *Prepare, Embrace, Attend, Communicate, and Empower*, which represented some of the goals for the measures. Project directors identified possible measures from a number of sources, including measures endorsed by NQF for end-stage cancer patients; common, validated symptom assessment instruments; the NHPCO end-result outcome measures (Table 5–1); measures developed for a CMS hospice demonstration project; and the Family Evaluation of Hospice Care questionnaire (described later in this chapter.) The recommended measures (published on the Internet at www.medqic.org) address the domains of care identified by the National Quality Forum, as well as an indicator of adverse events to address patient safety.

SELECTED MEASURES AND TOOLS FOR ASSESSING OUTCOMES OF END-OF-LIFE CARE

As the foregoing discussion indicates, there have been many efforts to develop useful outcome measures and other quality indicators for end-of-life care. A discussion of all the applicable measures would be lengthy, so this chapter will focus on brief descriptions of clinical process and outcome measures that have proved useful in end-of-life care settings.

PATIENT COMFORT MEASURES

Patient comfort outcome measures are typically focused on specific symptoms, most often (but not exclusively) physical pain. The pain measure developed by the NHWG/NHPCO outcomes task force (described earlier in this chapter) uses two categorical variables rather than a severity rating scale. Patients are asked whether they are uncomfortable because of pain on an initial visit;

48 to 72 hours later, those who said "yes" are asked whether their pain was brought to an acceptable level within the first 72 hours of care. This measure has been endorsed by the National Quality Forum for use in quality improvement.

Use of a well-validated symptom assessment scale at periodic intervals over the course of care (on each visit, monthly, or more often for patients with particularly bothersome symptoms) provides longitudinal data that can be used to craft optimal interventions for an individual patient and to monitor outcomes for a patient population. Two examples are the Memorial Symptom Assessment Scale and the Edmonton Symptom Assessment Scale. The National Association for Home Care and Hospice developed tools for using the latter with hospice patients to meet Medicare requirements for quality assessment and performance improvement. An often overlooked but essential element of symptom severity measurement in end-of-life care is the issue of the patient's self-identified threshold for a specific symptom. Many terminally ill patients want to balance symptom relief against medication side effects that might affect their ability to interact with family or otherwise complete "unfinished business"; others may have cultural or religious reasons for rejecting medication. The most appropriate outcome measure for patient comfort, therefore, might be "percentage of patients who reach their self-identified threshold" for any specific symptom.

The American Pain Society has promulgated a measure of pain as a fifth vital sign. Patients are asked to rate pain severity on a scale from 0 (no pain at all) to 10 (worst pain imaginable) and, consistent with the concept of a self-identified threshold, to report the acceptability of the current pain level. Data collected using this measure can be used to determine the mean pain severity (and relief) over time for patients whose initial pain was mild (1–3), moderate (4–6), or severe (7–10).

The patient survey developed for the TIME project suggests another measurement strategy. Patients identify their two most bothersome symptoms, and then are asked three questions about these symptoms: (1) how often the symptom occurs, (2) the severity of the symptom, and (3) how much distress the symptom generates. The TIME survey also includes several other items concerning pain management most of which focus on patient experience of care including whether the patient ever had to wait too long for pain medication. This type of patient experience measure can often reveal process failures that directly affect outcomes.

PATIENT SAFETY

Although it has always been a critical part of healthcare quality, patient safety became a focus of quality improvement in the early twenty-first century partly as a result of two studies by the Institute of Medicine: *Crossing the Quality Chasm* and *To Err is Human*. The latter highlighted an astonishing prevalence of medical errors in the United States. The classic measures of patient safety, incidence and prevalence of adverse events, is applicable in end-of-life care. Adverse events that should be tracked for patients near the end of life include iatrogenic infections, medication errors, falls, and nonfall injuries, as well as dire events such as suicide, or unexpected loss of body function. In end-of-life care, patient safety also encompasses preservation of independence and ability to perform activities of daily living in ways that do not endanger the patient or caregivers, and education of family members to be confident and therefore more competent caregivers. As an indicator of the safe dying outcome, the NHWG/NHPCO Outcomes Taskforce devised the measure of family reported confidence in their ability to care for the dying patient safely at home (see Table 5–1).

AUTONOMY: MEETING PATIENT AND FAMILY PREFERENCES

Both the inclusion of an advance care planning measure as one of the limited number of PQRI measures from CMS and the identifica-

tion of "self-determined life closure" as the second end-result outcome in the *NHPCO Pathway for Patients and Families Facing Terminal Illness* attest to the central importance of autonomy and shared decision making for quality care at the end of life. The indicator drafted by the NHWG/NHPCO Outcomes Taskforce measures the frequency with which the choices of the patient (or legal representative) with respect to hospitalization and CPR were honored (see Table 5–1). The PQRI measure, which tracks the percentage of patients who have documented conversations regarding preferences and advance care planning, is a measure of process, not outcome; the conversations are correctly considered an essential prerequisite to achieving the outcome of self-determined life closure.

QUALITY OF LIFE

Quality-of-life measures are increasingly popular in healthcare, particularly as a way of evaluating the burdens and benefits of experimental therapies. For terminal patients, when quantity of life is known to be limited, quality of life becomes a primary goal of care.

Typically, health-related quality-of-life measures are designed to assess the impact of illness or treatment on the patient's role and functioning. In fact, many health-related quality of life instruments are constructed with the underlying assumption that functionality (physical, emotional, and social) and quality of life are directly proportional. For patients whose physical health and functional status are inexorably declining, however, quality of life becomes defined by other domains of living. For example, research with terminally ill patients has shown that the spiritual dimension is a major determinant of overall quality of life at the end of life. Appropriate tools for this population therefore must measure multiple dimensions of quality of life.

Rigorous qualitative and quantitative studies have identified critical components of quality of life for patients with life-limiting illness, and several instruments have been developed to quantify

TABLE 5–2. Critical Features of a Quality of Life Assessment Tool*
• A well-defined construct that has clinical applicability.
• Self-reported rather than observer-rated; a subjective assessment.
• Multidimensional, assessing relevant spheres of personhood including those related to health and function, as well as psychological, emotional, and spiritual dimensions of self.
• A scoring protocol that provides for weighting of dimensions by the person.
• Measurement of both negative and positive experiences at the end of life.
• "Sensibility" that includes measures of validity as well as "real world" applicability and utility, including ease of administration and scoring
• Use as both a discriminative tool, measuring differences between groups, and an evaluative tool, measuring changes in an individual over time.

*Adapted from Byock IR, Merriman MP: Measuring quality of life for patients with terminal illness: The Missoula-VITAS quality of life index. *Palliat Med* 12:231, 1998.

health-related quality of life at the end of life. Table 5–2 outlines the elements that characterize a valid and reliable quality of life scale. Two of these elements—subjectivity (report by the patient) and inclusion of a patient rating of the importance of various domains of quality of life—are critical from this author's perspective.

The Missoula-VITAS Quality of Life Index (MVQOLI) was designed specifically for terminally ill patients. It is based on Byock's theoretical framework of lifelong growth and development. Ira Byock, MD, has described the concept of landmarks and tasks to be completed before dying (Table 5–3) and posits that quality of life increases when these landmarks are reached. Results from the use of the instrument with hospice patients support the concept that quality of life for a terminal patient is not determined primarily by physical or functional status.

The MVQOLI is designed as a patient self-report questionnaire that gathers three kinds of information from patients in each of five dimensions of quality of life: symptoms, function, interpersonal relationships, emotional well-being, and transcendence. In each dimension, patients are asked questions that assess their subjective experience, their response to that experience, and the importance of the dimension to overall quality of life. A unique scoring protocol "weights" each dimensional score according to its importance. The MVQOLI has been used as a valuable

assessment tool that informs priorities and interventions during the care planning process. When the tool is used at periodic intervals over the course of care, the data also reveal outcomes in each domain for individual patients, or when aggregated, for defined patient populations.

The QUAL-E was developed based on qualitative research with patients, family members, and health care providers that identified elements of a "good death." Karen Steinhauser, Ph.D., and colleagues identified pain and symptom management, preparation for death, achieving a sense of completion, and being treated as a "whole person" as very important to all groups. Patients also identified being mentally aware, not being a burden, helping others and coming to peace with God as very important. The QUAL-E collects patient-reported information on physical symptoms or problems, participation in healthcare, concerns about the future, and life completion. An item in each area of inquiry asks patients how important that area is to overall quality of life.

CONTINUITY OF CARE AND CARE COORDINATION

One issue in measuring continuity of care is having a precise definition of the concept. The terms "care coordination" and "continuity of care" are

TABLE 5–3. Developmental Landmarks and Tasks for the End of Life

- Sense of completion with worldly affairs
  - Transfer of fiscal, legal, and formal social responsibilities
- Sense of completion in relationships with community
  - Closure of multiple social relationships (employment, commerce, organizational, congregational). Components include expressions of regret, expressions of forgiveness, acceptance of gratitude and appreciation
  - Leave taking; the saying of goodbye
- Sense of meaning about ones' individual life
  - Life review
  - The telling of "one's stories"
  - Transmission of knowledge and wisdom
- Experienced love of self
  - Self-acknowledgement
  - Self-forgiveness
- Experienced love of others
  - Acceptance of worthiness
- Sense of completion in relationships with family and friends
  - Reconciliation, fullness of communication, and closure in each of one's important relationships. Component tasks include expressions of regret, expressions of forgiveness and acceptance, expressions of gratitude and appreciation, *acceptance* of gratitude and appreciation, expressions of affection
  - Leave taking; the saying of goodbye
- Acceptance of the finality of life—of one's existence as an individual
  - Acknowledgement of the totality of personal loss represented by one's dying and experience of personal pain of existential loss
  - Expression of the depth of personal tragedy that dying represents
  - Decathexis (emotional withdrawal) from worldly affairs and cathexis (emotional connection) with an enduring construct
  - Acceptance of dependency
- Sense of a new self (personhood) beyond personal loss
- Sense of meaning about life in general
  - Achieving a sense of awe
  - Recognition of a transcendent realm
  - Developing/achieving a sense of comfort with chaos
- Surrender to the transcendent, to the unknown—"letting go"

Source: Reproduced, with permission, from Byock IR: The nature of suffering and the nature of opportunity at the end of life. *Clin Geriatr Med* 12:2, 1996.

often used interchangeably and are hard to distinguish in part because they are interdependent. Continuity has been described as a "thread" that connects episodes of care and distinguished from care coordination, which is the relationship between the various components of care. Building on this distinction, we suggest that care coordination refers to the processes, such as regular and parsimonious lines of communication, used to tie each provider and each episode into the continuous thread, which is continuity. The two are interdependent in that continuity cannot exist without coordination, and coordination is easier when there is continuity in terms of the individuals and organizations involved in delivering care. While both are critical components of high-quality care at any point in life, they become increasingly important for the terminally ill when length of life is decreasing more rapidly.

The American Society framework for quality of care at the end of life includes "sustained relationships with health care providers based on trust, reliability, and effective communication" as elements of continuity of care. (Lynn, 1997) Other elements of continuity are systems and processes that foster care coordination and cut down on duplicative data gathering, diagnostic procedures, and treatments. Indicators of continuity of care include both process measures and outcome measures. Process indicators might include (1) the presence of an electronic patient record accessible by various providers or a paper-based care plan that stays with the patient throughout care or (2) the number of duplicative laboratory tests. The best outcome indicator would be the patient's or family's perception of continuity as assessed through an experience questionnaire. The TIME family "after death" survey mentioned above includes items to assess continuity of care. In addition, Gerteis and coworkers have provided excellent descriptions of several continuity measures in their book *Through the Patient's Eyes*.

PATIENT AND FAMILY EXPERIENCE

Perhaps the most fundamental and critical outcome measure of care at the end of life is the nature of the patient and family experience of the care, the death, and the support after the death. Many healthcare providers utilize satisfaction surveys to capture patient perspectives on care, but the typical survey that asks patients to rate the quality of nursing care, or to indicate how satisfied they were with symptom management,

can be misleading. Satisfaction is closely linked to expectations and with respect to end-of-life care (specifically) and all health care (more generally) patient and family expectations tend to be relatively uninformed. Hence, satisfaction scores tend to be high even when the health care experience included less than optimal interventions or service components. For example, studies have shown that individuals who report that they are "satisfied" or "very satisfied" with a health care encounter will often describe aspects of the encounter that providers recognize as substandard care.

Since patient and family expectations, goals, and needs with respect to end-of-life care differ widely, the more accurate indicator of quality care is patient or family experience, rather than satisfaction. Gerteis, Cleary, and coworkers have described the use of patient-centered "reports" that allow the provider to measure how often preset standards of care are met (Fig. 5–2). Typical satisfaction surveys would ask consumers whether the patient and family were satisfied with pain management. This type of question requires that respondents (1) know what can be expected with respect to pain relief and (2) make a judgment

Have the doctors and nurses talked with you, in a way that you can understand, about treating your pain?

☐ YES   ☐ NO

Have you and your doctor made plans to ensure that your wishes for medical treatment will be followed?

☐ YES   ☐ NO

Figure 5–2. Two examples of patient-centered report questionnaire items that might be used to evaluate the patient's experience and perception of care. Note that the items do not ask patients to rate their care or express satisfaction or dissatisfaction. Instead, respondents simply indicate whether certain activities took place. (Modified from the "Patient Interview," Toolkit of Instruments to Measure End-of-Life Care, www.chcr.brown.edu/pcoc/toolkit. htm.)

about how well the provider implemented available treatments. A patient-centered report item would ask whether the patient experienced pain, and if so, how often and how bothersome it was. In this way, the provider learns whether pain was managed without asking the patient or family to make a judgment about the quality of care and without assuming what the consumer's expectation was.

The tools developed as part of the TIME project include a patient experience questionnaire designed for use while the patient is under care. For patients very near the end of life, administration of a questionnaire is often unrealistic for both ethical and practical reasons. Even if patients are able to answer, the burden must be weighed against the value of the information to be gathered. More commonly, experience questionnaires are administered to close family or friends who were involved in end-of-life care.

The Family Evaluation of Hospice Care (FEHC) developed through a collaboration of NHPCO and researchers at Brown University uses "patient-centered report" questions to assess the quality of care processes and outcomes specifically related to end-of-life care. The items in the questionnaire are based on questions first developed for the "after death" survey as part of the TIME project described above. The FEHC items were cognitively tested and assessed for reliability and validity. Notwithstanding the name of the tool, the questions are applicable outside of hospice, and some of the items were used in a national research study to compare the experiences of end-of-life care in a variety of settings, including individual medical practices. The FEHC has been endorsed by the National Quality Forum for public accountability use.

The FEHC is used by hospices across the United States and is typically sent to family 8 to 12 weeks after the death. Providers who are members of NHPCO can enter the data from their returned questionnaires into an Internet-based system that provides reports on individual agency performance along with comparative data based on all agencies reporting.

BEREAVEMENT OUTCOMES

Measuring bereavement outcomes is under-addressed in part because bereavement is not well-recognized as a care responsibility by practitioners outside of hospices and those who specialize in grief counseling. Like all outcomes, bereavement outcomes depend on the care provided and so the process of improving these outcomes begins with good assessment of risks for complicated grief both before and after the death (see Chapter 17).

In the NHPCO *Pathway for Patients and Families Facing Terminal Illness*, "effective grieving" is the end-result outcome that focuses on bereavement. This outcome encompasses the grieving of the family and the patient, both of whom experience loss. The focus, however, is on the family and on the task of continuing life without the loved one who has died. Desired bereavement outcomes include return to work or to one's social role. The outcome measure developed by the NHWG/NHPCO taskforce is family member self-report on coping with changes following the loss of a loved one. The data are collected via an after-death survey of family. Other excellent tools for evaluating the impact of grief on an individual and their "recovery" from grieving include The Grief Experience Inventory (Sanders and colleagues) and The Grief Resolution Index (Remondet and colleagues).

EXAMPLES: OUTCOMES AND QUALITY OF LIFE MEASUREMENT AT WORK

In looking at a provider's strategy for measuring outcomes and quality of life in the context of end-of-life care, simplicity should be seen as a plus. Successful programs have featured a small number of measures chosen because they are both meaningful—to patients, families, and professional caregivers—and actionable, providing information that will facilitate better care. A provider's choice of measures will be based on the primary goals of the end-of-life care program under evaluation, and thus reveal the program's underlying values.

The following examples illustrate outcomes measurement for terminally ill patients in hospice, palliative care, and other settings. The examples describe providers that have made a commitment to measuring outcomes of end-of-life care and designed successful strategies for collecting and using data.

HOSPICE PROVIDERS

Several hospice providers began measuring outcomes related to clinical status, quality of life, and satisfaction in the mid-1990s. As a measure of symptom management outcomes, providers have typically used patient-reported pain severity and/or patient satisfaction with pain management. As a quality of life measure, versions of the Missoula-VITAS Quality-of-Life Index have been favored, though several different tools have been used. The FEHC is the most widely used measure of experience of care.

In two different hospice organizations, protocols were designed to assure that all competent patients reported on pain management in the same way and at the same points in time following admission. The staff were taught language to use in asking the pain management question and primary nurses informed patients about the measures upon admission. At one agency, patient-reported pain severity (on the 0–10 scale recommended by the World Health Organization) was entered into a central database daily using a telephone voice-response data entry system. At another agency, pain was reported by patients using the 10-point scale along with the patient's answer to one item about whether pain relief was acceptable. In both cases, the data were collected by nurses in the course of their usual visits to patients and in the context of their routine assessment process. At the agency using telephone data entry, information on individual patients was available instantly to all staff, including those who may hear from the patient via phone on nights or weekends. At the other agency, scannable forms were used to record the data and these were sent to a contracted firm for data input, storage, and analysis services. For both hospices, the data could be analyzed for the entire patient population quarterly in order to determine how well pain was managed overall. Clinical managers used this quarterly performance measure data to determine whether performance improvement efforts were required. In the case of data collection by a contracted firm, the reports were used to set benchmarks for performance, and the agency could compare their performance with other agencies using the same data collection vendor.

These same hospice agencies implemented the Missoula-VITAS Quality of Life to measure quality of life during end-of-life care. The index was administered to patients who could complete it on admission and was repeated at approximately one-month intervals thereafter. If patients were unwilling or unable to complete the index, this information was also recorded. The index is designed to be administered in the course of routine visits to patients. Often, discussions following patient completion of the index led to important therapeutic interactions (see Chapter 14).

One agency chose a short version of the MVQOLI that generates a single overall quality of life score. This group analyzed data on the entire patient population on a quarterly basis. The other group used a longer version of the MVQOLI that generates sub-scores for the five quality of life dimensions. The dimensional sub-scores were plotted on a bar graph called the "quality-of-life profile" (Fig. 5–3) that shows which of the five domains are having the most impact on the patient and which are detracting from or adding to quality of life. The hospice care team could use this information for care planning, an example of outcomes management for individual patients.

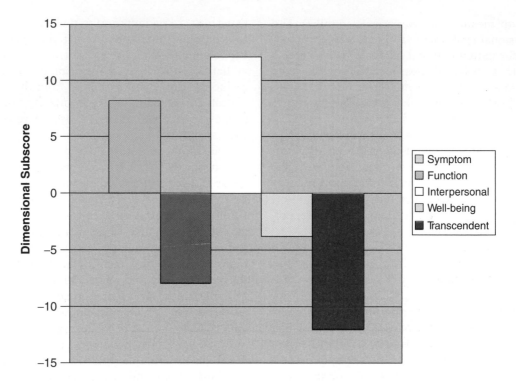

Figure 5–3. The profile generated by graphing dimensional scores from the Missoula-VITAS Quality of Life Index. The longer bars indicate dimensions that are contributing the most to the patient's overall quality of life; generally, these are the domains that are most important to the patient. Positive bars (above zero) are adding to good quality of life; negative bars (below zero) are detracting from good quality of life.

For measuring satisfaction or perception of care, both hospice groups chose surveys that were mailed to family members after the patient's death. In one group, the surveys were printed on scannable forms and were returned by mail to a central processing department. Survey scanning hardware and software were used to produce monthly and quarterly summaries of results. The data were used to provide feedback to staff and for performance improvement.

HOSPITALS AND MEDICAL CENTERS

In an impressive national effort to improve palliative care for terminally ill patients, one national group of medical centers included palliative care indicators in its quality performance measures beginning in 1997–1998. Most of these measures evaluated processes (Was there an advance care planning document in the file? Was there evidence of a pain management care plan?), but the focus was on processes that drive desired outcomes.

Between October 2002 and September 2003, 35 hospitals in the United Health System Consortium (UHC) conducted a benchmarking study to assess compliance with 11 "key performance measures" for palliative care. The measures included symptom assessment, reduction in symptom severity, use of a bowel regimen for patients prescribed opioid analgesics, documentation of patient status, psychosocial assessment, patient/family meeting to discuss care, and discharge planning. The data were collected via retrospective medical record review. The authors concluded that meeting the performance measure targets "was associated with improved quality, reduced costs, and length of stay" (Twaddle et al., 2007).

Beginning in 2004, another national healthcare provider organization with hospitals in several states launched an initiative to improve access to and quality of palliative care for inpatients. As part of the initiative, the organization identified several palliative care outcomes as well as protocols for data collection and reporting to be implemented in selected pilot sites. The measures were applied to all patients referred for palliative care consultation in the participating hospitals. The process and outcome measures included percentage of patients for whom a family meeting was convened within 48 hours of referral, percentage of patients reaching a pain level of 3 or less (on a 0 to 10 scale) within 48 hours of consultation, and percentage of patients receiving a spiritual care assessment by a qualified staff member. Data for all of the pilot sites was collected and compared, along with feedback about the usefulness of the measures and the burden of data collection. The results of the pilot were used to revise the measures and measurement processes for implementation across the healthcare system.

INDIVIDUAL HEALTHCARE PRACTITIONERS

Practitioners in a university clinic-based oncology practice implemented a symptom assessment scale completed by each patient on each visit prior to seeing the physician or nurse practitioner. Symptom severity could be reviewed over time to assure that individual patients were kept as comfortable as possible. In addition, population data were used to identify high-frequency symptoms for specific patient populations.

In two other community-based physician practices, symptom data collected as part of clinical trial participation were used to assess symptom management outcomes for participating patients.

SUMMARY AND CONCLUSIONS

Death is not the only outcome of end-of-life care. Even when disease cannot be cured and the prognosis is limited, much can be done for patients and the family and friends involved in the care of the terminally ill. Professionals providing end-of-life care have an obligation to help patients and families set realistic goals and then to assess how well those goals are achieved. Despite the many challenges discussed above, it is possible to measure quality of life and other outcomes of terminal care in a variety of healthcare settings. Widespread implementation of reliable and valid outcome measures will serve many purposes. The data will assure the best course of care for individual patients and will provide the means to demonstrate the value of end-of-life care to consumers and payers. The data will also contribute to the evidence base for palliative care and the identification of best practices. Finally, there is a potential for impact at a societal level. As more patients get better care at the end of life, defined as care that meets their individual needs and contributes to quality of life as they define it, the next generation of the dying may develop increased confidence in the ability of the medical community to deliver excellence in end-of-life care.

BIBLIOGRAPHY

Bandura, A: Self-efficacy determinants of anticipated fears and calamities. *J Pers Soc Psychol* 45:464, 1983.

Bruera E, Kuehn N, Miller MJ, Selmser P, Macmillan K: The Edmonton symptom assessment system (ESAS): A simple method for the assessment of palliative care patients. *J Palliat Care* 7(2):6-9, 1991.

Byock IR, Merriman MP: Measuring quality of life for patients with terminal illness: The Missoula-VITAS quality of life index. *Palliat Med* 12:231, 1998.

Byock IR: *Dying Well*. New York, Riverhead Books, 1997.

Byock IR: Growth: The essence of hospice. *Am J Hospice Care* 3:16, 1986.

Byock IR: The nature of suffering and the nature of opportunity at the end of life. *Clinics Geriatr Med* 12:2, 1996.

Carolinas Center for Hospice and Palliative Care (Cary, NC). *PEACE Project Summary (and hospice quality measures)*. www.medqic.org (click on hospice). Accessed November 14, 2008.

Cleary PD, Edgman-Levitan S, Roberts M, et al: Patients evaluate their hospital care: A national survey. *Health Aff* 10:254, 1991.

Cohen SR, Mount B: Quality of life in terminal illness: Defining and measuring subjective well-being in the dying. *J Palliat Care* 8:40, 1992.

Cohen SR, Mount BM, Tomas JJN, Mount LF: Existential well-being is an important determinant of quality of life. *Cancer* 77:576, 1996.

Connor SR, Teno JM, Spence C, Smith N: Family evaluation of hospice care: Results from voluntary submission of data via website. *J Pain Symptom Manage* 30(1):9, 2005.

Fletcher R, O'Malley M, Fletcher S, Earp J, Alexander J: Measuring the continuity and coordination of medical care in a system involving multiple providers. *Med Care* 22(5):403-411, 1984.

Fowler FJ, Coppola KM, Teno JM: Methodological challenges for measuring quality of care at the end of life. *J Pain Symptom Manage* 17:93, 1999.

Gerteis M, Edgeman-Levitan S, Daley J, et al: *Through the Patient's Eyes*. San Francisco, Jossey-Bass Publishers, 1993.

Gill TM, Feinstein AR: A critical appraisal of the quality of quality-of-life instruments. *JAMA* 272:619, 1994.

Haggerty J, Reid R, Freeman G, Starfield B, Adair C, McKendry R: Continuity of care: A multidisciplinary review. *BMJ* 327(7425):1219-1221, 2003.

Hearn J, Higginson IJ: Outcome measures in palliative care for advanced cancer patients: A review. *J Public Health Med* 19:193, 1997.

IOM (Institute of Medicine), Committee on Quality Health Care in America Quality Health Care in America: *Crossing the quality chasm: A new health system for the 21st century*. New York, National Academies Press, 2001.

Kohn LT, Corrigan JM, Donaldson MS, eds; IOM (Institute of Medicine), Committee on Quality Health Care in America Quality Health Care in America: *To Err is Human: Building a Better Healthcare System*. New York, National Academies Press, 2001.

Lev E, Munro BH, McCorkle R: A shortened version of an instrument measuring bereavement. *Int J Nurs Stud* 30(3):213-226, 1993.

Lynn J: Measuring quality of care at the end of life: A statement of principles. *J Am Geriatr Soc* 45:526-527, 1997.

MacMillan SC, Mahon M: Measuring quality of life in hospice patients using a newly developed hospice quality of life index. *Qual Life Res* 3:437, 1994.

National Hospice and Palliative Care Organization Standards and Accreditation Committee: *A Pathway for Patients and Families Facing Terminal Disease*. Alexandria, VA, National Hospice and Palliative Care Organization, 1997.

National Quality Forum (NQF): *A National Framework and Preferred Practices for Palliative and Hospice Care Quality*.Washington, DC, NQF, 2004.

Portenoy RK, Thaler HT, Kornblith AB, et al: The Memorial symptom assessment scale: An instrument for the evaluation of symptom prevalence, characteristics and distress. *Eur J Cancer* 30A(9):1326-1336, 1994.

Reid RJ, Haggerty J, McKendry R: Canadian Health Services Research Foundation, Canadian Institute for Health Information Advisory Committee on Health Services of the Federal/Provincial/Territorial Ministers of Health: *Defusing the Confusion: Concepts and Measures of Continuity of Healthcare*. Ottawa, Canadian Health Services Research Foundation, 2002.

Remondet JH, Hanson RO: Assessing widow's grief—A short index. *J Gerontol Nurs* 13:30-34, 1987.

Saultz JW: Defining and measuring interpersonal continuity of care. *Ann Fam Med* 1(3):134-143, 2003.

Schwartz CE, Merriman MP, Reed G, Byock IR: Evaluation of the Missoula-VITAS quality of life index—revised: Research tool or clinical tool? *J Palliat Med* 8(1):121-135, 2005.

Solberg LI, Moser G, McDonald S: The three faces of performance measurement (improvement, accountability, and research). *Jt Comm J Qual Improv* 23(3):135-147, 1997.

Steinhauser KE, Bosworth HB, Clipp EC, et al: Initial assessment of a new measure of quality of life at the end of life (QUAL-E). *J Palliat Med* 5(6):829-842, 2002.

Steinhauser KE, Clipp EC, Bosworth HB, et al: Measuring quality of life at the end of life: Validation of the QUAL-E. *Palliat Support Care* 2(2):3-14, 2004.

Stewart AL, Teno JM, Patrick DL, Lynn J: The concept of quality of life of dying persons in the context of health care. *J Pain Symptom Manage* 17:93-108, 1999.

Teno JM, et al: *Toolkit of Instruments to Measure End-of-Life Care*. http://www.chcr.brown.edu/pcoc/toolkit.htm. Accessed November 12, 2008.

Teno JM, Clarridge BR, Casey V, et al: Family perspectives on the last place of care. *JAMA* 291(1):88-93, 2004.

Teno JM, Coppola KM: For every numerator, you need a denominator: A simple statement but key to measuring the quality of care of the "dying". *J Pain Symptom Manage* 17:109-113, 1999.

The SUPPORT Principal Investigators: A controlled trial to improve care for seriously ill hospitalized patients. *JAMA* 274:1591-1598, 1995.

Twaddle ML, Maxwell TL, Cassel JB, et al: Palliative care benchmarks from academic medical centers. *J Palliat Med* 10(1):86-98, 2007.

Williams AL, Selwyn PA, Molde S, et al: A randomized controlled trial of meditation and massage effects on quality of life in people with late-stage disease: A pilot study. *J Palliat Med* 8(5):939-952, 2005.

SELF-ASSESSMENT QUESTIONS

1. Which of the following outcome measures, commonly used in multiple heath care settings to assess a provider's quality of care is LEAST useful for evaluating the quality of care of an end-of-life care provider?

   A. Patient mortality
   B. Adequate pain control
   C. Satisfaction with staff communication
   D. Recommend the end-of-life care provider to others
   E. Infection control rates

2. Regarding the National Hospice Work Group and National Hospice and Palliative Care Association outcome measure "self-determined life closure," which of the following represents the patient preferences used as indicators for this measure?

   A. Artificial feeding and CPR
   B. Artificial feeding and hospitalization
   C. Artificial feeding, CPR, and hospitalization
   D. CPR and hospitalization
   E. CPR only

3. For the outcome measure "percentage of patients who reach an identified threshold" for pain or any other symptom, who is the person who identifies the threshold?

   A. The nurse
   B. The physician
   C. The patient
   D. The primary care giver
   E. The social worker

4. Which of the following domains of quality of life measurement is LEAST useful in assessing quality of life in end-of-life care?

   A. Spiritual well-being
   B. Psychosocial well-being
   C. Emotional well-being
   D. Symptom control
   E. Functional status

5. All of the following are elements that characterize a valid and reliable quality of life scale, EXCEPT

   A. Multidimensional in nature
   B. Observer-rated
   C. Measurement of negative and positive experiences
   D. Weighting score by importance
   E. Ease of administration and scoring

6. Which of the following is best defined as "the processes, such as regular and parsimonious lines of communication, used to tie each provider and each episode" of care together?

   A. Continuity of care
   B. Coordination of care
   C. Components of care
   D. Quality of care
   E. Quality of life

7. Which one of the following statements about measures of the patient/family experience is true?

   A. Patient/family satisfaction surveys allow the provider to measure how often preset standards of care are met.
   B. Patient/family satisfaction scores accurately reflect the healthcare experience of the patient or family.
   C. Patient/family satisfaction surveys are more accurate indicators of quality of care than a "patient-centered" report.
   D. A "patient-centered" report requires respondents to make a judgment about the quality of care.
   E. Patient/family satisfaction surveys require respondents to know what should be expected regarding services provided.

8. In Byock's "Developmental Landmarks and Tasks for the End of Life," which of the landmarks includes tasks including life review, the telling of "one's stories," and the transmission of knowledge and wisdom?

A. Experienced love of self
B. Sense of meaning about one's individual life
C. Acceptance of the finality of life
D. Sense of meaning about life in general
E. Sense of completion in relationships with family and friends

9. Features of the MVQOLI include all of the following EXCEPT

A. Measures five dimensions of quality of life
B. Weights each dimension according to its importance
C. Should not be administered during a routine patient visit.
D. May be used to inform priorities and interventions during care planning.
E. It is based on Byock's theoretical framework of lifelong growth and development.

Management of Symptoms

CHAPTER

6

Management of Pain at the End of Life

Tara C. Friedman, Barry M. Kinzbrunner,
Neal J. Weinreb, and Michael Clark

INTRODUCTION

Uncontrolled pain is a substantial issue for patients with life-limiting illnesses. Studies reveal that the prevalence of "important pain problems" is as high as 50% among community-dwelling older people at the end of life, and that the prevalence of "substantial pain" ranges from 45% to 80% among nursing home residents. It is estimated that one in four elderly cancer patients in nursing homes receives no treatment at all for daily pain. Acute or chronic pain is reported among 30% of newly diagnosed cancer patients and increases from 60% to 80% among patients with advanced disease. Based on the aforementioned statistics, it is not surprising that adequate relief of pain is among the top five concerns that patients have about the quality of end-of-life care.

Although cancer is the illness that is most often associated with pain at the end of life, patients with nonmalignant terminal illnesses including AIDS; end-stage cardiac, pulmonary, and cerebrovascular diseases; and Alzheimer's disease and other neurodegenerative diseases often suffer from pain as well. A large study by the World Health Organization (WHO) found that 22% of primary care patients across Asia, Africa, Europe, and the Americas report persistent pain. Notably, pain sufferers are more likely to have an anxiety or depressive disorder. A study of chronic nonmalignant pain sufferers found 74% with limitation of social or recreational activities. A recent survey of Canadian physicians who had written prescriptions for patients with moderate to severe pain revealed that 35% of general practitioners and 23% of physicians who identified themselves as having a palliative care interest would "never" use opioids for noncancer pain, even when the pain was described as severe. With the "graying" of the "baby boomer" generation, the prevalence of these illnesses will inevitably increase. Primary care physicians will therefore need to assume a growing and formidable responsibility for the adequate management of pain at the end of life.

Concern for the enormity of the problem has prompted legislative and other regulatory remedies for pain at the end of life. In 2001, the Joint Commission on Accreditation of Healthcare Organizations enforced new standards in hospitals, nursing homes, and outpatient clinics ensuring that "patients have the right" to proper pain assessment and treatment, and that patients' pain be measured and recorded regularly from the time they are admitted. Numerous other health care organizations have developed national and international pain treatment guidelines and published position and policy statements. However, uncontrolled pain remains one of the most feared and undertreated symptom in terminally ill patients.

BARRIERS TO EFFECTIVE PAIN MANAGEMENT AT THE END OF LIFE

Although valid pain treatment guidelines are widely available, there are several recognized barriers to pain management at the end of life, listed in Table 6–1 and discussed below.

PATIENT RELUCTANCE TO REPORT PAIN

Patients are sometimes reluctant to inform physicians that they are in pain because of the fear of being regarded as complainers or malingerers.

TABLE 6–1. Barriers to Effective Pain Management

Patient barriers	Patient reluctance to report pain
	Patient reluctance to take opioid analgesics
	Fear of medication side effects
	Fear of addiction
	Stigma of medication
	Cost of medications and revisits to physician
	Stoicism/cultural issues
	Cognitive/language impairments
	Acceptance of pain/hopelessness
Clinician barriers	Inadequate pain assessment and reassessment
	Inadequate education and training in pain management
	Physician reluctance to prescribe opioids (i.e., "opiophobia")
	Undertreatment of specific populations of patients
	Minorities 3:1 compared with nonminorities
	Nonsurgical patients to surgical patients 2:1
	Women to men 1.5:1
	Elderly to younger patients 2.4:1
	Concerns of causing premature death from respiratory depression
Organizational and regulatory barriers	Pharmacy reluctance to refill opioid prescriptions earlier than the interval prescribed
	Limited pharmacy stock of opioid analgesics
	DEA and state-specific prescription constraints

Older patients may fear being involuntarily hospitalized, institutionalized, or having additional tests or procedures if they truthfully report pain. Some patients also consider that pain is an indicator of progressive illness or that treatment they are receiving for the illness is ineffective. In these circumstances, denial may be a defense mechanism to avoid confronting the prognostic implications of increasing pain. Finally, patients with neurological, mechanical, or cognitive deficits may be unable to verbalize pain.

PATIENT RELUCTANCE TO USE OPIOID ANALGESICS

Patients often associate opioid analgesics (especially morphine) with approaching and proximate death. Many patients and families associate opioids with a high risk of addiction and fear the social implications of taking medications that are akin to "street drugs." This has been particularly true in recent years with the increased public attention on diversion of prescribed opioids. The use of methadone as an analgesic has a unique association with addiction that requires special counseling. Many patients also believe that opioid use is associated with unpleasant or unmanageable side effects, particularly sedation and constipation. Finally, some patients may fear that if opioids are started "too soon," there will be no other medication to help them when the pain becomes "really bad."

INADEQUATE PHYSICIAN EDUCATION AND TRAINING

Studies and surveys of physicians indicate that education and training, beginning with medical school and extending through residency and continuing medical education curricula, have traditionally failed to adequately address techniques for pain assessment and treatment. A review of four widely used general medical textbooks found little helpful information on end-of-life care, and the authors concluded that physicians should seek guidance from other sources when dealing with end-of-life care. In 2003, the Liaison Committee on Medical Education mandated medical schools implement formal teaching in end-of-life care, and a recent study of graduating medical students revealed an improved perception of their schools' attention to end-of-life care curriculum. Over the past 10 years, the fraction of medical students who perceived that their school spent at least adequate time teaching pain management improved from 34.8% to 55.3%. This improvement represents important but still incomplete progress. Primary care physicians need to be competent in managing pain in the terminally ill. Evidence suggests that by applying the pain management techniques described in this chapter, clinicians should be able to relieve or substantially reduce pain for at least 90% of patients at the last phases of life.

INADEQUATE PAIN ASSESSMENT BY CLINICIANS

It is expected that 80% to 90% of all information about a patient can be obtained via a thorough assessment (history and physical examination). Evaluating pain is no exception. A proper pain assessment provides the baseline data that will determine selection of treatment modalities, medication dosage and intervals, and the need for adjunctive interventions. Unfortunately, an increased reliance on technology has diminished the importance of the patient encounter and eroded the clinical skills necessary for physicians and other health care professionals to perform adequate assessments for pain and other subjective symptoms that are not quantifiable by machine. Prolonged face-to-face assessments are also discouraged by a medical system that rewards volume over quality and comprehensiveness of the patient visit.

UNDERTREATMENT OF SPECIFIC PATIENT POPULATIONS

Medical literature demonstrates that certain patient groups are at a higher risk for poor pain control than the general population. Unfortunately, the most cogent explanation for this phenomenon is overt or subliminal stereotyping by health care providers and other caregivers.

Minority patients are three times more likely to have uncontrolled pain than nonminority patients. Postoperative patients with advanced dementia were found to receive one-third of the opioid analgesia of cognitively intact patients receiving the same surgical hip fracture repair. And, because surgical patients have a more obvious source for pain, patients with medical pain syndromes are twice as likely to have uncontrolled pain as postoperative patients. Gender biases, which assume that women exaggerate pain more than men, may account for the fact that women are 1.5 times more likely than men to have uncontrolled pain. This bias holds true whether the caregivers questioned are male or female. Elderly patients are almost 2.5 times more likely to have uncontrolled pain as younger patients. This may be due to underreporting of pain by elderly patients, the perception by healthcare providers that elderly patients are less credible informants, or concerns by providers that analgesics may not be well-tolerated in the elderly.

PHYSICIAN RELUCTANCE TO PRESCRIBE OPIOIDS

Many physicians still have a poor understanding of opioid pharmacology and are fearful of causing addiction, clinically significant respiratory depression, or premature patient death. However, when knowledgeable prescribers follow opioid prescribing guidelines, these fears are unwarranted. An exaggerated fear of the development of analgesic tolerance often prompts physicians to withhold opioids from patients with severe pain until the patients are near death, thinking that premature use of opioids will obviate their efficacy near the end of life when patients need it most. Still, other physicians are simply opiophobic. The heightened regulatory scrutiny surrounding opioids and other controlled substances has also discouraged the prescription of these agents, especially in states with expensive and burdensome triplicate prescription programs. Repeated official statements of reassurance that practitioners who appropriately prescribe opioids for pain control will not be subject to special examination and punitive review have been received with skepticism. Physicians remember incidents such as that occurred in Florida in 1998 when a medical examiner accused a hospice program of routinely killing patients with what was subsequently found to be normal therapeutic doses of morphine. On the other hand, in the last several years, physicians have been successfully sued for failing to provide adequate pain management for dying patients. Such litigation has shed light on the need for ongoing education in pain management so that several states now require continuing medical education in pain management and end-of-life care as a requirement for physician licensure reregistration.

FEAR OF ADDICTION

Concerns about addiction should be of little concern to the vast majority of terminally ill patients. However, many physicians continue to confuse physical dependence with addiction. Physical dependence is the universal, unavoidable altered physiologic adaptation to opioid use that requires continued use of the opioid to avoid withdrawal reactions. It usually occurs within days to weeks of starting the chronic use of opioids. For patients in whom the source of pain is removed, opioids may be rapidly and safely tapered without residual need for the medication.

In contrast, addiction represents a state of psychological dependence in which the patient exhibits a behavioral pattern of drug craving and an overwhelming involvement in obtaining and using the drug for reasons other than pain relief. The lifestyle of the addicted patient is geared to acquisition of the desired drug despite the legal, financial, and psychosocial difficulties entailed. Psychological dependence is a rare phenomenon among patients who have a medical need for opioid analgesics, with studies showing that it occurs in less than 0.1% of patients. Patients at highest risk for psychological dependence usually have a history of alcoholism or other substance abuse, and/or a history of mental illness, especially depression. Even these patients, although requiring careful and sometimes specialized management, should NOT be deprived of needed analgesia especially when they experience pain near the end of life.

FEAR OF OPIOID-INDUCED RESPIRATORY DEPRESSION AND PREMATURE DEATH

Although opioids have suppressant effects on the respiratory center, tolerance to the respiratory depressant effects of opioid analgesics develops rapidly and early in the course of treatment. Within a few days of initiation of opioid therapy, the threshold dose for respiratory depression far exceeds the analgesic threshold. In fact, because of their vasodilatory and preload reducing effects, opioids have traditionally been used to treat cardiopulmonary problems such as acute pulmonary edema. Opioids are highly effective in reducing subjective dyspnea across various advanced medical diagnoses, including chronic obstructive pulmonary disease (COPD) and lung cancer. At controlled doses of 25% to 50% of 4-hour opioid dose, opioids have been shown to significantly reduce dyspnea without decreasing respiratory rate or peripheral arterial oxygen saturation. Thus, there is no evidence that chronic opioid use negatively affects respiratory status,

and fear of hastening death by giving the next scheduled opioid dose to an actively dying patient is unfounded.

EFFECTIVE PAIN MANAGEMENT AT THE END OF LIFE

Despite the barriers to good pain control discussed above, and despite the daunting challenge posed by the high prevalence of pain in patients with advanced illnesses, sufficient relief can be achieved for most patients (up to 90%) if adequate treatment is provided. Suggested guidelines for effective pain management are outlined in Table 6–2, which will also serve as the organizational chart for the remainder of this chapter. Using these guidelines, the clinician should be able to abolish or significantly reduce pain, prevent its return, and positively influence quality of life even as that life draws to an end.

DEFINITIONS

The first step in understanding how to manage pain effectively is to develop a common language. To accomplish that, it is important to clearly define the various terms that are used when assessing and treating patients with pain.

Definition of Pain

The International Association for the Study of Pain (IASP) defines pain as "an unpleasant sensory and emotional experience associated with actual or potential tissue damage or described in terms of such damage." Clarifying this definition further, the IASP notes that pain is subjective, and that each individual creates his own definition for pain on the basis of his own experiences. This means that the way a patient defines or expresses pain may be very different from how

TABLE 6–2. Guidelines for Effective Pain Management

1. Always perform a thorough assessment of the patient's pain to identify and differentiate the various types and degrees of pain the patient may be experiencing.
2. Use medication and dosage schedules based on the characteristics of the patient's pain.
   a. Follow the World Health Organization (WHO) step ladder approach (see the section entitled Selection of the Appropriate Analgesic) to choose the right drug for the appropriate degree of pain severity.
   b. For acute, intermittent pain, the appropriate dose of an analgesic with a rapid onset of action should be used, with dosing on an as-needed or PRN basis.
   c. For chronic, continuous pain, the appropriate dose of analgesic, individually titrated for the patient's needs, should be used. A long duration of action is preferred and should be given on an around-the-clock basis to prevent pain recurrence. Use breakthrough medication to treat incident pain or acute exacerbation of chronic pain.
   d. Use appropriate adjunctive analgesics for specific types of pain, such as bone pain or neuropathic pain.
   e. Consider appropriate nonpharmacological forms of intervention, when indicated.
3. Choose the appropriate, least invasive route of therapy to meet the patient's needs. According to the literature, more than 90% of patients with chronic pain may be managed with oral medications.
4. Reassess the patient frequently. Routine monitoring and reassessment is the best way to maintain good pain control.

family members or professional caregivers perceive the patient's pain. This inherent subjectivity leads to a simpler and more practical definition:

Pain is whatever the experiencing person says it is, existing whenever the experiencing person says it does.

Believing the patient, accepting the patient's pain for what it is, and abstaining from superimposing one's own biases upon the patient are the first steps to effective pain management. With those steps accomplished, methodical assessment of the cause of the pain will lead the clinician, with the help of the patient, family, and other members of the end-of-life care team, to develop the plan of care and interventions that are necessary for effective treatment.

Nociceptive and Neuropathic Pain

Using pathophysiology to categorize pain helps to better understand the etiology of a patient's symptoms and to choose the most appropriate interventions. Pain is divided into two major physiologic types, nociceptive and neuropathic. Nociceptive pain is further subdivided into somatic and visceral subtypes. Table 6–3 presents differential characteristics of somatic and visceral nociceptive pain and neuropathic pain.

SOMATIC NOCICEPTIVE PAIN   Somatic nociceptive pain is caused by tissue injury that results in direct stimulation of intact afferent nerve endings. Somatic pain is usually described in the following terms: sharp, dull, aching, throbbing, or gnawing in quality. It occurs in bones, joints, and soft tissues and tends to be well localized. Causes for somatic pain include fractures, arthritis, burns, abrasions, abscesses, and tumor invasion of soft tissue. Somatic nociceptive pain typically responds well to nonopioid and opioid analgesics, in accordance with the WHO analgesic ladder. Bone pain due to tumor metastases is a subcategory of somatic nociceptive pain that is largely mediated by prostaglandins, and therefore amenable to treatment not only with opioids but also with anti-inflammatory agents.

TABLE 6–3. Characteristics of Nociceptive and Neuropathic Pain

	NOCICEPTIVE		NEUROPATHIC
	SOMATIC	VISCERAL	
Pathophysiology	Tissue injury resulting in direct stimulation of intact afferent nerve endings A subset of somatic pain is caused by direct cancerous infiltration of the bone, mediated by prostaglandins	Activation of nociceptors resulting from stretching, distension, or inflammation of the internal organs of the body	Injury to peripheral nerves or central nervous system structures
Description	Usually, well localized, and may be described as sharp, dull, aching, throbbing, or gnawing	Poorly localized and may be described as deep, aching, cramping, or a sensation of pressure	May be described as burning, shooting, tingling, stabbing, or like a vise or electric shock. It may be constant or paroxysmal and it is often associated with paresthesias or dysesthesias
Affected organs	Typically affected parts of the body include bones, joints, and soft tissues	Internal organs	Brain, central nervous system, nerve plexi, nerve roots, and peripheral nerves
Examples	Metastatic cancer to bone Fractures Tumors or erosive ulcers invading soft tissues Arthritis	Periumbilical pain of bowel obstruction Shoulder pain secondary to liver or lung metastases Jaw and/or left arm pain secondary to coronary insufficiency	Brachial or lumbosacral plexopathy Herpes zoster Diabetic neuropathy Alcoholic neuropathy Postherpetic neuralgia

Pharmacological management	NSAIDs
	Steroids (bone pain)
	Opioids
		Opioids
		Steroids (peritumoral edema)
			Less responsive to opioids
			Requires adjuvant medications
			  Tricyclic antidepressants
			  Steroids
			  Anticonvulsants (see Table 6–20)

VISCERAL NOCICEPTIVE PAIN As with somatic pain, visceral nociceptive pain is caused by tissue injury, inflammation, or stretching that results in direct stimulation of intact afferent nerve endings. Visceral pain affects internal organs and is, therefore, poorly localized and often referred to various somatic sites. Visceral pain is usually described as a deep ache, cramp, or sensation of pressure. Examples of referred visceral pain include shoulder pain caused by liver metastases or

TABLE 6–4. Characteristics of Acute and Chronic Pain

	ACUTE PAIN	CHRONIC PAIN
Onset	Usually sudden	Usually of long duration
Signs and symptoms	Physiologic response: Increased blood pressure and heart rate, sweating, pallor	Physiologic response: Often absent
	Emotional response: Increased anxiety and restlessness	Emotional response: Patient may be depressed, withdrawn, expressionless, and/or fatigued
Therapeutic goals	Relief of pain	Prevention of pain
	Sedation often desirable	Sedation not desirable
Timing	As needed (PRN) or upon request	Routine preventive schedule
Dosing	Often standardized	Individualized
		Based upon patient needs
Route of administration	Parenteral/intramuscular/ oral/sublingual	Oral preferred

SOURCE: Adapted, with permission, from Kinzbrunner BM: *Vitas Pain Management Guidelines*. Miami, FL, Vitas Healthcare Corporation, 1999.

cholecystitis, and the left arm and jaw pain that is classical for coronary insufficiency. An example of poorly localized visceral pain is the periumbilical discomfort that may be associated with multiple inflammatory or obstructive gastrointestinal conditions. Visceral nociceptive pain also tends to respond well to opioid analgesics.

NEUROPATHIC PAIN Neuropathic pain is caused by direct injury to peripheral nerves and/or the central nervous system (CNS) resulting in aberrant neural discharges unrelated to external noxious stimuli. Neuropathic pain is usually described with the following terms: burning, shooting, tingling, vice-like, electric. The pain may be constant or paroxysmal, and it is often associated with paresthesias, dysesthesia, or allodynia. Causes of neuropathic pain include spinal cord compression, plexopathy, neurotoxicity secondary to cancer chemotherapy, chemical and metabolic neuropathies such as diabetes mellitus, postherpetic neuralgia (PHN), tic douloureux, postmastectomy syndrome, and phantom limb pain. Unlike nociceptive pain, neuropathic pain is commonly less responsive to opioid analgesics

and optimal treatment requires the prescription of adjuvant agents such as corticosteroids, tricyclic antidepressants (TCAs), N-methyl-D-aspartate (NMDA) antagonists and anticonvulsants in addition to opioid analgesics (see Table 6–20)

Acute and Chronic Pain

Pain is also categorized as acute or chronic on the basis of the nature of its onset and its duration. The characteristics of acute and chronic pain are summarized in Table 6–4.

Acute pain is defined as a pain that occurs suddenly, usually with an identifiable cause. The acuity of onset causes the patient to develop subjective and objective physical signs associated with hyperactivity of the autonomic nervous system, such as tachycardia, hypertension, and diaphoresis. The patient usually exhibits overt signs of pain including facial grimacing, groaning, crying, or even screaming. Classical examples of acute pain include that associated with a fracture immediately after a fall, kidney stones, and postoperative pain.

Chronic pain is best defined as a pain that has been persistent and unremitting for some time. Although the literature typically refers to a time frame of 6 months, this seems unnecessarily restrictive and unrealistic in the context of end-of-life care. Unlike patients with acute pain, patients with chronic pain do not exhibit the typical autonomic or physical signs commonly associated with pain. Rather, they often seem apathetic, withdrawn, and depressed, leading the untrained or insensitive observer to doubt that the patient is experiencing pain at all. It is precisely this group of patients, whose credibility is questioned, that is at the greatest risk for inadequate pain management.

Distinguishing acute from chronic pain is essential to choosing an appropriate therapeutic approach (see Table 6–4). Acute pain should be treated with analgesia as needed, with the expectation that the painful stimulus will remit over time. In contrast, chronic pain must be treated with scheduled dosing to prevent recurring pain that will persist or worsen. Sedation is usually desirable when patients have acute pain as this will alleviate anxiety, promote rest, and allow healing to occur. Sustained sedation is undesirable for patients with chronic pain because one of the major goals of pain relief is to allow resumption of maximal activities of daily living. Because treatment of acute pain is expected to be transient, standard "one size fits all" analgesic doses are common, and parenteral routes of administration are not objectionable. For patients with chronic pain, treatment is likely to be sustained for the duration of the underlying illness. Analgesic doses must be titrated to the needs of the individual patient and should be administered by the least invasive route possible, preferably by mouth.

Terminally ill patients with chronic pain often have acute exacerbations, particularly as the disease process progresses and new complications ensue. When this occurs, the clinician must be careful not to overlook a potential new painful stimulus as a cause of the acute exacerbation. Each new flare of pain presents an opportunity to initiate a new pain assessment, and, if indicated, adjust or modify the treatment plan.

TABLE 6–5. Performing a Thorough Pain Assessment

1. Always obtain a complete history, preferably from the patient, paying specific attention to:
   a. Full pain history (see Table 6–6).
   b. Psychosocial, spiritual, and family history.
   c. Medication history, including over-the-counter medications.
2. Perform a physical examination focused on:
   a. Painful areas.
   b. A thorough neurological examination.
3. Establish a pain diagnosis or diagnoses.
4. Institute an appropriate plan of care based on the pain assessment.
5. Directly involve the patient and/or primary caregivers.
   a. Explain your findings to the patient (or to the primary caregivers).
   b. Involve the patient directly in his or her own management.
   c. Establish realistic time frames to achieve goals.
   d. Reassess the patient's pain frequently.
   e. Monitor for adverse side effects and treat in anticipation.
6. Document the pain assessment.

THE PAIN ASSESSMENT

The principal components of a thorough pain assessment are outlined in Table 6–5. The importance of developing and exercising good assessment skills is underscored by a survey of oncologists in which 75% identified clinical inadequacy in performing pain assessments as the leading barrier to effective pain management.

Always Obtain a Complete History, Preferably from the Patient

By nature, pain is a subjective experience; therefore, a detailed history obtained directly from the patient is the most critical aspect of a productive pain assessment. The goal of the pain assessment for a patient at the end of life is to reach a "pain diagnosis," rather than the usual "disease diagnosis." Thus, although the history of present illness is important to understanding the contextual basis of the complaint of pain, and the past history may identify potential pain etiologies that may not be directly related to the terminal illness, the primary history of the pain itself is critical and should not be overlooked. Questions about the characteristics of the patient's pain help to determine whether the pain is nociceptive, neuropathic, or mixed, and whether the pain is acute, chronic, or an exacerbation of acute pain superimposed on a chronic pain syndrome. Patients may have more than one site or cause for pain, with each pain having its own characteristics and therapeutic needs. As patients may be unaware of this complexity, the physician must maintain a high index of suspicion and interview the patient in sufficient detail to identify all painful areas.

HISTORY OF THE PAIN The mnemonic device *PQRST* has proven to be a useful reminder of what questions need to be asked to complete an adequate pain history (Table 6–6):

P: The "P" stands for both Palliative and Provocative, that is, what conditions affect the perception of pain? Ask whether movement, rest, position, weight bearing, or activities such as bathing, dressing, eating, swallowing, etc. have a positive or negative effect. Determine what interventions, including current or past medications, make the pain better or worse.

Q: The "Q" stands for Quality, that is, what are the properties and characteristics of the pain as perceived by the patient and how do they relate to the pathophysiology? Ask the patient to describe the pain in the patient's own words. Because patients may have difficulty with this task, clinicians must become skilled at guiding the patient without being overly suggestive. Open-ended questions are preferable, but, at times, it may be necessary to ask directly whether the pain is sharp, dull, aching, or throbbing (suggesting nociceptive pain) or shooting, piercing, burning, tingling (suggesting neuropathic pain).

R: The "R" stands for Radiation. Attempt to localize the pain if possible. Determining patterns of radiation and whether the pain appears to be referred helps to differentiate somatic from visceral nociceptive pain and provides clues to the origins of visceral pain. In the case of neuropathic pain, patterns of radiation help distinguish peripheral from CNS lesions and identify specific affected nerve roots, plexi, and dermatomes.

S: The "S" stands for Severity. Although pain is inherently subjective, for initial assessment, selection of treatment, and serial monitoring of response, it is useful to create a more objective and reproducible measurement system to quantify what the patient is experiencing. For this purpose, pain is rated by the patient according to its severity on a

TABLE 6–6. The PQRST's of Pain Assessment

	MEANING	EXAMPLE
P	Palliative	What makes the pain better?
	Provocative	What makes the pain worse?
Q	Quality	How would you describe the pain?
R	Radiation	Where is the pain and to where does it spread or travel?
S	Severity	On a scale of 0–10, how bad is the pain?
T	Temporal	Is the pain constant, or does it come and go?

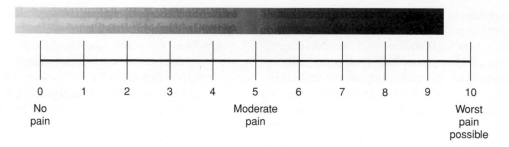

Figure 6–1. 0 to 10 Numerical Pain Intensity Scale: This is the gold standard for assessing pain severity. Patients should be asked about the severity of their pain, with 0 representing no pain, 5 representing moderate pain, and 10 representing the worst pain possible.

SOURCE: Acute Pain Management Guideline Panel: *Acute Pain Management: Operative or Medical Procedures and Trauma. Clinical Practice Guideline.* AHCPR Pub. No. 92–0032. Rockville, MD, Agency for Health Care Policy and Research, Public Health Service, US Department of Health and Human Services, 1992.

numerical 0 to 10 scale, with 0 representing no pain, and 10 representing the worst pain imaginable. The utility of this method has been validated in a number of studies.

When quantifying pain, the clinician should inquire not only about the current pain intensity, but also about the best and worst levels of pain during the past 24 hours and during the past several days. This gives the clinician a more complete assessment of pain control throughout the day rather than just one snapshot of time and allows one to judge whether there have been improvements since the last assessment or therapeutic intervention.

Figures 6–1 and 6–2 illustrate some of the tools that are helpful for assessing pain severity. Visual analog scales are particularly useful for patients who have difficulty verbally responding, children, and those with cognitive limitations that hinder comprehension. The most common tool used is a linear scale (Fig. 6–1) consisting of a line 10 cm in

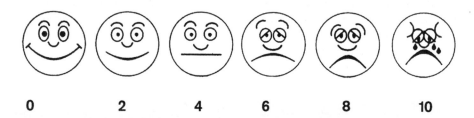

Figure 6–2. Wong/Baker Faces Rating Scale. This measure uses faces to pictorially represent the severity of a patient's pain. This was originally developed for pediatric patients, and has also been found to be very useful in the elderly as well as patients who have difficulty reading. Numerical values (0–10) have been assigned to each face to allow for compatibility with the 0 to 10 Numerical Scale.

SOURCE: Reproduced, with permission, from Hockenbury MJ, Wilson D: *Wong's Essentials of Pediatric Nursing*, 8th ed. St. Louis, MO, Mosby, 2009.

length with or without marked gradations (0–10). The line may be augmented by a color chart with cool colors (blue) representing the lowest levels of pain and hot colors (red) the highest pain levels. Patients who are able to write mark the line at the point that corresponds to their perception of the severity of the pain. Alternatively, patients may verbally express their estimate of pain severity using the line scale to guide their response.

For children, or for patients with difficulty reading numbers or understanding numerical concepts, the Wong/Baker Faces Rating Scale (Fig. 6–2) allows the patient to point to the face that best represents the severity of the pain. The clinician may then correlate the face with the 0 to 10 numerical scale.

Regardless of the method used to rate the severity of pain, it is essential that pain severity be measured as regularly as any other vital sign. All clinicians within an institution or group practice should use the same scale and criteria to promote consistency and continuity of care.

T: The "T" stands for Temporal. Understanding the pattern of pain experienced over time helps differentiate acute from chronic pain, provides clues to the etiology and a framework for scheduling specific interventions. For example, a patient who complains of muscle stiffness and pain on awakening may require extra medication at bedtime and benefit from a new mattress or from a different sleeping position. Increased pain late in the afternoon, coincident with the return home of a spouse or caregiver, might suggest that the pain has psychosocial components that require exploration and counseling rather than an increase in analgesia.

PSYCHOSOCIAL, SPIRITUAL, AND FAMILY HISTORY A social history and a family history adapted to the special circumstances of terminal illness can add valuable information to the pain assessment. Knowledge about the patient's occupation or recreational interests might help the clinician better understand, for example, why a man with meticulous habits who loved opera, stopped attending performances after undergoing a colostomy, with the explanation that he now suffers from constant abdominal pain. A family history emphasizing relationships can be instrumental in analyzing the difficult to control symptoms of a patient who, dying of advanced alcoholic cirrhosis, has not talked to his estranged daughter since her wedding years earlier, which he had missed due to a drinking binge.

The perception of pain can be influenced by a wide variety of psychosocial, familial, and spiritual issues, which, if left unaddressed, can interfere with the efficacy of analgesics. There is ample evidence that anxiety, sleeplessness, anger, fear, fright, depression, discomfort, isolation, and loneliness can all lower the pain threshold and decrease the patient's ability to cope with discomfort that might be tolerable under other circumstances (see Table 6–7).

MEDICATION HISTORY A complete medication history is crucial. Knowledge of all medications currently or previously in use, assessment of their efficacy and potential for drug interactions, and a determination as to whether treatment meets proper standards of care are critical for deciding the next steps in the patient's pharmacological management. The medication history should include over-the-counter (OTC) medications and information about recreational drug use and substance abuse.

Physical Examination

For the purposes of pain assessment, the physical examination should focus on painful areas and potential etiologies and include a thorough neurological evaluation. Assessment of pain in the neck or back requires a full motor, sensory, and reflex examination to identify spinal cord lesions and plexopathies. Patients with headaches or skull pain should be checked for possible cranial nerve defects that are characteristically found in certain well-defined cranial pain syndromes. Dermatological inspection should be performed to look for herpes zoster or skin breakdown. A

TABLE 6–7. Factors Affecting the Pain Threshold

EFFECT ON THRESHOLD	EFFECT ON PATIENT'S PERCEPTION OF PAIN	FACTORS
Lower	Increased severity	Poor pain control
		Depression
		Anxiety
		Sleeplessness
		Anger
		Fear
		Fright
		Isolation
		Loneliness
Raise	Decreased severity	Good pain control
		Treatment of depression
		Reduced anxiety
		Sleep
		Rest
		Distraction
		Empathy
		Sympathy

complaint of oral pain should prompt a dental examination (dentures also) as well as inspection of the oropharyngeal mucosa. The patient's environment should be inspected to identify uncomfortable furniture or other factors that may contribute to the patient's pain.

The physical examination is particularly important when evaluating pain in patients with cognitive impairment and in patients who are unwilling or unable to communicate verbally. Nonverbal phenomena such as gestures, facial expressions, guarding, restricted movement, and flinching that are observed in the course of physical contact with the patient may signal the presence of pain even in confused and disoriented individuals.

Establish a Pain Diagnosis or Diagnoses

Pain may be of single or multifocal origin and may be attributable to the primary disease process it-

self or the result of previous treatment such as chemotherapy or radiotherapy. If the pain diagnosis is not evident from the history and physical examination, it is occasionally necessary to perform various diagnostic studies, even in patients with advanced illnesses. Indications for the use of diagnostic studies in end-of-life care are discussed in Chapter 18. A complete pain diagnosis also identifies those psychosocial, emotional, spiritual, and financial issues that may modulate the patient's perception of pain.

Institute an Appropriate Plan of Care Based on the Pain Assessment

Although the remainder of this chapter is devoted to treatment strategies for physical pain, it is important to note that there are significant nonphysical influences on the perception of pain. Palliative care clinicians have redefined what is commonly referred to as "pain" with terms such

TABLE 6–8. Factors that Affect a Patient's Perception of Total Pain and Suffering

An individual's basic psychological make-up

Loss of work

Social isolation

Physical disability

Change in social and familial roles and relationships

Fear of death

Cultural, ethnic, and religious beliefs and morés

Financial concerns

as "total pain" or "suffering." These latter terms refer to the combination of physical, psychosocial, financial, and spiritual components that converge to produce the sensation that the patient complains of as "pain."

Some components of "total pain" or "suffering" that influence a patient's perception of pain can be found in Table 6–8. Addressing these issues can help increase a patient's pain threshold and render the physical pain more responsive to both the pharmacological and nonpharmacological interventions in the plan of care.

In light of the complexity of the challenge, it is prudent to acknowledge that no single health care professional possesses the expertise and skills needed to manage all of the physical and non-physical causes of pain. This is confirmed by the success of the hospice model of care. The structure of the hospice interdisciplinary team, which includes not only physicians, nurses, pharmacists, and home health aides (to address the physical symptoms and provide pharmacological management) but also social workers, chaplains, and volunteers (to address the psychosocial and spiritual needs), increases the likelihood the patient will benefit from "total pain" management. (See Chapter 4 for a discussion of how the interdisciplinary team functions to provide care to patients at the end of life.)

Directly Involve the Patient and/or Primary Caregivers

Regardless of the details of the treatment program, be careful to fully explain your findings and recommendations to the patient and/or to the primary caregivers and involve the patient directly in the management effort. Instead of just telling the patient what to do, ask whether the proposed plan makes sense, and seek the patient's consent to be a partner in its implementation. By asking the patient for permission to treat, you are offering a degree of control, an action that may in itself be therapeutic.

Reach agreement with the patient on the goals of the treatment plan, and establish a realistic time frame for their accomplishment. For example, to avoid discouragement and premature abandonment of the course of treatment, patients should be aware that neuropathic pain usually responds less quickly to analgesic therapy than nociceptive pain. Establish a schedule for regular follow-up visits. Reassess the patient's pain frequently; anticipate incident pain (e.g., increased pain associated with a particular activity); and monitor the patient for breakthrough pain, loss of pain control, or the development of new pain due to other causes. Be on the alert for side effects of therapy and initiate prophylactic treatment for expected adverse effects, such as opioid-related constipation.

Document the Pain Assessment

Detailed and comprehensive documentation of the pain assessment is essential to ensure effective communication with other caregivers and to create a baseline reference for future assessments. Using a standard pain assessment tool (Fig. 6–3) is a good way to ensure uniform documentation. The body chart is an important component of the pain assessment tool because it clearly illustrates the loci of pain and allows for the depiction of pain radiation. Furthermore, by asking the patient to help complete or review the body chart, the clinician creates an opportunity to involve the patient in his or her own care.

PAIN

	LOCATION:	1._____	2._____
P	PALLIATION:	1._____	2._____
	PROVOCATON:	1._____	2._____
Q	QUALITY:	1._____	2._____
R	RADIATION:	1._____	2._____
S	SEVERITY (0–10):	1._____	2._____
T	TEMPORAL: ONSET	1._____	2._____
	PATTERN	1._____	2._____

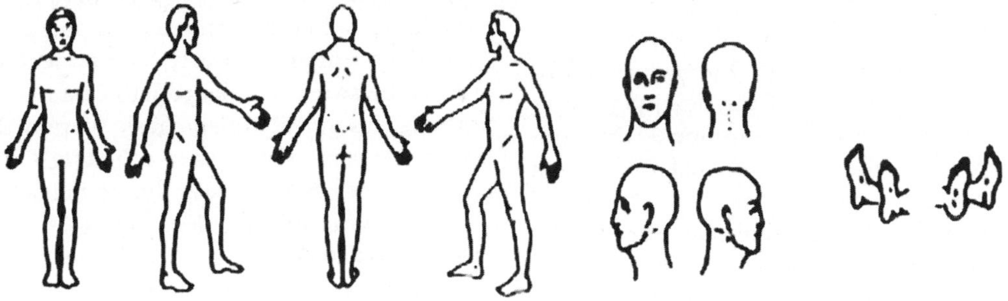

PATIENT'S PERCEPTION OF PAIN: _____

PRESENT MED.: _____ AMOUNT:_____ SCHEDULE: ____ STARTED: _____ ADEQUATE: ☐ YES ☐ NO

PAST MED.: _____ AMOUNT:_____ SCHEDULE: ____ HOW LONG TRIED: _____

REASON FOR STOPPING: ☐ NAUSEA ☐ CONSTIPATION ☐ SEDATION ☐ ITCHING ☐ DIDN'T CONTROL PAIN

HISTORY OF DRUG OR ALCOHOL USE: ☐ YES ☐ NO

Figure 6–3. Pain assessment tool.

Source: Adapted, with permission, from Kinzbrunner BM: *Vitas Pain Management Guidelines*. Miami, FL, Vitas Healthcare Corporation, 1999.

PHARMACOLOGICAL TREATMENT OF PAIN

Although nonpharmacological interventions deserve careful consideration in a comprehensive treatment plan for pain (see below), in Western medicine these techniques are generally regarded as complementary to pharmacological intervention, particularly in the context of end-of-life care. Expert knowledge in the use of analgesic drugs is essential for any clinician who cares for terminally ill patients, and alacrity in seeking appropriate consultation for difficult cases is highly recommended. Hospice medical directors, physicians who are certified in hospice and palliative medicine, and other trained pain specialists are available for consultation in most communities in the United States.

GUIDELINES FOR PHARMACOLOGICAL TREATMENT OF PAIN

Guidelines for the pharmacological treatment of pain are listed in Table 6–9 and are discussed below.

Develop a Medication Armamentarium

Effective pain management is best served by developing expert familiarity with two to three drugs within each class of analgesic agents and building on a base of personal clinical experience with this limited drug armamentarium.

Medication Selection: Patient-Specific Considerations

PRIOR EXPERIENCES AND MEDICATION HISTORY The choice of an optimal analgesic regimen must be adapted to meet the needs and requirements

TABLE 6–9. Guidelines for the Pharmacological Treatment of Pain

I. Develop a basic, generally applicable, drug armamentarium.
II. Drug selection should be based on consideration of the individual patient as well as the type and degree of pain.
  A. Patient considerations
    1. Prior experiences and drug history
      a. Prior response and adverse effects
      b. Allergies
      c. Substance abuse
    2. Physical condition and metabolic state
    3. Prognostic assessment
    4. Acceptability to patient and family
    5. Logistical considerations
    6. Expense
  B. Drug-specific considerations
    1. Use specific type of drug for a specific type of pain.
    2. Know the pharmacology of the drug(s) prescribed.
      a. Achieve maximum benefit at lowest effective dose with fewest side effects.
      b. Titrate to effect.
      c. Choose the least invasive and most physiologically sound route of administration.
      d. Select the most convenient schedule of administration.
    3. Anticipate and treat complications and side effects.
    4. Prevent acute withdrawal and the development of tolerance.
    5. Use adjuvant drug combinations to provide additive analgesia and to reduce side effects.
    6. Be aware of drug interactions.
    7. Believe the patient:
      a. Work with the patient with a history of substance abuse.
      b. Avoid pseudoaddiction.

of each individual patient. Information about the patient's prior experiences and a complete medication history should have been obtained during the process of pain assessment. Crucial information includes identification of agents that have been effective, as well as their dosages, routes, and schedules. The assessment should also identify allegedly ineffective agents, reasons for lack of efficacy, and a record of adverse reactions and side effects. A detailed investigation of medication "allergies" is important as patients frequently attribute adverse side effects such as opioid-induced constipation and nausea, or morphine-associated, histamine-mediated pruritus to "allergy," although true immunologic hypersensitivity to opioids is rare. It is very important to properly educate patients and their families so that unfounded concern about allergic reactions does not become a barrier to optimal pain management.

Although the incidence of iatrogenic addiction in patients with no prior personal or family history of substance abuse is negligible, significant numbers of patients in need of pain management may be active or recovered substance abusers. (The challenges of managing these patients will be addressed in the section entitled "Pain Management in the Patient with Previous or Current Substance Abuse.")

PHYSICAL CONDITION AND METABOLIC IMPAIRMENT   The overall physical condition of the patient may restrict and limit pharmacological options. The oral route, for example, may not be suitable when patients have severe dysphagia; a high risk of aspiration; or suffer from esophageal, gastric, or small bowel obstruction. Transdermal fentanyl may be a poor choice in severely cachectic patients who lack subcutaneous fat depots. Renal impairment often precludes the use of nonsteroidal anti-inflammatory drugs (NSAIDs) and may affect the dose and schedule of administration for opioids such as morphine and oxycodone whose active metabolites are renally excreted. For patients with severe renal insufficiency, hydromorphone, rather than morphine, may be the opioid of choice. On the other hand, morphine is preferable to other opioids for patients with hepatic impairment. Methadone, levorphanol, pentazocine, propoxyphene, and meperidine (Demerol) can cause CNS depression that mimics hepatic encephalopathy in patients with poor liver function, and oxycodone must be used with caution when patients have severe liver impairment. Nonopioid analgesics or adjuvant drugs that should be avoided when patients have liver disease include acetaminophen and TCAs.

In dying patients, the use of morphine for the palliation of terminal dyspnea is well documented in the literature. (See Chapter 7 for further discussion.) As already discussed (in the section "Fear of Opioid-Induced Respiratory Depression and Premature Death") above, concern for clinically significant respiratory depression should not generally be an obstacle to effective pain management with opioid agonist agents, even for patients with severe chronic hypoxia whose ventilatory drive depends heavily on the response to CO_2. Clinical experience with COPD patients shows that when low starting doses of morphine are gradually titrated upward as needed to control pain, the risk of respiratory depression or arrest is negligible. Recent studies using strong opioids in palliative care patients with dyspnea demonstrated the efficacy of relieving dyspnea in this patient population without causing respiratory depression.

PROGNOSTIC FACTORS   During the last few days of life, the principle that pain management should aim at maximal analgesia with minimal sedation may not necessarily be relevant. At this point in the patient's course, when pain and multiple other symptoms may be particularly difficult to control, and may be accompanied by marked agitation, the balance between competing desires for alertness and pain control may shift. As patients near death, and systemic organ dysfunction and metabolic failure ensue, dosage requirements for opioid medications may decrease, with a corresponding increase in opioid side effects. In these circumstances, fractional decreases in opioid dose or treatment of opioid-induced side effects are appropriate. However, opioids should not be abruptly or totally discontinued. Because of physiological dependence, abrupt cessation of opioids will almost certainly provoke significant withdrawal symptoms that will compound terminal suffering.

ACCEPTABILITY TO PATIENT AND FAMILY As previously discussed, patient resistance to the use of opioids is a significant barrier to optimal pain management. This behavior, known as "opiophobia," may sometimes be restricted to a single agent (most commonly morphine), in which case, selection of other opioid agonists may enhance patient acceptance. However, some patients may refuse all pharmacological analgesia because of fear of side effects, denial, or due to a belief that pain is, in some way, either deserved or ennobling. These patients require intensive education and psychosocial interventions.

Input from primary caregivers and family members may also be critical to the choice of analgesic agents. Family members may sometimes minimize pain and other symptoms, even to the point of disbelieving the patient's complaints. Caregivers may withhold prescribed analgesics, decrease the dosage, or prolong the interval between doses. Regimens that call for frequent administration of short-acting analgesics may interfere with sleep, disrupt family schedules, and be challenging to maintain. In these circumstances, sustained-release analgesics may offer a compliance advantage. Knowledge or suspicion of drug diversion by relatives or friends may also influence the choice and route of administration of analgesics, particularly those that are regulated as controlled substances.

EXPENSE Although expense should not be the prime element in choosing medication or other interventions at the end of life, neither should it be ignored, particularly when less expensive equipotent regimens are available. Although a cost-analysis of opioid analgesics is outside the scope of this chapter, prescribers should

be aware of the availability of generic formulations and have a general understanding of cost-effectiveness. Prudent pharmacoeconomic management can conserve limited resources, expand the circle of patients receiving optimal end-of-life care, and alleviate a major source of anxiety for terminal patients and their families who are, all too often, under considerable financial pressure.

Medication Selection: Medication-Specific Considerations

USE A SPECIFIC TYPE OF DRUG FOR A SPECIFIC TYPE OF PAIN The WHO recommends a three-step "ladder" guideline that provides for incremental analgesic increases based on the severity of a patient's pain (Fig. 6–4). This approach was included in the 1994 clinical practice guidelines of the Agency for Health Care Policy Research (AHCPR) for the management of cancer pain and is generally accepted as a guideline for treating pain in patients with terminal nonmalignant diseases as well. Following a thorough pain assessment (see earlier), patients may rate their pain as either mild (severity scale 1–3), moderate (severity scale 4–6), or severe (severity scale 7–10). Appropriate analgesic medication is then selected on the basis of this determination. Unlike a traditional "step ladder" (e.g., for hypertension), where treatment is usually started at the lowest rung and progressively intensified until the desired level of response is achieved, the WHO analgesic ladder is accessed at whatever level best represents the patient's pain on presentation. If a patient presents with a pain severity level of 9, treatment is initiated with a strong opioid per step 3 of the ladder, rather than with medications that are appropriate for step 1.

The WHO analgesic ladder favors the least invasive routes of administration and presupposes that appropriate nonopioid analgesics and adjuvant medications (e.g., acetaminophen, NSAIDs, corticosteroids, antidepressants, anticonvulsants) will be continued, if indicated, at all levels of the ladder. Should a patient advance from step 1 to step 3 because of progressive pain,

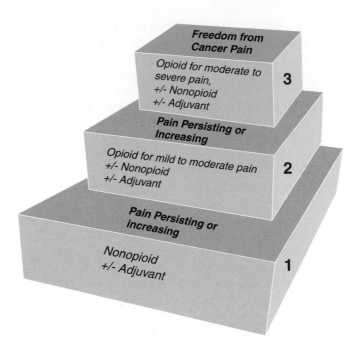

Figure 6–4. The World Health Organization (WHO) analgesic ladder.

Source: WHO's pain ladder. World Health Organization. http://www.who.int/cancer/palliative/painladder/en/. Accessed March 16, 2010.

nonopioid and adjuvant medications should not be discontinued (unless for reasons of toxicity) merely because a strong opioid is now prescribed. Step 2 is considered "weaker" than step 3 because it includes fixed combinations of an opioid and a nonopioid (e.g., oxycodone and acetaminophen) that cannot be significantly escalated because of toxicity attributable to the nonopioid component.

Step 1: Mild Pain (Severity Scale 1–3) Nonopioid analgesics, recommended for the treatment of mild pain, include acetaminophen and the NSAIDs, of which aspirin is the prototype. Some of the agents more commonly used to treat patients near the end of life are listed in Table 6–10.

Acetaminophen Acetaminophen is currently the most widely recommended nonopioid analgesic for mild pain and is often used in combination with opioid analgesics such as codeine, oxycodone, and hydrocodone for patients with moderate pain. Acetaminophen has analgesic and antipyretic properties. However, it is not an anti-inflammatory agent, a point that should be remembered when selecting medication for patients whose pain is largely mediated by inflammatory cytokines (e.g., bone metastases). Acetaminophen is generally well tolerated and has a safety profile sufficient to allow government authorized use as a nonprescription drug. It is frequently found in combination with other medications and packaged as a component of multiple OTC preparations for colds, nasal congestion, cough, gastrointestinal upset, and insomnia. Because the public regards these widespread acetaminophen combination products as innocuous, patients may use multiple preparations

TABLE 6–10. Step 1 Analgesics		
MEDICATION	**ROUTES OF ADMINISTRATION**	**DOSAGE RANGE**
Acetaminophen	PO, PR	325–650 mg q 4–6 h
Choline magnesium trisalicylate	PO	500–1,500 mg 2–3 times/d
Ibuprofen	PO	200–800 mg q 4–6 h
Indomethacin	PO, PR	25–50 mg 2–4 times/d
Naproxen	PO	250 mg q 6–8 h
Piroxicam	PO	20 mg daily

simultaneously and in conjunction with prescribed medications. Therefore, to avoid acetaminophen toxicity, it is important to have full knowledge of *all* medications taken by the patient.

Hepatotoxicity, including progressive, irreversible hepatic failure, is the major dose-limiting toxicity. For patients with normal liver function, it is usually recommended that the total daily acetaminophen dose should not exceed 4 g. For patients with impaired liver function, a lower total daily allowance may be advisable, especially when prolonged chronic use is compounded by alcohol abuse. With prolonged use, acetaminophen may also cause phenacetin-like nephrotoxicity. Although this is unusual, particularly in the context of terminal illness, it is a point worth considering for patients with a relatively long prognosis and marginal renal function.

NSAIDs   NSAIDs are the other major class of agents used to treat mild pain. As the name suggests, in addition to analgesic and antipyretic properties, NSAIDs have anti-inflammatory effects due to their inhibition of cyclooxygenase (COX)-mediated prostaglandin synthesis. Among these agents, aspirin, like acetaminophen, is often combined with codeine or oxycodone to treat moderate pain. However, in terminally ill patients, aspirin and aspirin-containing preparations are usually avoided because of an enhanced likelihood of gastrointestinal toxicity and bleed-

ing. A more generalized bleeding diathesis associated with aspirin treatment is attributed to impaired platelet function caused by irreversible acetylation of platelet surface glycoproteins. At analgesic doses, this effect supersedes aspirin-induced reversible inhibition of platelet COX-1, a phenomenon responsible for the vascular cardioprotective effects of low-dose aspirin therapy and one that is common to all NSAIDs. Because of the risk of clinically significant bleeding, aspirin is particularly to be avoided in patients with thrombocytopenia, whether due to advanced disease or secondary to prior chemotherapy or radiotherapy.

The nonacetylated salicylates, including salsalate, choline magnesium trisalicylate, and diflunisal, have less gastrointestinal toxicity than do aspirin and are less inhibitory to platelet function. Some of these products are inconvenient because of large tablet size and the need to ingest many tablets with each dose.

Other commonly used NSAIDs, some of which are available OTC in doses usually lower than those restricted to prescription only, include ibuprofen, naproxen, and indomethacin. Although most of these short-acting NSAIDs exert analgesic effects within hours of initiating treatment, it may require 1 to 2 weeks of sustained therapy to achieve a maximal effect. Because of structural biochemical differences, one should not assume crossresistance among different NSAID classes, and, should the patient fail to respond positively to one NSAID, trial of another from a different category should not be precluded. However, combination therapy with more than one NSAID is not recommended because of additive adverse reactions.

Ibuprofen and naproxen are generally better tolerated than aspirin and are also available in fixed combinations with opioid analgesics. Indomethacin and naproxen are available as sustained-release preparations suitable for twice a day and three times a day dosing. Piroxicam is an NSAID in capsule form that is long-acting and may be given in one daily dose. Ketorolac is often effective for managing acute inflammatory pain, especially when given parenterally. However, because of the high risk of gastrointestinal and renal toxicity, ketorolac is contraindicated for chronic use, and it should be administered for not more than 5 consecutive days or in not more than 20 doses. For patients who cannot swallow pills, there are liquid preparations of choline magnesium trisalicylate, ibuprofen, naproxen, and acetaminophen. Indomethacin, aspirin, and acetaminophen may also be administered as rectal suppositories.

Although individuals may respond variably to different NSAIDs, there is little evidence that any one of the estimated 20 to 30 NSAID products available has greater analgesic efficacy than any other, when prescribed in equivalent dosage. However, there may be significant differences in toxicity profiles, presumably based on differential inhibition of the COX isoforms, COX-1 and COX-2. COX-1 is a ubiquitous, constitutive isoenzyme producing prostaglandins necessary for homeostatic functions, such as maintenance of gastrointestinal mucosal integrity. COX-2 is believed to be largely induced and upregulated by inflammatory cytokines, producing prostaglandins that mediate pain and inflammation. However, COX-2 is also thought to have significant constitutive, noninflammatory functions including ulcer healing, intravascular volume regulation, and regulation of bone remodeling. It is believed that the therapeutic effects of all conventional NSAIDs relate to inhibition of COX-2, whereas the adverse effects, particularly gastrointestinal toxicity, are caused by inhibition of COX-1 activity.

Early studies of the specific COX-2 inhibitor NSAIDs rofecoxib and celecoxib suggested a significant decrease in NSAID gastrointestinal and renal toxicity without loss of therapeutic efficacy. However, in recent years, significant concerns about increased risk of cardiovascular events led both rofecoxib and valdecoxib to be taken off the market. The Food and Drug Administration (FDA) also required a black box warning for celecoxib, and trials of newer COX-2 inhibitors have been extended to investigate cardiovascular safety.

Regardless of toxicity profiles, NSAIDs, even those with COX-2 specificity, appear to have ceiling effects regarding analgesic efficacy. Thus, as chronic pain becomes increasingly severe, acetaminophen and NSAIDs, which relieve pain primarily through peripheral mechanisms, are employed best when combined synergistically with opioid analgesics that have both central and peripheral activity.

Step 2: Moderate Pain (Severity Scale 4–6)
Most agents used to treat moderate pain are combinations of opioids and step 1 agents. The agents most commonly used to treat patients near the end of life are listed in Table 6–11 and are dominated by combinations of acetaminophen with codeine, oxycodone, or hydrocodone. The popularity of these agents stems from the fact that unlike their single-agent opioid counterparts, the combination products are not schedule II controlled substances and, therefore, are not subject to the same prescribing regulations as single opioid preparations are in states with triplicate prescription programs.

Along with the acetaminophen combinations, opioids are available in combination with aspirin and ibuprofen. Aspirin combination products are generally not prescribed to patients near the end of life because of the increased risk of gastrointestinal toxicity and bleeding regarding aspirin (see above). Ibuprofen combination products

TABLE 6–11. Step 2 Analgesics

MEDICATION	COMPONENTS	DOSAGE RANGE
Codeine with acetaminophen	Acetaminophen 300 mg (cap) or 325 mg (tab) with: #2 Codeine 15 mg #3 Codeine 30 mg #4 Codeine 60 mg	One to two tablets or capsules every 4–6 h
	Acetaminophen 500 mg or 600 mg with codeine 30 mg (tab)	One to two tablets or capsules every 4–6 h
	Acetaminophen 120 mg with codeine 12 mg per 5 mL	10–20 mL every 4–6 h
Oxycodone with acetaminophen	Acetaminophen 325 mg with: Oxycodone 2.5 mg Oxycodone 5 mg	One to two tablets or capsules every 4–6 h
	Acetaminophen 325 or 500 mg with Oxycodone 7.5 mg Acetaminophen 325 or 600 mg with Oxycodone 10 mg	One to two tablets or capsules every 4–6 h
	Acetaminophen 325 mg with Oxycodone 5 mg per 5 mL	5–10 mL every 4–6 h
Oxycodone with ibuprofen	Ibuprofen 400 mg with oxycodone 5 mg	
Hydrocodone with acetaminophen	Acetaminophen 500 mg with: Hydrocodone 2.5 mg Hydrocodone 5 mg Hydrocodone 7.5 mg Hydrocodone 10 mg	One to two tablets or capsules every 4–6 h
	Acetaminophen 650 mg with: Hydrocodone 7.5 mg Hydrocodone 10 mg	One to two tablets or capsules every 4–6 h
	Acetaminophen 167 mg with hydrocodone 2.5 mg per 5 mL	5–10 mL every 4–6 h
Hydrocodone with ibuprofen	Ibuprofen 200 mg with hydrocodone 7.5 mg	One tablet every 4–6 h
Tramadol	Extended-release 100, 200, and 300 mg tablets (Ultram)	Up to 300 mg PO daily

(with hydrocodone and oxycodone) were created to take advantage of the anti-inflammatory effects common to both aspirin and ibuprofen while avoiding the increased risk of bleeding associated with aspirin.

The dose-limiting property of these products generally relates to the acetaminophen, aspirin, or ibuprofen, not the opioid component. In view of the potential for acetaminophen toxicity (see above), dosing of the acetaminophen-containing agents should be limited to not more than two tablets every 4 hours. Patients should also be warned to avoid other acetaminophen-containing products (which are commonly available OTC). In addition, a ceiling effect further limits the use of codeine combination products. When codeine is administered in doses greater than 65 mg every 4 hours, side effects increase without any gain in analgesic efficacy. In addition to concerns about acetaminophen toxicity, these combination agents can cause typical opioid side effects including constipation, nausea, vomiting, drowsiness, and dysphoria, especially in opioid-naïve patients. (See section entitled Anticipate and Treat Complications and Side Effects.)

Propoxyphene is a synthetic analgesic, structurally related to methadone, and often prescribed, typically in combination with acetaminophen, for the treatment of mild to moderate pain. Propoxyphene binds to opioid receptors but was originally believed to be free of potential for substance abuse. This has not proven to be the case. Furthermore, 65 mg of propoxyphene is, at best, equivalent in analgesic potency to 650 mg of acetaminophen, although there may be some synergy when used in combination. Propoxyphene crosses the blood–brain barrier and is also metabolized by the liver to norpropoxyphene, a highly neuroexcitatory, proconvulsant compound. Furthermore, propoxyphene has the potential to cause lidocaine-like cardiotoxic effects. Because there are ample equivalent or better analgesic alternatives with fewer side effects, propoxyphene combinations are not recommended for the management of pain in terminally ill patients, especially for elderly patients for whom propoxyphene may be particularly dangerous.

Tramadol is a synthetic, centrally acting, analgesic that possesses both opioid and nonopioid properties. It is a nonscheduled drug and available in oral and injectable formulations as well as in combination with acetaminophen. For chronic pain, tramadol has analgesic potency roughly equivalent to codeine on a per milligram basis. Because of reports of seizures in patients receiving tramadol even within the recommended dosage range, the use of immediate-release tramadol preparations is limited to acute pain, when less than five days of treatment is required. Thus, there is little role for immediate-release tramadol in patients at the end of life. However, extended-release tramadol may be appropriate for patients with moderate pain. Daily doses of tramadol exceeding 300 mg are not recommended for patients older than 75 years. Tramadol is not recommended for patients with creatinine clearance of less than 30 mL/min or severe hepatic impairment.

Step 3: Severe Pain (Severity Scale 7–10)

For treatment of severe pain, opioid agonist drugs, such as morphine, are the medications of choice. It is important to remember that to achieve pain control, adjunctive medications and other measures may be required in addition to opioid analgesics.

Mechanism of opioid action   The mechanism of opioid analgesia is related to the binding of opioid molecules to specific receptors in the brain, spinal cord, intestinal tract, and peripheral nervous system. Opioid receptors are embedded within synaptic membranes. Formation of the opioid–receptor complex influences a number of neurotransmitter events including decreased levels of norepinephrine and dopamine.

The opioid receptors, classified as *mu* (μ), *kappa* (κ), and *delta* (δ) are targets for the endogenous opioid peptides (enkephalins, dynorphins, β-endorphins) as well as the exogenous opioid analgesic drugs. Although analgesia is associated with *mu, kappa,* and *delta* receptors, only *mu* and *kappa* binding appear relevant to analgesic drugs used in clinical practice. Responses to activation of the *kappa* receptor include spinal analgesia as well as sedation, dysphoria, and miosis. *Mu* receptors are found at the spinal and supraspinal levels and peripherally in skin, joints, and gastrointestinal tract. Activation of the *mu* receptor produces analgesia as well as dysphoria, euphoria, respiratory depression, sedation, constipation, urinary retention, and drug dependence. In laboratory mice lacking a specific opioid recep-

TABLE 6–12. Classification of Opioids Based on Receptor Interactions

RECEPTOR	CLASSIFICATION	MEDICATIONS	RESPONSES
Mu	Agonist	Fentanyl Hydromorphone Methadone Morphine Oxycodone Oxymorphone	Supraspinal analgesia, constipation, urinary retention, dysphoria, euphoria, sedation, respiratory depression, drug dependence
	Partial agonist	Buprenorphine	
	Weak agonist	Meperidine	
	Antagonist	Naloxone Nalbuphine Pentazocine	Reverses opioid effects Withdrawal reaction in patients with physiologic opioid dependency
Kappa	Agonist	Nalbuphine Oxycodone Pentazocine	Spinal analgesia, sedation, dysphoria, miosis
	Weak agonist	Levorphanol Meperidine Methadone Morphine	
	Antagonist	Naloxone Buprenorphine	Reverses opioid effects Withdrawal reaction in patients with physiologic opioid dependency

tor (gene "knock-outs"), analgesia and all other effects associated with that receptor are not observed. Curiously, these knock-out mice appear to develop and live normally despite their lack of opioid receptors, leading to the paradox that although opioid receptors may not be necessary for functional living (at least in mice!), they are nonetheless instrumental in achieving pain control at the end of life.

Table 6–12 lists many of the commonly available opioids on the basis of their primary site of action. Opioids are classified as agonist, partial agonist, or mixed agonist–antagonist medications. An agonist drug, such as morphine, binds with its receptor(s) to activate and elicit a maximum response, whereas a partial agonist produces only a partial response. A mixed agonist–antagonist substance produces mixed effects; that is, it will activate one type of receptor but will block another type of receptor. Opioid agonist–antagonist drugs, such as pentazocine, have analgesic activity by virtue of binding to the *kappa* receptor but also have *sigma* receptor activity associated with undesirable psychotomimetic effects such as dysphoria, hallucinations, and confusion. Because of this dual activity, mixed agonist–antagonist drugs have a dose-related ceiling. Agonist–antagonist medications may also cause an acute withdrawal reaction and reverse opioid analgesia causing enhanced pain if administered to opioid-dependent patients or if given concurrently with an opioid agonist. For these reasons, partial agonist and agonist–antagonist opioid drugs are not recommended for managing chronic pain, particularly in terminally ill patients.

Morphine Among the opioid agonists, morphine is the prototypical agent and the standard to which others are compared. Morphine continues to be the drug of choice for the treatment of severe pain for most terminally ill patients because its pharmacology and pharmacokinetics are very well defined, and it may be administered by one of several routes. These include (a) orally as immediate-release liquid solution, tablets, and capsules, or as sustained-release tablets or capsules; (b) rectally as a suppository or in gelatin capsules; (c) subcutaneously or intravenously; or (d) via epidural, intrathecal, or intraventricular routes. (Morphine may also be administered in a nebulized form via inhalation for the treatment of dyspnea, as discussed in Chapter 7. However, due to poor systemic absorption [16% bioavailability] by this route, it is not an effective route of administration for the treatment of pain.)

Morphine is rapidly absorbed via the gastrointestinal tract with peak plasma concentrations of free morphine occurring 15 to 30 minutes after oral administration of immediate-release products. The rapidity of absorption means that it is rarely necessary for patients with chronic pain to receive morphine intravenously solely for the purpose of accelerating the onset of analgesia. Because of first-pass metabolism by the liver and intestine following an oral dose, only approximately 40% of ingested morphine reaches the systemic circulation. As a result of differences in presystemic elimination, marked variations in bioavailability occur from patient to patient and dosage titration must be individualized. Therefore, there is no standard effective dose for oral morphine. Some patients may achieve pain relief with milligram doses, whereas others may require tens, hundreds, or rarely, even thousands of milligrams with each dose.

Morphine is metabolized by the liver into morphine-3-glucuronide (M3G) (80%) and morphine-6-glucuronide (M6G) (15%). M3G is inactive at opioid receptors and provides no analgesic activity. However, it has been reported to have CNS stimulatory effects that contribute to opioid toxicity, side effects, and the development of tolerance, although these findings have not been consistently reproducible. The other by-product of glucuronidation, M6G, is pharmacologically active with significant analgesic potency, with some authors suggesting that M6G contributes up to 85% of the analgesic effects of morphine. Morphine blood levels are virtually undetectable 6 hours after a single oral dose, and the elimination of free morphine is unchanged in patients with impaired renal function. However, M3G and M6G blood levels remain elevated 12 hours after a single morphine dose, creating a risk of toxicity because of the accumulation of M6G. The elimination of these metabolites is markedly prolonged with renal insufficiency. Other metabolites of morphine, including normorphine and 6-monoacetylmorphine, bind to opioid receptors and may play smaller roles in the development of opioid toxicity.

Other opioids   As mentioned above, morphine is the classical opioid agonist and the prototype to which all others are compared. In addition to morphine, the clinician should be familiar with the pharmacology of several other commonly available opioid analgesics. This will allow for the effective pain management of patients who have allergic reactions, or develop intolerable side effects (see below) or tolerance (see below) to morphine. Like morphine, some opioids, including oxycodone and hydrocodone, are hydrophilic and are metabolized by the liver (undergoing significant first-pass effects) and predominantly excreted by the kidney. Lipophilic opioids, such as fentanyl and methadone, are also metabolized by the liver but have no known active metabolites. Fentanyl and its metabolites are primarily excreted by the kidney, whereas methadone and its metabolites are equally excreted by the kidney and in the stool.

Table 6–13 lists some of the most commonly used alternative opioids and compares each to morphine. Included in this table are the bioequivalence ratios between oral and parenteral forms of the different medications (where applicable) as well the ratios between the oral form of each medication and oral morphine. The use of these

TABLE 6–13. Equianalgesic Conversion Table

ANALGESIC	ORAL DOSE (mg)	PARENTERAL DOSE (mg)	DURATION OF ACTION (h)	HALF-LIFE (h)	ORAL TO PARENTERAL RATIO	ORAL MORPHINE TO ANALGESIC RATIO
Agonists						
Morphine	30*	10	4–6	2–4	3:1*	1:1
Oxycodone	20†	—	3–5	4–5	—	1.5:1†
Hydromorphone	7.5	1.5	3–4	2–3	5:1	4:1
Fentanyl	—					See Table 6–16
Levorphanol	4	2	4–6	12–16	2:1	7.5:1
Methadone	Variable‡,§					See Table 6–17
Codeine	200¶	130	4–6	3	1.5:1	1:7
Hydrocodone	200	—	3–6	3–4	—	1:7
Oxymorphone	6**	1	3–6	2–3	6:1	5:1
Meperidine††	300	75	2–4	2–3	4:1	1:10

*This dose of morphine is based on chronic use.

†There are some investigators who have reported that 30 mg of oxycodone is equivalent to 30 mg of morphine (ratio 1:1).

‡The equivalent dose of methadone in chronic use has been shown to vary according to previously administered opioid doses.

§Recent studies indicate that methadone's potency increases as previous total daily morphine doses increase. Dose ratios from 8:1 to 14:1 have been reported when previous daily morphine doses exceeded 300 mg. Lower equivalent dose ratios of 3:1 to 6:1 have been demonstrated with lower morphine doses and individual titration at all doses is therefore recommended.

¶Codeine has a ceiling dose of 360 mg/24 h.

**Oxymorphone comes in suppository form only. There is no oral product available.

††Meperidine is not recommended for the treatment of patients with chronic pain and is included here for comparison purposes and so conversions to more appropriate analgesics can be made. With chronic usage, meperidine may cause significant toxicity, including seizures and myoclonus, due to accumulation of toxic metabolites such as normeperidine.

ratios in titrating and managing the various opioid analgesics is discussed below.

Oxycodone Oxycodone is indicated for the treatment of moderate to severe pain. It is most familiar to clinicians when used in fixed combinations with acetaminophen, ibuprofen, or aspirin (see step 2 above). However, oxycodone in uncombined form is available as immediate-release tablets and capsules, as a liquid solution, and as sustained-release tablets, making it an ideal step 3 agent as well. Oxycodone gained public attention in the 1990s when the extended-release formulation, OxyContin, became a popular drug of abuse. Under Drug Enforcement Administration (DEA) scrutiny, the manufacturer discontinued production of the highest dose tablets (160 mg) in 2001. No parenteral forms of oxycodone are currently available in the United States.

Like morphine, oxycodone as a single agent has no ceiling effect, allowing upward titration as needed. Unlike morphine, whose major effects are expressed via the μ-opioid receptor, oxycodone has effects at the *kappa* opioid receptor, which may explain some reports that oxycodone causes less dysphoria and fewer nightmares and hallucinations than equipotent doses of morphine. However, not all investigators agree that oxycodone is *kappa* specific, especially since, as with morphine, oxycodone may cause side effects including euphoria, constipation, nausea, miosis, pruritus, orthostatic hypotension, suppression of the cough reflex, and respiratory depression.

The onset of action for immediate-release oxycodone is 30 to 60 minutes, and the recommended frequency of administration is every 4 hours. With a high oral bioavailability (>60%), oxycodone is metabolized by the liver to noroxycodone, oxymorphone, noroxymorphone, and their glucuronides and then excreted in the urine. Although noroxycodone is the major circulating metabolite, it has very weak analgesic activity. Oxymorphone, on the other hand, does possess significant analgesic potency, but it is present in the plasma in only small quantities. Therefore, the analgesic effect of oxycodone comes almost entirely from the parent compound. Oxycodone metabolites have not been associated with neuroexcitatory effects such as those that occur with normorphine or normeperidine. Oxycodone should be dosed conservatively in patients with severe renal or hepatic impairment.

Extended-release oxycodone (OxyContin) demonstrates biphasic absorption with an initial rapid phase half-life of 0.6 hours and a slow phase half-life of 6.9 hours. Use of OxyContin rectally is not recommended, since rectal administration results in greater absorption and poses a significant risk of side effects.

On a weight basis, oral oxycodone is generally considered to be more potent than oral morphine. Although equianalgesic potency ratios ranging from 1:1 to 1:2 have been reported, for conversion purposes (see Table 6–13) in patients with chronic pain, 1 mg of oral oxycodone is roughly equivalent to 1.5 mg of oral morphine. The variance in potency ratios may reflect the variable and unpredictable bioavailability of oral morphine.

Oxymorphone Oxymorphone, the major product of oxycodone hepatic metabolism, is available as suppositories and ampoules for hospital use and now available in the United States for oral use, as Opana and Opana ER in multiple dose options. Initially sold in the United States as Numorphan, the oral formulation was removed from the US market as a result of regulatory pressures and other considerations when it became a popular drug of abuse. The TIMERx system of Opana ER appears to have made the extended-release tablets resistant to abuse as an injectable formulation. Oxymorphone has high affinity for the μ-opioid receptor but negligible affinity for kappa and delta. A nasal spray is currently in development for use in severe episodes of breakthrough pain.

Hydromorphone Hydromorphone (Dilaudid) is another familiar μ-opioid receptor agonist that is available in multiple dosage forms: oral immediate-release tablets, oral liquid, rectal suppository, and parenteral. There is currently no sustained-release formulation available in the United States. The onset of action of oral hydromorphone is 30 minutes. Because of its short half-life, hydromorphone must be administered every 3 to 4 hours, limiting its use in chronic pain management as an oral agent due to patient and caregiver inconvenience. Hydromorphone is more lipid soluble than morphine, enhancing its ability to cross the blood–brain barrier and, as an oral agent, has a potency ratio of 1:4 compared with oral morphine. Hydromorphine is extensively metabolized by the liver to hydromorphone-3-glucuronide, which has no analgesic activity but can evoke a range of dose-dependent neuroexcitatory side effects, although toxicity is more rarely seen than with morphine. However, because hydromorphone toxicity is much more rarely experienced, it is generally considered preferable to morphine for patients with renal insufficiency, especially those with high opioid requirements. Because hydromorphone is highly water soluble, it can be administered parenterally in small volumes and is approximately seven times more potent than parenteral morphine, making it a suitable choice for continuous subcutaneous infusion.

Fentanyl Fentanyl is a highly lipid soluble opioid analgesic whose use in chronic pain and in end-of-life care is significant because of its availability as a transdermal patch system and as an oral transmucosal preparation. Fentanyl's analgesic potency lies mainly in its binding to μ-opioid receptors, yielding a potency approximately 80 times that of morphine. Fentanyl solution is used intravenously for analgesia prior to surgery, as an adjunct for anesthesia, and in the immediate postoperative period but has little relevance for chronic pain management. Fentanyl is metabolized in the liver and excreted in the urine.

Fentanyl is most commonly used at end of life as a transdermal patch. The patch releases fentanyl continuously by absorption through the skin into the subcutaneous tissue, where it accumulates and is then absorbed into the systemic circulation via capillary networks. The reservoir in the subcutaneous tissue is responsible for the 17- to 24-hour half-life of this preparation and produces steady fentanyl blood levels over a period of approximately 72 hours. It is also responsible for the fact that following patch application, 17 to 24 hours must elapse before a significant medication effect is detected, thus rendering the fentanyl transdermal system inappropriate for the treatment of acute pain. The reservoir effect also explains the wash out period of 17 to 24 hours after a patch is removed, such that toxic effects will not quickly dissipate after patch removal. Because of the delayed onset of analgesia, short-acting analgesics should be provided for the first 12 to 24 hours after initial patch application. Transdermal fentanyl takes 3 to 6 days to reach steady state, making it appropriate only for patients with known opioid requirements and tolerance.

Transdermal fentanyl requires intact superficial layers of skin (epidermis and stratum corneum) and should not be used on broken, irritated, or irradiated skin. It is not recommended for those younger than 18 years weighing less than 110 pounds. For many years, hospice physicians and nurses have noted that patients who are elderly and cachectic, with limited adipose tissue, seem to have less of a response to transdermal fentanyl. This observation has not been scientifically proven, but has led many hospice and palliative care clinicians to avoid the use of transdermal fentanyl in patients with low body mass indexes. It is absorbed into the blood supply, for systemic distribution and across the blood–brain barrier. Thus, variations in capillary permeability can affect absorption rates, so that exposure to external heat sources (i.e., hot tubs,

TABLE 6–14. Duragesic:Oral Morphine Equianalgesic Table	
MORPHINE (mg IN 24)	**DURAGESIC (μg/h)**
50	25
100	50
150	75
200	100
Additional 50 mg/24 h	Additional 25 μg/h

Transdermal fentanyl is available in the following formulations: 12, 25, 50, 75, and 100 μg/h.

saunas, and sunbathing heating pads) should be avoided. Transdermal fentanyl absorption is also thought to increase approximately 30% in patients with fever of 104°F or more; therefore, it should be used cautiously in patients who are prone to fevers. Patients at the end of life who have fluctuating blood pressures may also experience altered rates of absorption. Finally, according to the full prescribing information, transdermal fentanyl (Duragesic) should be used with caution in the elderly, cachectic, or debilitated patients as they may have altered pharmacokinetics due to poor fat stores, muscle wasting, or altered clearance, thus severely limiting its role in patients who are terminally ill. Transdermal fentanyl patches come in several dosage strengths, expressed in micrograms per hour, with corresponding morphine equivalents expressed as a 24-hour total dose (see Table 6–14). (Further discussion of how to use transdermal fentanyl can be found in the section on the transdermal route of administration.) Drug interactions and adverse effects are similar to those of the other opioid agonists (see below).

Oral transmucosal fentanyl citrate (Actiq) was designed to take advantage of the lipophilic nature of fentanyl and its ability to be absorbed across mucus membranes. It is formulated as a solid drug matrix on an applicator handle (i.e., a lollipop-like device), and is designed to dissolve slowly against the oral mucous membranes. Dosage strengths range from 200 to 1,600 μg. It is approved only for the management of breakthrough cancer pain for patients who are already receiving and who are tolerant to opioid therapy. Opioid tolerance is defined by the package insert as those taking at least 25 μg of transdermal fentanyl/hour or its equianalgesic equivalent for a week or longer (www.actiq.com, accessed August 21, 2008). The patient or caregiver places the Actiq unit in the mouth between the cheek and the lower gum, and the unit is occasionally moved from side to side. The unit must be sucked and not chewed. It requires at least 15 minutes for a full dose to be consumed. Unlike other opioids used for breakthrough pain, the dose of Actiq is not related to the dose of the around-the-clock maintenance opioid. Titration is empirical for each individual beginning with the lowest 200 μg unit with advancement in 200 μg increments every 30 to 60 minutes until an effective dose is achieved.

Although marketed as a transmucosal agent, only 25% of each dose is absorbed by the transbuccal route, with the remaining 75% being swallowed with the saliva and absorbed slowly from the gastrointestinal tract and undergoing first-pass effects in the liver. Therefore, for patients with chronic pain, it is unclear whether Actiq has a significant advantage for breakthrough pain over concentrated opioid solutions administered sublingually. Given the significant cost, its utility remains limited to relieving cancer-related incident pain when quick onset and offset are required.

The FDA recently approved the fentanyl buccal tablet (Fentora) for the treatment of breakthrough cancer pain in patients who are opioid tolerant (see definition earlier). The tablet is placed in the buccal cavity and left there for 15 to 30 minutes, until the tablet completely dissolves and is absorbed across the buccal mucosa. Fentora employs OraVescent drug delivery technology, which generates a reaction that releases carbon dioxide when the tablet comes in contact with saliva. This fizzing reaction is accompanied by a transient change in pH that is thought to promote dissolution and absorption across the buccal mucosa. This accounts for approximately

50% of absorption of the total dose administered and is represented by a peak plasma concentration achieved at approximately 45 minutes. The remaining 50% of the dose is swallowed leading to a second somewhat slower second phase of absorption. Chewing, sucking, or swallowing the tablets prevents the drug from achieving adequate plasma concentrations. Fentora is available in several 100 μg increments between 100 and 800. The starting dose of Fentora is 100 μg and is **not** dose-equivalent to Actiq, so care must be taken if switching patients between the two products. Curiously, the number of tablets administered may alter the dose equivalency. For example, four 100 μg Fentora tablets were found to deliver 12% to 13% higher plasma concentration values, compared with one 400 μg Fentora tablet. The clinical significance of this is not yet fully understood. (www.fentora.com, accessed August 21, 2008)

Methadone   Methadone was developed as a synthetic opioid agonist in Germany in 1937 and brought to the United States after WWII. It is currently available in the United States as methadone hydrochloride powder, which is prepared for oral (tablet/concentrated solution), rectal, and parenteral use. Methadone is a broad-spectrum opioid, which not only binds to *mu* and *delta* opioid receptors, but also antagonizes the NMDA receptor. It is this unique NMDA receptor antagonism that is thought to make it an effective treatment of neuropathic pain when other opioids are often inadequate. Other features that make methadone an attractive opioid analgesic are its low cost and lower incidence of constipation.

Until recently, oral methadone has been used primarily for drug detoxification rather than as an analgesic for chronic pain. Its use as a daily agent by methadone maintenance treatment (MMT) clinics reflects its long blood half-life that extends well beyond its ability to sustain analgesia. To control pain, methadone should be dosed every 6 to 12 hours, but progressive drug accumulation to toxic levels is not uncommon, particularly in elderly and debilitated patients. In addition, there are large individual variations in dose equivalency ratios and titration periods, and time to stabilization may be prolonged.

Methadone's role in the treatment of chronic pain in the terminally ill is evolving. In the past, methadone was reserved as a last-resort opioid for patients with severe side effects of other opioids (including opioid toxicity), neuropathic pain syndromes unresponsive to other opioids in combination with adjuvants, and those with renal failure. Today, pain and palliative care experts often use methadone as a first-line agent for patients with neuropathic pain. However, methadone prescribers should have comprehensive knowledge of its unique pharmacokinetic and pharmacodynamic properties.

The unique characteristics associated with methadone are primarily related to a biphasic elimination process with a prolonged terminal half-life. Methadone analgesia occurs within 30 to 60 minutes and peaks between 2.5 and 4 hours after administration. However, methadone has a very long and variable elimination half-life ranging between 4.2 and 190 hours. Initially, methadone's analgesia lasts 3 to 6 hours, making it necessary to redose several times per day.

Reflecting this, for patients who are opioid-naïve and who are starting methadone *de novo*, some experts recommend starting with 5 mg q3 hour as needed (PRN). However, with repeated dosing, methadone's analgesia lasts 8 to 12 hours, allowing it function like a long-acting opioid. Therefore, the need for PRN dosing typically drops off as steady state is achieved and a scheduled regimen of q8- to 12-hour dosing can be identified after 4 to 8 days of PRN dosing. This differs from morphine analgesia, which typically lasts 4 to 6 hours and does not change with repeated dosing. Because of the potential for a prolonged half-life, methadone carries a high risk of drug accumulation, which can cause toxicity after days or even weeks of effective analgesia. Therefore, methadone should not be rapidly titrated like other opioids, rather at least 4 to 6 days should be allowed between titrations, and careful monitoring for drug toxicity is essential.

With such a long and variable half-life, initiating an analgesic methadone regimen must be undertaken with care. Two approaches to initiating methadone in patients not currently on opioid regimens are presented in Table 6–15. It

---

TABLE 6–15. Protocol for Instituting Methadone for Patients Receiving Morphine or Other Strong Opioid Agonists

Conservative approach:

(1) Begin fixed dose methadone 5–10 mg orally two or three times per day for 4–7 d.

(2) If incomplete pain relief, increase the dose by 50% *and continue for* 4–7 d.

(3) Continue increasing dose every 4–7 d until stable pain relief achieved.

(4) Breakthrough pain: use an alternative short-acting oral opioid with short half-life every hour as needed for breakthrough pain and to provide pain relief during titration phase.

Loading dose approach:

(1) Load: start methadone at fixed oral dose (5–10 mg) q 4 h PRN only.

(2) Calculate maintenance dose: On day 8, calculate the total methadone dosage taken over last 24-h period and give in divided doses BID or TID.

(3) Breakthrough pain: Give 10% of total daily methadone as PRN drug q 1 h PRN for breakthrough pain. Instruct the patient to call you if they need to use more than five breakthrough doses per day.

SOURCE: Adapted from Von Gunten C: Methadone: starting dose information, fast fact and concepts #86. *J Palliat Med* 7(2):304–305, 2004.

TABLE 6–16. Dose-Related Conversion Ratios of Oral Morphine to Oral Methadone

DAILY ORAL MORPHINE DOSE EQUIVALENTS (mg)	CONVERSION RATIO OF ORAL MORPHINE TO ORAL METHADONE
<100	3:1 (3 mg morphine: 1 mg methadone)
101–300	5:1
301–600	10:1
601–800	12:1
801–1,000	15:1
>1,000	20:1

SOURCE: Data from Gazelle G, Fine PG. *Methadone for the Treatment of Pain*, 2nd ed. Wisconsin, EPERC, End of Life/Palliative Care Education Resource Center. http://www.mcw.edu/fastFact/ff_75.htm. Accessed March 15, 2010.

should be noted that the use of PRN methadone should be offered selectively to patients who understand the limitations of dosing frequency. For opioid-tolerant patients, the analgesic potency of methadone increases with increasing exposure to other opioids. Hence, methadone appears to provoke a more potent response for patients on higher oral morphine equivalents (OMEs). Methadone to morphine dose equivalency ratios varying from 1:8 to 1:20 have been reported when previous total daily morphine doses exceed 300 mg. Lower dose potency ratios of 1:3 to 1:6 have been reported with lower total daily morphine doses. One widely accepted conversion ratio is presented in Table 6–16. Although there is no consensus in the literature, pain and palliative care experts often make additional adjustments for patients being converted from extremely high OMEs, for example, using ratios of 40:1 or more for patients on >5,000 OMEs.

Once the total daily methadone equivalence of the existing regimen is established, the substitution of methadone is undertaken one of two ways. A straight conversion method involves discontinuing the existing opioid and initiating a methadone regimen in one process. The reduce and replace method involves stepwise reductions of the existing opioid and replacement with methadone over a series of days. For example, on day 1, the existing opioid is reduced by one-third and replaced with one-third the calculated methadone divided BID or TID. On day 2, replace another third of the opioid dose. On day 3, discontinue the initial opioid and replace with the last third of methadone if the pain is still rated at moderate to severe. Palliative care practitioners have noted that many patients achieve significant pain relief by the end of day 2 and are able to discontinue the existing opioid on day 3 without additional methadone increase.

Additional issues arise in rotating patients off methadone to other opioid regimens. Conversion ratios from morphine to methadone cannot be reversed. The existing literature is largely limited to case reports, and there is no commonly accepted method of achieving this. Attempts to rotate from methadone are often ineffective, with escalating pain following discontinuation of methadone. Many patients are rotated back to methadone after short trials of rapid opioid escalation fail. Patients who are enrolled in MMT programs who develop pain syndromes requiring opioid therapy do poorly when methadone is discontinued. Rather, many palliative care physicians use methadone as the opioid analgesic of choice in terminally ill patients who have been chronically exposed to methadone (see section below on Pain Management in Patients with Previous or Current Substance Abuse).

Methadone has been associated with numerous drug interactions. Although a discussion of potential interactions is beyond the scope of this chapter, it is worth noting that the existing literature on methadone relates largely to the MMT population. Medical literature describes both potential and actual interactions, but the clinical implications for patients at the end of life remain undefined. The risk for drug interactions primarily occurs through the risk of cytochrome P450 (CYP) interactions and the potential for QT prolongation. Inducers and inhibitors of the CYP enzyme system may affect methadone metabolism. Inhibitors (i.e., ciprofloxacin, fluoxetine, paroxetine, fluvoxamine, ketoconazole, fluconazole, desipramine, and dextromethorphan) may increase systemic methadone levels and inducers (such as rifampin, fluoroquinolones, phenobarbital, phenytoin, and St. John's wort) may decrease methadone levels, in some cases to the point of inducing an opioid withdrawal reaction. Antiretroviral therapies, including protease inhibitors, non-nucleoside reverse transcriptase inhibitors (nNRTIs) and nucleoside/nucleotide reverse transcriptase inhibitors (NRTIs), commonly interact with methadone, but there are conflicting reports regarding the metabolic pathways involved in either induction or inhibition. Methadone carries similar risks for CNS depression as other opioids, especially when used in combination with alcohol and neuroleptics. A unique pharmacodynamic property may induce a risk of QT prolongation, especially at doses greater than 300 mg/d. This risk may be exacerbated by the concomitant use of other QT-prolonging drugs, including clarithromycin, fluconazole, amitriptyline, trazodone, and some protease inhibitors. Weschules et al. provide a thorough review of the literature detailing drug interactions with methadone in their 2008 *Pain Medicine* article.

Between 1998 and 2002, methadone prescriptions increased 250%, due to an increased awareness of methadone's analgesic effectiveness and its unique affordability. Simultaneously, between 1999 and 2005, the number of poisoning deaths in the United States mentioning methadone increased 468% to 4,462. In 2004 to 2005 alone, all poisoning deaths increased 8%, whereas those mentioning methadone increased 16%. This rapid rise of methadone-related fatalities is likely due to a combination of specific prescribing practices, improper taking of the medication by patients, drug diversion, and other means. Because of its considerable complexities, clinicians are advised to consult with pain and palliative care experts and to review appropriate references before prescribing methadone for patients with chronic pain.

Opioids to avoid　Some opioid analgesics should be avoided. The disadvantages and hazards of the partial agonist and mixed agonist–antagonist opioids have been previously discussed. Meperidine, which is widely prescribed for acute pain, should not be used to treat chronic pain. Meperidine has a very short analgesic half-life and should be dosed every 2 to 4 hours to effectively control recurrent or continuous pain. It has poor and unpredictable oral bioavailability resulting in frequent underdosing, particularly after conversion from parenteral administration. Most important, meperidine is metabolized to normeperidine, which, with repeated dosing, can accumulate and precipitate dangerous toxic effects. Meperidine toxicity may present as distressing mood changes, CNS stimulation, tremors, multifocal myoclonus, and even seizures. Normeperidine accumulation is particularly marked when meperidine administration is prolonged, in high doses, and in patients with impaired renal or hepatic function.

Propoxyphene is a very weak opioid marketed in combination with acetaminophen (Darvocet) or aspirin/caffeine (Darvon). Propoxyphene provides little analgesia beyond the acetaminophen component and yet has significantly neurotoxic metabolites that can be clinically significant especially in the elderly and in those with impaired creatinine clearance. Thus, propoxyphene-based agents have a very limited role in the treatment of chronic pain. Patients, who use multiple doses per day, but not enough to predispose to hepatic toxicity, may benefit from acetaminophen dosed as a single agent, rather than in combination with propoxyphene.

USE OF ANALGESICS IN THE TREATMENT OF PAIN

Around-the-Clock-Dosing　As noted above in the section on acute and chronic pain (also see Table 6–4), analgesia for the treatment of chronic pain should be provided on a regular, preventive schedule. Patients with incident pain may be treated with PRN medications. However, patients who experience multiple episodes of pain each day or who have continuous pain should

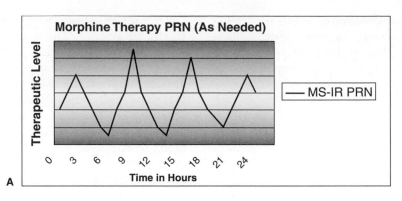

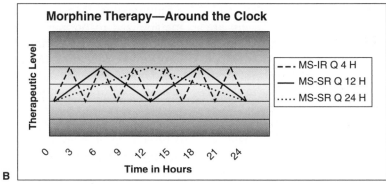

Figure 6–5. Morphine administered PRN (as needed) versus ATC (around-the-clock). **A.** Morphine therapy provided PRN. Therapeutic levels are hectic, falling below pain threshold (*lower blue area*), indicating that the patient is experiencing pain prior to next dose, and rising to toxic levels (*upper blue area*). **B.** Morphine therapy provided ATC. Therapeutic levels remain within the therapeutic range, and out of the blue areas, indicating that the patient does not experience either pain or toxicity between doses. (MS-IR, immediate-release morphine; MS-SR, sustained-release morphine.)

have analgesics scheduled to prevent pain—in other words, around-the-clock. Figure 6–5 illustrates the pharmacokinetics associated with around-the-clock treatment versus "as needed" or PRN dosing. Patients on a PRN schedule (Fig. 6–5A) will receive medication only when they complain of and are experiencing pain. In contrast, when analgesic medication is provided on a regular basis, in anticipation of recurring pain, the establishment and maintenance of drug blood levels within a therapeutic range will effectively prevent the recurrence of pain (Fig. 6–5B). In addition, around-the-clock dosing avoids or minimizes the peaks and valleys in blood levels that result in uneven pain control punctuated by periods of drug toxicity.

Routes of Administration

Oral route For patients with chronic pain who can take oral medication, oral administration of analgesics is the preferred route. Effective pain

TABLE 6–17. Titration of Immediate-Release Opioids for the Treatment of Uncontrolled Pain

1. Provide immediate-release analgesia around-the-clock. Recommended starting doses for opioid-naïve patients:

    Morphine 5–10 mg PO q 4 h around-the-clock
    Oxycodone 5–7.5 mg PO q 4 h around-the-clock
    Hydromorphone 1–2 mg PO q 3 h around-the-clock

2. Provide as needed additional doses at 50% of starting dose every 2 h.
3. If pain is nearly controlled with the present regimen, but the patient still has some mild discomfort, the drug dose may be increased by 10–20%.
4. If pain is only partially controlled, and the patient still complains for moderate pain, increase the dosage by 25–50%.
5. If pain is severe, and little or no pain relief has been noted with the current dose, an increase of 50–100% may be appropriate.
6. Upward titration should continue until pain relief is achieved or until unacceptable side effects intervene.

control may be accomplished using oral medications in 90% of patients. Orally administered analgesics are relatively safe, cost effective, and, with the availability of sustained-release preparations, convenient for patients and caregivers.

When patients who are opioid naïve present with pain that is severe and uncontrolled, there are two generally accepted approaches to achieving rapid pain control. Both methods utilize an immediate-release opioid, such as immediate-release morphine, immediate-release oxycodone, or hydromorphone. In the first method (see Table 6–17), a starting dose of oral morphine 5 or 10 mg every 4 hours, oxycodone 5 or 7.5 mg every 4 hours, or hydromorphone 2 or 4 mg every 3 hours is administered to the patient around-the-clock (RTC). Incremental increases in dose should be provided as necessary to achieve pain control. Additional doses at 50% of the around-the-clock (i.e., basal) dose should be provided every 2 hours on an as needed basis to achieve adequate analgesia. Lower starting doses may be prudent in very elderly patients or when patients are known to have renal impairment. The second, more conservative method utilizes the same medications but on an as needed basis only, every 2 to 4 hours.

With either method, after 24 to 48 hours, total opioid consumption and pain reassessment are performed and an appropriate standing opioid regimen is prescribed. The first method provides the potential of a sustained level of analgesia similar to the use of a long-acting preparation for chronic pain, preventing the peaks and valleys associated with PRN medication, although increasing the risk of toxicity for some patients who are opioid naïve. The latter method allows for patients to use as little or as much of the opioid as they need, but if not taken regularly, may demonstrate the unevenness of PRN opioid dosing and may impair the potential effectiveness of the analgesia in the short term. Dosing and method should be individualized, noting the degree of pain, social circumstance (i.e., patient's ability to self-medicate or the availability of a caregiver to administer medication as needed), cognitive status (i.e., ability of the patient to request the medication), and prognosis.

For patients who have been managed on another opioid agonist or a step 2 opioid/nonopioid combination analgesic, the starting dose of morphine should be based on the equianalgesic dose of the prior medication. Keep in mind, however, that if the reason for switching the patient to morphine is uncontrolled pain, the starting dose should generally be higher than that calculated by the conversion formula (see Table 6–13).

Dosage adjustments are based on the patient's response, and the dose should be increased as necessary. Upward titration of the dose should continue until pain relief is achieved or until unacceptable side effects are encountered.

Sustained-release opioid products   Around-the-clock dosing at 3 to 4 hour intervals is often burdensome for both patients and caregivers and is particularly disruptive to needed sleep and rest. Therefore, with the exception of patients who are actively dying, once pain has been controlled with a stable dose of an immediate-release opioid, conversion to a sustained-release preparation should be accomplished whenever possible.

Sustained-release oral opioid products that are currently available in the United States can be found listed in Table 6–18. They include the sustained-release morphine products MS Contin (q12-hour schedule), its generic equivalent, "morphine extended-release tablets," Oramorph SR (q12-hour schedule) (note: MS Contin and Oramorph SR are NOT considered generic equivalents), and morphine (Avinza) and morphine sulfate (Kadian) (q24-hour schedule), as well as the sustained-release oxycodone product, OxyContin.

To convert patients from immediate-release to sustained-release morphine products, the total amount of immediate-release morphine that is required in a 24-hour period is determined. The entire dose is then prescribed every 24 hours when Kadian or Avinza is ordered, or the dose is divided in half, with 50% of the dose ordered every 12 hours for MS Contin and Oramorph.

It is important to remind the patient and caregivers that sustained-release tablets should not be broken or chewed as this can result in a rapid and unintended release of a potentially toxic dose of morphine. However, Avinza and Kadian capsules

may be opened and the contents sprinkled into food or administered via a feeding tube, provided that the morphine-containing pellets themselves are not chewed.

For patients taking Avinza or Kadian, morphine blood levels peak at 8 to 12 hours. Some patients have reported somnolence during the period of peak blood levels at what is their therapeutic dose. One potential solution to this problem is to administer the medication in the late afternoon so that peak blood levels will occur during regular sleeping hours when somnolence is desired.

Some patients find that the sustained-release medication seems to lose its effectiveness 2 to 4 hours before the next dose of the product is due (20–22 hours for 24-hour preparations, 10 hours for the 12-hour products). This phenomenon, called "end of dose failure," can be resolved by either increasing the 12- or 24-hour dose of medication, or by providing the same total 24-hour dose as before, but increasing the interval of administration to every 12 hours for the 24-hour preparations and every 8 hours for the other products. In no instance, however, should any sustained-release opioids be administered more frequently than these intervals.

Unlike sustained-release morphine preparations, sustained-release oxycodone (OxyContin) exhibits a biphasic absorption pattern suggesting an initial immediate-release of oxycodone from the tablet followed by a prolonged phase of release. Whether this affords patients with an advantage is unclear, since, if one is following a proper dosage schedule, there should be no therapeutic need for immediate-release of medication on a routine basis. Food has no significant effect on the absorption of oxycodone from OxyContin but does affect absorption of immediate-release oxycodone, a point to remember when using the latter for breakthrough pain. As with sustained-release morphine, OxyContin tablets must be swallowed intact and may not be broken, chewed, or crushed without high risk of toxic effects. With reference to the commonly accepted oxycodone to morphine potency ratio of

TABLE 6–18. Oral Sustained-Release Opioid Products

1. MS Contin:	Analgesic:	Morphine
	Frequency:	Every 12 h
	Dosage form:	Tablet
	Dosage strengths:	15, 30, 60, 100, and 200 mg
2. MS Extended-release:	Analgesic:	Morphine
	Frequency:	Every 12 h
	Dosage form:	Tablet
	Dosage strengths:	15, 30, and 60 mg
3. Oramorph SR:	Analgesic:	Morphine
	Frequency:	Every 12 h
	Dosage form:	Tablet
	Dosage strengths:	30, 60, and 100 mg
4. Kadian:	Analgesic:	Morphine
	Frequency:	Every 12–24 h
	Dosage forms:	Capsule
		Sprinkle (Capsule may be broken open and sprinkled on applesauce or into water and flushed down a G-tube)
	Dosage strengths:	10, 20, 30, 50, 60, and 100 mg
5. Avinza:	Analgesic:	Morphine
	Frequency:	Every 24 h
	Dosage form:	Capsule
		Sprinkle (Capsule may be broken open and sprinkled on applesauce or into water and flushed down a G-tube)
	Dosage strengths:	30, 60, 90, and 120 mg
6. OxyContin:	Analgesic:	Oxycodone
	Frequency:	Every 12 h
	Dosage form:	Tablet
	Dosage strengths:	10, 20, 40, and 80 mg
7. Opana ER	Analgesic:	Oxymorphone
	Frequency:	Every 12 h
	Dosage form:	Tablet
	Dosage strengths:	5, 7.5, 10, 15, 20, 30, and 40 mg

1:1.5, extended-release oxycodone is significantly more expensive than the sustained-release morphine preparations, since at the time of writing this chapter, there are no generic formulations of extended-release oxycodone available on the market.

Treatment of breakthrough and incident pain Regardless of whether the patient is maintained on around-the-clock short-acting opioid preparations or is converted to a sustained-release opioid, the availability of an immediate-release opioid of proportionate dose for the treatment of breakthrough or incident pain is essential. Breakthrough pain refers to sporadic, self-limited episodes of acute pain due to the primary disease or to unrelated processes in a patient whose chronic pain is adequately controlled. Incident pain refers to an expected exacerbation of pain due to unusual physical activity, transfers, turning, or various diagnostic or therapeutic procedures.

For ease of titration of the sustained-release medication and to avoid polypharmacy, it is generally recommended that the breakthrough medication should be a short-acting/immediate-release version of the opioid being used to provide around-the-clock pain relief. In other words, immediate-release morphine should be used for any of the sustained-release morphine products, and immediate-release oxycodone should be used for OxyContin. Recommended doses of immediate-release opioid for breakthrough or incident pain are calculated at approximately 10% of the 24-hour total opioid dose given every 1 to 2 hours PRN, or 25% of the dose of opioid administered over 12 hours given at intervals of 3 to 4 hours. Remember, whenever the dosage of the sustained-release product is increased, the dose of immediate-release medication for breakthrough or incident pain should be increased proportionately.

Should pain increase to the point that the patient is frequently requesting "rescue" medication for breakthrough pain, the patient requires re-evaluation and titration of the sustained-release basal regimen. Titrations of the sustained-release product are suggested when the patient consistently has three or more episodes of breakthrough pain in a 24-hour period. It makes little sense to use a short-acting/immediate-release preparation RTC if the patient requires medication every 2 to 4 hours. The use of oral, sustained-release products for chronic pain relief and prevention supplemented as needed by oral, immediate-release opioids is conceptually similar to the parenteral patient-controlled analgesia (PCA) that is typically used to manage acute postoperative pain. Patients should be included

in discussions regarding any change in treatment regimen, to ensure that they understand why changes are being recommended and that they are in agreement with the adjustments.

Noninvasive alternative routes of analgesic administration Some patients cannot tolerate oral agents at some time during their illness because of disease-related nausea and vomiting; dysphagia due to oral or esophageal cancer, severe mucositis, or neurological deficits; or depressed consciousness close to the end of life. In one retrospective study, 59% of patients with advanced cancer used more than one route of drug administration during the last 4 weeks of life. Although it is commonplace in these circumstances to consider invasive, parenteral methods of drug delivery, a number of less invasive alternatives are available including buccal, sublingual, transdermal, and rectal routes of administration.

Buccal and sublingual With the exception of fentanyl, all commonly used opioid analgesics that are available in the United States are hydrophilic and, as such, are not substantially absorbed across the lipid membranes of the buccal and sublingual mucosa. Nevertheless, it is fairly common practice in hospice and palliative medicine to medicate patients who are unable to swallow with high concentration (20 mg/mL) morphine or oxycodone liquid either buccally or sublingually. The medication is absorbed via the gastrointestinal tract by "trickle down" swallowing and is widely accepted because it is noninvasive, has recognized efficacy, and is easy to administer. Fentanyl transmucosal and buccal formulations are described in detail in the fentanyl section above but have a limited role in terminally ill patients.

Transdermal Fentanyl transdermal (Duragesic) is particularly useful for managing chronic pain in patients with difficulty swallowing or complying with a schedule of oral medications. The latter problem includes situations in which either the patient or family members are unable or unwilling to administer oral doses reliably and on schedule. It also has been used to address drug diversion issues, although it now has a "street value" that diminishes its potential utility in these cases.

The fentanyl transdermal system is manufactured in five patch strengths: 12, 25, 50, 75, and 100 µg/h. The 12-µg/h patch is not intended to serve as a starting dose but rather to allow smaller titrations between doses. In most instances, a patch will provide analgesia for 72 hours, although in some patients, "end of dose failure" similar to the sustained-release oral opioids has been reported, with adequate pain relief lasting for only 48 to 60 hours. Because transdermal fentanyl has such a long time to analgesic onset and has a long half-life, it is safe to initiate it only after pain control has been essentially established. Therefore, it is not recommended for patients who are opioid naïve. For this reason, many hospice and palliative care specialists advocate a "fentanyl patch strength to 24-hour oral morphine" ratio of 1 µg/h:2 mg/d rather than the approximately 1:4 ratio recommended by the manufacturer in the product insert. Bioequivalent doses for transdermal fentanyl using the 1:2 ratio are shown in Table 6–14. When converting a patient to fentanyl transdermal from an opioid other than morphine, first calculate the 24-hour oral morphine dose equivalent using standard conversion tables (Table 6–13). Then, select the appropriate patch dose based on Table 6–16.

Fentanyl patch doses in excess of 300 µg/h (3–100 µg patches) are difficult to sustain because the amount of body surface area required to effectively place the patches, especially with the need for regular site rotation, presents a formidable obstacle. After applying the patch or patches for the first time, the existing analgesic regimen should be maintained for 24 hours to allow fentanyl blood levels to reach the therapeutic range. As with any sustained-release opioid product, provision must be made for breakthrough pain by prescribing an immediate-release opioid for "rescue." Patch dosage adjustments are best made at 6-day intervals, making it inappropriate for patients whose pain is not adequately controlled and who need more rapid dose titration.

When converting from the fentanyl patch to another opioid, begin treatment with the successor opioid 12 to 18 hours after removing the patch. Use 50% of the equivalent analgesic dose of the new opioid and then titrate the dose on the basis of the patient's need and clinical response. Because of the half-life of 17 to 24 hours, any supportive care for adverse effects of transdermal fentanyl should be maintained for at least 24 hours after patch removal.

The use of transdermal fentanyl in combination with other sustained-release opioids lacks clinical rationale, promotes polypharmacy, and should be discouraged. Used fentanyl patches must be disposed of with care. They can pose a significant, even fatal, hazard for young children.

Topical administration of opioid agents is an attractive option for patients at the end of life who lose the ability to swallow or have gastrointestinal obstructions. However, because of morphine's hydrophilic properties, it is not absorbable across intact skin. Compounding pharmacies have attempted to assist morphine across the skin in carrier agents such as pluronic lecithin organogel, but in a randomized double-blind clinical study serum morphine levels remain undetectable or negligible. Therefore, its use as a transdermal agent cannot be recommended. Alternatively, when applied to areas of broken skin, topical morphine has been shown to be an effective local analgesic. Hospice practitioners often use morphine gel formulations in painful wound beds for local pain relief to decrease the need for systemic analgesia.

Rectal route   Administration of opioids by rectal suppository is effective, although not necessarily perceived as noninvasive. Although rectal absorption of morphine is weaker than small intestinal absorption, rectal blood flow bypasses the liver and first-pass metabolism. Therefore, blood levels after rectal administration are about the same as after oral ingestion. The efficacy of rectal morphine in terminally ill patients makes rectal morphine a viable alternative during the last several days of life. With the use of gelatin capsules and hydrophilic morphine tablets, virtually any dosage level of morphine can be administered via the rectal route. Although not approved by the FDA, sustained-release morphine may be placed in a gelatin capsule and provide prolonged effects as long as the sustained-release morphine remains in contact with the rectal mucosa. This method reduces the frequency of suppository insertion. Other agents that may be used rectally include hydromorphone, acetaminophen, and several NSAIDs, including aspirin and indomethacin.

Parenteral analgesia   Initiation of parenteral analgesia, which permits rapid attainment of analgesic blood levels, may be appropriate for patients with severe, uncontrolled pain. The intravenous route is preferable when venous access is present. Subcutaneous injections and continuous infusions are good alternatives for patients without venous access. Intramuscular injections should be avoided because of pain at the injection site and unreliable absorption of the medication. Continuous intravenous or subcutaneous infusion is preferable to intermittent boluses that provide only 45 to 60 minutes of analgesia.

Continuous infusion provides patients with consistent blood levels and can be titrated to effect with ease. Infusion control devices, either mechanical (e.g., syringe driver pump) or computerized, ensure proper drug delivery. Computerized delivery systems enable PCA, with patients having the option of self-administering predetermined bolus doses for breakthrough or incident pain. Continuous subcutaneous infusion with a PCA is particularly effective for ambulatory, terminally ill patients who are unable to tolerate oral analgesia and who require opioid doses that are too large for practical administration by the transdermal route. These subcutaneous infusions utilize a small gauge silastic needle that needs to be replaced only every 3 to 5 days. Local irritation at the injection site may require more frequent site rotation but otherwise subcutaneous infusions are very well tolerated. Adjunctive agents such as antiemetic and anxiolytic drugs that are compatible in solution with parenteral opioids can often be mixed together and administered with one syringe driver or pump.

When converting patients from oral to parenteral medication, and vice versa, it is essential to remember that the relative potency of opioids is route-dependent. Equianalgesic conversion doses for oral and parenteral opioids are depicted in Table 6–13. Except for opioid-naïve patients, in whom the ratio of oral to parenteral morphine is 6:1 mg, most pain experts accept a conversion ratio of 3:1. For opioid-naïve patients, opioid infusions should be initiated at a low dose (i.e., morphine at 1–2 mg/h and hydromorphone at 0.1–0.2 mg/h). Intravenous PRN opioid doses are typically provided every 10 to 15 minutes and should be proportionate to the hourly rate. Although there are multiple models for determining the appropriate PRN dose, 50% to 100% is a generally accepted calculation. For example, patients on morphine 10 mg continuous IV infusion per hour might be prescribed 6 mg q15 minutes IV push PRN. Patients on subcutaneous infusions are generally provided with PRN doses every 20 minutes as needed for pain relief. Subcutaneous tissue can generally absorb about 3 cc/h but doses much higher than this have been reported in the medical literature and are typically well-tolerated. Three to four hours after initiating or titrating an infusion, a thorough pain assessment including the number of PRN doses requested and administered should be determined. New hourly rates and PRN doses may be prescribed if patients have inadequate pain relief or are requesting frequent PRN dosing.

Other invasive routes of analgesia administration
For end-of-life care, epidural, intrathecal, and intraventricular routes of analgesia should be reserved for the rare patients whose pain cannot be controlled noninvasively or parenterally. For patients with cancer, intraspinal therapy is most effective for pain related to pelvic tumors or

lumbosacral plexopathies. Although intraspinal opioid analgesia sometimes achieves effective pain relief with fewer side effects than with systemic routes of administration, respiratory depression and sedation may still occur. With disease progression, patients may also need to resume systemic therapy. Intraspinal analgesia is contraindicated for patients with musculoskeletal or spinal deformities, for patients with bleeding diatheses or coagulopathies, for patients with severe respiratory diseases, and in the presence of infections, increased intracranial pressure, or drug allergy. Rare cases of epidural hematomas associated with catheter placement have resulted in paraplegia. Infection associated with indwelling catheters is also a potential risk that may be minimized by total internalization of the catheter and pump. Comprehensive information about intraspinal analgesia may be found in review articles such as Bennett et al. (2000).

Anticipate and Treat Complications and Side Effects

Chronic opioid therapy predictably causes constipation. Nausea and vomiting occur in about 30% of patients starting opioid therapy, but unlike constipation, usually resolve within several days because of the development of tolerance. Transient sedation and confusion are also common. Less frequent side effects include dry mouth, myoclonus, urinary retention, pruritus, sleep disturbances, dysphoria, and inappropriate secretion of antidiuretic hormone. Respiratory depression, although a potential side effect in opioid-naïve patients who are being treated for acute pain, is generally not a factor in chronic pain management of terminally ill patients when proper titration guidelines are followed. The recommended treatment for the most common opioid-induced side effects such as, constipation, nausea, and sedation, are summarized in Table 6–19 and discussed below.

TABLE 6–19. Opioid Side Effects

SIDE EFFECTS	TREATMENT	
Constipation (see Chapter 8)	1. Increased hydration	
	2. Stimulant laxatives (senna or bisacodyl)	
	3. Osmotic laxatives (lactulose or sorbitol)	
	4. Stool softener (docusate)	
	5. The last option is to use castor oil or magnesium-containing products	
Nausea and vomiting (see Chapter 8)	Phenothiazines, such as:	
	Prochlorperazine	5–10 mg PO TID–QID
		25 mg PR BID
	Promethazine	25 mg PO/PR q 4–6 h.
	Chlorpromazine	10–25 mg PO q 4–6 h
		50–100 mg PR q 6–8 h.
	Metoclopramide	5–10 mg four times daily
Sedation	Dextroamphetamine	2.5–5 mg BID
	Methylphenidate	2.5–5 mg BID

SOURCE: Data from Levy M. Pharmacologic treatment of cancer pain. *N Engl J Med* 335:1124-1132, 1996; Jacox A, Carr DB, Payne R, et al: *Management of Cancer Pain. Clinical Practice Guideline No. 9.* AHCPR publication No. 94-0592. Rockville, MD, Agency for Health Care Policy and Research, US Department of Health and Human Services, Public Health Service, 1994.

CONSTIPATION Constipation occurs in nearly all patients receiving opioid analgesics. Therefore, any patient who is being treated with opioids should be started prophylactically on a bowel regimen with the objective of achieving a bowel movement at least every 2 to 3 days. Along with increased hydration, a stool softener (docusate) and a mild laxative (senna or biscodyl) are usually adequate as primary therapy. In principle, patients should be encouraged to add fiber to the diet, to avoid caffeinated beverages, and to increase exercise. However, these recommendations may be impractical or irrelevant for many end-of-life patients who are often weak, bedbound, anorectic, or require fluid restriction. Patients who cannot increase fluids should not use bulk laxatives because of the risk of obstruction and bolus formation. The use of biscodyl may sometimes be associated with fecal leakage due to excess colonic relaxation.

For resistant constipation, a strong laxative (lactulose, polyethylene glycol, citrate of magnesia) is required. Enemas may be indicated when stool is lodged in the rectum too proximal for digital disimpaction and the patient is unable to evacuate. For opioid-induced constipation that is refractory despite the above interventions, oral administration of the opioid antagonist naloxone may be effective. The use of naloxone to reverse opioid-induced constipation may be appropriate in extremely rare situations as it will usually result in uncontrolled pain. The recommended dose is 3 mg three times a day, escalated daily in 3 mg increments as needed, up to 9 mg three times a day. With this regimen, patients usually complain of abdominal cramps, and some patients, especially with the higher doses, experience sweating or shivering presumably due to an induced withdrawal reaction due to systemic absorption.

At the time of the writing of this chapter, methylnaltrexone has just been introduced to the market. As a quaternary amine, it has limited ability to cross the blood–brain barrier and, therefore, antagonizes peripheral gastrointestinal μ-opioid receptors, reversing opioid-induced constipation without reversing systemic analgesia or precipitating withdrawal. It is available as a subcutaneous injection. At this time, given the subcutaneous route and cost-effectiveness, its use would best be considered for patients with refractory and distressing opioid-induced constipation. A full discussion of constipation can be found in Chapter 8.

NAUSEA AND VOMITING Opioids cause nausea and vomiting via a number of mechanisms including inhibition of gastric motility, stimulation of the chemoreceptor trigger zone (CTZ) in the brain stem, and stimulation of the vestibular nerve. Opioid-induced nausea and vomiting usually subside spontaneously within a few days. When nausea and vomiting persist, alternative etiologies unrelated to opioids should be considered such as electrolyte abnormalities, hypercalcemia, gastritis, obstruction, increased intracranial pressure, and other medications. Because nausea does not occur in all patients receiving opioids, prophylactic antiemetic treatment is not recommended except for patients with a prior history of opioid-induced nausea.

Nonpharmacological interventions helpful to patients with opioid-related nausea and vomiting include elimination of provocative environmental stimuli (e.g., smells), providing adequate oral care, dietary consultation, and reassurance that the nausea will likely be transitory. Primary pharmacological interventions include CTZ inhibitors (phenothiazines, haloperidol) and agents that promote gastric emptying (metoclopramide), rather than antihistamines, which are often less-well tolerated. The newer 5HT3-receptor antagonists (ondansetron, granisetron, dolasetron) were developed primarily for treating acute nausea caused by cancer chemotherapy. Although these agents are generally not necessary for patients with opioid-induced nausea, they are sometimes effective for refractory cases. A sublingual ondansetron preparation may be an effective alternative to parenteral antiemetics in patients with severe nausea and vomiting who are unable to tolerate or who fail to respond to an oral agent. For patients who do not respond to the above measures, opioid rotation (discussed later) is often effective. A full discussion of nausea and vomiting can be found in Chapter 8.

SEDATION Opioid-related sedation, when it occurs, can be troublesome for patients and their loved ones and may result in poor compliance with the prescribed pain control regimen, leading to therapeutic failure. It is thus very important to inform patients and caregivers that tolerance to sedation usually occurs within several days. They also need to be reminded that, due to the stimulant effect that pain exerts, patients in pain often suffer from sleep deprivation. With initial pain relief, patients may be finally able to "catch up" on much-needed sleep, creating the false impression that they are improperly and overly sedated. Careful observation and a review of the medication regimen, as well as determination of what medications are actually being taken, and in what dosage, should allow distinction between a patient in deep sleep and one who is experiencing medication-induced sedation. For those patients with sustained opioid-related sedation, small doses of methylphenidate (2.5 mg at 8 AM and 12 noon with dose escalation to effect) may be prescribed, often with good results.

Confusion, difficulty concentrating, mood changes, and hallucinations may occur with initiation of opioids or after dose escalation. These symptoms, especially hallucinations, can be extremely disturbing both for patients and for their families. Dysphoria is most common. Euphoria, in the absence of concomitant use of other medications such as corticosteroids, is uncommon when opioids are prescribed for pain control. Tolerance to these side effects occurs rapidly in most patients, but there is considerable individual variation. If confusion or dysphoria persists, opioid rotation is recommended. Oxycodone appears to cause hallucinations less frequently than does morphine. When assessing persistent confusion, it is also important to rule out causes other than opioids, especially terminal delirium associated with systemic and metabolic failure as the patient approaches death.

OTHER OPIOID-RELATED SIDE EFFECTS Pruritus and flushing are primarily, but not exclusively, related to opioid-induced histamine release. Pruritus is most common in patients who are receiving intraspinal opioids, although it may occur with any route of administration. Pruritus is usually treated with antihistamines. Should this prove ineffective, paroxetine and mirtazapine have antipruritic properties. For severe cases, small doses of naloxone may offer relief.

Myoclonus and jerking movements may occur in conjunction with high doses of any opioid but are most commonly encountered in patients receiving high doses of meperidine or morphine, whose metabolites normeperidine and normorphine, respectively, are particularly neuroexcitatory. "Opioid neuro toxicity" consists of a constellation of symptoms including myoclonus, hyperalgesia, allodynia, and altered mental status. It is more likely to occur when patients have concurrent renal insufficiency, are dehydrated, or are on continuous infusions of high-dose morphine. When possible, opioid neuro toxicity is most effectively managed with opioid rotation. When rotating to another opioid, it is important to consider whether the offending opioid (usually, morphine) dose was escalated for uncontrolled pain before the hyperalgesic syndrome was recognized. Therefore, reductions of at least 50% of the equianalgesic morphine dose should be considered when rotating to another opioid. For patients who are actively dying and for whom opioid rotation is not possible, continuation of the offending opioid should be done at the lowest therapeutic dose possible, and side effects should be aggressively treated with other agents. Antipsychotics for opioid-induced psychosis and benzodiazepines for controlling myoclonus are generally effective treatments when the existing opioid and dose are necessary to maintain analgesic control.

Myoclonus may sometimes be a prodrome to seizures. Should seizures occur, patients should be managed with dose reduction, opioid substitution, and benzodiazepine and/or nonbenzodiazepine anticonvulsants that should be continued for the several days usually necessary for clearance of the neuroexcitatory metabolites. Administration of naloxone should be avoided because this opioid antagonist can paradoxically aggravate CNS hyperactivity and will cause an opioid withdrawal syndrome and the return of pain.

OPIOID WITHDRAWAL In rare circumstances, terminally ill patients with chronic pain may improve sufficiently so that opioid analgesics are no longer required. An example might be a patient with lung cancer and advanced bone metastases whose bone pain has responded to palliative radiotherapy. Because chronic opioid treatment results in physical dependence, opioids must be tapered and never discontinued abruptly. There are two recommended methods for tapering opioid therapy:

(1) Reduce the total daily dose by 10% per day over a 10-day period, or by 5% per day over 20 days.
(2) Provide 50% of the previous daily opioid dose for 2 days, and continue to reduce the dose by 50% every 2 days until the patient is receiving 10 to 15 mg of morphine (or equivalent) per day. Administer this low dose for 2 days and then discontinue.

The second method allows for rapid initial reduction of the opioid dose. Reductions of more than 50% are likely to cause withdrawal symptoms including generalized aches and pains, sweating, and chills.

When death is imminent, patients often exhibit evidence of multisystem failure, hypotension, poor tissue perfusion, decreasing renal function, and a depressed level of consciousness. At this stage, patients may appear to have a diminished sense of pain, and families (and even some physicians and other health care professionals) sometimes incorrectly attribute the patient's deterioration to opioid medication. In these circumstances, it may be appropriate to reduce opioid doses and/or increase the interval between doses. However, precipitous discontinuation may provoke withdrawal symptoms even in actively dying patients. Therefore, the opioid dosage needs to be maintained at no less than 25% of the chronic daily dose to avoid additional discomfort for the patient, a goal with which most family members will readily identify after adequate explanation.

OPIOID TOLERANCE The concept of opioid tolerance refers to the need to increase the dose of an analgesic medication to maintain the desired level of pain control in the absence of disease progression or other exacerbating cause. The development of tolerance appears to be dependent on a number of neurochemical adaptations to opioid administration including changes in neuronal concentrations of cyclic adenosine monophosphate, opioid effects on calcium ion channels, upregulation of endogenous endorphins, and competitive binding for opioid receptors. As a result of these multiple biochemical mechanisms, tolerance to the various opioid-induced physiological effects develops differentially, and sometimes selectively. For this reason, most patients with chronic pain may be titrated to amounts of opioid medication sufficient to control pain without experiencing respiratory depression or sustained nausea or excessive sedation. In fact, the onset of analgesic tolerance in patients who are receiving opioids for chronic pain is unusual when the pain has an identifiable physical cause such as tumor growth and invasion or other sustained tissue injury. The increased need for opioid analgesics in patients with advanced cancer, for example, is most commonly due to disease progression rather than to the development of tolerance. Clinicians and patients should be aware of this observation because the concept that strong opioids will become ineffective if started too early, and should be held in reserve until "really needed," continues to be one of the prevalent barriers to effective pain management.

Nevertheless, analgesic tolerance to a previously effective opioid may occur in some patients so that new pain relief is not achieved despite even rapid dosage escalation to high levels. In this circumstance, and after a thorough reassessment, it is advisable to switch to an alternate opioid. The justification for this approach, sometimes referred to as "opioid rotation," is that crosstolerance among the various opioid agonist analgesics is frequently incomplete. Because of incomplete crosstolerance, when converting such a patient to another opioid, the new analgesic should generally be started at no higher than 50% of the calculated bioequivalent dose (see Table 6–13), and, at times, even lower doses may prove to be effective.

Although similar from a practical and conceptual viewpoint, opioid rotation, which addresses the issue of analgesic tolerance, should be distinguished from opioid substitution, which refers to the practice of changing patients with unacceptable, refractory adverse effects from one opioid to another member of the class. The purpose of this practice, which is based on the concept of individual, differential tolerance among opioids to various nonanalgesic effects, is to improve the adverse effect profile while maintaining equianalgesia. Perhaps because its use is most prevalent, morphine is the opioid most often associated with uncontrolled adverse effects. In a recent study, substitution produced partial or complete relief from refractory opioid-related confusion in 18 out of 25 cases, from refractory opioid-induced nausea and vomiting in 13 out of 19 cases, and from drowsiness in 8 out of 15 cases. Unlike opioid rotation for analgesic tolerance, in which the effective analgesic dose of the new opioid is often less than that predicted from standard conversion tables, the effective analgesic dose of the new opioid when there is substitution for adverse effects is at least bioequivalent to the drug being replaced.

Adjuvant Medications

Although opioid analgesics are the mainstay of effective pain management, other medications, used in conjunction with opioids, are frequently necessary to achieve effective pain control. Indications for these medications, termed coanalgesics or adjuvants, are determined according to the classification and etiology of the pain. The purpose of using drug combinations is to provide additive or synergistic analgesia and to reduce side effects. Failure to prescribe adjuvant medication, especially when patients have pain that responds incompletely to opioids, is one of the major causes for inadequate pain control.

BONE PAIN   Bone pain due to metastatic cancer is largely mediated by prostaglandins whose synthesis is catalyzed by COX. Therefore, NSAIDs, which inhibit COX and decrease prostaglandin production, are often effective, in conjunction with opioid analgesics, in reducing the pain and inflammation associated with bone pain.

Corticosteroids are also sometimes effective for skeletal pain. In terminally ill patients, especially those with a very short life expectancy, the adverse effects of chronic corticosteroid therapy are relatively inconsequential. Other than pain relief, patients treated with corticosteroids may realize an increased sense of well-being, or even euphoria. Another possible adjuvant treatment for bone pain is calcitonin. However, because calcitonin is expensive, and its effect appears to be mediated by increases in endogenous β-endorphins, it is not clear that adding calcitonin is more advantageous than merely increasing the exogenous opioid dose to achieve the necessary effect. Other adjunctive modalities for bone pain, including bisphosphonates, radiopharmaceuticals, and radiotherapy, may be selectively useful for end-of-life care and are discussed in Chapter 19.

NEUROPATHIC PAIN   Neuropathic pain is sometimes described as being opioid resistant. This description is not entirely accurate because response rates up to 33% have been reported. Oxycodone appears to be useful for treating postherpetic neuralgia (PHN), tramadol is reported to ease the pain of diabetic neuropathy, and methadone has known activity for neuropathic pain. In addition, patients often have mixed pain

TABLE 6–20. Neuropathic Pain Medications

CLASS OF MEDICATION	MEDICATION	DOSE
Steroids	Dexamethasone	16–96 mg PO daily in two to four divided doses
Tricyclic antidepressant	Amitriptyline	10–150 mg PO daily
	Nortriptyline	10–150 mg PO daily
	Desipramine	25–100 mg PO daily or in divided doses
Anticonvulsants	Gabapentin	300–2,400 mg PO daily in two to four divided doses
	Carbamazepine	200–1,600 mg PO daily in three to four divided doses
	Phenytoin	300–500 mg PO daily
	Clonazepam	0.5–1 mg PO three to four times a day
	Valproic acid	500–1,500 mg PO/day in two divided doses
	Lamotrigine	Start 25 mg PO QOD, titrate up to 50–200 mg PO/day in two divided doses
Others	Clonidine	0.1–0.3 mg PO or transdermally daily
	Baclofen	10–30 mg PO daily
	Mexiletine	Start 200 PO qhs, titrate up to 300–1200 mg PO daily in divided doses
Local anesthetics	Lidocaine	5% apply to affected area for 12 h/d
NMDA antagonists	Ketamine	0.3–0.5 mg/kg PO three times daily
	Methadone	See Table 6–17
	Amantadine	100 PO daily to twice daily

NMDA, N-methyl-D-aspartate.

syndromes with nociceptive as well as neuropathic components. Therefore, it is reasonable to include opioids when treating neuropathic pain, but almost always in conjunction with other adjuvant medications.

Agents commonly used for the treatment of neuropathic pain are listed in Table 6–20. Unfortunately, no single agent or combination regimen is successful all of the time, and the treatment of neuropathic pain must be both empirical and individualized. A suggested stepwise schema, similar to the WHO step ladder is illustrated in Figure 6–6 and will now be discussed.

Step 1: Neuropathic Pain   As the first step in the treatment of neuropathic pain, the clinician should combine an opioid with either corticosteroids or an NSAID.

Corticosteroids are especially effective in treating neuropathic symptoms accompanied by

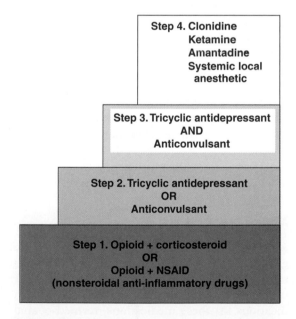

Step 4. Clonidine
       Ketamine
       Amantadine
       Systemic local
       anesthetic

Step 3. Tricyclic antidepressant
       AND
       Anticonvulsant

Step 2. Tricyclic antidepressant
       OR
       Anticonvulsant

Step 1. Opioid + corticosteroid
       OR
       Opioid + NSAID
       (nonsteroidal anti-inflammatory drugs)

Figure 6–6. Neuropathic pain analgesic ladder.

inflammation and edema. Headaches due to increased intracranial pressure and the pain and neurological deficits of spinal cord compression are examples of neuropathic symptoms that may be alleviated with corticosteroids. Dexamethasone in high doses is generally the steroid medication of choice. Corticosteroids may also be helpful in treating other forms of neuropathic pain and plexopathy. They are especially effective when there is a significant component of inflammation and soft tissue swelling. Corticosteroids may also be useful in the early management of herpes zoster and may possibly mitigate the later severity of PHN.

Combinations of opioids and NSAIDs are also sometimes effective for cancer-related neuropathic pain. NSAIDs were discussed in detail earlier.

Step 2: Neuropathic Pain In the proposed schema for treating neuropathic pain (Fig. 6–6), either a tri-cyclic antidepressant (TCA) or an anticonvulsant should be added as step 2.

Antidepressants The TCAs address neuropathic pain by three different mechanisms: mood elevation, potentiation or enhancement of opioid analgesics, and direct analgesic effects. Some palliative care experts have noted that TCAs are particularly effective for dysesthetic neuropathy in which patients complain of burning, cold, or vice-like sensations. In general, TCAs provide some relief in 40% of patients with neuropathic pain.

Amitriptyline is a tertiary tricyclic amine that has been extensively studied. Although some patients achieve analgesia with doses that are lower than those needed to treat depression, doses as high as 150 mg may sometimes be necessary. Patients are usually begun on 10 to 25 mg orally daily at bedtime and titrated up as tolerated. Analgesic effects may occur within 1 to 2 weeks, but the peak effect may not occur for 4 to 6 weeks; therefore, titrating TCAs more rapidly than weekly is not recommended. Patients need

to be aware of this time response to avoid disappointment and frustration.

Other TCAs that are useful for neuropathic pain include nortriptyline and desipramine. As secondary tricyclic amines, these medications may have fewer adverse effects than those associated with amitriptyline, including sedation, dry mouth, constipation, and urinary retention. Doxepin, a psychotropic medication with tricyclic properties may also have utility for neuropathic pain although it has a significant side effect profile.

The selective serotonin reuptake inhibitors (SSRIs) have limited usefulness as analgesics for neuropathic pain due to their selectivity for the serotonin pathway. It has been reported that paroxitene has alleviated symptoms of diabetic neuropathy in approximately one-third of patients treated, while fluoxetine, nefazodone, and sertraline have also been reported to be effective in treating symptoms of neuropathic pain for a small number of patients.

Venlafaxine, which shares properties of both SSRIs and TCAs, is reported to have enhanced activity against neuropathic pain. It is thought to inhibit norepinephrine, 5HT, and dopamine reuptake. Although renal and hepatic function must be considered, typical starting doses are 37.5 to 75 mg orally twice daily and titrated no more rapidly than every 3 or 4 days. Duloxetine is now FDA approved for the treatment of painful diabetic neuropathy. Like venlafaxine, it inhibits norepinephrine, 5HT, and dopamine reuptake in the brain. Doses less than 60 mg/d are not efficacious; therefore, the starting dose is generally 60 mg/d. It may not be crushed, chewed, or cut. Reduced dosing is indicated for patients with renal impairment, and extra caution should be exercised with patients with hepatic impairment. Mirtazapine has activity on both noradrenergic and serotonergic transmission and blocks 5HT2 and 5HT3 receptors. This biochemical profile reduces the likelihood of side effects related to nonselective serotonin activation and decreases the risk of cardiotoxicity. Mirtazapine is relatively safe for elderly patients, has beneficial effects on sleep, and has anxiolytic and antipruritic properties. It is anecdotally reported to have analgesic properties beyond its antidepressant effects, but it has not yet been tested in a controlled clinical trial. Thus, although there may well be an emerging role for SSRIs and SNRIs for the treatment of neuropathic pain, there is insufficient information to justify their routine substitution for TCAs.

Anticonvulsants   Older anticonvulsant medications, such as gabapentin, phenytoin, carbamazepine, valproic acid, and clonazepam, may be effective treatment options for neuropathic pain. Anecdotal evidence suggests that anticonvulsant therapy may be more valuable in treating episodic neuropathic pain that is lancinating or burning in nature. This type of pain is typically associated with nerve injury, trigeminal neuralgia, or PHN.

Anticonvulsant drugs reduce or prevent pathologically altered neurons from excessive discharge and reduce the spread of excitation from abnormal foci to normal neurons. One of the major limiting factors in the use of the various anticonvulsants is the high incidence of side effects. Therefore, as with TCAs, the initial dose should be low and upward titration should be slow and cautious. For example, a starting dose of carbamazepine can be as low as 50 mg at bedtime in elderly patients or 100 mg in younger patients. Side effects may occur before any therapeutic benefit is realized.

Gabapentin has a lower incidence of side effects than the other anticonvulsants and has been reported to effectively treat neuropathic pain in doses as low as 300 mg/d, up to the more commonly used doses of 600 to 1,800 mg/d. Doses as high as 3,600 mg/d have been reported, although patients who do not receive pain relief from 2,400 mg/d are unlikely to achieve pain relief from higher doses. To achieve these doses, patients are generally started at 300 mg/d, usually in divided doses three times daily. Titrations of 100 mg per dose may be made every 3 days,

allowing the patient time to accommodate to sedating side effects. Titration to effective doses, usually 600 to 2,400 mg/d, may not always be attained because of excess sedation and onset of dysequilibrium. Gabapentin may be especially useful for patients with AIDS neuropathies because it does not interact with antiretroviral medications and, unlike carbamazepine, it does not cause bone marrow toxicity. Gabapentin may be administered orally or rectally. The time necessary to titrate to an effective dose may limit the usefulness of gabapentin in those close to death.

A relative newcomer to the market for treating PHN and diabetic peripheral neuropathy is pregabalin (Lyrica). The recommended starting dose is 50 mg three times daily or 75 mg twice daily. A response may be seen as quickly as within 24 hours of initiating the drug. The maximum recommended dose is 300 mg/d, but clinical studies have demonstrated enhanced response when given in doses as large as 600 mg/d in divided doses. Higher doses should be restricted to patients with normal creatinine clearance.

Step 3: Neuropathic Pain   If there is an inadequate analgesic response to the addition of either a TCA or an anticonvulsant, concurrent use of both medications together is recommended as step 3. Anticonvulsants that work by different mechanisms (e.g., carbamazepine, phenytoin, valproic acid vs. clonazepam, phenobarbital, gabapentin) may also be tried concurrently, although with increased risk of adverse side effects.

Step 4: Neuropathic Pain

Clonidine and local anesthetics   Other agents with anecdotal success in the treatment of neuropathic pain include clonidine and systemically administered local anesthetic agents such as intravenous lidocaine and oral mexiletine and tocainide. Clonidine is a centrally acting α_2-adrenergic agonist that has been used successfully to treat phantom pain and pain associated with diabetic neuropathy, PHN, and spinal cord injury. Despite enthusiasm for these drugs as anesthetics, in larger studies their effectiveness as systemic analgesics has been disappointing, with only about 10% of patients studied reporting significant improvements in pain control.

Baclofen and tizanidine Baclofen and tizanidine are best known as muscle relaxants and have been found to be effective in the treatment of both neuropathic pain and the muscle spasm that so often accompanies neurologic injury. In cases of spinal cord compression or other CNS impairment that is associated with spastic paraparesis, for example, baclofen in gradually escalating doses from 10 to 30 mg/d may be very effective, whereas tizanidine has been used to relieve severe muscle spasms for patients with multiple sclerosis.

NMDA antagonists Interest in the treatment of neuropathic pain has most recently focused on agents that inhibit the NMDA receptor channel complex. The simplest NMDA receptor inhibitor is magnesium. Magnesium sulfate, 0.5 to 1.0 g intravenously, was effective in completely or partially alleviating pain for up to 4 hours in 10 out of 12 cancer patients with neuropathic pain that was poorly responsive to opioids. The practical clinical application of this finding is limited because of the short duration of response and the necessity for intravenous administration. However, it has also been postulated that hypomagnesemia may cause activation of the NMDA receptor, potentiate chronic pain, and blunt the response to opioids. For this reason, it may be worthwhile to identify and correct hypomagnesemia in terminal patients with intractable pain.

Primarily because of a high incidence of toxic effects, the use of NMDA receptor antagonists in humans has been restricted to a small number of clinical trials. These agents include methadone (see above), ketamine, dextromethorphan, and amantadine. Ketamine has been widely used as an anesthetic agent, producing analgesia in doses much lower than those required for anesthesia. Traditionally, it has been administered as a continuous intravenous infusion, and its utility for treating chronic pain has been limited by adverse side effects including excess sedation, psychotomimetic manifestations, and delirium. A number of studies have shown that ketamine, 10 mg TID to 20 mg QID, may be successfully used via the oral or sublingual route to treat PHN pain as well as other neuropathic conditions including postlaminectomy radicular pain.

Dextromethorphan is an antitussive medication that is a component of many cough syrup formulations. It can be administered in a slow-release preparation, in doses of 15 to 500 mg BID. Its major side effect is sedation. In combination with morphine, dextromethorphan can potentiate pain relief and allow a reduction in the total daily morphine dose, although it is not clear that this effect alone is sufficient reason for the commercial development of morphine–dextromethorphan combination products.

Amantadine, used as an anti-influenza medication, is also an NMDA antagonist. In one report, three patients achieved complete and sustained relief of neuropathic pain after a single 200 mg intravenous infusion. A follow-up, randomized trial in 13 patients confirmed that intravenous amantadine acutely relieves neuropathic pain, but that sustained, long-term relief after a single dose is unusual. Oral amantadine may also have some activity and may deserve a trial in patients with refractory neuropathic pain because it is less toxic, more easily available, and less expensive than oral ketamine.

ALIMENTARY TRACT PAIN SYNDROMES A discussion on the treatment of pain related to mucositis and stomatitis can be found in Chapter 10 in the section entitled "Disorders of the Mucus Membranes." A discussion of the etiologies and treatments of various forms of abdominal pain can be found in Chapter 8, in the section entitled "Abdominal Pain and Dyspepsia."

TABLE 6–21. Characteristics of Addictive Behavior

Overwhelming concerns about drug availability
Unsanctioned dose escalation
Continued use despite significant side effects
Manipulation of physicians to obtain additional drug supplies
Alterations of prescriptions
Drug acquisition from multiple medical or nonmedical sources
Drug hoarding or selling

Pharmacological Pain Management in the Patient with Previous or Current Substance Abuse

It is particularly important to be aware of a history of previous or current substance abuse when patients present with chronic pain. Because of the complex neurophysiologic interplay between pain and addiction pathways, it may be neccssary to modify pharmacological interventions in such patients to achieve effective pain control and avoid toxicity. Characterizations of addictive behavior are listed in Table 6–21.

The complexities inherent in the management of pain in currently addicted patients and in recovered or recovering patients have led to the development of guidelines that are delineated in Tables 6–22 and 6–23, respectively. It should be noted that these guidelines are not always appropriate or successful and require frequent adaptation and modification to meet the needs of individual patients. For patients enrolled in MMT programs, it is helpful to work closely with the MMT prescriber to determine the most effective analgesic prescription and ensure compliance. Patients with a prior history of heroin or prescription opioid drug abuse will likely have significant opioid tolerance, which can make their pain difficult to treat. Although methadone itself may be a useful analgesic in patients with opioid tolerance, the use of methadone as an analgesic should be coordinated directly with the patient's MMT program physician. Methadone is dosed daily by MMT programs to prevent withdrawal reactions but will need to be dosed two to four times daily as an analgesic. How the maintenance dose is incorporated into the methadone analgesic regimen must be synchronized with the MMT program. Some MMT programs prefer analgesic regimens not include methadone, but they should be informed if the patient is prescribed other opioids so as not to avoid misplaced suspicions when spot drug testing is performed.

Patients who are on MMT present a unique challenge when they approach the end of life and are physically unable to go to MMT centers. Although any licensed physician with a DEA number is legally allowed to prescribe methadone as an analgesic, a specific license is required to prescribe methadone for opioid maintenance. When the patient is too ill to go to the MMT center, prescribers will need to communicate with the MMT program and find creative solutions to prevent withdrawal. Often, patients at the end of life are on opioid analgesic regimens, but they may be insufficient to prevent withdrawal reactions, especially for those on high-dose MMT.

PSEUDOADDICTION Clinicians should be aware of a related phenomenon known as pseudoaddiction. This may occur in patients with or without a prior history of substance abuse. The natural history of this syndrome includes three characteristic phases:

1. Inadequate prescription of analgesics to meet the primary pain stimulus, resulting in persistent uncontrolled pain.
2. Escalation of analgesic demands by the patient associated with behavioral changes (similar to those listed in Table 6–21) to convince others of the pain's severity. Patients in this phase are often characterized as having a substance abuse problem, whether or not there was any prior history of substance abuse.

TABLE 6–22. Guidelines for Treatment of Currently Addicted Patients

1. Encourage open communication with the patient.
2. Avoid charting comments about drug use behaviors unless you have discussed your concerns with the patient. (May be required under current Federal Privacy Protection rules).
3. Remember that denial is a cardinal feature of addiction.
4. Within legal guidelines, obtain information about the patient's drug use from sources other than the patient.
5. Do not withhold opioids from patients with moderate or severe pain; doing so will only encourage craving and drug-seeking behavior.
6. Accept and respect the report of pain in spite of the possibility of being duped.
7. Assure patients that they will receive as much medication as needed to relieve pain.
8. Establish a written treatment plan or contract, negotiated with and agreed to by the patient to include:
   a. Allowable medications and doses
   b. Amounts of medication to be dispensed
   c. Policies regarding refills and "lost medications"
   d. Frequency of office or home-care visits
   e. Consequences of failure to follow the plan.
9. Arrange for all opioids and other adjunctive and psychotropic medications to be prescribed by the same physician.
10. Encourage participation of nurse addiction specialists and designate a nurse as coordinator for the management team, as traditionally done in hospice care.
11. These patients have often developed drug tolerance and may require much larger doses of opioids than the average patient. Therefore:
    a. Titrate to effect.
    b. Estimate the patient's usual daily intake and provide therapeutic dosing above this baseline dose to obtain effective analgesia.
12. Use regularly scheduled, long-acting opioids for baseline pain management. Avoid PRN schedules except as indicated for intermittent or breakthrough pain.
13. Use adjunctive medications liberally, but appropriately. Do not use them as replacements for opioids.
14. Encourage the use of nonpharmacological interventions.
15. Should the patient demand rapid or unexpected escalation in dosage requirements disproportional to the apparent extent or progression of the underlying disease, do not be too hasty to attribute this to the coexistent addictive disorder. Take the time to identify other potential areas of distress and suffering, including emotional, social, and spiritual pain.
16. Remember that relief of pain and maximization of quality of life are the common goals that should motivate the patient, family, caregivers, and health care team alike.

3. A crisis of mistrust between the patient and members of the health care team, resulting in the precipitation of a painful crisis.

Clinicians must always be alert to the possibility of inducing pseudoaddiction through inadequate treatment of chronic pain. To avoid contributing to the suffering of patients who are near the end of life, it is crucial to remember that "Pain is whatever the patient says it is, existing whenever the patient says it does."

TABLE 6–23. Guidelines for Managing Pain in Recovered and Recovering Patients

1. Distinguish between abstinence and recovery.
   a. The abstinent person who is struggling with his or her abstinence is often still in denial, socially dysfunctional, and actively fighting drug craving.
   b. Pain in these patients is best managed similarly to actively addicted patients.
2. Believe the patient's complaint of pain.
3. Determine whether pain control techniques other than opioids are preferable.
4. Address patient and family concerns about dependence and relapse. Explain that physical dependency, which will occur, is not the same as addiction.
5. Reassure the patient and family that opioid use will be structured. Formulate and obtain patient agreement to a treatment plan contract.
6. One caretaker should be designated as responsible for pain management.
7. Use drugs in effective doses and titrate the doses to achieve adequate analgesia. Do not underdose, as this may lead to anxiety and drug craving.
8. Prescribe on a scheduled (around-the-clock) basis.
9. Limit quantities per prescription and do not allow refills.
10. Have spouse, friend, other caregiver, or pharmacist dispense each dose.
11. Maintain frequent contact with the patient and caregiver.
12. Remember that stress may increase the patient's request for analgesics.
13. Be alert for and address aberrant drug use behavior suggestive of true addiction, such as acquisition of drugs from multiple sources, repeated claims of lost medications, unsanctioned dose increases, and prescription fraud.

NONPHARMACOLOGICAL INTERVENTIONS FOR THE TREATMENT OF PAIN

A total pain assessment that evaluates the physical, psychological, social, and spiritual causes of pain allows the clinician to formulate a holistic plan of care that targets each manifestation of a patient's overall experience of pain. This integrated approach to pain management extends treatment choices to include alternative therapies and nonpharmacological interventions. Although the medical literature on complementary and alternative medicine therapies is scanty, combining these techniques and treatment modalities with traditional analgesic medications allows the patient, caregivers, and physician to select from the full range of pain management strategies that might be needed to adequately address pain's physical, mental, and emotional components. Table 6–24 lists these interventions and categorizes them into four approaches.

PHYSICAL INVASIVE APPROACHES

Anesthetic and surgical procedures are used predominantly for managing cancer pain refractory to other less invasive modalities. Realistic goals and expectations for these interventions should take into account not only the ability of the patient with advanced disease to tolerate the surgery or therapy but also patient preference. The guiding principle for all of these interventions should be that they have a high probability of success, they lack side effects that exact too high a price

TABLE 6–24. Nonpharmacological Interventions for Pain Management

APPROACH	INTERVENTION/TECHNIQUE	ADVANTAGES	DISADVANTAGES
Physical— invasive	*Anesthetic procedures* • Nerve Blocks: e.g., celiac plexus • Infusions: intraspinal clonidine • CNS stimulation *Surgical procedures* • Neurologic: rhizotomy • Orthopedic: spinal decompression • Oncologic: debulking *Radiation therapy* • Localized, wide-field • Radiopharmaceuticals *Chemotherapy* • Cytotoxic, hormonal	Can provide rapid pain relief. Useful for pain that has not responded to less invasive measures. Effective for pain relief with certain diagnoses. Can allow dosage reduction (and side effects) of systemic drugs. Direct treatment of tumor.	Possible infection at catheter site. Requires special expertise, careful monitoring. May require expensive infusion pumps, specialized care, and/or costs. Procedures are irreversible.
Physical— nonin- vasive	*Physical rehabilitation* • Immobilization, movement, positioning • Hydrotherapy *Massage/manipulation/stimulation* • Superficial heat/cold applications • TENS, ultrasound • Acupuncture, Acupressure, Shiatsu • Myofascial, craniosacral therapy • Chiropractic, therapeutic massage • Rolfing, Pruden, Feldenkrais, Trager • Reflexology	May decrease pain and anxiety without drug-related side effects. Can be used as adjuvant therapy with most other interventions. Can be administered by patients or families.	Heat and cold may sometimes be contraindicated. Skilled therapist required for some interventions.
Cognitive/ mind— body	*Interpersonal/spiritual* • Therapeutic healing touch • Prayer • Bibliotherapy *Attention/diversion* • Music, humor, art, pet *Imagery* • Guided, incompatible, transformative *Education* • Information and instructions on care *Psychologic–physiologic* • Self-talk, distraction • Meditation, relaxation, Yoga	May decrease pain and anxiety for patients who have pain that is difficult to manage. May increase patient's coping skills. Gives patients sense of control over pain. Can be used as adjuvant therapy with most other interventions. Most are inexpensive, require no special equipment, and are easily administered.	Patient must be motivated to use self-management strategies. Some interventions require professional time to teach.

TENS, transcutaneous electrical nerve stimulation.

(Continued)

TABLE 6–24. Nonpharmacological Interventions for Pain Management (*Continued*)

APPROACH	INTERVENTION/TECHNIQUE	ADVANTAGES	DISADVANTAGES
Cognitive/ mind— body (cont'd)	• Guided imagery • Biofeedback, hypnotherapy • Autogenic training, cognitive restructuring • Rhythmic cognitive activity, problem solving		
Alternative/ natural Remedies	Herbal remedies Neutraceuticals Aromatherapy Homeopathy	Gives patient sense of control over pain. Some interventions demonstrate analgesic efficacy.	Some herbal remedies have the potential to cause drug interactions.

on the quality of life, and that the benefit will be evident within the time frame of the patient's anticipated survival.

PHYSICAL NONINVASIVE APPROACHES

Physical medicine techniques include immobilization, range-of-motion exercises, hydrotherapy, massage, acupuncture, application of heat or cold, and transcutaneous electrical nerve stimulation (TENS). Incorporating traditional therapies delivered by physical therapists, nurses, and other rehabilitation therapists with alternative interventions that can be administered by the patient or caregivers will provide more opportunities and choices for the patient. These interventions achieve pain relief directly, by means of manipulation or stimulation of the musculoskeletal, nervous, and integumentary systems or indirectly, by producing a generalized relaxation response.

Physical rehabilitation techniques may be used in limited settings for specific indications. Immobilization methods include use of a corset to help support the vertebral bodies and control back pain, a shoulder support to reduce pain sec-

ondary to brachial plexopathy, or splinting for a patient with a pathological fracture in whom surgery is not contemplated or desired. Range-of-motion exercises may help reduce discomfort for patients with spastic paraparesis or prevent the development of contractures. The benefits of hydrotherapy are attributable to the buoyancy of water. They include increased strength and flexibility for patients whose joints are stiff and whose limbs are weak. TENS may occasionally benefit a small subset of patients, but it has generally not been successful for treating pain in terminal patients. The utility of superficial cold/heat treatments and ultrasound is restricted to localized somatic pain.

Acupuncture has been used for the treatment of pain for more than 2,500 years, and its effectiveness for pain management has been documented in scientific studies. Acupuncture appears to elicit endorphin release at the level of the spinal cord and midbrain and may also lead to the release of anti-inflammatory cytokines. Its usefulness in managing for patients at the end of life is uncertain and should be evaluated on an individual patient basis.

The medical literature on massage therapy, although not robust, suggests an overall benefit.

Studies of massage therapy indicate an improvement in fatigue, nausea, quality of life, anxiety, and pain. Positive outcomes also include enhancing the patient's sense of control and satisfaction with medical care.

A detailed description of other alternative noninvasive physical techniques listed is beyond the scope of the chapter. Information about these techniques and the extent to which claims for efficacy have been validated scientifically is available from the Office of Alternative Medicine of the United States National Institutes of Health.

COGNITIVE/MIND–BODY APPROACH

For terminally ill patients, achieving a perception of personal control over pain is a key component of quality of life, which becomes most evident when pain is defined as a multidimensional experience. This conceptual framework includes sensory, cognitive, affective, and behavioral parameters that are ultimately defined in terms of neurophysiology as well as a spiritual dimension, which, although metaphysical, appears to affect the processing of pain in people from widely disparate backgrounds and cultures. The Cognitive/Mind–Body approach incorporates interventions such as prayer, therapeutic healing and touch, music, art, humor, and pet therapy that help the patient cope with pain and provide a means by which a sense of personal control can be restored. These techniques are especially useful for patients who have strong psychosocial and spiritual issues that are influencing their perception and reaction to pain. Helping a patient understand that pain can exist both objectively (i.e., physical) and subjectively (i.e., emotional, mental, spiritual) will increase receptiveness to these interventions.

For the clinician, the Cognitive/Mind–Body method requires a commitment to "total pain" management and the existence of a personalized therapeutic relationship with individual patients, caregivers, and family members. These techniques are compatible with both primary care and with the hospice interdisciplinary model of care in which physicians, nurses, social workers, chaplains, home health aides, and lay volunteers work together with the patient and family to provide a therapeutic environment that encourages the concept of "total pain" control. Hospices are committed to the principle that even dying patients should be given every opportunity to experience the maximal fullness of life possible. The extent to which this goal may be enhanced with Cognitive/Mind–Body interventions such as music therapy is apparent in the following quote: "At a time when I felt at the mercy of a situation and dependent on others for help, I was being offered a degree of self-determination. I was being challenged to take up with the tricky business of life again."

ALTERNATIVE/NATURAL REMEDIES

Although herbal remedies contain physiologically active ingredients, the FDA classifies these products as dietary supplements rather than as controlled or regulated drugs. As dietary supplements, they need not have substantial research proving safety and efficacy before they are released to the market; therefore, we are unable to recommend specific herbal therapies at the time of the writing of this book. Based on anecdotal evidence, however, some of these products (e.g., feverfew, ginseng, green tea extract) have been promoted for the treatment of headaches and fibromyalgia. Clinicians need to be aware of this usage, not necessarily because of efficacy, but rather because of their growing popularity and the occurrence of documented herbal-related drug interactions (e.g., "serotonin syndrome" due to the combination of St. John's wort and meperidine).

Neutraceuticals, or foods that are used therapeutically, may have possible analgesic effects. Amino acid precursors to neurotransmitters such as serotonin and endogenous opioid peptides

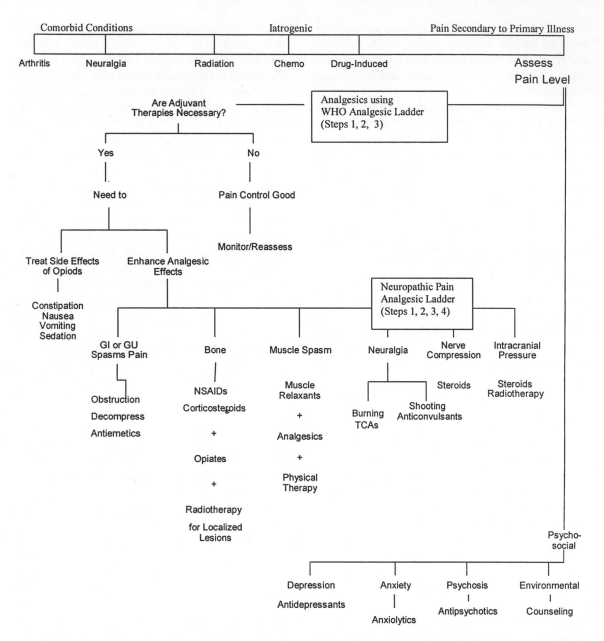

Figure 6–7. Pain management algorithm. *Abbreviations*: GI, gastrointestinal; GU, genitourinary; NSAIDs, nonsteroidal anti-inflammatory drugs; TCAs, tricyclic antidepressants.

Source: Reprinted, with permission, from Kinzbrunner BM: *Vitas Pain Management Guidelines*. Miami, FL, Vitas Healthcare Corporation, 1999.

include tryptophan, phenylalanine, and leucine. Foods high in these amino acids such as protein, legumes, and certain nuts and vegetables have been reported to provide pain relief.

The benefits of aromatherapy and homeopathy for treating pain are unproven and unsubstantiated at this time. Purported analgesia from aromatherapy may be due to local absorption of aromatherapy oils or from a feeling of well-being associated with their fragrance. Homeopathic preparations are based on the premise behind vaccines—"like cures like." These extremely diluted forms of substances might include products such as belladonna and chamomile and have not been shown to be of significant clinical value in managing pain.

CONCLUSION

In end-of-life care, the key objectives in the treatment of pain include achieving relief of pain, preventing pain recurrences, optimizing the patient's sense of well-being, and restoring a modicum of hope and belief in the value of life, however chronologically limited. These goals are enhanced by comprehensive pain assessment and by choosing the least obtrusive, least sedating, and most effective analgesic techniques.

Pharmacological intervention should incorporate the concepts of the analgesic ladder and appropriate use of adjuvant medications on the basis of the pathophysiology of the patient's pain. For patients with severe pain, non–ceiling-effect opioid agonist analgesics should be used in functionally effective doses, titrated according to individual need and response, and prescribed on a regular schedule with provision for additional "as needed" doses for breakthrough and incident pain. Nonpharmacological modalities and psychosocial and spiritual interventions should be integrated into the plan of care with the objective of addressing all dimensions of suffering. Par-

enteral and spinal analgesics and other aggressive "invasive" techniques should be offered to refractory patients with appropriate clinical and prognostic indications. Figure 6–7 presents the strategies for successful pain management in algorithmic fashion.

With the successful application of these concepts and principles, it may be theoretically possible to reduce the percentage of patients with truly intractable pain to less than 1% of the total population at risk. However, until data are available from further research and investigation, and more significantly, until the basic and well-founded principles of pain management described above are widely disseminated and effectively applied, apparently intractable pain will continue to be a major source of suffering for patients and their loved ones. Physician competency in pain management is essential to enable patients with advanced illness and those at the end of life to retain hope that they will not have to die in pain, and that dying does not have to be associated with unrelieved suffering.

BIBLIOGRAPHY

Actiq (oral transmucosal fentanyl citrate). Reference 58-0645-R2, Abbott Laboratories, North Chicago, IL, 1999.

Abrahm J: *A Physician's Guide to Pain and Symptom Management in Cancer Patients*, 2nd ed. Baltimore, MD, Johns Hopkins University Press, 2005.

Acute Pain Management Guideline Panel: *Acute Pain Management: Operative or Medical Procedures and Trauma.Clinical Practice Guideline*. AHCPR Pub. No. 92–0032. Rockville, MD, Agency for Health Care Policy and Research, Public Health Service, US Department of Health and Human Services, February 1992.

Alvarez MP, Agra Y: Systematic review of educational interventions in palliative care for primary care physicians. *Palliat Med* 20(7):673-683, 2006.

Anderson SL, Shreve ST: Continuous subcutaneous infusion of opiates at end-of-life. *Ann Pharmacother* 88:1015-1023, 2004.

Ashby M: The role of radiotherapy in palliative care. *J Pain Symptom Manage* 6:380, 1991.

Auret K, Schug SA: Underutilisation of opioids in elderly patients with chronic pain: Approaches to correcting the problem. *Drugs Aging* 22(8):641-654, 2005.

Bardia A, Barton DL, Prokop LJ, et al: Efficacy of complimentary and alternative medicine therapies in relieving cancer pain: A systematic review. *J Clin Oncol* 24:5457-5464, 2006.

Bennett G, Burchiel K, Buchser E, et al: Clinical guidelines for intraspinal infusion: Report of an expert panel. Polyanalgesic Consensus Conference 2000. *J Pain Symptom Manage* 20:S37-S43, 2000.

Bennett G, Serafini M, Burchiel K, et al: Evidence-based review of the literature on intrathecal delivery of pain medication. *J Pain Symptom Manage* 2:S12-S36, 2000.

Berger A, Schuster J, von Roenn J, eds. *Principles and Practice of Palliative Care and Supportive Oncology*, 3rd ed. Philadelphia, PA, Lippincott Williams & Wilkins, 2007.

Biancofiore G: Oxycodone controlled release in cancer pain management. *Ther Clin Risk Manag* 2(3):229-234, 2006.

Bolger J, Dearnly D, Kirk D, et al: Strontium-89 (metastron) versus external beam radiotherapy in patients with painful bony metastases secondary to prostate carcinoma. Preliminary report of a multicenter trial. *Semin Oncol* 20(3, Suppl 2):32-33, 1993.

Brannon GE, Stone KD: The use of mirtazapine in a patient with chronic pain. *J Pain Symptom Manage* 18:382-385, 1999.

Brater DC: Effects of nonsteroidal anti-inflammatory drugs on renal function: Focus on cyclooxygenase-2-selective inhibition. *Am J Med* 107:65S-70S; discussion 70S-71S, 1999.

Bruera E, Breinneis C, Paterson AH, MacDonald RN: Use of methylphenidate as an adjuvant to narcotic analgesics in patients with advanced cancer. *J Pain Symptom Manage* 4:3, 1989.

Bruera E, MachEachern T, Ripamonti C, Hanson J: Subcutaneous morphine for dyspnea in cancer patients. *Ann Intern Med* 119:906, 1993.

Bruera E, Macmillan K, Pither J, MacDonald RN: Effects of morphine on the dyspnea of terminally ill cancer patients. *J Pain Symptom Manage* 5:341, 1993.

Bruera E, Sweeney C: Methadone use in cancer patients with pain: A review. *J Palliat Med* 5(1):127-138, 2002.

Caraceni A, Zecca E, Martini C, Conno F: Gabapentin as an adjuvant to opioid analgesia for neuropathic cancer pain. *J Pain Symptom Manage* 17:441-445, 1999.

Carron AT, Lynn J, Keaney P: End-of-life care in medical textbooks. *Ann Intern Med* 130(1):82-86, 1999.

Cassileth BR, Deng GE, Gomez JE, et al: Complementary therapies and integrative oncology in lung cancer: ACCP evidence-based clinical practice guidelines (2nd ed.). *Chest* 132:340-354, 2007.

Cassileth BR, Vickers AJ: Massage therapy for symptom control: Outcome study at a major cancer center. *J Pain Symptom Manage* 28:244-249, 2004.

Center for Disease Control Web site. http://www.cdc.gov/nchs/products/pubs/pubd/hestats/poisoning/poisoning.htm. Accessed May 8, 2008.

Cherny NJ: The assessment of cancer pain. In: McMillan SC, Koltzenburg J eds. *Wall and Melzack's Textbook of Pain*. London, Elsevier, 1998, pp. 1099-1125.

Clark JM, Lurie JD, Claessens MT, et al: Factors associated with palliative care knowledge among internal medicine house staff. *J Palliat Care* 19(4):253-257, 2003.

Cleeland CS, Gonin R, Hatfield AK, et al: Pain and its treatment in outpatients with metastatic cancer. *N Engl J Med* 330:592, 1994.

Clemens KE, Klaschik E: Symptomatic therapy of dyspnea with strong opioids and its effect on ventilation in palliative care patients. *J Pain Symptom Manage* 33(4):473-481, 2007.

Clemens KE, Quednau I, Klaschik E: Is there a higher risk of respiratory depression in opioid-naïve palliative care patients during symptomatic therapy of dyspnea with strong opioids? *J Palliat Med* 11(2):204-216, 2008.

Cole L, Hanning CD: Review of the rectal use of opioids. *J Pain Symptom Manage* 5:118, 1990.

Courts NF: Nonpharmacologic approaches to pain. In: Salerno E, Willens JS, eds. *Pain Management Handbook, An Interdisciplinary Approach*. St. Louis, MO, Mosby, 1996, pp. 137-178.

Crosby V, Wilcock A, Corcoran R: The safety and efficacy of a single dose (500 mg or 1 g) of intravenous magnesium sulfate in neuropathic pain poorly responsive to strong opioid analgesics in patients with cancer. *J Pain Symptom Manage* 19:35-39, 2000.

de Leon-Casasola OA: Current developments in opioid therapy for management of cancer pain. *Clin J Pain* 24(4):S3-S7, 2008.

Dellemijn PL: Are opioids effective in relieving neuropathic pain? *Pain* 80:453-462, 1999.

Duong BD, Kerns RD, Towle V, Reid MC: Identifying the activities affected by chronic nonmalignant pain in older veterans receiving primary care. *J Am Geriatr Soc* 53:687-694, 2005.

Duragesic [package insert]. Janssen Pharmaceutica, Titusville, NJ, 2008.

Durand JP, Goldwasser F: Dramatic recovery of paclitaxel-disabling neurosensory toxicity following treatment with venlafaxine. *Anticancer Drugs* 13: 777-780, 2002.

Dworkin RH, Corbin AE, Young JP, et al: Pregabalin for the treatment of postherpetic neuralgia: A randomized, placebo-controlled trial. *Neurology* 60(8):1274-1283, 2003.

Edmundson EA, Simpson RK, Stubler DK, Beric A: Systemic lidocaine therapy for post-stroke pain. *South Med J* 86:1093, 1993.

Eisenberg E, Pud D: Can patients with chronic neuropathic pain be cured by acute administration of the NMDA receptor antagonist amantadine? *Pain* 74:337-339, 1998.

Enarson MC, Hays H, Woodroffe MA: Clinical experience with oral ketamine. *J Pain Symptom Manage* 17:384-386, 1999.

Enck RE: Adjuvant analgesic drugs. *Am J Hosp Care* 6(2):9, 1989.

Enck RE: Understanding and managing bone metastases. *Am J Hosp Palliat Care* 3(3):3, 1991.

Ettinger AB, Portenoy RK: The use of corticosteroids in the treatment of symptoms associated with cancer. *J Pain Symptom Manage* 3:99, 1988.

Farr WC: The use of corticosteroids for symptom management in terminally ill patients. *Am J Hosp Care* 5(1):41, 1990.

Felsby S, Nielson J, Arendt-Nielsen L, Jensen RS: NMDA receptor blockade in chronic neuropathic pain: A comparison of ketamine and magnesium chloride. *Pain* 64:283-291, 1995.

Ferrell B, Virani R, Grant M, et al: Analysis of pain content in nursing textbooks. *J Pain Symptom Manage* 19(3):216-228, 2000.

Ferrell BR, Virani R, Grant M: Analysis of symptom assessment and management content in nursing textbooks. *J Palliat Med* 2(2):161-172, 1999.

Fine PG: Low-dose ketamine in the management of opioid nonresponsive terminal cancer pain. *J Pain Symptom Manage* 17:296-300, 1999.

Fingerhut LA: *Increases in Poisoning and Methadone-Related Deaths: United States, 1999-2005.* Department of Health and Human Services, Centers for Disease Control and Prevention, National Center for Health Statistics Hyattsville, MD. http://www.cdc.gov/nhcs/products/pubs/pubd/hestats/poisoning/poisoning.htm. Accessed May 8, 2008.

Fingerhut LA: *Increases in Methadone-Related Deaths: 1999-2004.* National Center for Health Statistics. U.S. Department of Health and Human Services, Center for Disease Control and Prevention, National Center for Health Statistics, Hyattsville, MD, 2007.

Finlay I: Ketamine and its role in cancer pain. *Pain Rev* 6:303-313, 1999.

Fisher Wilson J: The pain divide between men and women. *Arch Intern Med* 144(6):461-464, 2006.

Fukui S, Komoda Y, Nosaka S: Clinical application of amantadine, an NMDA antagonist for neuropathic pain. *J Anesth* 15:179-181, 2001.

Galer BS, Harle J, Rowbotham MC: Response to intravenous lidocaine infusion predicts subsequent response to oral mexiletine: A prospective study. *J Pain Symptom Manage* 12:161, 1996.

Gazelle G, Fine PG. *Methadone for the Treatment of Pain,* 2nd ed. Wisconsin, EPERC, End of Life/Palliative Care Education Resource Center. http://www.mcw.edu/fastFact/ff 75.htm. Accessed March 15, 2010.

Green CR, Wheeler JRC, Marchant B, et al: Analysis of the physician variable in pain management. *Pain Med* 2(4):317-327, 2001.

Green CR, Wheeler JRC, LaPorte F, et al: How well is chronic pain managed? Who does it well. *Pain Med* 3(1):56-65, 2002.

Gureje O, Von Korff M, Simon GE, Gater R: Persistent pain and well-being: A World Health Organization study in primary care. *JAMA* 280(2):147-151, 1998.

Gurian B, Rosowsky E: Low dose methylphenidate in the very old. *J Geriatr Psychiatry Neurol* 3:152, 1990.

Hernon P: Hospice helps dull pain of dying patients (interview with Dr. C. Stratton Hill). *Montgomery Texas Advertiser,* March 17, 1992.

Herfindal ET, Gourley DR, Hart LL: *Clinical Pharmacy and Therapeutics,* 4th ed. Baltimore, MD, William and Wilkins, 1988.

Hockenbury MJ, Wilson D: *Wong's Essentials of Pediatric Nursing,* 8th ed. St. Louis, MO, Mosby, 2009.

International Association for the Study of Pain 1979. International Association for the Study of Pain, Subcommittee on Taxonomy. Pain terms: a list with definitions and notes on usage. *Pain* 6:249-252, 1979.

Jacobsen R, Sjogren P, Moldrup C, Christrup L: Physician-related barriers to cancer pain management with opioid analgesics: A systematic review. *J Opioid Manag* 3(4):207-214, 2007.

Jacox A, Carr DB, Payne R, et al: *Management of Cancer Pain. Clinical Practice Guideline No. 9.* AHCPR publication No. 94-0592. Rockville, MD, Agency for Health Care Policy and Research, US Department of Health and Human Services, Public Health Service, 1994.

Jaffe JH, Martin WR: Opioid analgesics and antagonists. In: Gillman AG, Rall TW, Nies AS, Taylor P, eds. *Goodman and Gilman's The Pharmacological Basis of Therapeutics*, 8th ed. Elmsford, NY, Pergamon Press, 1990, p. 502.

Jones R, Hale E, Talomsin L, Phillips R: Kapanol capsules. Pellet formulation provides alternative methods of administration of sustained release morphine sulfate. *Clin Drug Invest* 12(2):88, 1996.

Kaiko RF, Foley KM, Grabinski PY, ct al: Central nervous system excitatory effects of meperidine in cancer patients. *Ann Neurol* 13:180, 1983.

Katz N: MorphiDex (MS:DM) double-blind, multiple-dose studies in chronic pain patients. *J Pain Symptom Manage* 19(Suppl):S37-S41, 2000.

Kent JM: SnaRIs, NaSSAs, and NaRIs: new agents for the treatment of depression. *Lancet* 355:911-918, 2000.

Kinzbrunner BM: The terminally ill patient. In: Abeloff MD, Armitage JO, Lichter AS, Niederhuber JE, eds. *Clinical Oncology*. New York, Churchill Livingstone, 2000, p. 597.

Kinzbrunner BM, McGough JP: Cancer pain management. In: Salerno E, Willens JS, eds. *Pain Management Handbook, An Interdisciplinary Approach*. St. Louis, MO, Mosby, 1996, pp. 293-341.

Kinzbrunner BM, Policzer, J, Miller B, Neiber L: Noninvasive pain control in the terminally ill patient. *Am J Hosp Palliat Care* 7(4):26, 1990.

Kinzbrunner BM: *Vitas Pain Management Guidelines*, 3rd ed. Miami, FL, Vitas Healthcare Corporation, 1999.

Kollas CD, Boyer-Kollas B: Evolving medicolegal issues in palliative medicine. *J Palliat Med* 10(6):1395-1401, 2007.

Kreeger L, Hutton-Potts J: The use of calcitonin in the treatment of metastatic bone pain. *J Pain Symptom Manage* 17:2-5, 1999.

Kumar KS, Rajagopal MR, Naseema AM: Intravenous morphine for emergency treatment of cancer pain. *Palliat Med* 14:183-188, 2000.

Lasch K, Greenhill A, Wilkes G, et al: Why study pain? A qualitative analysis of medical and nursing faculty and students' knowledge of and attitudes to cancer pain management. *J Palliat Med* 5(1):57-71, 2002.

Lesser H, Sharma U, LaMoreaux L, Poole RM: Pregabalin relieves symptoms of painful diabetic neuropathy: a randomized controlled trial. *Neurology* 63(11):2104-2110, 2004.

Levy MH: Pharmacologic management of cancer pain. *Semin Oncol* 21:718, 1994.

Levy MH: Pharmacologic treatment of cancer pain. *N Engl J Med* 335:1124, 1996.

Liaison Committee on Medical Education. Functions and structure of a medical school. Standards for accreditation of medical education programs leading to the M.D. degree. http://www.lcme.org/functions2003march.pdf, p. 12, ED-13. Accessed July 8, 2008.

Lipsky LPE, Abramson SB, Crofford L, et al: The classification of cyclooxygenase inhibitors. *J Rheumatol* 25:2298-2803, 1998.

Lotsch J: Opioid metabolites. *J Pain Symptom Manage* 29(5 Suppl):S10-S24, 2005.

Lusher J, Elander J, Bevan D, et al: Analgesic addiction and pseudoaddiction in painful chronic illness. *Clin J Pain* 22(3):316-324, 2006.

Maloney CM, Kesner RK, Klein G, Bockenstette J: Rectal administration of MS Contin: Clinical implications of use in end-stage cancer. *Am J Hosp Care* 6(7):34, 1989.

Manfredi PL, Gonzales GR, CHeville AL, Kornick C, Payne R: Methadone analgesia in cancer pain patients on chronic methadone maintenance therapy. *J Pain Symptom Manage* 21:169-174, 2001.

McCaffrey M, Ferrell BR: Does the gender gap affect your pain control decisions? *Nursing* 22(8):48, 1992.

McKenna F: COX-2: separating myth from reality. *Scand J Rheumatol* 28(Suppl 109):19-29, 1999.

McCracken AL, Gersden L: Sharing the legacy: Hospice care principles for terminally ill elders. *J Gerentol Nurs* 17(2):4, 1991.

McKenry L, Salerno E: *Mosby's Pharmacology in Nursing*, 18th ed. St. Louis, MO, Mosby Yearbook, 1992.

McQuay HJ, Moore RA: Opioid problems, and morphine metabolism and excretion. In: Dickenson

AH, Besson J-M, eds. *Handbook of Experimental Pharmacology*, Vol. 130. Berlin, Germany, Springer-Verlag, 1997, pp. 335-360.

Mercadante S, Casuccio A, Calderone L: Rapid switching from morphine to methadone in cancer patients with poor response to morphine. *J Clin Oncol* 17:3307-3312, 1999.

Miser AW, Narang PK, Dothage JA, et al: Transdermal fentanyl for pain control in patients with cancer. *Pain* 37:15, 1989.

Mitchinson AR, Kerr EA, Krein SL: Management of chronic noncancer pain by VA primary care providers: When is pain control a priority? *Am J Manage Care* 14(2):77-84, 2008.

Morley-Forster PK, Clark AJ, Speechley M, Moulin DE: Attitudes toward opioid use for chronic pain: A Canadian physician survey. *Pain Res Manage* 8(4):189-194, 2003.

Morley JS, Makin MS: The use of methadone in cancer pain poorly responsive to other opioids. *Pain Rev* 5:51-58, 1998.

Morrison RS, Siu AL: A comparison of pain and its treatment in advanced dementia and cognitively intact patients with hip fracture. *J Pain Symptom Manage* 19(4):240-248, 2000.

Mystakidou K, Befon S, Hondros K, et al: Continuous subcutaneous administration of high-dose salmon calcitonin in bone metastasis: Pain control and beta-endorphin plasma levels. *J Pain Symptom Manage* 18:323-330, 1999.

Mystakidou K, Katsouda E, Parpa E, Vlahos L, Tsiatas ML: Oral transmucosal fentanyl citrate: Overview of pharmacological and clinical characteristics. *Drug Deliv* 13(4):269-276, 2006.

Nelson KA, Walsh TD: Metoclopramide in anorexia caused by cancer associated dyspepsia syndrome. *J Palliat Care* 9(2):14, 1993.

Ordonez GA, Gonazalez BM, Espinosa AE: Oxycodone: A pharmacological and clinical review. *Clin Transl Oncol* 9(5):298-307, 2007.

Paice JA, Von Roenn JH, Hudgins JC, et al: Morphine bioavailability from a topical gel formulation in volunteers. *J Pain Symptom Manage* 35(3):314-320, 2008.

Pain & The Law. Undermedicating Cases. http://www.painandthelaw.org/malpractice/undermedicating_cases.php. Accessed August 7, 2008.

Patt RB, Proper G, Reddy S: The neuroleptics as adjuvant analgesics. *J Pain Symptom Manage* 9:446, 1994.

Payne R: Novel routes of opioid administration in the management of cancer pain. *Oncology* 1(2 Suppl): 10-18, 1987.

Payne R: Cancer pain: Anatomy, physiology, and pharmacology. *Cancer* 63:2273, 1989.

Penson RT, Joel SP, Gloyne A, Slark S, Slevin ML: Morphine analgesia in cancer pain: Role of the glucuronides. *J Opioid Manag* 1(2):83-90, 2005.

Periyakoil VS: Opioid conversion. In: *The Stanford University End-of-Life Online Curriculum*. http://endoflife.stanford.edu/M11_pain_control/intro_m01.html. Accessed August 16, 2010.

Plaisance L, Logan C: Nursing students' knowledge and attitudes regarding pain. *Pain Manage Nurs* 7(4):167-175, 2006.

Pletcher MJ, Kertesz SG, Kohn MA, Gonzales R: Trends in opioid prescribing by race/ethnicity for patients seeks care in US emergency departments. *JAMA* 299(1):70-78, 2008.

Plezia PM, Kramer TH, Linford J, Hameroff SR: Transdermal fentanyl: Pharmacokinetics and preliminary clinical evaluation. *Pharmacotherapy* 9:2, 1989.

Portenoy RK: Drug therapy for cancer pain. *Am J Hosp Palliat Care* 7(6):10, 1990.

Portenoy RK, Coyle N: Controversies in the long-term management of analgesic therapy in patients with advanced cancer. *J Pain Symptom Manage* 5:307, 1990.

Portenoy RK, Hagen NA: Breakthrough pain: Definition, prevalence, and characteristics. *Pain* 41:273, 1990.

Portenoy RK, Thaler HT, Inturrise CE, et al: The metabolite morphine-6-glucuronide contributes to the analgesia produced by morphine infusion in patients with pain and normal renal function. *Clin Pharmacol Ther* 51:422-431, 1992.

Porter J, Jick H: Addiction rare in patients treated with narcotics. Correspondence. *N Engl J Med* 302:123, 1980.

Prommer E: Rotating methadone to other opioids: A lesson in the mechanisms of opioid tolerance and opioid-induced pain. *J Palliat Med* 9(2):488-493, 2006.

Pud D, Eisenberg E, Spitzer A, et al: The NMDA receptor antagonist amantadine reduces surgical neuropathic pain in cancer patients: A double-blind, randomized, placebo-controlled trial. *Pain* 75:349-354, 1998.

Rhodin A: The rise of opiophobia: Is history a barrier to prescribing? *J Pain Palliat Care Pharmacother* 20(3):31-32, 2006.

Riley J, Eisenberg E, Muller-Schwefe G, Drewess AM, Arendt-Nielsen L: Oxycodone: A review of its use in the management of pain. *Curr Med Res Opin* 24(1):175-192, 2008.

Ripamonti C, Groff L, Brunelli C, et al: Switching from morphine to oral methadone in treating cancer pain: What is the equianalgesic dose ratio? *J Clin Oncol* 16:3216, 1998.

Robinson CL: Relieving pain in the elderly. Health Progress 88(1):48-53, 2007.

Robinson RG, Preston DF, Baxter KG, et al: Clinical experience with strontium-89 in prostatic and breast cancer patients. *Semin Oncol* 20(3):44, 1993.

Rosner H, Rubin L, Kestenbaum A: Gabapentin adjunctive therapy in neuropathic pain states. *Clin J Pain* 12:56-68, 1996.

Ross FB, Smith MT: The intrinsic antinociceptive effects of oxycodone appear to be kappa-opioid receptor mediated. *Pain* 73:151-157, 1997.

Ross FB, Wallis SC, Smith MT: Co-administration of sub-nociceptive doses of oxycodone and morphine produces marked antinociceptive synergy with reduced CNS side-effects in rats. *Pain* 84:421-428, 2000.

Rupniak N, Kramer M: Discovery of the antidepressant and anti-emetic efficacy of substance P receptor (NK1) antagonists. *Trends Pharmacol Sci* 20: 485-490, 1999.

Rabow MW, Hardie GE, Fair JM, et al: End-of-life care content in 50 textbooks from multiple specialties. *JAMA* 283(6):771-778, 2000.

Sindrup SH, Jensen TS: Efficacy of pharmacological treatments of neuropathic pain: An update and effect related to mechanism of drug action. *Pain* 83: 389-400, 1999.

Slatkin Ne, Xie F, Messian J, Segal T: Fentayl buccal tablet for relief of breakthrough pain in opioid-tolerant patients with cancer-related chronic pain. *Suppor Oncol* 5(7):327-334, 2007.

Smith H, Barton A: Tizanidine in the management of spasticity and musculoskeletal complaints in the palliative care population. *Am J Hosp Palliat Care* 17:50-58, 2000.

Smith MT: Neuroexcitatory effects of morphine and hydromorphone: Evidence implicating the 3-glucuronide metabolites. *Clin Exp Pharmacol Physiol* 27(7):524-528, 2000.

State Medical Licensure Requirements and Statistics, 2008, Continuing Medical Education for Licensure Reregistration, pp. 51-55. www.aad.org/education/relicensure/doc/statelicensurerequirementsrevised.pdf. Accessed July 8, 2008.

Storey P, Hill HH, St Louis RH, Tarver EE: Subcutaneous infusions for control of cancer symptoms. *J Pain Symptom Manage* 5:33, 1990.

Sulmasy DP, Cimino JE, He MK, Frishman WH: U.S. medical students' perceptions of the adequacy of their schools' curricular attention to care at the end of life: 1998-2006. *J Palliat Med* 11(5):707-716, 2008.

Syrjala KO, Cleeland CS: How to assess cancer pain. In: Turk DC, Melzack R, eds. *Handbook of Pain Assessment*. New York, The Guilford Press, 2001, pp. 579-600. and Zech Dr, Grond S, Lynch J, et al: Validation of World Health Organization Guidelines for cancer pain relief: A 10-year prospective study. *Pain* 63(1):65-76, 1995.

Tanelian DL, Brose WG: Neuropathic pain can be relieved by drugs that are use-dependent sodium channel blockers: Lidocaine, carbamazepine, and mexiletine. *Anesthesiology* 74:949, 1991.

Tarzian AJ, Hoffmann DE: Barriers to managing pain in the nursing home: Findings from a statewide survey. *J Am Med Dir Assoc* 6(3 Suppl):S13-S19, 2005.

Taylor AL, Gostin LO, Pagnois KA: Ensuring effective pain treatment: A national and global perspective. *JAMA* 299(1):89-91, 2008.

Taylor DR: Fentanyl buccal tablet: Rapid relief from breakthrough pain. *Opin Pharmacother* 8(17):3043-3051, 2007.

Thomas J, Karver S, Cooney GA, et al: Methylnaltrexone for opioid-induced constipation in advanced illness. *N Engl J Med* 358(22):2332-2342, 2008.

Tolle T, Freynhagen R, Versavel M, et al: Pregabalin for relief of neuropathic pain associated with diabetic neuropathy: A randomized, double-blind study. *Eur J Pain* 12(2):203-213, 2008.

Trescot AM, Datta S, Lee M, Hansen H: Opioid pharmacology. *Pain Physician* 11:S133-S153, 2008.

Trescot AM, Helm S, Hansen H, et al: Opioids in the management of chronic non-cancer pain: An update of American Society of the Interventional Pain Physicians' (ASIPP) guidelines. *Pain Physician* 11:S5-S62, 2008.

US Dept of Health and Human Services. http://www.dpt.samhsa.gov/medications/methadonemortality

2003/methadone_mortality-05.aspx. Accessed May 8, 2008.

USPDI: *Drug Information for the Health Care Professional*, Vol. 1. Rockville, MD, United States Pharmacopeial Convention, 1994.

von Gunten C: Methadone: Starting dose information, fast fact and concepts #86. *J Palliat Med.* 7(2):304-305, 2004.

von Roenn JH, Cleeland CS, Gonin RS, et al: Physician attitudes and practice in cancer pain management. A survey from the Eastern Cooperative Oncology Group. *Ann Intern Med* 119:121, 1993.

Watanabe S, Bruera E: Corticosteroids as adjuvant analgesics. *J Pain Symptom Manage* 9:442, 1994.

Warner TD, Giuliano F, Vojnovic I, et al: Nonsteroidal drug selectivities for cyclo-oxygenase-1 rather than cyclo-oxygenase-2 are associated with human gastrointestinal toxicity: A full in vitro analysis. *Proc Natl Acad Sci U S A* 96:7563-7568, 1999.

Watson CPN: Antidepressant drugs as adjuvant analgesics. *J Pain Symptom Manage* 9:392, 1994.

Watson CPN: Topical capsaicin as an adjuvant analgesic. *J Pain Symptom Manage* 9:423, 1994.

Weinreb NJ: Pain management in special situations. In: Salerno E, Willens JS, eds. *Pain Management Handbook, An Interdisciplinary Approach*. St. Louis, MO, Mosby, 1996, pp. 465-523.

Weinstein E, Arnold R, Weissman DE: Fast Facts and Concepts #54. End-of-Life/Palliative Education Resource Center. September 2006. http://www.eperc.mcw.edu/fastFact/ff_54.htm. Accessed August 16, 2010.

Weinstein SM, Laux LF, Thornby JI, et al: Medical students' attitudes toward pain and the use of opioid analgesics: Implications for changing medical school curriculum. *South Med J* 33(5):472-478, 2000.

Weissman DE, Haddox JD: Opioid pseudoaddiction—An iatrogenic syndrome. *Pain* 36:363, 1989.

Weschules DJ, Bain KT, Richeimer S: Actual and potential drug interactions associated with methadone. *Pain Med* 9(3):315-344, 2008.

Whedon M, Ferrell BR: Professional and ethical considerations in the use of high-tech pain management. *Oncol Nurs Forum* 18(7):1135, 1991.

Wheeler WL, Dickerson ED: Pharmaceutical update: Clinical applications of methadone. *Am J Hosp Palliat Care* 17:196-203, 2000.

Whelton A, Schulman G, Wallemark C, et al: Effects of celecoxib and naproxen on renal function in the elderly. *Arch Intern Med* 160:1465-1470, 2000.

WHO Expert Committee: *Cancer Pain Relief and Palliative Care*. Geneva, World Health Organization, 1990.

Wikipedia. http://en.wikipedia.org/wiki/Rofecoxib. Accessed April 8, 2008.

Wilkinson TJ, Robinson BA, Begg E, et al: Pharmacokinetics and efficacy of rectal versus oral sustained release morphine in cancer patients. *Cancer Chemother Pharmacol* 31:251, 1992.

Wilson RK, Weissman DE: Neuroexcitatory effects of opioids: Treatment. Fast fact and concepts, #58. End-of-Life/Palliative Education Resource Center. July 2006. http://www.mcw.edu/fastFact/ff_58.htm Accessed August 16, 2010.

Wittwer E, Kern SE: Role of morphine's metabolites in analgesia: Concepts and controversies. *AAPS J* 8(2):E348-E352, 2006.

Wong D, Whaley L: *Clinical Handbook of Pediatric Nursing*, 2nd ed. St. Louis, MO, CV Mosby, 1986.

Xue Y, Schulman-Green D, Czaplinski C, et al: Pain attitudes and knowledge among RNs, pharmacists and physicians on an inpatient oncology service. *Clin J Oncol Nurs* 11(5):687-695, 2007.

Yung WT, Kwong SM: Pain management with oral ketamine in patients with advanced cancer. *Rev de Cienc da Saud de Macau* 5(2):116-118, 2005.

Zhukovsky DS, Walsh D, Doona M: The relative potency between high dose oral oxycodone and intravenous morphine: A case illustration. *J Pain Symptom Manage* 18:53-55, 1999.

Zylicz Z, Smits C, Krajnik M: Paroxetine for pruritus in advanced cancer. *J Pain Symptom Manage* 16:121-124, 1998.

SELF-ASSESSMENT QUESTIONS

1. Which one of the following barriers to pain management is unique to clinicians?

   A. Reluctance to report pain
   B. Inadequate knowledge base
   C. Fear of addiction
   D. Inadequate pain assessment
   E. Fear of premature death

2. You are treating a 63-year-old male with lung cancer who is complaining of pain that starts in the area of his left clavicle and radiates down his left arm. He describes the pain as an electric shock–like sensation that comes and goes in waves. He also says that at times he experiences numbness and tingling along the outer aspect of his left upper arm and left forearm. The best way to define this pain would be

   A. Visceral nociceptive pain secondary to coronary insufficiency
   B. Somatic nociceptive pain secondary to bone metastases
   C. Neuropathic pain secondary to brachial plexopathy
   D. Visceral nociceptive pain secondary to pleural metastases
   E. Neuropathic pain secondary to brain metastases

3. When assessing pain and instituting a treatment plan for a patient, all of the following elements are important, EXCEPT

   A. A thorough medication history, including OTC medications.
   B. Psychosocial and spiritual history
   C. History of the primary illness, including prior treatments
   D. A physical examination, specifically including the painful area or areas
   E. Telling the patient what medication he or she is to take

4. Which of the following is the major limitation to the prescribing of the acetaminophen/oxycodone combination analgesic in the treatment of moderate pain (step 2 on the WHO Analgesic Ladder)?

   A. Ceiling effects of the oxycodone
   B. Dose-limiting toxicity of the oxycodone
   C. Ceiling effects of the acetaminophen
   D. Dose-limiting toxicity of the acetaminophen
   E. Federal regulation by the DEA

5. Which one of the following opioid receptors is found at the spinal and supraspinal levels and peripherally in skin, joints, and gastrointestinal tract, and, when activated, may cause dysphoria, euphoria, respiratory depression, sedation, constipation, urinary retention, and drug dependence in addition to analgesia?

   A. *mu*
   B. *kappa*
   C. *delta*
   D. *sigma*

6. All of the following routes of morphine administration can provide acceptable levels of systemic analgesia, EXCEPT

   A. The oral route
   B. The nebulized inhaled route
   C. The subcutaneous route
   D. The intravenous route
   E. The epidural route

7. You are treating a 70-year-old female with severe mixed nociceptive and neuropathic pain secondary to metastatic breast cancer. She is on 1,500 mg a day of morphine in divided doses and still complains of severe pain. She is suffering from significant opioid toxicity including intermittent myoclonus. You decide to give her a trial of methadone. What would

be the proper conversion ratio of morphine to methadone that would you utilize?

A. 3:1
B. 5:1
C. 10:1
D. 15:1
E. 20:1

8. Which class of drug used to treat neuropathic pain is believed to be most effective for dysesthetic neuropathy in which patients complain of burning, cold, or vice-like sensations?

A. Steroids
B. Tricyclic antidepressants
C. Anticonvulsants
D. Local anesthetics
E. NMDA receptor antagonists

9. You have a patient whose pain is controlled on sustained-release oxycodone 100 mg every 12 hours. Which of the following would be the most reasonable immediate-release medication to provide to the patient for breakthrough or incident pain?

A. Oxycodone immediate-release 10 mg every 1 to 2 hours as needed
B. Oxycodone immediate-release 20 mg every 1 to 2 hours as needed
C. Oxycodone/acetaminophen combination, one tablet every 3 to 4 hours as needed
D. Oxycodone/acetaminophen combination, two tablets every 3 to 4 hours as needed

E. The patient does not need immediate-release medication as sustained-release oxycodone contains an immediate-release component.

10. You are treating a 75-year-old male with metastatic prostate cancer. He was in your office earlier this week complaining of severe pain, rated as 8 on a 0 to 10 severity scale. You are concerned as he has been complaining of this level of pain for a number of weeks despite the fact that you have been increasing his dose of opioid analgesia at each visit. At the visit, despite the severity of his pain, he appeared to have a very flat affect, and you decided that based on this observation you would not increase his analgesia any further. Today, you receive a call from the pharmacy letting you know that the patient was in to try and refill his opioid prescription prematurely and that this has actually happened several times over the past month. Based on the above description, from which of the following is this patient most likely suffering from?

A. Tolerance
B. Addiction
C. Pseudoaddiction
D. Withdrawal
E. Physical dependence

CHAPTER

7

Dyspnea and Other Respiratory Symptoms

Freddie J. Negron and Elizabeth A. McKinnis

INTRODUCTION

Irrespective of diagnosis, respiratory symptoms are common among patients at the end of life. The most common respiratory symptoms are dyspnea, cough, and hemoptysis. These symptoms can be very distressing for patients and families, and may have a profound effect on their quality of life. Therefore, it is vital for the practitioner to have an understanding of the definition, etiology, epidemiology, pathophysiology, clinical presentation, and appropriate palliative treatment for the most common respiratory symptoms at the end of life.

DYSPNEA

Dyspnea is the uncomfortable awareness of labored breathing (breathlessness). Fifty-five to seventy percent of patients who are near the end of life experience this symptom and it can be distressing to both the patient and family. Breathlessness is often more distressing than pain, and, like pain, dyspnea is most often multidimensional in its presentation. Nonetheless, the optimal treatment of dyspnea should be directed at a reversible cause, and this may not be feasible in the terminal stages of disease. However, since dyspnea can lead to significant suffering, immediate palliation of the symptom should always be the primary goal.

CAUSES OF DYSPNEA NEAR THE END OF LIFE

There are many causes of dyspnea in the terminal patient, and these are outlined in Table 7–1. Primary pulmonary diseases responsible for dyspnea at the end of life include chronic obstructive pulmonary disease (COPD), pulmonary fibrosis, and lung cancer. Pneumonia, severe congestive

TABLE 7–1. Causes of Dyspnea

Pulmonary
  Chronic obstructive pulmonary disease
  Asthma
  Pulmonary fibrosis
  Pneumothorax
  Pneumonia
  Pulmonary embolism
Cardiac
  Congestive heart failure
  Pericardial effusion
  Myocardial infarction
  Cardiac arrhythmia
Cancer-related
  Superior vena cava syndrome
  Lymphangitic carcinomatosis
  Metastatic disease from any primary site
  Obstruction of bronchus
  Malignant ascites
  Pneumonectomy
Constitutional
  Generalized weakness
  Anorexia and/or cachexia
  Anemia
Psychological
  Hyperventilation
  Anxiety
  Uncontrolled pain
Neuromuscular
  Motor neuron disease
Metabolic
  Hyperthyroidism
  Metabolic acidosis
Miscellaneous
  Severe kyphoscoliosis
  Restrictive ventilatory impairment
  Exogenous mechanical factors

heart failure, pulmonary embolism, superior vena cava syndrome, and metastatic cancer to the lung from other primary sites are common secondary causes of shortness of breath in patients near the end of life. Asthenia (see Chapter 13), anorexia and cachexia (see Chapter 24), and motor neuron disease may contribute to dyspnea due to weakness of muscles involved in the respiratory effort. Malignant ascites may cause dyspnea by diminishing movement of the diaphragm and decreasing vital lung capacity, while breathlessness from tachypnea may occur secondary to metabolic acidosis, hypoxia, anemia, or hypercapnia. The coexistence of pain can worsen dyspnea due to increased anxiety and guarded respiratory movements. In addition, the dyspneic patient with depression or anxiety may have increased manifestation and subjective sensitivity to pain.

Patients may have one or a combination of etiologies responsible for the symptom of breathlessness. A differential diagnosis for the causes of dyspnea in a hospice and palliative care setting can usually be determined by performing a thorough history and physical examination, and, when indicated, with a limited number of diagnostic tests.

CLINICAL PRESENTATION

Patients complaining of dyspnea typically describe the symptom as "shortness of breath," "tightness in the chest," "can't take a deep breath," or "smothering." The timing of dyspnea is often a clue to its cause. The terminally ill patient may present with sudden onset of dyspnea leading to consideration of an acute process such as pulmonary embolus, acute coronary syndrome with congestive heart failure, or cardiac dysrhythmia. Dyspnea that occurs within hours or days may be related to the development of a pleural effusion (malignant or parapneumonic) or pneumonitis. Gradual onset of dyspnea may be indicative of anemia, debilitated state, or growth of primary or metastatic tumor resulting in gradual obstruction of the airway. Chronic dyspnea is most likely related to the patient's primary illness.

Physical findings that may be important in assessing symptoms of breathlessness include the respiratory rate and pattern of respiration, presence of circumoral or nail bed cyanosis, the use of accessory muscles of respiration, and abnormal breath sounds, such as rales, rhonchi, and wheezes. Secondary physical findings that may help evaluate dyspnea near the end of life may include the presence of ascites, neck, facial, and upper body venous engorgement (suggestive of superior vena cava syndrome), and lower extremity signs of deep venous thrombosis (suggestive of pulmonary embolism).

Laboratory and diagnostic tools used to assess dyspnea, such as pulse oxymetry, bedside spirometry, arterial blood gases, imaging, and scans may be useful at times. However, the results of these tests frequently do not correlate with the patient's perception of distress and, therefore, their utility at the end of life is limited, and should only be performed after taking into consideration prognosis, the goals of therapy, and the risk versus benefit ratio. More often than not, it is possible to palliate a patient's dyspnea without relying on the aforementioned studies.

Psychosocial factors can significantly affect the perceived severity of breathlessness. For example, the fear of suffocating or choking (implying that increasing dyspnea may be signaling disease progression or approaching death) often leads to increased anxiety, which can further exacerbate the severity of the symptom.

Simple assessment tools are available to assist in measuring the level of distress the patient is experiencing. Verbal numeric (0–10) scales, verbal categorical scales such as none–mild–moderate–severe, and visual analog scales can be used to allow patients to self-report their level of shortness of breath. These scales have been validated and can also be used to evaluate the effectiveness of any interventions.

TREATMENT

The primary therapeutic goal when confronted with a patient experiencing dyspnea is the palliation of the breathlessness. The development of the treatment plan should involve the patient and family and reflect their goals and expectations. As previously mentioned, when it is feasible, an attempt should be made to assess and eliminate any reversible causes of the symptom.

Dyspnea, like pain, is a subjective experience and involves not only physical aspects but also psychological and social aspects. Since dyspnea can be multifactorial and multidimensional in nature, the optimal treatment combines measures to relieve symptoms, using pharmacologic and nonpharmacologic approaches, as well as specific treatments aimed at the underlying cause when possible and practical.

Table 7–2 summarizes treatments for dyspnea, categorized by the etiology of the symptom. The more common ones are discussed below. As al-

ready stated, these treatments should be based on the goals of therapy, prognosis, and the potential benefit and burden of those specific treatments.

Treatment of Dyspnea Based on Etiology

CHRONIC OBSTRUCTIVE PULMONARY DISEASE COPD may be a cause of dyspnea at the end of life, either as the primary terminal disease or as a comorbid condition in the terminally ill patient suffering from another life-limiting illness. The dyspnea is usually chronic in nature, and often

TABLE 7–2. Treatment of Dyspnea by Specific Etiology

ETIOLOGY	TREATMENT
Chronic obstructive pulmonary disease	Bronchodilators
Asthma	Corticosteroids
Pulmonary fibrosis	Opioids
Congestive heart failure with	Diuretics
pulmonary edema	Opioids
Pneumonia	Antibiotics appropriate for pathogenic organism
Superior vena cava syndrome	High-dose corticosteroids
	Radiotherapy
	Chemotherapy
Pleural effusion	Thoracocentesis
Pericardial effusion	Pericardiocentesis
	Pericardial window
Ascites	Paracentesis
	Diuretics
	Chemotherapy
Lymphangitic carcinomatosis	Corticosteroids
	Anxiolytics
Obstruction from primary tumor	Corticosteroids
or related	Radiotherapy
	Stent placement
	Cryotherapy
	Laser therapy
Pulmonary embolism	Anticoagulant
	Oxygen
	Benzodiazepines
Anemia	Transfusion of packed red blood cells

no longer responds well to bronchodilators, although the patient generally continues any COPD maintenance medications. Exacerbation of COPD, often due to infection (see below) may require adjustment of bronchodilators, treatment with antibiotics, initiation or addition of corticosteroids, and adjustments in oxygen therapy. Opioids, whether oral or nebulized, play an important role in the management of dyspnea, and are discussed in more detail below.

Similar therapeutic options exist for patients suffering from various forms of primary or secondary chronic asthma near the end of life, as well as from primary or secondary pulmonary fibrosis, with the only caveat being the decreased utility for bronchodilators in the latter.

CONGESTIVE HEART FAILURE Congestive heart failure is another common cause of breathlessness in terminally ill patients. Fluid restriction, decreased sodium intake, diuretic therapy, oxygen, and morphine may all be initiated to relieve acute symptoms. On a more chronic basis, left ventricular failure and volume overload may be treated with adjustments in the patient's current diuretics, positive inotropic therapy, and/or angiotensin-converting enzyme inhibitors, or with the addition of one or more these agents if tolerated and not currently being taken by the patient. The ongoing assessment of the clinical signs and symptoms such as auscultation of the lung and heart, jugular venous distention, peripheral edema, and measurement of urinary output will provide the clinician with sufficient information to properly manage the patient with congestive heart failure and ensure optimal patient comfort.

RESPIRATORY INFECTIONS Pulmonary infections including pneumonia, bronchitis, tuberculosis, or fungal infections occur in patients near the end of life who suffer from COPD, cancer, heart disease, HIV/AIDS, dementia, and numerous other terminal illnesses. Decisions as to whether to use antibiotics near the end of life should be individualized, based on such factors as the type of infection, the patient's current condi-

tion, life expectancy and quality of life, the potential reversibility or irreversibility of the infection, and the desires of the patient or family. When a decision is made to treat a patient near the end of life with antimicrobial agents, the oral route of administration is preferable whenever possible. However, a parenteral route of administration may be considered appropriate on an individual patient basis.

SUPERIOR VENA CAVA SYNDROME Superior vena cava syndrome is a clinical syndrome characterized by dyspnea; head, neck, and facial edema; headache; cough; and upper extremity edema. It results from obstruction of the superior vena cava, usually by a cancer, with the most common cancers being bronchogenic carcinoma and non-Hodgkin's lymphoma. A variety of other metastatic cancers may also be responsible for superior vena cava syndrome, as can fibrosis from prior chest radiation or the long-term presence of indwelling catheters.

Superior vena cava syndrome due to underlying neoplastic disease usually responds to a combination of high-dose corticosteroids and radiation therapy. At the end of life, however, patient life expectancy and the ability of the patient to physically tolerate radiation therapy should be considered when determining therapeutic options.

PLEURAL EFFUSION Pleural effusion is the excessive collection of fluid in the pleural space. In the patient with a life-limiting illness, the etiology may be paramalignant, parapneumonic (noncancer illness), or a combination of both. Malignancies commonly presenting with a pleural effusion are lung cancer, breast cancer, and lymphoma. Congestive heart failure, hepatic cirrhosis, and renal failure are common nonmalignant cause for pleural effusion.

Patients with pleural effusions generally present with one or more of the following symptoms, depending on the etiology and severity of the effusion: dyspnea, chest pain, cough, tachypnea, and/or hemoptysis. Physical findings may include dullness to percussion, a pleural friction rub, diminished breath sounds, or decreased tactile fremitus.

Pleural effusion may or may not need intervention depending on the degree of dyspnea, life expectancy, and the patient's desires regarding invasive therapy. Usually, by the time the patient has been referred to hospice, the options for disease-directed therapy to reduce the effusion, such as chemotherapy or radiotherapy, have been exhausted. Thoracentesis may provide symptomatic relief for patients with malignant pleural effusion but relief may be transient (1 month or sometimes only days). Patients with symptomatic persistent reaccumulation of pleural fluid may benefit from pleurodesis, with or without chest tube drainage, with a sclerosing agent to prevent the fluid from returning. In certain selected cases, consideration of a pleuroperitoneal shunt (e.g., a Denver® shunt) could be useful for a homebound patient with limited quality of life. (For further discussion of thoracentesis as a procedure at the end of life, see Chapter 18.)

ASCITES Ascites near the end of life is most often associated with end-stage liver disease, neoplasms that invade the abdominal cavity (ovary, endometrium, breast, stomach, colon, and pancreas), and, in some cases, cor pulmonale due to COPD or other causes of irreversible pulmonary hypertension. Ascites can cause breathlessness through decreased lung capacity resulting in a restrictive ventilatory impairment and discomfort due to abdominal distension as well as due to the sympathetic development of a pleural effusion.

Treatment of ascites at the end of life is primarily symptomatic, aimed at reducing the abdominal accumulation of fluid in sufficient quantities to provide comfort and relief from dyspnea. Diuretic therapy, using spironolactone combined with furosemide or another loop diuretic is somewhat controversial, but is commonly employed and is shown to be effective in reducing ascites in some patients. Paracentesis, a minimally invasive procedure, can offer immediate albeit temporary

symptom relief, even at the end of life. Fluid reaccumulation is common, sometimes forcing patients to undergo multiple repeat procedures. For such patients the placement of a catheter, either a temporary percutaneous or indwelling catheter with a three-way stopcock valve (the latter for patients with a sufficiently long life expectancy) may allow for more convenient maintenance of comfort at home without the burden of multiple invasive procedures. (For further discussion of paracentesis as a procedure at the end of life, see Chapter 18.)

LYMPHANGITIC CARCINOMATOSIS Lymphangitic carcinomatosis is caused by extensive lymphatic invasion of the lung by tumor cells, with surrounding fibrosis. It occurs most often in patients suffering from primary lung cancer or metastatic breast cancer to the lung. It is associated with severe dyspnea, cough, and sometimes bronchorrhea. It is frequently undiagnosed or incorrectly diagnosed. In chemotherapy-sensitive neoplasms, symptoms may improve as a result of primary disease-directed therapy. For patients near the end of life, when chemotherapy is unlikely to be of benefit, some temporary symptomatic improvement may be obtained with the use of high-dose corticosteroids.

OTHER CAUSES OF DYSPNEA There are several other causes for dyspnea that may be amenable to primary disease-directed therapy for selected patients. Symptoms from bronchial obstruction from a primary bronchial tumor may be ameliorated by such interventions as corticosteroids, radiation therapy, cryotherapy, laser therapy, or stent placement, depending of course on the clinical condition and life expectancy of the patient. (These interventions are discussed further in Chapter 18.)

Patients near the end of life are at high risk for dyspnea secondary to pulmonary emboli, due to their lack of mobility and, in patients with malignant disease, a hypercoaguable state. Treatment of these patients may include anticoagulation, oxygen, and anxiolytics.

Finally, patients may become dyspneic from progressive anemia, and for symptomatic patients who will benefit with relief of breathlessness, transfusion of packed red blood cells to alleviate symptoms (and not to a specific hemoglobin or hematocrit level) may be considered.

Pharmacologic Interventions for the Treatment of Dyspnea Near the End of Life

Pharmacologic interventions are the mainstay for providing symptomatic relief of dyspnea. As alluded to earlier, the use of these medications is dependent on the cause of the dyspnea. Commonly used medications for the treatment of dyspnea at the end of life include opioids, bronchodilators, corticosteroids, and anxiolytics (Table 7–3).

OPIOIDS Very near the end of life, especially when other commonly used medications such as bronchodilators and steroids in patients with end-stage COPD or diuretics in patients with congestive heart failure have limited benefit, opioids such as morphine are the medications of choice for rapid palliation of dyspnea. Opioids reduce breathlessness in several ways. They decrease the sensitivity of the medullary respiratory center to carbon dioxide and they reduce the response of the carotid body to hypoxia. Opioids have been shown to cause bradycardia and hypotension due to peripheral vasodilation and to reduce preload, which is responsible for their effectiveness in the treatment of pulmonary edema. Finally, opioids also have anxiolytic effects.

Systemic Opioids Opioid-naive patients who require therapy with systemic opioids for dyspnea should be started on low doses of an immediate-release opioid, typically morphine 2.5 to 5 mg. For patients receiving a chronic opioid for pain, it is recommended that the patient receive a dose of an immediate release opioid that is approximately 25 to 50% higher than the baseline dose they are receiving for pain to successfully palli-

ate the breathlessness. This is due to the tolerance that patients develop to respiratory depression when receiving opioids on a chronic basis. The opioid may be administered orally, or, if the patient is unable to swallow, parenteral morphine may be given at one-third of the oral dose.

Although immediate-acting morphine is generally used to control acute breathlessness, some patients with chronic dyspnea have anecdotally benefited from the combination of a sustained release opioid product to maintain baseline level of comfort, combined with an immediate release opioid for acute exacerbations of dyspnea. For patients who do not tolerate morphine, other opioids such as oxycodone and hydromorphone may be used. (A complete discussion of how to use morphine and other opioids for the treatment of pain, which can be applied to the treatment of dyspnea as well, can be found in Chapter 6.)

Nebulized Opioids Nebulization is another approach to the delivery of opioids to treat dyspnea near the end of life. Opioid receptors are located throughout the respiratory tract and are the likely target for nebulized opioids, although the exact mechanism of action by which nebulized opioids work is unclear.

Typically, the starting dose of nebulized morphine is 2.5 to 10 mg, generally repeated every 4 hours as needed. Most reported studies have used injectable preservative-free morphine in 2 mL of normal saline, although anecdotal reports have also demonstrated efficacy and safety with nebulization of preservative-containing injectable solutions and even oral morphine solution.

Morphine has been known to cause paradoxical bronchospasm when nebulized due to histamine release in the airways; hence, professional observation during administration of the first dose is appropriate. Some palliative care practitioners also add dexamethasone 2 to 4 mg to the nebulized morphine to reduce the risk of bronchospasm. It should be noted that in view of the fact that only 16% to 19% of inhaled morphine is absorbed systemically, the nebulized route of administration is recommended only for the

TABLE 7–3. Medications for the Treatment of Dyspnea

MEDICATIONS	ROUTE	DOSAGE
Opioids		
Morphine	Oral, PR, IV, SC	Starting oral or rectal dose 2.5–5 mg q 4 h
Nebulized morphine	Nebulized parenteral or oral solution	Starting dose 2.5–10 mg q 4 h (either alone or with dexamethasone 5 mg)
Bronchodilators		
β₂-Adrenergic	Nebulized (0.083%)	2.5 mg q 4–6 h
Albuterol	MDI (90 µg/puff)	2–3 puffs q 4–6 h
Lev-albuterol	Nebulized (0.63 mg)	0.63–1.25 mg tid
Anticholinergic		
Atropine	Nebulized 1%	0.5–2.5 mg q 4–6 h
Ipratropium	MDI (18 µg/puff)	2 puffs q 4–6 h
Combination		
Ipratropium and Albuterol	MDI (120 µg and 21 µg/puff)	2 puffs q 4–6 h
Methylxanthines		
Theophylline	Oral (sustained release)	Starting dose 10 mg/kg/d, titrate to effect and drug level
Aminophylline	IV	Loading dose 0.6 mg/kg, then 0.3 mg/kg/h*
Anxiolytics		
Benzodiazepines		
Lorazepam	Oral, IV	Starting oral dose 1–2 mg/d, 2–3 divided doses, adjust as needed*
Diazepam	Oral, IV	Starting oral dose 2–2.5 mg qd or bid; titrate as needed*
Alprazolam	Oral	0.25 mg bid-tid; adjust as needed*
Chlordiazepoxide	Oral, IV	5 mg bid-qid
Miscellaneous		
Buspirone	Oral	75–150 mg/d in divided doses
Corticosteroids		
Oral		
Prednisone	Oral	5–60 mg/d†
Prednisilone	Oral, IV	Oral dose: 5–60 mg/d
Dexamethasone	Oral, IV	Oral dose: 0.5–8 mg/d
Inhaled		
Beclomethasone	MDI (42 µg/puff)	2 puffs tid-qid
Flunisolide	MDI (250 µg/puff)	2 puffs bid
Fluticasone	MDI (110 µg/puff)	1–2 puffs bid

MDI, metered dose inhaler.

*Dosages should be adjusted for older patients based on consideration of all conditions that may affect clearance.

†Liver disease will impair clearance.

treatment of dyspnea, not for the treatment of pain.

Although the biology of inhaled medications makes sense, the research evaluating the use of nebulized opioids are conflicting. Review of recent studies with small patient populations revealed effectiveness relieving breathlessness in approximately half of the studies, and the other half showed no difference between morphine and placebo. Thus, there is a need for large-scale randomized trials on nebulized opioids for the treatment of dyspnea, and the nebulized route of morphine administration for the treatment of dyspnea cannot be considered standard of care. However, its effectiveness in at least some patients warrants its use on a case-by-case basis for patients near the end of life.

BRONCHODILATORS

Inhaled Bronchodilators Inhaled bronchodilators are available in two classes: β-adrenergics such as albuterol sulfate, and anticholinergics such as ipratropium bromide. Either class can be delivered via aerosol inhaler or nebulizer. These medications are primarily used for patients near the end of life who suffer from advanced COPD, and they may be utilized either alone or in combination. Occasionally, patients with malignant pulmonary disease may benefit from the short-acting β-adrenergic bronchodilators when experiencing bronchospasm. Proper dosing of these medications can be found in Table 7–3. Levalbuterol does not confer any specific benefits in the care of patients near the end of life, and therefore, it is not cost-effective when compared with albuterol.

Oral Bronchodilators Oral bronchodilators include the methylxanthines, and oral β-adrenergic agents. In addition to their bronchodilatory effects, methylxanthines can affect dyspnea centrally through the medulla via stimulation of respiration, and peripherally by increasing the contractility of the diaphragm and other muscles involved in respiration, resulting in decreased sensation of breathlessness. Methylxanthines that are most commonly used are theophylline and aminophylline. It should be noted, however, that due to significant cardiac side effects, a narrow toxic:therapeutic ratio and the availability of safer drugs, such as the combination of inhaled β-adrenergic agents and anticholinergic agents in patients with advanced COPD, the use of methylxanthines has fallen out of favor.

The most commonly utilized oral bronchodilator in the β-adrenergic class is albuterol sulfate. Unfortunately, systemic administration can cause undesirable side effects such as anxiety, restlessness, tachycardia, insomnia, and tremors, which may adversely effect the quality of life of the patient. Therefore, its use is not recommended because the readily available inhalation route has fewer side effects and similar efficacy.

CORTICOSTEROIDS Corticosteroids may be helpful as an anti-inflammatory adjunct in patients with dyspnea due to exacerbation of COPD, lymphangitic carcinomatosis, or with superior vena cava syndrome. By decreasing inflammation, the obstruction, whether bronchial or vascular, may be diminished and breathlessness may be relieved.

Corticosteroids can also enhance well-being and improve appetite thereby affecting dyspnea by reducing anxiety of the patient and family. Corticosteroids may be administered orally, or, for patients with chronic inflammation secondary to COPD, inhaled corticosteroids may be used. It is important to remember, however, that inhaled corticosteroids are not indicated for the treatment of acute dyspnea. Recommended corticosteroids that can be used for the treatment of dyspnea can be found in Table 7–3.

ANXIOLYTICS Anxiolytics of the benzodiazepine class can be helpful in patients with the concurrent presentation of anxiety with dyspnea. Like pain, anxiety increases the sensitivity to dyspnea. The dyspneic patient is often fearful of suffocating or smothering to death, thus precipitating anxiety. The resulting anxiety worsens the perception of dyspnea, which leads to a cyclical pattern of response. Recommended anxiolytics to treat dyspnea can be found in Table 7–3.

OTHER PHARMACOLOGICAL MEASURES   For patients with advanced congestive heart failure who develop acute dyspnea, the judicious use of diuretic agents such as furosemide, either orally or parenterally, may be of symptomatic benefit. In addition, diuretic therapy with the combination of furosemide and aldactone may be indicated for patients with ascites.

Oxygen   Another pharmacological measure that may have benefit for patients with dyspnea is oxygen therapy, although its actual efficacy is questionable. Correction of hypoxia has not been found to correlate with the degree of symptomatic benefit the patient experiences with oxygen therapy. A reason why oxygen therapy is able to palliate dyspnea, despite the lack of improvement in oxygen saturation, may be that airflow through the nasal cannula stimulates feedback to the respiratory center and thereby decreases the sensation of breathlessness. In addition, oxygen therapy may have a psychological benefit to patients and families as it is associated with active (though not resuscitative) treatment, thus aiding in patient and family comfort.

Nonpharmacological Measures Utilized to Treat Dyspnea

Nonpharmacological interventions are critically important in the treatment of dyspnea and can significantly improve a patient's quality of life. Many of these interventions are listed in Table 7–4, and include modification of the environment (e.g., an exhaust fan for cooling and circulating the air), position changes, breathing techniques, diet, and physiotherapy (massage). Meditation, relaxation techniques, and psychotherapy also may reduce dyspnea-associated anxiety. As mentioned earlier in the section on etiology-specific therapies, radiation therapy and procedures such as thoracentesis and paracentesis may also play a significant role in managing dyspnea. Careful

TABLE 7–4. Nonpharmacologic Interventions for Dyspnea
Environment
Cool air, low humidity
Fan circulating air
Quiet room
Lightweight clothing and bedding
Reduce pollen, dust, pet hair, etc.
Physical
Positioning
Sitting upright 45°
Breathing techniques
Pursed lip breathing
Diaphragmatic breathing
Energy conservation
Plan activities
Relaxation techniques
Progressive muscle relaxation
Guided imagery
Meditation
Music therapy
Massage therapy
Therapeutic touch
Psychosocial support
Active listening
Reassurance
Emotional support
Education

consideration of these interventions, by collaboration between the clinician and the hospice interdisciplinary team, can support the goals and expectations of the patient and family, significantly improving the quality of life in the terminal stages.

COUGH

Cough is defined as a sudden explosive forcing of air through the glottis, occurring immediately on opening the previously closed glottis. Cough is stimulated by mechanical or chemical irritation of the trachea or bronchi or by pressure from adjacent structures.

Cough occurs in 30% to 50% of all patients at the end of life, involving both cancer and noncancer diagnoses. Approximately 80% of lung cancer patients and patients prior to immediate death will have cough as a major symptom.

In the palliative care setting, cough requires aggressive management to prevent complications that may adversely affect quality of life. An inadequately treated cough may lead to laryngeal irritation, loss of sleep, soreness of the chest-wall muscles, cough-induced fractures, syncope, or headaches. The persistent cough can also result in the development or exacerbation of anxiety involving both the patient and family. Therefore, the importance of prompt assessment and appropriate treatment is essential to the care of the patient in the terminal phase of disease.

ETIOLOGY

Similar to dyspnea, the common causes for cough in patients at the end of life are usually related to their terminal illnesses, especially lung cancer, COPD, and cardiac disease, or to aspiration related to progressive weakness (see Table 7–5). However, it must be remembered that patients near the end of life are also susceptible to the more common causes of cough such as postnasal drip syndrome, gastroesophageal reflux, and asthma. These other causes should be taken into consideration when evaluating terminally ill patients who are troubled by cough.

CLINICAL PRESENTATION

The terminal patient may present with an acute cough related to an upper or lower respiratory tract infection, or may give a history of chronic cough associated with the terminal illness as mentioned earlier. If the cough is exacerbated by supine position, this could be indicative of pulmonary edema, the presence of an endobronchial tumor, gastroesophageal reflux disease, or a postnasal drip syndrome. Chronic cough occurring at night might correlate with postnasal drip syndrome, congestive heart failure, or gastroesophageal reflux disease, while a predominantly daytime cough could represent a habitual or psychogenic cough.

TREATMENT

The optimal therapy for cough in patients near the end of life is to treat the underlying condition, if possible. Most often, however, as with dyspnea, the underlying condition is either not identified, not easily treatable, or the patient does not wish to undergo aggressive treatment. For most patients, therefore, the treatment strategy will be to palliate the cough symptomatically.

Pharmacological Treatment of Cough

Medications that may be effective in the management and control of cough near the end of life includes cough suppressants, bronchodilators, inhaled lidocaine, and corticosteroids.

COUGH SUPPRESSANTS Cough suppressants are the mainstay of treatment for cough. They include soothing elixirs, dextromethorphan, local anesthetics, and opioids.

A soothing elixir provides first-line therapy and comfort without undesirable side effects. This first-line therapy works by forming a protective barrier over the pharyngeal sensory receptors; thus, inhibiting the activation of the cough relief. Caution is essential when administering such elixirs to patients with diabetes due to their high sugar content.

Dextromethorphan hydrobromide, available over-the-counter, is one of the most widely used cough suppressants worldwide. The drug acts centrally, raising the threshold for cough, and is almost equiantitussive to codeine. Dextromethorphan is available in combination with antihistamines, decongestants, and expectorants, to meet the specific need of the patient.

Opioids are the most effective cough suppressants available today and they appear to act

TABLE 7–5. Causes of Cough

Neoplasms and related conditions	Primary bronchogenic carcinomas
	Metastatic lung tumors
	Mediastinal tumors
	Superior vena cava syndrome
	Lymphangitic carcinomatosis
	Pleural effusion
Cardiovascular disorders	Acute pulmonary edema
	Pulmonary infarction
	Aortic aneurysm
Respiratory infections and diseases	Acute pharyngitis/laryngitis
	Acute tracheobronchitis
	Chronic bronchitis
	Lung abscess
	Pulmonary tuberculosis
	Fungal infections
	Bronchopneumonia
	Bronchiectasis
	Chronic obstructive pulmonary disease
Trauma and physical agents	Irritant gases
	Pneumoconioses
Allergic disorders	Bronchial asthma
	Seasonal allergies
	Allergic rhinitis
	Postnasal drip syndrome
Treatment related	Chemotherapy-induced interstitial disease
	Radiation pneumonitis
Miscellaneous	Pulmonary aspiration
	Gastroesophageal reflux
	Diaphragmatic irritation
	Tracheoesophageal fistula
	Vocal cord paralysis
	Drug-induced (i.e., ACE-inhibitor)
	Air quality
	Psychogenic

centrally. Codeine and hydrocodone are the two most commonly prescribed antitussives, usually in the elixir formulation. They are often used in combination with a decongestant, an antihistamine, or an expectorant, depending on the need of the patient. Recommended doses of these various elixirs is 5 to 10 cc by mouth every 4 hours. If the patient is already on an opioid, the current dosage should be increased, in lieu of adding a different opioid. The recommended dose increase in these patients should be an increase of approximately 25% over the routine dose to effectively suppress the cough. Remember, however, that cough suppressants, by causing mucus retention, can be problematic when patients are having difficulty with copious mucus production.

Anesthetic agents may be effective in the suppression of chronic cough. A commercially available product, benzonatate, is a peripheral anesthetic that affects the J-receptors located in the respiratory passages, lungs, and pleura. This product is available in the form of "perles" and the standard dose is one 100-mg perle taken three times a day, with a maximum dose of 600 mg/d.

For more difficult to control chronic cough caused by endobronchial malignancy, anecdotal reports suggest that inhaled lidocaine may be effective. The lidocaine inhibits the afferent nerve impulses from cough receptors in the pharynx that mediate the cough. The recommended dose is 5 mL of 2% lidocaine solution every 4 hours, nebulized and carefully titrated to effect, with the total dose not to exceed 300 mg of lidocaine per day. As there is a risk of bronchospasm when this treatment is initiated, close monitoring is imperative. Albuterol may be useful in this setting as well. Food and thick drinks should be avoided, to minimize the risk of aspiration, for approximately 1 hour after the treatment is provided, although small sips of water may be given. Patients should be made aware that injury to the oropharyngeal cavity may occur more easily when anesthetics are used.

OTHER PHARMACOLOGICAL MEASURES   Other medications, including expectorants, antihistamines, decongestants, bronchodilators, and corticosteroids may be useful in the treatment of cough. Guaifenesin is an expectorant found to be safe and mildly effective. Nebulized saline may assist in mobilizing thick secretions, especially when a patient's cough is too weak to expectorate the secretions without assistance. Antihistamines and decongestants, either alone or in combination, are effective for the patient with postnasal drip related to seasonal allergies or allergic rhinitis. Oral corticosteroids may be appropriate, when the cough is due to tumor compression of the bronchus; in such patients the steroids will decrease the edema from the tumor and thereby reduce the compression on the bronchus. Oral or inhaled corticosteroids are ef-

fective in asthma, bronchiectasis, chronic bronchitis, radiation pneumonitis or any other cause for inflammation of the airways. In these situations, treatment should be initiated with oral corticosteroids, which can be tapered to the dose effective to control the cough, and/or switch to inhaled corticosteroids. Bronchodilators, such as albuterol or ipratropium, may be necessary for cough related to bronchospasm (refer to treatment of dyspnea, above).

For the patient with gastroesophageal reflux disease, treatment may include H_2 antagonists or a proton-pump inhibitor with a prokinetic agent and elimination of any medications or foods that be contributing to an exacerbation of the symptoms (see Chapter 8).

Nonpharmacological Measures to Treat Cough

Nonpharmacologic approaches to the treatment of cough include positioning, chest physiotherapy, changes in air quality, and oral suctioning. These can be used to keep the patient comfortable. Positioning can improve the patient's ability to cough up secretions. The optimal position for most patients is upright, whenever possible, to maximize mobilization of secretions. For the patient with pleural effusion, the best position is lying on the side of the effusion, thereby preventing mediastinal shift and tension on the bronchial tree. This position will avert the stimulation of cough.

Chest physiotherapy, involving breathing exercises and postural drainage, may be beneficial to some patients. Chest pounding and vibration, however, are not recommended in terminally ill patients, because of the propensity for pathologic fractures related to osteoporosis or bone metastasis. Chest physiotherapy may also result in decreasing lung function by atelectasis or bronchoconstriction.

Consideration of air quality in the patient's environment can also assist in the palliation of the cough. Adjusting the environment can help if the air is either too hot or too cold. The air quality may be too dry causing pharyngeal irritation that allows stimulation of the cough reflex. The use of a humidifier will aid in the alleviation of the stimulus for cough.

HEMOPTYSIS

Hemoptysis is the expectoration of blood derived from the lungs or bronchial tubes as a result of pulmonary or bronchial hemorrhage. It is one of the most frightening of all symptoms at the end of life. Hemoptysis can be extremely alarming both to terminally ill patients and their caregivers. True hemoptysis is defined as the expectoration of some quantity of blood, usually more than 2 mL. Massive hemoptysis is defined as blood loss of more than 200 mL/24 h.

INCIDENCE

Patients with primary lung cancers at diagnosis present with hemoptysis 30% to 50% of the time. The most common cause for massive hemoptysis is bronchogenic carcinoma, while nonmalignant conditions such as acute bronchitis and pulmonary embolus are most often associated with mild to moderate hemoptysis.

ETIOLOGY

The causes of hemoptysis are listed in Table 7–6. They include neoplasms, infections, cardiac or pulmonary diseases, vascular diseases, hematologic diseases, trauma, or may be secondary to medication. Unfortunately, no cause can be determined in up to 40% of the cases.

It is important to differentiate true hemoptysis from blood coming from the nose, oropharyngeal cavity, or gastrointestinal tract. Therefore, a thorough examination of those areas should be performed to rule out other causes for bleeding.

The patient's description of sputum may help to determine the etiology. Pink, frothy sputum

TABLE 7–6. Causes of Hemoptysis

Neoplasm
　Bronchogenic carcinoma
　Metastatic carcinoma
　Tracheal tumors
Infection
　Bacterial pneumonia
　Fungal pneumonia
　Tuberculosis
　Parasitic
　Lung abscess
Cardiovascular disease
　Pulmonary edema
Pulmonary
　Pulmonary embolism
　Bronchiectasis
　Bronchitis
Vascular
　Arteriovenous fistula
　Pulmonary hypertension
Hematologic
　Thrombocytopenia
　Coagulopathy
　Disseminated intravascular coagulation
Trauma
　Bronchoscopy or secondary to lung biopsy
　Lung contusion
Medication
　Anticoagulant therapy
　Aspirin
Miscellaneous
　Foreign body

may indicate pulmonary edema. Copious amounts of blood-streaked sputum may point to bronchiectasis. Malodorous, purulent sputum may be consistent with a lung abscess.

TREATMENT

Once bleeding has been established as true hemoptysis, a treatment plan can be established (see Table 7–7). The management of hemoptysis

TABLE 7–7. Treatment of Hemoptysis

Mild hemoptysis	Cough suppressant
	Reassurance
Moderate hemoptysis	Oral hemostatic agent
	Radiation therapy
	Laser therapy
Massive hemoptysis	Anxiolytics
	Opioids
	Proper positioning to minimize bleeding
	Family counseling and support

is dependent on the cause, severity of bleeding, and life expectancy. Radiotherapy, laser therapy, and bronchial artery embolization have all been found effective in controlling bleeding from endobronchial tumors. When respiratory infection is the cause, antimicrobial therapy should be considered.

Mild to Moderate Hemoptysis

Mild hemoptysis usually warrants treatments with cough suppressants and the provision of psychosocial support in order to reassure the patient and family.

If a patient is experiencing moderate hemoptysis from an endobronchial lesion, visualization and therapy via bronchoscopy may be indicated if the patient's overall clinical condition and life expectancy warrant. Moderate hemoptysis due to endobronchial lesions is responsive to palliative radiotherapy in approximately 80% of cases. Alternative therapies to radiation may include bronchial artery embolization, laser coagulation, or cryotherapy.

Unfortunately, for most patients near the end of life, these interventions may not be realistic therapeutic options. Noninvasive therapeutic options for these patients include oral hemostatic agents such as tranexamic acid (1,000–1,500 mg PO three to four times a day), combined with

psychosocial support and education to the patient and family as to the possibilities of massive hemoptysis (see below).

Massive Hemoptysis

Massive hemoptysis is a rare condition occurring in approximately 1% to 4% of all patients presenting with hemoptysis. It is found more frequently with primary endobronchial tumors invading into a bronchial artery, and is rare with lung metastases because metastatic lesions remain intrapulmonary.

Death from massive hemoptysis may occur very suddenly. Patients will classically cough up massive amounts of blood, leading to rapid and generally, physically painless exsanguination. For the family, however, this event can be an exceedingly traumatic experience that will require all the skill of the hospice interdisciplinary team to support the family through a most difficult time.

When patients experience severe degrees of hemoptysis without rapid death, palliation is crucial to providing patients with comfort and to reduce awareness and anxiety related to fear. Opioids and benzodiazepines should be provided by the oral, rectal, or parenteral route, depending on the clinical situation. Patient positioning may be helpful, with the optimal position for patients with severe hemoptysis being to place the bleeding lung, if known, downward. Dark-colored towels are helpful at the bedside to reduce patient and caregiver anxiety.

"DEATH RATTLE"

Approximately 60% to 90% of patients who are within several days of death will develop noisy and moist breathing called the "death rattle." The patient usually appears unaffected by the noisy breathing, but family and staff may be distressed by its presence.

There are two types of death rattle. One type may be due to excessive oral secretions, and the other may be due to excessive bronchial secretions. Patients who receive artificial hydration or nutrition before death experience more excessive secretions than patients who are slightly dehydrated and are allowed a more comfortable, natural death.

Sometimes, simply repositioning the patient from a supine to a lateral recumbent position may allow the patient to breath easier. Suctioning has been noted to be ineffective and unnecessarily invasive, and should be avoided in the dying patient. Anticholinergic medications are effective in most patients. Transdermal scopolamine patches are an effective, noninvasive method of administering a drying agent. Generally, one transdermal patch every 3 days suffices to control symptoms, but there are case reports of using as many as three patches at once. Lower doses of scopolamine have been found to be effective for oral secretions, while higher doses have been found to be beneficial for bronchial secretions.

Another effective agent for the treatment of death rattle is atropine. It may be administered via nebulizer in normal saline at a usual dose of 2 mg. (For patients with dyspnea in addition to death rattle, nebulized morphine with or without dexamethasone may be given with the atropine.) Another route of atropine administration is to utilize atropine 1% ophthalmic drops sublingually.

Hyoscyamine 0.125 mg sublingual three to four times a day is another therapeutic alternative that may be used to decrease excessive secretions in actively dying patients. When using any of these medications, periodic moistening of the patient's oral cavity is important. The judicious palliation of excessive oral or bronchial secretions can help reduce the anxiety of the caregiver and family, and make the patient more comfortable.

Lastly, glycopyrrolate is very useful when all other options do not appear to be effective. A dose of 0.2 mg subcutaneously every 6 hours as needed may be very effective, even in patients with severe or dramatic symptoms of death rattle.

BIBLIOGRAPHY

Allard P, Lamontagne C, Bernard P, Tremblay C: How effective are supplementary doses of opioids for dyspnea in terminally ill cancer patients? A randomized continuous sequential clinical trial. *J Pain Symptom Manage* 17(4):256-265, 1999.

Berger AM, Shuster JL, von Roenn JH: *Principles and Practice of Palliative Care and Supportive Oncology*, 3rd ed. Philadelphia, PA, Lippincott William & Wilkins, 2006.

Booth S, Kelly MJ, Cox NP, Adams L, Guz A: Does oxygen help dyspnea in patients with cancer? *Am J Respir Crit Care Med* 153(5):1515-1518, 1996.

Boyd KJ, Kelly M: Oral morphine as symptomatic treatment of dyspnoea in patients with advanced cancer. *Palliat Med* 11(4):277-281, 1997.

Bruera E, Sweeney C, Ripamonti C: Management of dyspnea. In: Berger AM, Portenoy RK, Weissman De, eds. *Principles and Practice of Palliative Care and Supportive Oncology*, 2nd ed. Philadelphia, PA, Lippincott Williams & Wilkins, 2002, pp. 220-232.

Capodaglio EM: Comparison between the CR10 Borg's scale and the VAS (visual analogue scale) during an arm-cranking exercise. *J Occup Rehabil* 11(2):69-74, 2001.

Chandler S: Nebulized opioids to treat dyspnea [see comments]. *Am J Hosp Palliat Care* 16(1):418-422, 1999.

Cooley ME: Symptoms in adults with lung cancer. A systematic research review. *J Pain Symptom Manage* 19(2):137-153, 2000.

Corr DM, Corr CA: *Hospice Care: Principles and Practice*. New York, Springer, 1983.

Doyle D: *Palliative Care: The Management of Far-Advanced Ilness*. London, Croom Helm, 1984.

Doyle D: *Domiciliary Palliative Care: A Handbook for Family Doctors and Community Nurses*. Oxford/New York, Oxford University Press, 1994.

Doyle D, Hanks GWC, et al: *Oxford Textbook of Palliative Medicine*. Oxford/New York, Oxford University Press, 1998.

Dudgeon DJ, Lertzman M: Dyspnea in the advanced cancer patient [see comments]. *J Pain Symptom Manage* 16(4):212-219, 1998.

Dunlop R: *Cancer: Palliative Care*. London/New York: Springer, 1998.

Duthie EH, Katz PR: *Practice of Geriatrics*. Philadelphia, PA, Saunders, 1998.

Enck RE: *The Medical Care of Terminally Ill Patients.* Baltimore, MD, Johns Hopkins University Press, 1993

Enck RE: The role of nebulized morphine in managing dyspnea [editorial; comment]. *Am J Hosp Palliat Care* 16(1):373-374, 1999.

Fallon M, Neill BO: *ABC of Palliative Care.* London, BMJ, 1998.

Faull C, Carter Y, Woof R: *Handbook of Palliative Care.* Oxford/Malden, MA, Blackwell Science, 1998.

Genc O, Petrou M, Lada G, Goldstraw P: The long-term morbidity of pleuroperitoneal shunts in the management of recurrent malignant effusions. *Eur J Cardiothorac Surg* 18(2):143-146, 2000.

Goroll AH, May LA, Mulley A: *Primary Care Medicine: Office Evaluation and Management of the Adult Patient.* Philadelphia, PA, Lippincott William & Wilkins, 1995.

Hoegler D: Radiotherapy for palliation of symptoms in incurable cancer. *Curr Probl Cancer* 21(3):129-183, 1997.

Hoskin PJ, Makin W: *Oncology for Palliative Medicine.* Oxford/New York, Oxford University Press, 1998.

Kaye P; and Hospice Education Institute: *Notes on Symptom Control in Hospice & Palliative Care.* Essex, CT, Hospice Education Institute, 1990.

Kemp C: Palliative care for respiratory problems in terminal illness. *Am J Hosp Palliat Care* 14(1):26-30, 1997.

Kemp C: *Terminal Illness : A Guide to Nursing Care.* Philadelphia, PA, Lippincott William & Wilkins, 1999.

Kinzbrunner BM, Copeland J, Kinzbrunner E: Nebulized morphine using oral morphine solution. Paper presented at: A poster presentation at the Annual Assembly of the American Academy of Hospice and Palliative Medicine, Atlanta, GA, 2000.

Lalloo UG, Barnes PJ, et al: Pathophysiology and clinical presentations of cough. *J Allergy Clin Immunol* 98(5, Pt 2):S91-S96; discussion S96-S97, 1996.

Leung R, Hill P, et al: Effect of inhaled morphine on the development of breathlessness during exercise in patients with chronic lung disease. *Thorax* 51(6): 596-600, 1996.

MacBryde CM, Blacklow RS: *MacBryde's Signs and Symptoms: Applied and Pathologic Physiology and Clinical Interpretation.* Philadelphia, PA, Lippincott William & Wilkins, 1983.

Manning HL, Schwartzstein RM: Pathophysiology of dyspnea. *N Engl J Med* 333(23):1547-1553, 1995.

Patz EF Jr: Malignant pleural effusions: Recent advances and ambulatory sclerotherapy. *Chest* 113 (suppl 1):74S-77S, 1998.

Polosa R, Simidchiev A, Walters EH: Nebulised Morphine for severe interstitial lung disease. *Cochrane Database Syst Rev* (3), Art No.:CD002872, 2002.

Ripamonti C, Bruera E: Dyspnea: Pathophysiology and assessment. *J Pain Symptom Manage* 13(4): 220-232, 1997.

Saunders CM: *The Management of Terminal Malignant Disease.* London, Edward Arnold, 1984.

Saunders CM, Sykes N: *The Management of Terminal Malignant Disease.* London, E. Arnold (a division of Hodder & Stoughton), 1993.

Stein WM, Min YK: Nebulized morphine for paroxysmal cough and dyspnea in a nursing home resident with metastatic cancer. *Am J Hosp Palliat Care* 14(2):52-56, 1997.

Thomas JR, Von Gunten CF: Clinical management of dyspnoea. *Lancet Oncol* 3(4):223-228, 2002.

Twycross RG, Wilcock A, et al: *Palliative Care Formulary.* Oxford, Radcliffe Medical Press, 1998.

Vainio A, Auvinen A: Prevalence of symptoms among patients with advanced cancer: An international collaborative study. Symptom Prevalence Group. *J Pain Symptom Manage* 12(1):3-10, 1996.

von Gunten CF, Twaddle ML: Terminal care for non-cancer patients. *Clin Geriatr Med* 12(2):349-358, 1996.

Waller A, Caroline NL: *Handbook of Palliative Care in Cancer.* Boston, Butterworth-Heinemann, 1996.

Webb M, Moody LE, Mason LA: Dyspnea assessment and management in hospice patients with pulmonary disorders. *Am J Hosp Palliat Med* 17(4): 259-264, 2000.

World Health Organization: *Symptom Relief in Terminal Illness.* Geneva, World Health Organization, 1998.

Zeppetella G: Nebulized morphine in the palliation of dyspnoea. *Palliat Med* 11(4):267-275, 1997.

SELF-ASSESSMENT QUESTIONS

1. A patient who is already on chronic morphine for pain develops significant shortness of breath. What is the most appropriate adjustment to the morphine dose that should be made to help treat the dyspnea?

    A. Increase the morphine dose by 10%
    B. Decrease the morphine dose by 10%
    C. Increase the morphine dose by 50%
    D. Decrease the morphine dose by 50%
    E. Stop the morphine, as this is causing the shortness of breath

2. You are evaluating a hospice patient with lung cancer who developed sudden onset of shortness of breath approximately 2 hours ago. Which of the following is the most likely cause of this patient's dyspnea?

    A. Anemia
    B. Pulmonary embolus
    C. Progression of the patient's cancer
    D. Malignant pleural effusion
    E. Progressive ascites

3. You are caring for a 72-year-old male with advanced chronic obstructive disease complaining of increasing shortness of breath. He is already receiving the maximum doses of bronchodilators and steroids, so you have recommended treatment with an opioid. The patient and his attending physician are both very concerned that the opioid will suppress respirations. All of the following are true statements about the use of opioids to treat dyspnea that you provide to the physician EXCEPT:

    A. They reduce breathlessness by decreasing the sensitivity of the medullary respiratory center to carbon dioxide.
    B. They reduce breathlessness by reducing the carotid body's response to hypoxia.
    C. They are effective in the treatment of breathlessness secondary to pulmonary edema.

    D. Patients who are opioid naïve require a minimum of 20 mg of morphine to start in order to affect breathlessness.
    E. Patients on chronic opioid therapy require 25% to 50% more morphine than their baseline dose to affect breathlessness.

4. As the patient and his attending physician are both very concerned that the opioid will suppress respirations, you have offered a trial of nebulized morphine, which has been agreed to. Which of the following is true regarding the use of nebulized morphine to treat dyspnea?

    A. The typical starting dose is 20 mg
    B. It should be administered no more often than every 8 hours
    C. Virtually all studies have demonstrated the efficacy of nebulized morphine
    D. 50% to 60% of the morphine is absorbed systemically
    E. The patient should be observed when receiving the first dose

5. Concerning the treatment of dyspnea with bronchodilators, which of the following statements is true?

    A. Methylxanthines are not commonly used due to cardiac side effects and a narrow toxic:therapeutic ratio.
    B. Levalbuterol is the preferred inhaled bronchodilator to treat patients near the end of life.
    C. Patients with malignant pulmonary disease and bronchospasm do not benefit from inhaled short-acting bronchodilators.
    D. Oral β-adrenergic agents are well tolerated by patients, with minimal side effects.
    E. Inhaled ipratropium and albuterol should not be used together in combination.

6. You are asked to visit a 70-year-old female hospice patient with advanced chronic obstructive pulmonary disease (COPD) who is becoming increasingly short of breath at

home. When you arrive, you are taken into the patient's bedroom to see her. The window is open but the air in the room is warm and stagnant. She is dressed in a very light nightgown with no blanket. The room is carpeted and her two cats, both of whom she is petting affectionately, are laying next to her. She is listening to her favorite classical music while her head rests on her favorite goose-down pillow. Which of the following would be the most reasonable environmental change that you could make to possibly make her breathing easier?

A. Remove the pets to reduce pet dander
B. Remove the carpet to reduce dust and dirt
C. Bring in a small fan to better circulate the air
D. Stop playing the music to quiet the room
E. Get her a nonallergenic foam rubber pillow

7. Which of the following statements regarding treating terminally ill patients with oxygen is true?

A. Correction of hypoxia correlates with the degree of symptomatic benefit the patient experiences with oxygen therapy
B. A pulse oximetry measurement is required prior to initiating oxygen therapy in hospice patients
C. Patients and families benefit psychologically when oxygen therapy is utilized
D. Improved oxygen saturation affects the respiratory center, decreasing the sensation of breathlessness

8. You are treating a 70-year-old male with terminal metastatic lung cancer and COPD who has been experiencing chronic debilitating cough for several days and nights, secondary to copious secretions. In addition to various medications, which of the following nonpharmacologic techniques to help manage his cough would be most appropriate?

A. Lying on his left side as much as possible
B. Being in an upright position as much as possible
C. Chest pounding three to four times a day
D. Dehumidifying the air to keep it as dry as possible

9. Which of the following conditions is most commonly associated with massive hemoptysis?

A. Primary lung cancer
B. Metastatic lung cancer
C. Chronic obstructive pulmonary disease
D. Pulmonary edema
E. Pulmonary embolus

10. All of the following may be appropriate in treating "death rattle" in terminally ill patients EXCEPT:

A. Transdermal scopolamine patch
B. Atropine eye drops sublingually
C. Hyoscyamine sublingually
D. Oral suctioning
E. Reduce or discontinue tube feedings

CHAPTER

8

Gastrointestinal Symptoms
Near the End of Life

Barry M. Kinzbrunner and Elizabeth A. McKinnis

INTRODUCTION

The normal functioning of the gastrointestinal tract is something that occupies even healthy individuals. That is because the ingestion and digestion of food, as well as the excretion of its waste products, are central to the maintenance of a healthy life. The ingestion of food is an activity that pervades human existence, and serves a major social function in addition to its biological purpose. Therefore, it is no wonder that, when facing the end of life, symptoms related to dysfunction of the gastrointestinal tract can be extremely distressing to patients and families. For not only do the symptoms cause physical distress, they often cause psychological distress as well by interfering with the patient's ability to socially interact with family members and others at a time when these interpersonal relationships are crucial.

This chapter examines some of the more common gastrointestinal symptoms that occur when patients are approaching the end of life. Nausea and vomiting are discussed first, followed by perhaps the most troubling gastrointestinal symptom of all, constipation. Other symptoms, including diarrhea, dysphagia, dyspepsia and abdominal pain, bowel obstruction, and ascites, are then reviewed. Anorexia and cachexia, two other common symptoms related to the gastrointestinal system, are reviewed separately in Chapter 24 along with a discussion of the ethical issues involved with treatment of these symptoms. As with most other symptoms near the end of life, it is important to have knowledge of the etiology of these symptoms when possible, as the most appropriate treatment that leads to symptom relief is often dependent on the cause of the symptom.

NAUSEA AND VOMITING

Nausea is an unpleasant sensation in the region of the stomach, usually associated with an aversion to food, which may or may not be followed by vomiting. Vomiting, or emesis, is the sudden forceful peroral expulsion of the contents of the stomach, often, but not always, preceded by nausea. Retching, or dry heaves, is to be differentiated from vomiting by the fact that while muscular contractions of the stomach and respiratory muscles occur with both, retching occurs without expulsion of gastric contents.

Nausea, with or without vomiting, occurs commonly near the end of life, being reported in more than half of all terminal cancer patients as well as in many terminal patients without cancer. That nausea and vomiting are troublesome symptoms goes almost without saying. It can prevent patients from not only taking in nutritional support, but, perhaps more importantly, from ingesting the very medication that they need to prevent pain and other symptoms.

To manage nausea and vomiting effectively, it is important to identify the specific cause and to correct or remove it whenever possible. When it is not possible to remove or correct the cause, or while assessing the patient for the specific cause, various pharmacological and nonpharmacological treatments can be used to effectively control the symptoms.

THE VOMITING PROCESS

Understanding the mechanisms by which various stimuli cause nausea and vomiting is crucial to effectively treat these symptoms. To accomplish this, the vomiting process will be reviewed. As illustrated in Figure 8–1, the pathophysiological process that results in nausea and vomiting is a complex one, involving the central nervous system, peripheral and central nerves, the gastrointestinal tract, and motor efferent nerves that stimulate the diaphragm and abdominal muscles.

Central to the process is the vomiting center (VC), thought to be located in the lateral reticular formation of the medulla. The VC contains both histaminic and muscarinic cholinergic receptors. Vomiting occurs when the VC is stimulated by afferent impulses from one or more areas

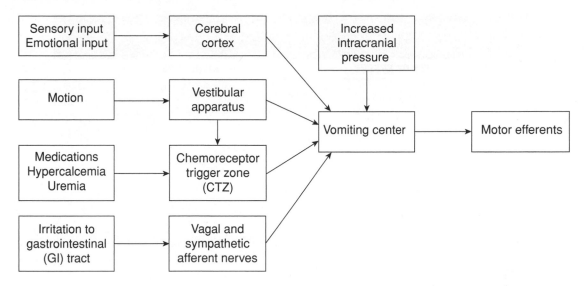

Figure 8–1. Pathophysiological mechanisms of nausea and vomiting.

of the nervous system: the cerebral cortex, the vestibular apparatus, the chemoreceptor trigger zone (CTZ), and vagal and sympathetic afferent nerves from stimuli originating in the gastrointestinal tract. The many varied etiological factors responsible for nausea and vomiting, as shown in Figure 8–1, will stimulate one (or sometimes more than one) of these areas, causing activation of the VC and the symptom of nausea. If the stimulus to the VC is sufficiently strong to stimulate motor efferents, actual vomiting will result.

With this basic outline of the process, some of the more common causes of nausea and vomiting seen in patients who are near the end of life can be examined in association with the specific sites of the nervous system that each one most directly affects (see Table 8–1).

Cerebral Cortex

Nausea and vomiting near the end of life that is caused by stimulation of the cerebral cortex is often the result of noxious inputs from the senses of smell, taste, or sight. Strong odors and strange or unusual tastes can sometimes invoke nausea and emesis even in healthy individuals, and they are more likely to cause symptoms in individuals who are terminally ill who often have a preexisting aversion to oral intake. Even the sight of food may be enough to invoke vomiting in these patients.

Anticipatory nausea and vomiting is an interesting form of sensory-mediated nausea and vomiting. Patients who have previously been exposed to a particularly noxious stimulus that resulted in severe symptoms of nausea and vomiting may develop recurrent symptoms by being exposed to something that reminds them of the primary stimulus, even in the absence of the stimulus itself. A well-described example of anticipatory nausea and vomiting is the cancer patient who has had particular difficulty with nausea and vomiting following chemotherapy. Such patients may experience recurrent nausea and/or emesis when, for example, they hear music similar to that played in the oncologist's office where and/or when the chemotherapy was administered or when they merely drive by the office in which they received the chemotherapy.

Anxiety without other sensory input may lead to symptoms of nausea and vomiting under certain circumstances. Common examples of

TABLE 8–1. Causes of Nausea and Vomiting in Patients Near the End of Life

PRIMARY SITE OF EFFECT	EXAMPLES
Cerebral cortex (CC)	Sensory inputs
	Anticipatory nausea and vomiting
	Anxiety
Vestibular apparatus (VA)	Motion sickness
	Vertigo
Chemoreceptor trigger zone (CTZ)	
Medications	Opioid analgesics
	Nonsteroidal anti-inflammatory drugs (NSAIDs)
	Antibiotics
	Chemotherapeutic agents
	Other chronic medications
Metabolic	Uremia
	Hypercalcemia
Gastrointestinal tract (GI)	Constipation
	Bowel obstruction
	Gastric outlet obstruction
	Gastroparesis
Direct effect on vomiting center (VC)	Increased intracranial pressure

anxiety-related nausea might include the provocation of the symptom prior to the delivery of a major speech or before final exams.

Vestibular Apparatus

The vestibular apparatus, located in the inner ear contains both histaminic and muscarinic cholinergic receptors. It causes nausea by signaling both the CTZ and the VC (see Fig. 8–1). The role of the vestibular apparatus as a direct pathway to cause nausea and emesis near the end of life is somewhat limited. With the exception of patients suffering from advanced cerebrovascular disease with vertebrobasilar insufficiency, pre-existent vertigo, or a malignancy affecting the vestibular apparatus, it is not that common for patients at the end of life to suffer from nausea primarily related to vestibular stimulation. Nevertheless, it is important to rule these causes out when assessing terminally ill patients for symptoms of nausea and vomiting.

Chemoreceptor Trigger Zone

The CTZ is an important mediator of symptoms of nausea and vomiting in patients near the end of life. The CTZ is located in the area postrema at the ventral aspect of the fourth ventricle, and consists of dopamine receptors, as well as 5-HT3 (serotonin) receptors. As the CTZ is outside the blood–brain barrier, it can be stimulated by various noxious substances that do not normally enter into the central nervous system.

The noxious substances that mediate nausea and vomiting by stimulation of the CTZ are many, with the majority being medications. For patients near the end of life, opioid analgesics are among the most common medications that cause nausea and vomiting through CTZ stimulation. However, one should consider other medications that patients are taking as well, such as nonsteroidal anti-inflammatory agents, antibiotics, and chronic medications for comorbid conditions such as heart or lung disease. Chemotherapy agents also produce nausea primarily through stimulation of the CTZ, with cisplatinum and related compounds more specifically stimulating the 5-HT3 receptors in the CTZ. This receptor specificity has led to the development of anti-emetic therapy that effectively counteracts the emetogenic effects of these chemotherapy agents by specifically blocking the stimulation of the 5 HT3 receptor.

In addition to the effects of medications, metabolic abnormalities associated with nausea are mediated through stimulation of the CTZ. For example, uremia and hypercalcemia, two conditions commonly associated with patients who are near the end of life, cause nausea and emesis by this mechanism, and should be considered whenever patients near the end of life are symptomatic.

Vagal and Sympathetic Afferent Nerve Stimulation from the Gastrointestinal Tract

The main neural pathway from the gastrointestinal tract to the VC in the central nervous system is via the vagus nerve. Nausea and vomiting mediated by the vagus nerve comes by stimulation of chemoreceptors and mechanoreceptors located in the serosa and viscera of the gastrointestinal tract. Conditions commonly seen at the end life that may cause nausea and emesis mediated by vagal nerve stimulation include constipation, gastric outlet obstruction, gastroparesis, and bowel obstruction.

ASSESSMENT

As with most symptoms, a thorough assessment of the patient is key to determining the best therapeutic approaches to treat nausea and vomiting. Questions regarding the nature of the symptoms themselves are important. For example, projectile emesis with little or no nausea may be indicative of increased intracranial pressure, although increased intracranial pressure can also be associated with nausea and nonprojectile emesis. Gastric outlet obstruction often presents with vomiting after eating and the expelled material

may include undigested food, while vomiting associated with intestinal obstruction may be associated with fecaloid emesis.

Querying the patient as to activities that occurred prior to the symptoms might provide additional clues to potential causes. This could be especially important in evaluating the potential for anticipatory nausea and vomiting, or symptoms associated with sensory input such as sight, smell, or taste.

Historical information may lead one toward the consideration of, for example, bowel obstruction from recurrent tumor or adhesions if the patient had prior abdominal surgery, or hypercalcemia if the patient is suffering from a progressive malignancy with bone metastases. Alternatively, it might lead to the uncovering of pre-existent vertigo, unrelated to the patient's terminal illness, which would not have been suspected if specific inquiry was not made.

A key component to the assessment of the patient near the end of life with nausea and vomiting is a full medication review, searching for emetogenic medications, including opioid analgesics and antibiotics. Blood levels of medications that can cause nausea when toxicity is present should be checked even if the patient has not had recent dosage changes, as alterations in drug metabolism and clearance often occur as renal and liver function change during the dying process. Since patients are often on multiple emetogenic medications, looking for an association between the taking of the medication and the onset of nausea may be an important clue as to which medication may be responsible. Polypharmacy itself, a common problem among chronically ill elderly patients, including those near the end of life, can contribute to nausea, not only due to the increased likelihood that one or more of the multitude of agents being taken will be emetogenic, but also due to the sheer number of pills and capsules patients may be asked to swallow at one time.

The physical assessment can provide additional information as to potential etiologies for symptoms of nausea and emesis. For example, abdominal distension with high-pitched, tinkling

TABLE 8–2. Guidelines in the Treatment of Nausea and Vomiting in Patients Near the End of Life

1. Treat reversible causes when indicated and appropriate.
   a. Remove and/or avoid noxious stimuli.
   b. Discontinue unnecessary emetogenic medications.
   c. Reduce dose of medications at toxic levels or discontinue if unnecessary.
   d. Assess for and treat constipation if present.
   e. Decisions on whether to attempt to surgically correct bowel obstruction or to reverse metabolic abnormalities should be based on patient's clinical condition, quality of life, and life expectancy.
2. Provide appropriate nonpharmacological measures to ensure patient comfort (see Table 8–3).
3. Pharmacological therapy should be utilized for irreversible causes and emetogenic medications (i.e., opioid analgesics) must be continued.
   a. Choose an initial anti-emetic therapy based on potency and the primary site through which the nausea is being mediated (i.e., CTZ, vagal stimulation of GI tract).
   b. Avoid the oral route of administration when the patient is actively vomiting.
   c. If symptoms persist, do not start a second agent unless certain that use of the first agent has been optimal in dose, route of administration, and frequency.
   d. If symptoms persist after optimal use of a single agent, a second medication may be needed. Consider using an agent with site specificity that is synergistic with the first medication.
   e. If the addition of a second medication is not successful in ameliorating symptoms, the patient should be reevaluated. A third medication may be necessary to palliative symptoms while reassessing the patient.

bowel sounds would be suggestive of intestinal obstruction while the presence of a succussion splash in the gastric region would point toward gastric outlet obstruction. The presence of a fecal impaction might suggest constipation. Nystagmus or the reproduction of vertiginous symptoms when the patient changes positions would point to a vestibular problem, while the presence of papilledema could indicate the presence of increased intracranial pressure.

TREATMENT OF NAUSEA AND VOMITING

The majority of patients near the end of life have multiple coexistent causes of nausea and vomit-

ing. Therefore, a combination of both nonpharmacological and pharmacological interventions is necessary for successful palliation. The following guidelines, which are summarized in Table 8–2, are designed to assist the clinician in deciding how to utilize the various interventions available to treat nausea and vomiting.

Treat Reversible Causes When Indicated and Appropriate

The first step in the treatment of nausea and vomiting is to remove and/or avoid the cause when possible. When removal or avoidance is impossible, for example, if the patient has a malodorous fungating skin lesion or cannot tolerate the taste of a necessary medication, masking the odor or the taste of the medication is an alternative way of addressing the patient's symptoms.

As noted, medications often cause nausea and vomiting, either as a primary side effect of the medication, or when blood levels of the medication are at toxic levels. When possible, especially with chronic medications not directed at symptom management near the end of life, the offending medication should be discontinued. If the medication is essential for the management of symptoms, dosage adjustments should be considered if the blood levels are in or near the toxic range. A trial of an alternative medication with a similar action should be attempted, as patients may not have the same reactions to different medications in the same therapeutic class. Finally, if the medication is essential, and there is no other alternative, pharmacological therapy with an anti-emetic should be provided (see below).

A sometimes overlooked cause of nausea and emesis, especially in patients near the end of life, is constipation. By evaluating and treating for this common symptom, one can sometimes provide a simple solution to the patients' nausea and resolve the constipation as well. (A discussion on the treatment of constipation may be found below.)

Finally, when patients are near the end of life, one must consider whether or not potentially reversible causes of nausea and vomiting can or should be reversed. For some patients, clinical condition, quality of life, and/or life expectancy, might dictate whether or not a bowel obstruction can be surgically reversed, or whether or not it is feasible to reverse a metabolic abnormality such as uremia or hypercalcemia. As always, these decisions are made on an individual patient basis after discussion of the issues between the patient and family, and the members of the palliative care or hospice interdisciplinary team, and based on the patient's current clinical condition, short-term prognosis, and goals of care.

Nonpharmacological Measures

There are many nonpharmacological interventions that can help ameliorate symptoms of nau-

---

TABLE 8–3. Nonpharmacological Interventions for Nausea and Vomiting

Create a comfortable environment
    Encourage patient to sit in fresh air
    Loosen clothing
    Apply a cool damp cloth to patient's forehead, neck, and wrists
    Discourage staff and family from wearing strong perfume, deodorants, etc.
Working with the patient
    Relaxation and visualization
    Practice deep breathing and voluntary swallowing to suppress vomiting reflex
    Avoid patient lying supine for 2 h after eating
    Oral care after each episode
Modify the patient's diet
    Small, frequent meals encouraged
    Restrict fluids with meals
    Serve cold food (lessens the odor that may stimulate nausea)

---

sea and vomiting in patients near the end of life. Some of the more common ones are listed in Table 8–3. As already mentioned earlier, removal of noxious olfactory and visual stimuli, the discontinuation of unnecessary medications, and the avoidance of emotional or physical stressors are of great importance.

Creating a comfortable environment for the patient is of great assistance. Such measures include encouraging the patient to sit in fresh air, loosening clothing, and applying cool compresses to the patient's forehead, neck, and wrists. Staff and family should be discouraged from wearing strong perfumes, after-shave lotions, and deodorants.

Patients should be taught relaxation and visualization techniques and should be encouraged to practice deep breathing and voluntary swallowing, each of which helps suppress the vomiting reflex. Patients should also be instructed to avoid lying in the supine position for at least 2 hours after eating. If emesis should occur, oral care should be provided after each episode.

The nature of food served to the patient may also have an ameliorating affect. If early satiety is a problem, small frequent meals should be encouraged and fluids should be restricted to avoid the sensation of bloating. Reducing food odor can be accomplished by serving food that is at room temperature or cooler.

An interesting noninvasive technique for the treatment of nausea that may have a limited role in patients near the end of life is acupressure. This technique, commonly used to help avoid motion sickness at sea and in other nausea-producing environments by the use of special bands that apply pressure to the wrist area, has been the subject of several studies assessing its role as an adjunct to the pharmaceutical treatment of chemotherapy-induced nausea. Results have been mixed, with several randomized trial reporting positive results, while several others studies were negative. There has also been one positive study using acu-

pressure bands to treat radiation-induced nausea. How this may or may not translate into symptom relief for patients near the end of life is not clear and might be an interesting area for further study. Meanwhile, in hospice or palliative care patients with symptoms of nausea refractory to standard forms of therapy, a therapeutic trial of acupressure would not be unreasonable due to its noninvasive nature and lack of significant side effects.

Pharmacological Therapy for Nausea and Vomiting

Despite application of many of the interventions outlined earlier, the irreversible nature of the patient's clinical condition and/or the need to continue medications, such as opioids for pain, make continued nausea and vomiting irreversible. For such patients near the end of life, the appropriate and judicious use of anti-emetic medications is critical for effective symptom management.

STANDARD THERAPY   Table 8–4 lists many of the commonly used anti-emetic agents, classified

TABLE 8–4. Standard Pharmacological Interventions for Nausea and Vomiting for Patients Near the End of Life

MEDICATION	SITES OF ACTION	DOSAGE
Phenothiazines		
Prochlorperazine	CTZ, VC	10 mg PO q 6–8 h
		25 mg PR q 6–8 h
Promethazine	CTZ, VC	25 mg PO/PR q 4–6 h
Chlorpromazine	CTZ, VC	10–25 mg PO q 4–6 h
		50–100 mg PR q 6–8 h
Metoclopramide	GI, CTZ	5–10 mg PO/SC AC & HS
Dexamethasone	CC, GI	4–8 mg PO/SC qd-q 6 h
Haloperidol	CC, CTZ	0.5–1 mg PO/SC q 4–6 h
Lorazepam	CC	0.5–2 mg PO/SC q 4–6 h
Hydroxyzine	VA, VC	10–25 mg PO/SC q 4–6 h
Scopolamine	VA, VC	Apply one patch transdermally to the postauricular area q 72 h
Glycopyrrolate	VA, VC	1–2 mg PO/SL q 8 h
Meclizine	VA, VC	12.5–25 mg PO q 6–12 h

by the primary sites of action of the individual agents. By performing a good clinical assessment and having a good idea of the etiology or etiologies of the symptoms, the clinician can choose the best agent or agents to use, based on the site or sites through which the nausea and emesis are most likely being mediated. For example, patients who are experiencing nausea from a medication, such as morphine, which is primarily mediated via the CTZ, are best treated initially with a phenothiazine such as prochlorperazine, as these medications act on the CTZ. If olfactory or visual stimuli are causing nausea secondary to affects on the cerebral cortex, lorazepam might be a good primary agent because of its cortical effects. Nausea due to delayed gastric agent without gastric outlet obstruction may respond best to metoclopramide, while that caused by increased intracranial pressure or a partial bowel obstruction with bowel wall edema generally will respond best to dexamethasone.

When the primary symptom is nausea with little or no emesis, the oral route of administration is preferred. However, the clinician should be aware that when active vomiting occurs, an alternative route, which can be either rectal or parenteral, should be prescribed until the vomiting subsides, when oral medication can then be provided.

If symptoms persist, do not start a second agent unless certain that use of the first agent has been optimal in dose, route of administration, and frequency. If this has been assured then choose a second agent that has a complementary primary site of action, based on the cause of the patient's symptoms. If the addition of a second medication is not successful in ameliorating symptoms, the patient should be reassessed to ensure that no other potential cause of nausea and emesis has been overlooked, and that the medications prescribed are being taken appropriately. While the reassessment is being completed and/or if no new information is uncovered, a third medication, again with a complementary primary site of action, should be used to help palliate symptoms.

THERAPY OF REFRACTORY NAUSEA AND VOMITING Once the clinician is forced to consider a third anti-emetic agent, it is reasonable to consider the nausea and vomiting to be refractory. When this point is reached, there are several reasonable alternative agents that may be considered. They are listed in Table 8–5.

Compounded Agents As one of the hallmarks of refractory nausea is that patients are already receiving two, or possibly, three agents, one of the more popular approaches to this problem has been to compound several agents together. The most common anti-emetic agents that are compounded together to treat refractory nausea are lorazepam, diphenhydramine, haloperidol, and metoclopramide, better known by the initials of their brand names, ABHR. This combination was arrived at based on the different anti-emetic locations of action of each of the agents as well as their use for many years in combination parenterally as primary anti-emetic therapy for cisplatinum chemotherapy. (The combination has been supplanted to a great extent in the treatment of chemotherapy-induced nausea by the 5 HT3 antagonists that will be discussed shortly.) The compounded product is available in an oral form, a rectal suppository form, and more recently in a gel. There are various permutations of the ABHR compound in which one or more of the agents are omitted (i.e., ABH or ABR) and sometimes another agent, usually dexamethasone, may be added or substituted (i.e., BDR). Although there are standard formulations for each of the dosage forms (see Table 8–4), individual pharmacy providers may have their own formulation that varies from the standard. Therefore, it is important for practitioners who choose to utilize ABHR or related compounds in any of its dosage forms to make sure that they are aware of the component medications and dosages of each component in the compound they are prescribing.

A retrospective analysis published in 2005 demonstrated that after over a decade of use, the compound appeared to be well tolerated by hospice patients (Weschules). As of the writing

TABLE 8–5. Pharmacological Interventions for Refractory Nausea and Vomiting for Patients Near the End of Life

MEDICATION	SITES OF ACTION	DOSAGE
Compounds		
ABHR oral/PR*	CC, CTZ, VA, GI	1 cap or supp q 4–6 h
ABH (w/o R)*		Components of ABHR
ABR (w/o H)*		A: Lorazepam 0.5 mg
		B: Diphenhydramine 12.5 mg
		H: Haloperidol 0.5 mg
		R: Metoclopramide 10 mg
BDR oral/PR*	CC, CTZ, VA, GI	1 cap or supp q 6 h
		B: Diphenhydramine 20 mg
		D: Dexamethasone 4 mg
		R: Metoclopramide 4 mg
ABHR gel*	CC, CTZ, VA, GI	Apply 1 mL topically q 4–6 h
ABH (w/o R)*		Components of ABHR gel/mL
ABR (w/o H)*		A: Lorazepam 1 mg
		B: Diphenhydramine 25 mg
		H: Haloperidol 1 mg
		R: Metoclopramide 10 mg
BDR gel*	CC, CTZ, VA, GI	Apply 1 mL topically q 6 h
		B: Diphenhydramine 20 mg
		D: Dexamethasone 4 mg
		R: Metoclopramide 4 mg
5-HT3 receptor antagonists		
Ondansetron*	CTZ, GI	8–24 mg PO/d in 2–3 divided doses[†]
Granisetron*	CTZ, GI	3–9 mg IV or SC infusion over 24 hours[†]
Other agents		
Olanzapine*	CC, CTZ, VA, GI	2.5 mg PO HS as initial dose[†]
		Dose titrated to as high as 10 mg PO HS[†]
Dronabinol*	CC	2.5–5 mg PO q 4–6 h and titrated

*These medications should only be considered for use in patients with symptoms refractory to two or more agents listed in Table 8–4 and are not recommended for use as primary therapy.
[†]There are no standard dose recommendations for these agents in palliative medicine. Dose recommendations and routes of administration are based on published case reports and studies only.

of this chapter, there were no randomized controlled trials proving the efficacy of ABHR. However, there are a number of case reports in the literature supporting the efficacy of the compound, even when administered by gel, in the treatment of refractory nausea and emesis in palliative care (Moon, 2006). Another retrospective analysis demonstrated the efficacy of ABH (lorazepam, diphenhydramine, and haloperidol) gel in the treatment of breakthrough nausea and emesis following chemotherapy (Bleicher et al., 2008).

5 HT3 Antagonists   One group of agents that might be considered in refractory nausea is the

5 HT3 antagonists that are primarily utilized in the treatment of chemotherapy-induced nausea and vomiting (CINV). There are a number of agents available today, all of which function by antagonizing the 5 HT3 receptors in the CTZ, and to a lesser extent, the gastrointestinal tract. Ondansetron, the first of these agents to become available, was reported in a small retrospective analysis to control refractory nausea (13 of 16 patients, 80%) and emesis (10 of 14 patients, 71%) within 48 hours of starting the medication (Currow et al., 1997). More recently, a series of 23 patients with refractory nausea and emesis secondary to inoperable malignant bowel obstruction were treated with parenteral granisetron, with control of symptoms being achieved in 20 patients (87%) (Tuca et al., 2009). Regarding other 5 HT3 antagonists used to treat CINV, such as dolasetron, palonosetron, or tropisetron, no case reports or studies have been published to date to support their use in the palliative care setting.

Other Agents　Olanzepine, an atypical antipsychotic agent, has been shown to relieve refractory nausea and emesis in eight palliative care patients as reported in two separate articles in 2003 (Srivastava et al.; Jackson and Tavernier). Starting dose was reported to be 2.5 mg at bedtime, with escalation to as high as 10 mg.

Cannabinoids, such as dronabinol, have antiemetic effects that, according to some, are at least on par with the more standard agents. However, their high incidence of toxic effects, such as dizziness, dysphoria, and hallucinations, which are particularly prevalent in the elderly, make them difficult agents to utilize in patients near the end of life, and should be avoided.

The NK_1 receptor inhibitor aprepitant is an extremely effective agent in the treatment of nausea and emesis induced by highly emetogenic chemotherapy agents. However, to date, no studies using this medication to treat non-CINV have been performed. Therefore, at the present time it would not appear to have a significant role in

the treatment of refractory nausea and emesis in patients near the end of life.

CONSTIPATION

Constipation is a subjective term describing the symptom of unsatisfactory defecation. Chronic constipation is a common complaint, with a prevalence of 4% to 30% among the elderly patient, and a significantly higher prevalence for patients near the end of life.

ETIOLOGIES

The terminal patient is at increased risk for constipation for a number of reasons, many of which are listed in Table 8–6.

Medications commonly used by patients near the end of life are major causes of constipation, with the opioid analgesics leading the way. Opioids are believed to cause constipation by several different mechanisms including the suppression of forward peristalsis of the intestines, an increase in intestinal fluid absorption, and a reduction of intestinal secretions. The prevalence of opioid-induced constipation is so great (reported in 15–90% of noncancer patients and approximately 50% of cancer patients receiving opioids) that it is highly recommended that virtually all patients receiving analgesics should be preemptively treated for constipation at the time the analgesic is started.

Other medications that may contribute to symptoms of constipation include aluminum-containing antacids, anticholinergic agents, calcium-channel blockers, and other calcium-containing supplements.

A number of advanced neurological disorders commonly afflicting patients near the end of life, including Parkinson's disease, cerebral infarction, and multiple sclerosis, may have a high risk of constipation. Patients with spinal cord

TABLE 8–6. Causes of Constipation

ETIOLOGY	EXAMPLES
Medications	Opioid analgesics
	Aluminum-containing antacids
	Anticholinergic agents
	Calcium-channel blockers
	Calcium-containing supplements
Neurological disorders	Spinal cord compression
	Parkinson's disease
	Multiple sclerosis
	Cerebral infarction
Mechanical obstruction	Various malignancies
	Adhesions
Metabolic and endocrine disorders	Uremia
	Hypercalcemia
	Hypokalemia
	Hypothyroidism
	Diabetes mellitus with autonomic neuropathy
Changes in lifestyle	Dehydration due to lack of oral intake
	Lack of activity and exercise
	Low-fiber diet
	Inability to go to bathroom
	Unwillingness to use bedside commode or bedpan

compression may suffer from constipation as well. Although they are more commonly perceived as having incontinence and loose stools due to loss of sphincter control, lack of peristalsis may actually lead to fecal impaction, with soft stool seeping around the impaction leaving the false impression that the patient has diarrhea rather than constipation. Therefore, patients with diarrhea and fecal incontinence should be routinely assessed for the presence of fecal impaction.

Bowel obstruction, due to various malignancies or adhesions in the patient with prior abdominal surgery, often presents with constipation as one of the initial complaints. Various metabolic disorders often associated with patients near the end of life, including uremia and hypercalcemia, may cause constipation as can other metabolic abnormalities including hypokalemia

and hypothyroidism. Patients suffering from advanced diabetes mellitus with autonomic neuropathy may suffer from lack of bowel movements due to a decrease in the peristaltic activity of the colon.

Patients near the end of life experience changes in lifestyle that may adversely affect their ability to move their bowels on a regular basis. As a life-limiting illness progresses, patients often eat and drink less, leading to dehydration, which results in increased fluid absorption from the colon and harder stools. A decrease in dietary fiber is another contributing factor. Exercise has positive effects on the propulsion of bowel content and the decreased activity that accompanies progressive illness near the end of life further complicates the situation. Finally, as patients lose their ability to ambulate to the bathroom, bowel function is inhibited by the lack of privacy and perceived lack of dignity often associated with a bedpan or a bedside commode, leading to a marked decrease in the frequency of bowel movements.

CLINICAL PRESENTATION

Patients vary in their description of normal bowel movements, both as to the frequency and the degree of difficulty of defecation, which are the two basic parameters that define constipation. Studies suggest that most individuals have three or more bowel movements per week, while difficulty in defecation is almost entirely subjective. From this discussion it is clear that constipation may be perceived differently by different patients, highlighting once again the importance of an individual assessment as to the nature of the specific patient's symptoms.

Most patients who complain of constipation will note a decrease in what they perceive to be their normal bowel movement frequency and/or complain of hard stools with or without pain on defecation. Some patients, however, especially those who have experienced a marked decrease in oral intake due to their terminal illness, may not complain at all as they believe that the decrease in frequency of bowel movements and/or hard stools are simply the natural result of not eating and does not need attention. Therefore, clinicians must question patients at every visit regarding the frequency and consistency of their bowel movements. If constipation persists untreated over a prolonged period of time, patients may become progressively confused, develop a decreased level of consciousness, complain of progressive abdominal pain, and even experience fever, severe abdominal distention, nausea and vomiting, and leukocytosis, depending on the severity.

As noted already, the clinician must be alert to constipation presenting as loose stool or diarrhea as a result of fecal impaction. Although fecal impaction usually causes complaints of constipation, sometimes, especially if stool softeners are started without concomitant laxatives, soft stool is able to pass around the fecal impaction, resulting in what the patient perceives as diarrhea, while, in fact, the constipation remains the major problem.

TREATMENT

The goal of treatment is evacuation of soft fecal material without straining and optimally, to have evacuation occur at least every 3 days. Nonpharmacological measures that can be used to treat or prevent chronic constipation include increasing mobility and improving the state of hydration to the extent possible. Patients who are no longer able to ambulate to the bathroom should be provided with maximum privacy during defecation even when needing assistance with a bedside commode or a bedpan. Another nonpharmacological intervention that is occasionally required is a manual disimpaction, if the patient is suffering from the complication of a fecal impaction.

Pharmacological Treatment

STANDARD THERAPY The hallmark of the treatment of constipation is pharmacological, and as alluded to earlier, therapy should be initiated prophylactically when patients are at high risk, such as when started on opioid analgesics. Table 8–7 lists commonly used medications for constipation.

The pharmacological therapy of constipation has two major components, stool softeners and laxatives. Stool softeners, such as docusate sodium, are surfactants and act via detergent activity to facilitate the admixture of fat and water to soften stool, and laxatives promote fecal evacuation. Stool softeners and laxatives should be used together (either as two separate preparations or in a combination tablet) to allow softer stool to more easily be evacuated.

There are several different types of laxatives including saline laxatives, irritant or stimulant laxatives, bulk-producing laxatives, lubricant laxatives, and hyperosmolar agents. An algorithm illustrating how these different medications may be used is presented in Figure 8–2.

TABLE 8–7. Pharmacological Treatment of Constipation

MEDICATION	DOSAGE
Stool softeners	
Docusate sodium*	50–500 mg PO bid
Docusate calcium*	240 mg PO qd
Laxatives	
Saline	
Magnesium hydroxide	15–30 mL PO as needed
Citrate of magnesium	300 mL PO as needed
Stimulants	
Bisacodyl	5 mg tab PO or 10 mg suppository PR as needed
Senna	1–2 tabs PO HS
	2 tabs PO qid maximum dose
Cascara	325 mg tablets or 5 mL PO as needed
Castor oil	15–60 mL PO as needed
Bulk producing	
Psyllium	1 rounded teaspoon or a 7 g packet of granules PO three times a day
Lubricant	
Mineral oil[†]	5–45 mL PO as needed
Hyperosmolar agents	
Lactulose	15–30 mL PO qd–tid
Sorbitol	15–30 mL PO qd–tid
Glycerin suppository	One suppository PR as needed
Combination laxative/stool softener	
Senna/docusate sodium	2 tabs PO at bedtime or bid
Enemas	
Fleet (hypertonic phosphate)	PR as needed
Mineral oil	PR as needed
Opioid antagonist	
Methylnaltrexone bromide[‡]	Weight <38 kg: 0.15 mg/kg SC qod
	38–62 kg: 8 mg SC qod
	62–114 kg: 12 mg SC qod
	>114 kg: 0.15 mg/kg SC qod

Note: Preparations containing sodium should not be used by individuals on a sodium-restricted diet or in the presence of edema, congestive heart failure, or hypertension.

*Should not be used concurrently with mineral oil.

[†]May cause lipid pneumonitis in dysphagic patients and chronic use may interfere with absorption of lipid-soluble vitamins.

[‡]The role of methylnaltrexone in the treatment of opioid-induced constipation is not yet defined and should be reserved for patients refractory to standard therapies.

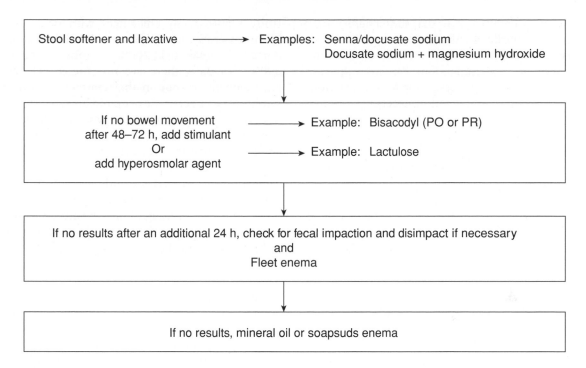

Figure 8–2. The treatment of constipation.

Saline laxatives, such as magnesium hydroxide, attract and retain water in intestinal lumen, increasing intraluminal pressure and stimulating the release of cholecystokinin. The irritant and stimulant laxatives, such as senna and bisacodyl, have both motor and secretory effects on the colon, acting directly on intestinal mucosa to stimulate the myenteric plexus and altering water and electrolyte secretion.

Methylcellulose-psyllium is an example of a bulk-producing laxative, which acts by holding water in the stool and causing mechanical distention. The use of bulk-producing laxatives should be limited in palliative care due to the poor state of hydration experienced by most patients near the end of life, which, when combined with a bulk-producing laxative, can place the patient at an increased risk for intestinal obstruction.

Lubricants, such as mineral oil, retard colonic absorption of fecal water and also soften stool. However, one must be aware of certain issues when using mineral oil. Chronic use of mineral oil can affect the absorption of lipid-soluble vitamins, though this is not often a concern near the end of life. On the other hand, aspiration of mineral oil can cause a lipoid pneumonitis, and this should be avoided when patients suffer from dysphagia. Use of docusate sodium in combination with mineral oil increases the absorption of the mineral oil, thus increasing the potential for mineral oil toxicity.

Hyperosmotic agents, such as lactulose and sorbitol, deliver osmotically active molecules to the colon to promote bowel function and also soften the stool. Glycerin suppositories cause local irritation and have hyperosmotic action resulting in rapid action after administration.

Finally, when oral stool softeners combined with oral or rectal laxatives are not achieving the desired results, enemas may be used. The most common type of enema provided to patients is hypertonic phosphate. When results are still not achieved, mineral oil or soapsuds enemas may need to be utilized. As already mentioned, one must be ever alert to and concerned about the problem of fecal impaction. Patients requiring enemas should be assessed for fecal impaction, and manually disimpacted, if necessary, prior to receiving an enema.

OPIOID-INDUCED BOWEL DYSFUNCTION AND THE OPIOID ANTAGONIST-METHYLNALTREXONE Opioid-induced bowel dysfunction is a term that has recently appeared in the palliative medicine literature. The term has been coined to describe the myriad of gastrointestinal side effects of opioids related to its direct effects on the gastrointestinal tract including constipation, delayed gastric emptying resulting in increased esophageal reflux, abdominal pain, cramps, and bloating. Unlike the common opioid side effect of nausea and vomiting to which many patients develop tolerance, patients do not become tolerant to constipation and the other symptoms associated with opioid-induced bowel dysfunction.

A medication designed to specifically treat opioid-induced constipation, and perhaps other symptoms characteristic of opioid-induced bowel dysfunction has recently become available. Methylnaltrexone bromide is a peripheral μ-receptor antagonist that, unlike its well-known relative naltrexone, does not cross the blood–brain barrier, and, hence, its opioid antagonistic effects are limited to the periphery. Methylnaltrexone binds to the μ-receptors in the gastrointestinal tract, blocking the decreased motility, fluid secretion, and blood flow, and increased water absorption that opioids normally cause.

Two recent randomized clinical trials have demonstrated that subcutaneous methylnaltrexone was safe and significantly more effective than placebo in its ability to induce laxation when administered to hospice and palliative care patients suffering from opioid-induced constipation and being treated with stable doses of opioids and laxatives and stool softeners. Reported side effects included abdominal pain, flatulence, nausea, dizziness, and diarrhea. Neither study reported any challenges with pain control nor were symptoms of opioid withdrawal reported (Thomas et al., 2008; Chamberlain et al., 2009). To date, there are no studies evaluating methylnaltrexone in the treatment of other symptoms characteristic of opioid bowel dysfunction, although studies in healthy volunteers have demonstrated that the medication reduces the delay in oral–fecal transit times that is induced by morphine (Yuan, 2004).

Methylnaltrexone is currently available by subcutaneous injection and is generally administered every other day, although it may be administered as often but no more than once daily. Dosing is weight based and the recommended dosing can be found in Table 8–6. The role of methylnaltrexone in the treatment of opioid-induced constipation or any other symptoms associated with "opioid-induced bowel dysfunction" is as yet unclear for patients near the end of life. Therefore, its use at present should be reserved for patients who have constipation or other gastrointestinal symptoms and are not having acceptable symptom relief from standard therapy.

DIARRHEA

Diarrhea is usually defined as the passage of more than three unformed stools within a 24-hour period. It can be a troubling symptom for patients near the end of life, and can lead to a number of associated problems, including fecal incontinence, skin breakdown, dehydration, electrolyte imbalance, and a painful rectum and perirectal skin. Caregivers of patients with diarrhea will have the additional burden of providing more frequent personal care to the patient as well having to make frequent bedding changes, adding to patient distress because of the patient's awareness of the increased burden of care. Therefore, diarrhea should be resolved as quickly as possible by identifying the cause and initiating a plan to treat or palliate the symptom.

TABLE 8–8. Causes of Diarrhea	
ETIOLOGY	**EXAMPLES**
Constipation with fecal impaction	
Dietary intake	Supplemental drinks
	Increase in fruit, bran, hot spices, or alcohol
Medication and treatment	Laxatives
	Magnesium-containing antacids
	Antibiotics
	NSAIDs
	Chemotherapy
	Radiation therapy
Disease related	Pancreatic insufficiency
	Malignant bowel obstruction—partial
	Carcinoid
	AIDS related
	Infection
	Inflammatory bowel disease
	Irritable bowel disease
	Excess bile salts

ETIOLOGY

The more common causes of diarrhea that occur in patients near the end of life are listed in Table 8–8, with most frequent cause being the overuse of laxatives. This problem should resolve within 24 to 48 hours of discontinuing the offending agent. The laxative can then be resumed if necessary, at a lower dose and titrated to the desired effect.

A thorough review of all other medications should be done and medications that may cause diarrhea, such as magnesium-containing antacids or antibiotics, should be discontinued or changed immediately. Certain chemotherapeutic agents that may occasionally be provided to patients near the end of life, such as the combination of 5-flurouracil and leucovorin and the single agent ironotecan, may also result in severe diarrhea. (See Chapter 19 for further discussion of the role of chemotherapy in the treatment of patients near the end of life.)

As discussed in the section on constipation earlier, fecal impaction may present with diarrhea and should not be overlooked. A complete history regarding bowel movements, including their frequency, consistency, and amount, in addition to an examination of the rectal vault will help to avoid missing this diagnosis.

Dietary habits that may contribute to diarrhea include excessive ingestion of fiber, fruits, and nonabsorbable sugars. Radiotherapy can cause diarrhea 2 to 3 weeks after treatment is completed, due to damage to the intestinal mucosa, which releases prostaglandins that lead to increased bowel motility, and also leads to malabsorption of bile salts. Malignancies of the pancreas and gastrointestinal tract, as well as other diseases of the small bowel, may result in diarrhea secondary to malabsorption. Gastrointestinal infections that may occur in patients near the end of life, especially those suffering from AIDS, may be bacterial, viral, fungal, or protozoan in nature. (See Chapter 25 for further discussion of AIDS-related diarrhea.) Patients on chronic antibiotics therapy for other infections may also develop diarrhea secondary to antibiotic-related pseudomembranous colitis.

TREATMENT

The initial step in the treatment of diarrhea should be to address any reversible causes of the symptom. Laxatives should be withheld and/or modified if necessary, and other potentially offending medications should be discontinued if possible. Fecal impaction should be considered and treated if found. Diet should be modified to avoid high fiber content foods as well as fruits and other offending agents, and foods low in fiber should be substituted.

Medications used to treat diarrhea are listed in Table 8–9. For some patients, specific agents should be chosen based on the cause of the diarrhea. If an infectious cause of diarrhea is suspected, then appropriate antimicrobials should be prescribed. (See Chapter 25 for a discussion of appropriate antimicrobial agents used in the treatment of infectious diarrhea secondary to AIDS.) If pseudomembranous colitis from antibiotic therapy is suspected, then the offending antibiotic agent should be discontinued, and the patient should be treated with metronidazole or vancomycin. Diarrhea secondary to malabsorption, which may occur in patients with pancreatic and other gastrointestinal malignancies, may respond to pancreatic enzymes or cholestyramine. Cholestyramine combined with aspirin and/or bulk-forming agents such as psyllium may help reduce diarrhea secondary to radiation-induced enteritis. Secretory diarrhea, secondary to AIDS and carcinoid tumors, may require therapy with octreotide.

TABLE 8–9. Treatment for Diarrhea

TYPE OF MEDICATION	MEDICATION	DOSAGE
Adsorbents	Bismuth subsalicylate	30 mL or 2 tablet every $^1\!/_2$ to 1 h Max 240 mL or 16 tabs/24 h
Adsorbent + bulk-forming agent	Kaolin with pectin: 90 g kaolin and 2 g pectin/30 mL	60–120 mL PO q bowel movement
Hypomotility agents	Loperamide	4 mg PO initial dose; 2 mg PO after each loose movement, not to exceed 16 mg/d
	Diphenoxylate with atropine	1 tablet (5 mg) PO qid Max 8 tablets/24 h
	Codeine	15–60 mg PO qid
Bile salt binder	Cholestyramine	1 packet (4 g) PO bid-qid before meals Max 24 g (6 packets)/24 h
Antibiotics for pseudomembranous colitis*	Metronidazole	250 mg PO qid or 500 mg PO tid for 10–14 d
	Vancomycin	125–250 mg PO qid for 10–14 d
Pancreatic enzyme replacement	Pancrelipase	1–2 tabs PO with meals or snacks individualized to control steatorrhea
Synthetic somatostatin analog	Octreotide	10–80 μg/h by continuous subcu infusion

*In patients with pseudomembranous colitis, administration of hypomotility agents is not recommended as it may exacerbate infection.

Patients near the end of life who do not have an identifiable or reversible cause of diarrhea should be treated symptomatically with antidiarrheal agents. Kaolin–pectin suspension or bismuth subsalicylate may be used if the diarrhea is mild to moderate. In more severe cases, or if there is no response to the kaolin–pectin suspension or bismuth, then medications that slow bowel motility, such as loperamide or diphenoxylate with atropine, should be prescribed.

DYSPHAGIA

Dysphagia is technically defined as difficulty in transferring liquids or solids from the mouth to the stomach, but in more practical terms, the term is used to describe difficulties with swallowing. Dysphagia occurs in approximately 10% to 20% of patients with advanced cancer, and also occurs in patients near the end of life who suffer from advanced dementia and other advanced neurodegenerative disorders.

Common causes of dysphagia are listed in Table 8–10. Dysphagia in cancer patients is usually either due to mechanical obstruction from direct tumor growth, inflammation caused by radiation therapy or chemotherapy, or by infection, such as candidiasis, in the immunocompromised patient. Xerostomia secondary to medications, especially opioid analgesics, may also contribute to the patient's complaints of difficulty swallowing. (See Chapter 11 for a discussion of the treatment of xerostomia.)

Patients suffering from nonmalignant illness near the end of life who complain of or exhibit dysphagia may have abnormalities in the swallowing mechanism on a neuromuscular basis, caused by their primary neurodegenerative

TABLE 8–10. Causes of Dysphagia in Patients Near the End of Life

ETIOLOGY	EXAMPLES
Mechanical obstruction	Carcinomas of the head and neck
	Carcinoma of the esophagus
	Carcinoma of the upper stomach
	Thyroid carcinomas
Neurological and neuromuscular disorders	Amyotrophic lateral sclerosis
	Alzheimer's disease
	Parkinson's disease
	Huntington's Chorea
	Multiple sclerosis
	Cerebrovascular disease
	Head trauma
	Myasthenia gravis
Pain	Tumor related
	Candidiasis and other infections
	Radiation and/or chemotherapy-induced stomatitis
Pharmacologic agents	Anticholinergics
	Antihistamines
	Phenothiazines

disorder. Patients near the end of life, irrespective of diagnosis, may also have difficulty swallowing secondary to various commonly used medications, including anticholinergics, antihistamines, and phenothiazines.

CLINICAL PRESENTATION

Patients with dysphagia may exhibit drooling, hesitancy in swallowing, holding food in the mouth, pain with swallowing, coughing, and/or choking or nasal regurgitation. Drooling is often associated with pain on swallowing or obstruction, while hesitancy in swallowing may be caused by a neurological disorder. Coughing, especially after swallowing, may be a sign of a tracheoesophageal fistula. Patients with a mechanical obstruction, if they are alert, may be able to point to the location of the blockage. Patients with dysphagia from either mechanical or neurological causes may also present with aspiration pneumonia.

TREATMENT

Conservative treatment for dysphagia includes good oral hygiene and providing food of the type and consistency that the patient can swallow. Small meals served at room temperature may be of benefit. The head of the bed should be elevated during eating and for at least approximately 1 to 2 hours after eating, as this will facilitate food moving down the esophagus and reduce the risk of aspiration. Another physical maneuver that may help reduce aspiration risk is to keep the chin down toward the chest during swallowing, as this will close off the airway and decrease pressure in the throat.

Medications for the treatment of dysphagia, listed in Table 8–11, may include topical or systemic antimicrobials for oropharyngeal or esophageal infection. Nystatin suspension 400,000 U via a swish and swallow technique, or clotrimazole lozenges five times a day may be effective in mild cases of oropharyngeal candidiasis. However, if topical treatment is not effective, or when the infection extends into the esophagus, oral therapy with fluconazole 50 to 150 mg daily should be used. Viral esophagitis, caused by organisms such as cytomegalovirus, may be treated with acyclovir, 1,000 mg a day in divided doses. For esophagitis secondary to noninfectious inflammation, agents that coat the mucosa, including liquid antacids and sucralfate suspension are sometimes helpful. If swallowing

TABLE 8–11. Pharmacological Treatment of Dysphagia		
ETIOLOGY	**MEDICATION**	**DOSAGE AND ROUTE**
Candidiasis	Nystatin suspension	400,000 U, 4–5 times/d via swish and swallow
	Clotrimazole lozenges	Dissolve in mouth 4–5 times/d
	Fluconazole	50–150 mg PO daily
Viral	Acyclovir	200 mg PO 5 times a day
Noninfectious inflammation or as an adjunct to antimicrobials	Liquid antacids	30 cc PO 3–4 times a day
	Sucralfate suspension	10 cc PO 4 times a day
	Ranitidine	75–150 mg PO 1–2 times/d
	Famotidine	10–20 mg PO 1–2 times/d
	Omeprazole	20 mg PO daily
Mechanical obstruction	Prednisone	20–40 mg PO daily
	Dexamethasone	2–4 mg PO 2–4 times/d

problems are caused by gastroesophageal reflux, H_2-blockers, such as ranitidine or famotidine, or proton-pump inhibitors, such as omeprazole, may be prescribed.

When there is a mechanical obstruction caused by tumor, corticosteroids may be helpful in improving symptoms by decreasing edema and hence tumor size, or reducing the size of mediastinal lymph nodes that may be interfering with swallowing. For patients near the end of life with appropriate prognoses and life expectancies, definitive treatment to alleviate the obstruction with radiation therapy, esophageal dilatation, stent placement, and/or laser therapy may be considered. (See Chapter 18 for a discussion of the utility of invasive therapies for patients near the end of life.) Finally, for patients with mechanical obstruction who are not candidates for more definitive treatment, and for patients with neurological problems who have swallowing difficulties, gastrostomy tube placement may need to

be considered under appropriate circumstances. (See Chapter 24 for further discussion of the indications and ethical considerations of gastrostomy tubes in patients near the end of life.)

ABDOMINAL PAIN AND DYSPEPSIA

Although the subject of pain is discussed elsewhere (Chapter 6), it is important to pay some specific attention to abdominal pain as a symptom, due to the multiplicity of causes and potential interventions other then analgesics that may be used to treat abdominal pain. Table 8–12 lists some of the more common causes of abdominal pain, as well as the various medications associated with the treatment of each specific cause.

TABLE 8–12. Abdominal Pain: Etiologies and Pharmacologial Therapies

ETIOLOGY	MEDICATION	DOSE AND ROUTE
Dyspepsia	Liquid antacids	15–30 cc PO 3–4 times/d
	Ranitidine	75–150 mg PO bid
	Famotidine	10–20 mg PO 1–2 times/d
	Omeprazole	20 mg PO qd
	Misoprostol	100–200 µg PO qid with food
Delayed gastric emptying without obstruction	Metoclopramide	5–10 mg PO/SC AC & HS
Gastric distention	Simethicone	40–125 mg PO qid
Abdominal cramping with or without partial bowel obstruction	Stool softeners	See Table 8–7
	Dexamethasone	2–4 mg PO 2–4 times a day
	Hyoscyamine	0.125–0.25 mg PO q 4 h
		Max 12 tabs in 24 h
	Antidiarrheals*	See Table 8–9
Constipation	Stool softeners and laxatives	See Table 8–7
Bladder spasms	Belladonna/opium suppositories	1 every 4 h as needed
	Hyoscyamine	0.125–0.25 mg PO q 4 h
		Max 12 tabs in 24 h

*Antidiarrheals should generally be avoided in patients with partial bowel obstruction, as they may aggravate symptoms.

One of the more frequent abdominal complaints that patients experience near the end of life is, not surprisingly, dyspepsia, more commonly known as an "upset stomach." Dyspepsia is characterized by epigastric pain that is sometimes described as burning, nausea, and/or gaseous eructation.

There are two main types of dyspepsia: organic and functional. Organic dyspepsia is due to a specific lesion such as gastritis, peptic ulcer disease, gastroesophageal reflux disease, gastric carcinoma, or cholelithiasis. Signs of organic dyspepsia may include organomegaly, one or more abdominal masses, ascites, fecal occult blood, dysphagia, weight loss, constant or severe pain, pain that radiates to the back, recurrent vomiting, hematemesis, melena, or jaundice. Functional dyspepsia is dyspepsia with no identifiable focal or structural cause and accounts for approximately 40% of dyspepsia.

Patients near the end of life may have abdominal pain for reasons other than dyspepsia. These include gaseous distention, diarrhea (with or without infection) associated with abdominal cramping, partial or complete bowel obstruction, and, perhaps, most commonly, constipation (see above). Hepatomegaly due to metastatic cancer may cause abdominal discomfort secondary to stretching of the liver capsule, which contains pain receptors. Finally, abdominal pain in patients near the end of life is often due to bladder spasms or urinary retention.

TREATMENT

There are a number of nonpharmacological interventions that should be attempted to address symptoms of abdominal pain, based on the identified or suspected cause. Dyspepsia accompanied by reflux may respond to elevation of the head of the bed and avoiding foods such as mint, coffee, and fatty foods all of which decrease lower esophageal sphincter (LES) tone. Other foods that should be avoided include tomatoes, citrus fruits, and alcohol because of their direct irritating effect on the esophageal mucosa.

The patient's medication profile should be reviewed, and medications that may contribute to dyspepsia, such as nonsteroidal anti-inflammatory drugs (NSAIDs) and steroids, should be discontinued if possible. If the patient has symptoms of reflux, medications that decrease LES tone, such as calcium-channel blockers, anticholingerics, and benzodiazepines should be avoided.

Patients should always be assessed and treated for constipation, including manual disimpaction if a fecal impaction is identified. If urinary retention is suspected, placement of a catheter to drain the bladder might be a simple, nonpharmacological way to resolve a troubling symptom.

Recommendations for the pharmacological management of abdominal pain can be found in Table 8–12. For dyspepsia, antacids, H_2-blockers, or proton pump inhibitors may be used. If a patient is complaining of early satiety suggestive of poor gastric emptying, and there is no evidence of gastric outlet obstruction, metoclopramide might be a good agent to try. Be aware, however, that if there is gastric outlet obstruction, metoclopramide will worsen rather than improve symptoms.

For gaseous distention, simethicone products, either alone or in combination with antacids if the gas is accompanied by dyspepsia, may be helpful. Constipation, if present, should be appropriately managed with stool softeners and laxatives and other measures as necessary (see Table 8–7). Patients with abdominal cramps and diarrhea who have an infectious or inflammatory diarrhea may require appropriate antibiotics and antidiarrheal agents (see Table 8–9). Antispasmodics, such as hyoscyamine, either alone or in combination with phenobarbital, atropine, or scopolamine may provide relief.

One must be aware of the possibility that abdominal cramps accompanied by diarrhea may be a sign of partial bowel obstruction, in which case the antidiarrheals and antispasmodic agents could aggravate rather than reduce symptoms. However, if the patient is suffering from an insoluble terminal bowel obstruction, antispasmodic agents combined with steroids may be able to palliate specific symptoms by reducing cramps and keeping the bowels as open as possible. (Bowel obstruction is discussed in more detail later in the chapter.) Antispasmodics, including belladonna/opium suppositories and hyoscyamine, have also been found useful in the palliation of bladder spasms.

GASTROINTESTINAL BLEEDING

Patients near the end of life are susceptible to gastrointestinal bleeding from many causes, with some of the more common ones listed in Table 8–13. Upper gastrointestinal (GI) bleeding may be related to ulcer disease or gastritis, which near the end of life is often due to medication, with NSAIDs and steroids being the most common offending agents. Patients with esophageal or gastric malignancies may, of course, have bleeding directly from these lesions, while patients with end-stage liver disease and portal hypertension may develop bleeding esophageal varices.

In terminally ill patients, bleeding from colorectal and anal neoplasms is often obvious, but one must also be alert to common potential causes of lower GI bleeding seen in the general population, including hemorrhoids, diverticulosis, and arteriovenous malformations. Comorbid inflammatory bowel disease may also give rise to bleeding at times. Finally, patients near the end of life may bleed from ischemic or infectious lower bowel diseases.

The treatment of GI bleeding near the end of life depends on the cause, the severity of the bleeding, and the patients' overall clinical condition. If the bleeding is limited, symptomatic therapy may be all that is warranted. Discontin-

TABLE 8–13. Causes of Gastrointestinal Bleeding in Patients Near the End of Life

LOCATION	EXAMPLES
Upper GI bleeding	Gastritis
	Malignant gastric ulcer disease
	Benign peptic ulcer disease
	Esophageal varices
	Erosive esophagitis
	Mallory–Weiss tear
	Esophageal carcinoma
Lower GI bleeding	Colorectal cancer
	Anal neoplasm
	Diverticulosis
	Hemorrhoids
	Angiodysplasia
	Inflammatory bowel disease
	Ischemic colitis
	Infectious colitis

uation of any potentially offending medications and the use of antacids and/or other anti-ulcer preparations (see Table 8–12) may be effective in ameliorating upper GI bleeding related to gastritis or ulcer disease. Patients with limited lower GI blood loss may be observed, provided with iron replacement therapy, and, if indicated based on symptoms, receive periodic red blood cell transfusions. (See Chapter 18 for further discussion on the indications for transfusion therapy near the end of life.) If blood loss is not adequately controlled by these relatively conservative measures, then consideration for further evaluation, including the potential of upper or lower GI endoscopy with possible laser coagulation therapy, may be considered on a case-by-case basis. (See Chapter 18 for further discussion.)

Although acute bleeding may warrant replacement of blood products, fluids, and endoscopy, for some patients near the end of life, prognosis and clinical condition may dictate a more conservative approach, with comfort measures being provided, allowing the patient's life to end in a relatively painless way.

JAUNDICE AND BILIARY OBSTRUCTION

Jaundice and/or biliary obstruction occur in patients who are near the end of life suffering from primary and metastatic malignancies directly affecting the liver or gallbladder, from pancreatic carcinoma or lymphoma that obstruct the bile ducts, or from primary hepatic failure. Although jaundice itself is not necessarily dangerous, jaundice can cause severe pruritus. Pruritus can be treated symptomatically with antihistamines, such as diphenhydramine 25 mg or cyproheptadine 4 mg given every 4 to 6 hours. Cholestyramine 4 g given three times a day before meals may also reduce itching by binding and reducing the absorption of excess bile salts in the GI tract, which are responsible for the pruritus.

In some patients with obstructive jaundice, the placement of a biliary stent to relieve the obstruction may be indicated. This is discussed in more detail in Chapter 18.

BOWEL OBSTRUCTION

Bowel obstruction is an unfortunate complication occurring in patients near the end of life, the majority of whom suffer from advanced abdominal or pelvic cancers. Some of the more common etiologies of bowel obstruction in patients near the end of life are listed in Table 8–14. Bowel obstruction near the end of life may be complete or partial, and its severity may fluctuate during the patient's clinical course.

TABLE 8–14. Causes of Bowel Obstruction Near the End of Life

Malignancy
    Intraluminal obstruction secondary to primary tumor or recurrence
    Peritoneal carcinomatosis
    Fibrosis secondary to prior radiation therapy
Adhesions secondary to prior surgery
Constipation with or without fecal impaction
Medications
    Anticholinergics
    Opioids
    Tricyclics
    Neuroleptics

Recurrent tumor is the most common reason for bowel obstruction, with the nature of the malignancy varying from a recurrent intraluminal mass to the more likely possibility of extraluminal metastatic implants. Nonmalignant causes of obstruction in patients with terminal neoplastic disease may include radiation-related strictures and fibrosis. Terminally ill patients with or without malignant disease who have a prior history of abdominal surgery may develop obstruction from adhesions. And, as already mentioned earlier, constipation with or without fecal impaction, if allowed to become severe enough, may present with frank bowel obstruction. Medications that may contribute to symptoms of functional bowel obstruction include anticholinergics, opioid analgesics, tricyclic antidepressants, and neuroleptic agents.

Although the treatment of bowel obstruction is traditionally surgical, patients near the end of life are often not considered surgical candidates. A discussion of the indications for surgery to relieve bowel obstruction near the end of life can be found in Chapter 18. Patients with obstruction who are not surgical candidates generally suffer from symptoms of abdominal pain, intestinal colic, and nausea and vomiting. Obstructed patients may present with constipation, however, especially when the obstruction is partial, diarrhea may sometimes be a major complaint. When the obstruction is partial, interventions may include a liquid diet along with stool softeners to reduce complaints of constipation (Table 8–7), anti-emetics to reduce nausea (Tables 8–4 and 8–5), and antispasmodics to reduce abdominal pain and cramps (Table 8–12). Stimulant laxatives should be avoided as they may worsen symptoms of intestinal colic. Steroids, such as dexamethasone (Table 8–12), may be useful as an adjunctive agent by reducing the edema or inflammation of bowel wall in the area of the obstruction, hopefully resulting in at least a partial opening of the intestinal lumen.

Despite these measures, emesis may be more difficult to control due to the natural secretion of fluids that accumulate in the obstructed GI tract. For some patients, a once-a-day bout of emesis, with relative comfort the rest of the time, is acceptable. For others, the placement of a nasogastric tube (or a percutaneous gastrostomy tube) may need to be considered to provide periodic decompression without emesis. Patients who elect treatment with a tube may still be permitted to take oral food and fluids by mouth to allow them to experience the pleasure of eating if they so desire. Another approach to reduce the incidence of emesis in these patients is with the use of the agent octreotide (see Table 8–9), which reduces gastric and intestinal secretions and hence the need for vomiting or tube decompression.

ASCITES

Ascites is the pathologic accumulation of fluid in the peritoneal cavity that causes abdominal distention. Common causes of ascites that occur in patients near the end of life are listed in Table 8–15. Ascites occurs in 15% to 50% of patients with cancer, with the most common primary sites

TABLE 8–15. Common Causes of Ascites Near the End of Life

Peritoneal carcinomatosis
   Gynecological malignancies: ovary, endometrium
   Gastrointestinal malignancies: colon, stomach, pancreas
   Other malignancies: breast, lung
Liver metastases
Cor pulmonale
   End-stage chronic obstructive pulmonary disease
   Primary pulmonary hypertension
End-stage congestive heart failure
End-stage nonmalignant liver disease

being the ovary, colon, stomach, endometrium, pancreas, breast, and lung. Ascites near the end of life may also occur in patients with nonmalignant conditions such as end-stage liver disease, cor pulmonale secondary to advanced chronic obstructive pulmonary disease or primary pulmonary hypertension, and end-stage congestive heart failure.

Peritoneal carcinomatosis produces ascites by obstructing lymphatic flow and accounts for more than 50% of patients with malignant ascites. Primary and metastatic malignancies involving the liver cause ascites by obstructing the hepatic venous circulation. In cirrhosis with portal hypertension, abnormal renal function characterized by sodium and water retention is responsible for ascitic fluid accumulation.

Symptoms due to ascites are the result of increased abdominal pressure created by the accumulation of fluid. These symptoms include abdominal pressure or discomfort, anorexia, dyspepsia, dyspnea, and edema of the lower extremities. When the ascites is tense, the physical finding of shifting dullness to percussion may help differentiate ascites from abdominal distention due to obstruction. Measurement of the abdominal girth is an important way to assess the degree of fluid accumulation and the effectiveness of treatments.

Primary treatment of ascites includes a salt-restricted diet (<1,000 mg/d) when possible, with fluid restriction (<1,500 mL/d) if the patient becomes hyponatremic. Diuretic therapy is often attempted, with spironolactone 25 mg four times a day, either alone or in combination with furosemide 40 mg/d. It must be remembered that despite the large amount of fluid in the peritoneal space, many of these patients are intravascularly dehydrated, so both fluid restriction and diuretics should be used with care. With the aforementioned diuretic regimen, it has been found that approximately 70% of patients will have resolution of ascites in 2 to 4 weeks. If patients remain symptomatic despite treatment with diuretic therapy and salt and fluid restriction if necessary, then an abdominal paracentesis may be helpful. A full discussion of the indications for abdominal paracentesis for patients near the end of life, as well as the option of a peritovenous shunt for patients with chronic ascites who have a sufficiently long life expectancy, can be found in Chapter 18.

BIBLIOGRAPHY

Aberra FN, Gronczewski CA, Katz JP: Clostridium difficile colitis: Treatment and medications. eMedicine Gastroenterology. http://emedicine.medscape.com/article/186458-treatment. Updated August 4, 2009. Accessed October 9, 2009.

Alderman J: Fast facts and concepts: Diarrhea in palliative care. *J Palliat Med* 8:449-450, 2005.

Baron TH, Dean PA, et al: Expandable metal stents for the treatment of colonic obstruction: Techniques and outcomes. *Gastrointest Endosc* 47(3):277-286, 1998.

Baumrucker SJ: Management of intestinal obstruction in hospice care [published erratum appears in *Am J Hosp Palliat Care* 15(5):137, 1998]. *Am J Hosp Palliat Care* 15(4):232-235, 1998.

Becker G, Galandi D, Blum H: Peripherally acting opioid antagonists in the treatment of opiate-related constipation: A systematic review. *J Pain Symptom Manage* 35:547-565, 2007.

Berger AM, Portenoy RK, Weissman DE: *Principles and Practice of Supportive Oncology.* Philadelphia, PA, Lippincott-Raven, 1998.

Bleicher J, Bhaskara A, Hyuck T, et al: Lorazepam, diphenhydramine, and haloperidol transdermal gel for rescue from chemotherapy induced nausea/vomiting: Results of two pilot trials. *J Support Oncol* 6:27-32, 2008.

Buchanan D, Muirhead K: Letter to the editor: Intractable nausea and vomiting successfully treated with granisetron 5-hydroxytryptamine type 3 receptor antagonists in palliative medicine. *Palliat Med* 21:725-726, 2007.

Chamberlain BH, Cross K, Winston JL, et al: Methylnaltrexone treatment of opioid-induced constipation in patients with advanced illness. *J Pain Symptom Manage* 38(5):683-690, 2009. http://download.journals.elsevierhealth.com/pdfs/journals/0885-3924/PIIS0885392409006411.pdf. Accessed October 8, 2009.

Conn HF, Rakel RE: *Conn's Current Therapy.* Philadelphia, PA, W.B. Saunders, 1984.

Currow DC, Couglan M, Fardell B, Cooney NJ: Use of ondansetron in palliative medicine. *J Pain Symptom Manage* 13:302-307, 1997.

Doyle D: *Domiciliary Palliative Care: A Handbook for Family Doctors and Community Nurses.* Oxford/New York, Oxford University Press, 1994.

Doyle D, Hanks GWC, MacDonald N: *Oxford Textbook of Palliative Medicine.* Oxford/New York, Oxford University Press, 1998.

Dunlop R: *Cancer : Palliative Care.* London/New York, Springer, 1998.

Duthie EH, Katz PR: *Practice of Geriatrics.* Philadelphia, PA, W.B. Saunders, 1998.

Enck RE: *The Medical Care of Terminally Ill Patients.* Baltimore, MD, Johns Hopkins University Press, 1993.

Fainsinger R: Integrating medical and surgical treatments in gastrointestinal, genitourinary, and biliary obstruction in patients with cancer. *Hematol Oncol Clin North Am* 10(1):173-188, 1996.

Fallon BG: Nausea and vomiting unrelated to cancer treatment. In: Berger A, Portenoy RK, Weissman DE, eds. *Principles and Practice of Supportive Oncology.* Philadelphia, PA, Lippincott-Raven, 1998, pp. 179-189. Chapter 12.

Fallon M, O'Neill B: ABC of palliative care. Constipation and diarrhoea. *BMJ* 315(7118):1293-1296, 1997.

Fernandes JR, Seymour RJ, et al: Bowel obstruction in patients with ovarian cancer: A search for prognostic factors. *Am J Obstet Gynecol* 158(2):244-249, 1988.

Finlay I: End-of-life care in patients dying of gynecologic cancer. *Hematol Oncol Clin North Am* 13(1):77-108, viii, 1999.

Fischer DS: Abdominal paracentesis for malignant ascites. *Arch Intern Med* 139(2):235, 1979.

Gilbar PJ: A guide to enteral drug administration in palliative care. *J Pain Symptom Manage* 17(3):197-207, 1999.

Gines P, Arroyo V, et al: Comparison of paracentesis and diuretics in the treatment of cirrhotics with tense ascites. Results of a randomized study. *Gastroenterology* 93(2):234-241, 1987.

Goroll AH, May LA, et al: *Primary Care Medicine: Office Evaluation and Management of the Adult Patient.* Philadelphia, PA, Lippincott Williams & Wilkins, 1995.

Hajjar ER, Caffero AC, Hanlon JT: Polypharmacy in elderly patients. *Am J Geriatr Pharmacother* 5:345-351, 2007.

Hoegler D: Radiotherapy for palliation of symptoms in incurable cancer. *Curr Probl Cancer* 21(3):129-183, 1997.

Hospice Pharmacia Pharmacy and Therapeutics Committee: *Hospice Pharmacia Medication Use Guidelines*, 7th ed. Philadelphia, PA, excell RX, Inc., 2005.

Hurdon V, Viola R, et al: How useful is docusate in patients at risk for constipation? A systematic review of the evidence in the chronically ill. *J Pain Symptom Manage* 19(2):130-136, 2000.

Jackson WC, Tavernier L: Olanzapine for intractable nausea in palliative care patients. *J Palliat Med* 6:251-255, 2003.

Jordan K, Sippel C, Schmoll H: Guidelines for antiemetic treatment of chemotherapy induced nausea and vomiting: Past, present and future recommendations. *Oncologist* 12:1143-1150, 2007.

Kaye P; Hospice Education Institute: *Notes on Symptom Control in Hospice & Palliative Care.* Essex, CT, Hospice Education Institute, 1990.

Kemp C: *Terminal Illness: A Guide to Nursing Care.* Philadelphia, PA, Lippincott Williams & Wilkins, 1999.

Kinzbrunner BM: *Vitas Pain Management Guidelines*, 3rd ed. Miami, FL, Vitas Healthcare Corporation, 1999.

Kinzbrunner BM, Policzer JS: *Vitas Guidelines for Intensive Palliative Care*, 2nd ed. Miami, FL, Vitas Healthcare Corporation, 2008.

Kornblau S, Benson AB, et al: Management of cancer treatment-related diarrhea. Issues and therapeutic strategies. *J Pain Symptom Manage* 19(2):118-129, 2000.

Lee J, Dodd M, Dibble S, Abrams D: Review of acupressure studies for chemotherapy-induced nausea and vomiting control. *J Pain Symptom Manage* 36:529-544, 2008.

Legg JJ, Balano KB: Symptom management in HIV-infected patients. *Prim Care* 24(3):597-606, 1997.

MacBryde CM, Blacklow RS: *MacBryde's Signs and Symptoms: Applied and Pathologic Physiology and Clinical Interpretation.* Philadelphia, PA, Lippincott Williams & Wilkins, 1983.

MacDonald N. *Palliative Medicine: A Case-Based Manual.* Oxford/Toronto, Oxford University Press, 1998.

Maguire P, Faulkner A, et al: Eliciting the current problems of the patient with cancer—a flow diagram. *Palliat Med* 7(2):151-156, 1993.

McGann KP. *Griffith's 5-Minute Clinical Consult.* Philadelphia, Lippincott, 1999.

Mercadante S, Casuccio A, Mangione S: Medical treatment of inoperable malignant bowel obstruction: A qualitative systemic review. *J Pain Symptom Manage* 33:217-223, 2007.

Moon RB. ABHR gel in the treatment of nausea and vomiting in the hospice patient. *Int J Pharm Compound* 10(2):95-98, 2006.

Morita T, Tsunoda J, et al: Contributing factors to physical symptoms in terminally-ill cancer patients. *J Pain Symptom Manage* 18(5):338-346, 1999.

Nevitt AW, Vida F, et al: Expandable metallic prostheses for malignant obstructions of gastric outlet and proximal small bowel. *Gastrointest Endosc* 47(3):271-276, 1998.

Oderda K, Peterson D: New drug bulletin: Methylnaltrexone bromide (Relistor™—Wyeth). University of Utah Hospitals & Clinic, August 14, 2008. http://healthcare.utah.edu/pharmacy/bulletins/NDB_166.pdf. Accessed August 8, 2009.

Ottery FD: Cancer cachexia: Prevention, early diagnosis, and management [published erratum appears in Cancer Pract 2(4):263, 1994]. *Cancer Pract* 2(2):123-131, 1994.

Panchal SJ, Muller-Schwefe P, Wurzelmann JI: Opioid-induced bowel dysfunction: Prevalence, pathophysiology and burden. *Int J Clin Pract* 61: 1181-1187, 2007.

Passik SD, Kirsh KL, Theobald DE, et al: A retrospective chart review of the use of olanzapine for the prevention of delayed emesis in cancer patients. *J Pain Symptom Manage* 25:485-489, 2003.

Philip J, Depczynski B: The role of total parenteral nutrition for patients with irreversible bowel obstruction secondary to gynecological malignancy. *J Pain Symptom Manage* 13(2):104-111, 1997.

Portenoy RK, Thomas J, Boatwright MLM, et al: Subcutaneous methylnaltrexone for the treatment of opioid-induced constipation in patients with advanced illness: A double-blind, randomized, parallel group, dose-ranging study. *J Pain Sympt Manage* 25:458-468, 2008.

Raijman I, Siddique I, et al: Palliation of malignant dysphagia and fistulae with coated expandable metal stents: Experience with 101 patients. *Gastrointest Endosc* 48(2):172-179, 1998.

Ripamonti C, Bruera E. Pain and symptom management in palliative care. *Cancer Control* 3(3):204-213, 1996.

Ripamonti C, Mercadante S, et al: Role of octreotide, scopolamine butylbromide, and hydration in symptom control of patients with inoperable bowel obstruction and nasogastric tubes: A prospective randomized trial. *J Pain Symptom Manage* 19(1): 23-34, 2000.

Roscoe JA, Bushunow P, Jean-Pierre J, et al: Acupressure bands are effective in reducing radiation therapy-related nausea. *J Pain Symptom Manage* 38:381-389, 2009.

Roscoe JA, Morrow GR, Hickok JT, et al: The efficacy of acupressure and acustimulation wrist bands for the relief of chemotherapy-induced nausea and vomiting. A university of Rochester cancer center community clinical oncology program multicenter study. *J Pain Symptom Manage* 26:731-742, 2003.

Rossi RL, Traverso LW, et al: Malignant obstructive jaundice. Evaluation and management. *Surg Clin North Am* 76(1):63-70, 1996.

Saunders CM, Baines M., et al: *Living with Dying: A Guide for Palliative Carers.* Oxford/New York, Oxford University Press, 1995.

Saunders CM, Sykes N: *The Management of Terminal Malignant Disease.* London, E. Arnold (a division of Hodder & Stoughton), 1993.

Sharma S, Walsh D: Management of symptomatic malignant ascites with diuretics: Two case reports and a review of the literature. *J Pain Symptom Manage* 10(3):237-242, 1995.

Sleisenger MH, Fordtran JS, et al: *Sleisenger & Fordtran's Gastrointestinal and Liver Disease: Pathophysiology, Diagnosis, Management.* Philadelphia, PA, W.B. Saunders, 1998.

Soetikno R: Palliation of malignant gastric outlet obstruction using an endoscopically placed Wallstent. *Gastrointest Endosc* 47(3):267-270, 1998.

Souter RG, Wells C, et al: Surgical and pathologic complications associated with peritoneovenous shunts in management of malignant ascites. *Cancer* 55(9):1973-1978, 1985.

Srivastava M, Brito-Dellan N, Davis MP, et al: Olanzapine as an antiemetic in refractory nausea and vomiting in advanced cancer. *J Pain Symptom Manage* 25:578-582, 2003.

Sykes NP: An investigation of the ability of oral naloxone to correct opioid-related constipation in patients with advanced cancer. *Palliat Med* 10(2):135-144, 1996.

Talmi YP, Bercovici M, et al: Home and inpatient hospice care of terminal head and neck cancer patients. *J Palliat Care* 13(1):9-14, 1997.

Thomas J. Opioid-induced bowel dysfunction. *J Pain Symptom Manage* 35:103-113, 2008.

Thomas J, Austin Cooney G: Palliative care and pain: New strategies for managing opioid bowel dysfunction. *J Palliat Med* 11(S1):S1-S19, 2008.

Thomas J, Karver S, Austin Cooney G, et al: Methylnaltrexone for opioid-induced constipation in advanced illness. *N Engl J Med* 358:2332-2343, 2008.

Tuca A, Roca R, Sala C, et al: Efficacy of granisetron in the antiemetic control of nonsurgical intestinal obstruction in advanced cancer: A phase II clinical trial. *J Pain Symptom Manage* 37:259-270, 2009.

Twycross RG, Wilcock A, et al: *Palliative Care Formulary.* Oxford, Radcliffe Medical Press, 1998.

Vainio A, Auvinen A: Prevalence of symptoms among patients with advanced cancer: An international collaborative study. Symptom Prevalence Group. *J Pain Symptom Manage* 12(1):3-10, 1996.

Veehof LJG, Stewart RE, Meyboom-de Jong B, Haaijer-Ruskamp FM: Adverse drug reactions and polypharmacy in the elderly in general practice. *Eur J Clin Pharmacol* 55:533-536, 1999.

von Gunten C, Muir JC. Fast facts and concepts: Medical management of bowel obstruction. *J Palliat Med* 5:739-740, 2002.

von Gunten CF, Twaddle ML: Terminal care for non-cancer patients. *Clin Geriatr Med* 12(2):349-358, 1996.

Walsh D, Doona M, et al: Symptom control in advanced cancer: Important drugs and routes of administration. *Semin Oncol* 27(1):69-83, 2000.

Watanabe S, Bruera E: Anorexia and cachexia, asthenia, and lethargy. *Hematol Oncol Clin North Am* 10(1):189-206, 1996.

Weschules DJ. Tolerability of the compound ABHR in hospice patients. *J Palliat Med* 8:1135-1143, 2005.

World Health Organization: *Cancer Pain Relief and Palliative Care in Children.* Geneva, World Health Organization, 1998.

World Health Organization: *Symptom Relief in Terminal Illness.* Geneva, World Health Organization, 1998.

Wrede-Seaman L: Symptom management algorithms for palliative care. *Am J Hosp Palliat Care* 16(3): 517-526, 1999.

Yuan C. Clinical status of methylnaltrexone, a new agent to prevent and manage opioid-induced side effects. *J Support Oncol* 2(2):111-122, 2004.

Yuan C, Foss JF, O'Connor M, et al: Methylnaltrexone for reversal of constipation due to chronic methadone use. A randomized control trial. *J Am Med Assoc* 283:367-372, 2000.

SELF-ASSESSMENT QUESTIONS

1. Which of the following areas of the nervous system that stimulate the vomiting center (VC) is the one that is most responsible for causing nausea and vomiting due to medications such as opioids and chemotherapeutic agents?
   A. Cerebral cortex
   B. Vestibular apparatus
   C. Chemoreceptor trigger zone (CTZ)
   D. Vagal and sympathetic afferent nerve stimulation

2. All of the following are nonpharmacological interventions that may be used to attempt to ameliorate symptoms of nausea and vomiting EXCEPT:
   A. Acupressure
   B. Discontinuation of emetogenic medication
   C. Deep breathing and voluntary swallowing
   D. Wearing of strong perfume or after-shave lotion
   E. Apply cold compresses to forehead, neck, and wrists

3. All of the following medications are recommended as standard pharmacological therapy of nausea and vomiting in patients near the end of life EXCEPT:
   A. ABHR gel
   B. Prochlorperazine
   C. Haloperidol
   D. Lorazepam
   E. Dexamethasone

4. Each of the following can be a cause of constipation in patients near the end of life EXCEPT:
   A. Opioid analgesics
   B. High-fiber diet
   C. Spinal cord compression
   D. Dehydration due to poor oral intake
   E. Hypercalcemia

5. When starting a patient on an opioid analgesic, it is recommended that medication to prevent constipation be started at the same time. Of the following agents, which would be the best choice as an initial agent in the prevention of opioid-induced constipation?
   A. Methylnaltrexone
   B. Senna/docusate sodium combination
   C. Bisacodyl
   D. Lactulose
   E. Fleet enema every 3 days if no bowel movement

6. Which of the following symptoms is NOT considered to be part of the syndrome known as "opioid-induced bowel dysfunction?"
   A. Constipation
   B. Esophageal reflux
   C. Nausea and vomiting
   D. Delayed gastric emptying
   E. Abdominal cramps

7. All of the following may be causes of diarrhea EXCEPT:
   A. Laxatives
   B. Fecal impaction
   C. Aluminum-containing antacids
   D. Antibiotics
   E. Radiation therapy

8. Nonpharmacologic interventions for the treatment of dysphagia may include all of the following EXCEPT:
   A. Serving small meals at room temperature
   B. Keeping the head of the bed elevated for up to 2 hours after eating
   C. Provide food of the type and consistency the patient can swallow
   D. Keep the chin elevated and away from the chest during swallowing
   E. Provide good oral hygiene

9. All of the following may reduce lower esophageal sphincter (LES) tone and

contribute to symptoms of dyspepsia secondary to gastroesophageal reflux EXCEPT:

A. Nonsteroidal anti-inflammatory drugs (NSAIDs)
B. Alcohol
C. Benzodiazepines
D. Coffee
E. Calcium-channel blockers

10. Which of the following medications will be most useful in treating symptoms related to bowel obstruction?

A. Dexamethasone
B. Metoclopramide
C. Bisacodyl
D. Omeprazole
E. Loperamide

CHAPTER

9

Neurological Symptoms at the End of Life

Barry M. Kinzbrunner, Tina Maluso-Bolton, and Bruce Schlecter

INTRODUCTION

Neurological symptoms are extremely common at the end of life. Some of the most frequent neurological syndromes are presented in Table 9–1. In terminal care, the complex nature of multisystem failure and extensive disease processes may render extensive, invasive, diagnostic work ups inappropriate. Rather, the focus in palliative care is the symptomatic management of neurological symptoms, regardless of their cause. This chapter discusses management of end-of-life neurological symptoms, which frequently present challenging management issues for the patient, family, and palliative care clinicians.

NEUROCOGNITIVE DISORDERS

DELIRIUM AND TERMINAL AGITATION

A full discussion of these symptoms can be found in Chapter 10.

DEMENTIA AND OTHER NEURODEGENERATIVE DISORDERS

Dementias and other neurodegenerative disorders are becoming increasingly important in end-of-life care. On the basis of 2007 data from the National Hospice and Palliative Care Organization, more than 10% of the over 1 million patients cared for by hospice programs in 2007 suffered from either dementia or a related neurodegenerative disorder. Therefore, it is important for hospice and palliative care providers to be intimately familiar with these clinical syndromes that cause a loss of cognitive and emotional abilities severe enough to interfere with daily functioning.

Dementias

On the basis of Diagnostic and Statistical Manual of Mental Disorders (DSM)-IV criteria, the diagnosis of dementia may be established in a patient by the presence of memory impairment characterized by either the impaired ability to learn new information or to recall previously learned information. In addition, the patient must have at least one of the following cognitive deficits: aphasia, apraxia, agnosia, and/or disturbances in executive functioning. These cognitive defects must cause significant impairment in social or occupational functioning, represent a significant decline from previous functional levels, and not occur only during an episode of delirium.

Alzheimer's dementia is the most prevalent, accounting for between one-half and two-thirds of dementia patients. In order to classify the dementia as primary Alzheimer's disease, the patient must be between 40 and 90 years of age, the cognitive deficits must be progressive, not accompanied by any disturbance of consciousness, and

TABLE 9–1. Common Neurological Symptoms at the End of Life

Delirium or acute confusion	Neuropathic pain syndromes
Terminal agitation	Mononeuropathies
Dementias	Plexopathies
Seizures	Cervical
Headaches	Brachial
Primary brain tumors	Lumbosacral
Metastatic brain lesions	Radiculopathy
Meningeal carcinomatosis	Epidural spinal cord compression

TABLE 9–2. FAST Classification for Alzheimer's Disease

STAGE	DESCRIPTION
1.	No difficulties, either subjective or objective
2.	Complains of forgetting location of objects; subjective word finding difficulties only
3.	Decreased job functioning evident to coworker; difficulty traveling to new locations
4.	Decreased ability to perform complex tasks (i.e., finances, marketing)
5.	Requires assistance in choosing proper clothing for season or location
6.	A. Difficulty putting on clothing properly without assistance
	B. Unable to bathe properly; includes adjusting water temperature
	C. Inability to handle mechanics of toileting
	D. Urinary incontinence; occasional or more frequent
	E. Fecal incontinence; occasional or more frequent
7.	A. Ability to speak limited to approximately six words in an average day
	B. Intelligible vocabulary limited to a single word in an average day
	C. Nonambulatory (unable to walk without assistance)
	D. Unable to sit up independently
	E. Unable to smile
	F. Unable to hold up head

SOURCE: From Reisberg B: Dementia: A systematic way to identifying reversible causes. *Geriatrics* 41(4):30, 1986.

there should be an absence of any other systemic or neurological disorders to account for the progressive cognitive deficits. To better know where patients are in the course of Alzheimer's dementia, a staging system, known as the FAST (*F*unctional *A*ssessment *St*aging) system, was developed by Reisberg in the mid-1980s. A summary of the entire staging system can be found in Table 9–2. As discussed in Chapter 1, this staging system has been instrumental in helping identify patients who are eligible for hospice care under the provisions of the Medicare Hospice Benefit.

Non-Alzheimer's dementias include frontotemporal dementia, dementia with Lewy bodies, and vascular dementia, each of which are found in approximately 10% to 15% of dementia patients, sometimes superimposed on Alzheimer's disease. Although there are ways of establishing the diagnosis of each of these other forms of dementia, they are beyond the scope of this discussion as all dementia patients receiving end-of-life care, irrespective of the etiology of the dementia, have severe cognitive impairment that is irreversible.

In addition to the primary causes of dementia, there are a number of secondary causes of dementia, including sedative, hypnotic, and anticholinergic medications, depression, febrile illnesses, dehydration, and a variety of other metabolic disorders. These etiological factors may also be responsible for causing patients with pre-existing dementia to experience sudden progression of cognitive impairment. Therefore, it is always important, even in patients near the end of life, to determine whether a patient's dementia or its progression is secondary and potentially reversible. If this possibility exists then, as in all end-of-life care situations, it is important to consider whether reversing the situation is compatible with a specific patient's life expectancy and goals of care.

Treatment of Dementia

A discussion of how to determine when patients with various forms of dementia and other neurodegenerative diseases should be receiving hospice and end-of-life care can be found in Chapter 1 and will not be discussed further here. Likewise, various ethical issues related to providing these patients with interventional therapies, such as artificial nutrition and hydration, are discussed elsewhere. However, one issue that affects dementia patients, primarily those suffering from Alzheimer's disease, that does need to be addressed here is the question of whether it is appropriate to provide or to continue to provide primary therapy with cholinesterase inhibitors, such as donepezil and/or the glutamate antagonist memantine, in patients with severe Alzheimer's disease, who are near the end of life.

CHOLINESTERASE INHIBITORS   The cholinesterase inhibitors are now considered to be standard therapy for Alzheimer's disease, based on the fact that they have been shown to improve cognition and global function in patients with mild to moderate dementia. Although the improvement lasts for at least 1 year, therapy does not change overall prognosis and treatment with these agents has not been shown to delay either nursing home placement or death. The available agents in this class include donepezil, galantamine, rivastigmine, and tacrine. Tacrine is avoided because of severe hepatotoxicity. The other three agents are all considered about equally effective and have similar side-effect profiles.

Regarding the care of Alzheimer's patients near the end of life, the cholinesterase inhibitors have not been shown to be effective in the treatment of severe dementia. Additionally, trials of these agents in nursing home patients have shown no significant benefit. Therefore, a recent review states that "it is appropriate to discontinue cholinergic therapy in institutionalized patients. In addition, there is no compelling evidence that patients may develop irreversible clinical setbacks if therapy with cholinesterase inhibitors is discontinued and then resumed" (Lewis et al., 2006a).

On the basis of these statements, it would appear that the cholinesterase inhibitors by themselves have little role to play in the treatment of advanced Alzheimer's disease patients who are near the end of life and being cared for by a hospice or palliative care program, especially if the patient is a resident of a long-term care facility.

GLUTAMATE ANTAGONISTS   In a placebo-controlled trial published in 2003 (Reisberg et al.), the N-methyl-D-aspartate (NMDA) glutamate antagonist memantine was found to improve global function and cognition in patients with moderate to severe Alzheimer's disease. Additionally, another trial demonstrated improvement in cognitive and global functioning in patients with moderate to severe Alzheimer's disease when memantine was combined with donepezil (Tariot et al., 2004). Although both studies do suggest benefits to memantine in patients with severe Alzheimer's disease, whether this can be applied to dementia patients near the end of life remains to be seen. For in the first study, the investigators did not report results that were segregated by disease severity and only reported average results, while in the latter study, patients with severe disease had to be "ambulatory or ambulatory-aided (i.e., walker or cane)" to be study eligible. Therefore, neither study would seem to be applicable to the population of advanced dementia patients receiving hospice and palliative care services, and hence, the role of memantine, either alone or in combination with donepezil in patients with severe dementia near the end of life, remains unclear at best.

OTHER AGENTS   There are several other agents that have been shown to have some activity in the treatment of Alzheimer's disease. Vitamin E is among the more popular of these other agents based on one trial showing a delay in nursing home placement or death in patients with moderately advanced Alzheimer's disease (Sano et al., 1997). Another agent, selegiline, which is primarily used in Parkinson's disease, was reported to have similar effects to vitamin E in the same study. Unfortunately, these findings have not been able to be confirmed in other studies. Finally, ginkgo biloba has been shown to modestly improve cognitive function without any benefit in global function, but it tends to be avoided as a first-line agent because it is not as effective as the cholinesterase inhibitors and increases bleeding risks in patients taking vitamin E and/or aspirin, which is common in dementia patients. As with the more commonly utilized agents for the treatment of Alzheimer's disease, these agents have, at best, a very limited role in the treatment of dementia patients near the end of life receiving hospice and palliative care.

Other Neurodegenerative Disorders

In addition to caring for patients suffering from Alzheimer's disease and other forms of dementia, patients with a host of other neurodegenerative disorders will benefit from hospice and palliative care services as their lives are coming to a close. Parkinson's disease and amyotrophic lateral sclerosis are the two diseases most commonly seen, but there are many others. Although it is beyond the scope of this book to discuss each illness individually, and instead to focus on the management of symptoms, these illnesses present patients and families with many of the same dilemmas around treatment and goals of care decisions that occur in patients with advanced dementia. And, as in all things related to the care of patients near the end of life receiving hospice and/or palliative care, these decisions are made on an individual patient basis based on each patient's goals of care and wishes.

OTHER SYMPTOMS OF THE CENTRAL NERVOUS SYSTEM

SEIZURES

Classification

Seizures differ in their characteristic and presentation according to the area of brain involved, behaviors elicited, level of consciousness, length of seizure, and postictal manifestations. The international classification of seizures is used most frequently to classify seizures according to whether they involve all or part of the brain from the beginning of the seizure (i.e., primary generalized seizure vs. partial seizure). Further, there is a different distribution of seizure types according to age. With few exceptions, seizures in older individuals are of focal origin, with complex partial seizures being most common in persons aged 65 and older. Secondary generalized tonic clonic convulsions and simple partial seizures with motor manifestations may also occur.

Causes

The etiology of seizures varies with age. For older patients near the end of life, the causes are similar to those seen in elderly persons in general, and most commonly include cerebrovascular disorders, brain tumors, metabolic disorders, and cerebral degeneration. Many physicians are not aware that seizures are a common complication of progressive end-stage Alzheimer's disease, occurring in an estimated 20% of patients with advanced disease. Seizures can also be precipitated by medications, including tricyclic antidepressants and phenothiazines, which are commonly used at the end of life.

The differential diagnosis of seizures also includes disorders that may mimic seizures including, but not limited to, cardiovascular disease in the elderly, transient ischemic attacks including transient global amnesia, movement disorders, migraine, and various psychological disorders. Despite the many known causes of seizures, it is important to note that epidemiologic studies suggest that seizures have an unknown cause in approximately 50% of older patients.

Treatment

Medications used to treat seizures are listed in Table 9–3, and some, such as gabapentin, phenytoin, and carbamazepine are also effective in treating neuropathic pain (see below and Chapter 6). Although the preferred route of

TABLE 9–3. Anticonvulsant Drugs

DRUG	SEIZURE TYPES	USUAL STARTING ADULT DOSAGES	USUAL ADULT DOSE (mg)	THERAPEUTIC RANGE (mg/dL)	USUAL ROUTES OF ADMINISTRATION	SIDE EFFECTS
Phenytoin	Generalized tonic clonic Partial seizure	300 mg/d	300–400/d	10–20	Oral/IV	Ataxia, gingival hypertrophy, acneiform rash, hirsutism, hepatic failure, lymphadenopathy
Carbamazepine	Partial seizures Generalized tonic clonic	200 mg BID	800–1,600/d	4–12	Oral	Drowsiness, blurred vision, diplopia, ataxia, leukopenia, hepatic failure
Valproate	Absence Myoclonic Partial seizure Generalized tonic clonic	250 mg TID	1,000–3,000/d	50–100	Oral/IV	Weight gain, hair loss, tremor, thrombocytopenia, hepatic failure
Phenobarbital	Generalized seizures Partial seizures	3 mg/kg/d	90–180/d	10–40	Oral/IM/IV	Sedation, hyperactivity, decreased concentration, depression
Gabapentin	Adjunct for partial seizures	300 mg TID	900–1,800/d	None established	Oral	Lethargy, dizziness, ataxia, fatigue

248

administration is typically oral, an individual with a seizure disorder who, near the end of life, can no longer swallow will still need seizure prophylaxis by some other route of administration. Thus, consideration should be given to using the medications that allow for the greatest number of routes of administration. The fewest daily doses and the least invasive route of administration will greatly enhance the comfort of a dying patient.

Because early aggressive treatment of prolonged seizures is thought to result in a higher percentage of termination of the seizure with smaller doses of medication and less risk to the patient, aggressive intervention to terminate the seizure should be instituted, even when patients are near the end of life. In an inpatient setting, parenteral benzodiazepines, such as lorazepam 2 to 4 mg or diazepam 5 to 10 mg administered intravenously, are the medications of choice to terminate seizure activity. The maximum duration of the anticonvulsant effects of these medications is approximately 20 minutes. Either medication may be repeated every 5 to 15 minutes (or less frequently if warranted) up to a maximum dose of 8 mg of lorazepam or 80 mg of diazepam if seizures have not abated after the initial dose, or recur after the initial dose wears off. In the home or hospice setting, reasonably good anti-seizure effects have been achieved administering either of these agents by the rectal route if there is no parenteral access available.

Status Epilepticus

At some point during prolonged or repetitive seizures, the seizures are unlikely to end spontaneously. This point is the defining characteristic of status epilepticus. De facto criteria for the diagnosis of status epilepticus have been 30 minutes of continuous seizure activity or two or more discrete seizures without recovering consciousness in between. The focus of most discussions on treatment of status epilepticus has been generalized convulsive status epilepticus, but, clearly, other types exist (complex partial, epilepsy partialis continua).

Because prolonged seizures have a substantial risk of neurologic, cardiac, respiratory, renal, and orthopedic disorders, once the determination of status epilepticus is made, aggressive therapy should be instituted, even when patients are near the end of life. This is true whether the seizures are generalized or of a complex partial nature. It is recommended that status epilepticus be treated initially with lorazepam, 0.1 mg/kg intravenously, diluted with an equal volume of IV solution. Diazepam 0.15 mg/kg is a second-line alternative. The overall success rate in suppressing status epilepticus using lorazepam is approximately 65%. It is recommended that, concurrently, the patient should receive phenytoin 18 mg/kg, also intravenously. If the seizures persist, then phenobarbital 15 mg/kg IV should be administered. If seizure activity does not subside, then it is recommended that pharmacological coma be induced. Although for patients with a reasonable life expectancy, induction of coma in this situation generally includes mechanical ventilatory support and is beyond the scope of this discussion, for patients receiving hospice and palliative care and approaching death, palliative sedation without ventilatory support may be a viable option if it is compatible with patient/family goals of care and wishes. A full discussion of palliative sedation can be found in Chapter 23.

HEADACHES

Headaches are among the most frequent of all pain disorders near the end of life. For patients with advanced malignant diseases, headaches may result from direct progression of the malignancy. For example, growth of primary or metastatic brain tumors and meningeal carcinomatosis will cause headache because of increased intracranial pressure, while progressive skull metastases from multiple myeloma or breast cancer will result in headache from bone pain.

Whether caused by a malignant or nonmalignant terminal illness, patients near the end of life may develop a cervical radiculopathy and may develop severe muscle spasm in the neck and the head resulting in the complaint of headache. These patients may also suffer headaches from causes not directly related to their terminal illness, such as migraine headaches, tension headaches, and headache due to fever.

Treatment of headache is directly dependent on the cause. For patients with suspected malignant disease of the brain or spinal cord with increased intracranial pressure, steroids may be an effective way of ameliorating symptoms. Such patients are commonly started on dexamethasone 4 mg orally or intravenously four times a day. Once symptomatic improvement occurs, the dexamethasone may be tapered slowly to the lowest dose that maintains the patient free of symptoms. For patients expected to live several months or more, antineoplastic therapy, such as radiation therapy or intrathecal chemotherapy, may be considered in addition to the steroids. Nonsteroidal anti-inflammatory medications, opioid analgesics, and other measures that are effective against bone pain may be used for patients with headache caused by skull metastases (see Chapter 6). Other interventions may include antispasmodics for muscle spasms, and nonpharmacologic interventions, such as heat, ice, or traction.

SYMPTOMS OF THE PERIPHERAL NERVOUS SYSTEM

The peripheral nervous system consists of the anterior horn cells, dorsal root ganglia, dorsal and ventral nerve roots, nerve plexi, peripheral nerves, and myoneural junctions. Damage to any part of the nervous system may result in neuropathic pain that is widely accepted to be, at best, only partially responsive to opioid analgesia. Though the exact nature of neuropathic pain is unknown, its lack of sensitivity to opioid analgesics is thought to be due to a variety of factors including the mechanism of injury. Some commonly held theories to explain neuropathic pain include: (a) inflammatory mediators at the injured nerve site, which lower nociceptive thresholds, (b) increased neuronal membrane excitability, (c) altered processing of neural impulses by the central spinal cord neurons resulting in activation of NMDA receptors, (d) stunted axonal regrowth resulting in hypersensitive neuromas, and (e) a down regulation of nociceptive inhibitory transmitters. Though knowledge of the exact pathway is unnecessary in the clinical setting, acquaintance with the variety of causal mechanisms will enhance the understanding of the need for serial trials of adjuvant medications to relieve neuropathic pain in individual patients.

A discussion of the general evaluation and treatment of neuropathic pain is presented in Chapter 6. In this chapter, the discussion primarily focuses on the different neuropathic pain syndromes that must often occur when patients are near the end of life. After reviewing the various causes of neuropathic pain, recommendations for treatment will be provided.

FOCAL NEUROPATHIES

Mononeuropathies

Mononeuropathies occur as a result of compression or infiltration of nerves by bony or soft tissues in the extremities. Common mononeuropathies include intercostal nerve injury from rib metastasis or local extension of chest tumors, and peroneal neuropathies at the fibular head that are more common in cachectic, bedbound patients and patients with malignant lesions in the area of the popliteal fossa. Mononeuropathies of the cranial nerves can arise from tumors found at the base of the skull. Obturator and femoral neuropathies are seen when the tumor involves the soft tissues of the pelvis and thighs. Ulnar and radial neuropathies may result from bony lesions in the elbow or humerus.

Mononeuropathies can also result from nerve entrapment that refers to peripheral nerve injuries that occur at specific locations where the nerve is constricted in a fibrous band or osseous tunnel. Some examples of entrapment neuropathies are carpal tunnel syndrome, ulnar neuropathy, thoracic outlet syndrome, femoral entrapment neuropathies from retroperitoneal or pelvic tumor masses, iliolingual neuropathy from tumors of the anterior superior spine, and sciatic entrapment neuropathy. Regardless of the exact mechanism or nerve involved, mononeuropathies frequently present with a combination of focal weakness, focal pain, and/or dysesthesia.

Plexopathies

Metastatic cancers can infiltrate peripheral nerves and plexi, resulting in severe pain and neuromuscular weakness. The most common plexopathies seen in cancer patients are cervical plexopathy, brachial plexopathy, and lumbosacral plexopathy. Low back pain is the most prevalent presenting symptom, followed by thoracic pain and cervical spine pain.

BRACHIAL PLEXOPATHY Metastatic brachial plexopathy is usually associated with spread from the supraclavicular lymph nodes, as in breast cancer or lymphoma, or from a superior sulcus (Pancoast's) tumor of the lungs. The most frequent presenting symptoms are pain, located in the shoulder and axilla that radiates down the medial arm and forearm to the fourth and fifth fingers, and weakness. Pain is generally constant and severe and may be accompanied by areas of numbness and dysesthesias. Associated findings may include the presence of Horner's syndrome (ptosis, miosis, and anhidrosis due to tumor invasion of the cervical sympathetic plexus) and/or associated vertebral disc disease.

CERVICAL PLEXOPATHY Infiltration of the cervical plexus usually results from head and neck cancers, lymphoma, or metastasis from systemic tumors to the cervical lymph nodes or vertebrae. Pain frequently presents in the preauricular, postauricular, or anterior shoulder or neck area. Pain has been described as being both constant and intermittent with a lancinating component that may be exacerbated with swallowing or head movement. Associated findings may include an ipsilateral Horner's syndrome and/or hemidiaphragmatic paralysis if the phrenic nerve is involved.

LUMBOSACRAL PLEXOPATHY Invasion of the lumbosacral plexus usually results from direct extension of pelvic tumors or from metastasis to the regional lymph nodes, sacrum, iliacus, or vertebrae. Lumbosacral plexopathies are most frequently associated with colorectal cancer, gynecologic malignancies, retroperitoneal sarcomas, lymphoma, or breast cancer. Pain is generally the presenting symptom and may be dull, aching, boring, or burning in nature and is generally unilateral, although bilateral plexopathies can occur. Pain may worsen following a bowel movement. Clinical symptoms will depend on the level of nerve involvement. Upper lumbosacral plexopathies generally present with pain in the low back, flank, iliac crest, or anterior thigh and have associated L1-L4 dermatomal distribution deficits. Involvement of the lower plexus frequently present with pain in the buttocks, perineum, and posterolateral leg and thigh with associated L4-S1 deficits including leg edema.

Radiculopathies

A radiculopathy is characterized by pain or numbness in a dermatomal distribution in a region innervated by the spinal nerve roots. In cancer patients, radicular pain is most commonly caused by an epidural tumor mass, leptomeningeal carcinomatosis, or compression due to metastatic tumor arising from the vertebral body. Pain may be constant or intermittent, achy or dysesthetic, and may be localized or experienced anywhere throughout the dermatome. Radicular pain is frequently exacerbated by cough, sneezing, strain, or being in a recumbent position. Herpes zoster and postherpetic neuralgias are common in cancer patients and frequently present in a classic, radicular pain pattern. Other implications of radicular pain include potential emergencies such as epidural spinal cord compression.

Phantom Pain

Phantom pain is manifested by symptoms of neuropathic pain in a limb that has been amputated. It may occur in patients who have amputation of a limb due to a malignancy or due to vascular disease. It has also been described in the chest wall area in women who have undergone mastectomy. Although it is thought to be of central nervous system origin, it tends to respond best to tricyclic antidepressants, as is true of peripheral neuropathies.

POLYNEUROPATHIES

Polyneuropathies are a group of disorders that affect motor, sensory, or autonomic nerves by damaging the nerve axon, myelin sheath, or, in some cases, the small to medium-sized blood vessels that supply the affected nerves. The major causes of polyneuropathies seen in patients near the end of life are listed in Table 9–4, and in-

---

TABLE 9–4. Causes of Polyneuorpathies in Patients Near the End of Life

Paraneoplastic syndromes
Medication-induced toxic polyneuropathy
    secondary to chemotherapy
Ascending polyneuropathy associated with:
    Guillain–Barre syndrome
    Hodgkin's disease
    Non-Hodgkin's lymphoma
Autoimmune-mediated dorsal root ganglionitis
    associated with thoracic cancers
Autonomic neuropathy accompanied by
    lymphocytic infiltration
Metabolic disorders

---

clude direct and indirect effects of the primary terminal illness, side effects of medications (i.e., chemotherapy agents) used to treat the terminal illness, paraneoplastic syndromes, and comorbid metabolic neuropathies most often related to diabetes mellitus or alcohol abuse.

Symptoms depend on the area of the nervous system affected. Muscle weakness suggests motor neuron involvement, while numbness, tingling, and/or pain occurring in the hands and feet, the "stocking/glove" distribution, are typical of sensory neuropathy. Involvement of the autonomic nervous system usually manifests with symptoms of orthostatic hypotension, cardiac arrhythmia, impotence, and/or bladder dysfunction.

In patients near the end of life, the diagnosis has often already been established, but, even if it has not, given the prognosis of these patients, an approach based on the treatment of symptoms is usually appropriate with neuropathic pain generally being the most pressing problem. Treatment is discussed below and in greater detail in Chapter 6.

EPIDURAL SPINAL CORD COMPRESSION

Epidural metastasis is the most ominous complication of bony mctastastic disease to the vertebral spine. It is a common complication in patients with cancer of the breast, prostate, and lung; multiple myeloma, melanoma, and renal cell carcinoma. Epidural spinal cord compression (ESCC) almost always presents with back or neck pain, either focally or in a radicular distribution, which then progresses over a period of several weeks until neurologic deficits appears. Pain is usually in the midline but sharp, shooting, radicular pain is frequently present in patients with nerve root involvement. Progressive back pain, which is aggravated by the Valsalva maneuver, accompanied by a positive straight leg raise and/or positive Lhermitte's sign (shooting pain on neck flexion), and exacerbated by recumbency, should alert the clinician to the possibility of pending ESCC.

Neurological symptoms usually begin in the lower extremities with motor weakness, paresthesias, sensory loss, and reduced or absent reflexes. The pain progressively travels proximally and patients eventually develop urinary retention and constipation. Once urinary or bowel problems appear, neurologic progression may be rapid and result in permanent dysfunction. Early recognition of symptoms and prompt initiation of treatment, generally with high-dose steroids and radiation therapy, may reduce pain, minimize neurologic deficits, and preserve sphincter function, thereby, improving the quality of life of terminally ill patients with ESCC. A full discussion of the treatment of spinal cord compression can be found in Chapter 19.

TREATMENT OF NEUROPATHIC PAIN

The treatment for neuropathic pain presenting as a mononeuropathy, plexopathy, or polyneuropathy is primarily directed at decreasing the inflammation, preserving neurological function, and aggressive management of pain. In patients with a reasonable life expectancy, diagnostic evaluation including a CT scan or MRI, and radiation therapy if the etiology is malignant may be considered an appropriate palliative intervention. Nearer to end-of-life, these invasive, costly, and energy draining interventions may no longer be appropriate or desired.

The most appropriate pharmacological intervention will often consist of oral steroids such as prednisone 20 mg two to three times a day or dexamethasone 4 mg four times a day. Steroids will reduce the edema that is at least partially responsible for the symptoms of increased intracranial pressure and spinal cord compression, as well as the management of pain due to perineural edema from infiltration or compression. An acute episode of very severe radicular pain related to a neuropathic lesion such as a plexopathy or spinal cord compression may respond dramatically to intravenous steroids followed by oral administration with dosage tapering over time. It is important to methodically reduce steroids to the lowest effective dosage to minimize the associated potential side effects such as steroid-induced myopathy, gastrointestinal distress, and neuropsychiatric manifestations including confusion, mental clouding, depression, and psychosis.

In addition to the use of steroids, most patients with neuropathic pain will require opioids, with methadone, which partly functions as an NMDA receptor antagonist, being particularly effective. Adjuvant medications are generally also required and a list of the agents most commonly used in hospice and palliative care are listed in Table 9–5. Although the tricyclic antidepressants are the agents that have been studied most extensively, due to their side effects, many practitioners

TABLE 9–5. Medications for the Treatment of Neuropathic Pain

DRUGS	ROUTES OF ADMINISTRATION	USUAL ADULT DOSE (mg)	MAXIMUM DOSE
Dexamethasone	PO	16–96/d	
Gabapentin	PO	300–1,800/d in 3 divided doses	1,800/d
Amitriptyline	PO	10–150/d	300/d
Nortriptyline	PO	10–150/d	150/d
Carbamazepine	PO	200–1,600/d in 3–4 divided doses	1,600/d
Clonidine	PO	0.1 PO HS	2.4/d
	Topical	0.1/d	
Mexiletine	PO	300/d in divided doses	1,200/d
Pregabalin	PO	150–300/d in 3 divided doses	300/d

now prefer gabapentin as first-line therapy, with the other medications listed being reserved for second-line use, either alone or in combination with gabapentin, or for specific pain syndromes (i.e., carbamazepine for trigeminal neuralgia). Pregabalin, a fairly new agent approved for the treatment of diabetic peripheral neuropathy, has not found a significant role in treating patients near the end of life, although it is sometimes used as a second or third-line agent, and also may be appropriately continued in end-of-life care patients with neuropathic pain that has responded to the medication. In addition to the oral medications, topical preparations of lidocaine and capsaicin have been found to be useful in certain types of radicular pain. A complete discussion of the treatment of neuropathic pain can be found in Chapter 6.

CONCLUSION

Neurological symptoms present unusual challenges in end-of-life care. The manifestation of physical as well as cognitive symptoms may threaten quality of life, devastate caregivers, and tax physical, emotional, and financial resources. Furthermore, what constitutes "appropriate management" may be difficult to define, as the neurological symptoms are complicated by progressive disease and multisystem failure. Symptom control is frequently complex as self-care skills and activities of daily living are progressively compromised.

Management strategies must be based on a complete history, accurate physical assessment skills, prudent pharmacologic and interventional modalities, and comprehensive interdisciplinary support. Interventions should reflect the prognosis and life expectancy as well as the patient/family informed desires. In addition, management strategies should be guided by caring clinicians who, through conscientious application of

ethical principles, acknowledge the limitations of our understanding, and support the patient and family through compassionate, individualized interventions.

BIBLIOGRAPHY

Adams RD, Victor M, Ropper AH: Intracranial neoplasms and paraneoplastic disorders. In: *Principals of Neurology*, 6th ed. New York: McGraw-Hill, 1997, pp. 642-690.

Allen RR: Neuropathic pain in the cancer patient. *Neurol Clin* 16(4):869-887, 1998.

American Pain Society: *Principles of Analgesic Use in the Treatment of Acute Pain and Cancer Pain*, 4th ed. Glenview, IL, American Pain Society, 1999.

American Psychiatric Association: *Diagnostic and Statistical Manual of Mental Disorders*, 4th ed. Washington, DC, American Psychiatric Association, 1994.

Argoff C, Wheeler A: Spinal and radicular disorders. *Neurol Clin* 16(4):833-849, 1998.

Ashby M, Fleming B, Wood M, Somogyi S: Plasma morphine and glucuronide (M3G and M6G) concentration on hospice patients. *J Pain Symptom Manage* 14:157-167, 1997.

Bennett G: Update on the neurophysiology of pain transmission and the modulation: Focus on NMDA-receptor. *J Pain Symptom Manage* 19(1):2-6, 2000.

Bleck TP: Management approaches to prolonged seizures and status epilepticus. *Epilepsia* 40 (suppl 1):S49-S53, 1999.

Bleck TP: Seizures in the critically ill. In: Parrillo JE, Bone RC, eds. *Critical Care Medicine: Principles of Diagnosis and Management*. Chicago, IL, Mosby-Year Book, 1995, pp. 1217-1233.

Bruera E, Neumann CM: Opioid toxicities: Assessment and management. In: Max M, ed. *Pain 1999: An Updated Review*. Seattle, WA: IASP Press, 1999a, pp. 443-457.

Bruera E, Neumann CM: Cancer pain. In: Max M, ed. *Pain 1999; An Updated Review*. Seattle, WA, International Association for the Study of Pain (IASP) Press, 1999b, pp. 25-35.

Cairncross JG, Kim JH, Posner JB: Radiation therapy for brain metastases. *Ann Neurol* 7:529-541, 1980.

Cameron RB: *Practical Oncology*. Norwalk, CT, Appleton & Lange, 1994.

Caraceni A, Martini C: Neurological problems. In: Doyle D, Hanks G, MacDonald N, eds. *Oxford Textbook of Palliative Medicine*, 2nd ed. New York, Oxford University Press Inc, 1998, pp. 728-749.

Chad D, Recht D: Neuromuscular complications of systemic cancer. *Neurol Clin* 9(4):901-918, 1991.

Chamberlain MC, Friedman HS: Leptomeningeal metastases: Presentation, diagnosis, and management considerations. In: Levin VA, ed. *Cancer in the Nervous System*. New York, Churchill Livingstone, 1996, 281-301.

Cherny N, Foley K: Current approaches to the management of cancer pain: A review. *Ann Acad Med* 23(2):139-159, 1994.

Cherny N, Thaler HT, Friedlander-Klar H, et al: Opioid responsiveness of cancer pain syndromes caused by neuropathic or nociceptive mechanisms: A combined analysis of controlled, single-dose studies. *Neurology* 44:857-861, 1994.

Christrup L: Morphine metabolites. *Acta Anaesthesiol Scand* 41:116-122, 1997.

Classen J, Hirsch LJ, Mayer SA. Treatment of status epilepticus: A survey of neurologists. *J Neurol Sci* 211:37-41, 2003.

Commission on classification and terminology of the international league against epilepsy: Proposal for revised classification of epilepsies and epileptic syndromes. *Epilepsia* 30:389-399, 1989.

Courtney C, Farrell D, Gray R, et al: Long-term donepezil treatment in 565 patients with Alzheimer's disease (AD 2000): Randomized double-blind trial. *Lancet* 363:2105-2115, 2004.

Cummings JL. Current perspectives in Alzheimer's disease. *Neurology* 51(suppl 1):S1, 1998.

Delattre JY, Krol G, Thaler HT, et al: Distribution of brain metastases. *Arch Neurol* 45:741, 1988.

Dreifuss FE, Rosman NP, Cloyd JC, et al: A comparison of rectal diazepam gel and placebo for acute repetitive seizures. *N Engl J Med* 338:1869-1875, 1998.

England J: Entrapment neuropathies. *Curr Opin Neurol* 12:597-602, 1999.

Fabiszewski KJ, Volicer B, Volicer L: Effect of antibiotic treatment on outcome of fevers in institutionalized Alzheimer patients. *JAMA* 263(23):3168-3172, 1990.

Ferrante FM: Principles of opioid pharmacotherapy: Practical implications of basic mechanisms. *J Pain Symptom Manage* 11(5):265-273, 1996.

Fine P: Conflicts in medical care at the end of life. In: Slatkin N, Rhoda G, Bernard G, eds. *Sarnat Symposium for Supportive Care of the Patient with Cancer and Other Life-Threatening Diseases*. Conducted at City of Hope National Medical Center, Duarte, CA, 1999.

Fitzgibbon D, Ready L: Intravenous high-dose methadone administered by patient controlled analgesia and continuous infusion for the treatment of cancer pain refractory to high-dose morphine. *Pain* 73:259-261, 1997.

Flores-Terrazas JE, Torres-Salazar JJ, Campos-Salcedo JG, et al: Meralgia paresthetica as a urological surgery complication: A case presentation and literature review. *Rev Mex Urol* 68:132-137, 2008.

Galer B: Neuropathic pain of peripheral origin: Advances in pharmacologic treatment. *Neurology* 45(suppl 9):S17-S25, 1995.

Galicich JH, Sundaresan N, Thaler HT: Surgical treatment of single brain metastases. Factors associated with survival. *Cancer* 45:381, 1980.

Geldmacher DS, Whitehouse PJ: Evaluation of dementia. *N Engl J Med* 335:330-336, 1996.

Greig NH, Ries LG, Yancik R, et al: Increasing annual incidence of primary malignant brain tumors in the elderly. *J Natl Cancer Inst* 82:1621-1624, 1990.

Grond S, Radbruch L, Meuser T, Sabatowski R, Loick G, Lehmann K: Assessment and treatment of neuropathic cancer pain following WHO guidelines. *Pain* 79:15-20, 1999.

Hanks G, Forbes K: Opioid responsiveness. *Acta Anaesthesiol Scand* 41:154-158, 1997.

Hauser WA: Epidemiology of seizures in the elderly. In: Rowan AJ, Ramsay RE, eds. *Seizures and Epilepsy in the Elderly*. New York: Butterworth-Heinemann, 1997, pp. 7-18.

Hewitt D, Portenoy R: Adjuvant drugs for neuropathic cancer pain. In: Bruera E, Portenoy R, eds. *Topics in Palliative Care*, Vol 2. New York, Oxford University Press, Inc, 1998, pp. 41-62.

Hospice Pharmacia Medication Use Guidelines, 7th ed. Philadelphia, PA, ExcellRX, Inc., 2005.

Iscoe N, Bruera E, Choo R: Prostate cancer: Palliative care. *Can Med Assoc J* 160(3):365-371, 1999.

Jacox A, Carr DB, Payne R, et al: Management of cancer pain. In: *Clinical Practice Guideline #9*. AHCPR Publication No. 94-0592. Rockville, MD, Public Health Service, 1994.

Jaeckle KA: 1991 Nerve plexus metastases. *Neurol Clin* 9(4):857-953, 1991.

Kelly JB, Payne R: Pain syndromes in cancer patients. *Neurol Clin* 9(4):937-953, 1991.

Kokkoris CP: Leptomeningeal carcinomatosis: How does cancer reach the pia-arachnoid? *Cancer* 51:154, 1983.

Lewis SL, Ende J, Grabowski TJ, et al: Dementia. In: Alguire PC & Epstein PE, eds. *MKSAP 14: Neurology*. Philadelphia, PA, American College of Physicians, 2006a, pp. 1-10.

Lewis SL, Ende J, Grabowski TJ, et al: Epilepsy. In: Alguire PC & Epstein PE, eds. *MKSAP 14: Neurology*. Philadelphia, PA, American College of Physicians, 2006b, pp. 45-52.

Lewis SL, Ende J, Grabowski TJ, et al: Peripheral neuropathies. In: Alguire PC & Epstein PE, eds. *MKSAP 14: Neurology*. Philadelphia, PA, American College of Physicians, 2006c, pp. 28-37.

Lipton RB, Stewart WF: Epidemiology and comorbidity of migraine. In: Goadsby PJ, Siberstein SD, eds. *Headache: Blue Books of Practical Neurology*. Boston, MA, Butterworth-Heinemann, 1997, pp. 75-94.

Lloyd-Williams M: A survey of palliative care given to patients with end-stage dementia (abstract). *Palliat Med* 10:63, 1996.

MacDonald N, Der L, Allan S, Champion P: Opioid hyperexcitability: The application of alternate opioid therapy. *Pain* 53(3):353-355, 1993.

Mailis A, Bennett G: Painful neurological disorders: Clinical aspects. In: Aronoff GM, ed. *Evaluation and Treatment of Chronic Pain*, 3rd ed. Baltimore, MD, Williams & Wilkins, 1999, pp. 93-114.

Martin LA, Hagen N: Neuropathic pain in cancer patients: Mechanisms, syndromes, and clinical controversies. *J Pain Symptom Manage* 14(2):99-117, 1997.

Mayeux R, Sano M: Treatment of Alzheimer's disease. *N Engl J Med* 341:1670-1679, 1999.

National Hospice and Palliative Care Organization. *NHPCO Facts and Figures: Hospice Care in America*. Alexandria, VA, National Hospice and Palliative Care Organization, 2008.

O'Brien T, Kelly M, Saunders C: Motor neuron disease: A hospice perspective. *BMJ* 304:471-473, 1992.

Payne R, Gonzales G: Pathophysiology of pain in cancer and other terminal diseases. In: Doyle D, Hanks G, MacDonald N, eds. *Oxford Textbook of Palliative Medicine*, 2nd ed. New York: Oxford University Press, Inc, 1998, pp. 299-310.

Portenoy R: Neuropathic pain. In: Portenoy R, Kanner R, eds. *Pain Management: Theory and Practice*. Philadelphia, PA, F.A. Davis Co, 1996, pp. 83-125.

Portenoy R: Adjuvant analgesics in pain management. In: Doyle D, Hanks M, MacDonald N, eds. *Oxford Textbook of Palliative Medicine*, 2nd ed. New York, Oxford University Press Inc, 1998a, pp. 361-390.

Portenoy R: *Contemporary Diagnosis and Management of Pain in Oncologic and AIDS Patients*, 2nd ed. Newtown, PA, Handbooks in Health Care Co, 1998b.

Portenoy R: Opioid and adjuvant analgesics. In: Max M, ed. *Pain 1999; An Updated Review*. Seattle, WA, International Association for the Study of Pain (IASP) Press, 1999, pp. 25-35.

Portenoy R: Current pharmacotherapy of chronic pain. *J Pain Symptom Manage* 19(1):16-20, 2000.

Posner JB: Clinical manifestations of brain metastasis. In: Weiss L, Gilbert HA, Posner JB. eds. *Brain Metastasis*. Boston, MA, GK Hall, 1980, p. 207.

Posner JB: Management of brain metastases. *Rev Neurol* 148:477, 1992.

Rall TW, Schleifer LS: Drugs effective in the therapy of the epilepsies. In: Gilman AG, ed. *The Pharmacological Basis of Therapeutics*, 8th ed. Maidstone, McGraw Hill, 1993.

Ray BS, Wolff HG: Experimental studies on headache: Pain sensitive structures of the head and their significance in headache. *Arch Surg* 41:813, 1940.

Reisberg B: Dementia: A systematic way to identifying reversible causes. *Geriatrics* 41(4):30, 1986.

Reisberg B, Doody R, Stoffler A, et al: Memantine in moderate to severe Alzheimer's disease. *N Engl J Med* 348:1333-1341, 2003.

Rhiner MI, Coluzzi P: Managing breakthrough pain. *Adv Nurse Pract* 6(1):41-43, 68, 1998.

Riggaud J, Labat JJ, Riant T, et al: Obturator nerve entrapment: Diagnosis and laparoscopic treatment: Technical case report. *Neurosurgery* 61:E175, 2007.

Ripamonti C, Zecca E, Bruera E: An update on the clinical use of methadone for cancer pain. *Pain* 70:109-115, 1997.

Rowan AJ: Reflections on the treatment of seizures in the elderly population. *Neurology* 51:3, 1998.

Sandyk R: Sodium valproate-induced analgesia: Possible role of the GABA-ergic system in pain mechanism. *J Clin Psychopharmacol* 6(6):388-389, 1986.

Sano M, Ernesto C, Thomas RG, et al: A controlled trial of selegiline, alpha-tocopherol, or both as treatment for Alzheimer's disease. The Alzheimer's disease cooperative study. *N Engl J Med* 336:1216-1222, 1997.

Saper JR: Headache disorders. *Med Clin North Am* 83:663-689, 1999.

Scheuer ML, Pedley TA: The evaluation and treatment of seizures. *N Engl J Med* 323(21):1468-1474, 1990.

Shafer PO: Epilepsy and seizures. *Nurs Clin North Am* 34:3, 1999.

Sindrup S, Jensen T: Efficacy of pharmacological treatments of neuropathic pain: An update and effect related to mechanism of drug action. *Pain* 83, 389-400, 1999.

Sjogren P, Thunedborg L, Christrup L, Hansen S, Franks J: Is the development of hyperalgesia, allodynia and myoclonus related to morphine metabolism during long-term administration. *Acta Anaesthesiol Scand* 42:1070-1075, 1998.

Stiefel F, Fainsinger R, Bruera E: Acute confusional states in patients with advanced cancer. *J Pain Symptom Manage* 7(2):94-98, 1992.

Stone P, Phillips C, Spruit O, Waight C: A comparison of the use of sedatives in a hospital support team and in hospice. *Palliat Med* 11:140-144, 1997.

Tariot PN, Farlow MR, Grossberg GT, et al: Memantine treatment in patients with moderate to severe Alzheimer's disease already receiving donepezil. A randomized controlled trial. *J Am Med Assoc* 291: 317-324, 2004.

Teasell RW: Managing advanced multiple sclerosis. *Can Fam Physician* 39:1127-1141, 1993.

Teener J, Farrar J: Neuromuscular dysfunction and supportive care. In: Berger A, Portenoy R, Weissman D, eds. *Principles and Practices of Supportive Oncology.* Philadelphia, PA, Lippincott-Raven, 1998, pp. 465-476.

Thapar K, Laws ER: Tumors of the central nervous system: Diagnosis and therapy of brain tumors. In: Murphy GP, Lawrence W, Lenhard RE, eds. *Clinical Oncology,* 2nd ed. Atlanta, GA, American Cancer Society, 1995, p. 382.

Thomas Z, Bruera E: Use of methadone in highly tolerant patients receiving parenteral hydromorphone. *J Pain Symptom Manage* 10(4):315-317, 1995.

Treiman DM, Meyers PD, Walton NY, et al: A comparison of four treatments for generalized convulsive status epilepticus. Veterans Affairs Status Epilepticus Cooperative Study Group. *N Engl J Med* 339:792-798, 1998.

Twycross R: Symptom control: The problem areas. *Palliat Med* 7(suppl 1):1-8, 1993.

Ventafridda V, Ripamonti C, De Conno F, Tamburini M, Cassileth B: Symptom prevalence and control during cancer patients' last days of life. *J Palliat Care* 6(3):7-11, 1990.

Vigano A, Fan D, Bruera E: Individualized use of methadone and opioid rotation in the comprehensive management of cancer pain associated with poor prognostic indicators. *Pain* 67:115-119, 1996.

Walker MD, Green SB, Byar DP, et al: Randomized comparisons of radiotherapy and nitrosoureas for the treatment of malignant glioma after surgery. *N Engl J Med* 303:1323-1329, 1980.

Walton NY, Treiman DM: Rational polytherapy in the treatment of status epilepticus. *Epilepsy Res* 11(suppl):123-139, 1996.

Wasserstrom WR, Glass JP, Posner JB: Diagnosis and treatment of leptomeningeal metastasis from solid tumors: Experience with 90 patients. *Cancer* 49:759, 1982.

Watson CP, Babul N: Efficacy of oxycodone in neuropathic pain. *Neurology* 50:1837-1841, 1998.

Weinberger J, Nicklas WJ, Berl S: Mechanism of action of anticonvulsants. *Neurology* 26:162-173, 1976.

Woodruff R: *Symptom Control in Advanced Cancer.* Victoria, Australia, Asperula Pty. Ltd, 1997.

Woolf C, Decosterd I: Implications of recent advances in the understanding of pain pathophysiology for the assessment of pain in patients. *Pain* 6:141-147, 1999.

Woolf C, Mannion R: Neuropathic pain: Aetiology, symptoms, mechanisms, and management. *Lancet* 353:1954-1964, 1999.

Yaksh TL, Chaplan SR: Physiology and pharmacology of neuropathic pain. *Anesthesiol Clin North America* 15(2):335-352, 1997.

SELF-ASSESSMENT QUESTIONS

1. On the basis of Diagnostic and Statistical Manual of Mental Disorders (DSM)-IV criteria, in order to make a diagnosis of dementia, a patient must have memory impairment characterized by each of the following EXCEPT:
   A. A cognitive defect such as apraxia or aphasia
   B. The inability to recall previously learned information
   C. The memory impairment is only associated with delirium
   D. The inability to learn new information
   E. The memory impairment must represent a significant decline from previous functional levels

2. On the basis of the FAST Classification for Alzheimer's disease, which of the following functional deficits is associated with a patient with Stage 7 disease?
   A. Inability to put on clothing without assistance
   B. Inability to bathe properly
   C. Urinary and/or fecal incontinence
   D. Inability to ambulate without assistance
   E. Inability to handle mechanics of toileting

3. You are caring for an 80-year-old male nursing home patient with moderate Alzheimer's dementia, who is unable to dress by himself and is incontinent of urine, but has been able to communicate his needs and receive sufficient nourishment by mouth. You are called to the facility because the patient has suddenly become unable to ambulate, unable to communicate, and refuses to swallow. The patient has an advance directive stating that he does not want cardiopulmonary resuscitation (CPR) or a feeding tube. At this point, you would institute all of the following measures EXCEPT:
   A. Refer the patient to a hospice program with terminal dementia
   B. Obtain blood and urine cultures and start empirical antibiotics
   C. Do a medication review
   D. Obtain serum electrolytes and a chemistry profile
   E. Start parenteral fluids either intravenously or subcutaneously

4. All of the following statements regarding the use of cholinesterase inhibitors in the treatment of Alzheimer's disease are true EXCEPT:
   A. Therapy does not change overall prognosis
   B. They improve cognition in moderate to severe Alzheimer's disease
   C. Therapy should be discontinued in institutionalized patients
   D. Improvement lasts for at least one year
   E. Of the available agents, tacrine is generally avoided due to severe hepatotoxicity

5. All of the following statements regarding various agents used in the treatment of Alzheimer's disease are true EXCEPT:
   A. One unconfirmed study showed that vitamin E delayed nursing home placement and death in patients with moderately advanced dementia.
   B. The combination of memantine and donepezil was shown to improve cognitive impairment in patients with severe Alzheimer's disease who are eligible for care under the Medicare Hospice Benefit.
   C. Ginkgo biloba increases the risk of bleeding in patients taking vitamin E and/or aspirin.
   D. One unconfirmed study showed that selegiline delayed nursing home placement and death in patients with moderately advanced dementia.
   E. There is no compelling evidence that patients may develop irreversible setbacks if cholinesterase inhibitor therapy is discontinued and then resumed.

6. All of the following statements regarding the diagnosis and treatment of seizures in patients near the end of life are true EXCEPT:

   A. Seizures occur as a complication in approximately 20% of patients with end-stage Alzheimer's disease.

   B. Parenteral benzodiazepines such as lorazepam are generally used to terminate acute seizures.

   C. When patients with a seizure history are near the end of life and can longer swallow, anti-seizure medications can be discontinued.

   D. Intravenous lorazepam will effectively suppress status epilepticus approximately 65% of the time.

   E. Seizures in patients near the end of life may be precipitated by medications including tricyclic antidepressants and phenothiazines.

7. All of the following are pathophysiological mechanisms believed to contribute to causing neuropathic pain EXCEPT:

   A. Inflammatory mediators that function at the site of nerve injury

   B. Increased neuronal membrane excitability

   C. Altered processing of neural impulses by central spinal cord neurons resulting in suppression of N-methyl-D-aspartate (NMDA) receptors

   D. Stunted axonal regrowth resulting in hypersensitive neuromas

   E. Down regulation of nociceptive inhibitory transmitters

8. Which of the following focal neuropathies is characterized by pain in the buttocks, perineum, and posterolateral leg and thigh?

   A. Femoral entrapment neuropathy
   B. Iliolingual neuropathy
   C. Upper lumbosacral plexopathy
   D. Lower lumbosacral plexopathy
   E. Obturator neuropathy

9. Phantom pain syndrome typically responds best to which of the following medication used to treat neuropathic pain?

   A. Nortriptyline
   B. Dexamethasone
   C. Gabapentin
   D. Clonidine
   E. Mexiletine

10. Which type of polyneuropathy is associated with symptoms of orthostatic hypotension, cardiac arrhythmia, impotence, and/or bladder dysfunction?

    A. Diabetic peripheral neuropathy
    B. Autonomic neuropathy
    C. Guillain–Barre syndrome
    D. Chemotherapy-induced peripheral polyneuropathy
    E. Paraneoplastic sensory neuropathy

CHAPTER

Delirium, Depression, and Anxiety

Barry M. Kinzbrunner, James B. Wright, Bruce Schlecter,
and Tina Maluso-Bolton

INTRODUCTION

When life is approaching its end, alterations in the mental functioning of patients can be distressing to families as well to patients themselves. When a patient's mental status begins to deteriorate, it is important to determine what the nature of the change is to be able to properly palliate symptoms. This can often be a challenge as family and medical personnel may frequently confuse delirium with depression, anxiety, or even progressive dementia. In addition, the fact that two or more of these conditions can often coexist in the same patient who is approaching death adds to the challenge of the situation.

The earliest signs and symptoms suggesting a change in the patient's mental status may be subtle, and the most obvious reactions may be identified as the primary process. Consider the following case:

Mr. M is a 70-year-old retired Navy Chief who has a primary brain tumor. Six months have elapsed since his last oncologic treatment. He is not having pain or any overt symptoms of disease except for a right hemiparesis. He was receiving sleep medication for insomnia, an H₂ blocker for reflux, and two anticonvulsants.

After many days of nocturnal wakefulness and daytime sleep, he began to refuse medications. He stated that he was fearful that the staff was trying to poison him.

When pressed to take his medications, he became angry and belligerent. Antianxiety medications were ordered in large enough dosages to cause sedation and sleep. Unwilling but persuaded by family members, the patient took the new medication. After initially sleeping for several hours, Mr. M awoke and became even more agitated. He also began to experience visual hallucinations.

At this point, the hospice physician was consulted. All medications that had psychotrophic effects were discontinued and the patient was started on haloperidol. Within 24 hours he returned to his prior mental status.

In this case, believing that the patient was suffering from anxiety and failure to recognize early evidence of drug-induced delirium resulted in interventions that exacerbated, rather than improved, the patient's condition.

As already noted, depression, anxiety and dementia can often coexist with delirium, so it is incumbent on hospice and palliative care physicians and other caregivers to be able to distinguish between these processes, as outlined in Table 10–1. Delirium and dementia may significantly affect cognitive skills such as short-term memory, judgment, and the ability to think, whereas depression and anxiety do not. Delirium is generally of acute onset, anxiety and depression can be acute, subacute, or chronic, whereas dementia does not manifest acutely, but tends to occurs gradually over months and year.

The course of dementia is one of progressive loss in the ability to perform activities of daily living and the loss of mental functionality. Delirium

TABLE 10–1. Comparison of Depression, Anxiety, Delirium, and Dementia

	HALLUCINATION PRESENT	ONSET	SPEECH LOSS PRESENT	AWARENESS AFFECTED	LABILE EMOTIONAL RESPONSE PRESENT	AFFECT MEMORY JUDGMENT AND THINKING
Depression	−	Possible acute	−	−	Occasional	−
Anxiety	−	Possible acute	−	−	++	−
Delirium	+++	Acute	−	++	++	+
Dementia	−	Gradual	+	++	−	+

on the other hand, has a course that waxes and wanes, with exacerbations in symptoms often occurring at night and improving during the day. Dementia results in a limitation in speech content with progression to loss of vocabulary, whereas delirium is associated with occasional incoherent word usage but no actual verbal loss. There are no actual verbal deficits with depression or anxiety.

Delirium is a state of hyperawareness and may be associated with increased emotional liability, from apathy to anxiety, and from fear to rage. Dementia patients progress slowly toward the unaware and unconcerned. Hallucinations are not associated with anxiety or depression, and are seldom seen in dementia. However, hallucinations are common in delirium, because delirium is a state of altered wakefulness. The cerebral cortex is not fully aroused by the reticular-activating system. Hence, the patient is rendered half-awake in a dream-like stupor. There are reversals of normal sleep patterns and inadequate rest when the patient does sleep.

To differentiate delirium from anxiety, depression, and dementia, a history is most important. If the patient has or had hallucinations, speech loss, affected awareness, labile emotional responses, and problems with memory, judgment, or thinking, and the symptoms are of acute onset, delirium is most likely the cause. The history should be obtained from people who know the patient the best. One must remember that a patient with delirium may not be blatantly abnormal at first appearance. For example, in mid afternoon a delirious individual can appear quite normal. However, at night, usually when the physician is not present, the patient will exhibit diagnostic features. Thus, a careful recounting of the patient's behavior for more than 24 hours is necessary to avoid a missed diagnosis, the consequences of which might result in serious patient harm.

With this background, the chapter now discusses the subjects of delirium, along with terminal agitation, and then moves to depression and anxiety. Dementia has already been discussed in Chapter 9.

DELIRIUM AND TERMINAL AGITATION

DEFINITIONS

Delirium is a common occurrence in end-of-life care, although the exact prevalence of delirium at the end of life is difficult to determine, partly because of the variety of terms used to refer to similar phenomena. For example, confusion, encephalopathy, cognitive failure, and impaired mental status are only a few of the terms used to describe what most experts refer to as delirium. Delirium is a disorder characterized by a fluctuating cognitive disturbance and change in mental status that develops over a short period of time and which can be associated with a known medical illness. Studies on delirium in cancer patients show this disorder to be experienced by 25% to 85% of patients, with rates as high as 77 to 90% in those who are near death. One prospective study from an inpatient palliative care unit reported delirium in 42% of 44 patients on admission, with a total of 68% developing delirium at some time during their stay (Lawlor et al., 2000).

The occurrence of delirium is particularly disturbing to caregivers, both lay and professional, as difficult decisions regarding informed consent and what constitutes appropriate treatment must be confronted without coherent input from the patient. Delirium is especially devastating to the families and friends of patients as the onset of delirium frequently precludes hopes for a meaningful goodbye and emotional closure. Furthermore, delirium, particularly if accompanied by agitation, marks a situation in palliative care in which passive observation is no longer a viable option. Rather, intervention is essential because delirium may be easier to reverse in its earlier stages than in the final days of life when rapid disease progression and multisystem failure further make reversal of delirium almost impossible. For in patients near the end of life, once delirium is established, it frequently progresses to severe "terminal agitation."

Terminal agitation is a particularly distressing variant of delirium that is characterized by anguish, restlessness, agitation, and cognitive failure. It has a profound effect on the anguish and suffering experienced by families and caregivers and, therefore, treatment of terminal agitation should be considered a palliative care emergency. As in delirium, terminal agitation is generally accepted to be multicausal and is complicated by coexisting multisystem failure, polypharmacy, and physical, emotional, spiritual, and psychologic factors. If terminal agitation cannot be controlled, palliative sedation is often the only effective treatment alternative.

Given the aforementioned background, it is clear that the implications of assessment and management of delirium have profound consequence. Assessment should rapidly identify and treat medical disorders that may be causing delirium. Treatment, in turn should be based on rational, evidence-based studies with careful consideration of the patient's life expectancy, comorbid conditions, goals of treatment, and patient/family desires. In addition, the treatment team should be guided by a commitment to the ethical principles of autonomy, beneficence, and nonmaleficence as well as the hospice principles to "neither hasten nor prolong death." Careful consideration must be given to quality of life and the burden of intervention and treatment. There is mounting clinical evidence that can guide decision making by exploration of the common reversible causes of delirium and terminal agitation.

CAUSES

Delirium and terminal agitation are generally accepted to be multicausal in nature and often complicated by the polypharmacy and multisystem failure generally seen in patients near the end of life. Some of the most common causes are presented in Table 10–2. Despite the reputation of delirium being a potentially fatal disorder, studies have indicated that delirium and terminal agitation may be reversible in approximately 50% of patients without the extensive diagnostic interventions that would be incongruous with end-of-life care treatment goals. Therefore, the focus of assessment should be on identifying the most common reversible causes of delirium and agitation.

Pharmacologic Causes of Delirium

There are a plethora of medications that can cause delirium and terminal agitation, with the most common ones listed in the left-hand column of Table 10–2. One of the primary treatable causes of delirium and agitation in end-of-life care is prolonged or high-dose opioid administration. This is frequently seen with the use of morphine, which has active glucuronide metabolites that can cause neuroexcitation, myoclonus, hyperalgesia, allodynia (pain from a nonnoxious stimulus to normal skin), and terminal agitation. Neurotoxic effects are thought to be caused when these metabolites accumulate in end-of-life patients because of diminished renal excretion due to of multisystem failure, dehydration, and prolonged administration.

Medications other than opioids that can cause delirium and terminal agitation include the psychoactive drugs, anticholinergics, and benzodiazepines. The anticholinergic drugs have been long associated with the risk of delirium in terminal care and should be used cautiously. Tricyclic antidepressants (TCAs) are known to increase plasma morphine levels as well as induce anticholinergic side effects. Fluoxetine, as well as other selective serotonin reuptake inhibitors (SSRIs), are known to be potent inhibitors of cytochrome P450 hepatic enzymes, which may result in multiple drug interactions that may underlie delirium especially when used in conjunction with cisapride or the anticonvulsants. Fluoxetine, can also cause plasma levels of TCAs to rise by three to five times, which may induce delirium as well as seizures.

Other medications frequently prescribed to patients near the end of life that can contribute to symptoms of delirium include the nonsteroidal

TABLE 10–2. Potential Etiologies of Delirium and Terminal Agitation

DRUG-RELATED CAUSES	NONDRUG RELATED
Opioids	Dehydration
Hypnotics	Hypoxia/dyspnea
Antimuscarinic drugs	Anemia
Anticonvulsants	Infection
H_2 antagonists	Fever
Furosemide	Cerebral metastasis
NSAIDs	Increased intracranial pressure
Digoxin	Pain
Steroids	Urinary retention
Psychotropic drugs	Fecal impaction/constipation
Anticholinergic side effects	Fear, anxiety, spiritual turmoil
Neuroleptics	Environmental causes
Antihistamines	CA treatments (chemotherapy, radiation)
Antidepressants	Metabolic disturbances
Anti-parkinsonian agents	Hypercalcemia
Substance withdrawal	Renal failure
Alcohol	Hypoglycemia
Nicotine	Liver failure
Steroids	Hyponatremia
Anticonvulsants	
Benzodiazepines	
Opioids	

Source: Reprinted, with permission, from Maluso-Bolton T: Terminal agitation. *J Hosp Palliat Nurs* 2(1):9, 2000.

anti-inflammatory drugs (NSAIDs), steroids, digoxin, furosemide, anticonvulsants, and the H_2 antagonists. Almost paradoxically, withdrawal of some of these same agents including opioids, steroids, benzodiazepines, and anticonvulsants may also cause delirium, as may withdrawal of nicotine and alcohol. Alcohol withdrawal, in particular, is a sometimes overlooked cause of delirium in this population. In addition to thinking about this in a patient with a history of excess alcohol consumption, one must also consider the patient with no overt alcohol abuse history who has been innocently drinking a glass of wine with dinner every night for many years, and who now is removed from the home environment to a hospital, long-term care facility, or hospice or palliative care unit.

Clearly, when reversal of delirium is the goal, the review of medications must take into account the most likely causative agents as well as the risk/benefit ratio of discontinuation. This challenges the palliative care professional to draw on a complex understanding of pharmacokinetics and pharmacodynamics in the midst of multisystem failure and unpredictable metabolite clearance.

Nonpharmacologic Causes of Delirium

Causes of delirium and terminal agitation not related to medications are delineated in the right-hand column of Table 10–2. Some, such as uncontrolled pain, fecal impaction, and urinary retention should always be looked for. The environment should be checked as well to make sure that nothing in the surroundings is creating discomfort for the patient. Although hypoglycemia should always be looked for, especially in diabetic patients on oral agents who have reduced oral intake, whether one should evaluate a patient for other metabolic disorders, such as hypercalcemia or renal failure for example, would depend on the patient's current life expectancy and goals of care. This would also hold true for evaluation and treatment of anemia, fever and infection, hypoxia, and the possibility of increased intracranial pressure from cerebral metastases or other intracerebral causes.

Probably the most intriguing cause of delirium, at least in terms of end-of-life care, is dehydration. Dehydration may be a primary cause of delirium and may also contribute further to delirium by causing increased opioid toxicity due to build-up of toxic metabolites and by contributing to electrolyte and metabolic abnormalities. As with many of other potentially reversible causes of delirium mentioned earlier, the key question with dehydration is determining under what clinical circumstances one should attempt to treat the dehydrated patient with parenteral fluid replacement.

EVALUATION AND TREATMENT

Table 10–3 provides strategies for the treatment of delirium and terminal agitation based on the most likely and potentially treatable causes. When delirium is suspected, it is important to provide an orderly, calm environment free of stress or stimulation. Adherence to a routine daily schedule provides a coherent framework for the patient to hold on to. The presence of friends and familiar care providers are also beneficial. Hospice team members, particularly home health aides, who have established relationships with the patients, can be very supportive and provide a sense of comfort and stability.

If uncontrolled pain, constipation or fecal impaction, and/or urinary retention are present, attempts should be made to remedy these symptoms as a way of trying to reduce patient agitation. Antipyretics for reduction of fever, and possibly obtaining a urine culture and initiating antibiotics may be considered in appropriate patients if urinary tract infection is contributing to the patient's delirium. As already stated, whether one would assess for and, if present, treat one or more of the various electrolyte and metabolic disturbances that are associated with delirium would depend on the patient's clinical condition, prognosis, and goals of care.

A thorough medication review is essential. In addition to the patient's current medication, including over-the-counter medications, past medications that have been discontinued, and other substances recently ingested should also be documented to evaluate the role of substance withdrawal or medication interactions in the evolution of delirium. After considering the relative risk/benefit ratio, potentially offending medications should be appropriately reduced, discontinued, or changed to an alternative agent whenever possible.

The development of delirium in the presence of high-dose or sustained opioid administration should be treated as opioid-induced neurotoxicity and opioid rotation should be undertaken. Opioid rotation is the process of switching from one opioid to another when tolerance or intolerable side effects develop. Research evidence supports opioid rotation as a sound, efficacious practice for alleviating side effects as well as for potentially improving analgesia (see Chapter 6 for further discussion).

Lawlor et al. (2000) demonstrated that delirium caused by opiate toxicity, psychoactive drugs, and dehydration was most often associated with reversible delirium; hypoxic and metabolic encephalopathy were, on the other hand, associated with irreversibility. Other studies have demonstrated similar results, with reversal of delirium associated with discontinuation of various medications, opioid rotation, and hydration to facilitate the excretion of toxic metabolites.

Given that dehydration is one of the correctable causes of delirium, one of the key questions

TABLE 10–3. Checklist for Evaluation and Treatment of Delirium and Terminal Agitation

ASSESS FOR:	INTERVENTION:
Constipation	Medicate/disimpact,/prevent with aggressive management of bowel regimen.
Urinary retention	Catheterize and manage retention
Check hydration and urine output	Consider a liter of fluids/day*
Urosepsis	Urine dipstick/treat if symptomatic
High dose or prolonged opioid treatment	If pain is well managed, consider reduction of 25% of opioid delivered. If ineffective or in presence of pain, rotate opioid, consider fluids to excrete metabolites*
Dyspnea	Elevate head of bed. Remove environmental irritants. Use fan for comfort. Consider use of O_2 and/or morphine. Treat anxiety if present.
Hypercalcemia	Consider hydration* or treat according to patient/family wishes
Drug side effects or polypharmacy effects	Review medications and discontinue or taper offending medications if possible.
Pain	If symptoms persist; rotate opioid with equianalgesic amount and monitor
Recent history of drug/alcohol/nicotine addiction	Consider treating with benzodiazepines for drug/alcohol withdrawal or nicotine patch for nicotine withdrawal
Hypoglycemia	Consider glucose replacement
Liver/renal failure	Take this into account when ordering all medications
Metabolic abnormalities	Monitor for hypercalcemia and hyponatremia. Treat if desired by patient and/or family
Fever	Cooling measures and antipyretics
Anxiety/fear	Involve interdisciplinary team for intensive psychosocial, spiritual and emotional support. Treat cautiously with anxiolytics as needed. Music therapy, therapeutic touch, and nonmedicinal nursing interventions should be considered
Environmental causes	Reduce environmental stimulus; Modify surroundings to provide orientation. Involve familiar social support system at bedside. Consider therapeutic use of aromatherapy to enhance soothing environment
If delirium or terminal agitation persists and patient is near death	Consider terminal sedation

*Consideration of fluids must always be weighed against the potential burden of fluid overload.

Source: Reprinted, with permission, from Maluso-Bolton T: Terminal agitation. *J Hosp Palliat Nurs* 2(1):9, 2000.

in hospice and palliative medicine regards under what circumstances it would be appropriate to treat dehydration. For in the early days of hospice and palliative care, it was generally the practice not to routinely hydrate patients who were very near the end of life, even with symptoms of delirium. In the last 10–15 years, however, there have been a growing number of articles in the palliative medicine literature that have been published suggesting that hydration of many, if not all patients, might significantly reduce the incidence of delirium during the final phases of life.

To try and answer this question, a randomized trial was designed to evaluate the effect of 2 days of parenteral hydration with 1,000 cc/day of parenteral fluid on various symptoms of dehydration including hallucinations, myoclonus, fatigue, sedation, global well-being, and overall effectiveness, as compared with a placebo of 100 cc of parenteral fluid administered over no more than 4 hours for 2 days. Preliminary results of the trial, which incorporated a relatively small number of patients, showed that significantly more patients who received hydration had improvement in myoclonus (83% vs. 47%, $p = 0.035$) and sedation (83% vs. 33%, $p = 0.005$) when compared with placebo. Although there was improvement in a higher percentage of patients with hallucinations who were hydrated (83% vs. 50%), this difference did not achieve statistical significance ($p = 0.208$), whereas there was no difference in the percentage of patients with fatigue who

improved (54% vs. 62%, $p = 0.767$) irrespective of whether they were hydrated or not. Although more patients and investigators perceived an increase in global well-being and overall benefit with hydration compared with placebo, these differences also did not reach statistical significance. Based on these results, the investigators concluded that although parenteral hydration decreased symptoms associated with dehydration, there was a definite placebo effect observed, and that further studies involving a larger number of patients with a longer follow-up period were warranted (Bruera et al., 2005). From these data, one can only conclude that at present, decisions regarding whether to hydrate patients with symptoms of delirium and agitation near the end of life must remain individualized and based on a patient's clinical circumstances and goals of care.

If measures to reverse potential primary causes of delirium or terminal agitation fail, or while waiting for toxic metabolites to clear, appropriate pharmacologic interventions should be instituted. The more commonly used agents are listed in Table 10–4. Haloperidol has generally been considered the standard medication for the treatment of acute delirium. More recently, however, due to the relatively high incidence of toxicity, especially in the elderly, haloperidol is being increasingly replaced by atypical antipsychotics such as respiridone. In a limited number of studies comparing haloperidol with respiradone or one of the other atypical antipsychotics, efficacy has been found to be similar, whereas the

TABLE 10–4. Medications for the Treatment of Delirium and Agitation Near the End of Life

DRUG	ROUTES OF ADMINISTRATION	USUAL ADULT DOSE (mg)	MAXIMUM DOSE
Haloperidol	Oral/SC	0.5–5 mg po bid to tid 2–5 mg IM q 4–8 h PRN	30–100 mg/d
Respiridone	Oral	0.5–1 mg qd to bid	4 mg/d
Lorazepam	Oral/IV	0.5–1 mg bid to qid	12 mg/d
Phenobarbital	Oral/SC/IV	90–180 mg tid in divided doses	320 mg/d
Chlorpromazine	Oral/rectal/IV	25–50 mg tid to qid	200 mg/d

percentage of adverse reactions for the atypical agents was reported to be lower. Other agents that are sometimes utilized for delirium and agitation include chlorpromazine, lorazepam, and phenobarbital.

For severe, refractory cases of terminal agitation, however, recovery may be impossible. In these instances, sedation is widely accepted as an act of benevolence. More commonly known as palliative sedation, intractable suffering is relieved through the titration of medications such as midazolam, high-dose phenobarbital, or propofol to the desired level of sedation. The palliative care professional has an important role in differentiating between difficult to manage symptoms and refractory symptoms thereby assuring that palliative sedation is accomplished with integrity (see Chapters 12 and 23 for further discussion on the role of palliative sedation in hospice and palliative care).

DEPRESSION AND ANXIETY

According to recent studies, there is a 39% prevalence of a depressed mood in patients with advanced cancer, whereas anxiety is seen in approximately 30% of these patients. Somewhere between 15% and 25% of these patients suffer from a major depressive disorder. Extrapolating these data to all causes of terminal illness, depression, and anxiety undoubtedly affect a significant number of patients at the end of life. These patients must be identified and offered appropriate medical and psychologic treatment.

Depression and anxiety often have similar causes, although they may occur concurrently or separately in the same patient at varying intervals during the process of dying. Therefore, as already discussed above and illustrated in Table 10–1, it is important to be able to distinguish the differences between depression and anxiety (as well as delirium and dementia) in order to en-

sure that appropriate interventions are applied, for the consequences of inappropriate treatment can often result in the worsening of symptoms.

DEPRESSION

Causes

Depression at the end of life may be related to changes in a patient's life situation as the terminal illness progresses and/or to direct or indirect effects of the illness. In patients with a prior history of depression, the above issues may cause an exacerbation of depressive symptoms that were previously controlled. Common causes of depression at the end of life are summarized in Table 10–5.

CHANGES IN LIFESTYLE

Loss of Control Control entails managing oneself and one's environment in a self-satisfying manner. In an acute, reversible illness, loss of control is generally viewed as a temporary impairment that will dissipate on return to normal health. Chronic illness, however, and particularly terminal illness, changes that outlook. As our society associates prestige and dignity with those who possess physical control and independence, progressive, irreversible disability due to illness or

TABLE 10–5. Causes of Depression near the End of Life

Changes in life situation
　Loss of control
　Loss of self-esteem or self-worth
　Loss of independence
　Alteration in environment
Direct or indirect effects of terminal illness
　Lack of knowledge concerning illness
　Unaddressed or uncontrolled symptoms
　　of disease
　Medications
　Metabolic abnormalities
Exacerbation of preexisting condition

injury inevitably leads to a loss of independence and the sense of control. Such a loss of control often results in anger and frustration. Loss of independence also fosters feelings of low self-esteem that may ultimately manifest as depression.

Loss of Self-Esteem or Self-Worth   Most terminally ill people experience changes in body image and/or their place in society. The sense of loss that accompanies these changes usually causes a realistic and expected grief reaction. "Normal" grieving usually reflects a number of losses, including the loss of physical prowess, the loss of one's station or role in the family and society at large, and loss of sufficient time that is needed to take care of unfinished business such as unresolved family problems and/or financial uncertainties. However, when grieving over these losses seems disproportionate and is accompanied by expressions of profound guilt or loss of self-worth, clinical depression should be suspected. Individuals most vulnerable to developing depression due to loss of self-esteem are often those who provide the main financial support or otherwise serve as the titular head of the household. Caregivers should be aware, however, that no one is immune.

Loss of Independence   Illness-induced dependency in activities of daily living is thought to contribute to the development of depression. However, its role in any given individual may be difficult to assess as it does not necessarily correlate with the physical state of the patient. Some physically dependent individuals can be very independent of mind, whereas individuals with apparently minimal physical problems can perceive themselves as being significantly dependent on others.

Patients who are unwilling to acknowledge the progression of their disease usually do not adjust well to progressive dependence. By using denial as an adaptive mechanism, patients sometimes readily discuss with the physician the signs and symptoms of their decline without focusing upon the existential meaning of these changes indicative of impending death. This intellectualization of the process of decline may create a false impression that the patient is actually coping with his or her illness and its attendant dependency. However, input obtained from family, friends, or the hospice team may reveal that the patient appears to resent or even abuse his or her care providers, and this will clearly indicate the extent of the patient's maladjustment and discontent. The clinician should also suspect maladaptive behavior when patients begin to discuss their disease using medical jargon or scientific terminology rather than in personal terms. An attempt to divert such stilted conversation to a more personal and interactive level may be valuable.

Alterations in Environment   Patients with serious illnesses, especially those near the end of life, are rarely popular and may sometimes even be shunned by others. Isolation of a patient from family and friends often occurs, contributing to a patient's feelings of loneliness and loss of self-worth. Isolation may occur even in the home environment as families seek to protect or even hide the patient from others. Patients will often give in to such measures due to physical or mental decline. Due to infirmity, or out of desire not to be a burden, patients may passively accept social isolation as an inevitable outcome of their illness, withdraw further into themselves, and sink into despair.

DIRECT OR INDIRECT EFFECTS OF THE ILLNESS

Lack of Knowledge Concerning Illness   A patient's lack of knowledge concerning the nature of the illness, the goals of therapy, or the reason why definitive therapy is not offered, can lead to depression. Physicians must be aware that telling a patient about his disease or its treatment and prognosis may not ensure that he will understand or be able to recall that information at a later time. Unfortunately, many patients referred to hospice programs do not understand the implications of the referral and why the referral was made. In the absence of understanding the purpose and scope of hospice and palliative care services, patients and families may erroneously interpret a referral to hospice as synonymous with abandonment of all hope. In this circumstance, the patient cannot avoid feeling like a helpless victim of disease or of the medical system, and if the patient discloses this feeling at all, it may well be to nurses or a social worker rather than to the physician. Depression in such patients is often attributed directly to knowledge of the terminal illness (hence, the common request: "Don't tell him he has cancer"). However, it is more likely that poor understanding of the disease process, fear of the unknown, fear of unrelieved physical and emotional suffering, and a conviction that there is no hope for a continued useful and fulfilling life are really the causative factors. From a position of first blaming his condition on the system, the patient may well begin to blame himself.

Unaddressed or Uncontrolled Symptoms of Disease
Promote depression. Although this is most commonly recognized when pain is poorly controlled, any symptom may lead to depression if not adequately treated. If the clinician fails to ask, listen, and act, symptoms may go unreported or inadequately treated. Forgetting to assess the response to a palliative intervention in a timely manner will increase the likelihood of therapeutic failure, and magnify the patient's sense of abandonment and hopelessness. Evasiveness and dishonesty about the limitations of treatment, whether curative or palliative, also often leads to disillusionment, anger, and despondency.

Medications and Metabolic Abnormalities
Signs and symptoms of depression may be evoked by medications prescribed for the patient, as well as by biologic or physiologic abnormalities associated with the terminal disease or other comorbid conditions. For patients with cancer, the rigors of radiation and chemotherapy treatments, especially when side effects are inadequately addressed, may provoke or potentiate a depressive reaction. Opioid analgesics, anxiolytic agents, corticosteroids, and antihypertensive medications are also known to produce depression.

Altered biologic states, either incidental to or as a consequence of terminal disease, and including, but not limited to, fluid and electrolyte abnormalities, hypercalcemia, infections, brain tumors, cerebrovascular accidents, hypoglycemia, or progressive organ failure must be considered as potential causes of depression as a patient's illness progresses. However, it is important to remember that organic mental disorders such as delirium, which alter mood and mimic depression, should be distinguished, as they require a different treatment approach.

EXACERBATION OF PRE-EXISTING DEPRESSION Patients with terminal disease may have a past history of significant depression or other psychiatric illness. In these patients, depression may recur or become more severe in the face of a terminal illness, even if all other predisposing or provocative factors are avoided or minimized.

Diagnosis

When assessing a terminally ill patient for depression, neurovegetative symptoms such as fatigue, anorexia, weight loss, and altered sleep patterns, which are often reliable indicators of depression in nonterminally ill patients, are nondiagnostic because these symptoms are often caused by the terminal disease itself. Therefore, psychologic features will serve as more reliable indicators and must be carefully evaluated. The depressed patient may exhibit loss of self-esteem, guilt, lack of interest in social interactions, suicidal ideation, sadness, crying, and mood disturbances. Although some of these phenomena are components of the normal grieving that is part of the dying process, assessing the sum and/or depth of these various manifestations should help identify the patient with true depression. The single question "Are you depressed?" has been shown to be a reliable indicator of depression in terminally ill patients when answered in the affirmative.

In any event, whether "normal" or "abnormal," psychologic distress must be identified and should be treated aggressively with appropriate pharmacologic and nonpharmacologic interventions. When the diagnosis is questionable, a therapeutic trial of antidepressant medication is usually justified.

Treatment

RECOMMENDED CLINICAL APPROACH TO THE TREATMENT OF DEPRESSION Patients who develop depressive symptoms should have a full medication review, as many medications can cause or exacerbate symptoms of depression. It may be possible to discontinue some medications, including beta-blockers and other antihypertensives, when patients are near the end of life. On the other hand, other medications, such as opioids, steroids, and anxiolytics may need to be continued to address symptoms such as pain and anxiety. However, changing to an equianalgesic dose of an alternative opioid, reducing the dose of steroids to the minimum needed for symptom relief, and choosing an anxiolytic that does not contribute to depression may alleviate some depressive symptoms without further measures.

The clinician must also consider whether direct progression of the terminal illness or a secondary metabolic disorder could be contributing to symptoms of depression. If a reversible cause of depression is suspected, and the patient's overall clinical condition suggests that correcting the problem will improve quality of life, then, even if the patient is on a hospice or palliative care program, appropriate diagnostic studies and therapeutic interventions should be undertaken. If the patient is close to death, or the problem is determined to be irreversible, then rapidly acting psychostimulant antidepressants and other symptomatic approaches should be provided. For severely depressed patients in whom the expected prognosis is several weeks or more, treatment should be started with a psychostimulant to achieve a rapid response. Thereafter, antidepressants of the SSRI class or TCA

may be added and titrated upward to a therapeutic level, allowing a gradual withdrawal of the psychostimulant. The various medications that are used to treat depression can be found listed in Table 10–6 and are discussed in "Pharmacologic Therapy" section. At the same time that medication is started, nonpharmacologic interventions for the treatment of depression, discussed below, should be initiated, based on patient needs as determined by assessments performed by the various members of the hospice or palliative care interdisciplinary team.

Other medications may be useful adjuncts in the treatment of depression. Trazadone, in low doses at bedtime, is useful for depressed patients with insomnia. Buspirone, an anxiolytic that does not possess antidepressant activity has been found to augment the effect of antidepressants in doses of 2.5 mg twice a day. It is contraindicated for patients with known convulsive disorders or who are at high risk of having seizures. Pindolol is a postsynaptic antagonist that, in doses of 2.5 to 7.5 mg/d for up to 6 weeks, accelerates the onset of benefit of SSRIs. Because new antidepressants, including many not mentioned here, are frequently introduced, hospice and palliative care specialists should be prepared to adapt these recommendations as evidence-based studies become available.

Exogenous thyroid hormones, both T3 (cytomel) and T4 (levo-thyroxine), can augment the effectiveness of both tricyclic antidepressants and SSRIs when administered during the first two to three weeks of therapy. The exact mechanism of action is not known, but may relate to potentiation of noradrenergic activity. T3 seems to be more effective than T4.

NONPHARMACOLOGICAL THERAPY FOR DEPRESSION Regardless of the cause, treatment for depression in the terminally ill should not be restricted to pharmacotherapy, but should also include various nonpharmacologic interventions (Table 10–7). In addition to the hospice or palliative care physician, all members of the hospice or palliative care interdisciplinary team, including

TABLE 10–6. Antidepressant Medications

MEDICATION	DOSAGE	CLINICAL APPLICATIONS
Tricyclic Antidepressants		
Amitriptyline	75–150 mg PO daily in divided doses	Better for neuropathic pain
Nortriptyline	25–250 mg PO daily in divided doses	Anticholinergic effects vary with compound
Desiprimine	10–150 mg PO daily	and dose
		Possibly more sedative and with slower onset of action than SSRIs
Selective Serotonin Reuptake Inhibitors (SSRIs)		
Fluoxetine	10–80 mg PO daily	Less anticholinergic side effects and more
Paroxetine	20–60 mg PO daily	rapid onset of action than tricyclic
Sertraline	25–200 mg PO daily	antidepressants
Escitalopram	10–20 mg PO daily	
Mirtazapine	15–45 mg PO daily	
Psychostimulants		
Methylphenidate	2.5–5 mg daily or in divided doses up to 20 mg/d. Up to 60 mg/d has been used.	Rapid onset of action
		May be most effective for end-of-life patients with short life expectancy.
		Can cause anxiety and restlessness

chaplains, social workers, and nursing personnel should assess for various issues in their areas of expertise that may be contributing to a patient's depressive symptoms. The most common nonmedical patient concerns that contribute to depression involve personal or family problems, as well as financial, social, and religious/spiritual distress. In addition to identifying possible etiologies for the depressive symptoms, these assessments often are the first step in treatment, as the conversations between patients and their professional caregivers help to relieve anxiety and stress.

Personal or family problems may be long-standing and are often not resolvable prior to death. However, the physician and members of a hospice team should try to be aware of such problems. Careful thought must be given as to how such problems are to be discussed with the patient. Good intentions aside, increased stress can be experienced when personal relationships are explored. When such stress is overwhelming, professional counseling by clinical psychologists or psychiatric consultants may be required in addition to the continued support provided by the end-of-life care chaplains and social workers.

Financial concerns are nearly always present as the end-of-life approaches. Even well-to-do individuals can be stressed by the cost of medical care. The financial stability of the family is

TABLE 10–7. Nonpharmacologic Therapy for Depression

Identify personal or family problems
Consider counseling
Address concerns about illness and therapy
Review level of care
Explore religious and spiritual concerns

threatened when the patient is the main source of family income. The patient may feel guilty about the cost of care. Loss of income and dependency affects self-esteem and precipitates suicidal intentions as well as depression. The physician and allied health professionals can help to identify and marshal community resources and bolster the patient's self-image.

The focus of palliative care is different than acute care, but the lay person may find the distinction unclear and unsettling. Some patients perceive a hospice referral as "giving up," and may believe that no treatment will be provided. It is necessary to emphasize that, although a cure seems to be out of reach, treatment will continue and symptoms will be controlled. An astute and caring clinician will realize that nonpharmacologic interventions such as listening, dialogue with the patient and family, careful exploration of the patient's concerns, and identification and reinforcement of adaptive mechanisms, although time-intensive, are a vital part of the therapeutic armamentarium for combating both depression and anxiety.

PHARMACOLOGICAL THERAPY There are a number of different pharmacologic agents available for the treatment of depression in advanced illness (Table 10–6). With the exception of the psychostimulants, for which there are published, small, prospective trials, there have been no controlled studies of antidepressant medications in terminal patients near the end of life.

Tricyclic Antidepressants (TCAs) Depression is associated with a relative decline in neuroactive chemical transmitters in the brain. TCAs, which were developed as derivatives of chlorpromazine, inhibit uptake of serotonin and norepinephrine at neural synaptic junctions, allowing for increased transmitter activity between nerves, thus enhancing neuronal activity. These agents, which include amitriptyline, imipramine, doxepin, and nortriptyline, have been standard antidepressant therapy for many years.

With specific reference to end-of-life care, depressed patients with terminal cancer often respond to lower TCA doses than those required in physically healthy patients with depression. Appetite and insomnia usually improve rapidly. TCAs are also frequently effective in treating neuropathic pain, which commonly coexists along with depression in patients with advanced or terminal cancer. Because the therapeutic dose for the treatment of neuropathic pain may be lower than for depression, patients on a TCA for neuropathic pain who develop depression may best be treated with an increased dose of the TCA rather than with addition of a new antidepressant from a different pharmacologic class. Other advantages include availability for oral, rectal, and parenteral routes, ability to monitor drug levels, and differential sedative effects and toxicity profiles.

Sedative TCAs, such as amitriptyline, are especially useful at bedtime for depressed patients with agitation and insomnia. Desipramine, which is less sedative, is more suitable for patients with apathetic depression and psychomotor slowing. Anticholinergic side effects such as dry mouth, blurred vision, constipation, urinary retention, and increased intraocular pressure can be particularly troublesome in elderly or debilitated patients, in whom there may be additional problems with drug interactions. In these patients, nortriptyline or desipramine may be preferred. TCAs can also cause postural hypotension, cardiac toxicity, seizures, extrapyramidal effects, and excess sedation. For this reason, many clinicians favor the use of newer, less toxic classes of antidepressant medications such as the SSRIs.

Selective Serotonin Reuptake Inhibitors (SSRIs) SSRIs (fluoxetine, paroxetine, sertraline, escitalopram, and mirtazipine) are being used more often in the terminally ill, primarily for patients who have several weeks or months to live. Compared with TCAs, they cause fewer side effects and have a more rapid onset of action. Thirty to fifty percent of all patients with a poor response to TCAs will respond positively to a switch to SSRIs. Furthermore, due to differences in chemical structure, "cross resistance" among the various SSRIs is less common than among TCAs, thus allowing intraclass switching for poorly responding patients. However, because SSRIs have relatively long half-lives, it may be necessary to allow a washout period before starting another SSRI. Abrupt cessation of SSRIs may lead to withdrawal symptoms that include dizziness, headaches, nausea, and mood changes, so clinicians should be alert to this, especially when end-of-life patients on one of these agents are no longer able to swallow oral medication.

Paroxetine and sertraline, which have shorter half-lives and fewer metabolites than fluoxetine, also have fewer side effects, which may include nausea, headache, somnolence, insomnia, a brief period of increased anxiety, anorexia, and transient weight loss. Escitalopram and sertraline have lower potential for drug–drug interactions, whereas fluoxetine is noted for being incompatible with codeine. Mirtazapine has antihistaminic-like effects similar to diphenhydramine and can cause increased sedation on its own as well as potentiate the sedating effects of opioid analgesics and benzodiazepines. When medication-related sedation or somnolence is a problem, central nervous system stimulants may be a better choice and more useful for patients in whom medication-related somnolence is a problem.

Psychostimulants Psychostimulants (methylphenidate, dextroamphetamine, and pemoline) have generally been supplanted by monoamine oxidase inhibitors (MAO) inhibitors, TCAs, and SSRIs for treatment of chronic depression. However, the rapid onset of action of psychostimulants makes them particularly valuable for end-of-life care. Methylphenidate is particularly appropriate in terminally ill patients with very short life expectancies, except for those with advanced, unstable heart disease. It is generally well tolerated even in elderly, debilitated patients and can rapidly increase energy and appetite. Methylphenidate counteracts opioid-induced fatigue and lethargy and has adjuvant analgesic effects. Psychostimulants may also be used to treat cognitive impairment in patients with AIDS. In the non–sustained-release form, a response can

occur in 1–2 hours and continue for 3–6 hours. The sustained release may take 4–7 hours to begin to have effect, but activity persists for approximately 8 hours. Methylphenidate can initially be combined with a longer-acting antidepressant. When the longer-acting antidepressant begins to take effect, the psychostimulant may be discontinued.

Monamine Oxidase Inhibitors (MAOs) and Electroconvulsive Therapy (ECT) MAOs and electroconvulsive therapy (ECT) are not recommended for end-of life care.

"Placebo Effect" of Antidepressant Medications Given the importance of nonpharmacologic interventions in the treatment of depression (and other symptoms as well), which primarily consists of professional caregivers interacting verbally with patients, there have always been questions as to whether antidepressant medications have a primary effect on the symptoms they are indicated to treat, or whether the positive effects are due to the patient's perception that the medication will work or other outside influences, in other words, a "placebo effect." In the palliative medicine literature, this placebo effect has been best demonstrated by Bruera et al. (2003, 2006) regarding the use of methylphenidate to treat asthenia and other symptoms in advanced cancer patients (see the section on Asthenia in Chapter 13 for a more detailed discussion of these studies).

In a recent meta-analysis, Rief et al. (2009) examined the placebo effect in 96 randomized clinical trials that compared various antidepressant medications with placebo controls. The investigators concluded that the placebo effect accounted for 68% of the improvement in symptoms in the antidepressant-treated groups of patients. Although trials that used observer ratings had a greater placebo effect than those using patient self-reports, the percentage of the response in the medication-treated group attributable to the placebo effect was 66.5%, regardless of who rated the response. Placebo response was greater in patients with major depression than those with less severe depressive symptoms, whereas the class of antidepressant used in a particular study did not influence the size of placebo effect.

From this analysis, one is forced to conclude that, although there may be a role for pharmacologic therapy in the treatment of depression, its role may be secondary or adjunctive. For, based on the strength of the "placebo effect" found in this recently published meta-analysis, it would appear that it is the time that end-of-life care professionals spend conversing with and listening to patients at the bedside, the hallmark of hospice and palliative care, that is of primary importance in the treatment of depression, and likely, many other difficult to manage symptoms that significantly affect patients near the end of life.

ANXIETY

Causes

The causes of anxiety in patients near the end of life are listed in Table 10–8. Although anxi-

TABLE 10–8. Causes of Anxiety Near the End of Life
Changes in life situations
Loss of control
Loss of self-esteem
Loss of independence
Alteration in environment
Direct or indirect effects of terminal illness
Lack of knowledge concerning illness
Unaddressed or uncontrolled symptoms
Drug interactions or medication effects
Delirium/depression
Hypoxemia
Sepsis
Impending cardiac or respiratory failure.
Exacerbation of preexisting conditions
Adjustment disorders
Psychiatric conditions

ety shares many root causes with depression, it may also present acutely due to an exacerbation of symptoms such as pain or dyspnea. In addition, chronic anxiety and depression often coexist. Therefore, when evaluating and treating an emotional reaction to terminal illness, it is best to anticipate the need to treat both symptoms. Pain has been described as "being what the patient says it is." To an extent, this dictum may be applied to anxiety and depression as well. Patients who complain of anxiety or depression need serious attention, and the physician must be alert to those patients who are suffering from anxiety and depression but who deny the presence of symptoms.

Anxiety may be viewed as denial or resistance to life changes, resulting in physiologic and emotional stress, whereas depression reflects an attitude of resignation and hopelessness. Anxiety may be provoked by a lack of knowledge about the illness and its expected course and symptoms. A patient may find some comfort in knowing that most people who share the same disease experience similar changes, and even more comfort in the knowledge that expert management will be offered. Listening to the patient's concerns may sometimes be the best form of therapy, and this holds true not only for the hospice or palliative care physician, but for the nurse, social worker, and chaplain as well.

Acute anxiety commonly accompanies hypoxemia, sepsis, and cardiorespiratory and other systemic organ failure. In these circumstances, it may be associated with delirium. As the stress of a terminal illness can reactivate or exacerbate latent or preexisting pathologic mental states such as adjustment disorders or other psychiatric conditions, these can also be a cause of uncontrolled anxiety. A delay in treating symptoms or inadequate treatment that results in poor symptom control will make patients anxious. Symptoms that particularly create anxiety are pain, dyspnea, nausea, and vomiting. Some drugs used to treat terminal illness such as neuroleptics, steroids, and psychotropic stimulants may cause anxiety as a side effect. Drug interactions may also play a role, especially when multiple

TABLE 10–9. Diagnosis of Anxiety

Psychologic reactions
  Insomnia
  Irritability
  Inability to concentrate
  Poor coping skills
Symptoms and physical features
  Anorexia
  Nausea
  Hyperventilation
  Palpitations
  Sweating

medications are prescribed, dosages are varied frequently, or medications are rapidly withdrawn, especially those such as opioids, which cause physiologic dependence.

Diagnosis

Psychologic expression of anxiety includes insomnia, irritability, poor coping skills, and poor concentration (Table 10–9). Poor concentration should be differentiated from disorientation, which is a feature of delirium. Poor concentration means distractibility and inability to focus. Anxious individuals do not lose awareness of self and their environment.

Physical features of anxiety include palpitations, sweating, hyperventilation, anorexia, and nausea. These physical symptoms represent reactions to psychologic stress. As stresses build, a decline in the ability of the patient to perform usual levels of activities of daily living may result. Although functional disability usually is indicative of progression of the terminal illness, in some instances, it may be attributable to undiagnosed anxiety.

Treatment

NONPHARMACOLOGICAL THERAPY As with depression, the use of nonpharmacologic interventions is key to relieving anxiety for many patients near the end of life. Following assessment, this starts with good psychosocial and spiritual counseling from the end-of-life care social worker and chaplain, as well as adjunctive conversations with the physician and nurse, with all caregivers using open-ended questions and a good dose of active listening. Relaxation through breathing exercises, listening to favorite music on CDs, guided imagery, or a variety of other interventions designed to put the patient more at ease may also be of great importance.

PHARMACOLOGICAL THERAPY Because anxiety and depression often coexist, and because depression may be worsened by the use of antianxiety agents, it is advisable to first initiate antidepressant therapy for patients with mixed symptoms. If antidepressant therapy is not successful, or depression is not present, benzodiazepines are usually first-choice agents for treatment of anxiety (Table 10–10), although there is no clinical evidence base in the medical literature to date regarding their efficacy. They can be grouped into short-acting (plasma half-lives of less than 5 hours), medium-acting (plasma half-lives of 5–24 hours), and long-acting (plasma half-lives of more than 24 hours). The short-acting benzodiazepines such as triazolam and midazolam are of little clinical value for treatment of anxiety. The medium-acting agents like lorazepam, temazepam, and oxazepam are preferred. Lorazepam tends to be preferred as it is shorter acting and has a better side effect profile than some of the other agents. The typical starting dose is 0.5 to 2 mg three or four times a day. It comes as a tablet or liquid, including a liquid with a highly concentrated formulation that can be placed "sublingually" when patients have difficulty swallowing. Although typically used to treat insomnia at a dose of 30 mg, temazepam, which has no active metabolites, given in lower doses of 10 mg twice a day to decrease somnolence and sedation has been found to be an acceptable alternative by the World Health Organization and others. Long-acting benzodiazepines such as

TABLE 10–10. Pharmacologic Treatment of Anxiety

MEDICATION	DOSAGE	CLINICAL FACTORS
Benzodiazepines		
Lorazepam	PO 0.5–1 mg bid to qid IV 0.5–1 mg bid to qid	Tablets, liquid concentrates, and IV forms available May be expensive
Temazepam	Initially given as 10 mg bid Titrate to effective dose Maximum daily dose 60 mg	No active metabolites that accumulate Causes somnolence and sedation especially in the elderly
Oxazepam	10–30 mg PO tid to qid titrate to effect Maximum daily dose 1–80 mg	Medium length of action Useful for alcohol withdrawal
Diazepam	2–4 mg PO bid to qid IV 2–10 mg Q 3–4 hours PRN Maximum daily dose 40 mg	Long-acting with accumulating active metabolites May be used for seizure control as well.
Alprazolam	0.25– 0.5 mg PO to tid	Long-term usage may cause dependence Useful as limited PRN medication.
Barbiturates		
Pentobarbital	PO 50–100 mg bid to qid Maximum daily dose 400 mg Rectal 30 mg, 200 mg bid or qid Higher dosage for terminal agitation only.	Useful in terminal agitation and rectally for seizure control when PO dosage not appropriate.
Thioridazine	25 mg tid	Useful in terminal agitation and rectally for seizure control when PO dosage not appropriate.

diazepam have accumulating active metabolites. As a consequence, blood levels may not reach a steady state for weeks. They are, therefore, not as useful as routine daily medication and side effects tend to persist after discontinuation of the drug. Diazepam is useful, however, for patients with anxiety and recurrent seizures.

Because anxiety does not necessarily persist from day to day with the same intensity, it is a mistake to assume that the terminally ill require sedation as they advance in their disease. Clinicians should address the causes of anxiety and only if the anxiety cannot be eliminated should extended sedation be considered.

Benzodiazepines have significant undesired effects such as sedation and confusion. Titration to effect is desirable. Sudden withdrawal should also be avoided as acute anxiety or an abstinence syndrome may result. Benzodiazepines should never be used with alcohol, as the effects are potentiated.

The literature suggests that alprazolam is not recommended in the terminally ill because of development of intense dependence and severe withdrawal reactions including seizures. However, with limited PRN (as needed) usage, these reactions are less significant and it may, therefore, have some utility in selected patients.

Barbiturates such as phenobarbital and pentobarbital can be useful if patients do not respond to benzodiazepines. Because benzodiazepines compete with endorphin-binding sites, barbiturates, which do not compete, may be a better choice for patients with pain control problems. Pentobarbital is particularly useful for patients who can no longer swallow, as it is available as a suppository.

Phenothizines also have a role in treating anxiety. Thioridazine is an older product, which is most effective when used to take advantage of its sedative side effects. In contrast, haloperidol can be given orally, intravenously, or subcutaneously, and it is not a sedative. In delirious patients with anxiety, it is the drug of choice.

BIBLIOGRAPHY

American Psychiatric Association: *Diagnostic and Statistical Manual of Mental Disorders,* 4th ed. Washington, DC, American Psychiatric Association, 1994.

Ashby M, Fleming B, Wood M, Somogyi S: Plasma morphine and glucuronide (M3G and M6G) concentration on hospice patients. *J Pain Symptom Manage* 14:157-167, 1997.

Bergevin P, Bergevin RM: Recognizing delirium in terminal patients. *Am J Hospice Palliat Care* 13(2):28-30, 1996.

Breitbart W, Bruera E, Chochinov H, Lynch M: Neuropsychiatric syndromes and psychological symptoms in patients with advanced cancer. *J Pain Symptom Manage* 10(2):131-141, 1995.

Block SD: Assessing and managing depression in the terminally ill patient. *Ann Intern Med* 132:209-218, 2000.

Bruera E, Driver L, Barnes EA, et al: Patient controlled methylphenidate for the management of fatigue in patients with advanced cancer: A preliminary report. *J Clin Oncol* 21:4439-4443, 2003.

Bruera E, Franco J, Maltoni M, Watanabe S, Suarez-Almazar M: Changing patterns of agitated impaired mental status in patients with advanced cancer: Association with cognitive monitoring, hydration, and opioid rotation. *J Pain Symptom Manage* 10(4):287-291, 1995.

Bruera E, Miller L, McCallion J, Macmillan K, Krefting L, Hanson J: Cognitive failure in patients with terminal cancer: A prospective study. *J Pain Symptom Manage* 7(4):192-195, 1992.

Bruera E, Neumann CM: Opioid toxicities: Assessment and management. In: Max M, ed. *Pain 1999: An Updated Review.* Seattle, WA, IASP Press, 1999, pp. 443-457.

Bruera E, Sala R, Rico MA, et al: Effects of parenteral hydration in terminally ill cancer patients: A preliminary study. *J Clin Oncol* 23:2366-2371, 2005.

Bruera E, Valero V, Driver L, et al: Patient-controlled methylphenidate for cancer fatigue: A double-blind, randomized, placebo-controlled trial. *J Clin Oncol* 24:2073-2078, 2006.

Burke A: Palliative care: An update on terminal restlessness. *Med J Aust* 166:39-42, 1997.

Cadieux RS: Practical management of treatment-resistant depression. *Am Fam Physician* 58:2059, 1998.

Caraceni A, Martini C: Neurological problems. In: Doyle D, Hanks G, MacDonald N, eds. *Oxford Textbook of Palliative Medicine,* 2nd ed. New York, Oxford University Press Inc, 1998, pp. 728-749.

Christrup L: Morphine metabolites. *Acta Anaesthesiol Scand* 41:116-122, 1997.

Davis M: Placebo response: Meta-analysis of placebo response in antidepressant trials. PC-FACS, American Academy of Hospice and Palliative Medicine, September, 2009.

Enck RE: *The Medical Care of Terminally Ill Patients.* London: Johns Hopkins, 1994.

Fainsinger R: Use of sedation by a hospital palliative care support team. *J Palliat Care* 14(1):51-54, 1998.

Fainsinger R, Miller M, Bruera E, Hanson J, Maceachern T: Symptom control during the last week of life on a palliative care unit. *J Palliat Care* 7(1):5-11, 1991.

Fainsinger R, Tapper M, Bruera E: A perspective on the management of delirium in terminally ill patients on a palliative care unit. *J Palliat Care* 9(3):4-8, 1993.

Fallon MT, Hanks GW: Control of common symptoms in advance cancer. *Ann Acad Med* 23:2, 1994.

Fine P: Conflicts in medical care at the end of life. In: Slatkin N, Chair, Rhoda G, Bernard G: *Sarnat Symposium for Supportive Care of the Patient with Cancer and Other Life-Threatening Diseases.* Duarte, CA, Conducted at City of Hope National Medical Center, 1999.

Gagnon PR: Treatment of delirium in supportive and palliative care. *Curr Opin Support Palliat Care* 2:60-66, 2008.

Hospice Pharmacia Pharmacy and Therapeutics Committee: *Hospice Pharmacia Medication Use Guidelines*, 7th ed. Philadelphia, PA, ExcelleRX, Inc., 2005.

Jacox A, Carr DB, Payne R, et al: *Management of Cancer Pain: Clinical Practice Guideline #9*. AHCPR Publication No. 94-0592. Rockville, MD, Public Health Service, 1994.

Jackson KC, Lipman AG: Drug therapy for anxiety in palliative care. *Cochrane Database Syst Rev* 1:CD004596, 2004.

Johanson GA: *Symptom Relief in Terminal Care*. Santa Rosa: Sonoma County Academic Foundation, 1994.

Lawlor P, Gagnon B, Mancini IL, et al: Occurrence, causes, and outcome of delirium in patients with advanced cancer. *Arch Intern Med* 160:786-794, 2000.

Lonergan E, Britton AM, Luxenberg J, Wyller T: Antipsychotics for delirium. *Cochrance Database Syst Rev* 2:CD005594, 2007.

Lovejoy N, Matteis M: Pharmacokinetics and pharmacodynamics of mood-altering drugs in patients with cancer. *Cancer Nurs* 19(6):407-418, 1996.

Maluso-Bolton T: Terminal agitation. *J Hosp Palliat Nurs* 2(1):9-20, 2000.

March PA: Terminal restlessness. *Am J Hosp Palliat Care* 15(1):51-55, 1998.

Marks J: Mirtazapine (remeron) drug information on MedicineNet.com. Accessed online on 9/2/09 at http://www.medicinenet.com/mirtazapine/article.htm. Assessed September 2, 2009.

Massie MG, Holland J, Glass E: Delirium in terminally ill cancer patients. *Am J Psychiatry* 1983:1048-1050, 1983.

Morita T: Hydration in the palliative care setting. *J Supp Oncol* 9:456-457, 2006.

Morita T, Inoue S, Chihara S: Sedation for symptom control in japan: The importance of intermittent use and communication with family members. *J Pain Symptom Manage* 12:32-38, 1996.

Olsen AK, Sjogren P: Neurotoxic effects of opioids. *Eur J Palliat Care* 3:139-142, 1996.

Omudhome O, Marks J: Lexapro (escitaloprim) drug information on MedicineNet.com. http://www.medicinenet.com/escitaloprim/article.htm. Assessed September 2, 2009.

Osborne R, Joel S, Slevin ML: Morphine intoxication in renal failure: The role of morphine-6-glucuronide. *Br Med J* 292:1548-1549, 1986.

Ozbolt LB, Paniagua MA, Kaiser RM: Atypical antipsychotics for the treatment of delirious elders. *J Am Med Dir Assoc* 9:18-28, 2008.

Paice JA: Managing psychological conditions in palliative care: Dying need not mean enduring uncontrollable anxiety, depression, or delirium. *Am J Nurs* 102(11):36-42, 2002.

Panerai A, Bianchi M, Sacerdote P, Ripamonti C, Ventafridda V, De Conno F: Antidepressants in cancer pain. *J Palliat Care* 7(4):42-43, 1991.

Pereira J, Hanson J, Bruera E: The frequency and clinical course of cognitive impairment in patients with terminal cancer. *Cancer* 79(4):835-842, 1997.

Rief W, Nestoriuc Y, Weiss S, et al: Meta-analysis of the placebo response in antidepressant trials. J Affect Disorders 2009, in press. [ePub ahead of print], Feb 25, 2009. http://www.ncbi.nlm.nih.gov/sites/entrez?orig_db=   PubMed&db=pubmed&cmd=Search&TransSchema=title&term=2009[pdat]%20AND%20Rief[author]%20AND%20meta-analysis%20of%20the%20placebo%20response. Accessed September 2, 2009.

Storey P, Knight C: *Management of Selected Non-pain Symptoms in the Terminally Ill*. Gainsville, FL, American Academy of Hospice and Palliative Medicine, 1996.

Teunissen SCCM, Wesker W, Kruitwagen C, et al: Symptom prevalence in patients with incurable cancer: A systematic review. *J Pain Symptom Manage* 34:94-104, 2007.

Ventafridda V, Ripamonti C, De Conno F, Tamburini M, Cassileth B: Symptom prevalence and control during cancer patients' last days of life. *J Palliat Care* 6(3):7-11, 1990.

Wilson KG, Chochinov HM, Skirko MG, et al: Depression and anxiety disorders in palliative cancer care. *J Pain Symptom Manage* 33:118-129, 2007.

World Health Organization: *Symptom Relief in Terminal Illness*. Geneva, World Health Organization, 1998.

Woodruff R: *Symptom Control in Advanced Cancer*. Victoria, Australia, Asperula Pty. Ltd., 1997.

SELF-ASSESSMENT QUESTIONS

1. When trying to differentiate delirium from anxiety, depression, and dementia, which of the following characteristics is unique to delirium and does not occur in the other conditions?

   A. Labile emotional responses
   B. Hallucinations
   C. Decreased level of awareness
   D. Impaired memory, judgment, and thinking
   E. Speech loss

2. Delirium may be reversed in about what percentage of patients near the end of life without resorting to extensive diagnostic interventions that would be inconsistent with end-of-life care treatment goals?

   A. 10%
   B. 20%
   C. 30%
   D. 40%
   E. 50%

3. You have been caring for an 80-year-old male with advanced prostate cancer. His pain has been difficult to control despite escalating doses of morphine. Finally, at a dose of 1,000 mg/day he achieved some degree of comfort. However, over the next several days he has developed cognitive symptoms consistent with delirium. In addition to initiating haloperidol to treat the acute symptoms of delirium, all of the following interventions would be considered appropriate EXCEPT:

   A. Provide an orderly, calm environment for the patient.
   B. Subcutaneous hydration by hypodermoclysis.
   C. Continue the morphine as this had his pain under control.
   D. Switch to an alternative opioid using the technique of opioid rotation.
   E. Check for hypercalcemia since he has advanced prostate cancer.

4. In a recently published randomized clinical trial evaluating the use of parenteral fluid replacement to treat various symptoms of dehydration, which of the following symptoms showed a statistically significant improvement after 2 days of hydration as compared to placebo?

   A. Hallucinations
   B. Sedation
   C. Fatigue
   D. Patient perception of global well-being
   E. Investigator perception of benefit

5. All of the following causes of depression in patients near the end of life are due to changes in a patient's life situation EXCEPT:

   A. Exacerbation of preexisting depression
   B. Loss of control
   C. Loss of self-esteem
   D. Loss of independence
   E. Alteration of environment

6. Which of the following questions put to a patient near the end of life has been shown to be a reliable indictor of depression?

   A. Are you depressed?
   B. Are you having more trouble sleeping?
   C. Have you ever thought of taking your own life?
   D. Do you have any interest in seeing friends anymore?
   E. Have you lost your appetite and have you lost weight?

7. In patients near the end of life, especially those with a life expectancy measured in weeks, which of the following antidepressant medications would provide the most rapid improvement in depressive symptoms?

   A. Amytriptyline
   B. Sertraline
   C. Methylphenidate
   D. Desipramine
   E. Escitalopram

8. Based on a recently published meta-analysis of placebo-controlled randomized clinical trials in the treatment of depression, what is the percentage of improvement in depressive symptoms that can be accounted for by the "placebo effect?"

   A. 13%
   B. 25%
   C. 32%
   D. 54%
   E. 68%

9. All of the following may be psychologic expressions of anxiety EXCEPT:

   A. Insomnia
   B. Distractibility
   C. Irritability
   D. Disorientation
   E. Poor coping skills

10. All of the following statements regarding the use of benzodiazepines for the treatment of anxiety are true EXCEPT:

    A. If anxiety and depression coexist, antidepressants should be initiated first as benzodiazepines can worsen depression.
    B. There is a good evidence base in the medical literature to support the efficacy of benzodiazepines in the treatment of anxiety.
    C. Lorazepam is the preferred benzodiazepine by many end-of-life care practitioners.
    D. Short-acting benzodiazepines such as midazolam are of little clinical value in treating anxiety.
    E. Long-acting benzodiazepines such as diazepam have accumulating active metabolites, making them less useful in the daily treatment of anxiety.

Wound Care and Other Dermatologic Problems at the End of Life

Andrea M. Adkins, Joel S. Policzer, and Domingo Gomez

INTRODUCTION

Caring for the skin and mucus membranes of patients near the end of life can be challenging. The skin is in full sight of both the patient and the caregiver, and new lesions are usually noted immediately. These lesions can be very troubling to patients, causing interference with comfort, interpersonal interactions, eating, and voiding. Skin lesions can cause symptoms ranging from minor irritation to recurrent bleeding to intense unremitting pain and itching. Lack of activity as the end of life approaches can lead to the development of skin breakdown, and foul-smelling drainage from secondarily infected wounds may keep both medical personnel and family at a distance.

Recognition of potential causes of skin and mucus membrane disorders is especially important as end-of-life patients do not have the luxury of waiting for diagnostic test and biopsies to return from the laboratory before therapy is started. Thus, treatment planning is based on clinical identification of the most likely diagnosis, and therapy is instituted rapidly to effect palliation of discomfort as soon as is possible.

The goal of this chapter is to review pressure ulcer prevention and treatments, as well as other common disorders of the skin and mucus membranes that occur in patients who are near the end of life. The all too common and challenging problems related to pressure ulcers are examined first, followed by a review of the treatment of complications of neoplastic diseases such as fistula formation and the fungating tumor mass. Pruritus and the various skin lesions that can cause it, including infections of the skin, drug reactions, and the dermatitides are then discussed. Finally, there is a discussion of the various lesions that can affect the mucus membranes of the mouth.

Paraneoplastic skin disorders (i.e., acanthosis nigricans, necrolytic migratory erythema) and other specific skin lesions (i.e., bullous pemphigus or pemphigoid) that occur uncommonly in terminally ill patients are not reviewed in this chapter. Rather, the focus of this chapter is to examine skin disorders that occur across the spectrum of patients at the end of life, irrespective of diagnosis. The interested reader is referred to any good medical or dermatological textbook for a review of uncommon disease-specific skin disorders.

PRESSURE ULCERS

Pressure ulcers are caused by unrelieved pressure to an area of skin over a prolonged period of time that results in damage of and to the underlying tissue. Pressure ulcers are staged based on the depth of tissue damage as outlined in Table 11–1 and discussed further on in the chapter.

Pressure ulcers have a high prevalence among patients who are near the end of life. One-third of

TABLE 11–1. Staging of Pressure Ulcers	
Stage I	Nonblanchable erythema of intact skin
Stage II	Partial-thickness skin loss involving epidermis, dermis, or both. This can appear as an abrasion, blister, or shallow crater
Stage III	Full-thickness skin loss involving damage to or necrosis of subcutaneous tissue; damage extends to, but no through, fascia
Stage IV	Full-thickness skin loss with extensive destruction or damage to muscle, bone or supporting structures
Unstageable	Presence of eschar and/or slough over the ulcer bed preventing assessment of depth
Deep Tissue Injury	Localized area of discolored intact skin or blood-filled blister

TABLE 11–2. Risk Factors for Development of Pressure Sores
Increasing age
Male gender
History of cerebrovascular accident
Diabetes mellitus
Altered level of consciousness
Poor tissue perfusion and low blood pressure
Decrease in skin fold thickness
Contractures
Urinary and fecal incontinence
Decrease in serum protein and albumin
Poor nutritional intake
Dehydration

hospice patients suffer from skin wounds. Fourteen to nineteen percent of hospice patients cared for at home and up to 28% of hospice patients cared for in long-term care facilities have Stage I pressure ulcers. Stage II pressure ulcers occur in approximately 8% of hospice home care patients and 11% of hospice patients living in nursing homes. Risk factors for pressure ulcers, listed in Table 11–2, are well established and include many of the common condition that are present when patients are near the end of life.

Pressure ulcers are associated with significant morbidity and mortality. Infection is the most serious complication. Infection may be localized, may spread subcutaneously causing cellulitis, may spread to the underlying bone causing osteomyelitis, or may result in septicemia. In fact, of patients who have pressure ulcers and bacteremia, the ulcer itself is the source of the organism in half the patients, and the mortality rate from sepsis associated with pressure ulcers is more than 50%. Pain is another major symptom associated with pressure ulcers, with approximately half of patients who are able to self-report pain indicating that there is pain in the affected area.

Pressure ulcers result from exposure of the skin to high pressure over a short period of time, or to lower pressure for prolonged periods. In most patients, the exposure of the skin to such pressure is a result of decreasing activity from the immobility that is associated with progressive illness. Primary conditions responsible for this immobility include muscle weakness from deconditioning, paralysis, and fatigue. Decreased movement may also occur in patients who are still somewhat mobile, but who have lost the motivation to change positions, such as, for example, where movement aggravates pain and patients will voluntarily decrease their activity. Depressed patients, as a symptom of the illness, also tend to remain in one position. Finally, conditions that block the perception of the pain that is evoked by pressure damage will prevent the pain stimulus from signaling the patient to move, thus allowing the pressure damage to continue. Examples of conditions in which this may occur, and which are common near the end of life, include damage to the central nervous system or peripheral nervous structures, and the use of medications such as sedatives or analgesics that can cloud the sensorium.

PREVENTION OF PRESSURE ULCERS

The key to the treatment of pressure ulcers is to try and prevent their occurrence, a sometimes daunting task given the high number of risk factors present in the end-of-life patient population. Activities that can be useful in reducing the risk of pressure ulcer development are outlined in Table 11–3 and discussed below.

Turning

Turning the patient is still believed to be the best preventive measure and it must be done frequently. The standard is to turn patients every 2 hours, based on the observational study that patients turned on this schedule had fewer pressure ulcers than those turned less often. However, as with all facets of care at the end of life, this standard needs to be individualized for each patient. Some patients will require turning more often, while other patients may be at a phase of

TABLE 11–3. Prevention of Pressure Ulcers

ACTIVITY	INSTRUCTIONS
Turning	Frequently: usually, every 2–3 h
Skin care	Wash with warm water, nondrying soaps
	Inspect skin daily and report changes
	Minimize exposure to moisture to incontinence, perspiration, or wound drainage
	Moisturize dry skin
	Avoid hot water, drying soaps
	Avoid overhydration
Positioning	Reposition at least every 2 h
	Use positioning devices, such as pillows
	Heel: Lift leg to suspend foot
	Sacrum and coccyx: Side position, less than 90 degrees
	Limit the amount of time the head of bed is elevated greater than 30 degrees
	Maintain the head of bed at the lowest degree possible with consideration of the medical condition and other restrictions
	Avoid use of donut devices
Lift patient without sliding	Undersheet
	Mechanical lift
Pressure-reducing surfaces	Air mattress or bed
	Water mattress or bed
	Low air loss mattress
Nutritional support	Encourage fluids as tolerated
	Small frequent meals as tolerated
	Assistance with feeding

life where they either choose to be or should be left alone and not moved at all.

Skin Care

A second key to the prevention of pressure ulcers is good skin care. The goal of such care is to maintain and improve tissue tolerance to pressure. The full skin surface, especially areas over bony prominences prone to pressure damage, must be inspected daily. The skin should be cleansed with warm water, nondrying soaps, and moisturizers; hot water and drying soaps should be avoided. The skin should be cleansed as quickly as possible after soiling to prevent the added damage of prolonged contact with acidic body waste. Although the skin needs to be kept moist, overhydration will also compromise the skin's ability to serve as a barrier. Moist, damp skin is more permeable to irritants, and bacteria will colonize such skin more readily. Therefore, moisture barriers should be used to prevent the accumulation of too much moisture.

Positioning

Positioning of various body areas susceptible to pressure ulcers is another important aspect of preventive care. The heels, which are the most common sites for pressure ulcers, should be protected by lifting the legs up onto a pillow to suspend the foot without putting pressure on the heels. To minimize the shear forces on tissues that result from patients sliding down in the bed, the head of the bed should not be elevated greater than 30 degrees. The risk of sacral and coccygeal ulcers may be reduced by placing patients in a side-lying position but this position should not place the body perpendicular to the bed, as placing the patient at a 90-degree angle places too much pressure over the greater trochanter of the hip, risking ulcer formation there.

Lifting to Avoid Sliding

Preventing frail and fragile skin from sliding and dragging across surfaces is another important preventative measure. Devices, ranging from simple undersheets to full mechanical lifts, should be used whenever patients need to be lifted and moved.

Pressure-Reducing Surfaces

Placing high-risk patients on pressure-reducing surfaces, such as air and water mattresses or full air or waterbeds, is another way to help prevent pressure ulcers. Studies do not seem to indicate that one system is superior to another: rather, any and all of these mattresses can produce benefit for some patients. In general, high-density foam mattresses are better than standard hospital mattresses and should be preferentially used. However, none of these surfaces are a substitute for frequent repositioning and proper care of the fragile skin, which must be provided to reduce the risk of pressure ulcers in patients near the end of life.

Nutritional Support

Finally, improvement in nutritional status is believed to assist in the prevention and treatment of pressure ulcers, although, in reality, the literature does not support this concept. It has been suggested that certain foods, such as citrus fruits, green leafy vegetables, grains, meat, fish, and eggs, may be helpful in the promotion of wound healing. However, for patients near the end of life, poor nutritional status is the norm, and it is unlikely that one will be able to reverse a patient from a state of poor nutrition. Therefore, aggressive nutritional support in this population in an effort to prevent or promote the healing of pressure ulcers is likely to be ineffective and may be more of a burden than a benefit.

PRESSURE ULCERS STAGING

When, despite preventive measures, a pressure ulcer develops, the stage of the ulcer must be determined, as treatments are very much dependent on the ulcer stage. The staging of pressure ulcers is outlined in Table 11–1, and is primarily based on the extent of the tissue damage and appearance of the wound. The National Pressure Advisory Panel has recently modified the staging system, supplementing the classical four stages with an additional stage focusing on deep tissue injury and another for classifying unstageable pressure ulcers. It should be noted that end-of-life patients do not always progress linearly from a lower to higher stage and a deep Stage III or IV lesion may be the first sign of a problem, as subcutaneous tissue can become necrotic before the dermis. Even a small ulcer should be looked at as the "tip of the iceberg," with a potentially deep base.

Stage I

Stage I lesions are characterized by nonblanchable redness of localized areas of skin, usually over bony prominences. The skin remains intact. The affected area may be painful, firm, soft, and either warmer or cooler than unaffected adjacent tissue. Stage I lesions may be difficult to detect in individuals with dark pigmented skin tones, as darkly pigmented skin may not have visible blanching; its color may differ from the surrounding area.

Stage II

A Stage II pressure ulcer is identified by a partial-thickness loss of dermis presenting as a shallow open ulcer with a pink wound bed, without slough. It also may present as an intact or open/ruptured serum-filled blister or as a shiny or dry shallow ulcer without slough or bruising (bruising indicates suspected deep tissue injury). This stage should not be used to describe skin tears, tape burns, perineal dermatitis, maceration, or excoriation.

Stage III

Stage III wounds are characterized by full-thickness tissue loss. Subcutaneous fat may be visible, but bone, tendon, or muscle is not exposed. Slough may be present, but does not obscure the depth of the tissue loss. It may include undermining and tunneling.

The depth of a Stage III pressure ulcer varies by anatomical location. In areas that do not have subcutaneous tissue, such as the bridge of the nose, ear, occiput, and malleolus, Stage III ulcers can be shallow. In contrast, areas with significant fatty tissue can develop extremely deep Stage III ulcers. In such situations, neither bone nor tendon is visible or directly palpable.

Stage IV

Stage IV pressure ulcers are characterized by full-thickness tissue loss with exposed bone, tendon or muscle. Slough or eschar may be present on some parts of the wound bed. It often includes undermining and tunneling. As with Stage III lesions, the depth of Stage IV ulcers varies by anatomical location. Unlike Stage III lesions, however, these ulcers can extend into muscle and/or supporting structures (e.g., fascia, tendon or joint capsule) making osteomyelitis possible. Bone or tendon in affected areas is visible and/or directly palpable.

Deep Tissue Injury

A deep tissue injury is defined as a purple or maroon localized area of discolored intact skin or a blood-filled blister due to damage of the underlying soft tissue from pressure and/or shear. The visible signs of deep tissue injury may be preceded by tissue that is painful, firm, mushy, boggy, and either warmer or cooler than unaffected adjacent tissue. Deep tissue injury may be difficult to detect in individuals with dark skin tones. Evolution of the lesion may include a thin blister over a dark wound bed, followed by the development of a thin eschar covering. Even with optimal treatment, rapid evolution of these lesions may occur, exposing additional layers of tissue.

Unstageable

Unstageable pressure ulcers are those lesions that have full-thickness tissue loss and the base of the ulcer is covered by slough and/or an eschar in the wound bed. Until enough slough and/or eschar is removed to expose the base of the wound, the true depth, and therefore stage, cannot be determined. Although it is usually desirable to remove enough eschar to stage lesions of this type, stable (dry, adherent, intact without erythema or fluctuance) eschar on the heels serves as "the body's natural biological cover" and should not be removed.

TREATMENT OF PRESSURE ULCERS

Although healing is the usual goal of pressure ulcer care, this goal may not be a realistic outcome for patients near the end of life. The potential for healing depends on the status of affected patients and their expected overall time of survival. For example, it may be possible to work toward the healing of a deep ulcer when a patient has a prognosis for survival of several months or more. The goal for wound care in such patients is to maintain a moist wound environment that promotes re-epithelialization and healing. On the other hand, if a patient has a life expectancy of days to a couple of weeks, the goal of care for even a shallow ulcer may be to simply keep the area clean and noninfected.

When choosing a dressing for the wound, one should consider the ability of the dressing to stay moist, so that when it is removed it does not disrupt the newly formed tissue. Although keeping a wound moist is vital for healing, too much moisture can delay healing and cause further tissue damage, therefore excess exudate must be absorbed. Once a treatment plan is implemented, it should be continued for at least 2 weeks before determining the potential success of the therapy, and whether the treatment plan will require any modification. The treatment strategy for pressure ulcers is based on the stage of the ulcer and amount of exudate, and is summarized in Table 11–4 and is discussed below.

Stage I

Despite the intactness of the skin, the patient is at increased risk for further skin breakdown and the development of higher stage lesions. Therefore, the treatment of choice is prevention, employing the techniques described above and in Table 11–3. Hydrocolloid dressings should be utilized for Stage I lesions that are subject to friction or incontinence to prevent further deterioration.

Stage II

In Stage II pressure ulcers, the goal of treatment is to maintain a moist, physiologic environment by keeping the area clean and noninfected, and by preventing damage to surrounding normal tissue. The wound should be gently cleansed with saline and scrubbing should be avoided. The area is then patted dry and covered with a dressing designed to keep the ulcer bed moist, keep the area clean, and reduce pain. A hydrofiber dressing covered by a hydrocolloid should be applied. If utilizing the hydrofiber dressing, premoisten it with normal saline if the wound is dry. The dressing should be changed every 3 to 7 days, or when drainage seeps out from under the dressing edge. Hydrogel preparations, semipermeable foams, and polyurethane films can also be utilized when appropriate.

Stage III and Stage IV

As already stated, Stage III ulcers penetrate through the dermis and into the subcutaneous tissue, while Stage IV lesions involve destruction through the subcutaneous tissue and involve fascia, muscle, joints, and/or bone. Therefore, healing of these ulcers is by secondary intent and can take many months, an unrealistic expectation for the overwhelming majority of patients near the end of life. Therefore, the maintenance of a clean, uninfected wound with minimization of pain is a much more reasonable and achievable goal in this population.

All Stage III and IV ulcers should be cleansed with saline and gently patted dry. Further treatment depends upon whether the wound has minimal drainage, copious amounts of drainage, or has an eschar or necrotic tissue present.

When there is minimal to no drainage, a hydrofiber or hydrogel dressing should be applied to the wound. Both can be covered with a secondary hydrocolloid dressing. This dressing should also be changed every 3 to 7 days, or when drainage seeps out from under the dressing edge.

For wounds with moderate to copious amounts of drainage, hydrofiber in the form of a pad or a rope should be applied into the wound. The wound should then be covered with hydrocolloid with an absorbent center or a foam dressing. Calcium alginate can be utilized for wounds with moderate bleeding. Change the dressing every 3 to 7 days. If leakage occurs, change the dressing immediately.

Unstageable/Necrotic Tissue

When there is an unstable eschar or necrotic tissue present, mechanical debridement is the preferred method of treatment. The wound should be covered with damp to dry normal saline dressings that are changed every 8 hours. It is important that necrotic tissue be removed to reduce the risk of infection, as necrotic tissue can support the growth of bacteria. Do not institute aggressive debridement if the eschar is stable, dry, nondraining, and odorless. For an intact eschar, it is important to relieve pressure on the area; however, no dressing or debridement is required.

TABLE 11–4. Treatment of Pressure Ulcers

STAGE	GOALS OF TREATMENT	RECOMMENDED TREATMENT
I	Maintain skin integrity	See Table 11–3
	Keep area clean and odor free	Irrigate wound with saline or wound cleanser
	Prevent further tissue damage	Apply hydrocolloid or transparent film if area of frequent incontinence or shearing
		Change every 5–7 d or as needed
II Shallow depth	Keep area clean	Irrigate wound with saline or wound cleanser
	Keep area infection free	Apply zinc oxide paste bandage (cut to size)
	Prevent further tissue damage	Cover with gauze and secure with tape
	Promote comfort	Change every 3 d and as needed
II, III, IV Dry to minimal exudate	Keep area clean	Irrigate wound with saline or wound cleanser
	Keep area infection free	Apply hydrofiber dressing or rope (Premoisten if wound bed is dry)
	Prevent further tissue damage	
	Promote comfort	Cover with a thin hydrocolloid dressing
	Promote moist wound environment	Change dressing every 5–7 d or when drainage occurs
II, III, IV Moderate exudate	Keep area clean	Irrigate wound with saline or wound cleanser
	Keep area infection free	Apply hydrofiber dressing or rope
	Prevent further tissue damage	Cover with a hydrocolloid or foam dressing
	Manage exudate	Change dressing every 3–7 d or when drainage occurs
	Promote comfort	
II, III, IV Copious Exudate	Keep area clean	Irrigate wound with saline or wound cleanser
	Keep area infection free	Apply hydrofiber dressing or rope
	Prevent further tissue damage	Cover with a dressing with absorbent center, or a foam dressing
	Promote comfort	
		Change dressing every 3–7 d or when drainage occurs
II, III, IV Infected	Keep area clean	Irrigate wound with saline or wound cleanser
	Minimize odor	Apply ionic silver hydrofiber dressing or rope
	Prevent further tissue damage	Cover with a hydrocolloid with absorbent center, or foam dressing
	Promote comfort	
		Change dressing every 3–7 d or when drainage occurs
		Once infection or symptoms resolve, revert to recommended treatment of wound stage and exudate amount
Unstageable eschar or necrotic tissue	Keep area clean	Do not institute debridement if eschar is stable, dry, nondraining, and odorless
	Keep area infection free	
	Minimize odor	**Mechanical debridement:**
	Prevent further tissue damage	Irrigate the ulcer bed with normal saline in 35 mL syringe and a 19-gauge needle to debride wound
	Debride necrotic tissue	Apply a damp to dry normal saline dressing
	Promote comfort	Change every 8 h

(continued)

STAGE	GOALS OF TREATMENT	RECOMMENDED TREATMENT
TABLE 11–4. Treatment of Pressure Ulcers (*Continued*)		
Unstageable eschar or necrotic tissue (cont'd)		**Autolytic debridement:** Apply an transparent film or hydrocolloid dressing Change every 5–7 d for optimal benefit Contraindicated for immunocompromised patients or patients with an infected ulcer **Enzymatic debridement:** Apply enzyme carefully to the necrotic tissue Discontinue when necrotic tissue is dissolved **Surgical debridement:** Utilize for patients with good healing potential
Imminent patient (days to 2 wks until death)	Keep area clean Keep area infection free Promote comfort	Irrigate wound with saline or wound cleanser Apply hydrocolloid or transparent film Change every 3–5 d or as needed
Imminent patient with infected wound	Keep area clean Promote comfort Minimize odor	Irrigate wound with saline or wound cleanser Apply triple antibiotic or Silvadene ointment Cover with gauze or ABD pad Change dressing daily and as needed

Autolytic debridement is another method of removing necrotic tissue. This is accomplished by covering the ulcer with a clear occlusive or semiocclusive dressing, such as Opsite or a hydrocolloid. Instead of changing the dressing as drainage increases, the tissue fluid is allowed to accumulate. Macrophages and white cells in the fluid remove bacteria and necrotic debris via a natural process. Debridement can also be accomplished enzymatically by utilizing topical enzyme creams such as collagenase or papain. Surgical debridement, using forceps and a blade, should be reserved for patients with a reasonable life expectancy and with good healing potential, making it a rarely used procedure in patients near the end of life.

Imminent Patient

If a patient is actively dying or is within weeks of dying the goal is not to heal the wound, but rather to minimize discomfort and keep the wound clean and free of infection. In such situations, the wound should be cleansed and covered with a bio-occlusive dressing such as a hydrocolloid or a transparent film. The dressing should be changed every 3 to 5 days unless leakage occurs, in which case the dressing should be changed immediately. If wound infection is suspected, the area should be irrigated with saline. Triple antibiotic or Silvadene ointment should be applied to the wound bed and then the wound should be covered with gauze or an ABD pad. This dressing should be changed daily and any time leakage occurs. When a patient is near death and the condition of a pressure ulcer suggests that altering the treatment plan may be necessary but would be disruptive to the patient and family, it may be appropriate to continue the current wound care treatment plan and avoid the potential of additional stress that a change in treatment might cause.

A fistula is defined as an abnormal communication between two hollow organs, or between a hollow organ and the skin. Patients who develop fistulas near the end of life are most often those suffering from complications of progressive, advanced malignant disease, although occasionally patients will develop fistulas from nonmalignant causes. Fistulas can be extremely distressing to patients due to interference with normal bodily functions, alteration in self-image, and the uncontrolled leakage of fluid that is often malodorous and can damage surrounding skin. As with pressure ulcers, management of these fistulas at the end of life requires a systematic approach and the recognition that these patients often will not have healing as a goal.

ENTEROCUTANEOUS FISTULAS

Enterocutaneous fistulas occur between the gastrointestinal tract and the skin, usually as the result of progressive malignant disease affecting the gastrointestinal tract and/or as a complication of prior radiation therapy.

Due to the acidic nature of intestinal fluid, discharge of intestinal contents through the fistula will cause skin breakdown and concomitant pain. Proper skin protection needs to be planned so that irritated skin is soothed and further breakdown prevented. The affected area of the skin should be cleansed with warm water, avoiding soaps and irritant cleansers. An appliance, such as an ostomy bag, should then be placed to both capture the leaking fluid and to protect the surrounding skin. Application of the stoma adhesive as close as possible to the fistula borders is desirable to afford maximal protection to the skin. To make the best seal, the adhesive area of the appliance must be placed on as flat a surface as possi-

ble, which may be difficult when fistula sites are located on irregular anatomic areas. In such circumstances, anatomic creases may be filled with an ostomy sealing agent. The hole in the adhesive of the bag must be cut as closely as possible to the shape of the stoma. Once applied, the bag should be emptied and changed frequently to avoid having the weight of the effluent pull on the adhesive and cause leakage.

If the fistula is very large or the skin is so excoriated that the appliance will not adhere, low-pressure suction may be applied to control the fistula output and allow the skin to heal. Carboxymethylcellulose or another barrier cream should be applied around the tube site.

A well-fitting appliance with a tight seal will prevent the other complication of fistulas—the malodorous nature of the discharge. These odors are embarrassing to the patient and often limit contact between the patient and family or other caregivers. Activated charcoal, 4 to 8 g per day, or chlorophyll tablets, taken by mouth, may help to control the odor, though charcoal may also affect the absorption of other medication and, therefore, must be used with caution. In addition, use of scented candles and aromatherapy oil in the patient's room can serve to mask odor if necessary.

URINARY FISTULAS

Vesicoenteric Fistulas

Formation of a fistula between the urinary bladder and the gastrointestinal (GI) tract can occur at any level of the bowel. The problem almost always derives from pathology of the GI tract such as malignancy, inflammatory bowel disease, or diverticulitis. Rarely does the original problem come from the bladder. Symptoms can range from pneumaturia (passage of gas and froth in the urine), to urine with a foul smell, to passage of frank fecal material in the urine.

Management is dependent on the overall clinical status of the patient. If symptoms are severe enough, the patient's prognosis for survival is sufficiently long, and the patient's clinical condition warrants, surgical correction of the fistula may be attempted. If the fistula is large or not surgically correctable, diversion of the fecal stream with a simple loop colostomy (operative externalization of a loop of colon proximal to the fistula) can be considered. Patients near the end of life who are not surgical candidates require compassionate supportive care. Urine should be removed as quickly as possible after voiding. If odor is the main problem, bladder catheterization and collection of urine into a closed system may be effective palliation.

Vesicovaginal Fistulas

Vesicovaginal fistulas are most often the result of gynecologic malignancy, surgery, or local trauma. Characteristically, there is leakage of urine from the bladder into the vagina. If there is only a small leak, this may be managed by vaginal packing or by bladder catherization. In situations where there is extensive damage to the pelvic organs, urinary diversion from the upper renal tracts may be needed to avoid a situation where the patient is continually incontinent.

CANCERS OF THE SKIN

Malignant involvement of the skin can occur from a variety of neoplastic disorders. Primary cancers of the skin include basal cell carcinoma, squamous cell carcinoma, and malignant melanoma. Many solid tumors and hematological malignancies will invade the skin secondarily, either through direct invasion or metastatic spread. As patients near the end of life, progressive malignant involvement of the skin, whether of primary or secondary origin, can be a troubling and distressing problem.

TREATMENT

At the end of life, treatment of malignant skin lesions is usually symptomatic. Therefore, asymptomatic, slow-growing lesions can often be left alone. In patients with hematological malignancies with skin involvement, small doses of oral antineoplastic agents such as hydroxyurea, or corticosteroids, may reduce tumor mass just enough to retard progression and keep the lesions from ulcerating and/or causing pain.

Rapidly enlarging, painful lesions, which often ulcerate or fungate over time, are much more difficult to treat. If the lesion is localized and the patient is a surgical candidate, then local excision may be indicated. If the malignancy is radiosensitive, then radiation therapy may be attempted. Occasionally, systemic chemotherapy may be effective as well. More often, however, the patient is not a surgical candidate, other antineoplastic therapies have been unsuccessful, and/or the size and location of the lesion prevents local excision with clear margins and a chance for healing. In such circumstances, local care of the lesion is the only treatment available. Treatment recommendations are listed in Table 11–5.

These lesions should be kept dry and uninfected if possible, and require dressings that must be changed frequently. As dressing changes may be painful, it is suggested that analgesics be given one-half to one-hour prior. The lesion should be irrigated with warm saline. If bleeding is noted, it may be controlled by using gauze soaked in a solution containing 1:1,000 epinephrine. (Reports suggest that, depending on the extent of bleeding, undiluted solutions as well as solutions diluting the epinephrine to as little as 1:200,000 have been effective. There is minimal risk of side effects, as topically applied epinephrine solutions are poorly absorbed systemically.) If the lesions are red, inflamed, and malodorous, irrigation with metronidazole solution or application of sterile metronidazole gel may be useful. The gel is preferred because it soothes, stays on the skin, and helps reduce infection and any odors. Natural (i.e.,

TABLE 11–5. Treatment of Fungating Lesions

- Administer analgesia $\frac{1}{2}$ to 1 h prior to dressing change
- Soak off prior dressing with warm saline, if dressing adheres
- Irrigate lesion with normal saline in 35 mL syringe and a 19-gauge needle or wound cleanser
- If lesion is NOT infected:
  - Apply a nonadherent gauze or zinc oxide paste dressing
  - If a moderate to copious amount of exudate is present, pack loosely with an absorbent nonadherent hydrophilic dressing
  - Cover with an ABD pad or an activated charcoal dressing. Hold dressing in place with tubular elastic netting when possible
- Necrotic tissue:
  - Enzymatic debridement may be useful. Discontinue when necrotic tissue is dissolved
- If lesion appears infected:
  - Apply topical antibiotic
  - If infection appears severe, use systemic antibiotics as well
- If bleeding noted, hold gauze soaked with 1:1,000 epinephrine or Atropine solution over bleeding points
- If lesions are red, inflamed, and/or malodorous apply one of the following:
  - Metronidazole gel
  - Metronidazole solution
  - Natural yogurt
- Nonpharmacological measures to control odor:
  - Place charcoal pads under the netting to absorb any odors
  - Place oil of wintergreen on a cotton ball and place in patient's room.
  - Place a dryer sheet over an air vent in patient's room

unflavored) yogurt may also be used, as it is soothing and reduces anaerobic infection as well. Oral metronidazole, 500 mg three times a day, may be administered to help reduce any odor caused by bacterial overgrowth.

If the lesion is large or deep and there are signs of local infection, topical antimicrobial agents can be applied. If infection is more severe, then systemic antibiotics may be helpful, with the choice of antibiotics depending on the organism or organisms cultured. If the lesion is not infected, enzymatic debridement can be attempted, or, if there is sufficient exudate, absorbent nonadherent hydrophilic packing can be placed.

After the lesion has been cared for, it should be covered with a nonadherent dressing. If an exudate is present, the dressing should be of an absorbent material. The dressing should be held in place with tubular elastic netting, and, to help reduce odor, charcoal pads may be placed under the netting.

SKIN LESIONS CAUSED BY PHYSICAL FACTORS

SKIN TEARS

Due to the effects of long-standing chronic illness and poor nutrition, the skin of patients near the end of life often deteriorates into a state marked by poor elasticity and lack of lubrication. Use of

TABLE 11–6. Treatment of Skin Tears

TYPE OF SKIN TEAR	RECOMMENDED THERAPY
Prevention	Keep area clean
	Keep area infection free
	Prevent further tissue damage
	Promote comfort
All skin tears	Irrigate wound with saline or wound cleanser, pat dry
	Further treatment depends on amount of exudate
Minimal exudate	Apply a nonadherent gauze dressing or transparent film (remove cautiously)
	Secure with elastic tubular paper or tape netting
	Change daily or as needed
Moderate exudate	Apply zinc oxide paste bandage (cut to size)
	Wrap with nonconforming gauze and secure with elastic tubular netting
	Change every 3 d and as needed
Copious exudate	Cover with a hydrocolloid with absorbent center or foam dressing
	Make sure dressing is $1\frac{1}{4}$ in. wider than the wound edge
	Secure with paper tape or tubular elastic netting
	Change every 5–7 d and as needed

steroids, as is common in many chronic illnesses, adds to deterioration of the supporting skin structures. As a result of these changes, any shear stress caused by moving the skin across sheets and bedclothes can cause a superficial tear.

Treatment of skin tears is summarized in Table 11–6. The best treatment of skin tears is, not surprisingly, prevention. Because the main cause is loss of natural skin oils for lubrication, emollients that will trap moisture after bathing are very effective. Harsh cleansers that can dry the skin further are to be avoided. Attempts should be made to move patients as carefully as possible, with lifting movements rather than dragging ones.

Once a tear has occurred, clean the skin and pat dry. For small, minimally weeping tears apply nonadherent gauze or transparent film dressing. For multiple skin tears with a moderate amount of exudate, apply zinc oxide impregnated gauze and cover with a nonconforming gauze wrap. Secure the dressing in place with a tubular elas-

tic netting to prevent further trauma to the surrounding tissue and change the dressing every 3 days or as needed. Large tears with copious exudate should be covered with either a hydrocolloid dressing with an absorbent center or a foam dressing and it should be changed every 5 to 7 days and as needed. Skin tears can also be treated as a superficial burn with topical ointments and dressings (see below). As these patients have compromised immune systems, tears are prone to infection and may require oral antibiotics if painful sequelae occur.

THERMAL BURNS

In an attempt to relieve the pain that can so often complicate end of life, caregivers commonly use heating pads as a form of nonpharmacological relief. Patients with altered mental status may not be able to complain of the heat and therefore, their frail skin may burn easily at settings that would be tolerated by otherwise healthy skin. These burns are usually first degree, involving the epidermis superficially and accompanied by tenderness and erythema, or second-degree, involving the epidermis and varying thicknesses of the dermis.

Treatment focuses on wound care, pain relief, and prevention of infection. For superficial burns, the affected area is soothed with cool compresses and then covered with an occlusive dressing. A hydrocolloid dressing is used if the burn is over a pressure site. Healing generally occurs within approximately 1 week. Analgesia can usually be provided by acetaminophen with or without a nonsteroidal anti-inflammatory agent. Infection is generally not a problem.

Burns that break the epithelium are exquisitely painful and usually require an opioid analgesic for management of the pain (see Chapter 6). Treatment involves cleansing the site with soap and sterile water to remove loose skin and debris, preventing these from becoming potential sources of infection. A topical antimicrobial agent is then applied. Silver sulfadiazine 1% is commonly used, but, bacitracin or polysporin can be used if the patient is sulfa allergic. Whereas bulky gauze dressings have classically been used, occlusive dressings are preferred, as they provide immediate pain relief, prevent drying of the wound, and speed healing. Dressings should be changed as necessary and once epithelialization begins, the lesions should be treated in a similar fashion to that recommended for first-degree burns.

PRURITUS

Both pain and itch occur due to activation of the unmyelinated C-fibers in the peripheral nerves. The same chemicals, histamines, proteases, and prostaglandins, mediate both of these sensations. However, the two sensations are perceived differently by patients. Pain induces withdrawal, while pruritus induces scratching; opioids palliate pain, but can cause pruritus secondary to histamine release. Pain can occur anywhere, but pruritus is limited to the skin. Therefore, the transmission of the sensation of pruritus is likely via pathways distinct from pain.

ETIOLOGIES AND TREATMENT

As with any other physical symptom, the primary therapy of pruritus is dependent on first identifying the underlying cause or causes. Near the end of life, these causes (listed in Table 11–7) may be related to the patient's primary illness, comorbid conditions, allergies to medications and other substances, infection, or may be psychogenic in origin.

Once the etiology of pruritus is identified, treatment can be planned appropriately. When the cause of pruritus is due to skin infection or infestation, or is secondary to a medication allergy, the most effective strategy will be to treat the primary cause. Specific treatment recommendations for treating various causes of itching are found in other sections of this chapter.

In many situations near the end of life, one cannot influence the underlying disease sufficiently to relieve pruritus and, therefore, effective palliation of the symptom is required. Skin dryness, which may be a primary cause of pruritus, is also present in most patients who have pruritus from another cause. Therefore, moisturizers are an essential basic treatment for patients who experience itching. Wet wraps placed over a liberal application of a topical moisturizer are very effective.

Medications that can help counteract pruritus are listed in Table 11–8. A nonspecific topical agent such as menthol (0.5–2.0%) in aqueous cream may be beneficial as a soothing agent and it can also act as a mild anesthetic or counterirritant. Another approach is the use of topical

TABLE 11–7. Causes of Pruritus

ETIOLOGY	EXAMPLES
Primary skin diseases	Xerosis (skin dryness)
	Many others
Metabolic	Hepatic dysfunction
	Renal impairment
	Hypo or hyperthyroidism
Hematologic	Iron deficiency
	Polycythemia vera
Cancer	Lymphoma (esp. Hodgkin's disease)
	Leukemia
	Cholestatic jaundice due to metastases from many solid tumors
Drugs	Opioid analgesics
	Allergic drug reaction
Infestations	Scabies
Infections	Candidiasis
Allergic reactions, urticaria	Laundry detergents and soaps
Psychogenic	

steroids, especially when there is an inflammatory component to the skin that accompanies the itch. Providing the topical steroid as an ointment rather than as a cream has the added benefit of keeping the skin moist, palliating the dryness that is often present, and avoiding the stinging sensation that sometimes accompanies application of creams.

For most patients with pruritus, however, oral antihistamines such as diphenhydramine or

TABLE 11–8. Medications to Treat Pruritus

MEDICATION	RECOMMENDED DOSE
Topical creams and ointments	
Menthol	Apply to affected areas 3–4 times per day as needed
Hydrocortisone	Apply to affected areas 2–4 times per day as needed
Oral medication (anti-histamines)	
Hydroxyzine	25–50 mg 3–4 times per day
Diphenhydramine	25–50 mg every 4–8 h as needed
Cyproheptidine	4 mg 3–4 times per day
For cholestatic jaundice	
Cholestyramine	4 g orally before meals and at bedtime

hydroxyzine are the mainstay of empiric therapy. One needs to be concerned about the side effect of drowsiness, which can sometimes be exaggerated when patients are also on opioid analgesics. In patients with pruritus secondary to cholestasis, reduction in itching may be accomplished with cholestyramine.

CUTANEOUS INFECTION

Due to the immunosuppression that is present in virtually all patients near the end of life, susceptibility to infections, including cutaneous infections, is quite high. There is often an area of prior skin injury that permits the infection to begin, although this is not always the case. In terminally ill patients, common lesions from which cutaneous infection develops include pressure ulcers, malignant lesions, and stasis ulcers, although even areas of dry, cracked skin can serve as a focus from which a skin infection begins.

Infecting organisms may include bacteria, fungi, and viruses, and any of these organisms can either be indigenous or externally acquired. Although decisions regarding the treatment of infection with antibiotics near the end of life are often individualized, antibiotics are commonly prescribed for the treatment of cutaneous infections, because effective antibiotic therapy will significantly palliate the pain and discomfort experienced from the inflammation and swelling that accompanies the infection.

BACTERIAL CUTANEOUS INFECTIONS

Cellulitis

Cellulitis is an acute inflammation of the skin associated with pain and swelling of the affected area. It can be caused by indigenous skin flora (generally, staphylococcus species) or by a wide range of exogenous flora. Bacteria gain access to the epidermis via cracks in the skin, abrasions, cuts, insect bites, and catheters.

Cellulitis due to *Staphylococcus aureus* spreads from a localized infection, such as an abscess or an infected foreign body. Recurrent cellulitis of the lower extremities commonly is due to streptococcal organisms associated with chronic venous stasis, or chronic lymphedema.

The primary treatment of cellulitis is with antibiotics. When patients are near the end of life, the choice of antibiotic therapy often needs to be empiric, based on the probably offending organism. This is because the ability to identify the organism by culture is possible in only a minimum of cases, as the yield of tissue aspiration cultures is too low to be useful and purulent drainage is not always present in sufficient quantity to permit obtaining cultures.

Impetigo

Impetigo is a more superficial bacterial infection than cellulitis and is usually due to either group A beta-hemolytic streptococcus or *S. aureus*. The primary lesion is a pustule that ruptures to form a honey-colored crust. Impetigo may occur on normal skin or in areas where other skin lesions are present

In view of the nature of the skin lesions, the treatment of impetigo includes topical therapy with soaks to debride the crusts together and topical antibiotics. Systemic antibiotics, usually oral, are often used as well.

Erysipelas

Erysipelas is the abrupt onset of fiery-red swelling of the face and extremities, typically with well-demarcated indurated margins that progress rapidly. It is accompanied by intense pain. The causative organism is group A beta-hemolytic streptococcus. As erysipelas is common in elderly, debilitated patient, it must be a consideration when patients develop a cutaneous infection near the end of life. Treatment with penicillin is effective, causing pain and other symptoms to rapidly resolve, followed by desquamation of the affected skin.

CUTANEOUS FUNGAL INFECTIONS

Fungal infections of the skin, hair, and nails can occur in the normal population, but, as with other types of cutaneous infection they are more common in immunocompromised patients, and, hence, in patients near the end of life. Common dermatophytoses, such as tinea pedis, cruris, capitis, corporis, and versicolor, are beyond the scope of this discussion, and, while they can occur in patients near the end of life, the reader is referred to any medical or dermatological textbook for further discussion of these common lesions.

Candida Albicans

The most common and troublesome fungal infections occurring in patients near the end of life are caused by *Candida Albicans*. Candida is a normal inhabitant of the GI tract, but can cause infection due to overgrowth secondary to antibiotic treatment, diabetes, chronic intertrigo, and other immune deficiencies. The organism has an affinity for areas that are chronically wet and macerated, such as the intertriginous areas under the breasts or in the perineum. Cutaneous lesions caused by candidiasis are usually edematous, erythematous, and scaly with scattered "satellite pustules." In contrast to other dermatophyte infections in which inflammation is minimal, there is frequently a marked inflammatory response in Candida infections.

Therapy involves removing predisposing factors such as wetness, as well as applying topical antifungal agents, such as nystatin or clotrimazole cream, two to three times a day to the affected areas. If a marked inflammatory response is present, the skin can be treated with hydrocortisone cream or lotion, or with a combination antifungal/steroid cream. When cutaneous candidiasis is recurrent or refractory, systemic therapy with oral antifungal agents such as fluconazole 150 mg one time (combined with ketoconazole 2% cream twice a day for 2 weeks) or itraconazole 200 mg daily for 7 to 10 days may be used. Therapy of oral candidiasis is discussed later in this chapter.

VIRAL INFECTIONS

Herpes Varicella/Zoster

VARICELLA (CHICKEN POX) The Herpes varicella-zoster virus causes two distinct clinical illnesses. First, infection with the virus causes varicella, commonly referred to as chicken pox, which is an acute illness highlighted by a prodromal febrile illness followed by the development of pruritic vesicular lesions, usually in a diffuse distribution. The lesions are often intensely pruritic, and if scratched off, may leave significant scarring. Varicella is typically a viral childhood illness that is well tolerated, although its course may be more virulent in previously unexposed adults, especially when the adult is immunocompromised. Therefore, although quite unusual, a patient at the end of life who has not been previously exposed to the varicella-zoster virus, is at risk of developing a severe case of chickenpox if exposed to, for example, a visiting child who is incubating or has active disease. In such a situation, treatment with varicella globulin could be provided at the time of exposure and before the development of active disease. If active disease occurs, treatment with acyclovir 4,000 mg per day in divided doses for 5 days may be provided.

ZOSTER (SHINGLES) The more common problem with the varicella-zoster virus at the end of life is the reactivation of infection, known as herpes zoster or shingles. Shingles presents as a very painful vesicular eruption classically in a dermatomal distribution. It most often occurs in the sixth to eighth decade of life. Although the definitive mechanism for reactivation of the virus is unknown, it is clearly associated with immunosuppression, and hence, can be a significant problem for patients who are near the end of life. Exposure of persons who were previously infected with the varicella virus to patients with active chickenpox has also been reported to be a risk factor for the development of shingles.

Pain of shingles may actually precede the skin eruption by several days to a week, and the duration of the skin lesions is usually 3 to 10 days, although it may sometimes take weeks for the skin to return to normal. The most distressing complication is postherpetic neuralgia, which can occur in more than 50% of patients older than 50 years and requires adjuvant medications that are effective for the treatment of neuropathic pain to provide the patient with adequate analgesia. (See Chapter 6 for recommendations on how to treat neuropathic pain). Treatment of the active infection consists of acyclovir 800 mg per day for 7 to 10 days. Although acyclovir therapy will speed healing of the skin lesions, it has no effect on the incidence of postherpetic pain.

Herpes Simplex

Another virus that can be troublesome to some patients at the end of life is herpes simplex virus. There are two subtypes of the virus, HSV-1 and HSV-2. As with varicella-zoster, this virus is usually acquired early in life, and the major concern near the end of life is the reactivation of infection, usually in the oropharyngeal area, the perineal area, and/or the perirectal areas. In immunocompromised and terminally ill patients, the infection may be severe, extending into the mucosal and deep cutaneous layer, and the lesions appear clinically similar to mucosal lesions caused by chemotherapy, fungal or bacterial infections. Systemic acyclovir can speed healing of the lesions and relief of symptoms.

CUTANEOUS INFESTATIONS: SCABIES

Scabies is the most common cause of pruritic dermatosis worldwide. It is caused by infestation of the skin with the mite, *Sarcoptes scabiei*. Person-to-person contact is the usual route of transmission and medical practitioners are at high risk of acquiring scabies. As outbreaks among patients living in nursing homes and hospitals are frequent, scabies can be a significant problem for patients who are near the end of life and institutionalized in a hospital, in-patient or live-in hospice, adult home, or nursing home.

The itch and rash of scabies derive from a sensitization reaction. Thus, even though scratching destroys the mite, symptoms persist even in its absence.

Patients report an intense pruritus, which is worse at night or after showering. Burrows may be difficult to find. They appear as wavy lines, 2 to 15 mm in length that end in a pearly bleb. They are common on volar wrist surfaces, between fingers, on elbows and on the penis. Papules, vesicles, pustules, and nodules are seen in these sites as well as under breasts, around the navel, in axillae, the belt line, buttocks, upper thighs, and scrotum. The face, palms, and soles are spared.

Treatment is topical, with 5% permethrin cream being recommended. Permethrin is much less toxic than the more commonly used 1% lindane cream. It is applied thinly behind ears and from the neck down, and washed off 8 hours later. Although patients become noninfectious within one day of treatment, symptoms of pruritus and rash may persist for weeks to months. The pruritus may be symptomatically treated as outlined in Table 11–8.

CUTANEOUS DRUG REACTIONS

Polypharmacy is common among patients near the end of life. Therefore, these patients are susceptible to adverse reactions to the myriad of medications used to help control symptoms. Whenever a patient who is near the end of life develops a new onset of pruritus associated with urticaria or maculopapular eruptions, a cutaneous drug reaction must be considered high on the list of possible causes, and a full review of all medication must be performed.

Urticarial drug eruptions are typically described as pruritic, red wheals that can vary from pinpoint to large in size, and usually last less than 24 hours. Involvement of the dermis and subcutaneous tissue can lead to more generalized swelling of the skin, termed angioedema. Uriticaria generally occur early in the course of treatment with a new medication. The urticaria may be allergic in origin, or, in the case of opioids, aspirin, and nonsteroidal anti-inflammatory drugs (NSAIDs) (medications commonly used in patients near the end of life) the reaction may be due to nonallergic release of histamine and other vasoactive mediators.

Maculopapular eruptions caused by medication tend to occur 1 to 2 weeks after the onset of therapy with a new medication. Erythematous macules and/or papules generally start on the trunk or on areas of pressure or prior trauma. They are frequently symmetrical and may become confluent.

The primary therapy for all cutaneous drug reactions is withdrawal of the offending medication. In the case of maculopapular eruptions, however, the eruptions may fade even if the offending agent is continued. In the absence of angioedema, primary treatment should include antihistamines (see Table 11–8), soothing baths, and emollients. If angioedema and/or anaphylaxis occurs, treatment must include epinephrine and/or corticosteroids, as needed, to halt the anaphylactic response.

PHOTOSENSITIVITY

A less typical cutaneous drug reaction may develop when the medication causes the skin to develop an increased sensitivity to light. Among the medications responsible for causing photosensitivity are sulfonamides, tetracyclines, thiazide diuretics, sulfonylurea and other hypoglycemic agents, phenothiazines and antihistamines. The skin reaction is very similar to the erythema of sunburn, but occasionally bullae may occur.

Primary treatment consists of breaking the connection between the medication and exposure of the skin to the sun. Depending on the needs and goals of the patient, either the medication is stopped or sunlight is avoided. Treatment of the skin lesions is identical to that of first-degree or second-degree thermal burns (see above).

DERMATITIS

ATOPIC DERMATITIS

Atopic dermatitis is an extremely common skin disorder described as superficial, inflammatory, erythematous, pruritic, and eruptive. In adults, it is usually localized and chronic. It is in many ways a cyclic disorder, starting as a constant pruritus causing scratching, which in turn causes a rash that is pruritic and causes more scratching, and so on. The causes of atopic dermatitis are unclear, although there is often intolerance to environmental irritants. Exacerbation of atopic dermatitis may be caused by conditions that are common to patients near the end of life including emotional stress, temperature changes, and bacterial skin infections, and for this reason it is important to consider these factors as a potential etiology of dermatitis in these patients.

Therapy involves avoidance of rubbing the skin, minimization of scratching, and decreasing exposure to triggering stimuli in the environment. The skin should be kept well lubricated. Medications that are useful in reducing symptoms are similar to those used for pruritus (see Table 11–8) and include hydroxyzine, diphenhydramine, and topical steroids. If lesions are resistant to empiric therapy then superimposed infection may be present. For such patients, antibiotic treatment directed against *S. aureus* may be of benefit.

CONTACT DERMATITIS

Contact dermatitis is an inflammatory process caused by agents that injure the skin by direct contact. It is due to an antigen-specific immune response that can either be acute (edematous and wet) or chronic (dry, thickened, and scaly). Acute contact dermatitis can present as mild erythema or as a more pronounced skin eruption with the presence of vesicles and ulcers. An important clue that the skin reaction is due to contact dermatitis is that the area involved is strictly demarcated and may be unilateral. Patients near the end of life may develop contact dermatitis from contact with substances such as laundry detergents used to clean linens.

Treatment involves removing the offending agent, providing physical barriers to avoid contact, and high-potency fluorinated topical steroids. The dermatitis typically resolves in 2 to 3 weeks after treatment begins.

STASIS DERMATITIS

Stasis dermatitis is a reaction that develops on the lower extremities due to vascular incompetence and chronic edema. Near the end of life it may be seen in patients who suffer from such illnesses as advanced congestive heart failure, advanced chronic obstructive pulmonary disease (COPD) with cor pulmonale, and advanced malignancies with obstruction of blood flow from the lower extremities due to tumor or radiation-induced fibrosis.

Early in the course of stasis dermatitis, one finds erythema and scaling with pruritus. Typically, this starts over the medial aspect of the ankle at the site of an engorged vein. Eventually, the area becomes pigmented due to hemosiderin deposition from extravasated red cells. The area can then become acutely inflamed with exudate and crusting. Chronic stasis dermatitis is associated with fibrosis, so-called brawny edema. Areas of brawny edema are highly susceptible to infection and superimposed contact dermatitis. In severe cases, ulceration can occur.

Treatment of early stasis changes is based on the use of emollients and midpotency topical steroids to reduce inflammation and elevation of the affected limb and use of compression stockings of at least 30 to 40 mm Hg to decrease chronic edema.

Ulcers from stasis dermatitis are difficult to treat. The optimal goal at end of life is to keep the ulcer clean and to avoid infection. This can involve gentle debridement of necrotic tissue with application of a semipermeable dressing under pressure. Antibiotics are used only for active infections

DISORDERS OF THE MUCUS MEMBRANES

XEROSTOMIA (DRY MOUTH)

Xerostomia is an all too common complaint among patients near the end of life. The most common causes of xerostomia in this population are outlined in Table 11–9. Patients with xerostomia usually complain of the need to continually do things to keep the mouth moist, the need to drink water at night, and difficulty with speech. If the dryness is severe, the patient may also complain of a burning sensation in the tongue or mouth. Other symptoms associated with xerostomia include halitosis, decreased taste acuity, and difficulty chewing and swallowing food. Difficulty chewing and swallowing may sometimes be aggravated by dentures that become ill-fitting due to insufficient saliva to help seal dentures to the oral mucosa.

Measures to reduce xerostomia include use of ice cubes, hard candy, or gum to maximally stimulate salivary flow. Frequent sips of cold liquids, frequent rinsing of the mouth with tap water, and use of a saliva substitute are also helpful. If there is any evidence of oral infection (see below), appropriate therapy should be prescribed. The oral

TABLE 11–9. Causes of Xerostomia	
ETIOLOGY	**EXAMPLE**
Medication	Opioid analgesics
	Tricyclic antidepressants
	Antihistamines
	Phenothiazines
	Anticholinergics
Dehydration	Local: mouth breathing, oxygen use
	Systemic
Reduced salivary flow	Complication of local malignancy, radiation therapy, or surgery
Erosion of the buccal cavity	Infection (viral or fungal)
	Stomatitis
Depression	
Anxiety	

cavity should be kept as clean as possible by cleansing with a toothbrush, foam stick, or cotton bud soaked with water, as frequently as every 1 to 2 hours if needed. Mouthwashes that are alcohol-based and astringent should be avoided to prevent further drying of the tissues. Patients who have xerostomia due to prior radiation therapy may benefit from pilocarpine tablets 5 mg three times a day.

ORAL INFECTIONS

The most common oral infections in terminally ill patients are fungal (oral candidiasis) and viral.

Oral Candidiasis

The presentation of oral candidiasis may vary. Patients can present with the typical white-yellow plaques that wipe off easily, generalized red lesions, or a diffuse red surface. Pain is present to a greater or lesser extent.

Treatment is available in both topical and systemic forms. Nystatin suspension is the classic topical treatment with 400,000 U applied via a swish and swallow technique to the infected mucosa four times daily. Treatment is often disappointing because antifungal action is limited to the time the agent has contact with the fungus. Clotrimazole lozenges used five times daily are often effective, and may have the advantage of increased contact time with the infected mucosa. If topical treatment is not effective and systemic treatment is indicated, fluconazole 50 to 150 mg daily is effective with few side effects. Its long half-life allows once daily dosing.

Oral Viral Infections

Viral infections of the oral mucosa are most commonly due to Herpes simplex and zoster, and may also be caused by cytomegalovirus and Epstein–Barr virus. They generally present as yellow lesions that are easily wiped from the mucosa and are exquisitely painful, often requiring treatment with systemic opioids for pain relief. Acyclovir, 1,000 mg a day in divided doses, is the treatment of choice. Topical agents that may help soothe the mucosa include viscous lidocaine solution, often mixed with equal part liquid antacid to allow better and longer adherence of the anesthetic to the mucosa.

STOMATITIS

Stomatitis is manifested in diffuse erythema, inflammation, and ulceration of the oral mucosa. It is most often a complication of chemotherapy and radiotherapy. The major risk factor is poor oral health and hygiene prior to initiation of these therapies. The inflammatory process most often affects the nonkeratinized oral mucosa, including the cheek, soft palate, lips, tongue, and floor of the mouth.

Treatment of stomatitis involves minimizing trauma to the mucosa and adequate pain management. Aggressive mouth care is needed to keep the mucosal surface clean, using soft brushes and hydrogen peroxide or chlorhexidine rinses. Lips should be kept moist with a petroleum-based jelly. The oral cavity can be cleansed with mouthwashes, but careful attention should be paid to avoiding alcohol-based preparations. Ice chips or popsicles can be very soothing, and topical anesthetics may also be of benefit.

An innovative technique is to make hard candy containing cayenne powder. Although the initial use of these candy lozenges may increase burning initially, the capsaicin in the pepper powder may well have an analgesic effect. Pain may be sufficiently severe to require systemic opioids.

BIBLIOGRAPHY

Allman RM: Pressure ulcer prevalence, incidence, risk factors, and impact. In: Thomas DR, Allman RM, eds. *Clinics in Geriatric Medicine* 13(3):421-436, 1997.

Arnold HL Jr, Odom RB, James WD: *Andrews' Diseases of the Skin*, 8th ed. Philadelphia, PA, W.B. Saunders Co, 1990.

Bergstrom NI: Strategies for preventing pressure ulcers. In: Thomas DR, Allman RM, eds. *Clinics in Geriatric Medicine* 13(3):437-454, 1997.

Baranoski S: Skin tears: The enemy of frail skin. *Adv Skin Wound Care* 13:223-226, 2000.

Brienza D: Understanding support surface technologies. *Adv Skin Wound Care* 13:237-244, 2000.

Bruera E: Skin disorders and their management. In: Portnoy RK, Bruera E, eds. *Topics in Palliative Care*, Vol 3. New York, Oxford University Press, 1998.

Doyle D, Hanks GWC, MacDonald N: *Oxford Textbook of Palliative Medicine*, 2nd ed. Oxford, Oxford University Press, 1998.

Dwyer S: Silver is precious in wound care. Wounds1. com October 2, 2001. http://www.wounds1.com/news/tech.cfm/4/1. Accessed August 24, 2010.

Fauci AS, Braunwald E, Isselbacher KJ, et al: *Harrison's Principles of Internal Medicine*, 14th ed. New York, McGraw-Hill, 1998.

Gaymar Industries. Medicare part B support surface guidelines. Wound Care Information Network July 5, 2001: 1-6. http://www.medicaledu.com/supportsurfacemedpartb.htm. Accessed August 24, 2010.

Goode PS, Thomas DR: Pressure ulcers: local wound care. In: Thomas DR, Allman RM, eds. *Clinics in Geriatric Medicine* 13(3):543-552, 1997.

Jaffe R: Atopic dermatitis. In: Zuber TJ, ed. *Primary Care: Dermatology.* Philadelphia, PA, W.B. Saunders Co, 2000.

Kinzbrunner BM, Pyron M, Coluzzi P, Gardner D: *Vitas Guidelines for Intensive Palliative Care.* Miami, FL, Vitas Healthcare Corporation, 1996.

Krasner DL, Rodeheaver GT, Sibbald RG: *Chronic Wound Care: A Clinical Sourcebook for Healthcare Professionals*, 3rd ed. Wayne, PA, HMP Communications, 2001.

Maklebust J, Sieggreen M: *Pressure Ulcers Guidelines for Prevention and Nursing Management*, 2nd ed. Springhouse, PA, Springhouse Corporation, 1996.

Mayer ME: The terminology of skin disorders. In: Zuber TJ, ed. *Primary Care* 27(2):277-288, 2000.

McEvoy GK, Litvak K, Welsh OH, et al, eds: *AHFS 98 Drug Information.* Bethesda, MD, American Society of Health-System Pharmacists, 1998.

Meyers D: *Client Teaching Guides for Home Health Care.* Rockville, MD, Aspen Publishers Inc, 1989.

Miller H: *Vitas Wound Care Best Practice Guidelines.* Miami, FL, Vitas Healthcare Corporation, 2007

Ovington L: "Wound care products: How to choose." *Adv Skin Wound Care* 14:259-266, 2001.

Pearson AS, Wolford RW: Management of skin trauma. In: Zuber TJ, ed. *Primary Care* 27(2):475-492, 2000.

Remsburg RE, Bennett RG: Pressure-relieving strategies for preventing and treating pressure sores.

In: Thomas DR, Allman RM, eds. *Clinics in Geriatric Medicine* 13(3):513-541, 1997.

Thomas S: A structured approach to the selection of dressings. World Wide Wounds, published 7/14/97 and accessed on 8/24/10 at http://www.worldwidewounds.com/1997/july/Thomas-Guide/Dress-Select.html.

Types of wound debridement. Wound Care Information Network http://www.medicaledu.com/ debridhp.htm. Published 1995 and accessed August 24, 2010.

Frequently asked questions. Wound infection and infection control. National Pressure Ulcer Advisory Panel July 28, 2000: 1-3. http://www.npuap.org/ woundinfection.htm. Accessed July 2, 2001.

WOCN society's CMS-reviewed wound care guidelines. Home Health Line EXTRA September 7, 2001: 1-4.

SELF-ASSESSMENT QUESTIONS

1. Pressure ulcers have a high prevalence among patients who are near the end of life.
   About what fraction of end-of-life patients have pressure ulcers?
   A. 1/4
   B. 1/3
   C. 1/2
   D. 2/3

2. You are treating a hospice patient who has a Stage III decubitus ulcer. Several days ago, the nurse caring for the patient notified you that the ulcer appeared infected, and a culture was ordered. The patient has now developed septicemia. What is the likelihood that the organism causing the septicemia is from the infected ulcer?
   A. 10%
   B. 25%
   C. 50%
   D. 70%

3. You are asked to examine an 80-year-old patient with terminal dementia who has a new pressure ulcer. When you examine the ulcer, you find that there is full-thickness tissue loss, and that the base of the ulcer is covered by an eschar. What would be the stage of this pressure ulcer?
   A. Stage I
   B. Stage II
   C. Stage III
   D. Stage IV
   E. Unstageable

4. Same patient as question 3. You decide to debride the wound to remove the eschar so it can be properly staged and treated. You choose the technique described as "autolytic" debridement. Which of the following best describes "autolytic" debridement?

A. Topically applied enzymes dissolve necrotic tissue
B. Macrophages and white blood cells self-digest necrotic tissue
C. Removal of necrotic tissue by irrigation and a damp to dry dressing
D. Dissection of necrotic tissue from the wound bed with a scalpel

5. An 85-year-old female with advanced dementia was recently admitted to your hospice program as she has recently become bedbound and can no longer communicate her needs. She has been eating only small amounts when fed and has lost 15% of her lean body weight in the last 6 months. The patient has an advance directive stating that she does not want to be fed artificially, and this desire is supported by the family. Her skin is currently intact, and the family is very concerned about the possibility that she will develop pressure ulcers in the future, and want everything done to prevent them. Which of the following would be the best way to prevent this patient from developing pressure ulcers?

A. Provide the patient with an air mattress
B. Have the patient turned approximately every 2 hours
C. Cleanse the skin daily with hot water and drying soaps
D. Convince the family to have a PEG tube placed for feeding

6. You are called by the hospice nurse for orders for an 82-year-old male with advanced dementia who has developed a skin tear that has a moderate amount of drainage. Which of the following treatment options should you order?

A. Zinc oxide paste dressing, covered with a nonconforming gauze
B. Nonadherent gauze dressing
C. Hydrocolloid with absorbent center or foam dressing
D. Transparent film dressing

7. You are caring for a 70-year-old male with advanced metastatic squamous cell carcinoma of the lung and advanced chronic obstructive pulmonary disease (COPD). The patient has a rather large metastatic lesion in the skin of the right upper leg that is fungating and malodorous. All of the following measures would be appropriate methods to control the odor of the fungating skin lesion EXCEPT

    A. Place a cotton ball saturated with oil of wintergreen in the patient's room
    B. Apply a charcoal pad over the dressing to absorb odor
    C. Place a scented dryer sheet over the air vent in the patient's room
    D. Spray air freshener in the patient's room

8. All of the following statements regarding the symptom of pruritus are true EXCEPT:

    A. When using oral anti-histamines in patients on opioids, there is an increased risk of drowsiness
    B. Moisturizing the skin is an essential part of the management of pruritus
    C. When using topical steroids, a cream is preferred over an ointment
    D. Topical menthol (0.5–2.0%) in aqueous cream can act as a mild anesthetic or counter-irritant

9. Recurrent cellulitis infections to the lower extremities are commonly due to which organism:

    A. Staphylococcus
    B. Streptococcus
    C. *Candida albicans*
    D. Herpes zoster

10. Treatment for xerostomia include all of the following EXCEPT:

    A. Chewing gum
    B. Rinse with an astringent mouthwash
    C. Sucking ice chips
    D. Frequent rinsing of the mouth with tap water

The Last Days: The Actively Dying Patient

Barry M. Kinzbrunner, Vincent D. Nguyen, and Jeanne Micklich Ash

INTRODUCTION

"There is an appointed time for everything, and a time for every affair under the heavens. A time to be born and a time to die."

Ecclesiastes 3:1–2

Death is inevitable; dying is the concluding stage of life and death. For many, especially those who work in the hospice and palliative care arenas, death is seen as part of life's natural cycle and often as an accepted friend. Just as one feels joy when embracing a newborn as it leaves its mother's womb, hospice and palliative care providers feel a sense of satisfaction when having the privilege of caring for a dying individual at the end of life.

Although the satisfaction that one experiences in caring for the terminally ill occurs throughout the course of a patient's final illness, it is perhaps greatest during the final days of the patient's life, when attention is specifically focused on ensuring patient comfort and dignity as that life draws to its inevitable conclusion. During the final days of life, patients and families are often confronted with a multitude of shifting emotions, from hope to despair, from fear to courage, from relief to guilt. For some patients and families, it is the first time that the realities of the dying process are recognized and acknowledged. End-of-life caregivers are equally challenged, often torn between attending to the ever-changing needs of the patients in their charge, while trying to support the patients' family through the final dying process.

In view of the special nature of the final days of life, this chapter focuses on the signs of impending death. It also offers contemporary palliative approaches to the most common challenging symptoms faced by the patients and families during the active-dying process.

THE CLINICAL SIGNS OF APPROACHING DEATH

Most patients die peacefully. The process is often described as a gentle withdrawing from the external stimuli and a slipping away into a very deep slumber. The multiple prominent cascading events that eventually occur before the patient's death will often include functional, cognitive, nutritional, and physical declines.

The actively dying process is divided into two phases, the "preactive phase," which begins around 7 to 14 days prior to death, and the active phase, which generally constitutes the last 2 to 3 days of life. The important clinical characteristics of each phase are outlined in Table 12–1, and described in detail below.

PREACTIVE PHASE

As patients enter the preactive phase of dying, they develop progressive weakness and lethargy, and become increasingly dependent on caregivers for the basic activities of daily living. Those patients who had previously been active are likely to become bedbound, and sleep occupies the majority of their time. Cognitively, patients may become progressively disoriented and their attention span is often limited. Some patients may withdraw from their surroundings while others may speak to external objects or persons that are not present. Restlessness is also not uncommon.

Regarding nutritional status, the combination of lack of interest in food and fluid and difficulty swallowing result in severely diminished oral intake. Not surprisingly, urine output is reduced, and the loss of involuntary muscle control may lead to incontinence of bowel and bladder of patients who had previously retained these functions.

TABLE 12–1. Characteristics of the Phases of the Active-Dying Process	
Preactive (7–14 d prior to death)	Weakness and lethargy
	Increased dependence on caregivers
	Bed bound status in formerly active patient
	Increased sleep
	Progressive disorientation
	Limited attention span or withdrawal
	Restlessness
	Decreased interest in food and fluid
	Difficulty swallowing
	Loss of bladder or bowel control in previously continent patient
Active (2–3 d prior to death)	Clouding of consciousness
	Decreased responsiveness to external stimuli
	Eyes glassy, pupils unfocused
	No interest in food or fluid
	Abnormal respiratory patterns
	Blood pressure and pulse difficult to obtain
	Hypotension
	Progressive cooling and mottling of extremities
	Terminal congestion
	"Surge of energy" during the period prior to death

ACTIVE PHASE

Patients are as unique in life as they are at the hours before their death. However, during the final phases of their dying process, patients will share similar clinical signs and symptoms. For example, patients generally remain in bed and lose any remaining interest in food or fluid. There is clouding of the consciousness, as the body no longer responds to external stimuli. The eyes may become glassy and the pupils appear to focus on unseen remote objects. The extremities, starting from the distal end, become progressively mottled, clammy, and cool to the touch. Blood pressure, heart sounds, and palpable pulses are often difficult to detect. Respiratory patterns can vary, from being slow, deep, and regular to more rapid and irregular. Upper and lower airway congestion is often apparent. Periods of apnea occur, and over time may progressively lengthen until breathing finally ceases.

It is not easy to predict the exact time of death based on the development of any particular signs or symptoms, as this process often varies from several hours to many days. It is well known that on occasion, for inexplicable reasons, some patients may have a transient improvement in physical, cognitive, or functional abilities during the dying process. Hospice and palliative care workers characterize this phenomenon as a "surge of energy." When this surge occurs, patients no longer appear to be imminently dying, instead, seem to have awakened from their deep sleep with a new sense of vitality. This transitory episode can last from hours to days before the patient returns to their previous dying state. This surge of energy often makes families and caregivers confused and distraught as they go through an "emotional roller coaster" of hope and despair. Sometimes, they will doubt that the patient is actually dying and may desire a shift to disease-directed interventions in the hope of reversing the patient's condition. It is important for the professional caregivers to assist the family in characterizing the temporary nature of this "surge" as a precious memento from the dying person to them. It should be explained to the family that any medical interventions made in an attempt to prolong this temporary phenomenon will not be beneficial, and may, in fact, be a painful and unnecessary intrusion on their loved one as life comes to an end.

As mentioned, however, most deaths are peaceful for the patient. The survivors often recall a nondramatic process. In a series of studies of dying patients, up to 98% of individuals died peacefully and 65% were peaceful 48 hours prior to death. However, in the final days, some patients may develop new symptoms or may experience a recurrence or an exacerbation of one or more previously well-controlled symptoms. Pain, restlessness, confusion, agitation, hallucinations,myoclonic jerks, seizures, hemorrhage, nausea, vomiting, shortness of breath, and dyspnea are common symptoms from which dying patients can suffer. Oftentimes, these symptoms can be terrifying for the witnessing friends and family members. The memories of the final moments will often linger in the mind and heart of the surviving members for many years to come. It is important, therefore, that health professionals know how to recognize and treat these terminal symptoms.

THE MANAGEMENT OF SYMPTOMS OF APPROACHING DEATH

PAIN MANAGEMENT AS LIFE CONCLUDES

The most important principle for pain management during the active-dying phase is that pain management practices employed in earlier stages do not change (see Chapter 6). Decreased levels of consciousness do not mean that earlier pain levels have lessened. Although there is some indication that metabolic changes induced by dehydration and diminished nutrition may have an analgesic effect, it cannot be assumed that pain abates as death approaches. In fact, pain during this stage of dying may actually increase. Therefore, pain management protocols established earlier in the course of the disease should be maintained.

The issues related to pain management during this final phase of life revolve around assessment, route of medication administration, an increased risk of opioid toxicity, fear of hastening death due to continued opioid administration, and opiate withdrawal in the patient whose pain has been managed by opioids.

Assessment

Fundamental to pain management is the need to identify pain etiology and provide interventions that relieve the source of pain. Pain assessment in the mentally alert and verbally responsive patient does not change. In evaluating the nonalert or nonverbal patient, however, the clinician may have to rely on visual signs such as facial grimacing and motor restlessness, and auditory cues such as moaning that may imply physical discomfort. To assist caregivers in caring for patients who may have pain and can no longer effectively communicate, various scales have been developed to objectify the various visual and auditory clues to discomfort observed. One of these, the FLACC Behavioral Scale, (see Figure 12–1) allows the caregiver to derive a pain severity score by observing the patient's facial expressions (F), leg movements (L), overall bodily activity (A), whether or not they are crying (C), and whether or not they can be consoled or comforted (C).

As patients enter the actively dying phase of their illnesses, caregivers and health care professionals have often observed pain with movement of the patient. This pain has been variously

FLACC Behavioral Scale

Categories	Scoring		
	0	**1**	**2**
Face	No particular expression or smile	Occasional grimace or frown, withdrawn, disinterested	Frequent to constant frown, clenched jaw, quivering chin
Legs	Normal position or relaxed	Uneasy, restless, tense	Kicking, or legs drawn up
Activity	Lying quietly, normal position, moves easily	Squirming, shifting back and forth, tense	Arched, rigid, or jerking
Cry	No cry (awake or asleep)	Moans or whimpers, occasional complaint	Crying steadily, screams or sobs, frequent complaints
Consolability	Content, relaxed	Reassured by occasional touching, hugging, or being talked to, distractable	Difficult to console or comfort
Each of the five categories (F) Face; (L) Legs; (A) Activity; (C) Cry; (C) Consolability is scored from 0 to 2, which results in a total score between 0 and 10.			

Figure 12–1. FLACC behavioral scale. To use the FLACC scale, the total points are added. The sum of 0 to 10 is the score used to assess the severity of the pain and guide the clinician to a choice of therapies. (Reproduced, with permission, from Merkel S, Voepel-Lewis T, Shayevitz J, Malviya S. The FLACC: A behavioral scale for scoring postoperative pain in young children. *Pediatr Nurs* 23:293–297, 1997.) © 2002, The Regents of the University of Michigan. All Rights reserved.

described as "disturbance pain" and as "incident pain." This type of episodic pain is brief in duration and apparently occurs when the patient is moved or disturbed. The patient may cry out, moan, or grimace. It is probably attributable to the stiffness that occurs with immobility, although researchers have described it as an "alarm response" that is particularly evident in the blind, deaf, and confused.

This type of pain can be a source of distress for the family or caregiver who may feel that they are causing their loved one extreme discomfort by touching them. It is therefore essential to teach the family and caregivers to expect this type of response and to ensure that they are comfortable with moving the patient. To this end, the patient caregivers must receive appropriate instruction in positioning techniques. Family communication with the patient should be en-

couraged even in the nonresponsive patient. Management of disturbance pain includes explaining procedures and treatments carefully before performing them in addition to deliberate, careful, and planned movement of the patient. For prolonged manipulation of the patient or when performing certain treatments (i.e., wound care or Foley catheter insertion), the patient should be premedicated with a short-acting analgesic, such as liquid morphine, approximately half an hour prior to such activities.

Other common causes of physical discomfort during the final days of life may relate to the genitourinary and gastrointestinal tracts as well as the integument and musculoskeletal systems. Urinary retention leading to a distended bladder or promoting infection can cause pain. Constipation can occur and be painful, and is complicated by the fact that many caregivers believe that with a lack of food intake, patients need not move their bowels. There is an increased incidence of pressure ulcers due to the immobility and incontinence associated with the last days of life. Although analgesics may be important in managing these symptoms, it is important to remember that interventions may also be nonpharmacologic in nature. Proper skin care, positioning, gentle range of motion, placement of a Foley catheter for bladder drainage, and maintenance of a bowel program are all examples of approaches that can increase comfort and decrease pain in the dying patient.

Routes of Medication Administration

ORAL ROUTE In certain cases, the oral route remains the optimal choice for the administration of pain medication at this stage of life. A concentrated form of liquid morphine or oxycodone (20 mg/mL), administered every 4 hours (or more often if needed), can be used safely, noninvasively, and effectively. These medications are actually given by placing the liquid medication in the sublingual or buccal space, leading to the mistaken belief by many caregivers that these medications are actually being absorbed directly through the mucosa. However, our best understanding about the absorption of sublingually administered liquid morphine and oxycodone suggests that these two opioids are actually absorbed in the gastrointestinal tract after they trickle past the pharynx. Fentanyl is the only orally available opioid analgesics that is truly absorbed sublingually and transmucosally (see discussion on the Oral Transmucosal Route below). By anecdotal reports, these orally administered medications do not appear to contribute to symptomatic aspiration when given in small amounts. This is especially true for those patients requiring less than 120 mg a day of concentrated liquid oral morphine or oxycodone.

RECTAL ROUTE In the patient with less than a few days left to live, the rectal route is an effective alternative, provided there is a willing caregiver who is comfortable medicating the patient via this route. Morphine and hydromorphone are the most common choices since they are readily available in suppository forms.

Absorption of rectally administered opioids can be affected by the presence of stool in the rectal vault, and defecation before complete absorption of the suppository can result in unreliable pain relief. Absorption and plasma levels of rectally administered opioids may differ from equivalent oral doses because the first-pass effect is diminished in rectal administration, although for most patients the ratio of oral to rectal opioid is 1:1. Careful assessment of level of consciousness, pain-related behaviors, and patient self-report of effectiveness, when possible, must be used to determine the efficacy of substituting the rectal for the oral route for pain medication delivery.

Continuous-release morphine and oxycodone preparations have been used as suppositories for rectal administration. On the basis of anecdotal reports, these are effective in sustaining patients' comfort, provided that the opioid suppositories are left in place. Theoretically, the vascular supply in the rectum is adequate for medication absorption, but there has been little research comparing the oral versus the rectal use of oral sustained release compounds in terms of efficacy, plasma levels, and absorption.

The rectal route is especially useful for patients experiencing nausea and vomiting, and in those with partial or complete bowel obstructions. However, the rectal route cannot be used for long periods of time because it will cause discomfort from the irritation of rectal mucosa. In the presence of diarrhea, hemorrhoids, anal fissures, and neutropenia, the rectal route must be avoided or its use considered carefully. In these instances, other modes of administration may be more suitable.

ORAL TRANSMUCOSAL ROUTE Fentanyl is lipophilic (lipid soluble), making it an ideal candidate for oral transmucosal use. There are two commercially available products, both primarily indicated for the treatment of breakthrough pain in patients already being treated with opioids. One, known as Actiq, incorporates fentanyl citrate into a lozenge that is on a stick resembling a "lollypop," and called an "oralet." This "oralet" is then placed in or rubbed against the buccal area for 15 minutes, where it dissolves and is absorbed into the bloodstream. Fentanyl delivered transmucosally in this manner is reported to provide pain relief in 5 to 10 minutes. It must be noted that only 25% of the medication is actually absorbed through the mucosa, while the remaining 75% of the medication is swallowed and is absorbed through the gastrointestinal (GI) tract.

The second product, known as Fentora, is a fentanyl buccal tablet, which is placed in the buccal cavity and is left to dissolve over a 15-minute time span. Approximately 50% of the medication is actually absorbed transmucosally, while the remaining 50% is swallowed and absorbed through the GI tract. Given the fact that these agents are not cost-effective when compared with concentrated liquid morphine, and with half to three-quarters of the active medication needing to be swallowed (just like the concentrated liquid morphine), it would appear that these agents do not have any significant advantage over concentrated liquid morphine in the management of pain in the actively dying and that their role in this setting should be extremely limited. Further discussion of these agents can be found in Chapter 6.

TRANSDERMAL ROUTE Patient whose pain has been adequately managed by transdermal fentanyl should continue to use this medication during the last hours of life. However, transdermal fentanyl by itself is seldom the drug or route of choice to initiate in the actively dying patient. Transdermal fentanyl takes approximately 12 to 24 hours to reach peak plasma levels, so that the patient would have to use other additional means of pain management until peak blood levels are reached. The other drawback to using this method is that rapid titration is difficult. For further discussion of the use of transdermal fentanyl, see Chapter 6.

PARENTERAL ROUTES Although noninvasive routes of administration are generally preferable, especially when the patient only has a short time to live, there may be times when it is necessary to provide analgesia via a parenteral route. For patients with an already existing venous access site, the intravenous (IV) route would be most appropriate, while for the majority of patients, in which no indwelling IV line is present, the subcutaneous route has been found to be an effective delivery system.

Subcutaneous Route A continuous subcutaneous infusion with bolus doses for breakthrough pain has been shown to provide good pain relief during the final stages of life, with stable blood levels and the ability for rapid titration. The subcutaneous route compares favorably with the IV route in terms of efficacy and plasma levels without the complexities inherent in an IV delivery system.

Although morphine may be used for subcutaneous pain management, hydromorphone may actually be a preferable agent, as it provides comparable pain relief and has the advantage of higher potency and concentration capabilities than morphine, meaning it can be delivered in a lesser volume. This is especially valuable for those patients who require substantial amounts of opioids to adequately manage pain. Methadone, fentanyl, and diamorphone may also be administered subcutaneously. Although administration of methadone by this route has been reported to cause significant cutaneous adverse reactions such as induration and erythema, these have been reported to be minimized by frequent site changes or concurrent use of dexamethasone or hyaluronidase. Two recent case reports also demonstrate that skin toxicity may be avoided by giving the methadone via a hypodermoclysis line. Fentanyl has also been reported in some case reports to be effective when administered subcutaneously, although little research has been conducted on its pharmacokinetics during administration. Diamorphone, which, like hydromorphone, has a higher potency and can be given in smaller volumes of fluid, is unavailable in the United States.

The biggest drawback to subcutaneous infusions for pain management is the limited volume that subcutaneous tissue can absorb without creating discomfort or side effects such as tissue damage. Subcutaneous tissue can absorb only approximately 2 to 3 mL/h, although the use of hyaluronidase can significantly increase the capacity of the subcutaneous tissue to absorb fluid (see Hydration During the Last Days of Life below).

Discomfort from needle placement is rarely an issue for this route. Butterfly needles are typically used, although there are also specialized needles designed specifically for subcutaneous infusion delivery. Typical subcutaneous infusion protocols call for needle and site changes every 72 hours to minimize the chance of infection and to promote fluid absorption.

For pain management by subcutaneous infusion to be effective, the patient must have adequate subcutaneous tissue. This means that cachectic patients are not ideal candidates for this method of pain management. Conversely, the grossly edematous patient is also not a good candidate for pain management via subcutaneous infusion. For immunosuppressed patients and those with coagulopathies, subcutaneous infusions must be carefully weighed against other choices since the possibility of side effects will increase.

Intravenous Route   IV pain management is very effective in providing stable plasma levels, rapid titration, and bolus dosing for breakthrough pain. Medications used in subcutaneous infusion can likewise be used for the IV administration. For the patient with a functional central venous access device, this route is an ideal alternative. It is often the route of choice when large volumes of opioids are necessary to maintain pain control. In the absence of a central line or port, particularly during the last hours of life, venous access may often be difficult and often illogical. The use of the subcutaneous route is frequently the better alternative.

Opioid Toxicity

As patients actively approach death, renal function tends to decline rapidly, increasing the risk for the accumulation of opioid metabolites that may be neurotoxic, resulting in a much greater risk of opioid toxicity. This most commonly man-

ifests in symptoms of opioid-induced delirium or myoclonus. Therefore, when patients being treated with opioids are actively moving toward life's end and these symptoms occur, opioid toxicity should be considered high on the list of possible causes. If a patient is not at a point where death is imminent, one should contemplate attempting to improve the situation by opioid rotation and/or subcutaneous hydration. If the patient is very close to death, then symptomatic treatment with haloperidol or risperidone for delirium or benzodiazepines for myoclonus may be the best alternatives. See Chapter 6 for further discussion of the management of opioid toxicity.

Fear of Premature Death

As discussed in Chapter 6, fear of causing premature death with administration of opioid analgesics is major barrier to good pain management. Even when patients nearing the end of life have been treated with opioids for pain control for prolonged periods of time, alterations in levels of consciousness and other changes that herald impending death are often interpreted by family members as being caused by the analgesics. As a reaction to this, family members may be unwilling to give the patient scheduled analgesic medication or request the professional caregiver to stop the medication. The holding of opioids in this setting has also been anecdotally described in hospital settings, although perhaps less frequently than in the past due to improvement in end-of-life care education among health care workers. As discussed in Chapter 6, these fears are for the most part unfounded, families should be reassured, and analgesics should be continued. If families are insistent that medication be held, administration of at least a small amount of opioid analgesic is advisable to prevent the unpleasant complications of opioid withdrawal.

Opioid Withdrawal

Suspending the use of opioids in patients whose pain has been controlled will result in recurrent pain as well as distressing withdrawal symptoms (i.e., restlessness, agitation, tremors, or seizures).

Withdrawal symptoms occur in patients taking oral medications and who become less responsive as death approaches and, therefore, are unable to swallow large quantities of oral medications, or, as described above, when medication is held by family or other caregivers for fear that it is causing the patient's premature demise. For patients unable to swallow, another route of opioid administration (i.e., rectal, subcutaneous, or IV) can be chosen to maintain controlled levels. Alternatively, as discussed above, pain control can be maintained and withdrawal symptoms can be avoided by treating patients with concentrated morphine or oxycodone preparations (20 mg/mL) into the sublingual or buccal space (where it is then swallowed). When there is fear of premature death or concern that a patient's altered level of consciousness is secondary to the opioid it is important that the patient receive at least 25% of the original opioid dose in order to avoid withdrawal symptoms.

DYSPNEA

Dyspnea is an uncomfortable awareness of breathlessness associated with shortness of breath. It is one of the most frequent and terrifying symptoms in the last days of a patient's life. Dyspnea may manifest as copious secretions, cough, fatigue, air hunger, anxiety, agitation, tachypnea, and/or chest pain. Some data suggest that dyspnea occurs in up to 70% of dying people, with the highest incidence in those with lung cancer, head and neck cancer, and degenerative neurological diseases.

Terminal dyspnea is often multifactorial, and it is rarely possible to treat the underlying cause of dyspnea during the final stage of life. Therefore, the treatment goal is aimed at relieving the perception of breathlessness and associated symptoms. Interventions that may be effective in the treatment of dyspnea in the last days of life are listed in Table 12–2.

TABLE 12–2. Treatment of Dyspnea During the Last Days of Life

NONPHARMACOLOGIC	INTERVENTION		
	Presence of caregiver		
	Soothing calm voice		
	Gentle touch		
	Relaxation techniques		
	Circulation of air by the use of a fan or opening a window		
	Oxygen		

PHARMACOLOGIC	MEDICATION	ROUTE OF ADMINISTRATION	DOSE
Benzodiazepines	Lorazepam	Oral, parenteral	0.5–2 mg q 4 h PM
	Alprazolam	Oral	0.25–2 mg q 4 h PM
	Diazepam	Oral, parenteral	2–20 mg q 4 h PM
Phenothiazines	Chlorpromazine	Oral, rectal, parenteral	30–100 mg q 4 h PM
	Thioridazine	Oral, parenteral	30–100 mg q 4 h PM
Opioids	Morphine	Oral*	5–10 mg q 2–4 h PM
		Parenteral*	2–5 mg q 2–4 h PM
		Already on opioids	Increase dose 50% over baseline
		Nebulized	5–20 mg q 4 h PM

*Opioid naïve patient.

Nonpharmacologically strategies include having the presence of a caregiver, a soothing calm voice, and added gentle touch to induce relaxation and relieve apprehension, especially when dyspnea is related to anxiety. In some circumstances, the use of a fan or opening of a window allows a cool draft of air to reach the cheek and nasal cavity that can be useful in relieving dyspnea because the perception of breathlessness is thought to be altered by stimulation of the areas innervated by the trigeminal nerve. A simple fan generally acts as well and provides as much relief as oxygen provided by nasal cannula. Oxygen may provide symptomatic relief for some patients, although whatever meager evidence there is in the literature suggests that it mainly benefits patients who are hypoxemic. Patients with cyanosis may benefit from the use of noninvasive, positive-pressure facemasks.

Pharmacologic strategies are usually part and parcel of the management of dyspnea during the dying process. Although bronchodilators (β_2-agonists and xanthines) and steroids may be effective treatments for those with airway obstruction and inflammation, especially earlier in the course of illness, respiratory sedatives such as the benzodiazepines, phenothiazines, and opioids are the mainstay of pharmacotherapy when patient are very close to death. (See Table 12–2 for appropriate dosing information.) They may be used alone or in conjunction with bronchodilators and steroids for added potency.

Opioids, in particular morphine sulfate, have an established role in the treatment of dyspnea by suppressing respiratory awareness and at the same time improve the efficiency of breathing. In relative "healthy" patients, morphine has been shown to improve exercise endurance. The precise mechanism for this is still unknown.

The overemphasized fear of potential for respiratory depression and hastening death has caused many health care professionals to withhold morphine for the treatment of dyspnea, especially for patients with lung pathology (i.e., COPD, lung cancer). This concern is not justified, and thus morphine should not be withheld. Rather, the dose should be titrated against the respiratory rate to achieve a rate of 12 to 20 per minute. For those patients already using opioids for pain control, a dose increase of 50% is needed to achieve adequate respiratory control. The route of delivery often recommended is oral; however, the subcutaneous (SQ), IV, and most recently the nebulized form are routes of delivery used to treat dyspnea in the last days of life.

The rationale for using nebulized morphine is based on the fact that opioid receptors have been found in the bronchial trees and along the sensory fibers of the vagus nerve. When effective, nebulized morphine works quickly, with initial onset of action on dyspnea occurring in 2 to 5 minutes. Additionally, morphine is very poorly absorbed through the lung, making this route of administrative especially attractive when there is concern about systemic opioid toxicity. Morphine solution, prepared for either parenteral or oral use, diluted in 2 cc of normal saline (NS) solution, at a starting dose of 5 to 10 mg every 4 hours as needed, is recommended for administration via the nebulized route. The most common side effect is bronchospasm; thus, the first treatment should be administered in a controlled setting.

Studies evaluating the efficacy of nebulized morphine in the treatment of dyspnea are mixed. A meta-analysis of nine studies on the efficacy of nebulized morphine in the treatment of dyspnea in patients with advanced chronic lung disease did not provide sufficient evidence to support the use of nebulized morphine in that population (Brown et al., 2005). In palliative care patients, however, a recent study by Bruera et al. (2005b) showed that nebulized morphine was as effective as SQ morphine in relieving dyspnea in 11 patients who were studied in a double-blind cross-over fashion. Although, due to the small sample size, further studies were recommended, this study, as well as scattered case reports in the medical literature, provide some support to the utilization of nebulized morphine in the management of terminal dyspnea.

When dyspnea during the active phase of dying cannot be controlled by any of the interventions already described, palliative sedation should be considered. This technique is discussed below.

TERMINAL CONGESTION (DEATH RATTLE)

Terminal congestion, exhibited by noisy moist breathing or "rattling", is commonly observed in patients nearing death. Although patients are not often troubled by it, the noise is often a source of distress to the family and caregivers.

This congestion, also known as the "death rattle," can simply be described as a collection of oscillating mucous secretion in the oropharynx and trachea during inspiration and expiration of the dying patient who is unable to clear the secretion. With empathetic explanation and assurance, positioning, and judicious usage of anticholinergic medication and occasional gentle aspiration of the secretion, this symptom can often be palliated. Hyoscyamine sulfate, atropine sulfate, glycopyrrolate, and scopolamine have been recommended and are available in oral, SQ and transdermal forms. As most patients experiencing terminal congestion are unable to swallow, liquid forms of hyoscyamine and glycopyrrolate, as well as atropine ophthalmic drops are often administered via the sub-lingual (SL) route, and have been observed to be effective. (See Table 12–3 for appropriate dosing information.) When utilizing any of these agents, one must be alert to the potential for significant anticholinergic side-

effects, most notably, the onset or exacerbation of delirium. Although delirium in this population is multi-factorial, the potential contribution of these agents should not be overlooked. (The management of Terminal Delirium is discussed further below, and full discussion of the topic can be found in Chapter 10.) Suctioning should be avoided whenever possible, and only used as an intervention of last resort.

It is important to note that this type of moist respiration is different from congestion related to pulmonary edema. Anticholinergics will have minimal to no effect in reducing congestion related to cardiac failure. Morphine and gentle diuresis with furosemide or bumetanide in these cases are often required.

XEROSTOMIA

It is believed by some that xerostomia (dry mouth) is a major cause of discomfort at the end of life, and is a primary reason for the desire to administer parenteral fluids to patients who have no fluid intake in the last days of life (see below). With fastidious oral care, however, discomfort from xerostomia can be relieved, obviating the need for fluids. Appropriate oral-care treatments include: (1) cleansing and swabbing the oral cavity with peroxide and water or glycerin swabs, (2) lubricating the oral mucosa by offering sips of liquid or using a spray bottle, (3) using

TABLE 12–3. Treatment of Terminal Congestion During the Last Days of Life

MEDICATION	ROUTE OF ADMINISTRATION	DOSE
Hyoscyamine	Oral, SL (liquid)	0.125–0.25 mg q 4 h PM
Atropine	Oral, SL (ophthalmic solution)	1–2% drops q 3 h PM
	Parenteral	0.4 mg q 1–2 h PM
Glycopyrrolate	Oral, SL (liquid)	1–2 mg q 4 h PM
	Parenteral	0.1–0.2 mg q 4 h PM
		0.4–1.2 mg/d by cont. infusion
Scopolamine	Transdermal	1 patch q3d

TABLE 12–4. Treatment of Confusion, Agitation, and Terminal Delirium During the Last Days of Life

MEDICATION	ROUTE OF ADMINISTRATION	DOSE
Lorazepam	Oral, parenteral	1–2 mg q 4 h PM
Chlorpromazine	Oral, parenteral	25–50 mg q 4 h PM
Haloperidol	Oral, parenteral	1–2 mg q 4 h PM
Risperidone	Oral	0.5–1 mg 1–2 times per day

saliva substitutes, (4) application of moisturizer or petroleum jelly to the lips, and (5) administration of vitamin C, lemon drops, or pilocarpine to stimulate salivary flow. (See Chapter 11 for further discussion of xerostomia).

CONFUSION, AGITATION, AND TERMINAL DELIRIUM

Confusion occurs in up to 10% of patients during the last hours of life. The spectrum of presentation can often be quite dramatic ranging from disorientation, to physical restlessness and agitation, to frank delirium. The causes of confusion include environmental changes, anxiety, pain or generalized physical discomfort, constipation or a distended bladder, dehydration, electrolyte imbalance, infection, and medications. (A full discussion of delirium can be found in Chapter 10.)

Treatment of confusion, agitation, and terminal delirium should begin by assessing and treating any correctable causes. Nonpharmacologic measures such as appropriate hygiene, positioning, calm reassurance, and keeping the room temperature at a comfortable setting should all be addressed. Eliminating unnecessary medications is also of great importance. As dehydration is often a major contributing factor to terminal agitation delirium, the question of providing patients with parenteral hydration, even when close to death, continues to be debated among hospice and palliative medicine professionals. (This will be discussed further below.) If there is no improvement in symptoms despite any efforts to treat correctable causes based on the patient's short-term prognosis and goals of care, medications are often required. For milder symptoms, benzodiazepines such as lorazepam, or phenothiazines such as chlorpromazine, are often used. When the agitation is more severe, or there is frank delirium, haloperidol or one of the atypical antipsychotics, such as risperidone may be required. (See Table 12–4) If symptoms are still not controlled, then palliative sedation may need to be considered (see below).

HEMORRHAGE

Occasionally, patients will develop uncontrolled hemorrhage as a terminal event. Although only seen in 6% to 10% of dying cancer patients, and a small percentage of hospice and palliative care patients with nonmalignant terminal illnesses (i.e., massive bleeding from esophageal varices secondary to end-stage cirrhosis of the liver with portal hypertension), this type of death, although not usually causing the patient any physical pain, can be emotionally devastating and extremely distressing to families, as well as to patients who are conscious and aware during the event.

In some patients at high risk for hemorrhage as the terminal event, there initially may be a period of chronic bleeding, during which attempts at control through the use of hemostatic dressings, and, if patients have a reasonable short-term prognosis, various invasive interventions described in Chapter 18 or radiation therapy described in Chapter 19, may be considered. However, whether there is chronic bleeding or not,

TABLE 12–5. Recommended Interventions for Uncontrolled Hemorrhage

- Cover the area with dark colored (i.e., blue or green) towels to limit visual exposure of the blood
- Keep the area as clean as possible
- Speak calmly and reassure the patient that he or she is not alone
- If patient is awake and distressed, consider sedation with a fast-acting sedative
- Provide support to family members

SOURCE: National Cancer Institute: Last Days of Life (PDQ®): Care during the final hours. http://www.cancer.gov/cancertopics/pdq/supportivecare/lasthours/HealthProfessional/page3. Modified September 3, 2009. Accessed September 9, 2009.

when patients who are at high risk for hemorrhage are identified, they and their families should be counseled and prepared for the possibility that this will occur.

Recommended interventions for uncontrolled hemorrhage can be found in Table 12–5. It is important to cover the area with dark towels to minimize visual exposure of the blood, which may be distressing to patients and family members. The area should also be cleaned quickly and frequently as blood often produces a distinctive foul odor. Speak calmly and reassure the patient that he or she is not alone. If patients are awake and aware and appear to be significantly distressed, sedating the patient may be considered, with midazolam being recommended because of its fast onset of action. Due to the extreme distress this causes to family members as well, they also need a great deal of attention and support from the end-of-life care professionals during this time.

HYDRATION DURING THE LAST DAYS OF LIFE

Despite the lack of evidence that artificial hydration is of significant benefit to patients near the end of life (see Chapter 24 for more discussion), families and medical professionals alike often feel compelled to provide fluids during the patients last days. There are many reasons. For the families, it may seem to be the loving thing to do. For the clinicians, it is basic "standard" medical care; to withhold or discontinue fluids seems like a break in the sacred bond of the patient–physician relationship. The implications of allowing a person to die from dehydration and/or starvation may be perceived as acts of omission on the physician's part. Thus, for all parties involved, withholding the ever so available medical therapeutic interventions of parenteral fluids may lead to guilt, frustration, and "loss of control" over death.

Another major reason why physician and families want to give fluids to dying patients is the notion that death by dehydration will cause pain and suffering. This suffering has been hypothesized to be caused by thirst, dry mouth, fatigue, lethargy, nausea, vomiting, confusion, and restlessness, as well as an increased risk of bedsores and constipation. In the presence of renal failure and accumulation of opioid metabolites, confusion, myoclonus, seizures, muscle cramping, and hastening of death may occur. Electrolyte imbalance, such as hypernatremia, may develop and cause confusion, weakness, lethargy, and eventual progression to obtundation, coma, and death.

However, several studies have examined the issue of pain and suffering and dehydration in the dying patients and have refuted some of the concern. Dehydration does not cause pain or discomfort because during dehydration, ketones are produced and serve as a natural anesthetic and euphorant. Ketones also cause a decreasing level of consciousness. Further, patients in end-state dehydration appear to experience less discomfort than do those receiving medical hydration.

Adverse effects of parenteral fluids are exhaustively long and include: repetitive venipuncture from infiltration or self-removal, decreased patient mobility, congestion, increased respiratory secretions and pleural effusion that leads to coughing, and the common distressing signs of choking and drowning. Further adverse effects include: fluid overload with resulting signs and symptoms of CHF (congestive heart failure); increased risk for intra-abdominal ascites;

increased urinary output that can contribute to skin breakdown, which may lessen if an invasive urinary catheter is placed; increased GI fluid that leads to an increased incidence of nausea and vomiting that may require a nasogastric tube (NGT) to suction for relief; increased peripheral edema which leads to an increased risk of pressure ulcers; increased tumor growth; and increased symptoms related to tumor size. Therefore, the many adverse affects if IV fluids and a lack of data suggesting that dehydration causes pain or discomfort for dying patients has led most experts in palliative care to continue to not recommend fluids by the IV route to prevent dehydration.

Hypodermoclysis

Hypodermoclysis (HDC) is a technique by which parenteral fluids are provided by SQ infusion, eliminating many of the logistic challenges that make providing IV fluids so challenging in end-of-life care. (Further discussion of HDC can be found in Chapter 24.)

In the last days of life, hydration by HDC may be provided via a continuous 24-hour infusion at 40 cc an hour, a 12-hour infusion at 80 cc an hour, or 3 times a day in 500 cc boluses over one hour each. The recommended solution used should contain electrolytes (i.e., NS or two-thirds 5% dextrose and one-third saline), since nonelectrolyte solutions (i.e., D5W) tend to draw fluid into the interstitial space that can lead to edema and swelling, and cause tissue sloughing. Hyaluronidase, 150 U per liter of solution or prior to the first of the three 500 cc infusions, is added to facilitate fluid absorption.

In a study using HDC, researchers found the majority of patients tolerated the procedure well. If the needle was placed properly, patients did not have any discomfort and some were not aware of the needle's presence. Needles used to administer fluids and medications are butterfly needles and Teflon cannula. The average duration of SQ sites using butterfly needles is 5.3 days versus 11.9 days using a Teflon cannula. The cannula however is reported to be 10 times the cost of the butterfly needles.

The ease and availability of providing hypodermoclysis to patients near the end of life has allowed hospice and palliative care providers to meet the needs of patients who are close to death and who have symptoms such as delirium or opioid toxicity that might improve with judicious hydration. Patients and families from diverse cultural, ethnic, or religious background who believe that hydration must be provided even when someone is approaching death can have those beliefs respected in a safe and appropriate fashion, without significant risk of the effects of fluid overload that often accompanied more traditional IV fluid replacement. Finally, the ease of administration of fluids by hypodermoclysis has raised the question among many palliative care clinicians as to whether the majority of patients should receive fluids as death approaches to reduce the risk of the more unpleasant effects of dehydration, most specifically, terminal agitation and delirium.

As already discussed in Chapter 10, a study by Bruera et al. (2005a) reported that a statistically significant percentage of patients receiving 2 days of hydration by hypodermoclysis had improvement in symptoms of myoclonus and sedation when compared with a group of patients treated with a placebo control. Hallucinations, one of the hallmark symptoms of delirium, improved in a higher percentage of hydrated patients than placebo patients, but the difference was not statistically significant. Although the primary conclusion of the investigation was that more studies needed to be performed, the study was not specifically designed to evaluate the use of hypodermoclysis to hydrate patients who were actively dying. Therefore, regarding this population of patients, no conclusion can be drawn, and decisions to hydrate patients who are in the dying phases of their illness should continue to be individualized based on patient symptoms and goals of care.

Proctoclysis

The use of proctoclysis, fluid administration via the rectal route, has been described in the literature and appears to be an alternative safe method for administering fluids. This mode of

TABLE 12–6. Palliative Sedation During the Last Days of Life

CLASS OF MEDICATION	MEDICATION	ROUTE OF ADMINISTRATION	DOSE
Barbiturates	Phenobarbital	Rectal	30–60 mg q 4 h
	Pentobarbital	Rectal	2–6 mg/kg q 4 h
		Parenteral	2.5 mg/kg q 15 min
Benzodiazepines	Diazepam	Rectal (gel)	10–20 mg q 4 h
	Midazolam	Parenteral	0.02–0.1 mg/kg/h
Anesthetics	Ketamine	Parenteral	0.1–0.5 mg/kg/h
	Propofol	Parenteral	1 mg/kg bolus; 0.05–0.1 mg/kg/min

administration is based on the fact that fluid absorption occurs after enemas in normal volunteers. Although most patients would prefer the SQ route, the proctoclysis technique is an effective means of hydrating patients who are unable to receive fluid by any other route—provided there is no tumor involvement of the colon.

Proctoclysis requires the insertion of a 22 French naso-gastric tube 40 cm into the rectum. NS or tap water can be administered at 100 to 400 cc an hour four to five times a day. The two most common side effects are leakage and tenesmus (spasm of anal sphincter).

PALLIATIVE SEDATION FOR THE ACTIVELY DYING PATIENT

The cardinal goal of medicine in caring for the dying is the relief of distressing symptoms and physical suffering. This obligation often brings about quandaries for physicians caring for those dying patients whose symptoms are recalcitrant to the aforementioned interventions and who require sedation to obtain symptom relief.

The ethical issues surrounding palliative sedation are discussed in Chapter 23. Suffice it to say that for patients who are actively dying and who have symptoms refractory to accepted palliative interventions, palliative sedation can be reasonably viewed as another treatment option geared at symptom control.

Refractory symptoms that may require sedation in the actively dying phase include intractable pain, dyspnea, agitated delirium, multifocal myoclonus, hemorrhage, and intractable emesis. It is crucial, however, when considering patients for palliative sedation, that all appropriate and reasonable therapeutic options have been considered or attempted prior to deciding to sedate the patient.

For patients already using opioids for pain and respiratory management, the dose of opioids can be titrated to the point of sedation. If the patient is not receiving opioids, is refractory to dosage escalation, or has developed neuroexcitatory side effects such as myoclonus or agitated delirium (which may be contributing to the decision to sedate the patient) the addition and titration of anesthetics, barbiturates, benzodiazepines, or phenothiazines have been effectively used. (See Table 12–6 for recommended agents and dosing information.)

CAREGIVER SUPPORT

Death rarely occurs as it is depicted on television. The actual period immediately preceding death is in reality, an evanescent phase—the dying individual gradually "fades" away. During this period, families and caregivers need information, emotional support, and concrete assistance with the physical as well as bureaucratic burdens that accompany death.

INFORMATION AND EDUCATION

First and foremost, family members need to be told that death is approaching and given a general idea as to how soon it will occur. Time frames can be given to families using "days versus weeks" or "hours versus days" types of terminology to give them an idea of when death is most likely to occur. Although it is often difficult for health care providers to predict exactly when death will occur, the signs and symptoms that signal approaching death are easily identified. The need to identify impending death is important because most patients and family members need the emotional closure of being able to say "goodbye." Family members and caregivers should be advised that an unresponsive patient might still be able to hear and comprehend.

Education as to what to expect during this phase should be given to the family at this time. Caregivers will require instruction regarding what to anticipate, physical care needs of their loved one, interventions to control expected symptoms, and medication administration. Families may need assistance with physical care on an intermittent or full time basis during this time of physical and emotional distress. This assistance can be provided via hospice or palliative care team, hired caregivers, and family and friends.

EMOTIONAL SUPPORT

It goes without saying that patients, family members, and caregivers will require increased emotional support as death approaches. The hours before death will probably be intensely emotional for the family, and will be remembered long after the patient has died. Managing symptoms around the time of death will visibly reduce patient suffering, thereby providing families and caregivers with positive memories during bereavement. Pa-

tients, families, and caregivers should be reassured that events are proceeding as expected, that the patient is comfortable, and that they are "doing the right thing" by allowing the patient to die in the chosen environment. Positive reinforcement regarding the caregiving efforts of family members should be given freely and often. Guilt at wishing for the patient's death, for example, needs to be addressed by assuring the family that it is natural to wish for an end to the patient's suffering and family turmoil that often surrounds death. Survivors often take comfort in the fact that they have provided hands-on care to their loved ones in the last days.

SPIRITUALITY

Spirituality is an individual concept. Patients and families may or may not welcome spiritual support as their loved one enters the last phase of life. It should, however, be offered with the emphasis that chaplain services are focused on spiritual issues and concerns of the patient and family, whatever those concerns and issues may be. The chaplain, in conjunction with the assistance of a social worker, can also provide structured emotional support and concrete assistance with funeral, mortuary, cremation, and burial services. Planning the final arrangements for the patient in advance will greatly assist in decreasing emotional turmoil at the time of death.

TIME OF DEATH

Families react in various ways at the time of death, often dictated by cultural or ethnic behavioral norms or expectations. These are so variable as to be beyond the scope of this discussion. What is important is for end-of-life care providers to be empathetic, understanding, and available to support the family through this period. Be sure that the body of the deceased is treated with the appropriate care and dignity, and that any cultural or religious customs are observed as requested by the family. Allow family members private time with the body, if desired, and reinforce the idea that the care they gave their loved one was appropriate and proper. If a family member gave a dose of sedating medication shortly before death, reassure the individual that the medication was not what ended the patient's life. Assist the family in calling the funeral home or other authorities if necessary.

TOWARD DEATH WITH DIGNITY

Death is an expected event that can be a positive experience for the survivors and a comfortable one for the dying person. By combining consistencies in the delivery of care to our patients and families, compassion balanced by rigorous scientific facts, knowledge, and skill, we can ensure that our patients will die a dignified and peaceful death. The last days of life need not be terrible, painful, or lonely, but rather an opportunity for growth, remembrance, and closure.

BIBLIOGRAPHY

AMA Council on Scientific Affairs: Good care of the dying patient [Council Report]. *JAMA* 275:474-478, 1996.

American Society of Clinical Oncology: Cancer care during the last phase of life. *J Clinic Oncol* 16:1986-1996, 1998.

Appleton M: Hospice medicine: A different perspective. *Am J Hospice Palliat Care* 13:7-9, 1996.

Baumrucker SJ: Management of intestinal obstruction in hospice care. *Am J Hosp Palliat Care* 15:232-235, 1998.

Baydur A: Nebulized morphine: A convenient and safe alternative to dyspnea relief? *Chest* 125:363-365, 2004.

Bennett M, Lucas V, Brennan M, et al: Using antimuscarinic drugs in the management of death rattle: Evidence-based guidelines for palliative care. *Palliat Med* 16:369-374, 2002.

Bergevin P, Bergevin RM: Recognizing delirium in terminal patients. *Am J Hosp Palliat Care* 13:28-29, 1996.

Bernat JL, Gert B, Mogielnicki RP: Patient refusal of hydration and nutrition: An alternative to physician-assisted suicide or voluntary active euthanasia [Commentary]. *Arch Intern Med* 153:2723-2728, 1993.

Block SD, Billings JA: Patient requests to hasten death: Evaluation and management in terminal care. *Arch Intern Med* 154:2039-2047, 1994.

Booth S, Wade R, Johnson M, et al: The use of oxygen in the palliation of breathlessness. A report of the expert working group of the Scientific Committee of the Association of Palliative Medicine. *Respir Med* 98:66-77, 2004.

Bottomley DM, Hanks GW: Subcutaneous midazolam infusion in palliative care. *J Pain Symptom Manage* 5:259-261, 1990.

Bozzetti F, et al: Guidelines on artificial nutrition versus hydration in terminal cancer patients. *Nutrition* 12:163-167, 1996.

Brant JM: The art of palliative care: Living with hope, dying with dignity. *Oncol Nurs Forum* 25:995-1004, 1998.

Breitbart W, Jacobsen PB: Psychiatric symptom management in terminal care. *Clin Geriatr Med* 12:329-347, 1996.

Brown SJ, Eichner SF, Jones JR: Nebulized morphine for relief of dyspnea due to chronic lung disease. *Ann Pharmacother* 39:1088-1092, 2005.

Bruera E, Pruvost M, Schoeller T, et al: Proctoclysis for hydration of terminally ill cancer patients. *J Pain Symptom Manage* 15:216-219, 1998.

Bruera E, Sala R, Rico MA, et al: Effects of parenteral hydration in terminally ill cancer patients: A preliminary study. *J Clin Oncol* 23:2366-2371, 2005a.

Bruera E, Sala R, Spruyt O, et al: Nebulized versus subcutaneous morphine for patients with cancer dyspnea: A preliminary study. *J Pain Symptom Manage* 29:613-618, 2005b.

Burge FI: Dehydration symptoms of palliative care cancer patients. *J Pain Symptom Manage* 8:454-464, 1993.

Byock I: Patient refusal of nutrition and hydration: Walking the ever-finer line. *Am J Hosp Palliat Care* 12(2):8-13, 1995.

Caruso-Herman D: Concerns for the dying patient and family. *Semin Oncol Nurs* 5:120-123, 1989.

Chandler S: Nebulized opioids to treat dyspnea. *Am J Hosp Palliat Care* 16:418-422, 1999.

Cherny NI: The use of sedation in the management of refractory pain. *Princ Prac Supporte Oncol Updates* 3(4):1-11, 2000.

Cherny NI, Portenoy RK: Sedation in the management of refractory symptoms: Guidelines for evaluation and treatment. *J Palliat Care* 10:31-38, 1994.

Cleary JF: Pharmacokinetic and pharmacodynamic issues in the treatment of breakthrough pain. *Semin Oncol* 24:S16-13-S16-19, 1997.

Coluzzi PH: Sublingual morphine: Efficacy reviewed. *J Pain Symptom Manage* 16:184-192, 1998.

Davis BD, Cowley SA, Ryland RK: The effects of terminal illness on patients and their carers. *J Adv Nurs* 23:512-520, 1996.

Doyle D, Hanks GW, MacDonald N, eds: *Oxford Textbook of Palliative Medicine.* New York, Oxford University Press, 1993.

Drickamer M, Lee MA, Ganzini L: Practical issues in physician-assisted suicide. *Ann Intern Med* 126:146-151, 1997.

Ellison NM, Lewis GO: Plasma concentrations following single doses of morphine sulfate in oral solution and rectal suppository. *Clin Pharm* 3:614-617, 1984.

Enck RE: The role of nebulized morphine in managing dyspnea [Editorial]. *Am J Hosp Palliat Care* 16:373-376, 1999.

Erlen JA: Issues at the end of life. *Orthop Nurs* 15(4):37-41, 1996.

Faisinger R, Bruera E: The management of dehydration in terminally ill patients. *J Palliat Care* 10:55-59, 1994.

Faisinger RL, Bruera E: When to treat dehydration in a terminally ill patient? *Support Care Cancer* 5:205-211, 1997.

Faisinger R, MacEachern T, Miller MJ, et al: The use of hypodermoclysis for rehydration in terminally ill cancer patients. *J Pain Symptom Manage* 9:298-302, 1994.

Fentora package insert. http://www.fentora.com/pdfs/pdf100_prescribing_info.pdf. Published in December, 2009 and accessed August 24, 2010.

Ferris FD: Last hours of living. *Clin Geriatr Med* 20:641-667, 2004.

Ferris FD, von Gunten CF, Emanuel LL: Competency in end-of-life care: Last hours of life. *J Palliat Med* 6:605-613, 2003.

Fine PG: Fentanyl in the treatment of cancer pain. *Semin Oncol* 104:694-700, 1997.

Foral PA, Malesker MA, Huerta G, et al: Nebulized opioids in COPD. *Chest* 125:691-694, 2004.

Gavrin J, Chapman R: Clinical management of dying patients. *West J Med* 163:268-277, 1995.

Gremaud G, Zulian GB: Indications and limitations of intravenous and subcutaneous midazolam in a palliative care center [Letter]. *J Pain Symptom Manage* 15:331-332, 1998.

Gordon D, Schroeder M: Fast facts and concepts # 103. In: *Oral Transmucosal Fentanyl Citrate-OTFC (Actiq®).* End-of-Life/Palliative Education Resource Center, 2003. http://www.eperc.mcw.edu/fastFact/ff_103.htm. Accessed September 11, 2009.

Hanks-Bell M, Paice J, Krammer L: The use of midazolam hydrochloride continuous infusion in palliative care. *Clin J Oncol Nurs* 6:367-369, 2002.

Hansen-Flaschen J: Advanced lung disease: Palliation and terminal care. *Clin Chest Med* 18:645-655, 1997.

Hanson LC, Danis M, Garrett J: What is wrong with end-of-life care? Opinions of bereaved family members. *J Am Geriatr Soc* 45:1339-1344, 1997.

Horn LW: Terminal dyspnea: A hospice approach. *Am J Hosp Palliat Care* 9(2):24-32, 1992.

Hum A, Fainsinger R, Bielech M: Subcutaneous methadone—An issue revisited, Letter to the editor. *J Pain Symptom Manage* 34:573-575, 2007.

Jecker NS: Medical futility and care of dying patients. *West J Med* 163:287-291, 1995.

Kemp C: Palliative care for respiratory problems in terminal illness. *Am J Hosp Palliat Care* 14(1):26-30, 1997.

Kinzbrunner BM, Copeland J, Kinzbrunner E: Nebulized morphine using oral morphine solution. Poster presented at: Annual Assembly of the American Academy of Hospice and Palliative Medicine, Atlanta, GA, June 30, 2000.

Kinzel T: Managing lung disease in late life: A new approach. *Geriatrics* 46:53-58, 1991.

Levy MH: Pain management in advanced cancer. *Semin Oncol* 12:394-410, 1985.

Lichter I: Home care in the last days of terminal illness. *Home Health Care Consult* 6(1):15-22, 1999.

Lichter I, Hunt E: The last 48 hours of life. *J Palliat Care* 6(4):7-15, 1990.

Lynn J, Teno JM, Phillips RS, et al: Perceptions by family members of the dying experience of older and seriously ill patients. *Ann Intern Med* 126:97-106, 1997.

MacDonald N: Suffering and dying in cancer patients: Research frontiers in controlling confusion, cachexia, and dyspnea. *West J Med* 163:278-286, 1995.

Macmillan K, Bruera E, Kuehn N, et al: A prospective comparison study between a butterfly needle and a Teflon cannula for subcutaneous narcotic administration. *J Pain Symptom Manage* 9:82-84, 1994.

Malone N: Hydration in the terminally ill patient. *Nurs Stand* 43(8):29-32, 1994.

March PA: Terminal restlessness. *Am J Hosp Palliat Care* 15:51-53, 1998.

Matthew P, Storey P: Subcutaneous methadone in terminally ill patients: Manageable local toxicity. *J Pain Symptom Manage* 18:49-52, 1999.

McCaffrey-Boyle D, Abernathy G, Baker L, Conover-Wall A: End-of-life confusion in patients with cancer. *Oncol Nurs Forum* 25:1335-1343, 1998.

McCann RM, Hall WJ, Groth-Juncker A: Comfort care for terminally ill patients: The appropriate use of nutrition and hydration. *JAMA* 272:1263-1266, 1994.

McIver B, Walsh D, Nelson K: The use of chlorpromazine for symptom control in dying cancer patients. *J Pain Symptom Manage* 9:341-345, 1994.

Mercadante SG: When oral morphine fails in cancer pain: The role of alternative routes. *Am J Hosp Palliat Care* 15:333-342, 1998.

Mercadante S, DeConno F, Ripamonti C: Propofol in terminal care. *J Pain Symptom Manage* 10:639-642, 1995.

Miller FG, Meier DE: Voluntary death: A comparison of terminal hydration and physician-assisted suicide. *Ann Intern Med* 128:559-562, 1998.

National Cancer Institute: Last Days of Life (PDQ®): Care during the final hours. http://www.cancer.gov/cancertopics/pdq/supportivecare/lasthours/Health Professional/page3. Modified September 3, 2009. Accessed September 9, 2009.

Nuland SB: *How We Die.* New York, Vintage Books, 1995.

Oneschuk D: Subcutaneous midazolam for acute hemorrhage in patients with advanced cancer. *Can Fam Physician* 44:1461-1462, 1998.

Paix A, Coleman A, Lees J, et al: Subcutaneous fentanyl and sufentanil infusion substitution for morphine intolerance in cancer pain management. *Pain* 63:263-269, 1995.

Pearlman RA: Forgoing medical nutrition and hydration: An area for fine-tuning clinical skills [Editorial]. *J Gen Intern Med* 8:225-227, 1993.

Portenoy RK: Treatment of temporal variations in chronic cancer pain. *Semin Oncol* 24: S16-7-S16-12, 1997.

Portenoy RK: Oral transmucosal fentanyl citrate (OTFC) for the treatment of breakthrough pain and cancer patients: A controlled dose titration study. *Pain* 79:303-312, 1999.

Ronan KP, Gallagher J, George B, Hamby B: Comparison of propofol and midazolam for sedation in intensive care unit patients. *Crit Care Med* 23:286-293, 1995.

Rousseau P: Terminal sedation in the care of dying patients [Commentary]. *Arch Intern Med* 156:1785-1786, 1996.

Simmonds MA: Pharmacotherapeutic management of cancer pain: Current practice. *Semin Oncol* 24:S16-1-S16-6, 1997.

Spitalnic S, Blazes C, Anderson AC: Conscious sedation: A primer for outpatient procedures. *Hosp Physician* 5:22-32, 2000.

Stein WM, Min YK: Nebulized morphine for paroxysmal cough and dyspnea in a nursing home resident with metastatic cancer. *Am J Hosp Palliat Care* 14:52-56, 1997.

Steiner N, Bruera E: Methods of hydration in palliative care patients. *J Palliat Care* 14:6-13, 1998.

Storey P: *Primer of Palliative Care.* Gainesville, FL, The Academy of Hospice Physicians, 1994.

Storey P, Hill HH, St Louis RH, Tarver EE: Subcutaneous infusions for control of cancer symptoms. *J Pain Symptom Manage* 5:33-41, 1990.

Sullivan RJ: Accepting death without artificial nutrition or hydration. *J Gen Intern Med* 8:220-224, 1993.

Taylor MA: Benefits of dehydration in terminally ill patients. *Geriatr Nurs* 16:271-272, 1995.

Thorns A, Sykes N: Opioid use in last week of life and implications for end-of-life decision making. *Lancet* 356(9227): 398-399, 2000.

Truog RD, Berde CB, Mitchell C, Grier HE: Barbiturates in the care of the terminally ill. *N Engl J Med* 327:1678-1682, 1992.

Ventafridda V, Ripamonti C, DeConno F, et al: Symptoms prevalence and control during cancer patients' last days of life. *J Palliat Care* 6(3):7-11,1990.

Wildiers H, Menten J: Death rattle: Prevalence, prevention, and treatment. *J Pain Symptom Manage* 23:310-317, 2002.

Zebraski SE, Kochenash SM, Raffa RB: Lung opioid receptors: Pharmacology and possible targets for nebulized morphine in dyspnea. *Life Sci* 66:2221-2231, 2000.

Zeppetella G: The palliation of dyspnea in terminal disease. *Am J Hosp Palliat Care* 15:322-330, 1998.

SELF-ASSESSMENT QUESTIONS

1. All of the following are characteristics of the "preactive" phase of dying EXCEPT:

   A. Increased dependence on caregivers
   B. Increased sleep
   C. Limited attention span or withdrawal
   D. Abnormal respiratory patterns
   E. Increased weakness and lethargy

2. All of the following are characteristics of the phenomenon known as the "surge of energy" EXCEPT:

   A. It occurs during the "active" phase of dying.
   B. Patients with this "surge" show improvement in physical, cognitive, or functional abilities during the dying process.
   C. It indicates that the patient is likely to live for several more weeks.
   D. The "surge" may last for several hours to several days.
   E. Families may want to shift goals of care to disease-directed interventions.

3. Patients who are in the "active" phase of dying, often have exacerbations of pain when they are moved or disturbed, a phenomenon known as "disturbance" or "incident" pain. All of the following are true regarding this type of pain, EXCEPT:

   A. The best way to treat this pain is to avoid moving the patient.
   B. Patients may moan, groan, or grimace when moved.
   C. It may be due to stiffness that occurs with immobility.
   D. It has been described as an "alarm" response that is particularly evident in the blind, deaf, or confused.
   E. Families need to be taught to expect this type of response if they move the patient.

4. All of the following statements regarding the administration of opioids by the sublingual or oral transmucosal route are true EXCEPT:

   A. 25% of the active drug in the fentanyl oralet, Actiq, is absorbed through the transmucosal route, while the remaining 75% of the drug needs to be swallowed and absorbed through the GI tract.
   B. 50% of the active drug in the fentanyl buccal tablet, Fentora, is absorbed through the transmucosal route, while the remaining 50% of the drug needs to be swallowed and absorbed through the GI tract.
   C. 75% of highly concentrated liquid morphine (20 mg/mL) administered sublingually is absorbed through the transmucosal route, while the remaining 25% of the drug needs to be swallowed and absorbed through the GI tract.
   D. The sublingual or oral transmucosal routes of administration are preferred over the rectal route in patients unable to swallow due, at least in part, to caregiver discomfort administering medications via the rectal route.
   E. The lipophilic nature of fentanyl makes it an ideal agent for the oral transmucosal route.

5. Regarding the continued use of opioids when patients are in the "active" dying phase, all of the following are true EXCEPT:

   A. Neurotoxic opioid metabolites may increase secondary to declining renal function.
   B. Family members may be fearful that continuing their loved one's opioid analgesia could result in premature death.
   C. If there is concern that a dying patient's change in level of consciousness is due to opioid toxicity, the dose may be reduced up to 75% in order to avoid withdrawal symptoms.

D. Actively dying patients on chronic opioids who develop myoclonus should have all opioid analgesics discontinued.

E. When patients are very close to death, symptomatic management of opioid-induced delirium with haloperidol may be the best option.

6. All of the following statements regarding the treatment of dyspnea in actively dying patients are true EXCEPT:

A. Oxygen provides symptomatic relief to patients with dyspnea irrespective of their level of oxygenation.

B. A fan or cool breeze from an open window will improve the perception of breathlessness via altered stimulation of areas innervated by the trigeminal nerve.

C. Patients who are dyspneic and on opioids for pain require a 50% increase in opioid dose to improve symptoms of breathlessness.

D. Nebulized morphine may work via the stimulation of opioid receptors in the bronchial tree and along sensory fibers of the vagus nerve.

E. Bronchodilators and steroids are most effectively used to treat dyspnea earlier than the actively dying phase.

7. All of the following statements regarding the treatment of terminal congestion (death rattle) in actively dying patients are true EXCEPT:

A. Terminal congestion is a collection of oscillating mucous secretion in the oropharynx and trachea during inspiration and expiration in the dying patient unable to clear secretions.

B. Families are often more troubled than patients by the presence of the "death rattle."

C. Atropine ophthalmic drops may be administered sublingually to treat terminal congestion.

D. Agents used to treat terminal congestion may precipitate or exacerbate terminal delirium.

E. Suctioning is preferred to anti-cholinergic medication for the treatment of terminal congestion.

8. All of the following statements regarding the evaluation and treatment of terminal confusion, agitation, and delirium are true EXCEPT:

A. Any unnecessary medications should be eliminated.

B. All patients should receive parenteral hydration.

C. Haloperidol or risperidone should be used for symptomatic therapy of delirium.

D. Confusion occurs in up to 10% of patients during the last hours of life.

E. Proper patient positioning and calm reassurance are important nonpharmacological interventions.

9. All of the following statements regarding the provision of hydration to patients who are in the active phase of dying are true EXCEPT:

A. 1–1.5 L of fluid a day can be safely administered to patients via hypodermoclysis.

B. Proctoclysis, the administration of fluid via the rectal route, has been shown to be a safe alternative to parenteral hydration.

C. D5W is the fluid of choice when hydrating patients via hypodermoclysis.

D. By using hypodermoclysis, patients who desire hydration for cultural or religious reasons may have their beliefs respected in a safe and appropriate fashion.

E. Many families of dying patients as well as many physicians believe that dying without parenteral hydration and dehydrated causes increased pain and suffering.

10. When providing caregiver support to the families of patients who are in the "active" phase of dying, all of the following are true EXCEPT:

   A. It is better to wait until after the death of the patient to make funeral arrangements, in order to not take away hope from the family.
   B. Giving families time frames as to when death is likely to occur, such as "hours versus days" or "days versus weeks," is generally acceptable.
   C. It is important to reassure the family that they are doing "the right thing," when allowing the patient to die in the chosen environment.
   D. When families feel guilty at wanting the death to occur to "get it over with," they need to be reassured that this is a natural feeling due to all the turmoil surrounding the event.
   E. Families should be educated on expected symptoms during the "active" dying process, and how to administer medication to control those symptoms.

Other Common Symptoms Near the End of Life

Barry M. Kinzbrunner and James B. Wright

INTRODUCTION

Previous chapters in this book have addressed major symptoms experienced by patients near the end of life. This chapter will discuss other symptoms commonly associated with terminal illness: asthenia, insomnia, hiccups, disorders of the urinary tract, venous thromboembolic disease, and edema.

ASTHENIA

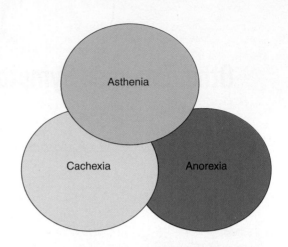

Figure 13–1. The intersection of asthenia, anorexia, and cachexia.

ASTHENIA DEFINED

Asthenia means a loss of energy or fatigue with an inability to maintain previous levels of performance or activities. Patients experiencing asthenia usually complain of a pervasive sense of generalized weakness. Described in patients having malignant disease is the "asthenia-fatigue syndrome" (AFS), which may be characterized by a pathologic degree of physical and psychological fatigue, poor endurance, the inability to initiate activity, and impaired cognitive function. It is estimated that more than 70% of cancer patients experience this syndrome during the course of their illness, and many perceive this as the most distressing symptom associated with their malignant disease.

To understand asthenia, it should be contextually related but also differentiated from anorexia and cachexia (Fig. 13–1). Anorexia may be defined as loss of appetite, while cachexia is the severe muscle wasting associated with loss of lean body mass. Anorexia is sometimes reversible, although rarely so in the terminally ill. Cachexia is a cytokine-mediated inability to maintain muscle proteins, and it is not reversed by increased food intake. Tumor products called cachectin are among the abnormal proteins that may be asso-

ciated with and responsible for cachexia. (Further discussion of anorexia and cachexia and the anorexia–cachexia syndrome can be found in Chapter 24.) In asthenia, although decreased food intake contributes to weakness, correction of nutritional losses usually does not improve the debility. Unlike cachexia, there are no specific markers that have been identified as being responsible for asthenia, although nonspecific inflammatory markers such as C-reactive proteins and ferritin are found at high levels in asthenic patients, and, therefore, they are thought to possibly have some relationship to asthenia.

Because asthenia can occur with general inactivity, it may be expressed through abnormality of the musculature. Although loss of muscle and lean body mass and function can exist with normal calorie intake, and elevation of lactic acid is not necessarily noted in asthenic cancer patients, studies have shown atrophy of type II muscle fibers in the adductor pollicis muscles in patients with advanced breast cancer, suggesting that muscle dysfunction may be an underlying feature in asthenic cancer patients.

To better understand the relationship between inflammatory markers and muscle abnormalities with asthenia, one can examine a recent study that was designed to define the asthenia–fatigue syndrome in more objective terms than just patient reported fatigue on a 0 to 10 VAS scale. The investigators found that the 97.7% of patients had abnormalities in one or more of the following variables: serum albumin levels below 3.8 g/dL (91.6%), C-reactive protein levels greater than 0.5 mg/dL (79.3%), hemoglobin levels below 12 gm/dL (78.6%), and/or BMI less than 20 kg/m^2 (15.3%). Multivariate analysis was unable to establish any of these as independent variables affecting variation in patient reported fatigue levels. However, the analysis did demonstrate that impaired motor function was the only variable that could be independently correlated with patients' reported VAS levels of fatigue (Scialla et al., 2006). This study seems to corroborate the nonspecific nature and/or the lack of understanding regarding the role of inflammatory proteins in AFS, while confirming that muscle weakness, expressed in the study as impaired motor function, correlates well with the level of patient-reported fatigue.

CAUSES OF ASTHENIA

Causes of asthenia are listed in Table 13–1. Asthenia in any individual patient is most often multifactorial, and as the interaction of these factors accounts for the severity of the symptom, it is important to try and identify whether any of the causes of the fatigue might be reversible. Irreversible causes of asthenia usually relate to the primary disease, which, whether malignant or nonmalignant in nature, is commonly associated with specific end-organ failure, such as the heart, kidneys, adrenal glands, and liver. Secondary effects of the primary disease process may lead to causes of asthenia such as anemia, hypocalcemia, hyponatremia, hypokalemia, Addison disease, and Cushing syndrome, which may or may not be considered reversible, depending on the nature of the patient's primary illness, as well the patient's clinical course, prognosis, and goals of care. Finally, there may be some reversible forms of asthenia, such as when the fatigue occurs in association with radiation and/or chemotherapy. In such situations, stopping the active treatment may see a lessening of the asthenia after several weeks have elapsed.

Medications may contribute to asthenia in the terminally ill. Polypharmacy may result in a general decline, but specific medications such as opioids, antidepressants, neuroleptics, benzodiazepines, diuretics, hypoglycemics, and antihypertensives are more specific contributors. Many of these drugs are commonly used to control symptoms in terminally ill patients. Opioids, for example, exact a direct affect upon the reticular activating system, which in turn produces a sensation of fatigue. Therefore, whether or not the contribution of specific medications to a patient's asthenic symptoms is reversible is dependent on whether or not the patient can do without the offending agents.

Anxiety, depression, and adjustment disorders have been reported to be associated with asthenia in 75% of terminally ill patients with noncancer diagnoses and may be amenable to treatment in many (see Chapter 10). Malnutrition or starvation also may contribute to asthenia, but, as noted earlier, better nutrition does not reverse asthenia in the terminally ill. The anorexia–cachexia syndrome, well described in patients with advanced cancer and advanced AIDS and alluded to above,

TABLE 13–1. Causes of Asthenia	
IRREVERSIBLE	**POTENTIALLY REVERSIBLE**
Primary disease process	Addison disease
Comorbid and secondary disease processes	Anemia
	Chemotherapy
End-organ failure	Cushing syndrome
Anorexia–cachexia syndrome	Hypocalcemia
	Hypokalemia
Malnutrition	Hyponatremia
Humoral factors not yet well described	Polypharmacy
	Radiation therapy

> **TABLE 13–2.** Treatment for Asthenia
>
> Nonpharmacological
> * Evaluate and attempt to correct reversible causes if consistent with patient clinical conditions and patient goals of care
> * Discontinue unnecessary medications
> * Regular exercise
>
> Pharmacological
> * Oral Steroids
>   * Prednisone 40–100 mg PO daily
>   * Dexamethasone 16–96 mg PO daily in 2–4 divided doses
> * Progestational agents
>   * Megestrol acetate 160–240 mg PO bid
> * Antidepressants when depression present
> * Methyphenidate 5 mg q 2 h PM, max 4 capsules per day

is a disturbance of carbohydrate, fat, and protein metabolism with endocrine dysfunction and anemia that results in asthenia and often contributes to patient death.

TREATMENT

Potential treatments for asthenia can be found in Table 13–2. As the causes of asthenia are multiple, and not always easily distinguished from the disease process, treatment will often be more general than specific. However, a reasonable initial step would be to evaluate the patient for any reversible causes and consider attempting to reverse them if appropriate and consistent with the patient's clinical condition and goals of care. If possible, correct any electrolyte or other metabolic abnormalities that are amenable to therapy. If anemia is playing a significant role in the patient's fatigue, and the patient is a potential candidate, consider a blood transfusion. If the patient is receiving anti-neoplastic therapy and the asthenia is overwhelming, a break in therapy under the appropriate circumstances may be warranted. It

is important, though, that one must remember that in these situations, interventions designed to reverse these abnormalities may be ineffective in correcting the abnormality, or, even if the abnormality is corrected, in improving the patient's level of fatigue.

When possible, discontinue antihypertensive agents, sedatives, tranquilizers, and any other unnecessary medications. Diabetes should be managed in a standard medical manner and oral hypoglycemics should be avoided whenever possible. Regular exercise limited to maintaining function and range of motion also helps. However, exercise should not be overdone as too strenuous a program could produce muscle fiber damage or exhaustion.

Future progress in treating asthenia may be dependent on a better understanding of cytokine interactions. For the present, pharmacological treatment options aimed at the general symptoms of asthenia are limited. Steroids are most often used, especially if the patient's prognosis can only be measured in a few weeks or months. For patients with a longer life expectancy, where untoward side effects of steroids may become a much more significant factor, progestational agents such as megestrol acetate, that exert anti-cytokine effects, stimulate appetite, and increase the sense of well being may be tried.

Antidepressants, whether of the tri-cyclic or SSRI variety, do not have much of an impact on asthenia, unless there is coexistent depression, nor do other general appetite stimulants. Psychostimulants such as methylphenidate may cause arousal and lessen fatigue, but whether they have any role to play in the treatment of asthenia remains questionable. A recent uncontrolled trial suggested that methylphenidate, 5 mg q 2 h as needed up to four capsules a day, improved fatigue, overall well-being, and depression in a group of patients with advanced cancer (Bruera et al., 2003), while a randomized control trial comparing methylphenidate to placebo showed improvement in fatigue in both the treatment and control arms. This finding suggested that the improvement was not due to the effects of methylphenidate but due to some other cause. The investigators hypothesize that the daily phone call from the research nurse, common to both study arms, may have been the intervention responsible for the improvement in fatigue and this is currently being investigated in another clinical trial (Bruera et al., 2006).

INSOMNIA

Insomnia is the subjective complaint of poor sleep. This problem includes insufficient sleep, difficulty initiating or maintaining sleep, interrupted sleep, or poor-quality sleep. The reported incidence of insomnia in palliative care patients varies from as low as 23% to as high 70%.

CAUSES OF INSOMNIA

Like many other symptoms that occur in patients near the end of life, insomnia is multifactorial. The more common causes are listed in Table 13–3. Uncontrolled or poorly controlled physical symptoms contribute to insomnia, with

the most prevalent uncontrolled symptoms reported in one study being pain (36%), urinary frequency (29%), and dyspnea (13%). Nonphysical symptoms that contribute to lack of sleep include anxiety, depression, and delirium. Commonly used medications in palliative care that may contribute to insomnia include steroids, antihypertensives, diuretics, sympathomimetics, anticholinergics, CNS stimulants, and SSRIs. Caffeine may also be an offending agent.

TREATMENT

The recommended approach to the treatment of insomnia is listed in Table 13–4. As with many symptoms in end-of-life care, the first line of treatment, prior to resorting to pharmacological intervention to ameliorate the symptom, is to try to identify the causes and treat those causes amenable to therapy. Specific problem-oriented interventions are much better than routinely prescribing sleep medication. For example, fear of dying is not relieved with temazepam. A psychosocial evaluation would be much more appropriate.

With this in mind, review the patient's medications and discontinue any suspected causative agents that are not necessary for control of other symptoms. Assess for and treat uncontrolled

TABLE 13–3. Causes of Insomnia

UNCONTROLLED SYMPTOMS	MEDICATIONS
Physical symptoms	Steroids
Pain	Antihypertensives
Urinary frequency	Diuretics
Dyspnea	Symphthomimetics
Leg cramps	Anitcholinergics
Nausea	CNS stimulants
Nonphysical symptoms	SSRIs
Anxiety	Caffeine
Depression	
Delirium	

TABLE 13–4. Therapeutic Approaches for Insomnia

- Review medications and discontinue any unnecessary medications.
- Assess for and treat uncontrolled physical symptoms.
- Assess for and treat anxiety, depression, and/or delirium.
- Encourage the patient to try and remain awake during the day.
- Use pharmacological therapy only when necessary (see Table 13–5).

physical symptoms as well as any evidence of anxiety, depression, and/or delirium. For patients not able to sleep because of pain, stiffness, or night sweats, adding a nonsteroidal antiinflammatory in the evening, 1 to 2 hours before bedtime may be helpful. Try not to schedule routine medications during normal sleeping hours. Many drugs come in long-acting form that can be used prior to bedtime. If using immediate release opiods to treat pain, an increase of the daytime dose may be used at bedtime to extend the hours of sleep without pain. Antidepressants are useful when depression is present. In particular, doxepin and amitryptyline may be better choices when insomnia is present, as they have sedative properties.

Encourage the patient to try and remain awake during the day. This can be difficult since oftentimes, daytime stimulation in the home environment for a sedentary patient can be lacking, causing such patients to doze throughout the day without even realizing how much sleeping they are doing. Daytime activities need to be enriched for such a person and naps, while often necessary, should be reduced in number and length.

Other measures that may be tried include recommending a relaxing activity at bedtime, like reading a book or listening to soft music, drinking warm milk, or a soothing back massage. If urinary frequency at night is a problem, the patient should be instructed to avoid drinking large amounts of water or other beverages prior to bedtime. Alcohol and caffeine should also be avoided.

Sedative/hypnotic medications should only be resorted to when the aforementioned treatments are ineffective, keeping in mind that terminal illness alone does not justify the need for sedation. Recommended medications are listed in Table 13–5. Although there is a lack of medcial evidence on the whether they are the drugs of first choice, benzodiazepines are most commonly used to treat insomnia, with the preferred medications in the class being lorazepam or oxazepam. If the patient is already on a benzodiazepine for the treatment of anxiety, rather than adding another medication for insomnia, it is recommended that a higher nighttime dose of the regular daytime anxiety medication be used. Some of the benzodiazepines commonly used for

TABLE 13–5. Pharmacological Therapy for Insomnia

MEDICATION	DOSAGE	CLINICAL	NOT RECOMMENDED
Lorazepam	0.5–4 mg PO hs Max dose 12 mg	May be given in large dose, at hs when used as routine daily antianxiety agent	Temazepam: slow onset of action Flurazepam: accumulation of metabolites
Oxazepam	15–30 mg PO hs Max dose 180 mg		Triazolam: withdrawal symptoms.
Amtriptyline	25–50 mg PO hs Max dose 300 mg	Also good for depression and pain control	
Diphenhydramine	25–50 mg PO hs Max dose 200 mg	May be too sedating the following day in the elderly	
Zolpidem	10 mg at hs Max dose 10 mg	Cannot titrate to response. Cost can be a limiting factor.	
Doxepin	75 mg PO hs Max dose 150 mg/d		

insomnia, including temazapam, flurazepam, and triazolam, should actually be avoided as they have a longer duration of effect, rebound effects, and increased anxiety or morning drowsiness than loazepam or oxazepam. If there is an element of depression or neuropathic pain overlaying the insomnia, amitriptyline may be used. Diphenhydramine, which is available over the counter, has always been a popular agent; however, over time, it has been found to be overly sedating in the elderly and should probably be avoided in that population. Zolpidem is another popular hypnotic, but is difficult to titrate and is less cost-effective than some of the other agents.

HICCUPS

Hiccups are a pathological respiratory reflex characterized by spasm of the diaphragm. This results in sudden inspiration (the "hic" portion) and then closure of the vocal cords (the "cup" portion).

CAUSES

The hiccup reflex is a result of irritation of the diaphragm, phrenic nerve, thoracic or upper lumbar spinal nerves, or the celiac plexus. In terminal patients, hiccups may occur due to a wide variety of causes. They may be associated with various malignancies, including esophageal and gastric cancers, colon cancer, lung cancer, pancreatic carcinoma, liver metastases from a variety of neoplasms, and with radiation therapy to the chest or neck. Metabolic abnormalities that cause hiccups include uremia and renal failure, uncontrolled diabetes, and various electrolyte imbalances. CNS lesions including brain tumors and cerebrovascular lesions, cardiovascular disorders including myocardial ischemia and pericardial disease, various pulmonary disorders, and disorders of the gastrointestinal tract including peptic ulcer disease, gall bladder disease, or pancreatitis have also been reported to cause hiccups.

TREATMENT

Treatment should focus on the underlying disease if possible. General principles include avoiding gastric loading, promoting gastric emptying, and avoiding foods and beverages that produce gas or irritation. Pharyngeal stimulation can disrupt spasms and suppress the reflex hiccups. This may be accomplished by drinking from the wrong side of the cup, rapid ingestion of granulated sugar or liquor, cold placed at the back of the neck, swallowing dry bread, and stimulation of the pharynx by an oral or nasal catheter. Breath holding or rebreathing to raise the levels of carbon dioxide in the lungs and blood may help as well.

Medications that may be useful are listed in Table 13–6 and include gabapentin, baclofen, chlorpromazine, metaclopramide, prednisone, simethicone, haloperidol, nifedipine, phenytoin, and carbamazepine. Of these agents, only chlorpromazine has been approved by the FDA for the treatment of hiccups. Over the years, baclofen has been the agent of choice for many experts in hospice and palliative care, although one has to be cautious when using this agent in the elderly due to an increased risk of sedation. Metaclopramide may be useful when the hiccups are believed to be secondary to disease involving the upper gastrointestinal tract, while prednisone may be effective for inflammatory or destructive lesions in the thorax or abdomen.

Finally, recent studies have suggested that gabapentin may be another effective agent in the treatment of hiccups. In one series of note, 15 patients with refractory hiccups secondary to ischemic lesions of the brainstem were treated with gabapentin 400 mg three times daily for 3 days, 400 mg daily for 3 days, and then the medication was discontinued, with only one patient requiring retreatment (Moretti et al., 2004). Due to the fact that gabapentin is well tolerated by most

TABLE 13–6. Pharmacological Therapy of Hiccups

MEDICATION	DOSE	CLINICAL NOTES
Gabapentin	400 mg tid for 3 d	No randomized trials
	400 mg qd for 3 d, then stop	Optimum dose and duration of therapy unknown
Baclofen	5–10 mg PO tid	Agent of choice by many palliative medicine clinicians
		May cause excess sedation in elderly
Chlorpromazine	10–20 mg PO bid to q 6 h	Calms CNS response
		Only agent approved by FDA for treatment of hiccups
Metoclopramide	10–20 mg PO bid to q 6 h	Promotes gastric emptying
		Useful with hiccups due to upper GI tract causes
Prednisone	10 mg PO q 8 h	Effective for inflammatory process from malignancies
Simethicone	40–120 mg PO after meals and hs PRN	Relieves gastric distention
	Max dose 500 mg	
Haloperidol	3–5 mg PO q 8 h	Calms CNS response
Nifedipine	10 mg PO tid or XL 30 mg qd	If no cardiac contraindications
Phenytoin	300–500 mg PO daily in divided doses	Decreases nerve hyperstimulation
Carbamazepine	200–1,600 mg PO daily in 3–4 divided doses	Decrease nerve hyperstimulation. Large dosages over time can cause bone marrow dysfunction

patients and also is used widely to treat neuropathic pain, it has been suggested that it may be the drug of choice for refractory hiccups (Marinella, 2009). However it must be cautioned that there are no randomized trials comparing gabapentin to any other agent in the treatment of hiccups, and optimum dosing schedules are as yet unknown.

DISORDERS OF THE URINARY TRACT

INTRODUCTION

Complications related to the urinary system commonly occur near the end of life. Early in the course of terminal illness, when a patient's overall functional abilities and performance score tend to be high, and life expectancy, although limited, is relatively long, most urinary tract problems are appropriately managed with conventional interventions such as would be offered to patients with nonterminal illnesses. In these circumstances, when failure to act will shorten life substantially, even invasive treatments such as surgical or radiological intervention for upper or lower urinary tract obstruction, or dialysis for renal failure, may properly be considered and discussed with patients and their families. Later in the course of terminal illness, when patients weaken and functional capacity declines, urinary complications such as incontinence, retention, bladder spasms, infection, and hematuria often contribute to patient discomfort and detract from the quality of living. This section discusses aspects of the management of these problems that are specifically relevant to the patient with terminal illness in whom death appears to be quite near.

URINARY INCONTINENCE

Urinary incontinence (oftentimes in conjunction with fecal incontinence) is one of the most common occurrences in end-of-life care and affects patients with both malignant and nonmalignant terminal diagnoses. For patients who remain mentally alert, the problem is not only physically but also psychologically distressing and is a tangible reminder of loss of control of bodily function and independence.

Urinary incontinence is caused by pathological, anatomical, or physiological factors that affect the pressure gradient from the bladder to the urethral sphincter (Table 13–7). Typically, patients experience either uncontrolled detrusor contraction, poor sphincter function (stress incontinence), or inability to empty the bladder (overflow incontinence). In malignancy, these abnormalities can be caused by a variety of lesions, including spinal cord compression and direct tumor invasion of the bladder, that disrupt the bladder's nerve supply and affects muscle function. Tumor invasion of the bladder and surrounding tissue may also cause urinary leakage from external fistulas.

Aging can lead to lax sphincter control, a phenomenon which is even more common in patients with debilitating, degenerative illnesses such as Alzheimer disease or end-stage cerebrovascular

TABLE 13–7. Causes of Urinary Incontinence
Pathological factors
Malignancy
Anatomical changes
Aging
Prostatic hypertrophy
Bladder displacement
Physiological factors
Medications
Trauma
Irritation

or cardiovascular disease. A variety of medications may also cause urinary incontinence by several mechanisms, and a careful review of medication history is mandatory for proper assessment of potential causes. Strong involuntary detrusor muscle contractions (overactive bladder) may be idiopathic or caused by bladder irritation from internal bladder tumors, extrinsic compression, radiation or chemical cystitis, or bacterial or fungal infection. Prostatic enlargement may affect flow dynamics. Causes for overflow incontinence include neurogenic bladder, shrunken bladder due to radiation or chemical cystitis, bladder outlet or urethral obstruction, and medications such as anticholinergics, phenothiazines, antihistamines, and opioids.

An appropriate treatment care plan depends on the stage of terminal illness. For patients with a relatively long prognosis, simple diagnostic evaluations such as urinalysis and/or urine culture may be indicated, while for others, more invasive procedures including cystoscopy, ultrasonography, computed tomography, and/or cystometrics may be considered when the information obtained will help direct specific therapy.

For patients closer to death, such a work-up is more intrusive than helpful, and treatment should be empiric and symptom-oriented. For some patients, discontinuing provocative medications may prove helpful. For patients with an "overactive bladder" and bladder spasms, anticholinergics such as oxybutinine can be used, but only to the point where troublesome anticholinergic side effects are not produced. Newer agents, such as tolterodine, have fewer systemic anticholinergic side effects and may be preferable treatment for older, debilitated patients. Nevertheless, one should be alert for problems such as dry mouth, constipation, and headache, especially when patients are receiving other palliative anticholinergic agents. For stress incontinence in alert mobile patients, agents that increase urethral sphincter tone such as pseudoephedrine and phenylpropanolamine can be tried, usually in conjunction with continence pads or adult diapers. For patients with overflow incontinence, catheterization is usually necessary, especially when the patients are immobilized and bedbound and/or are actively dying. It is important to remember that a markedly distended bladder should never be emptied precipitously after catheterization in order to avoid hypotension and bradycardia. Proper catheter care including irrigation with normal saline, when necessary, and rigorous perineal care are extremely important in order to minimize unnecessary discomfort for the patient. Some patients, even if they are confused and disoriented, may find a catheter annoying or otherwise objectionable. When such patients are managed with diapers or incontinence pads, scrupulous perineal and skin care, including the use of a skin barrier, is essential. Hospice programs have learned that willing family members are capable of providing this care, provided that they are properly instructed and supported.

URINARY RETENTION

Urinary retention is usually associated with a distended bladder that fails to empty completely. It can be detected with physical examination, ultrasonography, or by a postvoiding catheterization done to detect and measure residual urine. Urinary retention is typically caused by denervation disorders that lead to detrusor muscle failure or by bladder outlet obstruction at or distal to the bladder neck. Symptoms associated with detrusor muscle failure include hesitancy, impaired bladder sensation, longer time intervals to micturition, and decreased urgency. In contrast, patients with outlet obstruction usually complain of urinary frequency, urgency, nocturia, and a slow urinary stream. In the terminally ill, both mechanisms may sometimes coexist, and both may be exacerbated by exposure to various medications including opioids, antiemetics, antihistamines, antidepressants, and other anticholinergic agents that are commonly prescribed in hospice and palliative care.

Common causes of a neurogenic bladder in terminally ill patients include generally ir-

reversible conditions such as spinal cord compression and sacral plexopathy associated with invasive tumor, radiation myelopathy, vinca alkaloid neuropathy, nerve injury associated with abdominal–perineal resection, and diabetic neuropathy. Outlet obstruction in men is classically caused by benign prostatic hypertrophy (BPH) or prostatic cancer, but may also be caused by urethral stenosis or strictures associated with infections, including sexually transmitted diseases. In women, distal obstructive uropathy is associated with carcinoma of the cervix and vagina, meatal stenosis, urethral strictures, and tumors of the urethra.

From a pragmatic viewpoint, with the exception of urinary retention, which may be reversed through adjustment of concurrent medications, for patients near the end of life, the treatment of urinary retention, whatever the etiology, is primarily via chronic transurethral or suprapubic catheterization. For some mobile patients with outlet obstruction who wish to remain free of catheters, metal, self-expanding urethral stents may prove to be a satisfactory alternative. Rarely, terminally ill patients with concurrent BPH and sufficient expected longevity may respond to conservative measures such as bladder rest for 1 to 2 weeks and institution of treatment with alpha$_1$-blockers such as terazosin or doxazosin. Usually, however, deconditioning and debility associated with terminal illness make recovery of micturition highly unlikely, and, in the context of a short prognosis, also rule out, for all intents and purposes, surgical intervention. Patients terminally ill due to advanced prostate cancer are invariably refractory to hormonal therapy. However, androgen deprivation might reasonably be entertained for a patient with prostate cancer-related outlet obstruction and an unrelated terminal condition whose expected survival is thought to be measured in months rather than in weeks or days.

For a motivated, physically capable patient, clean intermittent catheterization is a preferable alternative to a chronic indwelling Foley catheter. Unfortunately, the majority of patients with advanced terminal illness do not fit this description, and the potential advantages in terms of decreased risk of infection, strictures, leakage, and bladder spasms are usually obviated by short life expectancy and other concurrent symptoms. Whether catheter use is intermittent or chronic, the risk of urosepsis relative to the risk of selecting progressively resistant microorganisms rarely justifies antibiotic prophylaxis or attempts to sterilize the urine in terminally ill patients.

BLADDER SPASM

Bladder spasms are primarily caused by irritation of the bladder trigone. In the terminally ill, irritation can result from radiation, infection, blood or clots, stones, catheters, or tumor invasion. Spasm can originate in the bladder wall due to tumor invasion or radiation. Spinal cord injury from tumor invasion can also produce bladder wall irritability.

Treatment is directed at the cause. Catheters can be withdrawn or their balloons deflated. Urinary infection should be treated with antibiotics with the clear purpose of alleviating discomfort. If bleeding is present due to a reversible cause, invasive interventions may sometimes be indicated, depending on the patient's overall condition and prognosis. Otherwise, nonspecific measures discussed below can sometimes help in decreasing hematuria and clot formation. Increased fluids help to relieve irritation from infection, blood, or retained stones. If a stone will not pass, a palliative urology referral may be needed.

Nonspecific measures include anticholinergics such as flavoxate, oxybutinin, and tolterodine. In addition to the side effects described earlier and the potential for drug interactions, these agents may cause anticholinergic side effects including dry mouth, drowsiness, and blurred vision, and, in noncatheterized patients, may cause urinary retention. Nonsteroidal antiinflammatory drugs may help to suppress spasms by inhibiting prostaglandin-related bladder irritation. However, NSAID's may also increase the risk of hematuria and further compromise renal func-

tion. For actively dying patients, or for those unable to swallow oral medications, "B & O" suppositories can be useful, and, in catheterized patients, irrigation with 0.25% acetic acid solution or bupivacaine 0.25%, 20 mL every 8 to 12 hours is sometimes effective. Finally, a case report published in 2003 described the use of diamorphine 10 mg in 20 mL of saline instilled intravescially every 4 hours to effectively treat a patient with refractory bladder spasms.

HEMATURIA

The significance of hematuria in patients near the end-of-life is often more psychological than physiological. Gross hematuria, whether from the upper or lower urinary tract, may often be asymptomatic, and even urine that is very red in color may, in fact, contain only a small volume of red blood cells. Nevertheless, patients and families are often very disturbed, even agitated, at the site of blood and are often convinced, despite the fact that it is highly unlikely, that the patient is bleeding to death. Therefore, controlling hematuria can be crucial for the relief of emotional suffering.

Of course, hematuria may cause significant physical symptoms as well, especially clot colic due to upper urinary tract bleeding, and dysuria and bladder spasms due to lower urinary tract bleeding. Persistent gross hematuria may also cause symptomatic anemia in debilitated terminal patients, especially those dying with cancers that were previously treated with myelosuppresive chemotherapy or radiotherapy.

At the end of life, hematuria is likely due to one or more of the following: urinary tract infections, tumors, radiotherapy or chemotherapy-induced cystitis, kidney stones, or an acquired bleeding diatheses. Upper urinary tract hematuria results most often from renal cell carcinoma, transitional cell carcinoma of the renal pelvis and/or ureter, other metastatic cancers, or stone formation. In the lower urinary tract, hemorrhagic cystitis is usually due to infection, previous radiotherapy or chemotherapy, or neoplasia. Bleeding may also emanate from the prostate or bladder neck. Drug-induced hematuria (e.g., NSAIDs, Coumadin) should also be considered if clinically relevant.

As has been repeatedly stressed throughout this book, the treatment plan is dictated by the patient's condition and prognosis, and ultimately, by the patient's goals and wishes. Some diagnostic tests such as urinalysis and culture or coagulation screening are minimally invasive and may prompt relatively simple and rapidly effective palliative interventions such as antibiotics or reversal of anticoagulation. Hemorrhage due to tumors may respond to radiotherapy or cauterization. These interventions may be appropriate for select patients with longer prognoses. Aggressive palliative surgery including nephrectomy, cystectomy, and hypogastric artery ligation is rarely relevant for terminal hospice patients.

In end-of-life care, gross hematuria, especially when asymptomatic, may sometimes call for nothing beyond reassurance. When treating symptomatic hemorrhagic cystitis, patients should be encouraged to decrease physical activity and, if possible, to increase fluid intake. For persistent bleeding causing urinary clot retention, clots may be evacuated through a large diameter Foley catheter. Further bleeding and clotting can be minimized via bladder irrigation with saline chilled to 4°C at a rate of 3 L/24 hours. Empiric treatments to control bleeding from the bladder include etamsylate 500 mg orally every 6 hours or epsilon-amino-caproic acid (Amicar) 5 gm orally as an initial loading dose and 1 gm every 1 to 4 hours as needed. Amicar is contraindicated for patients with disseminated intravascular coagulation or with advanced liver disease and should be avoided when hematuria originates in the upper urinary tract as it can cause intrarenal obstruction due to clot formation, which can lead to severe pain from renal colic as well as to renal failure. Amicar may also be administered intravenously or intravesically, although these routes are generally not preferred for hospice patients. Another relatively innocuous treatment for hemorrhagic cystitis is 1% alum in sterile water given by continuous bladder irriga-

tion. Formalin instillation, although highly effective, is also highly toxic, and requires general or regional anesthesia. It does not appear to have a place in palliative end-of-life care.

For terminal patients with symptomatic upper urinary tract bleeding and clot colic, treatment is best confined to fluid-induced diuresis and appropriate analgesics. As explained earlier, Amicar may be excessively risky and should be avoided. For ethical reasons, the physician may be obligated to discuss the option of a palliative unilateral nephrectomy with the patient, but it is difficult to foresee the circumstance in which such a procedure would be recommended in end-of-life care.

URINARY INFECTIONS

Urinary infections in the terminally ill may be difficult to identify. Many elderly or debilitated patients may not be febrile despite significant infection. The basal body temperatures in such people may be lower than in a healthy person in which case a normal temperature reading may actually represent a fever. In addition, the blunting of the febrile response to infection in these patients may delay the onset of a fever by one or more days following the onset of infection.

Other signs and symptoms of infection in end-of-life care patients may also be vague or attenuated. There may be some loss of appetite, a relative increase in fatigue or confusion, lower blood pressure, declining urine production, and tachycardia. Therefore, it is best to have a high index of suspicion for the presence of infection and sepsis.

Patients in long-term care facilities may have colonization of the urinary tract with one or more organisms usually responsible for infection. Therefore, without signs or symptoms consistent with a urinary infection, a positive culture in such an individual may not warrant aggressive management that could result in selective growth of organisms resistant to antibiotic therapy. In the severely debilitated and/or demented patient, discussion with the family regarding the pros and cons of aggressively treating urinary infections should be undertaken when formulating an overall plan of care. If the aim of treatment is primarily to relieve the symptoms of irritative voiding, acidification of the urine by drinking cranberry juice or the use of urinary analgesic drugs such as phenazopyridine (Pyridium) may be sufficient. The addition of anticholinergic drugs may also help to relieve symptoms.

If it is elected to prescribe antibiotics, treatment may be empirical pending culture results. Reasonably effective oral agents include amoxicillin, trimethoprim/sulfamethoxazole, and ciprofloxacin. Alternative, intravenous antibiotics may sometimes be indicated depending on the defined palliative goal.

PERIPHERAL EDEMA

Although not always focused on, the presence of lower extremity edema is a relatively common symptom for patients near the end of life and can result in a number of patient complaints, including leg weakness and/or heaviness, local discomfort or frank pain, leakage of fluid, skin lesions, and infection. The causes of peripheral edema in these patients is generally multi-factorial and may include heart failure and other causes of fluid retention, hypoalbuminemia, decreased mobility, neurological dysfunction, obstruction of venous flow secondary to deep vein thrombosis (which will be discussed in the next section), and obstruction of lymphatics due to metastatic disease in the inguinal or pelvic nodes or radiation induced fibrosis. Some patients may develop edema due to the release of neuropeptides from sensory nerves that cause an increase in vascular permeability, leading to plasma extravasation into the legs.

As most of the causes of peripheral edema are related to a patient's primary disease process and

irreversible when patients are near the end of life, treatment of peripheral edema is challenging at best. Keeping with the goal of only using pharmacological therapy when necessary, leg elevation is always a good first step. If the edema is confined to the lower part of the legs, antiembolic stockings or even regular socks may also be of benefit, keeping in mind that, since the stockings may only displace the fluid, where the sock ends the swelling will begin. Good skin care is important as well to reduce the risk of both stasis and pressure ulcer formation.

When the edema is troublesome and pharmacological treatment is required, diuretics remain the mainstay of treatment, although clinical evidence as to the efficacy of diuretics in the treatment of edema in the palliative care setting is lacking. Generally, small doses of thiazide diuretics or furosemide are utilized. Patients so treated will generally require periodic monitoring of serum electrolytes and often require potassium supplementation or the addition of small dose of spironolactone, which is potassium-sparing. As many patients near the end of life develop edema for reasons other than fluid overload, one runs the significant risk of salt and fluid depletion, despite the edema, when diuretics are used. Therefore, especially when patients can sit up or are ambulatory, blood pressure should be monitored and diuretics should be discontinued if there is any evidence of hypotension. Infusion of albumin combined with diuresis, which is sometimes used to treat patients with edema secondary to hypoalbuminemia, has generally been unsuccessful, and is not usually deemed appropriate for patients near the end of life. For the treatment of symptomatic severe edema refractory to diuretic therapy, two approaches have been suggested in the palliative care literature. One report has suggested that an infusion of a small amount of hypertonic saline with high-dose furosemide may significantly improve symptoms of leg weakness and heaviness in patients with refractory edema (Mercadante, 2009). In a second study, eight patients near the end of life with refractory edema had reduction in leg swelling and associated symptoms when treated by subcutaneous drainage using a series of small butterfly needles inserted into the lower extremities (Clein and Pugachev, 2004). Although these treatments may be effective, their use should not be considered routine, and these interventions should be confined to selected patients with symptomatic severe refractory peripheral edema.

VENOUS THROMBOEMBOLIC DISEASE

Cancer patients near the end of life are known to be at high risk for the development of venous thromboembolic disease, with estimates putting the risk with advanced disease at greater than 50%. In the noncancer population with advanced disease, the development of deep vein thrombosis may be the first sign of occult neoplasia, or in the sub-population of patients with nonmalignant terminal disease, it may be caused by the immobility that affects many of these patients as their diseases progress. Because of the multifactorial nature of edema in patients near the end of life (as discussed earlier), signs and symptoms that may suggest that swelling of the lower extremities may be due to venous thromboembolic disease are difficult to define. One clue may be found in a retrospective analysis, which suggests that patients with advanced cancer who present with bilateral asymmetric lower extremity edema of potentially multifactorial origin have a high incidence of deep vein thrombosis (Kirkova et al., 2005).

The decision of whether and how to best treat these patients has remained a challenge. In addition to leg elevation and warm compresses to relieve local symptoms, anticoagulation has always been the mainstay of therapy. Warfarin had generally been considered the treatment of choice in the past for all patients. However, the requirement for constant monitoring of the INR [international normalized ratio of the patient's prothrombin time (PT) to the control value],

the number of drug–drug interactions that affect warfarin dosing, a high incidence of bleeding complications in palliative care patients, patient discomfort, and the risk of medication side effects have all made management challenging. With the advent of the low molecular weight heparins (LMWHs), this has changed, as they require no INR monitoring and lack the drug–drug interactions that make warfarin management difficult. Therefore, for many patients, especially those not near the end of life, the LMWHs have replaced warfarin as the treatment of choice.

For patient near the end of life, however, the use of LMWHs has remained controversial, for despite the need for laboratory monitoring when using warfarin, it is an oral agent. The LMWHs, on the other hand, can only be given by daily subcutaneous injection, and there is significant concern among end-of-life care providers that the need for a daily injection will be extremely burdensome to patients and outweigh the less frequent venipunctures required when using warfarin. Despite these concerns among caregivers, a qualitative study of 40 palliative care patients demonstrated that for the majority of these patients, LMWH was an acceptable treatment as it allowed them freedom from blood tests. These patients also found it to be preferable to treatment with warfarin, which had a negative impact on their quality of life (Noble and Finlay, 2005). In another study, these same investigators found that the use of LMWH was safe and effective when administered to 62 palliative care patients (Noble et al., 2007), without any evidence of drug–drug interactions or significant bleeding complications. While optimum dosing schedules and duration of therapy in end-of-life care have yet to be defined, it would appear, that, at least for selected patients near the end of life, LMWHs may be appropriate therapy to treat venous thromboembolic disease.

BIBLIOGRAPHY

Bruera E, Driver L, Barnes EA, et al: Patient controlled methylphenidate for the management of fatigue in patients with advanced cancer: A preliminary report. *J Clin Oncol* 21:4439-4443, 2003.

Bruera E, Valero V, Driver L, et al: Patient-controlled methylphenidate for cancer fatigue: A double-blind, randomized, placebo-controlled trial. *J Clin Oncol* 24:2073-2078, 2006.

Clein LJ, Pugachev E: Reduction of edema of lower extremities by subcutaneous controlled drainage: Eight cases. *Am J Hosp Palliat Care* 21:228-232, 2004.

Doyle D, Hanks G, McDonald N: *The Oxford Textbook of Palliative Medicine*. New York, Oxford University Press, 1996.

Enck RE: *The Medical Care of Terminally Ill Patients*. London, Johns Hopkins, 1994.

Fallon MT, Hanks GW: Control of common symptoms in advance cancer. *Ann Acad Med* 23:2, 1994.

Harris A: Providing urinary continence care to adults at the end of life. *Nursing Times* 105:29, 2009. http://www.nursingtimes.net/nursing-practice-clinical-research/specialists/continence/providing-urinary-continence-care-to-adults-at-the-end-of-life/5004035.article. Accessed August 24, 2009.

Hirshberg SJ, Greenberg RE: Urologic issues of palliative care. In: Berger A, Portenoy RK, Weissman DE, eds. *Principles and Practice of Supportive Oncology*. Philadelphia, PA, Lippincott-Raven, 1998, pp. 371-383.

Hirst A, Sloan R: Benzodiazepines and related drugs for insomnia in palliative care. *Cochrane Database Syst Rev* (4):CD003346, 2002.

Hospice Pharmacia Pharmacy and Therapeutics Committee. *Hospice Pharmacia Medication Use Guidelines*, 7th ed. Philadelphia, PA, ExcellRX, Inc., 2005.

Hugel H, Ellershaw JE, Cook L, et al: The prevalence, key causes, and management of insomnia in palliative care patients. *J Pain Symptom Manage* 27:316-321, 2004.

Johanson, GA: *Symptom Relief in Terminal Care*. Santa Rosa, Sonoma County Academic Foundation, 1994.

Johnson MJ: Problems of anticoagulation within a palliative care setting: An audit of hospice patients taking warfarin. *Palliat Med* 11:306-312, 1997.

Kirkova J, Oneschuk D, Hanson J: Deep vein thrombosis (DVT) in advanced cancer patients with lower extremity edema referred for assessment. *Am J Hosp Palliat Med* 22:145-149, 2005.

Lee A, Levine M: Treatment of venous thromboembolism in cancer patients. *Cancer Control* 12(S1):17-21, 2005.

Levine M: Comment: Home-treatment of deep vein thrombosis in patients with cancer. *Haematologica* 90:150a, 2005.

Marinella MA: Diagnosis and management of hiccups in the patient with advanced cancer. *J Support Oncol* 7:122-130, 2009.

McCoubrie R, Jeffrey D: Letter: Intravesical diamorphine for bladder spasm. *J Pain Symptom Manage* 25:1-3, 2003.

Mercadante S, Villari P, Ferrara P, et al: High-dose furosemide and small-volume hypertonic saline solution infusin for the treatment of leg edema in advanced cancer patients. *J Pain Symptom Manage* 37:419-423, 2009.

Moretti R, Torre P, Antonello RM, et al: Gabapentin as drug therapy of intractable hiccups because of vascular lesion: A 3 year follow-up. *Neurologist* 10:102-106, 2004.

Noble SIR, Finlay IG: Is long-term low-molecular-weight heparin acceptable to palliative care patients in the treatment of cancer related venous thromboembolism? A qualitative study. *Palliat Med* 19:197-201, 2005.

Noble SIR, Finlay IG: Comment: Home treatment of deep vein thrombosis in patients with cancer: Quality of life impact of therapies. *Haematologica* 90:e65, 2005.

Noble SIR, Hood K, Finlay IG: The use of long-term low-molecular weight heparin for the treatment of venous thromboembolism in palliative care patients with advanced cancer: A case series of sixty two patients. *Palliat Med* 21:473-476, 2007.

Rousseau P: Asthenia in terminally Ill cancer patients. A brief review. *Am J Hospice Palliat Care* 14:258, 1997.

Scialla SJ, Cole RP, Bednarz L: Redefining cancer-related asthenia-fatigue syndrome. *J Pall Med* 9:866-872, 2006.

Storey P, Knight C: *Management of Selected Non-pain Symptoms in the Terminally Ill*. Gainsville, American Academy of Hospice and Palliative Medicine, 1996.

Tegeler ML, Baumrucker SJ: Gabapentin for intractable hiccups in palliative care. *Am J Hosp Palliat Med* 25:52-54, 2008.

World Health Organization: *Symptom Relief in Terminal Illness*. Geneva, World Health Organization, 1998.

SELF-ASSESSMENT QUESTIONS

1. Which of the following variables has been shown to independently correlate with patients' self-reported fatigue ratings on a VAS scale?

    A. Serum albumin levels
    B. C-reactive protein levels
    C. Hemoglobin levels
    D. BMI
    E. Motor function impairment

2. Mr. Smith is a 75-year-old male with advanced lung cancer. He completed a 1-week course of radiotherapy to the left femur due to a painful metastatic lesion approximately 4 weeks ago and his pain is improved. He has a history of hypertension for which he takes a diuretic and a calcium-channel blocker. He is also an insulin-dependent diabetic and his blood sugars have remained under good control. You are seeing him today for evaluation of severe fatigue. He also complains of lightheadedness sometimes when he sits up or stands. Remarkable physical findings include a blood pressure of 110/70 lying and 100/60 sitting upright and a regular pulse of 90. His mucus membranes are pink and dry and his conjunctivae show no pallor. Which of the following would be first step in approaching his complaint of fatigue?

    A. Do a CBC to check for anemia and transfuse if necessary.
    B. Change his insulin to an oral hypoglycemic agent.
    C. Discontinue his antihypertensive medication
    D. Reassure him the fatigue is from the radiation therapy and it will get better in a couple of more weeks.
    E. Start methylphenidate 5 mg every 4 hours as needed (maximum 4 tablets per day)

3. Mrs. Jones is an 82-year-old female who is on your hospice program with a diagnosis of debility. She is confined to bed at home due to paralysis from a prior stroke, has been losing weight, and does not want to be evaluated for the cause of the weight loss. She now is complaining of difficulty sleeping at night. This started several weeks ago when a dear friend of hers with whom she played gin rummy everyday became ill and could no longer come to spend time with her. Since then, she has been extremely bored, and despite watching TV, she has tended to doze during the day and has been unable to sleep at night. The only medication she takes is lorazepam 1 mg in the morning and 1 mg in the afternoon to reduce her anxiety and says that it is the "only thing that gets me through the day." Of the following, which would be the best first approach to try and improve her insomnia?

    A. Find a hospice volunteer who is willing to play gin rummy with the patient
    B. Discontinue the lorazepam
    C. Add a dose of lorezepam 1 mg at bedtime.
    D. Start zolpidem 10 mg at bedtime.
    E. Start diphenhydramine 25 mg at bedtime

4. All of the following are potential nonpharmacological interventions for the treatment of hiccups EXCEPT

    A. Rapid ingestion of granulated sugar
    B. Drinking from the wrong side of the cup
    C. Warm compress placed at the back of the neck
    D. Swallowing dry bread
    E. Stimulation of the pharynx with an oral or nasal catheter

5. Which of the following medications used to treat hiccups is approved by the FDA for this indication?

    A. Baclofen
    B. Gabapentin
    C. Metaclopramide
    D. Chlorpromazine
    E. Prednisone

6. All of the following are symptoms characteristic of urinary retention due to detrusor muscle failure EXCEPT

    A. Hesitancy
    B. Urgency
    C. Impaired bladder sensation
    D. Long time intervals to micturition

7. All of the following may be instilled intravesically to treat bladder spasms in patients near the end of life EXCEPT

    A. Acetic acid solution
    B. Bupivicaine
    C. Formalin
    D. Diamorphine
    E. Chilled saline solution

8. Which of the following statements regarding urinary tract infections in patients near the end of life is true?

    A. Patients will usually develop a fever as an early sign of infection.
    B. All patients living in a long-term care facility who have positive urine cultures should be treated with antibiotics.
    C. One should wait for the results of the urine culture before staring antibiotics.
    D. Cranberry juice can effectively reduce bacterial growth in the urine via urine acidification.
    E. Pyridium should be avoided as it masks symptoms of bladder irritation, which may be a sign of infection.

9. Which of the following causes of edema should be suspected in a patient with advanced cancer who has bilateral asymmetric swelling of the lower extremities?

    A. Hypoalbuminemia
    B. Deep vein thrombosis
    C. Congestive heart failure
    D. Plasma extravasation secondary to sensory nerve neuropeptides
    E. Neurologic dysfunction

10. All of the following are reasons why low-molecular weight heparins (LMWH) may be considered preferable to warfarin for the treatment of deep vein thrombosis in patients near the end of life EXCEPT

    A. Warfarin is taken orally
    B. Warfarin causes significant drug–drug interactions
    C. Warfarin requires monitoring of the INR
    D. Warfarin has been reported to negatively impact patient quality of life
    E. Warfarin has been reported to cause a high incidence of bleeding in palliative care patients

CHAPTER

14

Psychosocial and Spiritual Concerns at the End of Life

Sarah E. McKinnon and Bob Miller

INTRODUCTION

In our death-denying society, the opus of those going through the dying process has been muted, only to be heard, if at all, among those living with and caring for the dying on a daily basis. Although there has been a significant increase in energy and focus on caring for pain and other physical symptoms at the end of life, less emphasis has been placed on the management of psychosocial and spiritual issues, as well as their influences on patients' perceptions of pain and symptoms. In this chapter, therefore, the goal is to provide a basic overview of psychosocial and spiritual issues in end-of-life care while presenting a framework within which to discuss these subjects. The approach is not completely clinical in nature. We provide personal observations and share the opinions of dying persons and their families, as well as summarize literature that has been reviewed.

The understanding of psychosocial and spiritual issues that occur at the end of life is often of great importance to those who have received the least training about them, such as physicians and clinical nurses. In Buckman's book on *Breaking Bad News* (1992) he describes the paradox that occurs in healthcare. Those who have the most knowledge about psychosocial and spiritual issues (psychiatrists, psychologists, socials workers, and chaplains) are those who "do not perform this task in daily practice." Rather, physicians do. Too often the stories patients and families share of their perceptions of their doctor delivering a terminal prognosis include words like "cold" or "insensitive," "in a hurry" or "just doesn't care."

> In a great majority of cases, those doctors were not cold or insensitive (most doctor's aren't) but they were uncomfortable, edgy, and embarrassed. They may well have been aware that they did not know how to carry out the conversation effectively and supportively, and so may have backed off, attempting to end the interview quickly to reduce their own discomfort and sense of clumsiness. They may well have overused medical jargon to give an air of efficiency and professionalism to the proceedings, and thus may have added to the perception that they were impersonal or indifferent.

Much of this can be attributed to a physician's training. In the movie, *Patch Adams*, Dr. Hunter "Patch" Adams chronicles many of his real-life experiences in medical school. In one scene, the Dean of the School of Medicine, in an opening lecture to all first-year medical students, tells them "It is our mission here to rigorously and ruthlessly train the humanity out of you in order to make you into something better. We are going to make doctors out of you." The objectivity necessary to deal with the realities of medical practice serves physicians well, as does the focus on the treatment of the symptoms and the disease process. In addition, to be overly emotionally involved with each and every patient might bring about an inability to effectively treat patients over a lifetime of practice. Therefore, the challenge is to be able to include some subjectivity where and when it is truly "what is best for the patient." End-of-life care is just such a time.

Another piece of this puzzle is to attempt to fill the gap that exists between the professional role of the physician and the humanity of the individual who lives that role. In a recent gathering of community physicians, the issue of bereavement for doctors was discussed. It should come as no surprise that these physicians, who deal repeatedly with death, identified their need to grieve the loss of their patients in some structured way. Too often we fall under the influence of the myth of the "doctor as God." For many years, physicians have even contributed to that fable. Now it is not only the duty of doctors to move beyond this view, but it is also the responsibility of the general public to remove physicians from the uncomfortable pedestal on which we have placed them.

Another challenge that physicians face in properly addressing the psychosocial and spiritual needs of their patients at the end of life relates to the evolving and changing nature of the healthcare industry.

(Sarah): A patient I know, who was dealing with cancer, told a friend of his "My doctor is my best friend for the fifteen minutes a month I get to see him." This was no reflection on the humanity of the physician, simply a comment on the reality of a medical practice and an ability to make a living (and pay off medical school loans) in this day and age.

(Sarah): Recently, a volunteer I work with mentioned that her own physician told her "don't get me started" when she mentioned whether or not he referred to hospice. Further discussion unearthed the fact that he was under the mistaken assumption that he would have to turn over his patient to the hospice physician who would then become his patient's primary physician. He is a doctor who is connected and involved in his patient's care, to the point of making house calls when necessary. She educated him about a physician always being able to follow his/her patient on a hospice program and also his capability to continue to bill separately for his care of his patient. What resulted was a win-win: for the volunteer, the physician, and ultimately, his patients.

On the positive side, physicians are becoming increasingly aware of the psychosocial and spiritual issues that affect their patients near the end of life. However, what doctors seem to struggle with most is what to do about these problems when they manifest. More good news is that hospice care, which sets the standard in end-of-life care, addresses this struggle by including in its philosophy the need for psychosocial and spiritual components of care at the end of life. The hospice team includes trained social workers and chaplains to help the team address such issues. These team members can provide support for physicians in ensuring that patients receive appropriate psychosocial and spiritual care.

PSYCHOSOCIAL AND SPIRITUAL CHALLENGES AT THE END OF LIFE

Although the title of this chapter differentiates spiritual aspects from the psychosocial, in truth,

the range and depth of being human makes it impossible to know where one ends and the other begins. Therefore, psychosocial and spiritual concerns are addressed as a continuum.

What are some potential psychosocial and spiritual challenges a physician might encounter when caring for terminally ill patients and their families? There might be difficulty managing symptoms resulting from dysfunctional family situations or the patient's own need for autonomy. Dealing with patient/family emotional reactions related to the terminal illness and impending death: fear, depression, denial, anger, and anxiety are often common in these situations. They may be unable to effectively address the spiritual dimension of care which surfaces at the end of life.

Enhanced understanding of the common psychological concerns of patients with serious illness can improve not only the clinical care of the patient, but also the physician's sense of satisfaction and meaning in caring for the dying. (Block, 2001)

DYING'S INHERENT OPPORTUNITIES!

It is suggested that the first and most helpful resource for those traveling on the path toward the end of life is a new paradigm that reframes society's view of dying and brings to light the opportunities inherent in this end-of-life process. As stated by Dr. Ira Byock in his 1986 article on growth as the essence of hospice care:

Dying represents more than a set of problems to be solved. It represents an extraordinary opportunity. An opportunity for review, for restitution, for amends, for exploration, for development, for insight. In short it is an opportunity for growth.

Rather than looking at psychosocial and spiritual care at the end of life as problems to be solved, they should be viewed from the perspective of

TABLE 14–1. Psychosocial and Spiritual Opportunities at the End of Life

The Opportunity to...
Reframe society's view of dying: grow on
Expand our definition of quality of life
Focus on the individual, not the disease
Address as a whole physical pain, psychosocial issues and spiritual concerns
Move through fear to peace
Move through confusion to meaning
Mover through despair to hope
Move from isolation to community
Come to terms with your physical body
Move from loss to closure
Adjust to new roles
Get your affairs in order

opportunities they provide to the patients, families, and caregivers, when the end of life is near. A list of these opportunities are presented in Table 14–1.

OPPORTUNITY TO . . . REFRAME SOCIETY'S VIEW OF DYING: GROW ON!

One way to facilitate the shifting of the view of dying from problem to opportunity is to redefine the end of life as an identifiable stage of human development. Instead of growing up, growing old and dying, Dr. Byock suggests we grow up, grow old, and grow on.

Growing on takes place for both the aged and terminally ill and their families. And although patients and families will universally find growth producing deaths as important and positive, it may not be easy. Indeed, there are typically many obstacles that must be overcome if the process of dying is to unfold in a productive manner.

In this light, the dying process may be seen as an established experience, attributed with specific tasks attached to the unfolding of the process itself. Fostering this understanding will be the challenge of established cultural and religious teachings that imply that death is the enemy, a sign of personal failure, betrayal by one's body, or a shortfall in the promise held out by medical science. Those of us who have journeyed alongside the dying know the other side of the story, that the dying process can be a time of great achievement.

Ironically, although illness and death come into each life, we tend to resist seeing these processes as "normal" or as opportunities to learn. Illustrative of this fact is that many Quality of Life instruments tend to "imply that a good quality of life is the result of an absence of problems rather than a reflection of favorable balance between positive and negative influences." As with any new experience, there are aspects of what appear to be problems which, when you begin to address them, become more comfortable and understandable due to the context created by the "problem" itself.

(Sarah): I remember being in my sixth grade math class when the "smartest" boy in the class complained to the teacher about how long it was taking the rest of us to finish a problem. The teacher silently went to the board, wrote out a math problem, and asked Randy to solve it. I will never forget the look on Randy's face. "But Mr. Lentz, I don't know how to do that problem!" Mr. Lentz went to the board and within a minute, wrote out the answer. He then looked at Randy and said, "When you know how to do something, it is easy. The challenge is learning something new. You understand how to do the problems the rest of the class is working on just as I know how to do Calculus. Soon the rest of the class will know how to do what you have already learned just as someday you will learn to do what I know how to do now."

Unlike other experiences, the challenge in dying is that you don't really get any practice prior to doing it! However seeing the process of dying as a stage of life development, which, like every other life process, inherently contains both the good and the not so good, allows us a framework within which to comfortably explore this natural and expected life event. Then and only then will we be able to see the psychosocial and spiritual experiences of dying as opportunities rather than concerns.

OPPORTUNITY TO . . . EXPAND OUR DEFINITION OF QUALITY OF LIFE

Early in adulthood, quality of life (QOL) is typically thought of in terms of success in the world through work, family, friends, and personal activities. Rarely do people include health in describing their quality of life unless they have experienced the loss of it. Health has been defined by people with a life-threatening illness as a "sense of self-integrity encompassing physical, mental/emotional, and spiritual domains." When one's health is compromised, a larger definition of quality of life must be developed. Although many associate a lessening of functional status with a lessening of quality of life, it is not always the case because the evaluation is subjective. "Patients' appraisal of QOL is thus dynamic and changeable across time and perhaps even across situations."

When the first living will documents came into existence, they typically contained language that described the person's wish to be taken off life support when their "quality of life" was significantly diminished. Very soon, it was realized that more information was needed, specifically, what this unique individual meant by the phrase "quality of life." Each person's perception of quality will differ based on the importance and satisfaction the person gives each dimension or activity in life. For one person, that might mean the ability to get up every day and walk around the golf course, for another it might mean the ability to interact and communicate with loved ones, for another the feeling that they are still contributing something to society. It is the perception of the patient that defines quality of life for that individual. "For patients who are dying, appropriate care must respond to the patient's subjective and often changing quality of experience and needs."

Missoula–VITAS Quality-of-Life Index

The Missoula–VITAS Quality-of-Life Index has been an invaluable tool in exploring the patient's subjective experience of quality of life and the impact of illness on that perception. It also helps professional and family caregivers conceptualize broad concepts related to quality of life. The tool measures five dimensions of quality: symptom, interpersonal, functional, well-being, and transcendent, each of which is discussed here as it relates to psychosocial and spiritual care at the end of life (for a more thorough discussion of the MVQOLI and quality of life in general, please refer to Chapter 5).

The *symptom* section outlines the level of physical discomfort and distress experienced because of the progressive illness. For example, patients who have gone from having a few coughing fits throughout the day to one every time they speak is potentially going to have a lessened quality of life if they value social interaction and enjoy talking with others. This will not affect someone who prefers being alone to the same extent.

Function refers to the perceived ability to perform accustomed functions and activities of daily living (such as dressing, feeding, and bathing oneself) and the emotional response to this based on one's expectations.

(Sarah): My grandfather, as he grew more and more ill, had a terrible time with others having to dress him and take him to the bathroom. He had been a Vice-president of a major corporation and wore a suit and tie every day of his life, complete with an ironed, cloth handkerchief. In direct contrast, I often kid with my friends that once a woman goes through childbirth any sense of privacy regarding her body is gone, and as far as mothers are concerned, any type of help with anything is greatly appreciated, no matter how basic.

The *interpersonal* dimension deals with the degree of investment in personal relationships and the perceived quality of one's relations and interactions with family and friends. An illness may force, or provide an opportunity for, changes in one's significant relationships. These changes may be positive or negative in the eyes of the individual. The perception of satisfaction in this area may be dependent on the individual's ability to redefine and reframe important relationships, and the ability of the significant others in their life to do the same.

One's *well-being* is defined through a self-assessment of one's internal sense of wellness or "disease," and weighted for importance related to a sense of contentment or lack of contentment within each identified area.

Finally, *transcendence* refers to the experienced degree of connection with an enduring construct and the resulting sense of meaning and purpose given to life. Spiritual issues are inherent in the measuring of quality of life in the patient at the end of life. "The data suggest that the existential domain is at least as important as the physical, psychological, and support domains in determining quality of life and therefore cannot be ignored." Transcendence is about the connection to something beyond oneself, however one defines that "something." For some this is "God," for others it is simply a sense of meaning to the universe, and for others still, it is the legacy they will leave behind as a result of having lived.

These dimensions are reviewed here because, at the end of life, there are specific opportunities available within each of these dimensions. Although they will not form the outline of the remainder of this chapter, they underlie and inform much of the information that is to follow.

One "disclaimer" needs to be addressed at this point. Many professionals who care for patients near the end of life harbor the hope that the "perfect death" can happen for each patient and family. However, the reality is that many factors, both physical and psychologic, influence whether this actually happens or not. As noted earlier, in most cases, individuals will die the same way they lived.

This phenomenon is referred to as "remaining in character."

Typically, a kind, caring family man will be surrounded, supported, and loved by family members and his dying process will reflect his way of being. If a woman was angry, hurtful, and resentful in her lifetime, unless there is an epiphany during the dying process, the chances are her dying experience will reflect the same. A patient's skill at adapting to changes during life prior to the terminal illness will play a large part in the capacity to make changes affecting quality of life as death nears. For many, the definition of what constitutes a true problem versus a minor inconvenience is redefined.

OPPORTUNITY TO . . . FOCUS ON THE INDIVIDUAL, NOT THE DISEASE!

We all know that we are more than just our bodies. The mind–body connection, stress awareness, and caring for the "whole" self are becoming part and parcel of our understanding of ourselves rather than a fashionable part of the so-called "New Age" movement. However, this holistic view continues to find a great deal of resistance within the traditional medical model. In the traditional model, our bodies and psyches are "split." When someone has a physical problem, we address that problem with little regard for the rest of the person. Once they are healed physically, and if they so are inclined, they can work toward emotional or spiritual healing of those areas affected by their illnesses. It is our experience that most individuals simply try to get back to "the way it was" prior to the illness. The problem with this approach is that it ignores the physical and psychosocial changes which have occurred as a result of the illness, leaving individuals wondering why things aren't the same or "back to normal." The challenge is for them to embrace the fact that "normal" now has a new definition.

One of the results of emphasis on the traditional healthcare model, which tends to place importance only on the physical side of illness, is the reduction of the multidimensional nature of the individual into a single dimension, defined by the disease process. A patient loses his identity, and becomes "the lung cancer in Room 203." There is a unique terror, known only to those diagnosed with serious or life-limiting illness, that their humanity will somehow be lessened by their relationship with the medical establishment. They fear that they will be known as and, perhaps, become little more than, their disease in relationship to their doctors, the nurses providing care to them, and perhaps even to their families and friends.

Therefore, when caring for patients with terminal illnesses (and even with chronic longer term diseases), physicians must be sure that their focus shifts away from a preoccupation with the disease back to paying primary attention to the patient. Inclusion of the family as part of the unit of care, as promulgated by hospice and palliative care programs is also crucial. By viewing the patients and families that they care for from this perspective, physicians will be better able to recognize the importance of the psychosocial and spiritual needs of a person as essential elements of the treatment plan.

Of course, there is no reason to wait until someone has 6 or less months to live before addressing him/her as a whole person. For many persons, however, the dying process represents the first time in their lives in which they take the time to gain this awareness. There is much to be learned about life in general by examining this time, when, outside of the need for controlled pain and other symptoms, the overwhelmingly urgent issues are psychosocial and spiritual in nature.

OPPORTUNITY TO . . . ADDRESS AS A WHOLE, PHYSICAL PAIN, PSYCHOSOCIAL ISSUES, AND SPIRITUAL CONCERNS

Maslow's Hierarchy of Needs postulates that "higher" needs such as self-actualization cannot be met until more basic needs, such as food and shelter, are met. For example, a child who has not eaten will have a hard time studying ethics in school. Although life is rarely so neat or linear, this dynamic also applies to those dealing with a terminal illness. For example, when a patient is in physical pain, it may be difficult to focus on psychosocial or spiritual concerns. As Cella states: "Patients in severe or excruciating pain often cannot relate to general questions about mood, social functioning, or even less severe symptoms." However, it would be a mistake to assume that psychosocial or spiritual concerns will wait until the physical concerns are resolved. While experiencing the pain, the person may be wondering "What did I do to deserve this?" or "Who can help me get through this?" or "Why is God punishing me so?" These concerns may or may not be spoken during the crisis, but as the physical pain is controlled, the opportunity to address psychosocial and spiritual issues increases.

Although patients may not focus on psychosocial and spiritual issues when physical pain is poorly controlled, it is equally important to remember the significant effect unresolved psychosocial and spiritual issues may have on the perception of physical pain.

(Sarah): I remember a patient in a nursing home who spent hours and hours moaning as though she was in physical pain. The nursing home staff had warned me about her and she had received plenty of attention regarding medication to treat her pain, but she continued to engage in these behaviors. As a psychology student, she intrigued me. Everyday when I would visit Mrs. "Smith," I would hear her "complaining" down the hall and would gear myself up to see her. It would take about 10 minutes, but once she realized I was not going to come in and out and that I was going to stay with her for an extended period of time (1 hour), she quit her moaning. She simply wanted someone to be with her. Her "physical" complaints were "psychosocial" in origin. As our hospice care team worked with her, we were able to stop her groans completely.

Sometimes, it is the physical pain that leads to a psychosocial or spiritual symptom.

(Sarah): I remember a time when I dealt with an on-going, undiagnosed medical condition. After more than eight months with no relief, a friend said to me, "I think I know what the problem is, you're depressed." I remember telling her "Of course I'm depressed. I am in chronic pain."

In his article "An educational model for explaining hospice services," Welk expounds on the interaction between physical pain and the psychosocial and spiritual challenges that occur at the end of life. He uses the word "suffering" to describe what many terminally ill patients' experience, which should be distinguished from pain, even though the word "pain is frequently used interchangeably with suffering." Welk uses the word pain to describe physical pain only, and notes that someone may be in physical pain and may not be suffering. The corollary to that is true too; someone may be free of physical pain but suffering none the less. Areas in which suffering needs to be addressed are emotional, social, and spiritual. Without emotional support, one may experience fear, without social support, there may be conflict and disconnection, without spiritual support, many lose their source of hope. Although one may address these areas separately, it is only by addressing all areas— the physical, the emotional, the social, and the spiritual—that one may truly be successful in relieving "suffering" at the end of life.

OPPORTUNITY TO . . . MOVE THROUGH FEAR TO PEACE

During the dying process, we have the opportunity to look at the journey as one from fear to peace. Conversations with dying individuals show that there are a number of "unknowns" anticipated in this dying process that generate tremendous anxiety and fear, one of the greatest being the lack of knowledge as to what will happen physically as one nears death. In such circumstances, providing a roadmap so that patients and care-givers know what to expect from the physical experience may be necessary. For example, end-of-life caregivers may be called upon to explain the reason for decreased appetite and thirst during the dying process, or the desire for a darker environment. Patients and families may need reassurance that fear of uncontrolled symptoms, such as increasing pain or the sensation of suffocating near the end of life, is unwarranted, as these symptoms will be treated and controlled as the dying process continues. Family member's caregiving efforts may need to be directed away from cooking huge meals and toward providing simple mouth or skin care. Providing guidance to patients and families regarding these and other similar issues in a gentle and compassionate fashion, from the standpoint of experiences with others who have been through similar disease processes, will reduce fear and provide patients and families with the support and peace they seek as life draws to a close.

Paul Tournier, in his book *Learn to Grow Old* (1991), discusses life as a task to be accomplished. Within that task there is the paradox that one can never finish the task, and that the true task in the end becomes "acceptance of unfulfillment, acceptance of the unfulfilled." He goes on to say that that it is hard to accept the unfulfilled and that is one of the problems in dealing with death. He defines acceptance as an active choice, one which is decided upon rather than arrived at passively. "To accept is to choose the reality, choosing freely between the reality and the fiction . . . You make the unity of your life by accepting the reality." For many, that unity can help to bring a sense of peace.

The only way one will know how to comfort an individual patient or family is to listen to their concerns and address them as directly and sincerely as possible. Often, just having the information results in a greater level of comfort. Patients and families learn what is "normal" in the current situation. Remember, people do not get a chance to practice dying—it is a new experience for everyone.

Another aspect of the "unknown" is more existential in nature, and in this arena no one has ever "been there, done that." No one has been beyond death and come back to tell about it. No one can make the ultimate unknown known. Different people's "faith" systems will provide either comfort or create fear, depending on their orientation toward their faith. The crisis of facing death may cause some patients to be more open to the need for outside help, providing them with an opportunity to change a system of belief with which they are unhappy. It should be noted that there often needs to be a great deal of willingness and desire on the part of patients for this shift to occur.

The best that professional caregivers can offer in this circumstance is to be there and be present. To really listen to what is important to the patient, and if possible, build on the things that bring comfort. Even patients who reach what Elisabeth Kubler-Ross described as the "acceptance" stage outlined in her five stages of dying, often desire company as they make their transition.

> (Bob): I had one patient, Fran, who didn't seem like she'd ever come to terms with her sense that God had abandoned her to her illness. She constantly said, "I've lost my faith." During the months I visited her, she found no comfort in anything I offered. Then, on her deathbed, she told me that she now understood that God had not abandoned her because I had not abandoned her. Sometimes just being there can make all the difference in the world, and you never know what patients will make of your relationship. In Fran's case, it wasn't anything I said; it was simply my presence with her.

Kathleen Dowling Singh in her book *The Grace in Dying* (1998), builds upon the Kubler-Ross model by addressing spirituality in the dying process. She describes three stages of dying: chaos, surrender, and transcendence. She offers "a different theoretical structure to the nature of the profound inner changes which are taking place as the personality restructures on a deeper level in response to transpersonal forces." More and more people are coming to see themselves as spiritual beings living a human existence. Singh describes the process of letting go of one's "humanness" or one's ego connection to the world through the process of surrendering. The opportunity is then presented to acknowledge that part of one's self that is spiritual and eternal. This leads to a place of transcendence, a sense of unity with self and the world. The dying process takes on new meaning as the patient can see beyond the limits of the physical body and experience a sense of who they are beyond this singular life. These stages provide a framework within which to address the release of the struggle to hold on in the dying process and find tranquility.

OPPORTUNITY TO . . . MOVE THROUGH CONFUSION TO MEANING

One critical factor in the capacity to "die well" is one's belief about the meaning of the illness. Is the illness seen as a punishment for past wrongdoing, invoked either by God or by some "law of retribution?" Exploring the source of that guilt may be helpful, especially if reconciliation is possible.

> (Bob): One of the most difficult cases for me as a caregiver was a man who worked hard to develop a healthy form of detachment from his guilt regarding his illness. He tried to embrace the understanding that his disease was not a punishment from God. His last words to me were "I almost believed it." It took months for me to develop my own healthy form of detachment as a caregiver and to realize that although his journey didn't end up the way I wanted, it was his journey and my involvement was important just the same.

Perhaps the illness is seen as fate, a random occurrence that is the result of an impersonal, uncaring universe. Exploring some sense of love and purpose may be helpful. Simply opening up the possibility that God may be grieved by the suffering of people, for example, may produce an unexpected insight, or at least produce a reaction worth exploring!

Is the illness seen as a sign of some personal failure, such as the case of a person whose smoking has resulted in emphysema, or a person who believes that their anger has internalized in the form of a tumor? Exploring the cause and effect as well as the nature of the disease may be as helpful to a patient as is taking responsibility to make amends with oneself and one's family where appropriate. The variations on these themes are many; the responses need to be equally diverse.

Walter Wangerin in his book *Mourning into Dancing* (1992) makes an observation regarding the essence of tragedy and its meaning. He points to the time after an experience of despair, when there is awareness that "the griever *had* to suffer hopelessness in order to be astonished by her new life." Walter Brueggemann, a Biblical scholar, describes a similar dynamic as the basis of what we call pastoral care, which he describes as helping people enter into an experience of exile, to be in exile, and then to depart out of exile. He points out that, although the process is not as quick or easy as we'd like it to be, "only grief permits newness."

Victor Frankl wrote about the meaning of suffering in his work *Man's Search for Meaning* (1959). He describes suffering as one way to discover meaning in life and feels that "Man's main concern is not to gain pleasure or avoid pain but rather to see a meaning in his life. That is why man is even ready to suffer, on the condition, to be sure, that his suffering has meaning." This is not to say that it is necessary to suffer, but that when suffering there is an opportunity to transcend that suffering by attaching significance to it.

(Sarah): I will never forget a woman I'll call Anna. Anna was dying of cancer. The first time I met her she told me that her cancer was the best thing that had ever happened to her. Now, I am a positive person, but this threw even me. Anna went on to share with me how she had never taken the time to "stop and smell the roses". Because of her diagnosis, she had learned to do many things, play with her grand-

children, have deep conversations with her daughter, how to garden, to listen to an opera, and take naps; things she was certain she would never have done had she not become ill. She had truly used her "suffering" to create new meaning in her life.

OPPORTUNITY TO . . . MOVE THROUGH DESPAIR TO HOPE

How a patient will find hope, and in what, is entirely a unique experience. For one patient, it may mean living until he is able to take part in some significant family event. For another it may be the sense of a life well lived, a sense that she has contributed something to the world or to someone important to her. For another, it might be the hope that in the afterlife the wrongs of this world will be corrected. Whatever the source, our challenge is to support patients as they find, explore, redefine, or change the source of their hope, sometimes several times in the course of an illness (or in the course of a single day!).

Allowing patients to take the lead in identifying their unique and preferred source of hope is not always easy, especially if we're inclined to help by offering or suggesting our own values as an alternative to the patient's values.

(Bob): One of my patients, Otis, who was under the care of our local hospice for terminal cancer, was telling me about his brother who had previously died from cancer. He told me his brother had been increasingly weak and drowsy, developed a poor appetite, and shortly thereafter, died. Otis asked me if I could tell him whether or not he had cancer too. He said the doctor had told him he had a tumor. Evidently to Otis this didn't necessarily mean that he had cancer.

Then Otis proceeded to tell me that putting a "tube" down his throat had made the diagnosis. He scrunched up his nose. I said, "That must've been an uncomfortable procedure." He said, "They put me under for the procedure, but when I woke up, my throat was sure sore". Then he paused and a gleam came to his eye, "Come to think of it, my rectum was sore too. I think they put the tube up there to get a look at the tumor from the other side." He fixed me in his gaze and said, with a straight face, "I sure hope they put it down my throat first!"

We laughed and together experienced what was a sacred moment. I say the moment was sacred because it was then that Otis began to tell me about feeling weak and sleepy much of the time, and that he was losing his appetite. He was letting me know that he knew he was dying of cancer as he was sharing with me the same symptoms he remembered about his brother's death. In this way he could communicate with me indirectly without having to acknowledge the "c-word" or admit that he had cancer. We had an opportunity to laugh and let humor put some space between him and his tumor. My allowing him to do this, I believe, enhanced his sense of hope.

OPPORTUNITY TO . . . MOVE FROM ISOLATION TO COMMUNITY

The social conflict described by Welk refers to the changes that occur in our relationships with the onset of illness and terminality. In a perfect world, all individuals, upon death, would have full closure with all those they had connected with during their lifetime. Realistically, however, many come to this time in their life with much left undone. Often, there have been separations between family members. Many of these have gone on for years with no thought given to reconciliation until the onset of the terminal illness. Frequently, patients have been heard to say that they have forgotten what the argument was about in the first place. When a reconnection takes place, the internal conflict for the patient and family may be relieved.

The opposite also holds true.

(Sarah): I recently heard about a patient who had lost contact with his son. The hospice social worker tracked the son down only to hear from him a definite "no" in regards to visiting or even talking to his father on the telephone. This patient, had been an alcoholic, was physically abusive to his wife, and had abandoned his family when they were very young.

Sometimes, at the end of life the task is to come to terms with life's disappointments, and what they mean. There may literally be no way to "fix" or make amends with what has happened. When there is no opportunity for reconciliation, caregivers may need to get creative in assisting a patient in his search for closure, maybe role-playing the hurt son, helping write a final letter, or making a recording of the father's "confession." Even if it doesn't lead to reconciliation, there may be some opportunity for healing in the simple act of confession, some absolution in the gentle listening presence offered, and maybe even some previously unrealized sense of a community established by the interaction.

As in the above-mentioned situation, sometimes one's community of choice does not have the capacity to remain constant and supportive of one who is ill. It is heartbreaking to listen to some of those who have been shunned by friends or people in their condominium or neighborhood because of an illness, even one as "noncommunicable" as cancer. This forced isolation can cause the one who is ill to feel all the more abandoned. What is needed is someone who has the capacity to be close and not afraid: someone for whom the disease is not perceived as a threat; someone who can help patients understand that there is nothing wrong with them, that the distance their friends may establish says more about them than it does about those who are ill. It says that the friends are afraid of their own frailty, their own potential for loss or illness, or that they simply don't know what to say and because of that fear, they say and do nothing. That supportive "someone" is often a relative, or a best friend, or sometimes even a healthcare professional.

OPPORTUNITY TO . . . COME TO TERMS WITH YOUR PHYSICAL BODY

As discussed earlier, physical changes associated with chronic or terminal illness often "mean" something in the subjective experience of the patient. If independence or control is central to an individual's ego, then the process of giving up roles in one's family can threaten one's sense of self. Or worse, a family system can be thrown off balance if cherished roles are reversed, such as when the "breadwinner" becomes the one in need, or the parent needs to be the one cared for. Often, how it will go depends on the family's or the individual's adaptability.

Body image concerns can be devastating, especially when illness is disfiguring. Our society, as part of its denial of death, celebrates youth and beauty. Women have a standard against which they are measured; one that is unattainable by most. Many are unable to come to terms with the changes that treatments such as surgery may bring, even if the surgery saves their life.

(Sarah): I know of a woman whose husband walked out on her the night before her mastectomy because he couldn't handle it.

Dealing with one's own responses to physical changes is difficult enough. This difficulty is doubled when others around you have trouble managing their reactions.

(Sarah): Working in a cancer support community taught me about the ability to transcend this mindset. Through a gathering of people living with many of the same changes and challenges, a new model is created. I have seen women go into the bathroom together, five at a time, to look at a member's surgery results, to laugh and cheer and gather strength for themselves as a group. One member chose to have a tattoo of a smiley face put on her reconstructed breast rather than a nipple tattoo. She brought in cookies to her weekly support group decorated with, you guessed it, smiley faces.

There is also the issue of how an individual feels about his/her body.

(Sarah): My grandmother was raised during a time when certain areas of the body were not discussed, described, or explored. She, at 77, was still referring to her pubic area as "down there" and it presented a challenge when her cancer necessitated treatment, dressing changes, and a catheter "down there."

Education and a nonjudgmental attitude will make a significant difference when dealing with these patients. Reminding them that they are more than just their body and approaching this new experience in a light-hearted and gentle manner will help. Depending on the relationship, humor can often cut through the worst embarrassment.

(Sarah): My sister, who had cystic fibrosis, was a great teacher for me in this respect. She referred to her wheelchair and oxygen canister (which went everywhere with her toward the end of her life) by nickname. Once a woman on an elevator (who obviously had no idea she had this chronic and terminal illness) looked severely at her following one of her coughing spells. She proceeded to say to my mother "Gee, I guess it is about time I give up my two packs a day habit." Her responses to her realities paved the way for the rest of us.

OPPORTUNITY TO . . . MOVE FROM LOSS TO CLOSURE

One's response to dying and the reactions of those around them are often tied to how openly they have or have not dealt with prior losses in their life. A family member may shed a few tears and respond to bereavement follow up with "I am doing great, fine, no problem" only to emotionally break down 3 months later when their dog dies. The pet's death opens the door for her to openly acknowledge her grief around both losses.

(Sarah): I heard once of a woman who lived in a small house behind the larger, main house where her grandson and granddaughter-in-law lived. The grandson was on a hospice program and because of friction between the granddaughter-in-law and the grandmother, the older woman was not involved in her grandson's care. She would, however, talk with the hospice nurse when she came to care for him and one day asked her if she had any information on death and dying. At her next visit, the nurse brought some bereavement materials and the woman took them into her house to read them. Two days later when the nurse returned, the woman came running out of her house to greet her. She shared, in broken English, how grateful she was for the information the nurse had brought. It turned out that she had had a child who had died over 50 years ago of Sudden Infant Death Syndrome (SIDS). She had never taken the time to grieve this loss nor did she understand the importance of doing so. That hospice nurse is convinced to this day that had this woman been able to process that loss at that time, her role within her family and eventually in the life of her grandson, would have been different and better.

Attendant losses have been discussed as part of addressing the many changes that occur as one copes with the dying process. Already discussed was the subject of prior losses and their potential effects on someone in the present. Another area of loss revolves around the loss of someone's future. In general, when the death of a loved one occurs, most will grieve the life that person lived and the memories of the life that was shared between the deceased and those in mourning. In addition, there is also the actual missing of that person in the present moment. An area of loss that is sometimes overlooked, however, is the loss of the future that one had hoped to experience with the loved one. The younger someone is when he or she dies, the greater the opportunity for this kind of loss. Dreams and aspirations for that person's future and one's future with that person may be more elaborate simply because there are potentially more lost years to grieve when someone dies at a younger age. There are all the "what ifs" and the "I wonder whats" This is especially challenging for parents who lose a child, regardless of the child's age.

I wonder what she would have been had she had a chance to grow up." "I wonder if he would have gone to my alma mater if he had not gotten sick?" "She'll never get to turn 16 or get her driver's license". "I will never get to walk her down the aisle.

So many parents, particularly those who lose young children, see themselves living a lifetime in the grief of "what might have been?"

(Bob): I remember talking with a woman whose grown son was on our hospice program. She said to me "A mother is not supposed to bury her child. It's just not right." In our minds the natural order of death is parent first, then child.

Although one never completely recovers from the loss of a child, one can move on and continue with one's own life.

(Sarah): One mother I know talks now about the "meaning" behind her experience in losing her 14 year old daughter, which taught her to value life, love other people, and to stay connected to her faith. She remembers her child everyday and then uses that memory to fuel her life.

Other parents use their experience to rally behind a cause, hoping to provide for other families that which they did not have while honoring the life of their child at the same time.

The phrase "anticipatory grieving," defined as grieving that occurs prior to death in anticipation of a coming loss, may affect terminally ill patients as well as families. For some, the diagnosis of a terminal illness results in an emotional withdrawal, interfering with the ability of the patient, the family, or both to be present in the here and now. Many people feel that the knowledge of a terminal prognosis can be likened to an immediate death sentence, and revealing this information to patients may result in their withdrawal due to "loss of hope" and their no longer feeling a part of the "living" world. As previously mentioned, people, in general, have not prepared for the final stage of life or recognized the importance of "living until we die." Family members, trying to protect their dying loved ones, not only hide information, but, assuming that the patients are too fragile to deal with the intense emotional reactions that may result from family members' feelings, hide them as well.

> (Sarah): I have heard many a family member say that they cannot cry in front of the patient because they do not want to upset him. Sometimes the patient is anxiously awaiting those tears as a symbol of the love and connection between them; a validation of their relationship.

In these situations, the parties in a relationship prematurely treat each other as if the relationship were already over, and fail to see the importance of continuing to invest energy in this next, albeit probably final, stage of the relationship. When this occurs, tremendous opportunity for final closure is often lost.

Another aspect of loss is the "if onlys."

> "If only we had caught it sooner." "If only he had stopped smoking ten years earlier". "If only we had done this treatment instead of that treatment". "If only we had not had that treatment at all."

The best advice is that there is no advice. No matter what one might want to say in these instances, even if one has experienced similar situations, it is hard for the grieving individual to hear. For many, those are questions that they need to ask themselves as they make their way through their journey of grief. One can listen, support, and possibly connect them with others who have had a similar experience.

An important understanding that most experienced end-of-life care providers carry with them is that one can never take away someone's denial or patterns of coping. One simply joins the patient in his/her model of the world and offers unconditional support. Caregivers must trust the patient's and family's process as they would their own.

OPPORTUNITY . . . TO ADJUST TO NEW ROLES

So often, people define themselves and their relationships with others and to the world, based on what they do and the roles in which they participate. Upon first meeting a new person, after asking them their name and where they are from, one most commonly asks, "What do you do?" Our society emphasizes "doing" more than "being," and our societal structure often places worth or lack thereof on individuals based on what they do. As discussed earlier, when a patient is diagnosed with a terminal illness, he or she may ask, "Who am I if physically I can no longer fulfill those roles?" Most of us fulfill many roles.

> (Sarah): I am a mother, daughter, sister, friend, volunteer, spiritual student, athlete, employee and individual. Within each of these roles there are even more, smaller, yet essential roles.

Illness may bring on changes in societal, familial, and sexual roles. As with all the areas discussed, each area is interconnected to the other. Physical changes may affect social roles. For those who were active in the community, it may be impossible to attend activities outside of the home. This could include church or synagogue, Kiwanis or Rotary, or golf or tennis. Family roles change as well. For example, a man with a diagnosis of chronic obstructive pulmonary disease will eventually become too ill to work and no longer be able to hold the position of breadwinner. He also may no longer be able to fulfill his other roles such as driving the car, paying the bills, or even walking the dog. No longer is he the man his wife married. In long-term relationships, many of these roles have been assigned and fulfilled by only one of the partners for years. The wife may now need to take on several of her husband's roles, some of which she may be ill-equipped to handle. Over time, resentment may build in his wife, which may, in turn, negatively affect their intimacy.

Although intimacy takes on many forms, sexual contact is an integral part of most adult relationships. Long-term illness brings about many changes in the way a couple interacts sexually. Many times there are concerns around possibly hurting the infirm person. Are they too fragile to engage in the usual form of lovemaking? Will it tire them out? There is sometimes the illogical yet strong fear of contracting the illness that the partner has even when it is noncommunicable. The simple truth is that few individuals will feel sexy or desirable when ill, and it takes energy to engage in sexual activity. Many couples have been living with the illness for years and have stopped connecting physically due to the distractions involved with the disease process and treatment. If this couple is from the "old school", in which one did not discuss sex and sexuality, then a further gap occurs. Bridging this gap means finding small ways in which to reestablish intimacy. The benefit of the terminal diagnosis and the choice to no longer pursue aggressive treatment also allows a couple to refocus on each other and turn their attention away from the disease. Although sexual intercourse may no longer be an option, there are a myriad of ways for couples to connect: talking, holding hands, back rubs, baths, and any sexual activity that makes allowances for the abilities of the patient.

Some of the best support we can offer families whose roles are rapidly changing is training in practical "survival skills." An 80-year-old man may have to learn to boil an egg or use a microwave. Another caregiver may need to learn, for the first time, how to balance the checkbook.

(Sarah): One caregiver I knew, upon his first trip to the grocery store alone, was uncertain which kind of margarine to buy because he wasn't sure why his wife had chosen the one they had been using. He left the store without any margarine.

In these cases, concrete step-by-step instruction and joint participation during the first few trials can make all the difference.

It may also be very important to the one who is dying to know that someone will continue to be there for the survivor with practical or emotional support. In this way, the dying person may be able to die with confidence knowing that the caretaking responsibilities that they would normally assume will be followed up by someone else. Not being the one to fulfill that role may still be a loss, but perhaps not an inconsolable one.

Many family members and friends need reassurance to understand how these changes will affect them and their relationship to the dying person. In this case, the opportunity is more for the healthy individual than it is for the dying one. Fear about the dying process is understandable, and it takes someone with courage to cross that threshold to visit within someone's home. Sometimes, the challenge is due to the disconnection from the customary way of interacting. For instance, when you see someone at the mall in cutoff shorts and a T-shirt, someone that you have only seen in a suit at work, at first it seems strange and often it takes a moment before you can even identify them. Visiting a friend or family member who is now ill and homebound is similar in that it feels initially uncomfortable and strange because it is a similarly new and different experience. However, be reassured that once the "comfort zone" is extended, it is likely that they will discover different ways to connect. Wouldn't you want someone to visit with you if the situation were reversed?

Imagine how much more intensely the spouse or significant other experiences these changes. For example, a wife might have cooked large meals for her and her husband and maybe they had long conversations together over dinner about politics and world events. Maybe the husband can no longer eat large meals or talk for long periods of time. The couple might connect now by eating a smaller dinner together while *listening* to the news.

If you are a family member living out of state and your loved one can no longer use the phone, a new link may need to be created. Perhaps e-mailing letters for the caregiver to read to your family member would keep the connection. As the dying process continues, it is important to continue to adapt the bonding experiences as much as possible. Ultimately, this may lead to the simplest, yet most enduring form of connection—

the family member holding the hand of the patient as he/she takes the last breath.

There is also the dimension of one's relationships reflecting, in part, who we are as individuals. We make the assumption that if I have a compassionate, caring, committed support group who is with me throughout the dying process, then I must be all those things: compassionate, caring, committed, and supportive. However, if I don't, what does that say about me? Many of us assume we will receive from others all that we have extended to them, especially in our time of need. Often, however, this is not the case, and not because we weren't all those things to all those people. Many patients have simply outlived their families and friends and were at a time in their lives when creating new support relationships was less possible. Other patients have wonderful friends and family who live out of state or are too ill themselves to visit or offer much support. In many cases these dying patients have been ill with their disease for years and have been unable to maintain a viable network of connections.

There may be no way to "make this better" in terms of adding new people to their lives, but one can spend time reminiscing about prior relationships and honoring the time, energy, and fun that went into them. It is a beautiful way to practice the art of storytelling while passing on interesting and historical information. It also allows the patient to relive wonderful memories and actually "be" with these people from the past in the present.

The practice of life review actually has a long tradition. In one sense, life review is part of the venerable old tradition of storytelling. In the Jewish faith, this process is recognized as a part of the person's legacy, called an "ethical will." In their book *So That Your Values Live On—Ethical Wills and How to Prepare Them* (1991), Jack Riemer and Nathaniel Stampfer give a wonderful overview of ethical wills, examples of historic and modern ethical wills, and guidelines for creating one. They point out that the ethical will

does not have to be a written document—a voice or video recording can be an amazing legacy to leave behind.

OPPORTUNITY TO . . . GET YOUR AFFAIRS IN ORDER

(Sarah): I spoke recently with a woman who was told by her oncologist to "get her affairs in order" as she had been diagnosed with stage three ovarian cancer. A year and a half later, she is here and cancer free.

Although this is one of those success stories that one loves to hear, all too often, when the doctor tells a patient that "it is time to get your affairs in order," it is usually time to do so. "Affairs" in this context can include financial and medical matters, as well as more practical matters such as funeral arrangements and decisions that surround those who will still be here after the patient is gone.

Sometimes, the challenge is in addressing these "practical" matters while trying to cope with the overwhelming blow of being given a terminal prognosis. One might have to face up to the reality that efforts to combat the disease have been unsuccessful. It is hard enough to simply make it from minute to minute, hour to hour, much less decide who gets what and whether you want to be buried or cremated. Again, due to our "death-denying society," few of us take the time to consider these matters when we are healthy and when these discussions would carry much less emotional trauma.

In today's health care environment, many patients and families face a great deal of stress related to treatment costs as well as bureaucracy, resulting in what can be termed "bureaucratic pain." Challenges related to payment for incredibly expensive treatments, which may not be as successful as first hoped, coupled with negotiating through the red tape of insurance companies, doctors' offices, and hospitals, often contribute, together with the physical, social, and emotional challenges of being terminally ill, to what has been defined as "total or overwhelming pain."

(Sarah): The best example of how to handle this came from a woman I knew who was dying of lung cancer. She talked about having worried about paying her bills during the years she was ill and all the companies calling her for payment and the anxiety it brought to her already strained life. She was laughing now about their inability to get "blood from a stone" because she was dying. This was a woman who had worked up until her illness, paid her bills on time and in full, and spent everything she had to pay to treat her illness. She taught me, through her experience, that each of us needs to do the best that we can, but there are times when our best must be "good enough."

One way to deal with "bureaucratic pain" is by "chunking down" whatever it is that seems most overwhelming. If a problem seems too big to handle, then chunk it down into manageable parts. Even financially, small payments over time add up to bigger credits and less owed. Beyond that, there is only so much that it is in our control and it is our job, as the Serenity Prayer suggests, to accept what we cannot change, change what we can, and be clear on the difference between the two.

BEYOND BYOCK'S OPPORTUNITIES

Julie Patton, in her article on Jungian Spirituality: A Developmental Context for Late-Life Growth (2006) takes Byock's "opportunities for growth" and compares and contrasts them to other developmental theories. She states that, when combined with what we know about Jungian theories and Erik Erikson's stages of human development,

we can see "the progression toward wisdom as being a natural movement in late adulthood and old age." With Byock's opportunities, one is able to integrate a significant part's of oneself, allowing for an acceptance of death "without losing a sense of integrity and meaning". Erik Erickson's final developmental stage, Stage 8, identified the psychosocial crisis (from the psychologic or mind and social or relationships) as one of ego integrity versus despair. Can one look back on one's life with clarity? Embrace the joys, respect the challenges, and find meaning and purpose through their life's achievements? Did one's life have value and what is the contribution made as a result? What is one's legacy? If our responses to these questions result in a sense of fulfillment and contentment, then we form a more complete ego identity. Our strength comes from a "bigger picture" view of life, one in which we are an integral part of the greater world, at one with it, even as we are moving out of it. The result is wisdom. If not, if we perceive our life as one in which we failed, if our answer to the question "Was it worth it?" is no, we can be filled with despair and, as a result, rather than seeing death as the culmination of a good life, it becomes something to be feared.

This "wisdom" can start prior to the dying process. It is seen as the result of adults, as they age, developmentally turning their focus from an outward path to an inner journey as they begin to identify less with the body and more with the soul or spirit. This theory is referred to as *gerotranscendence*, a term coined by Lars Tornstam in his book of the same name, *Gerotranscendence: A Developmental Theory of Positive Aging* (2005). He suggests that "human aging, the very process of living into old age, includes a potential to mature . . . from a materialistic and rational view of the world to a more cosmic and transcendent one, normally accompanied by an increase in life satisfaction." Joan Erikson, Erik's wife, added a ninth stage to her husband's staging system and called it gerotranscendence. Inherent in this stage is a "feeling of cosmic communion with the spirit of the universe, and a redefinition of time, space, life and death." This process can go smoothly or ineptly based on one's family, friends, culture, or life experiences. Patton sees this as a "bridge between the universal or archetypal changes Jung considered characteristics of midlife and Byock's 'opportunities for growth' at the end."

Now that we have explored some of the theoretical issues involved with the psychosocial and spiritual stages of the dying, let's move on to some practical applications of this knowledge.

COMMON PSYCHOSOCIAL NEEDS OF TERMINALLY ILL PATIENTS AND THEIR FAMILIES

Psychosocial needs result from the physical, emotional, social, and spiritual changes that an individual and family face during a crisis such as a terminal illness. Persons faced with terminal illness encounter many challenges. Not only do they battle physical symptoms, they also deal with an onslaught of emotional/psychosocial needs. The goal of psychosocial care in hospice and palliative care is to positively assist the patient/family by helping them express and address their individual psychosocial needs.

Table 14–2 compares some of the more common psychosocial dynamics that may be present in short-term illnesses with those of long-term illnesses. Recognition of these differences is important so that professional caregivers can more effectively focus on the psychosocial needs of the patients and families under their care.

The next several tables will list some of the more common psychosocial needs identified in patients near the end of life and their families: conspiracy of silence (Table 14–3), isolation and alienation (Table 14–4); nearing death awareness (Table 14–5); fear (Table 14–6); loss (Table 14–7); and loss of sexuality (Table 14–8). For each of these needs, a desired outcome is included as are several characteristics signs and symptoms that help caregivers recognize the particular situation. Some possible interventions are also provided, although caregivers should never limit themselves to any list of suggested interventions. Rather, they should always feel free to be creative in order to achieve the best possible outcome for each patient and family under their care.

TABLE 14–2. Dynamics of Short-Term Versus Long-Term Illness

SHORT-TERM ILLNESS	LONG-TERM ILLNESS
Less time to adjust to illness	More time to adjust to illness
Less time to say "goodbye" and make arrangements	More time to say "goodbye" and discuss arrangements
Immobilization due to shock/denial, potential for a sense of chaos	Increased resentment of patient or caregiver due to long-time role reversal
Feeling pressure to get "unfinished business" in order	Stress disorder evident in caregiver
Support systems may not be developed	Abuse/neglect due to relationship being thrown off balance
Less "wear and tear" due to short duration of illness	Continued "ups and downs" taking toll on family members
Less likely to drain family finances	Increased financial hardship

SOURCE: VITAS Innovative Hospice Care: *Job Preparation Training: Social Worker Compass Guide.* Miami, 1995.

TABLE 14–3. Psychosocial Need: Conspiracy of Silence

Outcome	To facilitate communication regarding illness and the dying process
Possible signs/symptoms	Patient/family/friends avoid discussion of the terminal illness or the dying process
	Patient/family/friends remain silent because they do not want to upset others
	Patient/family/friends use half truths or simply lie outright in regards to the dying event
	Family/friends may appear overly busy to avoid feelings
Possible interventions	Encourage expression of feelings and fears—this decreases emotional isolation
	Discuss behavior—this reduces misunderstandings and helps reduce anger
	Encourage emotional closure-discuss last wishes/family traditions/favorite stories/questions
	Help put affairs in order for an easier transition for family at the time of death

SOURCE: VITAS Innovative Hospice Care: *Job Preparation Training: Social Worker Compass Guide*. Miami, 1995.

TABLE 14–4. Psychosocial Need: Isolation and Alienation

Outcome	Recognize the dynamics of and reduce isolation and alienation to the extent possible
Possible signs/symptoms	Community imposed isolation—less contact with community due to illness
	Decrease in desire/ability to go to work, parties, church, meetings, etc.
	Decrease in social stimulation—friends drift away not knowing what to say or do
	Self-imposed isolation—withdraw from contact with others
	Cease to have interest in outside world
	Friends and family contacts eventually fall to only family
	Patient draws further into him or herself in preparation for death
Possible interventions	Help family and friends understand the dynamics of isolation/alienation
	Help patient communicate with the family members

SOURCE: VITAS Innovative Hospice Care: *Job Preparation Training: Social Worker Compass Guide*. Miami, 1995.

TABLE 14–5. Psychosocial Need: Nearing Death Awareness

Outcome	To better understand and listen to what your patient is experiencing in order to be able to better prepare patient and family for approaching death
Possible signs/symptoms	Patient describes:
	Someone not alive seems to be present (uses various nonverbal cues: smiling, waving, nodding to communicate with them)
	The need to prepare for travel or a change
	Places only he or she can see
	Vivid dreams
	Patient states:
	Something or someone is needed so death can occur
	Desire to reconcile personal, spiritual, or moral relationships
	Desire to remove barriers in order to achieve peace
	Need for validation and permission to die
Possible Interventions	Let the person know you are there and listen
	Pay attention to everything the dying person says
	Analyze deeply what is being said to best understand what the person is trying to say
	Communicate with the family that dying people know they are dying
	Encourage communication—"Can you tell me more about what's happening?"
	Accept and validate what the dying person tells you
	Do not argue or challenge
	Be honest about having trouble understanding
	Do not push conversation—let the patient control the tempo of the conversation
	Instill a sense of pride in the patient—"I'm so proud that you shared these thoughts with me."
	Inform family that sometimes the patient may pick one confidant who he or she feels emotionally safe with, who won't get upset or rattled
	If you don't know what to say, don't say anything-just let them know you are there

SOURCE: VITAS Innovative Hospice Care: *Job Preparation Training: Social Worker Compass Guide.* Miami, 1995.

TABLE 14–6. Psychosocial Need: Fear

Outcome	To acknowledge and allay the patients' fear levels
Possible signs/symptoms	Fear of the unknown
	Fear of pain
	Fear of loss of control
	Fear of isolation
	Fear of poor physical care
Possible interventions	Provide comfort and continued reassurance that they will not be left alone
	Discuss that family members will be fine and manage well without them
	Remove irrational fears
	Acknowledge reasonable fears
	Provide truthful reassurance

SOURCE: VITAS Innovative Hospice Care: *Job Preparation Training: Social Worker Compass Guide.* Miami, 1995.

TABLE 14–7. Psychosocial Need: Loss

Outcome	To assist patients and families in coping with loss
Possible signs/symptoms	Loss of a sense of being invulnerable: patient loses the coping mechanism of the sense of being invulnerable-robbed forever of the carefree attitude of the healthy
	Loss of roles: Family members will begin to take on the roles of the dying patient. The greater the roles of the patient (mother, sister, communicator, peacemaker, bill payer, etc.), the greater the emotional reaction will be to the illness and death
Possible interventions	Be honest and make time to listen
	Encourage discussion on any issue that may arise
	Encourage story telling, journaling—listing positives about their loved one
	Encourage and expect introspection
	Consider complementary or creative interventions to reach feelings that are difficult to express, such as:
	Massage, light pressure reflexology, meditation, and art or music therapy

SOURCE: VITAS Innovative Hospice Care: *Job Preparation Training: Social Worker Compass Guide.* Miami, 1995.

TABLE 14–8. Psychosocial Need: Loss of Sexuality

Outcome	To understand and discuss potential loss of sexuality
Possible signs/symptoms	Altered body image due to illness
	Medications
	Loss of identity
	Isolation and alienation
Possible interventions	Encourage discussion on sexual issues
	Assist in construction of new alternatives for the couple
	Discuss touch (other than physical care) as an important role
	Discuss alternatives in order to boost self-image
	Assist in finding new and meaningful forms of sexual communication

Source: VITAS Innovative Hospice Care: *Job Preparation Training: Social Worker Compass Guide.* Miami, 1995.

COMMON SPIRITUAL NEEDS OF TERMINALLY ILL PATIENTS AND THEIR FAMILIES

Spirituality is that part of each individual which longs for meaning, integrity, beauty, dignity, hope, love and acceptance (VITAS concept of "spirituality").

Every member of the hospice team needs to be equipped with basic spiritual assessment and intervention skills. (See Chapter 16 for a full discussion of Psychosocial and Spiritual Assessments.) Although the hospice chaplain performs the spiritual assessment, input from each team member ensures the most effective interdisciplinary plan of care.

From experience hospice has learned that most patients, regardless of whether they consider themselves to be religious or not, have the following spiritual needs: meaning (Table 14–9); hope

TABLE 14–9. Spiritual Need: Meaning

Outcome	Recognize the purpose and value of the need for meaning and assist patient in finding meaning in life
Consider asking	To what degree are your relationships meaningful to you?
	What difficulties have you had in "making sense" out of what is happening to you?
	What gives your life meaning? Where do you find purpose?
	What would make life more meaningful for you?
Possible signs/symptoms	Lost the will to live
	Questions meaning and purpose of life
Possible interventions	Listen emphatically and avoid giving advice
	Accept the patient unconditionally
	Encourage the patient to discover his/her own meaning in living and dying
	Encourage discussion of past accomplishments
	Value the patient's accomplishments/insights

Source: VITAS Innovative Hospice Care: *Interdisciplinary Spiritual Care Compass Guide.* Miami, 1995.

TABLE 14–10. Spiritual Need: Hope	
Outcome	Recognize the purpose and value of the need for hope and assist patient in findings things to be hopeful for
Consider asking	What is it that you can count on or depend upon during the illness/loss?
	How would you describe your ability to be hopeful?
	How has the illness/loss affected your sense of well-being?
	In what ways, if any, has your hope changed during the illness/loss?
Possible signs/symptoms	Hopelessness
	Loss of well-being
	Despair
Possible interventions	Encourage discussion of the patient and family's well-being
	Discuss ways to preserve the patient's well-being, now and in the future
	Encourage discussion about ways hope has changed during illness
	Example: Cure or remission no longer realistic, therefore the hope may change to the hope of not suffering
	Discuss possible ambivalence regarding 'letting go of getting well' in the midst of remaining hopeful

SOURCE: VITAS Innovative Hospice Care: *Interdisciplinary Spiritual Care Compass Guide.* Miami, 1995.

(Table 14–10); sense of an ultimate spiritual source (Table 14–11); love and acceptance (Table 14–12); and dignity and humanity (Table 14–13). In addition to outcomes, signs and symptoms, and possible interventions, each table includes suggested questions that might assist the caregiver in identifying and getting to the root of the patient's need(s).

TABLE 14–11. Spiritual Need: Sense of an Ultimate Spiritual Source	
Outcome	Assist patient in developing a sense of an ultimate spiritual source in whatever form she or he desires
Consider asking	What is your concept, if any, of God?
	To what degree does your belief in God help you cope during the illness/loss?
	Are you struggling to be in control of certain things?
	What would be helpful to "let go" of?
Possible signs/symptoms	Anxious about losing control
	Feeling guilt or shame
	Desire for closure with family/friends/spiritual source
	Angry toward God or other spiritual source
Possible Interventions	Discuss patient's concept of an Ultimate Spiritual Source
	Recognize many may use other names besides "God"
	Discuss beliefs that something beyond ourselves gives direction and meaning
	Acknowledge the source may be found 'deep within' or outside of oneself
	Discuss struggles to be in control
	Discuss closure process(es) with family and friends

SOURCE: VITAS Innovative Hospice Care: *Interdisciplinary Spiritual Care Compass Guide.* Miami, 1995.

TABLE 14–12. Spiritual Need: Love and Acceptance

Outcome	Help patients and families experience love and acceptance more deeply
Consider asking	Are there persons from whom you feel isolated?
	To what degree do you feel loved and valued by others?
	Do you feel "at peace" with yourself, others, God? Is there anything that would help you obtain this? Are there things that feel "unfinished"?
	What would you like to say or have happen between you and your family/friends?
	Do you feel you can trust others and that others have your best interests at heart?
	In what sense do you feel obligated, if any, to God, your family, or friends?
Possible signs/symptoms	Inability to trust?
	Feeling alienated and isolated?
	Fear of abandonment
Possible Interventions	Accept patient unconditionally
	Communicate openly and honestly with the patient—this fosters trust
	Help patient/family express their love and emotions
	Ensure the patient that staff will "be there" for them
	Teach family to continue to relate to the patient as intimately as possible

SOURCE: VITAS Innovative Hospice Care: *Interdisciplinary Spiritual Care Compass Guide.* Miami, 1995.

TABLE 14–13. Spiritual Need: Dignity and Humanity

Outcome	Help the patient achieve and maintain a sense of dignity and humanity
Consider asking	Do you feel respected and treated with dignity? What would help you feel more respected as a person?
	To what extent are you allowed to make your own choices?
	What would help you to be more independent?
	Are there things you would like to do yourself?
	How has your illness/loss affected your self-worth and morale?
Possible signs/symptoms	Loss of identity
	Loss of control
	Feeling disrespected
Possible interventions	Allow the patient as much autonomy and independence as possible
	Allow the patient to make as many choices as possible
	Admit to the patient that you may be struggling with how best to help them achieve autonomy and independence

SOURCE: VITAS Innovative Hospice Care: *Interdisciplinary Spiritual Care Compass Guide.* Miami, 1995.

A BILL OF RIGHTS FOR A DYING PERSON

Hospice affirms that a dying person is still a person, no less human because they are dying. A sense of control is an important factor to a person who is terminally ill, as is the desire to continue to be part of life. Dame Cicely Saunders, founder of the modern hospice movement, said it most eloquently:

> You matter because you are you. You matter to the last moment of life, and we will do all we can, not only to help you die peacefully, but also to live until you die.

The "Dying Person's Bill of Rights" reminds both the patient and physician of the "bigger picture" involved when providing care at the end of life. It is presented in Table 14–14. Professional staff can work toward adhering to this "bill of rights" by following the suggested steps listed in Table 14–15.

IN CLOSING

In this chapter, we have explored a number of psychosocial and spiritual issues affecting care for those at the end of life. These issues affect everyone from the physician to hospice nurse to the patient's primary caregiver. With this knowledge leading to an increase in the physician's awareness of patient psychosocial or spiritual issues, earlier referrals to hospice or palliative care might be prompted and an interdisciplinary approach

---

TABLE 14–14. The Dying Person's Bill of Rights

- I have the right to be treated as a living human being until I die.
- I have the right to maintain a sense of hopefulness, however changing its focus may be.
- I have the right to be cared for by those who can maintain a sense of hopefulness, however changing this might be.
- I have the right to express my feelings and emotions about my approaching death in my own way.
- I have the right to participate in decisions concerning my care.
- I have the right to have any questions answered honestly.
- I have the right to have help from and for my family in accepting my death.
- I have the right to die in peace and dignity.
- I have the right to retain my individuality and not be judged for my decisions, which may be contrary to the beliefs of others.
- I have the right to expect that the sanctity of the human body will be respected after death.
- I have the right to discuss and enlarge my spiritual experiences, regardless of what they may mean to others.
- I have the right to be cared for by caring, sensitive, knowledgeable people who will attempt to understand my needs and will be able to gain some satisfaction in helping me face my death.

Note: This Bill of Rights was created at a workshop on "The Terminally Ill patient and the Helping Person" held in Lansing, Michigan, sponsored by the Southwestern Michigan Inservice Educational Council and conducted by Amelia J. Barbus, Associate Professor of Nursing, Wayne State University, in 1975.
SOURCE: Ferrell BR, Coyle N: An overview of palliative nursing care. *Am J Nursing* 102(5):26-31, 2002.

TABLE 14–15. Dying Persons Bill of Rights: Suggested Steps for Professional Staff

- Listen rather than give advice
- Do not impose your values and beliefs on patients and families but rather help them to explore the importance of their own
- Be nonjudgmental and tolerant of differing values and attitudes
- Respect and seek to understand the patient/family's cultural and ethnic aspects of their religious customs and beliefs
- Provide spiritual support but do not attempt to fix or solve spiritual issues
- Be aware of your limitations in assisting persons with spiritual needs
- Avoid answering tough questions, answer question "tentatively" so as to give as much latitude to the patient to explore his/her own feelings and needs
- Grow in your spirituality by listening to and learning from the patient
- Anger expressed by the patient or family member is often misplaced or misdirected toward anyone they come in contact with. The most important intervention is listening, and feeling comfortable with allowing the person to express and release his/her anger in an appropriate manner

SOURCE: VITAS Innovative Hospice Care: *Interdisciplinary Spiritual Care Compass Guide.* Miami, 1995.

to pain and symptom management may ensue. A hospice nurse might recognize that a patient or caregiver's anger, so distracting and frustrating in the past, is related to the dying process, freeing her up to use professional skills to address the true problem and provide comfort while managing physical symptoms. The family member who is caring for a loved one might have new tools to understand and bridge the gap the dying process creates.

Each person's end-of-life experience is unique and individual. It can be as a beautiful symphony, with numerous notes, instruments, and musicians coming together to create the exquisite final composition, or it can sound like a second grader's first piano lesson. The difference between the two often rest with those of us working with people at the end of life. We must remember that in our lives, as in music, the finale is as important as the overture. As Tournier put it, "I live differently, but not less." For those caring for the terminally ill, psychosocial and spiritual issues which in the past had been seen as problems can, with information and compassion, become opportunities,

opportunities which will allow each of us to live fully until we say goodbye.

In closing, the words of Henri J.M. Nouwen ring through.

> Is death something so terrible and absurd that we are better off not thinking or talking about it? Is death such an undesirable part of our existence that we are better off acting as if it were not real? Is death such an absolute end of all our thoughts and actions that we simply cannot face it? Or is it possible to befriend our dying gradually and live open to it, trusting that we have nothing to fear? Is it possible to prepare for our death with the same attentiveness that our parents had in preparing for our birth? Can we wait for our death as for a friend who wants to welcome us home?"

We think that the answer is yes! We hope the information in this chapter will help you to see that too.

BIBLIOGRAPHY

Becker E: *The Denial of Death.* New York, Free Press, 1973.

Block SD: Psychological considerations, growth, and transcendence at the end of life: The art of the possible. *JAMA* 285(22):2898-2905, 2001.

Brueggemann W: *Hopeful Imagination*. Fortress, Philadelphia, PA, 1986.

Buckman R: *How to Break Bad News*. Baltimore, MD, Johns Hopkins University Press, 1992.

Byock IR: Growth: the essence of hospice. *Am J Hosp Palliat Care* 3:16-21, 1986.

Byock IR, Merriman MP: Measuring quality of life for patients with terminal illness: The Missoula-VITAS quality of life index. *Palliat Med* 12:231-244, 1998.

Cella DF: Quality of life: Concepts and definition. *J Pain Symptom Manage* 9:186-192, 1994.

Cohen SR, Mount BM, Tomas JJN, et al: Existential well being is an important determinant of quality of life. *Cancer* 77:576-586, 1996.

Dowling Singh K: *The Grace in Dying*. San Francisco, Harbor Books, 1998.

Ferrell BR, Coyle N: An overview of palliative nursing care. *Am J Nursing* 102(5):26-31, 2002.

Frankl V: *Man's Search for Meaning*. New York, Touchstone, 1959.

International Work Group on Death, Dying and Bereavement: *Statements on Death, Dying and Bereavement*. Ontario, Kings College, 1994.

Kaplan HI, Sadock BJ, Grebb JA: *Kaplan and Sadock's Synopsis of Psychiatry*. Baltimore, MD, Lippincott Williams and Wilkins, 1994.

Kubler-Ross E: *On Death and Dying*. New York, Free Press, 1969.

Nouwen HJM: *Our Greatest Gift: A Meditation on Dying and Caring*. San Francisco, Harper San Francisco, 1994.

Patch Adams: The movie. Distributed by Universal Studios beginning on December 25, 1998.

Patton JF: Jungian Spirituality: A developmental context for late-life growth. *Am J Hosp Palliat Care* 23: 304-308, 2006.

Riemer J, Stampfer N: *So That Your Values Live On*. Woodstock, Vermont, Jewish Lights, 1991.

Sourkes BM: *The Deepening Shade*. Pittsburgh, PA, University of Pittsburgh Press, 1982.

Tornstam L: *Gerotranscendence: A Developmental Theory of Positive Aging*. New York, Springer Publishing, 2005.

Tournier P: *Learn to Grow Old*. Louisville, KY, Westminster/John Knox Press, 1991.

VITAS Innovative Hospice Care: *Job Preparation Training: Social Worker Compass Guide*. Miami, Vitas Healthcare Corporation, 1995.

VITAS Innovative Hospice Care: *Interdisciplinary Spiritual Care Compass Guide*. Miami, Vitas Healthcare Corporation, 1995.

Wangerin W: *Mourning Into Dancing*. Grand Rapids, Zondervon, 1992.

Welk TA: An educational model for explaining hospice services. *Am J Hosp Palliat Care* 8:14-18, 1991.

SELF-ASSESSMENT QUESTIONS

1. Based on Dr. Ira Byock's view that dying is an identifiable stage of human development, that one "grows on" during the end of one's life, which of the following best describes how one might view the dying process?

   A. An enemy
   B. A sign of personal failure
   C. A time of great achievement
   D. A betrayal of one's body
   E. A shortfall in the promises of medical science

2. Reassuring patients that concern about experiencing progressive symptoms near the end of life is unwarranted as these symptoms can and will be controlled is an illustration of which "opportunity" near the end of life?

   A. To move through confusion to meaning
   B. To move from fear to peace
   C. To move from isolation to community
   D. To adjust to new roles
   E. To expand our definition of quality of life

3. Assisting patients in working through feelings that their illness was a result of personal failure or punishment from God is an illustration of which "opportunity" near the end of life?

   A. To move through confusion to meaning
   B. To focus on the individual, not the disease
   C. To move from isolation to community
   D. To adjust to new roles
   E. To expand our definition of quality of life

4. Patients who are assisted in resetting their goals and aspirations as life is drawing to a close are being helped in working on which "opportunity" near the end of life?

   A. To move through fear to peace
   B. To focus on the individual, not the disease
   C. To move from loss to closure
   D. To come to terms with one's physical body
   E. To move through despair to hope

5. Assisting patients in trying to reconcile estranged relationships with family members helps patients work on which "opportunity" near the end of life?

   A. To move through fear to peace
   B. To focus on the individual, not the disease
   C. To move from isolation to community
   D. To adjust to new roles
   E. To expand our definition of quality of life

6. When patients are approaching the end of life, family members often try to protect their dying love ones by hiding their feelings from them. This often results in a lack of communication between patients and their loved ones, which often results in the parties prematurely treating each other as if their relationship were already over. When this occurs, patients and families are often prevented from working on which end of life "opportunity?"

   A. Focusing on the individual, not the disease
   B. Adjusting to new roles
   C. Expanding our definition of quality of life
   D. Moving from loss to closure
   E. Getting one's affairs in order

7. Which of the following best defines the term "Gerotranscendence?"

   A. A final task in life, which is the acceptance of unfulfillment and the acceptance of the unfulfilled.
   B. Adults, as they age, developmentally turn their focus from an outward path to an inner journey as they begin to identify less with the body and more with the spirit or soul.
   C. A theoretical structure to the nature of the profound inner changes which are taking

place as the personality restructures on a deeper level in response to transpersonal forces.

D. The ability to use suffering as way to discover meaning in life since when there is suffering there is an opportunity to transcend it by attaching significance to it.

E. A final developmental stage in life identified as a psychosocial crisis of ego integrity versus despair.

8. Which of the following psychosocial needs of patients and families may be addressed by interventions such as encouraging expressions of feelings and fears or encouraging emotional closure?

A. Conspiracy of silence
B. Isolation and alienation
C. Nearing Death Awareness
D. Fear
E. Loss

9. Which of the following spiritual needs of patients and families may be manifested by patients complaining of loss of control, loss of identity, or by feeling disrespected?

A. The Need for Meaning
B. The Need for Hope
C. The Need for a Sense of an Ultimate Spiritual Source
D. The Need for Love and Acceptance
E. The Need for Dignity and Humanity

10. Which of the following spiritual needs of patients and families may be addressed with interventions such as encouraging patients to discuss past accomplishments, and valuing patients' accomplishments and insights?

A. The Need for Meaning
B. The Need for Hope
C. The Need for a Sense of an Ultimate Spiritual Source
D. The Need for Love and Acceptance
E. The Need for Dignity and Humanity

The Physician's Role in Spiritual Care

Barry M. Kinzbrunner

INTRODUCTION

As has already been well established in earlier chapters in this volume, the treatment of patients near the end of life requires an interdisciplinary model of care to address not only the physical, but also the psychosocial and spiritual aspects of the myriad of symptoms these patients, and their families, experience. Of the various disciplines, the one that probably has the least attention paid to it is that of spiritual care. This is likely due to a number of factors including the difficulties seen in defining exactly what spiritual care truly means, and the lack of objectivity that is, to some extent, inherent in the nature of spiritual care and which causes physicians, who tend to focus on the concrete, to pay it less attention. This lack of attention can, perhaps, best be illustrated by the excellent model of "total pain" that was first published by a leading expert pain and palliative medicine physician in 1988, and continues to be in use to this day. Although he recognizes significant "psychosocial influences" to a patient's experience of "physical pain," and attributes many psychosocial issues to the "suffering" component of "total pain," including loss of work, financial concerns, and changes in one's social and family functioning, his only recognition of the spiritual components of "suffering" is the single element "fear of death."

To help physicians better understand the importance of spiritual care as a key component in end-of-life care, this chapter focuses on the role of physicians in ensuring that appropriate spiritual care is provided to their terminally ill patients and the families who care for them. To do so, an attempt will be made to better define spiritual care, following which a number of studies examining the potential importance of spiritual care to patients and the physicians who care for them will be explored. Next is an examination of the questions that physicians should include in their evaluation of patients to properly detect and assess spiritual needs, and finally, recommendations as to how physicians should participate in the spiritual care of patients under their care are discussed.

WHAT IS SPIRITUAL CARE?

The word spiritual is derived from the Latin "*spiritus*," which means "breath." Spirituality, which literally means "matters of the spirit," is the term most often used to describe an individual's association with the spiritual. In the context of end-of-life care, Keith Meador, Professor of the Practice of Pastoral Theology and Medicine at the Duke Institute on Care at the End of Life, defines spiritual care as something that "include(s) the spectrum from some sense of emotionally sensitive care of the 'human spirit' to a highly ritualized religious care incorporating very specific rites for the dying, and a multitude of possibilities in between." This inability to define spiritual care precisely, and to be forced to ascribe to it a broad spectrum of possible definitions, creates significant challenges for physicians being able to comfortably embrace spiritual care as a mainstream discipline in health care.

Looking further at the literature to achieve greater definitional precision only serves to further emphasize the imprecise nature of "spiritual care." A recent comprehensive literature review reported that there were at least 92 different definitions of spirituality presented in various forms in the articles reviewed. Fortunately, the authors of the review were able to cone the 92 definitions down to seven common definitional themes, which are outlined in Table 15–1 and can be used to begin to better delineate the elements the define spiritual care.

Of these themes, the two that produce the most contention and that need to be developed further are the first, "the relationship to a higher power," and the third, "a transcendence and connectedness without belief in a higher being." In other words, in our society, which is extremely diverse when it comes to questions of one's religion or

TABLE 15–1. Themes That Define Spiritual Care
• Relationship to a higher power or a reality greater than self
• Not of the self
• Transcendence or connectedness unrelated to belief in a higher being
• Not of the material world
• Meaning and purpose in life
• Life force of the person, integrating aspects of the person
• Summative definitions that combine two or more of the above themes

SOURCE: Unruh AM, Versnel J, Kerr N: Spirituality unplugged: A review of commonalities and contentions, and a resolution. *Can J Occup Ther* 69:5-19, 2002.

belief system, one must attempt to define the role of religious belief and faith, if any, in the context of spiritual care.

Kearney and Mount appear to define spirituality and religion separately. They state that spirituality is "a dimension of personhood . . . a part of our being" whereas religion is "a construct of human making that . . . enables conceptualization and expression of spirituality." However, as can be seen from their definition of religion, one could argue that they actually view religion as a way of expressing spirituality. This concept, that religion, whereas not the totality of spiritual care, may be one of several ways to express it, is, perhaps, best illustrated by the definitions provided by the Scottish National Health Service. In their "Guidelines on Chaplaincy and Spiritual Care" they state:

> Religious Care is given in the context of the shared religious beliefs, values, liturgies, and lifestyle of a faith community. Spiritual Care is usually given in a one to one relationship, is completely person centered and makes no assumptions about personal conviction or life orientation. Spiritual care is not necessarily religious. Religious care, at its best, should always be spiritual.

By viewing religion as part of spirituality without confining spirituality to religion, the potential

conflict between spirituality and religion in our diverse society can be resolved. This can then allow a definition of spirituality in palliative care to evolve in a neutral way, such as the one proposed by Cassidy and Davis.

> (Spirituality) . . . has come to describe the depth of human life, with individuals seeking significance in their experiences and in the relationships they share with family and friends, with others who experience illness, and with those engaged in their treatment and support.

By understanding that "religious" spiritual care is implicit in the definition, this definition can satisfy those who are religiously inclined, those who are entirely secular in their approach, and those in between without fear of offending any who feel strongly one way or another.

IS SPIRITUAL CARE IMPORTANT?

Although America has an extremely diverse society, the overwhelming majority of Americans, 84% in one recent study, consider themselves affiliated with one of the world's major religions. In addition, more than 90% believe in the existence of God or a universal spirit, although only 60% actually believe in God as a being with whom people have a relationship.

When illness strikes, these beliefs have significant influence over how patients react. In a recent study, two religious factors, "being at peace with God" (89%) and "prayer" (85%), and, one spiritual factor, "feeling one's life was complete" (80%), were among the factors considered most important by patients near the end of life. In another study, "faith in God" was considered the second most important of seven factors (only exceeded by the recommendations of the oncologist) considered by patients and their caregivers when making cancer treatment decisions. Most recently, in a survey examining the attitudes of the public toward potentially fatal traumatic injury, 57.4% of the respondents said they believed that divine intervention could save a person when the treating physician believed further treatment was futile.

Although it would appear that spirituality and, for many Americans, religion, are of great importance, can the same be said for the physicians who care for them? Studies suggest that family physicians are comparable to the general public regarding their religious characteristics, and are generally more religious than physicians from other specialties.

Overall, however, the attitudes of physicians toward religion and spirituality appear to significantly differ from the patients they serve. A 2005 survey of US physicians that examined the religious attitudes of physicians and compared them to data from a survey of the general public published in 1998 showed that the physicians were less likely to carry their religious beliefs over into other dealings in life (58% vs. 73%), more likely to consider themselves spiritual but not religious (20% vs. 9%), and more likely to cope with major problems without relying on God (61% vs. 29%).

These differences between physicians and their patients can be further supported by the same studies already discussed. For example, "being at peace with God" (66%), "prayer" (56%), and "feeling that one's life was complete" (68%) were significantly less important to the physicians surveyed than to the terminally ill patients they care for. Although cancer patients and their caregivers thought "faith in God" was second in importance out of seven factors used in decision making, their physicians ranked "faith in God" dead last. Finally, slightly less than 20% of trauma professionals (as opposed to 57.4% of the public) believed that divine intervention could save a trauma victim when the physicians believed further treatment was futile.

The practical consequences of this gap between the attitudes of patients and physicians regarding religion and spirituality in healthcare has been demonstrated in a recent study evaluating the question of whether patients believed their spiritual needs were being met. This study evaluated the care of 177 patients in a pulmonary outpatient clinic. Fifty-one percent of the patients were described as religious, and 90% believed that prayer may sometimes influence recovery from an illness. When the patients were asked whether spiritual or religious beliefs would influence their medical decisions if they became gravely ill, 45% (80 patients) responded in the affirmative. Of these patients, 94% (75 patients) agreed that their physicians should ask about this. In fact, two-thirds of all respondents, irrespective of whether or not their beliefs would affect medical decision making, indicated that they would welcome being asked about this as part of the medical history, but only 15% of patients recalled having ever been asked.

HEALTH OUTCOMES RELATED TO SPIRITUAL CARE

As has been demonstrated earlier, the data suggest that a majority of patients find religion and spirituality to be a very important element in their healthcare, whereas the physicians who care for them do not seem to share this attitude. As physicians profess to practice "evidence-based" medicine, one way to close this attitudinal gap would be to demonstrate to physicians that the health of their patients is improved by the addition of spiritual care to their treatment armamentarium.

To date, studies evaluating the efficacy of religious and spiritual care on health and illness have shown that spiritual care may have a protective effect against despair and depression in patients near the end of life. Patients with higher levels of what is described as "spiritual well-being" were shown in at least one study to exhibit less of a desire to have death hastened or express suicidal ideation, and to experience less of a sense of hopelessness in the context of their terminal illness. In this same study, the lack of "spiritual well-being" had a greater impact on "psychologic suffering" than did the level of depression, the burden of physical symptoms or functional disability, or the level of social support. Other studies have shown that quality of life for patients near the end of life is also influenced in a unique way by spiritual concerns that are independent and not compatible with other measures of psychosocial well-being and coping.

Studies evaluating the effects of religious and spiritual care on morbidity and mortality in the overall patient population are somewhat more controversial. In healthy individuals, it has been suggested that there is a reduction in adverse outcomes among individuals who attend church regularly as opposed to those who do not, whereas other forms of increased religiosity do not seem to be associated with improved health. For those suffering from illness, one study showed no positive effect of religious observance on progression of cancer, mortality from any cause, recovery from acute illness, or any clear effects of intercessory prayer on objective health outcomes, whereas another study demonstrated evidence for a possible physiologic relationship with religiosity or spirituality and desirable health states and processes. A recent study evaluating the effects of religiosity and spirituality on cognitive decline in patients meeting criteria for probable Alzheimer's disease showed that higher levels of spirituality (as determined by a standardized scale) and participation in private religious practices were significantly associated with slower rates of cognitive decline. A meta-analysis of several studies that evaluated more than 125,000 participants also suggested a beneficial relationship between spirituality or religiosity and health status, although the considerable amount of heterogeneity among the studies greatly limits any conclusions that one can draw.

Given the importance of pain control in managing end-of-life patients, a recent study published in 2008 by Wiech et al. on the potential effect of religious belief must be mentioned. This study, using functional MRI (fMRI) technology, evaluated the activity of the right ventrolateral prefrontal cortex (VLPFC) and the perceived intensity of pain in 12 religious subjects and 12 atheist or agnostic subjects (considered the control group) exposed to a painful stimulus. The religious subjects, when exposed to a religious image prior to the painful stimulus, showed increased activity of their right VLPFC on fMRI, and experienced less intense pain than when exposed to a nonreligious image, whereas the nonreligious subjects had the same level of VLPFC activity and pain intensity irrespective of which image they were exposed to prior to the painful stimulus. Although this study has a number of significant limitations, it raises the question of whether religious belief can affect the perception of pain intensity in at least some individuals, and lends credence to the validity of the "total pain" model that forms the basis of interdisciplinary end-of-life care and the need for spiritual care on a neurophysiologic level.

Finally, regarding the effects of spiritual support on religiousness on end-of-life treatment preferences and quality of life in advanced cancer patients, a number of studies have been generated from data collected as part of the federally funded "Coping with Cancer" study. Most of the study population (88%) considered religion to be at least somewhat important in their lives. However, almost half (47%) felt that their spiritual needs were only minimally met or not met at all by their religious community, whereas 72% felt the same lack of support from the medical community, despite the fact that for these patients there was found to be a significant association between quality of life and having their spiritual needs met. A significant direct correlation was also found between the level of patient religiousness and the desire for life extending therapies near the end of life. A follow-up study showed that patients who use religion in a positive way to cope with their terminal cancer were almost three times as likely to actually receive intensive life-prolonging medical care in the last few days of life.

THE PHYSICIAN'S ROLE IN SPIRITUAL CARE

With the understanding that patients believe that spiritual care (in whatever form they determine) is an integral part of the care that they desire to receive, with at least some evidence that this care may be beneficial (and with no evidence that it can be harmful), and with the indication that spirituality and religion may affect patient decision making near the end of life, how are physicians, who are traditionally not as comfortable or as focused on spiritual care, supposed to react? In order to assist physicians in better meeting patient and family needs in the area of spiritual and religious care, the "Working Group on Religious and Spiritual Issues at the End of Life" published a series of recommendations in 2002, which are summarized in Table 15–2 and are discussed below.

TABLE 15–2. Physician's Role in Spiritual Care

- Elicit and identify patients' spiritual and/or religious concerns
- Collaborate and connect with patients by listening carefully and acknowledging their concerns
- Respect patients' views and follow their lead while avoiding theologic discussions
- Maintain one's own integrity regarding one's own religious beliefs and practices and avoid engaging in specific religious rituals whenever possible
- Identify common goals for care
- Utilize appropriate professional resources of support for patients, such as referral to a chaplain or encouraging contact with patients' own clergy

SOURCE: Lo B, Ruston D, Kates LW, et al: Discussing religious and spiritual issues at the end of life. A practical guide for physicians. *JAMA* 287:749–754, 2002, and Okun T: Palliative care review. Spiritual, religious, and existential aspects of palliative care. *J Pall Med* 8:392–414, 2005.

ELICIT AND IDENTIFY PATIENTS' SPIRITUAL AND/OR RELIGIOUS CONCERNS

The first step in ensuring that patients receive appropriate spiritual care is to find out what their needs and issues are. In addition, it is important for the physician to understand how patients' spiritual and/or religious belief systems may affect the medical care they choose or do not choose to receive. This requires the physician to include questions regarding spiritual and religious needs as part of the patient's history. There are a number of different structured approaches to spiritual history taking that have been published in the medical literature, identified by mnemonics such as HOPE, FICA, and SPIRIT, to make the suggested questions easier for physicians to remember. The details of these structured assessments are listed in Table 15–3 and are discussed below.

HOPE

The HOPE model, developed by Anandarajah and Hight, is designed as an open-ended assessment system that allows for the physician to approach a person's spirituality in an indirect fashion. The developers recommend beginning with assessing the patient's resources for support, specifically in areas like **h**ope, strength, comfort and peace, to determine whether the patient has a spiritual belief system. During this time, the patient may also discuss the personal importance of God and religion in his or her life. This is the **H** of the HOPE mnemonic.

Once the physician establishes the patient's spiritual belief system or lack thereof, the next two areas, **O** and **P**, delve further into the person's involvement with **o**rganized religion and **p**ersonal practices. For example, the physician might ask: "For some people, their religious or spiritual beliefs act as a source of comfort and strength

TABLE 15–3. Mnemonic Methods of Spiritual History Taking	
HOPE*	
H	Sources of Hope
O	Organized religion: level of identification or participation
P	Personal spirituality and Practices
E	Effect on medical care and end-of-life issues
FICA†	
F	Faith
I	Importance/Influence of faith or spirituality
C	Community: identification or participation in spiritual or religious community
A	Address/Apply: how to address patients' spiritual or religious concerns
SPIRIT‡	
S	Spiritual belief system
P	Personal belief system
I	Integration with a spiritual community
R	Ritualized practices and restrictions if any
I	Implications for medical care
T	Terminal events planning

SOURCE: Adapted from Okon TR: Palliative care review: Spiritual, religious, and existential aspects of palliative care. *J Palliat Med* 8:392-414, 2005.

*Anandarajah G, Hight E: Spirituality and medical practice. Using the HOPE questions as a practical tool for spiritual assessment. *Am Fam Phys* 63:81-89, 2001.

†Puchalski CM, Romer AL: Taking a spiritual history allows clinicians to understand patients more fully. *J Palliat Med* 3:129-137, 2000.

‡Maugans, TA: The SPIRITual history. *Arch Fam Med* 5:11-16, 1996.

in dealing with life's ups and downs. Please tell me how this is or is not true for you." If the person does not find spirituality and religion important, the physician should try to ascertain whether it was ever important, for often one's spiritual and religious needs change during life.

The final letter, **E**, refers to how one's spirituality and religion effects one's view on medical care and end-of-life issues. The goal is to steer the conversation back to the clinical issues, learning from the patient how spiritual or religious beliefs may influence end-of-life choices.

FICA

Puchalski's spiritual assessment model, named **FICA**, is more focused and direct than the HOPE model already discussed above. **F** stands for **f**aith and beliefs, and Puchalski argues that directly questioning a person regarding one's faith or belief system is more appropriate and less agenda-filled than beginning the conversation by asking what helps the person cope. If the patient has neither spiritual nor religious beliefs, the physician should assess for other forms of meaning in life, and allow the patient to guide the conversation.

After establishing a general idea of the patient's level of faith, the physician should assess the level of **i**mportance (**I**) of those beliefs in the patient's life. Near the end of life, the key issue for many patients is to determine how their specific belief systems influence their ability to cope with their situation. A clue to the level of importance that a patient places on his or her faith can often be found in an individual's participation or lack of participation in spiritual or religious rituals.

The **C** in FICA is for **c**ommunity. The physician will want to assess what communal support systems are available to assist the patient, especially those that are associated with the patient's spiritual or religious beliefs, such as faith-based institutions and community clergy. Having gathered this information, the physician's must now **a**ddress (**A**) the patient's spiritual needs based on the assessment.

SPIRIT

Maugans' SPIRIT model is a six-step process that begins by identifying the patient's **s**piritual (**S**) belief system with its tenets and beliefs, which will allow the physician a first glimpse into the patient's spiritual life. Once the formal spiritual belief system is established, the physician asks patient how his or her or own **p**ersonal (**P**) spirituality is expressed within the context of that formal religious or spiritual belief system. Ensuring that each patient's spiritual beliefs are approached without making assumptions based on the formal spiritual background.

The physician should then ascertain to what degree the patient is **i**ntegrated (**I**) into the formal spiritual community by belonging to or participating in a faith institution. Included in this evaluation is establishing whether the patient has any relationship with one or more members of his or her faith's clergy, so that they can be involved in providing the patient with spiritual support when needed. Next, the physician should explore with the patient the roles of **r**itual (**R**) and religious practice, and what **i**mplications (**I**) these traditions and customs may have on how the patient views his or her current medical illness. Finally, the physician and patient should explore various advance care planning issues (i.e., artificial nutrition and hydration, resuscitation) that arise during the **t**erminal phase of the illness (**T**) in the context of the patient's spiritual or religious belief system, because many of these traditions have rules regarding whether patients may accept or reject such interventions.

COLLABORATE AND CONNECT WITH PATIENTS

Whether one chooses to use one of the structured approaches to taking a spiritual history or to question the patient in a less formal manner, it is important to avoid questions that require simple "yes/no" answers. Rather, one should use "open-ended" questions. One must also be careful not to cut-off conversation, but invite patients to elaborate on the spiritual issues and concerns that they raise. Active listening techniques, including reflecting back to patients what they have related, should be used to help better connect and show that their concerns are being acknowledged and understood. Asking patients about their own emotions and expressing empathy are other ways of ensuring that patients feel connected and part of the discussion.

RESPECT PATIENTS' VIEWS AND FOLLOW THEIR LEAD

Having elicited the appropriate spiritual and religious information from a patient, the physician must realize that the patient's views will significantly influence the therapeutic plan going forward. This is especially important when patients are making medical-decisions based on religious beliefs or observance. Although a patient's choice may not seem to make sense medically, simply discounting any religious or spiritual issues that are influencing the decision will not be an effective way to further the discussion. Nor is it appropriate for the physician to engage the patient in a theologic discussion to attempt and convince him or her that an alternative choice would be acceptable to his or her faith. By following the patient's lead and respecting his or her point of view, and using techniques of active listening to show the patient that his or her view is understood, the physician will have a much better chance to work with the patient to arrive at a treatment plan that will seem appropriate medically and still meet the religious needs of the patient. (Discussion of how different religious groups view certain end-of-life issues can be found in Chapter 32.)

MAINTAIN ONE'S OWN INTEGRITY

Although a physician's personal spiritual or religious beliefs and practices are generally considered off-limits (as are other aspects of his or her personal life), there are times when patients will ask about these beliefs, not to be intrusive, but as a way of raising their own spiritual or religious concerns. Rather than reject the inquiry out of hand, the physician should consider asking the patient why he or she is asking the question, potentially opening the door to a more fruitful dialogue that will have therapeutic benefit to the patient.

As discussed earlier, more than 80% of patients identified prayer as a very important aspect of care at the end of life. Sometimes, patients will request that, during the physician's visit, he or she participate in a prayer with the patient. This often causes great discomfort for the physician who may be of a different faith than the patient, or if from the same faith, at a different level of observance. Again, rather than rejecting the request out of hand, it is suggested that the physician choose from one of several optional responses, depending on his or her level of comfort with the request. The various options for how a physician might respond to a patient's request for prayer are listed in Table 15–4. Any support provided by the physician should be given without compromising his or her own beliefs or professional role and depends on the physician/patient relationship. By conducting himself or herself in such a thoughtful fashion, the physician can often provide spiritual support to a patient without feeling that he or she is compromising his or her own belief system.

TABLE 15–4. Responding to a Request for Prayer

OPTION	EXAMPLE
Remain and stand quietly without stating anything about prayer	
Disclosing an element of the physician's own beliefs	I am not of your faith
Offering passive support	I know that prayer is important to you, so allow me to leave so you can pray together with others
Offering active support	I understand how important prayer is to you and I will stand here quietly
Joining in prayer consistent with the physician's beliefs	I will quietly pray with you in a way I am comfortable
Joining actively in the prayer	I will be happy to participate with you in your prayer.

SOURCE: Adapted from Okon TR: Palliative care review: Spiritual, religious, and existential aspects of palliative care. *J Palliat Med* 8:392-414, 2005.

IDENTIFY COMMON GOALS FOR CARE

Once physicians have learned from patients about any spiritual or religious issues that are important to their care, they should, just as for any physical or psychosocial symptom, develop a treatment plan that reflects appropriate goals of care. As patients' needs drive the goals of care, it is important that physicians focus with their patients on those goals that they can agree on, especially when disagreements between the patient and physician are based on conflicts between spiritual/religious and medical needs.

UTILIZE APPROPRIATE PROFESSIONAL RESOURCES

Finally, and most importantly, although the information above has been meant to acquaint physicians with how to identify and understand the importance of spiritual and religious issues to their patients near the end of life, both in terms of the outcomes of their care and the medical decisions that they may choose to make, physicians need to realize that, as members of an interdisciplinary team, they are not alone. When it comes to meeting the spiritual needs of patients, physicians should be comfortable accessing members of the clergy to be the main providers of this aspect of their patients' care. If patients belong to a specific faith group and have their own spiritual leaders, then physicians should involve them in care at the earliest opportunity. When patients do not have their own clergy, then hospice/palliative care chaplains, as core members of the interdisciplinary team, are available as experts in assessing, identifying, and meeting the spiritual and religious needs of the patients near the end of life and their families. Although it is important for physicians to recognize the importance of spiritual care and be skilled at identifying the spiritual and/or religious concerns of their patients and families, they most importantly need to know when to consult the hospice or palliative care team chaplain,

and to feel comfortable doing so. In this fashion, physicians will be better able to ensure that their terminally ill patients and families receive the most comprehensive end of life care possible.

BIBLIOGRAPHY

Anandarajah G, Hight E: Spirituality and medical practice. Using the HOPE questions as a practical tool for spiritual assessment. *Am Fam Phys* 63:81-89, 2001.

Associaton of American Medical Colleges: Report III, Contemporary issues in medicine: communication in medicine. From Puchalski and Sandoval, "Spiritual Care" in A Clinical Guide to Supportive and Palliative Care for HIV/AIDS 2003 edition. http://hab.hrsa.gov/tools/pallitive/chap13.html. Accessed January, 2008.

Balboni T, Vanderwerker LC, Block SD, et al: Religiousness and spiritual support among advanced cancer patients and associations with end-of-life treatment preferences and quality of life. *J Clin Oncol* 25:555-560, 2007.

Brady MJ, Peterman AH, Fitchett G, et al: A case for including spirituality in quality of life measurement in oncology. *Psychooncology* 8:417-428, 1999.

Cassidy JP, Davies DJ: Cultural and spiritual aspects of palliative medicine. In: Doyle D, Hanks G, Cherny N, Calman K, eds. *Oxford Textbook of Palliative Medicine*, 3rd ed. New York, Oxford University Press, 2004, p. 954.

Chohinov HM, Cann B: Interventions to enhance the spiritual aspects of dying. *J Pall Med* 8(s1):S-103-S-115, 2005.

Cohen SR, Mount BM, Bruera E, et al: Validity of the McGill Quality of Life Questionnaire in the palliative care setting: A multi-centre Canadian study demonstrating the importance of the existential domain. *Palliat Med* 11:3-20, 1997.

Cohen SR, Mount BM, Tomas JJ, Mount LF: Existential well-being is an important determinant of quality of life. Evidence from the McGill Quality of Life Questionnaire. *Cancer* 77:576-586, 1996.

Costantini M, Mencaglia E, Giulio PD, et al: Cancer patients as 'experts' in defining quality of life domains. A multicentre survey by the Italian Group for the Evaluation of Outcomes in Oncology (IGEO). *Qual Life Res* 9:151-159, 2000.

Daaleman TP, Frey B: Spiritual and religious beliefs and practices of family physicians. *J Fam Prac* 49:98-104, 1999.

Ehman JW, Ott BB, Short TH, et al: Do patients want their physicians to inquire about their spiritual or religious beliefs if they become gravely ill? *Arch Int Med* 159:1803-1806, 1999.

Farr AC, Lantos JD, Roach CJ, et al: Religious characteristics of US physicians. A national survey. *J Gen Int Med* 20:629-634, 2005.

Ferrell B: Meeting spiritual needs: What is an oncologist to do? *J Clin Oncol* 25:467-468, 2007.

Frank E, Dell ML, Chopp R: Religious characteristics of US women physicians. *Soc Sci Med* 49:1717-1722, 1999.

George LK, Ellison CG, Larson DB: Exploring the relationships between religious involvement and health. *Psychol Inquiry* 13:190-200, 2002.

Guidelines on Chaplaincy and Spiritual Care in the NHS in Scotland SEHD, October 2002 from East Anglia's Children's Hospice. http://www.each.org.uk/index.php?option=com_content&task=view&id+170&Itemid=192. Accessed January, 2008.

Helm HM, Hays JC, Flint EP, et al: Does private religious activity prolong survival? A six-year follow-up study of 3,851 older adults. *J Gerontol A Biol Sci Med Sci* 55:M400-M405, 200.

Hermann CP: Spiritual needs of dying patients: A qualitative study. *Oncol Nurs Forum* 28:67-72, 2001.

Jacobs LM, Burns K, Jacobs BB: Trauma death: Views of the public and trauma professionals on death and dying from injuries. *Arch Surg* 143:730-735, 2008

Kaufman Y, Anaki D, Binns M, Freedman M: Cognitive decline in Alzeheimer disease. Impact of spirituality, religiosity, and QOL. *Neurology* 68:1509-1514, 2007.

Lo B, Ruston D, Kates LW, et al: Discussing religious and spiritual issues at the end of life. A practical guide for physicians. *JAMA* 287:749-754, 2002.

Lo B, Kates LW, Ruston D, et al: Responding to requests regarding prayer and religious ceremonies by patients near the end of life and their families. *J Palliat Med* 6:409-415, 2003.

Maugans TA: The SPIRITual history. *Arch Fam Med* 5:11-16, 1996.

Meador K: Spiritual care at the end of life. What is it and who does it? *NC Med J* 65(4):226-228, 2004.

McClain CS, Rosenfeld B, Breitbart W: Effect of spiritual well-being on end of life despair in terminally ill cancer patients. *Lancet* 361:1603-1607, 2003.

McCullough ME, Hoyt WT, Larson DB, et al: Religious involvement and mortality: A meta-analytic review. *Health Psychol* 19:211-222, 2000.

Nelson CJ, Rosenfeld B, Breitbart W, Galietta M: Spirituality, religion, and depression in the terminally ill. *Psychosomatics* 43:213-220, 2002.

Okon TR: Palliative Care Review: Spiritual, religious, and existential aspects of palliative care. *J Palliat Med* 8:392-414, 2005.

Peterman AH, Fitchett G, Brady MJ, et al: Measuring spiritual well-being in people with cancer: The functional assessment of chronic illness therapy—Spiritual Well-Being Scale (FACIT-Sp.). *Ann Behav Med* 24:49-58, 2002.

Pew Forum on Religious and Public Life: US Religious Landscape Survey, Part 1: Religious Affiliations, Summary of Key Findings. February 25, 2008. http://religions.pewforum.org/reports. Accessed January 26, 2009.

Pew Forum on Religious and Public Life: US Religious Landscape Survey, Part 2: Religious Beliefs and Practices, Social and Political Views, Summary of Key Findings. February 25, 2008. http://religions.pewforum.org/reports. Accessed January 26, 2009.

Phelps AC, Maciejewski PK, Nilsson M, et al: Religious coping and use of intensive life-prolonging care near death in patients with advanced cancer. *JAMA* 301:1140-1147, 2009.

Powell LH, Shahabi L, Thoresen CE: Religion and spirituality: Linkages to physical health. *Am Psychol* 58:36-52, 2003.

Puchalski CM, Romer AL: Taking a spiritual history allows clinicians to understand patients more fully. *J Palliat Med* 3:129-137, 2000.

Seeman TE, Dubin LF, Seeman M: Religiosity/spirituality and health. A critical review of the evidence for biological pathways. *Am Psychol* 58:53-63, 2003.

Silvestri GA, Knittig S, Zoller JS, Nietert PJ: Importance of faith on medical decisions regarding cancer care. *J Clin Oncol* 21:1379-1382, 2003.

Smith AK, McCarthy EP, Paulk E, et al: Racial and ethnic differences in advance care planning among patients with cancer: Impact of terminal illness acknowledgement, religiousness, and treatment preferences. *J Clin Oncol* 26:4131-4137, 2008.

Strawbridge WJ, Cohen RD, Shema SJ, Kaplan GA: Frequent attendance at religious services and mortality over 28 years. *Am J Public Health* 87:957-961, 1997.

Steinhauser KE, Christakis NA, Clipp EC, et al: Factors considered important at the end of life by patients, families, physicians, and other care providers. *JAMA* 284:2476-2482, 2000.

Thoresen CE: Spirituality and health: Is there a relationship? *J Health Psychol* 4:291-300, 1999.

Unruh AM, Versnel J, Kerr N: Spirituality unplugged: A review of commonalities and contentions, and a resolution. *Can J Occup Ther* 69:5-19, 2002.

Wiech K, Farias M, Kahane G, et al: An fMRI study measuring analgesia enhanced by religion as a belief system. *Pain* 139:467-476, 2008.

Williams AL, Selwyn PA, Liberti L, et al: A randomized controlled trial of meditation and massage effects on quality of life in people with late-stage disease: A pilot study. *J Palliat Med* 5:939-952, 2005.

SELF-ASSESSMENT QUESTIONS

1. In the model of "Total Pain," which component is the only one that specifically represents the spiritual influences on "suffering" and hence, on pain perception?

   A. Financial concerns
   B. Loss of work
   C. Changes in social and family functioning
   D. Fear of death
   E. Psychosocial influences on physical pain

2. Which of the following statements best defines the relationship between spiritual care and religious care?

   A. Spiritual care should always be religious.
   B. Religious care should always be spiritual.
   C. Spiritual care should never be religious.
   D. Religious care should never be spiritual.
   E. They actually are different terms for the same thing.

3. In a study in which oncology patients and physicians were asked to rank factors that influenced their medical decisions in order of importance, which of the following factors was ranked second in importance by patients, but last (seventh) by physicians?

   A. Oncologist's recommendation
   B. Family doctor's recommendation
   C. Faith in God
   D. Ability to cure
   E. Spouse's input

4. All of the following statements regarding physicians' attitudes toward spirituality and religion are true, EXCEPT:

   A. Family physicians are comparable to the general public regarding their religious characteristics.
   B. Physicians are less likely than the general public to cope with major problems without relying on God.
   C. Physicians are less likely than the general public to carry their religious beliefs over into other dealings in life.
   D. Physicians are more likely than the general public to consider themselves spiritual, but not religious.
   E. Only 20% of trauma physicians, as opposed to 57% of the public, believe that divine intervention could save a trauma victim when the physician believed further treatment was futile.

5. All of the following statements regarding health outcomes related to spiritual care are true, EXCEPT:

   A. A recent study of patients with probable Alzheimer's disease showed that higher levels of spirituality and participation in private religious practices had no effect on the rate of cognitive decline.
   B. Studies have shown that religious and spiritual care may have a protective effect against despair and depression in patients near the end of life.
   C. A meta-analysis of spiritual care studies suggested a beneficial relationship between spirituality or religion and health status, but study heterogeneity has limited any significant conclusions.
   D. One study showed that a lack of "spiritual well being" had a greater impact on "psychologic suffering" than did the level of depression, burden of physical symptoms or functional disability, or the level of social support.
   E. Spiritual concerns may influence quality of life in a unique way that is independent and not compatible with other measures of psychosocial well-being and coping.

6. When taking a spiritual history, which of following questions is most appropriate to ask?

   A. Do you go to church on Sunday?
   B. How has your faith affected your ability to cope with your illness?

C. Is your faith important to you?

D. Do you want to talk about anything else?

E. Do you believe in God?

7. When a patient desires an intervention that is not medically indicated for religious reasons, that you, as the physician, do not want to provide, what is the best way for you to manage the request?

A. Explain to the patient that the intervention is not appropriate because religion and science are often not compatible.

B. Explain to the patient that you are knowledgeable in his or her faith, and there are clergy who agree that is OK not to receive the intervention.

C. Ask the patient if he or she would be willing to discuss the situation with a chaplain of his or her faith who agrees with your position.

D. Tell the patient that you recognize his or her point of view and would like to work with

him or her to devise a mutually acceptable treatment plan.

E. Tell the patient that you will help him or her find another physician willing to provide the intervention that he or she is requesting.

8. While doing an assessment on a new patient with advanced congestive heart failure, the patient tells you that he or she would like to say a prayer with you. All of the following would be appropriate responses to the patient, except:

A. I know prayer is important to you, so I will leave the room while you pray.

B. I know prayer is important to you, so I will stand here with you while you pray.

C. I will participate in your prayer quietly with you in a way in which I am comfortable.

D. As we share a common faith, I will be happy to participate with you in your prayer.

E. I am sorry, but your prayer will have to wait until I have finished my assessment.

16

Psychosocial and Spiritual Assessments

Rabbi Bryan Kinzbrunner

INTRODUCTION

Upon admission into hospice care, in order to best meet the psychosocial and spiritual needs of terminally ill patients and their families that regularly arise during the dying process, social workers and chaplains, as active members of the interdisciplinary team, meet with these patients and families to assess the nonphysical aspects of their care. Various theoretical psychosocial and spiritual models have been utilized to create assessment methodology, and this chapter will explore these methods and how they have been incorporated into assessing the psychosocial and spiritual needs of patients near the end of life and their families.

DEFINING THE TERM ASSESSMENT

Assessment may be defined as the process of collecting information from an individual about a specific topic or situation that seeks out the meaning of the situation, puts the particulars of the issue into some order, and leads to appropriate interventions. It is a straightforward, distinctive cognitive process that involves using relevant (as determined by the practice model being used) knowledge and exercising informed judgments. In addition to being a process, it may also be considered a product, a statement that is the consequence of exploration of case data, use of inference, and definition of the problems to be treated.

PSYCHOSOCIAL ASSESSMENT MODELS

According to the National Association of Social Workers' (NASW) Standards for Palliative and End-of-Life Care, the goal of a psychosocial as-

sessment is to assess a client for the purpose of developing a case-specific treatment plan with appropriate interventions. In order for social workers to best determine the appropriate psychosocial plan of care, they are required to investigate and analyze the particular personal and communal dynamics of the patient and family.

Specifically regarding end-of-life and palliative care, the social work assessment must include the consideration of a myriad of relevant biopsychosocial factors that will reflect the needs of the patient and family. These factors are listed in Table 16–1 and include relevant current and past physical and mental health issues. Family issues that require exploration include its structure, the role of the patient and other family members within that structure, how decisions within the family are made, and the patient's and family's goals around palliative and end-of-life care. Cultural issues of importance include language preferences (and availability of an independent translator if indicated), ethnicity, spirituality, and faith. Prior experience with illness, disability, and death and loss, and the ability of family members to cope with crisis are crucial pieces of information to elicit as well.

ECOSYSTEMS THEORY AND PSYCHOSOCIAL ASSESSMENT

Much of the literature on psychosocial assessment models has its basis in social work theory, with the methodology being dependent upon the context of the patient encounter. Current social work practice is derived from an ecosystems theory, a unifying theory of all elements that encompass a person's life. The characteristics of an ecosystems approach to social reality are listed in Table 16–2. As stated by sociologist Max Siporin in his 1980 article on ecosystems in social work:

Ecological systems theory is such a general metatheory, one that provides for the many, and at the same time contradictory, purposes and activities of social workers. It constitutes an essential element of the generic core of social work knowledge, of its common person-in-situation and dialectical

TABLE 16–1. Areas for Consideration in the Comprehensive Assessment

- Relevant past and current health situations (including the impact of problems such as pain, depression, anxiety, delirium, decreased mobility)
- Family structure and roles
- Patterns/style of communication and decision making in the family
- Stage in the life cycle, relevant developmental issues
- Spirituality/faith
- Cultural values and beliefs
- Client's/family's language preferences and available translation services
- Client's/family's goals in palliative and end-of-life treatment
- Social supports, including support systems, informal and formal caregivers involved, resources available, and barriers to access
- Past experience with illness, disability, death, and loss
- Mental health functioning including history, coping style, crisis management skills, and risk of suicide/homicide
- Unique needs and issues relevant to special populations such as refugees and immigrants, children, individuals with severe and persistent mental illness, and homeless people
- Communicating the client's/family's psychosocial needs to the interdisciplinary team

SOURCE: National Association of Social Workers: *NASW Standards for Palliative and End of Life Care*. Washington, DC, 2004.

TABLE 16–2. Characteristics of Ecosystem Theory Based Assessment

- The environment is a complex environment–behavior–person whole, consisting of a continuous, interlocking process of relationships, not arbitrary dualism.
- The mutual interdependence among person, behavior, and environment.
- Systems concepts are used to analyze the complex interrelationships with the ecological whole.
- Behavior is recognized to be site-specific.
- Assessment and evaluation should be through the naturalistic, direct observation of the intact, undisturbed, natural organism–environment system.
- The relationships of the parts within the ecosystem are considered to be orderly, structured, lawful, and deterministic.
- Behavior results from mediated transactions between the person and the multivariate environment.
- The central task of behavioral science is to develop taxonomies of environments, behaviors, and behavior-environment linkages and to determine their distribution in the natural world.

SOURCE: Meares PA, Lane BA: Grounding social work practice in theory: ecosystems. In: Rauch JB, ed. *Assessment: A Sourcebook for Social Work Practice*. Milwaukee, WI: Families International Inc., 3-13, 1993.
Based on Sells SB: An interactionist looks at the environment. In: Moos RH, Insel PM, eds. *Issues in Social Ecology: Human Milieus*. Palo Alto, CA, National Press Books, 1974; Moos R, Brownstein R: *Environment and Utopia: A Synthesis*. New York, Plenum Publishing, 1977; and Schoggen P: Ecological psychology and mental retardation. In: Sackett GP, ed. *Observing Behavior: Theory and applications in Mental Retardation* Vol 1. Baltimore, MD, University Park Press, 1978.

perspective, and of its basic helping approach. It supports social work assessment and intervention focus.

Therefore, according to the ecological systems, or ecosystems, theory, it is the gathering of the patient's personal history during the assessment process that will give the social worker the most significant window into the patient's psychosocial needs. Such a personal history includes the significant moments of development, life events, family life, and the period during which the current challenges emerged. Understanding these various events in a person's life will assist the social worker in better understanding the patient's and family's reactions to the current situation and determining their current needs, as reactions to prior events often provide significant clues to a better understanding of the dynamics of the current situation.

In addition to using patient and family history to understand how the patient and family are coping with the present challenges, the assessing social worker must synthesize the gathered information in order to determine the interactive impact of these various factors, which include not only life history, socio–cultural ecology, environmental pressures and resources, but the patient's current affective, cognitive, and behavioral capacities and functioning as well. Determining the quality of the adaptive or maladaptive functioning of the patient and family to the present situation is also important, because, generally, clients who come to social agencies, clinics, and other helping centers, do so as a consequence of some breakdown in psychosocial functioning, or inability to manage some aspects of his or her life. In chronic care and end-of-life care situations, a somewhat unique aspect of the psychosocial assessment is to garner the information that will assist patients and families in sorting through the challenges of death and dying, both from a psychological perspective as well as a technical perspective. Inclusive in this are assessing the resources that the patient and family have available to them to han-

dle the various stressors associated with the dying process, from community groups to financial planning for funerals, from insurance challenges to organizing keepsakes of the dying.

On the basis of the goal of the assessment and the patient's and family's immediate needs, the social worker performing the psychosocial assessment will need to assess for the relevance of the data included, for known information is not always of the same level of importance when developing a plan of care. The goal is to assess the patient and family in relationship to how the person responds and reacts to the "environment situation." The issue of relevance is jointly determined by social worker and client. For example, a social worker might not encourage life review with the patient if the telling of the story is not salient to the support to be provided immediately. This allows the social worker to focus on handling the current problem without having to overstretch his/her boundaries.

When conducting a psychosocial assessment, time is always a significant factor. The pace of the assessment process may be dictated by the potential number of encounters that the social worker will have with the patient and family, which, in end-of-life care, may be a function of the patient's clinical condition and short-term prognosis. Since, given the short median and average lengths of stay of patients on hospice programs, it is not unusual for a social worker to have the opportunity for only one visit.

Carol Meyer presents a sample of a social work encounter that highlights this situation. Goals are generally short-term and must be specific either to the patient's desires or be preformulated, based on situations and potential outcomes common to patients and families with a very short life expectancy. The short-term encounter forces both the patient/family and social worker to focus on identifying relevant and nonrelevant information, and to make rapid inferences. While some care planning based on the psychosocial assessment can be accomplished during the visit, the lack of time and the patient's condition may require the professional to plan further interventions following the patient encounter.

Another short-term care model, termed single-session therapy, is described by Moishe Talman. During the "single session," the professional focuses on tapping into existing and potential levels of patient confidence and independence as well as available support systems, in order to give the patient a sense of autonomy and allow the patient to be able to fend for him or herself following the encounter. This approach obviously can only work well when a patient is still functional and has the requisite opportunities and personal resources to remain somewhat independent and is, therefore, of limited utility for patients near the end of life. The professional is also challenged to avoid overestimating the patient's ability to cope or rush to "move-on."

MULTIDIMENSIONAL ASSESSMENT OF THE ELDERLY CLIENT

Nancy Morrow-Howell argues that social work assessment for the elderly requires a unique blending of the biological, psychological, and social elements of one's life, for aging causes tremendous change in a person's life. Condensing the many elements of a psychosocial assessment described by the NASW (see Table 16–1), Howell presents an assessment model consisting of seven dimensions that take into account both physical and emotional concerns. These dimensions are listed in Table 16–3 and are discussed below.

Physical Health

As the elderly are generally comfortable talking about physical frailties, a discussion of physical health can create a comfort zone between the patient/family and the social worker that will ease the transition into the more intimate psychosocial and emotional issues to follow. This means that social workers must be knowledgeable in diseases

TABLE 16–3. Multidimensional Assessment of the Elderly Client

- Physical health
- Mental health
- Social support
- Physical environment
- Functioning
- Coping style
- Formal service usage

SOURCE: Morrow-Howell N: Multidimensional assessment of the elderly client. In: Rauch JB, ed. *Assessment: A Sourcebook for Social Work Practice.* Milwaukee, WI, Families International Inc., pp. 123-139, 1993.

that commonly occur in the elderly and how these illnesses manifest themselves. Part of the assessment of physical health is to inquire if the patient and family are able to properly utilize the health care system. The social worker will want to assess if the person is being compliant with taking medications and, if not, determine why the patient is not being compliant with the particular medication.

Although in end-of-life care, it is likely that the social worker will not be required to assess physical health, since this generally already has been done by the nurse on the interdisciplinary team, the social worker should be knowledgeable and conversant in the information gathered by the nurse during the physical assessment and be able to use and incorporate the information into the psychosocial assessment and any subsequent interventions recommended.

As end-of-life care includes caregivers and family as part of the unit of care, the social worker also must consider and advocate for the physical health of the caregiver during the assessment and care planning process. This is especially true in the common situation where both patient and caregiver are elderly, for more often than not, the caregiver is not taking proper care of himself or

TABLE 16–4. The Short Portable Mental Status Questionnaire (SPMSQ)

1. What are the date, month, and year?
2. What is the day of the week?
3. What is the name of this place?
4. What is your phone number?
5. How old are you?
6. When were you born?
7. Who is the current president?
8. Who was the president before him?
9. What was your mother's maiden name?
10. Can you count backward from 20 by 3's?

SCORING:*

0–2 errors: normal mental functioning

3–4 errors: mild cognitive impairment

5–7 errors: moderate cognitive impairment

8 or more errors: severe cognitive impairment

*One more error is allowed in the scoring if a patient has had a grade school education or less. One less error is allowed if the patient has had education beyond the high school level.

SOURCE: Pfeiffer E: A short portable mental status questionnaire for the assessment of organic brain deficit in elderly patients. *J Am Geriatr Soc* 23:433-441, 1975. http://www.npcrc.org/usr_doc/adhoc/psychosocial/SPMSQ.pdf.

herself due to the attention being paid to the patient.

Mental Health

The assessment of mental health begins with an evaluation of a patient's cognitive status, as emotional stress may contribute significantly to cognitive impairment in the population. In other words, does one's patient suffer from irreversible memory loss and confusion solely from an organic cause or is the impaired cognitive status at least partially the result of an underlying emotional problem? While it is often difficult to formally assess cognitive function when patients are near the end of life, when patients are intact enough to answer questions, social workers may utilize one of a variety of validated mental status exam tools that are available. One example of such a tool, the Short Portable Mental

Status Questionnaire (SPMSQ), is included as Table 16–4.

After establishing a patient's degree of cognitive impairment, the social worker should assess the patient's emotional health, primarily looking for signs and symptoms consistent with depressive disorders, including, but not limited to withdrawal, lack of energy, sadness, guilt, and/or hopelessness. These symptoms often occur in patients near the end of life as a result of grieving, loss of function, or from knowledge that one's life is coming to an end. As with cognitive function, assessment tools have been developed to evaluate patients for depressive symptoms, with one of more widely used tools, the Geriatric Depression Scale (GDS), illustrated as Table 16–5. One must be reminded that due to the nature of the condition of many patients who are near the end of life, the emotional assessment is often done by observing rather than questioning the patient

TABLE 16–5. Geriatric Depression Scale (GDS)

Choose the best answer for how you felt this past week
Circle one

*1.	Are you basically satisfied with your life?	yes NO
2.	Have you dropped many of your activities and interests?	YES no
3.	Do you feel that your life is empty?	YES no
4.	Do you often get bored?	YES no
*5.	Are you hopeful about the future?	yes NO
6.	Are you bothered by thoughts you can't get out of your head?	YES no
*7.	Are you in good spirits most of the time?	yes NO
8.	Are you afraid that something bad is going to happen to you?	YES no
*9.	Do you feel happy most of the time?	yes NO
10.	Do you often feel helpless?	YES no
11.	Do you often get restless and fidgety?	YES no
12.	Do you prefer to stay at home, rather than going out and doing new things?	YES no
13.	Do you frequently worry about the future?	YES no
14.	Do you feel you have more problems with memory than most?	YES no
*15.	Do you think it is wonderful to be alive now?	yes NO
16.	Do you often feel downhearted and blue?	YES no
17.	Do you feel pretty worthless the way you are now?	YES no
18.	Do you worry a lot about the past?	YES no
*19.	Do you find life very exciting?	yes NO
20.	Is it hard for you to get started on new projects?	YES no
*21.	Do you feel full of energy?	yes NO
22.	Do you feel that your situation is hopeless?	YES no
23.	Do you think that most people are better off than you are?	YES no
24.	Do you frequently get upset over little things?	YES no
25.	Do you frequently feel like crying?	YES no
26.	Do you have trouble concentrating?	YES no
*27.	Do you enjoy getting up in the morning?	yes NO
28.	Do you prefer to avoid social gatherings?	YES no
*29.	Is it easy for you to make decisions?	yes NO
*30.	Is your mind as clear as it used to be?	yes NO

*Appropriate (nondepressed) answers = yes, all others = no or count number of CAPITALIZED (depressed) answers
Score: _____ (Number of "depressed" answers)
Norms

Normal 5 ± 4
Mildly depressed 15 ± 6
Very depressed 23 ± 5

_____

_____

The Geriatric Depression Scale may be used freely for patient assessment according to the authors.
Source: http://www.acsu.buffalo.edu/~drstall/gds.txt.
Yesavage JA, Brink TL, Rose TL, et al: Development and validation of a geriatric depression rating scale: A preliminary report. *J Psych Res* 17:27, 1983.
Sheikh JI, Yesavage JA. Geriatric depression scale: recent evidence and development of a shorter version. *Clin Gerontol* 5:165-172, 1986.

and gathering additional information by evaluating the caregiver's perception of the patient's behaviors and emotional reactions.

Social Support

The social worker's third area for assessment is the patient's primary social structure, which includes both the quantity and quality of a person's social contacts. Evaluation of quantitative social support includes asking questions about one's living arrangements, who will be available for respite if the primary caregiver is in need of relief, and whether the patient or family are members of any outside institutions (such as religious or social institutions) that might be prevailed upon to provide additional support. On the other hand, when assessing qualitative social support, the professional must determine how the patient is interacting with those who are providing the support. For example, is the patient satisfied with the people available for help and with the help being provided, or are their needs not being met? Does the patient feel lonely or perceive that he or she is a burden to those providing care?

The social worker also needs to ask caregivers how they view their specific roles in caring for the patient to ensure that everyone involved, including the patient and all caregivers, share the same expectations. The caregiver's desire to care for the patient also needs to be ascertained to ensure that the caregiver is comfortable in the agreed upon role and not providing the help only out of a sense of obligation. The assessment should also take into account whether the patient is being treated well or being neglected or abused. A useful tool for assessing social support is the Lubben Social Network Index (LSNS), which may be found as Table 16–6.

Physical Environment

An often overlooked but critical part of the psychosocial assessment is the physical environment, which includes the patient's home as well as the surrounding neighborhood. It is important to ascertain whether the home environment is a safe and conducive place to provide the patient with proper care. For example a cluttered home or bathrooms without railings for support may significantly increase the risk of falls. Lack of room ventilation or air conditioning could result in increased symptoms of breathlessness for the patient. If a hospital bed is required, one must make sure that there is a room in the home large enough to accommodate it, and that it will fit through the doorways that lead to the room.

The surroundings of the home should also be assessed for safety, especially if the patient is going to spend time outdoors. As patients often need medications or other supplies quickly, one should be aware of the location of the nearest pharmacy and grocery store, their hours, and how easy or difficult it is for caregivers to go there. The safety of the neighborhood should also be assessed, both during the day and at night, to determine if a professional caregiver can visit alone or not in both routine and emergency situations.

Functioning

Functionality in the context of the assessment is defined by a patient's innate ability to interact with the psychosocial and physical environments on a day-to-day basis. For the social worker, when working in conjunction with a nurse, the concerns for assessing a person's activities of daily living (ADL) deficits are secondary to understanding how well the patient functions within the context of whatever those deficits are, including whether or not the patient has a realistic perception of the limits of his or her ability. A good method for performing a functionality assessment is to have the patient and/or caregiver describe the course of a typical day, as this will provide for a better sense of how the patient functions in the environment. As patients and families often have different perceptions of patient functionality, the social worker will commonly play the role of mediator between patient and family

TABLE 16–6. Lubben Social Network Scale—18 (LSNS-18)

Family: *Considering the people to whom you are related either by birth or marriage*

1. How many relatives do you see or hear from at least once a month?
   0 = none   1 = one   2 = two   3 = three or four   4 = five thru eight   5 = nine or more
2. *How often do you see or hear from relative with whom you have the most contact?*
   0 = never   1 = seldom   2 = sometimes   3 = often   4 = very often   5 = always
3. *How many relatives do you feel at ease with that you can talk about private matters?*
   0 = none   1 = one   2 = two   3 = three or four   4 = five thru eight   5 = nine or more
4. How many relatives do you feel close to such that you could call on them for help?
   0 = none   1 = one   2 = two   3 = three or four   4 = five thru eight   5 = nine or more
5. When one of your relatives has an important decision to make, how often do they talk to you about it?
   0 = never   1 = seldom   2 = sometimes   3 = often   4 = very often   5 = always
6. How often is one of your relatives available for you to talk to when you have an important decision to make?
   0 = never   1 = seldom   2 = sometimes   3 = often   4 = very often   5 = always

Neighbors: *Considering those people who live in your neighborhood. . . .*

7. How many of your neighbors do you see or hear from at least once a month?
   0 = none   1 = one   2 = two   3 = three or four   4 = five thru eight   5 = nine or more
8. How often do you see or hear from the neighbor with whom you have the most contact?
   0 = never   1 = seldom   2 = sometimes   3 = often   4 = very often   5 = always
9. How many neighbors do you feel at ease with that you can talk about private matters?
   0 = none   1 = one   2 = two   3 = three or four   4 = five thru eight   5 = nine or more
10. How many neighbors do you feel close to such that you could call on them for help?
    0 = none   1 = one   2 = two   3 = three or four   4 = five thru eight   5 = nine or more
11. *When one of your neighbors has an important decision to make, how often do they talk to you about it?*
    0 = never   1 = seldom   2 = sometimes   3 = often   4 = very often   5 = always
12. How often is one of your neighbors available for you to talk to when you have an important decision to make?
    0 = never   1 = seldom   2 = sometimes   3 = often   4 = very often   5 = always

Friendships: *Considering your friends who do not live in your neighborhood. . . .*

13. How many of your friends do you see or hear from at least once a month?
    0 = none   1 = one   2 = two   3 = three or four   4 = five thru eight   5 = nine or more
14. How often do you see or hear from the friend with whom you have the most contact?
    0 = never   1 = seldom   2 = sometimes   3 = often   4 = very often   5 = always
15. How many friends do you feel at ease with that you can talk about private matters?
    0 = none   1 = one   2 = two   3 = three or four   4 = five thru eight   5 = nine or more
16. How many friends do you feel close to such that you could call on them for help?
    0 = none   1 = one   2 = two   3 = three or four   4 = five thru eight   5 = nine or more
17. *When one of your friends has an important decision to make, how often do they talk to you about it?*
    0 = never   1 = seldom   2 = sometimes   3 = often   4 = very often   5 = always
18. How often is one of your friends available for you to talk to when you have an important decision to make?
    0 = never   1 = seldom   2 = sometimes   3 = often   4 = very often   5 = always

LSNS-18 total score is an equally weighted sum of these eighteen items. Scores range from 0 to 90

Source: http://www2.bc.edu/~norstraj/LSNS-18.htm.

in determining what the patient requires the family caregivers to provide in the way of support.

Coping Style

Perhaps the most challenging aspect of a psychosocial assessment is learning how the person and family are coping with the patient's life-limiting illness. What are the person's resources with regard to emotional stability? Is the person religious or spiritual? How does the person handle the stresses of dealing with a terminal illness? This would be an opportunity to introduce, for example, life review, for it will provide for better insight as to how one handles stress and crisis.

Formal Service Usage

In a standard social work assessment, the social worker will also investigate the person's concrete needs. Does the person need help in soliciting extra health care coverage, such as Medicaid, meals on wheels, and veterans' benefits? Is the caregiver in need of respite or support while caring for the terminally ill? The social worker will use this particular area of assessment as a means to pursue the additional formal services that the patient and family can utilize.

SPIRITUAL ASSESSMENTS

The purpose of a spiritual assessment is to investigate the spiritual needs and resources of people in the various contexts where spiritual care is provided and to be able to formulate a plan of care that includes nonphysical aspects and factors related to the disease process. According to Reverend Richard Gilbert, the four outcomes of a spiritual assessment should be to understand a person's beliefs about involvement with God and religious practices, to determine the extent to which a person's religious practices and spiritual understandings serve as a resource for faith

and life, to assess whether a person's resources for hope and strength are founded on reality, and to give a person an opportunity to accept spiritual support.

George Fitchett described eight factors that establish the importance of a spiritual assessment. According to Fichett, the assessment provides foundations for action, communication, contracting, personal accountability, quality assurance, research, and for the establishment of one's professional identity. (See Table 16–7 for further description of each of these factors.)

Reverend Simon Robinson presents an additional four reasons for spiritual assessment. First, he states that spirituality affects the prognosis of an illness and is a variable that may help to predict how patients will cope with illness. He views spirituality as an important part of patients' lived experience and believes that they will need to work through the impact of their illness on their belief systems to discover meaning. He notes that spiritual functioning is dynamic and, therefore, monitoring spiritual reflections shows how patients are progressing and adjusting to their illness. Finally, he maintains that spirituality may give indications about suitable interventions to treat problems.

CHARACTERISTIC APPROACHES TO PERFORMING A SPIRITUAL ASSESSMENT

Fitchett describes nine potential approaches that a spiritual care provider might take when performing a spiritual assessment, although both he and Handzo indicated that irrespective of the approach to the spiritual assessment, the key issues are usually gathered through semistructured or open-ended conversations. These nine different approaches are listed in Table 16–8 and discussed below.

Implicit Assessment

As its name suggests, the implicit assessment is a mutual process during which both parties

TABLE 16–7. Eight Factors Regarding the Importance of a Spiritual Assessment	
FACTOR	**EXPLANATION**
Foundation for action	Means to guide clinician in helping patient through development of individual plan of care
Foundation for communication	Focuses the conversation to gathering the pertinent information and data needed to create the plan of care.
Foundation for contracting	Establishes a mutually agreed upon approach as to how to best meet the specific needs of the patient.
Foundation for evaluation	Established parameters that allow the spiritual care provider to reassess the patient at each visit to determine the success of various interventions.
Foundation for personal accountability	Both the spiritual caregiver and patient are responsible to act based on the agreed upon plan of care and can be held accountable for success or failure.
Foundation for quality assurance	Agreed upon goals can be converted into measurable outcomes and their degree of achievement can be evaluated.
Foundation for research	The established outcomes can be used for evaluating the success of particular interventions and this can be shared with others in the field.
Touchstone of one's professional identity	The spiritual assessment is the tool through which the spiritual care giver established his or her professionalism.

SOURCE: Fitchett G: *Assessing Spiritual Needs: A Guide for Caregivers*. Lima, Ohio: Academic Renewal Press, 2002.

TABLE 16–8. Characteristic Approaches to the Spiritual Assessment
• Implicit assessment
• Inspired assessment
• Intuitive assessment
• Idiosyncratic assessment
• Assessments based on Traditional Pastoral Acts
• Assessments based on Normative Pastoral Stances
• Global assessment
• Psychological assessment
• Explicit Spiritual assessment

SOURCE: Fitchett G: *Assessing Spiritual Needs: A Guide for Caregivers*. Lima, OH, Academic Renewal Press, 2002.

involved recognize that an assessment is being performed without either party outwardly acknowledging the assessment. In other words, the patient and spiritual care provider engage in an informal conversation or discussion during which the spiritual care provider is learning the necessary information about the patient without the formality that generally accompanies the assessment process.

Inspired Assessment

An inspired assessment is one which incorporates the innate ability of the spiritual care adviser to recognize a particular situation and immediately provide the necessary spiritual or ritual care. Fitchett provides the example of a priest serving as a spiritual care provider who recognizes that the patient he is caring for is actively dying and performs the "Anointing of the Sick" ritual. Inspired assessments are most often time-sensitive, which allows the spiritual care provider to take charge of the situation and to be proactive. In end-of-life care, chaplain support to the patient and family often comes about only at this critical junction. In these situations, the spiritual care provider must possess the skill necessary to determine what areas need immediate attention and what areas can be left for post-death bereavement support.

Intuitive Assessment

As its name implies, an intuitive assessment is one which, as often described by spiritual caregivers, is based on "a gut feeling." It often comes about as a result of the spiritual care provider recognizing a situation based on verbal and nonverbal cues that would seem to be outside of the primary stated goal of the visit. By intuitively interpreting the clues to better understand the patient's needs, the spiritual care provider then tailors the plan of care and interventions to this heretofore unrecognized problem.

Idiosyncratic Assessment

Fitchett admits that spiritual care providers will often assess a patient without using a particular model of questioning and analysis, and when intentional, he calls this lack of formal questioning an idiosyncratic assessment. In end-of-life care, this may often occur in situations when a patient and/or family is reluctant to discuss the terminal nature of the patient's situation. The spiritual care provider, rather than resorting to formal questioning, will use casual conversation to gather the needed information. Although the idiosyncratic assessment has features in common with the implicit assessment described earlier, the lack of intent on the part of the patient and/or family sets the two apart.

Assessment Based on Traditional Pastoral Acts and/or Normal Pastoral Stances

As most spiritual care providers are clergy from a recognized faith body, assessments based on traditional pastoral acts and/or normal pastoral stances are the two most common forms of spiritual assessment. In end-of-life care, when the spiritual care provider encounters a family dealing with a dying loved one, the patient and family often find comfort in the traditional prayers and rituals from their specific religious tradition. By providing or arranging for the appropriate clergy to provide these "traditional pastoral acts," the spiritual care giver can assess the level of spiritual comfort that these interventions bring to the patient and family.

At other times, spiritual care givers initiate their assessment of patients and families via their own preconceived notions of an encounter, such as "being present" and "being available". The idea here is that if the patient and/or family know that the spiritual care giver is "present" or "available" and requests something, then the spiritual care provider "assesses" the patient/family need based on the nature of the request

Global Assessment

Global assessment is an assessment approach in which the spiritual care provider uses one or two broad diagnostic categories to support patient or family needs. For example, if the spiritual care provider determines that a patient is having spiritual distress related to loneliness and anxiety, rather than assessing the problem in greater depth, the provider will use the more general approach of encouragement.

Psychological Assessment

Spiritual care providers are sometimes called upon to perform a psychological assessment in order to provide psychological support in conjunction with spiritual support, which, of course, is their primary responsibility. Fitchett, as well as others, have found that there is an increased need for chaplains to have psychological training and the skills to assess the psychological needs of patients and families in order to provide the most comprehensive care. Paul Pruyser, author of *Minister as Diagnostician*, on the other hand, tends to dissuade spiritual care providers from using psychological categories for he believes that the goals of the patients/families and the care providers receiving spiritual care are different from those receiving psychological care and support. In end-of-life care, it would appear that spiritual care givers require the knowledge and skill to assess patients and families psychologically as the spiritual care provider is often the primary bereavement counselor. As discussed in depth in the chapter on bereavement care, bereavement counseling is built on a combination of spiritual and psychological counseling and requires the knowledge of both religious rituals and the knowledge of what is normal grief and what is complicated grief.

Explicit Spiritual Assessment

The last approach described by Fitchett is the explicit spiritual assessment. The spiritual care provider uses his or her skills to assess the needs of patients and families by evaluating both spiritual religious and nonreligious issues. These may include anything from the patient to God or whatever deity he or she believes in, to ways of finding meaning in life, suffering, and/or death in a purely secular way, without inclusion of a deity, based on the belief system of the patient or family member being cared for.

SPIRITUAL ASSESSMENT MODELS

Now that it is better understood why spiritual assessments are important and the various approaches to the assessment that the spiritual care provider may take, specific spiritual assessment models that have been developed will be examined. While there are a number of different models that a spiritual care provider may take advantage of, three specific ones, Paul Pruyser's "Guidelines for Pastoral Diagnosis" model, Fitchett's "7 × 7" model, and Hay's Spiritual Assessment Model for End-of-Life Care will be discussed in detail.

It must be noted that while these structured assessment models have been found useful in many situations, one must be aware that there are still occasions when the spiritual assessment will need to be conducted more informally, using general narrative and/or life review. It is up to the spiritual care provider to determine whether formal or informal methods will be most effective in planning for the care of any individual patient and family.

Paul Pruyser's "Guidelines for Pastoral Diagnosis"

Paul Pruyser, in his work, *Minister as Diagnostician*, presented the first thorough methodology for a focused spiritual assessment, "Guidelines for Pastoral Diagnosis." His primary purpose was to indicate to clergy the need for an in-depth spiritual understanding of their congregants. In addition, as he believed that spiritual support should be distinct from psychological support (as mentioned earlier) and as many nonfaith-specific chaplains working in noncongregational settings were diagnosing situations based on standard psychological terms, he also developed this tool as vehicle for changing this behavior. This model divides the assessment into seven distinct categories, which are listed in Table 16–9 and discussed below.

AWARENESS OF THE HOLY   The first goal is to characterize what specific transcendental relationships, if any, that a patient possesses provides meaning, irrespective of how one relates to them. The goal is to then define and understand the characteristics of the relationship. As Pruyser's frame of reference is that of a Christian minister, he also includes the question of whether the

TABLE 16–9. Pruyser's Guidelines for Pastoral Diagnosis

CATEGORY	CONTENT
Awareness of the Holy	What if anything is sacred, revered, untouchable, or inscrutable? Any experiences of awe or bliss, when, in what situation? Any sense of creatureliness, humility, awareness of own limitations? Any idolatry, reverence displaced to improper symbols?
Providence	What is God's intention toward me? What has God promised me? Related to capacity for trust. Extent of hoping versus wishing.
Faith	Affirming versus negating stance in life. Able to commit self, to engage. Open to world or constricted.
Grace or gratefulness	Kindness, generosity, the beauty of giving and receiving. No felt need for grace or gratefulness. Forced gratitude under any circumstances. Desire for versus resistance to blessing.
Repentance	The process of change from crookedness to rectitude. A sense of agency in one's own problems or one's response to them. Being a victim versus being too sorry for debatable sins. Feelings of contrition, remorse, regret. Willingness to do penance.
Communion	Feelings of kinship with the whole chain of being. Feelings embedded or estranged, united or separated in the world, in relations with one's faith group, one's faith institution.
Sense of vocation	Willingness to be a cheerful participant in creation. Signs of zest, vigor, liveliness, dedication. Aligned with divine benevolence and malevolence. Humorous and inventive involvement in life versus grim and dogmatic

Source: Adapted from Fitchett G, Handzo GF: Spiritual assessment, screening, and intervention. In: Holland JC, et al., eds. *Psycho-Oncology.* New York, Oxford University Press, pp. 790-808, 1998; Pruyser PW: *The Minister as Diagnostician: Personal Problems in Pastoral Perspective.* Philadelphia, PA, Westminster Press, 1976.

patient's relationship or "sense of the sacred" is "potentially misguided." Common assessment questions might include the following: Does the person recognize anything in life as sacred? Does the person imbue aspects of life with transcendent meaning?

PROVIDENCE   Providence examines the issue of what the patient perceives God's role is for him or her. Is the person searching for Divine meaning in life or expressing conflict regarding one's perceived sense of meaning versus the reality of the situation? Providence includes specific experiences of Divine benevolence and nurture. It examines the question of whether a person feels trust in God and, by extension, trust in the spiri-

tual care provider he or she is working with. It also explores the issues of patient hope, and whether he or she believes that there is something that was already promised by God.

FAITH   Faith examines the patient's feelings about his or her relationship with God. Does the person embrace a relationship with God or does the person question God's existence? Is the patient constricted by claiming "My faith" or is he or she open to expanding one's thinking? For the spiritual care provider, the assessment of openness or closedness can be difficult to maneuver around as goals for spiritual care do not include judging another's faith or attempting to impose one's own faith upon the patient. Rather, the goal is to help the patient understand or recognize how his or her "faith" helps or hinders the specific situation.

GRACE AND GRATEFULNESS   After establishing a patient's perspective on providence and faith, the spiritual care provider examines what the person believes he is giving to (gratefulness) or receiving from (grace) his relationship with God and others. In this area of assessment, Pruyser subsumes within the question of grace the issue of forgiveness; in other words, is the patient able to forgive and/or feel forgiven? When assessing one's sense of forgiveness, there is often an underlying sense of pride or ego that manifests itself.

Sometimes gratefulness is "forced" in the sense that one can feel the need to express gratitude, even when angered by situations or events leading to the need for spiritual counseling. In addition, Pruyser encourages the spiritual care provider to use blessings in many situations, as this allows one to gain a better perspective on a patient's sense of grace. Some patients might accept blessing in the form of tears or a smile, while others will express anger at receiving an unsolicited blessing because of skepticism in one's belief in the power of blessing.

REPENTANCE   Does the person see a problem in his or her life that needs fixing? Is there an "awareness of sin?" Does the person feel remorse or responsibility for past errors? How does a person correct these or other perceived "errors" in his or her life, especially near the end of life when time is short? When a person confronts challenging times during life, there is a tendency to take time out for introspection, which may result in a type of repentance, or the changing of one's former behaviors. Whether the behavioral changes are based on spiritual and religious traditions that have a litany of do's and don'ts that dictate how one lives, or whether the repentance is based on human–human interactions that are not spiritually or religiously based, one of the primary purposes of the spiritual care provider to assist patients by guiding them through the process of re-

pentance and behavioral change when desired, based on each patient's own expression of spirituality and religious belief system, if any.

COMMUNION   The category of communion evaluates the community resources that a patient might have available for additional spiritual support. This will help determine if the person may feel embedded or estranged, united or separated from the world at large, and whether or not these same feelings exist in the individual's relationships with his or her faith group or institution. The spiritual care provider would also assess what rituals, if any, help ground the patient and family within the community.

SENSE OF VOCATION   Finally, the spiritual assessment concludes by evaluating the patient's "sense of vocation," one's spiritual perceptions of his or her role in the world with respect to the divine. Does a person have a zest or vigor for life? While overlapping some with the category of "Providence," the "Sense of Vocation," rather than evaluating the speculative or perceived Divine purpose of one's life, examines the real and practical purpose of one's life.

The 7 × 7 Model for Spiritual Assessment

In the 1990s, George Fitchett developed what he described as a "functional approach" to spiritual assessments. He argued that the spiritual care provider was to be concerned both with meaning and purpose in life as well as the more general behavioral and emotional issues a person experiences. Fitchett's approach is multidimensional and covers a wide spectrum of spiritual systems, as it does not incorporate an established definition for spirituality. Rather it provides an opportunity for the patient to share information in the way in which he or she chooses with the spiritual care provider. The model, which he calls 7 × 7, divides the spiritual assessment into two areas, a holistic set of dimensions and a spiritual set of dimensions, which are listed in Table 16–10 and discussed in depth below.

TABLE 16–10. The 7 × 7 Model for Spiritual Assessment

HOLISTIC DIMENSIONS	SPIRITUAL DIMENSIONS
Medical	Beliefs and meaning
Psychological	Vocation and consequences
Family systems	Experience and emotion
Psychosocial	Courage and growth
Ethnic and cultural	Ritual and practice
Societal issues	Community
Spirituality	Authority and guidance

SOURCE: Fitchett G: *Assessing Spiritual Needs: A Guide for Caregivers.* Lima, OH, Academic Renewal Press, 2002.

HOLISTIC DIMENSIONS

Medical Before tackling spiritual issues, one must have a sense of the patient's physical health. For patients near the end of life, their physical health is often apparent and known to the spiritual care giver at the time of the spiritual assessment, although the presence or absence of acute physical symptoms can significantly impact the potential effectiveness of the spiritual evaluation. Therefore, most often, the role of the spiritual care provider is adjunctive. At times, the professional can serve as the patient's advocate or referral source if physical needs are of concern. In addition, since when dealing with terminally ill patients, there is often a resistance to discussing the terminal nature of the illness, the spiritual care provider can use the opportunity to broach these issues during this phase of the assessment.

Psychological The second dimension assesses the psychological make-up of the patient in order to gain an understanding of the patient's personality and his or her general approach to life. Knowledge of previous psychological problems should be sought, as oftentimes these may significantly impact one's spiritual well being. Fitchett

advocates for the spiritual care provider to be prepared to work in tandem with a mental health professional when necessary.

Family Systems An evaluation of the patient's interactions with and role within the family is another important window into a patient's spiritual needs. Emotional or spiritual challenges sometimes begin as a result of one's familial relationships, whether that be in the role of a child to a parent, a parent to a child, or through interactions with a spouse or significant other. Assessing the family dynamics, both past and present, can sometimes provide the spiritual care giver with important clues as to the nature of a patient's present psycho-spiritual problems.

Psychosocial Unlike assessing one's family system, which focuses on one's specific family dynamics, the psychosocial dimension is a broader assessment of the person's life and life experiences. Where was she/he born and raised? What was her/his educational level and what career does or did she/he have? What are the current living and financial conditions?

While this is predominantly the expertise of social workers, it is important for a spiritual care provider to gather relevant factual data about a patient to better understand the personal dynamics of the person.

Ethnic and Cultural People's behaviors are influenced by their race, ethnicity, and culture. Therefore, it is important to assess this area to determine if there are specific ethnic and/or cultural issues that are either helping or hindering a patient from dealing with spiritual issues. By recognizing the distinct cultural and ethnic dynamics of a person, the spiritual care worker will have a better ability to advocate for sensitivity toward the person.

Societal Issues Often, people do not recognize that distress can result from dysfunctional social and cultural systems. Is the person suffering as a result of being at a "power disadvantage," resulting from race, gender, or economic class? How do others perceive the person's illness? Are people avoiding supporting the family because of preconceived beliefs or ideas? There are situations where a person's ability to cope with a specific situation is significantly affected by their race, gender, economic class, or other societal classification. As Fitchett states regarding the societal issues dimension, "We include the societal issues perspective in our holistic assessment as a way to get the fullest possible picture of the person and his or her situation and to avoid creating a diagnostic perspective that forces us into individual-level explanations for social and cultural problems."

Spirituality   The final category, spirituality, or the spiritual dimension, links the 7 × 7 model, for the primary role of spiritual care providers is to evaluate and treat issues related to the spiritual aspects of the lives of the patients and families under their care.

As with the holistic dimensions, Fitchett divides the spiritual dimension into seven distinct categories in their own right, hence, the name of the model, 7 × 7.

SPIRITUAL DIMENSIONS

Belief and Meaning   The initial focus of the spiritual aspect of the assessment is to determine if the patient has a sense of meaning or purpose in life. Meaning may or may not be described using religious language and might not even be related to anything traditionally referred to as spiritual, such as a family heirloom or a favorite book. Some patients might not be able to directly state what life's meaning is to him or her, but will be better able to convey it through narrative. Others may talk about their faith institutions and attendance at services as a method of describing their sense of belief. Pertinent questions will include the following: Does a person's belief provide meaning in life? What is the person's belief system and how does it get expressed in his life?

In addition, while listening for meaning, the spiritual care provider should be aware of how the person describes his or her beliefs, for often what is stated and what is meant are noncon-

gruent. What is the language being used when talking about his purpose in life? Are one's beliefs specifically related to one's current situation, or are they long-standing beliefs imbued by religious tradition? The professional must also observe the patient and not just listen to what the he or she shares. Is the person energetic, uplifted, or neutral when talking? Important clues as to how significant the patient's beliefs are can often be derived not just from what is said, but by how the information is conveyed.

Vocation and Consequences   This dimension examines what a person believes are his duties and obligations in life. By assessing a patient's feelings or sense of duty, the spiritual care provider can be sensitive to the difficulties the person might be facing as a result of changes in life, which may interfere with the fulfillment of his or her obligations. Fitchett includes in this category the question of whether the patient's illness is serving as a spiritual atonement, leading the person to possibly believe that it is a duty to experience pain and suffering in order to receive a greater reward upon death. A further subdivision of the area of vocation is how one's faith tradition prescribes and prohibits behaviors and in what ways the permitted and the forbidden affect the individual.

Experience and Emotion   The third spiritual dimension evaluates how any direct experiences that the patient might have had with the sacred, whether divine or demonic, has affected the person's emotional expectations regarding the meaning of life. Perhaps a person has had a near-death experience or some other core spiritual experience, and despite the profound impact that the event had, the patient is reluctant to discuss the spiritual encounter for fear of being judged. As this dimension examines one's emotional reactions to meaning in life, it intersects with the "Belief and Meaning" dimension discussed earlier, asking questions such as what emotions or moods are associated with his contacts with the sacred and how does it relate to his general outlook in life?

Courage and Growth A person's spiritual courage can be assessed through examining how one handles spiritual doubt and how that doubt affects one's personal growth. Is a person able to enter a state of doubt without knowing what will come from questioning previously held beliefs about God and the universe? Courage also includes the ability to experience change. How does a person react when new life experiences challenge existing beliefs? During the assessment, the spiritual care provider should attempt to learn what events or feelings led to prior changes in the patient's life and whether one can take lessons from these prior periods of change and adapt them to the current situation.

Rituals and Practices People often ground important life experiences by using rituals that express the meaning of those experiences. These rituals may either be traditional practices from one's specific faith background or practices created by an individual and/or family for purpose of infusing meaning into specific events that are of importance and meaning to them. When assessing a patient's meaningful rituals, especially in an end-of-life care situation, it is important to evaluate whether the current situation will potentially force one or more changes in important rituals that the person desires to maintain, and whether there might be ways to adapt to the current circumstances so that the desired practice or practices may be continued.

Community This dimension evaluates the patient's involvement in various "communities." Community used in this context can include one's faith institution, veteran's associations or local senior groups, social or political clubs, any other organization that brings people together, or simply a group of friends who share a common focus. The spiritual care provider should determine the extent of the person's participation in these communities on both a formal and informal level and how these communities might be able to help provide support to the patient and family in times of crisis.

Authority and Guidance This final spiritual dimension examines whether and how well the patient and family will be able to submit to the guidance of the spiritual care provider. The first step, of course, is for the professional to determine whether the patient and family will allow for pastoral/spiritual support, following which the level of authority or control the patient (or, in some cases, the family) desires to exert over how the care is provided needs to be ascertained. Questions to be answered include the following: Where does the person find the authority for his or her beliefs, meaning in life, vocation, rituals, and practices? When faced with doubt, confusion, tragedy, or conflict, where does one look for guidance? Some people will find authority in their particular faith's sacred texts or members of their faith's clergy; others will find it within themselves, while for many, there is a middle ground between religious text and ritual and one's own interpretation of the specific belief system.

Spiritual Assessment Model for End-of-Life Care

The final spiritual assessment model that will be discussed in depth was one developed specifically for end-of-life care patients. In 1989, Milton Hay, a chaplain for San Diego Hospice, developed this model primarily as a tool for hospice social workers to help determine whether a patient required additional spiritual support, although it can certainly be used by spiritual care providers at the time of initial spiritual assessment.

Hay centers his assessment on five principles. First, one must recognize that spirituality encompasses both religious and nonreligious systems in order to avoid the potential hazard of seeming to impose specific beliefs upon the family. Second, the language of a spiritual assessment should combine religious and psychological languages to create a diagnostic language of spirituality. Third is the idea that psychosocial needs should be assessed first because some patients do not see spiritual needs as distinct from psychosocial concerns and, therefore, do not require distinct spiritual care services that compliment nursing or social work care. The fourth principle embodies the concept that the whole person, physical, spiritual, social, and psychological, can work together toward healing during disease. Finally, a spiritual assessment should account for how spiritual development occurs in three specific areas of the human experience: the communities to which one belongs, one's inner resources

for dealing with life's challenges (including dying), and how to give meaning to one's reality.

With these principles to guide him, Hay divided the spiritual assessment into four categories: spiritual suffering, inner resource deficiency, belief system problems, and religious needs. These categories, as well as suggested content for assessing each, can be found in Table 16–11.

TABLE 16–11. Spiritual Assessment Model for End-of-Life Care

PROBLEM	DEFINITION	ASSESSMENT
Spiritual suffering	Interpersonal and intrapsychic anguish of unspecified origin	1. Conscious awareness of factors in personal development 2. Nature and causes of spiritual support system breakdown 3. Relationship between interpersonal behavior and belief system 4. Whether suffering due to immediate circumstances or long-standing concerns of guilt and/or conflict 5. Religious history as causes, e.g., community conflict, spiritual leader relationship 6. Explore issues of guilt, blame, remorse, and forgiveness in personal context
Inner resource deficiency	Diminished spiritual capacity	1. Level of awareness of elements, which animate and empower 2. Level of aspiration to achieve goals 3. Willingness to carry out personal, community, and care plan goals 4. Past and present spiritual disciplines and adaptive techniques, e.g., meditation, prayer visualization, relaxation, guided imagery, reading, sharing, nature contact, laughter/humor, art, music, and poetry
Belief system problem	Lack of conscious awareness of personal meaning system	1. Nature of belief system, philosophy, or world view, which gives meaning to life 2. Perspective on meaning of diagnosis and prognosis 3. Consistency of relationship between belief system and interpersonal relationships 4. Past and present participation in communities that reflect belief system
Religious need	Specifically expressed religious request	1. Name and resource of religious belief system 2. Adequacy of local congregational resources in meeting needs and requests 3. Adequacy of clergy in meeting needs and requests 4. Presence of support system from local congregations

Source: Hay M: Principles in building spiritual assessment tools. *Am J Hosp Care* 6:25-31, 1989.

TABLE 16–12. Stoddard's Spiritual Assessment Instrument	
CATEGORY (PRUYSER EQUIVALENT)	**CONTENT**
Concept of God (Awareness of the Holy)	What has been most important for you in your life? What are the things that you have found most meaningful during the past year?
Subjective meaning of illness (providence, grace, repentance)	What does it mean to you that you've been ill? How have you been making sense of what has happened to you?
Approach to hoping (faith, vocation)	How have you kept a sense of hope in the past? What does having hope mean for you at the present time?
Relation to support systems (communion)	How have you felt your family has been doing with this illness? Who have you felt has been able to be most supportive of you in this time?

Source: Adapted from Fitchett G, Handzo GF: Spiritual assessment, screening, and intervention. In: Holland JC, et al., eds. *Psycho-Oncology.* New York, Oxford University Press, pp. 790-808, 1998.

Other Spiritual Assessment Models

In 1990, Gregory Stoddard designed a spiritual assessment instrument relying upon Pruyser's assessment model, which is illustrated in Table 16–12. Stoddard compresses Pruyser's seven categories into four primary areas for assessment: concept of God, subjective meaning of illness, approach to hoping, and relation to support system.

Erin Moss and Keith Dobson presented a paper in 2006 arguing for an integration of psychology and spirituality in the assessment of end-of-life needs. In their research, Moss and Dobson found evidence suggesting that in end-of-life situations, people with a stronger sense of faith/spirituality have a greater tolerance for the increased pain and suffering that often accompanies a terminal illness. They also argued that spiritual well-being indicates a decrease in the potential for suicidal ideation or the desire to hasten death among the dying. On the basis of their findings, they developed a seven section approach to spiritual assessment in order "to ethically provide these services in the context of contemporary health care." Although their primary audience was the psychological community, this model, illustrated in Table 16–13, can serve as another useful assessment guide for spiritual care providers.

Another model for spiritual assessment, proposed by Karen Skalla, MSN, ARNP, AOCN, and J. Patrick McCoy, MDiv, MPhil, ACPE in 2006, is the Mor-VAST model, and it was specifically designed for patients with cancer. Mor-VAST is an acronym for the *Mor*al *A*uthority,

TABLE 16–13. Seven Aspect Spiritual Assessment
• Religiosity
• Spiritual identity
• Spiritual coping and support
• Problem solving
• Well being
• Needs
• Appraisals

Source: Dobson KS, Moss EL: Psychology, spirituality and end-of-life Care: an ethical integration? *Can Psychol* 47:284-299, 2006.

TABLE 16–14. Mor-VAST Spiritual Assessment Model	
DIMENSION	**LEADING QUESTIONS**
Moral authority	Where does your sense of what to do come from? What principles of right and wrong guide you?
Vocational	What gives your life meaning? Has meaning changed for you? What kind of work has been important to you?
Aesthetic	What things do you enjoy doing? Are you doing them now?
Social	Are you part of a religious or spiritual community? Are there any others groups or people you enjoy spending time with?
Transcendent	What sustains you during difficult times? Who is in control?

SOURCE: Sample Clinical Assessment Questions Based on the Model. Skalla KS, McCoy JP: Spiritual assessment of patients with cancer: the moral authority, vocational, aesthetic, social, and transcendent model. *Oncol Nurs Forum* 33:745-751, 2006.

*V*ocational, *A*esthetic, *S*ocial, and *T*ranscendent, and the five domains of this assessment together with sample questions that are pertinent to each can be found Table 16–14.

CONCLUSION

One of the goals of psychosocial and spiritual assessments, as indicated by Fitchett, is the creation of a sense of professionalism in the nonphysical supportive aspects of patient care, placing them on a more equal footing with the well-accepted medical and nursing disciplines. This is especially critical in end-of-life care, which, by its very nature, is interdisciplinary.

Because of end-of-life care's interdisciplinary nature, patients receiving such care require multiple distinct assessments in order for caregivers to most effectively learn about the physical, emotional, social, and spiritual challenges the patient suffering from a terminal illness and their families are encountering. This chapter has presented a variety of assessments that spiritual care providers and social workers may utilize, with the choice being dependent in part on the discipline of the professional caregiver who first encounters and assesses the patient.

As nurses most commonly are the caregivers who perform comprehensive patient assessments, spiritual care providers and social workers often have the advantage of being able to use information that has already been gathered. In those situations, therefore, their assessments are able to be more limited and focused. However, in the less common situations when social workers or spiritual care providers are the first to encounter patients and families, it is their responsibility to perform a more comprehensive multidimensional assessment. By being facile in both comprehensive and more focused assessments as presented earlier, psychosocial and spiritual care professional will have the tools needed to provide holistic and diverse care to terminally ill patients and their families.

BIBLIOGRAPHY

Anandarajah G, Hight E: Spirituality and medical practice. Using the HOPE questions as a practical tool for spiritual assessment. *Am Fam Phys* 63:81-89, 2001.

Dobson KS, Moss EL: Psychology, spirituality and end–of–life care: an ethical integration? *Can Psychol* 47:284-299, 2006.

Fitchett G: *Assessing Spiritual Needs: A Guide for Caregivers*. Lima, Ohio, Academic Renewal Press, 2002.

Fitchett G, Handzo GF: Spiritual assessment, screening, and intervention. In: Holland JC, et al., eds. *Psycho-Oncology*. New York, Oxford University Press, 68:790-808, 1998.

Gilbert Rev R: A Chaplain's perspective: The challenge for today. In: Gilbert Rev R, ed. *Healthcare and Spirituality: Listening, Assessing, Caring*. Amityville, NY, Baywood Publishing, 2002.

Gilbert R: *Spiritual Assessment in Aspen Reference Group, Palliative Care: Patient and Family Counseling Manual*. Gaithersburg, MD, Aspen, 1996, p. 5.

Hay M: Principles in building spiritual assessment tools. *Am J Hosp Care* 6:25-31, 1989.

Kellehear A: Spirituality and palliative care: A model of needs. *Palliat Med* 14:149-155, 2000.

Maugans TA: The SPIRITual history. *Arch Fam Med* 5:11-16, 1996.

Meares PA, Lane BA: Grounding social work practice in theory: Ecosystems. In: Rauch JB, ed. *Assessment: A Sourcebook for Social Work Practice*. Milwaukee, WI, Families International Inc., 1993, p. 3-13.

Meyer C: *Assessment in Social Work Practice*. New York, Columbia UP, 1993.

Moos R, Brownstein R: *Environment and Utopia: A Synthesis*. New York, Plenum Publishing, 1977.

Morrow-Howell N: Multidimensional assessment of the elderly client. In: Rauch JB, ed. *Assessment: A Sourcebook for Social Work Practice*. Milwaukee, WI, Families International Inc., 1993, pp. 123-139.

National Association of Social Workers: *NASW Standards for Palliative and End of Life Care*. Washington, DC, 2004.

Okon TR: Palliative care review: Spiritual, religious, and existential aspects of palliative care. *J Palliat Med* 8:392-414, 2005.

Pargament K: *The Psychology of Religion and Coping*. New York: Guilford Press, 1997.

Pfeiffer E: A short portable mental status questionnaire for the assessment of organic brain deficit in elderly patients. *J Am Geriatr Soc* 23:433-441, 1975.

Power J: Spiritual assessment: Developing an assessment tool. *Nurs Older People* 18:16-18, 2006.

Pruyser PW: *The Minister as Diagnostician: Personal Problems in Pastoral Perspective*. Philadelphia, PA, Westminster Press, 1976.

Puchalski CM, Romer AL: Taking a spiritual history allows clinicians to understand patients more fully. *J Palliat Med* 3:129-137, 2000.

Robinson S, et al: *Spirituality and the Practice of Healthcare*. Basingstoke, UK, Palgrave Macmillan, 2003.

Schoggen P: Ecological psychology and mental retardation. In: Sackett GP, ed. *Observing Behavior: Theory and applications in Mental Retardation*, Vol 1. Baltimore, MD, University Park Press, 1978.

Sells SB: An interactionist looks at the environment. In: Moos RH, Insel PM, eds. *Issues in Social Ecology: Human Milieus*. Palo Alto, CA, National Press Books, 1974.

Siporin M: Ecological systems theory in social work. *J Sociol Soc Welf* 7:502-532, 1980.

Skalla KS, McCoy JP: Spiritual assessment of patients with cancer: The moral authority, vocational, aesthetic, social, and transcendent model. *Oncol Nurs Forum* 33:745-751, 2006.

SELF-ASSESSMENT QUESTIONS

1. The term "assessment" may be best defined as:
   A. Plan of professional clinical activities developed to implement the treatment plan
   B. The process of providing care or treatment to improve a clinical situation
   C. The process of collecting information from an individual about a specific situation
   D. A process that provides direction or advice regarding a course of action

2. According to the ecosystems theory of psychosocial practice, it is the gathering of what information that will provide the social worker with the most significant window into the patient's psychosocial needs?
   A. History of the patient's current illness
   B. The patient's past medical history
   C. The patient's current medications
   D. The patient's personal history
   E. History of familial medical illnesses

3. Reasons to have a social worker assess a patient's physical health include all of the following EXCEPT
   A. To confirm the information gathered by the nurse on the interdisciplinary team
   B. To create a comfort zone with the patient/family that will allow easier transition into the more intimate psychosocial issues to follow.
   C. To gain an understanding as to how well the patient and family are able to properly utilize the healthcare system.
   D. To be able to determine if there are psychosocial reasons why a patient is noncompliant with medication
   E. To be able to incorporate information on physical health into the psychosocial assessment when appropriate.

4. All of the following elements of the psychosocial assessment fall under the domain of social support EXCEPT
   A. Memberships in community or religious institutions
   B. Role and responsibility of the primary caregiver
   C. How satisfied the patient is with the support being provided
   D. Whether there is any possible neglect or abuse
   E. The safety of the patient's neighborhood

5. Of the following, which is the best way for a social worker to perform a functional assessment?
   A. Do a physical assessment
   B. Ask the patient to perform each of the ADL's and see how well s/he does
   C. Ask the patient and/or caregiver to describe the course of a typical day
   D. Utilize the nurse's functional assessment
   E. Ask the family to describe how the patient performs each ADL

6. George Fitchett suggests that there are eight factors that support the importance of the spiritual assessment. Which of the following of these factors is the one that "establishes a mutually agreed upon approach as to how to best meet the specific needs of the patient?"
   A. Foundation for action
   B. Foundation for contracting
   C. Foundation for personal accountability
   D. Foundation for evaluation
   E. Foundation for research

7. Which of the following of Fitchett's characteristic approaches to spiritual assessment can best be defined as "the innate ability of the spiritual care giver to recognize a particular situation and immediately provide the necessary spiritual or ritual care?"

A. Implicit assessment
B. Inspired assessment
C. Intuitive assessment
D. Idiosyncratic assessment
E. Explicit spiritual assessment

8. Of the following spiritual care experts who have developed spiritual assessment models, who tends to dissuade spiritual care providers from using psychological categories as he believes that spiritual care goals are different from psychological care goals?

A. Milton Hay
B. Erin Moss
C. George Fitchett
D. Paul Pruyser

9. Which of the assessment categories in Pruyser's "Guidelines for Pastoral Diagnosis" can be described as "kindness, generosity, and the beauty of giving and receiving?"

A. Providence
B. Faith
C. Grace or gratefulness
D. Repentance
E. Communion

10. In Hay's "Spiritual model for end-of-life care," which of the following items would be included in the assessment domain of "Spiritual suffering?"

A. Relationship between interpersonal behavior and belief system
B. Perspective on the meaning of diagnosis and prognosis
C. Level of aspiration to achieve goals
D. Adequacy of clergy in meeting needs and requests
E. Nature of world view which gives meaning to life

Grief and Bereavement

Robin Fiorelli

DEFINITION OF COMPLICATED GRIEF

Many post-modern grief theorists have attempted to delineate their perspective on what is complicated grief (sometimes called pathological or abnormal grief) and what causes it. Although grief theorists may differ on how to define complicated grief, there is some agreement that complicated grief is generally one (or both) of the following things:

- Complicated mourning is a result of the presence of specific high risk factors that can lead to an abnormal grief experience and lack of healthy adjustment.
- Complicated grief is the result of specific symptoms that are present in normal mourning, but have abnormal intensity and duration.

All agree, as Strobe and Gergen state, "The post-modern perspective on loss and bereavement suggests that there is a multiplicity of experience and expression of grief." There are factors that we know *tend* to make grief more complicated, but whether a grief reaction is complicated or not depends more on the mourner's *own* experience of his/her grief and ability to function after the loss. That is the vantage point that the clinician should start from in assessing whether the patient might benefit from professional help or not. This assessment and subsequent treatment is especially important in light of the debate over whether complicated grief should be categorized as a "disorder" in the *Diagnostic and Statistical Manual for Psychiatric Disorders*.

Defining complicated grief is difficult for several reasons:

- It is not a single syndrome with clear diagnostic criteria
- The cut off point between normal and complicated is hard to establish
- It is hard to distinguish pathological grief from other related disorders such as depression, anxiety, and Post-Traumatic Stress Disorder (PTSD).
- The definition of normal and pathological grief is constantly changing

PREVALENCE OF COMPLICATED GRIEF

There is significant variation of opinions about what percentage of mourners experience complicated grief with estimates varying between 3% and 25%. Marcia Lattanzi Licht, in describing her state-of-the-art assessment tool for bereavement risk, noted that after surveying 261 survivors of hospice patients one month after the death, she found that 5% of the survivors were at high risk, 22% were at moderate risk, and 70% were at low risk for complicated grief.

MYTHS ASSOCIATED WITH GRIEF

To understand what factors can lead to grief becoming complicated, one must first examine what constitutes "normal" grief. To do that, we will start by examining what grief *isn't*.

White, Anglo Saxon, Judeo-Christian culture tends to view grief in and of itself as a somewhat abnormal reaction to the loss of a loved one. In the United States, we tend to shun or deny emotional pain, and therefore we lack sufficient comfort to openly discuss needs and fears associated with death, dying, and bereavement

Our culture envisions healing from grief the same way we think about healing from the flu. First, that grief is something we "get over" completely, and second, that if we take a few days off, maybe even take some medication for our "nerves," then we should be "cured" in no time. The idea that grief should be approached in the

TABLE 17–1. Myths Associated with Grief	
Myth one	All bereaved persons grieve the same way.
Myth two	It takes about a year to "get over" a significant loss.
Myth three:	It's better to not think or talk about the pain.
Myth four:	The intensity and length of your grief reflects how much you loved the deceased.
Myth five:	Maybe I should leave the mourner alone and not bring up his/her loss.

same way as a minor infectious ailment is but one of a number of cultural myths that exists surrounding grief. These myths, listed in Table 17–1, will now be explored in order to better understand how they impact our understanding of complicated grief.

Myth One: All bereaved persons grieve the same way.

Truth: Although grief is a universal experience, there is tremendous variation between individuals in the style of grieving (instrumental vs. expressive), the length and intensity of grieving, and the customs of grieving based on different cultural norms. There is no right or wrong way to grieve nor is there a set time frame in which one must adjust to a loss. It is now well known that, while some adjust fairly quickly to a loss, usually within a year of the death, others may take several years

Myth Two: It takes about a year to "get over" a significant loss.

Truth: Survivors whose loved ones have died after a long history of Alzheimer's disease may have a relatively short grief response after the death, as they may believe that their loved ones' personality had "died" years before. Conversely, a parent who has lost a child years ago may have never truly "gotten over" the loss.

Myth Three: It's better to not think or talk about the pain.

Truth: On the contrary, it is known that avoiding the pain associated with grief can have negative consequences including physical complaints, anxiety, and depression. The important thing is for the bereaved person to honor the amount of time he or she needs to grieve, and try not to be influenced by internal expectations or outside pressure.

Myth Four: The intensity and length of your grief reflects how much you loved the deceased.

Truth: As mentioned earlier, there is tremendous variety in how an individual mourner grieves.

Myth Five: Maybe I should leave the mourner alone and not bring up his/her loss.

Truth: Studies have shown that social support is one of the most important factors in whether grief becomes complicated or not.

Having established what grief is not, it may be helpful to define some of the more common terms used when describing loss and bereavement. *Bereavement* is commonly understood as the objective situation or event in which an individual has suffered the loss of someone or something significant, while *grief* refers to the bereaved person's internal emotional response and subjective experience to the loss event. *Mourning* may be defined as the outward, public, cultural, and religious expressions of grieving, such as the recognition of a special date through visiting the gravesite. It may also take on more private expressions, such as keeping a journal, leafing through a photo album, finding new ways to relate to or think about the deceased, or finding healthy ways to integrate the loss into the present.

NORMAL GRIEF REACTIONS

Normal grief, also referred to as typical or uncomplicated grief, is the term used to describe the type of grief that is found in the vast majority

TABLE 17–2. Emotional and Social Experiences of Grief

- Sadness
- Loneliness
- Identity issues
- Recall of prior losses
- Guilt
- Anger
- Jealousy
- Idealization

of survivors. Given adequate support and time both before and after a loss, most individuals are able to eventually adjust to a loss even though the loss may have produced dramatic changes in one's life.

Often following a loss, the bereaved experience an initial numbness or disbelief that the death has occurred. However, this is usually only temporary and soon the bereaved begin to experience various aspects of grief, many of which are emotional and social in nature, but also may be physical or cognitive.

Emotional and social reactions to loss are listed in Table 17–2 and are discussed in more depth.

Sadness: When the reality of the loss sinks in, typically the mourner feels profound sadness and exhaustion. He/she cannot imagine life without the loved one, and may doubt even feeling OK again. Many find themselves crying at unexpected times or being irritable over seemingly nothing. Many are embarrassed that they are not feeling better.

Loneliness: The mourner may feel despair for dreams that will go unrealized. They may feel profound loneliness, that a part of *him/her* was lost along with the death. Difficulty being with others is common; small talk seems trivial. Relationships with family and friends change.

Identity Issues: Death shakes confidence in ourselves. The death of a spouse forces the mourner to establish an identity as a single person and take on roles/ tasks of their spouse.

Recall of prior losses: It is also common, while coping with the present loss, to re-experience prior losses (even loss due to divorce, pet loss, etc.).

Guilt: Some bereaved wonder if they could have done more to prevent the death or any suffering that occurred prior to death. Some feel guilty if they placed their loved one in a nursing home, or that they weren't there at the time of death. They may feel guilty that *they* survived. They may feel guilty because they are relieved their loved one died, or guilty if they feel no sorrow. The bereaved may feel guilty about things that did or did not happen in the relationship.

Anger: Almost all bereaved people feel angry at some point. They may feel angry at their loved one for leaving them; angry at the medical professionals; angry at themselves, at their family and friends, and even at God for letting their loved one die.

Jealousy: Jealousy at seeing other people's happiness is common.

Idealization: Sometimes, the mourner idealizes the deceased, possibly as an attempt to validate the pain of loss or yearning for that which cannot be recovered.

Physical and cognitive symptoms are as real to the bereaved as the heartache of emotional grief.

TABLE 17–3. Physical and Cognitive Reactions to Normal Grief

- Irritability, anxiety, dizziness, shortness of breath
- Difficulty sleeping or sleeping too much; having no appetite or eating too much
- Confusion, paranoia, memory gaps, difficulty concentrating, auditory, and/or visual hallucinations (often of their loved one)
- Odd and frightening dreams (often of their loved one)
- Extreme restlessness—or the opposite—sitting at length and doing nothing
- Searching behavior—looking for the loved one almost in a subconscious way

These symptoms may last just a few days or extend for several months, but generally do not last past a year. A list of the more common physical and cognitive grief reactions are listed in Table 17–3 and consist of a wide variety of symptoms, including shortness of breath and anxiety, disorders of appetite or sleep, confusion, hallucinations, odd or frightening dreams, or extreme restlessness or apathy.

FACTORS THAT MAKE THE GRIEF EXPERIENCE UNIQUE

According to Alan Wolfelt, there are factors that influence the way people grieve. They are listed in Table 17–4 and discussed below.

TABLE 17–4. Factors That Make the Grief Experience Unique (Alan Wolfelt)

FACTOR	
Nature of the relationship to the deceased	Attachment (strong, ambivalent, weak); conflicts and if/how they were resolved; any unfinished business. Special memories/recalling events
Circumstances surrounding the death	Unique circumstances—accidents, homicide, suicide; feelings of omnipotence/invulnerability; age of person who died; suddenness of loss; concern about ability to prevent death
Cultural, religious, or spiritual background	National—country's response to dying and grief; racial and ethnic traditions surrounding dying and grief; investment in faith community's doctrine about dying and mourning; support available from faith community
Gender	Men and women are treated differently; men are encouraged to repress grief and "be strong"; women may have a hard time expressing anger
Mourner's support	Stable support system—empathetic, caring; consistent ongoing social support—family, friends, grief groups, local, and faith communities
Mourner's personality/ attributes	Basic nature—quiet, moody, boisterous, outgoing; past coping skills—ability to confront crisis; history of other losses—openly expresses feelings and thoughts; level of self-esteem; values and beliefs; health history—mental and physical
Deceased's personality/ attributes	Soothing, stabilizing, difficult, disruptive; role the deceased played in mourner's life—best friend, spouse, child, etc.
Ritual or funeral experiences	Satisfaction with funeral can hinder or promote mourning; ability to assist with funeral planning; attendance at funeral; ongoing opportunities to ritualize the death
Other crises/stresses	Secondary losses—financial insecurity, social isolation; additional losses—deaths, other crises

NATURE OF THE RELATIONSHIP TO THE DECEASED

The relationship between the bereaved and the deceased often plays a significant role in grief reactions experienced by survivors of loss. Was the strength of the attachment between the bereaved and the deceased strong, ambivalent, or weak? How were conflicts in the relationship resolved or did any remain unresolved? Was there any other unfinished business?

A number of studies have been done that explore how the nature of the relationship between bereaved and deceased affect the grief response. It has been shown that the loss of a spouse will be grieved differently in terms of types of responses and intensity than the loss of a child. Bereaved parents have been shown to have more intense reactions than bereaved spouses, while bereaved spouses have been found to have more intense reactions than bereaved adult children. Male children appear to be affected more by the loss of a parent than by the loss of a sibling, whereas females seem to be more affected by sibling loss, especially the loss of a sister, than by the loss of a parent. One-third of children who lose a parent show high levels of emotional difficulty in their readjustment, with complicated grief reactions often not being evidenced until the second year of bereavement. Interestingly, one study found that children who lost a parent did not have any more significant school problems than those who hadn't lost a parent, suggesting that one must be cautious against assuming that all bereaved children need the same degree of intervention.

CIRCUMSTANCES SURROUNDING THE DEATH

The following circumstances can influence the survivor's reaction to the loss: whether the death was expected or sudden, the age of the deceased, and whether the death was due to a chronic disease, an accident, or a preventable cause. It has been demonstrated, for example, that those grieving victims of sudden death have a more difficult adjustment than individuals who have had adequate time to prepare for the loss of a loved one. However, the sudden death of an elderly individual, whose death was not unexpected due to advanced age, may not be highly traumatic to a survivor. Young survivors of loss by sudden death experience a more difficult time adjusting in the one or two years following the death than young survivors of losses that were expected, while family caregivers of patients who died following long-term illnesses were often too exhausted to completely grieve. In addition to the length of illness, the place of death will also influence the grief experience.

CULTURAL, RELIGIOUS, OR SPIRITUAL BACKGROUND

When working with mourners from different cultures or with those that have different religious or spiritual faith, it is important to show respect for and become willing to learn about the person's grief customs and practices and their potential for therapeutic value, and not to assume that everyone reacts in a predictable or expected way. Having cultural awareness, sensitivity and avoiding ethnocentrism and cultural stereotypes is paramount.

GENDER

Following a loss, men and women are often expected to have different grief reactions. Men are generally encouraged to repress grief and "be strong," while women may have a hard time expressing anger. This can translate into real differences in how males and females grieve. Women seem to express emotion more, to accept temporary regression, and to more often confide in others. Male mourners are reported to be more reluctant to attend support groups, go for counseling, or in general, acknowledge problems associated with their grief. Expecting men to cry or "open up" can be counter-productive. Instead, discovering practices that are acceptable to the male mourner may assist with his expression of grief.

The support available to a mourner, the mourner's basic personality as well as the personality attributes of the deceased, the experiences of the mourner at the funeral or memorial service and whether or not there are concurrent life crises in addition to the loss are among other factors that can make any grief experience unique. These factors are further delineated in Table 17–4 as well.

RELATIONSHIP OF THESE SYMPTOMS AND FACTORS TO COMPLICATED GRIEF

In trying to assess whether a mourner's grief is complicated or "abnormal," it is important to first realize that all of the symptoms/factors listed earlier are within the "normal limits" of the grief experience. It is when any of these factors (or combination of factors) become very intense, endure for an overly prolonged time, are uncomfortable to the mourner and/or cause significant disturbance in functioning, we might consider that the mourner's grief has become "complicated." It is in such circumstances that professional help would be warranted.

MAJOR POSTMODERN GRIEF THEORISTS

Since the early 1980s, much has been written about grief. In general, there has been a shift from viewing grief as a staged process that each mourner must go through in order to "complete" his or her "grief work" to viewing grief as a more cyclical process, one where the mourner does not

need to completely "sever" the tie with a loved one, but more that the nature of their relationship changes. In view of the number of valid theories proposed, Stroebe and Gergen, grief theorists themselves, have stated that in order to be most effective with mourners, the clinician should, "combine theories into a meaningful synthesis, recognizing the place of cultural richness in order to develop a therapeutic repertoire capable of responding to highly individual grief reactions." Therefore, before exploring the concepts of complicated grief and to help us better understand how to approach its treatment, we will examine a number of major postmodern theories of grief.

WILLIAM WORDEN

In his seminal work *Grief Counseling and Grief Psychotherapy,* William Worden exemplified the perspective that a mourner needs to go through somewhat defined steps in order to complete the grief process, which he terms the four tasks of mourning. Unlike "stages" or "phases" that imply that grief may go on at an unconscious level, the concept of tasks point out that effort is required to come to terms with the loss that occurred.

The first of the four tasks involves *accepting the reality of the loss* that the bereaved has come to recognize that the deceased loved one is gone and will not return. Without accepting that the loss has occurred, the bereaved cannot begin and continue through the mourning process. The second task involves *working through the pain of grief.* Once the loss has been recognized, the bereaved must acknowledge that there is pain associated with the loss and must deal with the pain, because to avoid or suppress it only prolongs the mourning process.

The third task involves *adjusting to an environment in which the deceased is missing.* This includes, for example, searching and adjusting to one's sense of self and identity such as beginning to think of oneself as a widow or single person rather than as a "couple." Finally, having accomplished the first three tasks, the bereaved is tasked with *emotionally relocating the deceased and moving on with life*. While not compelled to totally give up the relationship with the deceased, the bereaved must begin to be open to new relationships. This means that the bereaved needs to "find an appropriate place for the dead in his or her emotional life"—a place that will enable the bereaved to go on living effectively in the world." At the same time, the type of attachment that existed before the deceased passed on must be let go of so that new relationships can be formed. Worden defines complicated grief as "the intensification of grief to the level where the person is overwhelmed, resorts to maladaptive behavior, or remains interminably in the state of grief without progression of the mourning process to completion." He sees complicated grief as the inability to adapt to the loss. He states "These mourners work against themselves by promoting their own helplessness, by not developing the skills they need to cope, or by withdrawing from the world and not facing up to environmental requirements. Complicated grief is more related to the intensity of a reaction or the duration of a reaction rather than the presence or absence of a specific behavior."

THERESE RANDO

Therese Rando, in her book, *Grief, Dying, and Death* views grief as a process that one goes through to completion. In describing normal grief, she first discusses the *avoidance* of grief, which can be manifested in shock, denial, or disbelief. The next step in the grief process is described as *confrontation*. Once the grief is faced and recognized by the bereaved, intense emotions are experienced. Finally, the bereaved experiences *reestablishment (or accommodation)*, which is characterized by a general decline in the grief reaction and the beginning of an emotional and social reentry into the world.

Coinciding with these three phases, she believes that the mourner experiences six major mourning processes that she terms "The Six 'R' Processes: recognize the loss, react to the separation, recollect and re-experience the deceased and the relationship, relinquish the old attachments and the old assumptive world, readjust to the new world without forgetting the old, and reinvest in life."

Rando views complicated grief as a compromise, distortion, or failure in one or more of the "R"s. She defines the "syndromes of complicated mourning" as *absent mourning,* which includes complete denial or total state of shock (very rare); *delayed mourning* or procrastination; *inhibited mourning* (or partial mourning) where the grief process becomes restricted; *distorted mourning* where certain aspects of uncomplicated mourning are exaggerated and where other aspects are inhibited; *conflicted mourning,* which arises after the loss of a highly troubled, ambivalent relationship; *unanticipated mourning* from a sudden and unexpected death; and *chronic mourning* also known as prolonged or protracted mourning.

Rando states "Complicated mourning means that given the amount of time since the death, there is some compromise, distortion, or failure of one or more processes of mourning." Examples of complicated grief in this model include a denial or avoidance of the full realization of pain of living without the deceased, holding onto the deceased as though still alive, or various symptoms of grieving that do not resolve spontaneously and need active intervention.

In the past 10 years, there has been movement away from viewing the bereavement process as "moving on; letting go," in part because grief has no clear endpoint, and also because there is scant empirical evidence that "working through grief" has been a more effective process than not working through it. There also has been a shift away from defining grief as either complicated (symptomatic, pathological) or noncomplicated. Neimeyer states "There has been a deemphasis on universal syndromes of grieving and loss and a re-focus on 'local' practices among specific categories of the bereaved and within families."

STROEBE AND SCHUT

The challenge by Stroebe and her colleagues to the traditional "grief work" hypothesis has resulted in an alternative model of grief. The *Dual Process Model* suggests that there is a process of oscillation between rumination of painful emotions and attention to social adaptation of the loss. The former, known as *loss orientation,* can include grief work, the breaking of bonds, and a denial of restorative changes. The latter, sometimes called *restoration orientation,* includes attending to life changes, doing new things, distraction and avoidance, and the development of new roles and identities. This model is based on the premise that those who grieve take respites from their grieving to attend to other stressors and also experience a "fluctuation of attention in the coping process."

Stroebe and Schut define pathological grief as "a deviation from the cultural norm (that could be expected to pertain, according to the extremity of the particular bereavement event) in *time, course,* or *intensity* of symptoms of grief."

ROBERT NEIMEYER

Neimeyer focuses on the importance of the cognitive (rather than emotional) processes entailed in mourning. The main tenets of his viewpoint include the reconstruction of meaning, the rebuilding of previously held assumptions, and the creation or restoration of a cohesive life narrative. He also observed that mourners work to regulate their interpersonal emotions and evaluates the life and death of the deceased as it impacts their ongoing relationships. Grief is perceived as a major loss for an individual's self-identity, yet there can also be an appreciation of the life-enhancing nature of "posttraumatic growth."

MARTIN AND DOKA

Martin and Doka have developed a theory of grief, which distinguishes two distinct kinds of grieving: an intuitive response to loss character-

ized by an affective expression of grief and instrumental grief, which tends to be a more cognitive and active response to loss. These authors also see a blended pattern, which combines both the intuitive and instrumental styles of grieving.

MONICA McGOLDRICK

The impact of death on the family was first described by Monica McGoldrick in her book entitled *Living Beyond Loss—Death in the Family.* She describes how even though family members share a common loss, the death affects individual family members differently depending on where they are in their developmental cycle. She also describes how a family reorganizes itself to adapt to the death and has to find new ways of interacting with each other. Family members take on (or are assigned) different roles left vacant by the deceased.

GEORGE A. BONANNO

Instead of focusing on traumatic bereavement and pathological responses to loss, Bonanno focuses on the capacity to respond to loss with resilience. He states "Resilience is a process of positive adjustment to adversity and demands a capacity to appraise the positive within a situation, a willingness to confront the negative and an ability to make effective use of support." He sees that not every mourner experiences distress or grief and that this should not be viewed as absent or delayed grief. His social/ functional view suggests that when negative grief-related emotions are regulated and/or minimized and when positive emotions are instigated or enhanced, mourners may have a better outcome.

SELBY JACOBS

Selby Jacobs et al. termed the condition "Traumatic Grief." They believe this term avoids confusion with previous terms such as pathologic, neurotic, or morbid grief, which have negative connotations. They also think that traumatic grief is preferable to the terms complicated or unresolved grief, which they believe are vague or narrow in meaning. They state that traumatic grief captures the two underlying dimensions of the disorder, that is, *separation distress* and *traumatic distress*, two distinctly delineated domains of distress. The word "traumatic" refers in the new terminology to the phenomenology of the disorder, not the etiology, as the disorder can occur in the absence of an objectively traumatic death. Jacob's proposed four main diagnostic criteria for traumatic grief that distinguish it from other disorders and from normal grief.

HOLLY PRIGERSON

Prigerson and colleagues have included the range of traumatic as well as nontraumatic bereavement experiences in developing a framework for complicated grief. They have developed criteria for the classification for the DSM V, which views complicated grief as a mental disorder distinct from normal grief, bereavement-related depression, anxiety, and PTSD. Prigerson states "Complicated grief involves the presentation of certain grief-related symptoms at a time beyond that which is considered adaptive. We hypothesize that the presence of these symptoms after approximately 6 months puts the bereaved individual at heightened risk for enduring social, psychological, and medical impairment."

Prigerson points out that how a person is coping early on in his/her bereavement is a good indication of how they are going to cope later. She also sought to distinguish whether the presence of complicated grief would predict future functional impairments. She identified seven symptoms that constitute complicated grieving and they are searching, yearning, preoccupation with the deceased, crying, disbelief regarding the death, feeling stunned by the death, and lack of acceptance of the death. She found that complicated grief scores were significantly associated with impair-

ments in global functioning, mood, sleep, and self-esteem.

EVALUATING COMPLICATED GRIEF

There are two separate components that theorists and clinicians generally use in evaluating whether a mourner has complicated grief. They are *risk factors* and *symptoms*.

Stroebe and Schut define risk factors as "an aspect of personal behavior or lifestyle and environmental exposure or an inborn or inherited characteristic that is known to be associated with health-related conditions considered important to prevent." They categorize risk factors into those associated with the bereavement condition (i.e., mode of death), the person (e.g., personality, religiosity, age, and gender), and the interpersonal context (e.g., social support, kinship relationship).

There are a number of specific risk factors that practitioners generally note *can* predispose people to complicated grief, and they are listed in Table 17–5. These factors are sufficient but not necessary, and they *must* be seen with in the individual's specific bio-psycho-social-cultural and spiritual paradigm. For example, an individual at high risk for abnormal grief, based on having a history of psychiatric illness, might have that risk reduced somewhat if they have developed positive coping mechanisms during therapy and have a strong support system. In addition, while an increased risk of abnormal grief is intuitively associated with recent negative life events, it has also been demonstrated that positive events may also increase the risk of an abnormal grief response, since any change, whether positive or negative, can produce stress by requiring individual adaptation and adjustment.

Being able to recognize when the bereaved are at an increased risk for complicated grief allows practitioners to be on alert for the various

TABLE 17–5. Potential Risk Factors for Complicated Grief	
Unresolved past losses	Violent deaths from murder/suicide/accident
Sudden unexpected death	Other changes/stresses in life at the same time
Death from an overly lengthy illness	Mourner's perception of loss as preventable
Missing persons/absence of a body	Ambivalent, dependent, or stormy relationship with the deceased
Unintentional act	Secrets discovered after a death
Notoriety/news coverage	Pre-existing psychiatric illness and/or substance abuse
Death of a child	Inability to tolerate the extremes of emotional distress
Perceived lack of social support	Self-concept, role, and value of "being strong"
Shock of discovery	Socially "unspeakable" loss (e.g., suicide)

symptoms that may accompany complicated grief. These symptoms are listed in Table 17–6. By recognizing them early on, practitioners can better provide their bereaved patients with the proper support and intervention, especially when the symptoms have physical manifestations that might be confused with a medical illness.

TABLE 17–6. Potential Symptoms of Complicated Grief	
Verbalizing suicidal thoughts	Self-destructive or acting-out behavior
Substance abuse	Extreme idealization (or imitation) of the deceased
Ongoing numbness	Impulsive decision making
Chronic physical symptoms (even mirroring the deceased' symptoms)	Mental disorders that occur following loss (i.e., paranoia)
Extreme preoccupation with the deceased	Ongoing yearning/searching for the deceased
Extreme fear about one's own illness and/or death	Minor events trigger an intense grief reaction
Prolonged/extreme depression, anxiety anger, guilt, and/or lowered self-esteem	Themes of loss come into most discussions
Feeling out of control	Person unwilling to move physical possessions (Worden, 1992)
Long-term functional impairment	Inability to experience any emotional reactions typical of loss
Exaggerated, prolonged, and intense grief reactions	Self-destructive relationships; extreme fear of intimacy
Significant neglect of self-care	Isolation from self or others
Verbalizing suicidal thoughts	False euphoria

ASSESSMENT OF COMPLICATED GRIEF

The grief perspective of mourners reflects both their wider *social context* (including family, religious, and cultural influences) and the *history of losses* that they have experienced. According to Stroebe and Shut, the social context not only influences attitudes and behaviors toward loss but also is the arena in which collective social responses to the loss might be made (e.g., rituals) and within which support may or may not be provided.

When assessing for complicated grief, it is important for the practitioner to consider the following:

- Do the mourners have a history of coping well with adversity in the past and, therefore may be somewhat naturally resilient?
- Is s/he physically healthy?
- Does s/he have a positive, optimistic personality or a generally negative one?
- What kind of support system does the bereaved have?
- Are there other concurrent stressors affecting the bereaved, such as financial hardship?
- Does the mourner derive strength from some form of spirituality?

Therese Rando takes a similar approach to the assessment for complicated grief. She states that the factors that should be considered when assessing for complicated grief include

- The nature of the loss and the circumstances around it
- Whether the loss was expected or not
- The meaning of the loss to the mourner—degree it influences their life
- The mourner's prior losses and how they coped
- The mourner's current life circumstances—what resources/support are available

Worden explains that *in general*, normal grievers are more in touch with reality than those having complicated grief. Normal grievers may want to believe that the loss can be restored, but they know it cannot. Conversely, those having complicated grief continue to operate as if the person lost was still there, have chronic hope of reuniting with the deceased, and/or avoid situations that would remind them of their loss.

In its *Guidelines for Bereavement Care*, the National Hospice and Palliative Care Organization outlines the indicators that should be addressed in evaluating an individual's risk for complicated grief. These indicators, listed in Table 17–7, are divided into six specific domains: physical, emotional, social, spiritual, economic, and intrapersonal.

The importance of evaluating the socioeconomic and practical needs of the bereaved as part of a bereavement assessment cannot be underscored enough. At least one-third of survivors report financial problems due to post death economic sequelae of reduced income, disruption in their employment, and higher living expenses. Survivors, especially in the first few months following a loss, often report that dealing with the loss of the deceased spouse's income, or taking over the practical roles assumed by the deceased (such as the payment of bills, cooking, cleaning, driving) are of significant concern. For many, the need to address these issues may be as important as the psychological needs that are traditionally thought to be a primary concern.

MOURNING PATTERNS THAT CAN LEAD TO COMPLICATED GRIEF

Over the last 20 years, several grief theorists, including Kenneth Doka, Therese Rando, and William Worden have identified several different patterns of behavior that often result in complicated grief.

TABLE 17–7. NHPCO Evaluation of Risk of Complicated Grief

DOMAIN	FACTORS
Physical	Current health status and impact on grief
	Ability to care for self and perform activities of daily living
	Impairment as a result of substance abuse
	Change in sleeping and eating habits and in energy level
Emotional	Ability to engage in emotional expression
	Feelings of loss, sadness, hopelessness, conflict, frustration, anger, irritability, guilt, self-reproach, fear
	Suicidal ideation and risk
	History of mental health concerns
	History of loss/grief
Social	Family interaction and function
	Relationship with patient
	Degree of satisfaction with life closure tasks
	Support system
	Social outlets, work, meaningful activities
	Culture/ethnicity factors
Spiritual	Degree of spiritual distress
	Outlook (attitude), direction, and purpose in life
	Sense of community
	Role of faith and spirituality
	Ability to access hope for the future
Economic	Financial stability
	Employment status
	Dependents
	Debt status
Interpersonal	Self-esteem, self-worth, self-confidence, and self perception of competence
	Independence versus dependence
	Ability to adapt to new roles/responsibilities
	Personal strengths and weaknesses
	Coping resources and strategies

SOURCE: Reprinted with permission from National Hospice and Palliative Care Association: *Guidelines for Bereavement Care.*

The first of these is what is typically termed chronic grief. This refers to grief that is excessive in duration and does not reach a satisfactory conclusion. Chronic grief often coincides with an ambivalent or dependent relationship, an unwillingness to relinquish grief, or an intense yearning for the deceased. Behaviors that are typical of chronic grief may include obsessive trips to the grave site, continual sorting of the deceased's possessions, or constant memories of or conversations about the deceased. Often, an individual with chronic grief is unable to successfully integrate the loss into his/her life and return to normal activities even over an extended period of time.

Delayed grief can occur when the griever does not deal sufficiently with a loss at the time it happens. Grief is intentionally postponed to a later date, and is usually precipitated by other events or losses. At least one study has shown that caregivers whose caregiving role was prolonged, may, out of exhaustion, not have the emotional or mental energy to work through their grief process, and so put it off to a later time. Delayed grief is also sometimes seen when the mourner has other responsibilities at the time of death. Individuals with delayed grief may exhibit grief symptoms precipitated by other events or losses and may deny yearning for or remembering the deceased.

Disenfranchised grief is characterized by the griever being deprived of validation and recognition of a loss because of constraints in openly acknowledging the loss or of constraints in publicly grieving. Situations that may be associated with disenfranchised grief include relationships not based on traditional family and relationship ties such as friends, cohabitants, or partners; relationships that are not socially sanctioned such as gay relationships or extramarital affairs; deaths caused by socially unacceptable illnesses such as AIDS; relationships that existed in the past such as an ex-spouse; losses that may not be considered significant such as an abortion, a stillbirth, or the death of a pet; death of the personality of a loved one from Alzheimer's disease; or mourners that society might wrongly assume are incapable of grieving (children, elderly, and persons with developmental disabilities).

Exaggerated grief occurs when the mourner experiences an intensification of normal grief reactions and feels overwhelmed, typically resulting in emotional distress. Common symptoms of exaggerated grief include intense, frequent nightmares; frequent outbursts of anxiety or even panic attacks and phobias; anger, or delinquent behavior; consuming feelings of guilt related to the loss; or depression.

When the bereaved experience symptoms and behaviors that cause difficulty in coping but they are unable to associate them with the loss, the grief is said to be masked. Those who suffer from masked grief may develop medical symptoms similar to those of the deceased, develop another psychosomatic condition, or may develop psychiatric symptoms such as unexplained depression or paranoia. Sometimes, these mourners act out their grief through a maladaptive or delinquent behavior.

Finally, when death occurs with little or no warning, the mourner may experience what is termed sudden grief. With sudden grief, the mourner has little or no time to prepare for the loss, and there is an increase in the incidence of denial and numbness regarding the death. Those having sudden grief may experience increased regret about things they did not say or do before the death, or for not being able to do something to prevent the death. They may become angry at others because of feeling helpless and vulnerable. They may also experience prolonged grief intensified by the need to understand and find meaning in the death. When the circumstances of sudden death are of a traumatic nature (e.g., violent, random, or mutilating), bereavement reactions are more severe and complicated, sometimes resulting in PTSD.

GRIEF AND DEPRESSION

When evaluating mourners for evidence of complicated grief, it is important for the clinician to differentiate between grief and major depression. Depression can coexist with complicated grief and individuals having either one (or both simultaneously) may experience a number of similar symptoms including depressed mood, cathartic expressions such as crying, and somatic manifestations such as changes in eating and sleeping patterns, difficulty concentrating, and either fatigue or hyperactivity. Nevertheless, there are a number of significant differences that allow the observant clinician to differentiate between grief reactions and depression, and these differences can be found in Table 17–8.

TABLE 17–8. Differences between Depression and Grief		
DOMAIN	**DEPRESSION**	**GRIEF**
Self-esteem	Self-esteem decreases gradually over time	Self-esteem seems to decrease suddenly and is related to the timing of the loss
Social interactions	Social interactions are often not desired and patients do not report satisfaction from the interactions	Social interactions are often requested to assist with grief and are beneficial to the patients
Suicidal ideation	Depressed patients may have an active suicide plan because "it's not worth living anymore"	Bereaved patients may have vague thoughts of suicide in order to escape from the pain of loss or with hope of reuniting with their loved one, but they do not usually have an active plan
Mood	A depressed person's mood is usually consistently down and he or she may be regressed in appearance	It is more common to see a grieving person experience the typical "up and down" fluctuations of the grief process
Suffering	Suffering and emotional pain experienced by depressed patients is more chronic in nature. It is harder to identify the origin of the suffering	Suffering in grieving patients can generally be traced directly related to the loss experience

INTERVENTIONS FOR MOURNERS WITH COMPLICATED GRIEF

Effective treatment for *normal grief* requires assisting the bereaved through the crisis they are experiencing related to the loss. Normal grief work generally requires the presence of an ongoing supportive relationship and enough time for the bereaved to heal. Usually, there is only minimal intervention, if any, required from experienced professionals.

In contrast, mourners experiencing complicated grief often require significant intervention from experienced grief counselors, which may include social workers, chaplains, and other health care professionals. There are a fair number of interventions, both general and specific, that have been found to be effective with mourners whose grief is more complicated. These interventions may also be useful for working with mourners who have a normal grief reaction but are seeking

professional support. A list of general grief interventions can be found in Table 17–9 and specific grief interventions can be found in Table 17–10. A summarized discussion of some of these techniques is described below.

First, it is important to listen to the mourner's own account of the loss and the meaning of the loss to him or her. Generally, the mourner will indicate how s/he wishes to respond to the changing life situation. Goals for the various interventions that will be used should be set based on this objective. While working with mourners, it is important for the professional to keep in mind the distinction between the healthy processing of feelings and life review and negative ruminations that the bereaved may express. It is also important for the professional to distinguish between integrative resilience and superficial adaptation.

Once the interventions are selected, careful assessment and ongoing monitoring must be provided to ensure that the chosen intervention(s)

TABLE 17–9. General Grief Interventions

Provide education regarding the "normal" grief process	Suggest that they be patient not only with themselves, but also with others who may not understand what they are feeling.
Remind the mourner that many mourners say that the intense pain of grief eventually declines	Remind them to have realistic expectations about how quickly they will heal from the pain of grief.
Affirm their ability to survive their current loss	Suggest that they start slowly to return to their normal routine by doing small customary chores such as food shopping.
Affirm the persons current strengths and highlighting where they have succeeded in the past in coping with hardships	Doing small things for other people can also be helpful in that it takes attention off the bereaved and their pain for awhile.
Help the mourner set reasonable goals around fixable problems	Reassure them that it is also okay to set limits with people and to say "no".
When you speak of the deceased, use the past tense, use the deceased's name, and use words such as death, died, dead.	Validate the survivor as they develop new skills and take on new roles.
You can ask them to tell you about the death—what happened that day/night.	Affirm their right to feel joy and hope and to eventually have another relationship, without viewing these as being disloyal to the deceased.
Ask them about any funeral or memorial services.	When addressing fears about "letting go," it helps to focus on changing connections rather than separation
Ask them what has been happening since the death; how they have been functioning, interacting with others, etc.	Suggest that they be patient not only with themselves, but also with others who may not understand what they are feeling.
Ask them about their relationship with the deceased.	Remind them to have realistic expectations about how quickly they will heal from the pain of grief.
Help them examine their special qualities and talents that endeared them to the deceased	

are achieving the desired outcomes. At times, helping the bereaved individual become aware of the link between symptoms and the recent loss may sometimes be enough of an intervention to effect a remedy.

Robert Neimeyer has identified several favorable outcomes of bereavement interventions. They include the promoting of adaptive continuing bonds, the supporting of an adaptive search for meaning, and encouraging the bereaved to develop new goals.

He believes that "The life story disrupted by loss must be reorganized, rewritten, to find a new strand of continuity that bridges the past with the present."

William Worden differentiates grief counseling from grief therapy. According to Worden, grief counseling (provided by trained professionals or through self-help groups that are supportive and educational in nature) helps mourners with uncomplicated grief go through the various tasks of mourning. He believes that grief counseling

TABLE 17–10. Specific Grief Interventions

Encourage the use of symbols and "transitional objects" such as photos, audio or video tapes, articles of clothing/jewelry, or a special collection

Suggest writing a letter to the deceased (God, others)

Suggest keeping a journal of the grief experience; or of special thoughts, poems, and remembrances.

Reading about grief often helps to normalize it. Bookstores, libraries, hospices, and the Internet all have excellent grief resources.

Family members could put together a memory book that includes stories about family events, photos, poems, drawings, etc. They could also make a memory box, in which special items are kept and can be shared with others.

Suggest the use of art work to express grief feelings.

One grief therapist suggests that the bereaved person play out in their mind the "unfinished business" from the relationship with the deceased and try to come to some form of a resolution. It can be helpful to focus on what the survivor was able to do for the deceased instead of what they should have done.

The "empty chair" technique, where the bereaved person imagines the deceased and is encouraged to express whatever they need to say, is another effective method for "unfinished business."

helps the mourner talk about the loss, identify and express feelings, learn about normal grieving as well as differences in grieving styles amongst mourners. Counseling can also help the bereaved learn to make decisions and to live without the deceased, learn strategies on coping with grief during important holidays or anniversaries, understand their own personal methods of coping, and identify those coping strategies that may be dysfunctional.

In contrast to grief counseling, Worden believes that grief therapy (individual or group) may be useful when the bereaved experience more complicated grief reactions. He states that grief therapy tends to focus more on "intra-psychic conflict." The goals of grief therapy are to assist the mourner in developing the ability to experience, express, and adjust to the loss; to find effective ways to cope with difficult changes; to establish a continuing relationship with the deceased; to maintain a healthy self-image and to continue to function and reestablish relationships with others.

For individuals having *disenfranchised grief*, it is imperative to validate the significance of their loss, reassure them that you will be available to provide support, and assist them in accessing support from others who will understand the nature and intensity of their grief. When a sudden, devastating loss occurs, mourners usually feel vulnerable and out of control. These mourners are in need of professionals, who can provide them with stability and control rather than catharsis, can help them recognize the loss and remind them that there has been a drastic change in, what Therese Rando calls, their "assumptive world."

Finally, Shear, Frank, et al., in an article published *JAMA* in 2005, conducted a controlled clinical trial comparing complicated grief therapy to interpersonal psychotherapy. They found that while both treatments produced improvement in complicated grief symptoms, there was significantly greater response rate for those patients receiving complicated grief treatment (51%) than for those treated with interpersonal psychotherapy (28%; $P = 0.02$). The time to see a positive response was faster when complicated grief treatment was used ($P = 0.02$).

The complicated grief treatment that they used consisted of three phases. The first, or introductory phase, consisted of providing information about normal and complicated grief, describing the dual process model of adaptive coping (alternating attention to loss and restoration), and focused on establishing the personal life goals of the bereaved. During the middle phase, the therapist addressed all the processes identified in the introductory phase in tandem. The last phase, called the termination phase, allowed the therapist to review with the bereaved the progress made during therapy, plans for the future, and feelings about ending treatment.

Trauma-like symptoms are addressed by retelling the story of the death and included exercises to confront avoided situations. The story is taped and the mourner is periodically asked to report distress levels. Distress related to loss (yearning, longing, reveries, fear of losing the deceased forever) is targeted using techniques to promote a sense of connection to the deceased, using imagined conversation and completing a memory questionnaire. For personal life goals, the mourner is asked what they would like for themselves were their grief not so intense. The therapist then identifies ways they are working toward that goal. Concrete plans are discussed and put into action.

USE OF SUPPORT SYSTEM

The significance of a person's support system in adjustment to a loss cannot be emphasized enough. A person's family, friends, church or synagogue, community organizations, schoolmates, and coworkers all play major roles in helping a survivor feel loved, accepted, and supported. The support system can also assist the bereaved in participating again in life.

When working with the bereaved, it is important to encourage them to utilize members of their support system, especially those who are able to listen to their story and nurture memories of the deceased. Encourage the bereaved to reach out for help and to take people up on their offers to help and to be specific with their requests. Remind them not to isolate themselves from others, even if they have to make visits short. Let them know that some people may call less than they did at or just after the death, possibly because they do not know what to say or they might feel they are being intrusive. Educate the bereaved that they need not try to protect or provide support to others. They should also set limits if others tell them how to feel or what to do in their well-meaning but misguided attempts to be helpful.

USE OF MEDICATION

Much has been written concerning the use of medication during the bereavement process. With the bereaved often experiencing prolonged and intense anxiety and/or depression, the desire to prescribe anxiolytics and antidepressants can be quite strong. It is generally agreed, however, that such medications should be prescribed as an adjunct, and not as a replacement, for other interventions. In addition, these medications should be used sparingly both to avoid dependence and so as not to inhibit or circumvent the necessary process of mourning. The prescribing clinician needs to be aware of the potential for suicide in bereaved individuals receiving medication as well as the increase in the use of other prescription and nonprescription drugs and alcohol in the bereaved.

If medications are required, anxiolytics may be helpful to persons experiencing acute distress including posttraumatic stress symptoms manifested in the early stage of a loss. Antidepressants, on the other hand, are generally not indicated in persons with acute grief reactions, although they may sometimes be indicated if the bereaved experience a major depressive episode.

Reynolds et al., in studying 80 subjects, aged 50 years and older, with bereavement-related major depressive episodes, found that the use of the antidepressant nortriptyline was superior to placebo in achieving remission of these episodes. The combination of medication and psychotherapy, however, was associated with the highest rate of treatment completion, underscoring the importance of using grief therapy (or psychiatric therapy when indicated) and other supportive measures along with medications to properly manage complicated grief.

A WORD ABOUT SUICIDE

It is not uncommon for the bereaved to have suicidal thoughts. A wish to die can be a wish for reunion with a loved one. Thoughts of dying are also an imaginary way to gain relief from the pain of grief. As the bereaved come to accept the loss, however, suicidal thoughts usually disappear.

There are certain behaviors that, when being exhibited by the bereaved, could be an indication that the individual may be at risk for suicide. These include such actions as "putting one's affairs in order," giving away personal items, or asking others to care for people or pets for whom the bereaved is responsible. In addition, the person may ask questions about what it would be like to be dead, express extreme statements of hopelessness or helplessness, or experience a sudden change in attitude (often becoming inappropriately happy).

Mourners at low risk for suicide may have vague thoughts about suicide, but no specific plan. They may say something like, "I just don't feel like it's worth it anymore." Those at moderate risk express suicidal ideation, but the plan is vague in terms of means and time OR the plan is contingent on some event. They may say "If I'm not over my grief in 3 months . . . ." Those at high risk have a specific plan and the means available.

If a mourner is assessed at risk for suicide, it is important to intervene using the *least* restrictive method possible and also base the intervention level on the degree of risk.

CONCLUSION

Whether one views complicated grief as the presence of certain high risk factors that lead to an abnormal grief experience and an unhealthy grief reaction or as symptoms that are present in normal mourning that have abnormal intensity and duration, all can agree that defining whether a grief reaction is normal or not depends more on the mourner's *own* experience of his/her grief and ability to function after the loss. If any risk factors or symptoms described earlier become very intense, endure for prolonged time period, and/or are uncomfortable to the mourner and/or cause significant disturbance in functioning, then one might consider that the mourner's grief has become more complicated and professional help should be sought. It is important to remember that given adequate support and time, both before and after a loss, most individuals are able to eventually readjust to their loss even though the loss may have produced dramatic changes in one's life.

BIBLIOGRAPHY

Attig T: *How We Grieve: Relearning the World.* New York, Oxford University Press, 1996.

Bonnano GA: Loss, trauma and human resilience. *Am Psychol* 59:20-28, 2004.

Bradley EH, Prigerson HO, Carlson MDA, Cherlin E, Johnson-Hurzeler R, Kasl SV: Depression among surviving caregivers: does length of hospice enrollment matter? *Am J Psychiatry* 161(12):2257-2262, 2004.

Cook A, Dworkin D: *Helping the Bereaved: Therapeutic Interventions for Children, Adolescents and Adults.* New York, BasicBooks, 1998.

Doka K, ed: *Disenfranchised Grief: New Directions, Challenges, and Strategies for Practice.* Champaign, IL, Research Press, 2002.

Genevro J, Marshall T, Miller T: *Report on Bereavement and Grief Research.* The Center for the Advancement of Health, Washington, DC, 2003. http://www.cfah.org.

Hedtke L, Winslade J: *Re-membering Lives: Conversations with the Dying and the Bereaved.* Amityville, NY, Baywood Publishing, 2004.

Hogan NS, Worden JW, Schmidt LA: An empirical study of the proposed complicated grief disorder criteria. *Omega* 48(3):263-277, 2003-2004.

Horowitz MJ: Dr. Horowitz replies in letters to the editor. *Am J Psychiatry* 155:9, 1998.

Jacobs SC: Treating depression of bereavement with antidepressants: A pilot study. *Psychiatr Clin North Am* 10:501-510, 1987.

Jacobs SC: *Traumatic Grief: Diagnosis, Treatment, and Prevention.* Philadelphia, PA, Bruner-Mazel, 1999.

Jeffreys J: *Helping Grieving People: When Tears Are Not Enough: A Handbook for Care Providers.* New York, Brunner-Routledge, 2005.

Klass D, Silverman P, Nickman S: *Continuing Bonds: New Understandings of Grief.* Washington, DC, Taylor & Francis, 1996.

Licht ML: *Colorado Hospice Bereavement Services Project, Newsline.* Alexandria, VA, National Hospice and palliative Care Organization, 2000.

Martin T, Doka K: *Men Don't Cry . . . Women Do: Transcending Gender Stereotypes of Grief.* Philadelphia, PA, Brunner/Mazel, 2000.

Middleton W, Raphael B, Burnett P, Martinek N: A longitudinal study comparing bereavement phenomena in recently bereaved spouses, adult children and parents. *Aust N Z J Psychiatry* 32:235-241, 1998.

National Hospice and Palliative Care Organization, Evaluation of Risk of Complicated Grief; *Guidelines for Bereavement Care.* Alexandria, VA, 2002.

Neimeyer R, ed: *Meaning Reconstruction and the Experience of Loss.* Washington, DC, American Psychological Association, 2001.

Neimeyer R: *Lessons of Loss: A Guide to Coping.* Memphis, TN, Center for the study of loss and transition, 2006.

Ott C: The impact of complicated grief on mental and physical health at various points in the bereavement process. *Death Stud* 27:249-272, 2003.

Parkes CM: Risk factors in bereavement: implications for the prevention and treatment of pathologic grief. *Psychiatr Ann* 20:6, 1990.

Parkes C: *Bereavement: Studies of Grief in Adult Life,* 3rd ed. Philadelphia, PA, Taylor & Francis Inc., 2001.

Prigerson HG, Frank E, Kasl SV, et al: Complicated grief and bereavement-related depression as distinct disorders: Preliminary empirical validation in elderly bereaved spouses. *Am J Psychiatry* 152:22-30, 1995.

Prigerson HG, Shear MK, Newsom JT, et al: Anxiety among widowed elders: Is it distinct from depression and grief? *Anxiety* 2(1):1-12, 1996.

Prigerson H, Jacobs S: Diagnostic criteria for traumatic grief. In: Stroebe MS, Jansson RO, Stroebe W, Schut H, eds. *Handbook of Bereavement Research.* Washington, DC, American Psychological Association, 2001, pp. 614-646.

Rando T: *Grief, Dying, and Death.* Champaign, IL, Research Press, 1984.

Rando T: *Treatment of Complicated Mourning.* Champaign, IL, Research Press, 1993.

Rando T, ed. *Clinical Dimensions of Anticipatory Mourning: Theory and Practice in Working with the Dying, Their Loved Ones, and Their Caregivers.* Champaign, IL, Research Press, 2000.

Reynolds F, et al: Treatment of bereavement-related major depressive episodes in later life: A controlled study of acute and continuation treatment with nortriptyline and interpersonal psychotherapy. *Focus* 2(2):260-267, 2004.

Rosof B: *The Worst Loss: How Families Heal From the Death of a Child.* New York, Henry Holt & Company, 1995.

Sanders CM: A comparison of adult bereavement in the death of a spouse, child and parent. *Omega* 10:303-322, 1980.

Sanders CM: Effects of sudden vs. chronic illness death in bereavement outcome. *Omega* 13(3):227-266, 1982-1983.

Sanders CM: *Grief: The Mourning after. Dealing with Adult Bereavement.* New York, John Wiley & Sons, 2001.

Shear K, Frank E, et al: Treatment of complicated grief: A randomized controlled trial. *JAMA* 293:2601-2608, 2005.

Stroebe M, Schut H: The dual process model of coping with bereavement: Rationale and description. *Death Stud* 23:197-224, 1999.

Stroebe MS, Hansson RO, Stroebe W, Schut H: *Handbook of Bereavement Research: Consequences, Coping, and Care.* New York, American Psychological Association, 2001.

Stroebe M, Schut H: Complicated grief: A conceptual analysis of the field. *Omega* 52(1):53-70, 2005-2006.

Videka-Sherman L: Coping with the death of a child: A study over time. *Am J Orthopsychiatry* 52:688-699, 1982.

Walsh F, McGoldrick M: *Living beyond Loss: Death in the Family,* 2nd ed. New York, W.W. Norton and Company, 2004.

Wolfelt Alan D: The journey through grief. *Thanatos* 21:4-6, 1996.

Wolfelt A: *Healing Your Grieving Heart: 100 Practical Ideas.* Colarado, Companion Press, 2001.

Wolfelt Alan: *Understanding Your Grief: Ten Essential Touchstones for Finding Hope.* Colarado, Companion Press, 2004.

Worden W: *Grief Counseling and Grief Therapy: A Handbook for the Mental Health Practitioner.* 2nd ed. New York, Springer, 1991.

Worden JW, Davies B, McCown D: Comparing parent loss with sibling loss. *Death Stud* 23:1-15, 1999.

Wortman C, Silver R: The myths of coping with loss. *J Consult Clin Psychol* 57:349-357, 1989.

SELF-ASSESSMENT QUESTIONS

1. The following are myths associated with grief in this culture EXCEPT:
   A. It's better to not think or talk about the pain.
   B. Everyone has their own unique time table for grief and method for expressing grief.
   C. It takes about a year to get over a significant loss
   D. I should leave the mourner alone and not bring up his/her loss.
   E. The intensity and length of your grief reflects how much you loved the deceased.

2. All of the following are indications of normal grief EXCEPT
   A. Insomnia
   B. Nightmares
   C. Substance abuse
   D. Anger
   E. Searching behavior

3. All of the following are considered risk factors for complicated grief EXCEPT
   A. Deceased is a child
   B. History of psychiatric illness
   C. Close relationship with the deceased
   D. Concurrent life stressors in addition to the loss
   E. Multiple recent losses

4. Which of the following five grief theorists believes that grief affords an opportunity for the mourner to "reconstruct meaning" after a loss?
   A. Robert Neimeyer
   B. William Worden
   C. George Bonnano
   D. Holly Prigerson
   E. Kenneth Doka

5. All of the following regarding how different demographic groups react to loss is true EXCEPT
   A. Bereaved parents generally have more intense reactions than bereaved spouses.
   B. Bereaved spouses generally have more intense reactions than bereaved adult children.
   C. Male children generally are affected more by the loss of a parent than by the loss of a sibling.
   D. Survivors of sudden deaths have an easier time adjusting to loss than individuals whose loved one died after a protracted illness.
   E. One-third of children who lose a parent show high levels of emotional difficulty in their readjustment.

6. All of the following are symptoms that indicate that grief has become more complicated EXCEPT
   A. Searching behavior
   B. Extreme preoccupation with the deceased
   C. Significant neglect of self-care
   D. Themes of loss come into most discussions
   E. Person unwilling to move physical possessions

7. A 25-year-old male is referred to you for counseling for symptoms consistent with complicated grief. He tells you that a close male college friend died a few months ago. On further questioning, you learn that the relationship he had this friend was intimate and that he has not been able to discuss his loss with his parents or siblings because of they are not aware of his sexual orientation and of the relationship and he knows that they would react very negatively if they learned about this. The pattern of complicated grief being experienced by this patient is called

A. Chronic grief
B. Delayed grief
C. Exaggerated grief
D. Disenfranchised grief
E. Masked grief

8. Grief and depression have all of the following factors in common EXCEPT

A. Depressed mood
B. Cathartic expression like crying
C. Changes in eating and sleeping patterns
D. Difficulty concentrating
E. Desire for social contact

9. All of the following would be considered helpful interventions with someone who is grieving EXCEPT

A. Validate the significance of their loss
B. Provide education regarding the "normal" grief process

C. Suggest they move to a different house or even out of the area
D. Ask them about their relationship with the deceased.
E. Suggest writing a letter to the deceased

10. Which of the following is true about the use of medication during the bereavement process?

A. When necessary, anxiolytics and antidepressant medications should be used as an adjunct to counseling and not as a replacement.
B. Medication alone was no more effective than placebo in a study on the treatment of bereavement related major depressive episodes.
C. The risk of drug dependence and suicide are decreased when medication is used during the grief process.
D. Antidepressant medications may help control acute grief reactions.

Diagnostic and Invasive Interventions

CHAPTER

18

Diagnostic Tests and Invasive Procedures in End-of-Life Care

Barry M. Kinzbrunner and Neal J. Weinreb

INTRODUCTION

A 77-year-old man with advanced pancreatic carcinoma and obstructive jaundice is admitted to a hospice program for terminal, palliative care. In addition to anorexia and fatigue, he suffers from intractable pruritus, which has not responded to pharmacologic intervention. The patient is so distressed that he is contemplating suicide. In discussion with the hospice interdisciplinary team, the medical director suggests endoscopic or radiologic biliary stenting. The hospice nurse appears uncomfortable and comments "I thought that we don't do aggressive, invasive, life-prolonging procedures on hospice patients!" Nevertheless, after further explanation and discussion, the recommendation is presented to the patient and to his wife. To everyone's surprise and consternation, the patient categorically and repeatedly refuses the procedure, saying "All I want is to die as quickly as possible. Doc, why can't you just put me to sleep?"

This anecdote highlights a strange and frustrating paradox in modern medicine. Palliative care is fast becoming accepted as a broadly desired area of clinical expertise, and its practitioners have access, when appropriate, to a rapidly growing armamentarium of technologically sophisticated, symptom-oriented interventions capable of substantial enhancement of comfort, even at the end of life. On the other hand, public support for the legalization of physician-assisted suicide appears to be substantial throughout the United States, suggesting that there continues to be deep-rooted disbelief in the ability and willingness of modern medicine and technology to address and alleviate pain and suffering. Furthermore, knowledge of which outcomes are truly important for terminal patients continues to be incomplete, and defining and analyzing symptom palliation for any given intervention can be deceptively difficult. Few investigational trials define a standard of palliation on the basis of aspects of onset; duration and degree of pallia-

tion; and symptom improvement, control, and prevention.

The balance between the benefits and burdens of intervention is often evaluated in terms of quality of life (QOL). However, even with validated tools for QOL measurement, it may correlate poorly with other indicators of health status. A number of patients with significant physical and/or psychological symptoms report good global QOL, including 51% of patients with severe pain. Conversely, patients with less severe physical and psychological manifestations may describe their QOL as poor. A new endpoint, the clinical benefit response, which uses disease symptoms as clinical endpoints, also may correlate poorly with subjective evaluations of QOL by patients and physicians, and criteria designed for use in one diagnosis or study may not be applicable in other circumstances.

Thus, patient attitudes toward "aggressive," invasive palliative interventions are likely to be highly variable and unpredictable. Studies suggest that some patients with advanced disease are willing to put up with significant, but time-limited, toxicity for interventions, such as palliative chemotherapy, intravenous antibiotics, and limited mechanical ventilation, in return for even the hope of a modest benefit. Indeed, many patients, were they able, would trade months of even debilitating illness for a single month of "quality time." However, other patients might well identify with the attitude of the above anecdotal patient in eschewing any invasive intervention. Many more undoubtedly concur with the following instructions written by a physician in a model advanced directive: ". . . if there is little hope for recovery to my prior state of health, or if what hope exists requires prolonged and invasive medical treatments, I would prefer to receive care focused on my comfort rather than care focused on prolonging my life."

The purpose of this chapter, and several others to follow, is to identify various diagnostic procedures and invasive therapies that are potentially available to terminal patients; to examine the evidence that does or does not support the palliative value of these interventions near the end of life; and to consider the clinical circumstances in which these interventions can be appropriately recommended either to patients or to their health care surrogates. These interventions will be examined from the viewpoint of end-of-life care as a whole, without raising issues regarding the Medicare Hospice Benefit (i.e., a prognosis of 6 months or less) and without any references to cost-effectiveness or economic analysis. [The invasive interventions that will be addressed in their own chapters include chemotherapy and radiation therapy (Chapter 19); invasive cardiac interventions (Chapter 20); respiratory assist devices such as continuous positive airway pressure (CPAP), bilevel positive airway pressure (BiPAP), and ventilators (Chapter 21); and artificial nutrition and hydration (Chapter 24)].

TABLE 18–1. Determining Appropriateness of "Aggressive" Palliative Interventions at the End of Life

What is the goal or expected outcome of the proposed intervention?

Does the planned intervention have a high probability of efficacy?

How significant are potential toxicities, side effects, complications, or postintervention discomfort?

What is the patient's baseline level of function?

What is the life expectancy of the patient?

What does the patient want?

GENERAL PRINCIPLES

The goal of palliative care at the end of life, as defined by the World Health Organization, is achievement of the best possible QOL for patients and their families. Control of pain, of other physical symptoms and of psychological, social, and spiritual issues, is paramount. This goal includes optimizing function and making the best of each patient's remaining time. It does not necessarily preclude other goals such as remission or even cure, and some patients may wish to seek aggressive or experimental treatments for the primary terminal process until the very end. These patients are obviously no less entitled to optimal symptom management than those patients who are seeking comfort measures only, but the tolerance for risk and discomfort associated with invasive interventions may be considerably greater for the former group of patients as compared to the latter. For this reason, this discussion will be directed to those patients whose primary goal at the end of life is total symptom control and maximal functional capacity as long as possible.

In pursuit of this goal, it has been proposed that "palliative care must embrace all the high-tech, expensive, aggressive measures that can enhance patient and family care at the end of life." Several key factors that can assist the clinician in determining whether such palliative interventions are appropriate for patients near the end of life are summarized in Table 18–1 and discussed below.

WHAT IS THE GOAL OR EXPECTED OUTCOME OF THE PROPOSED INTERVENTION?

Suppose, for example, that a patient with advanced metastatic carcinoma suffers a pathologic fracture of the head of the femur. The proposed intervention is orthopedic stabilization via intramedullary rod fixation. Is the goal to restore ambulation, or, purely to alleviate pain with turning and positioning? If the former, is the goal realistic? Will the patient be able to accomplish a postoperative rehabilitation program? If the latter, would a lesser procedure achieve the same outcome?

DOES THE PLANNED INTERVENTION HAVE A HIGH PROBABILITY OF EFFICACY?

Efficacy needs to be defined in terms of rapidity of onset, degree of palliation, and the durability of the response. The assessment of efficacy must be applied both toward the proposed intervention in general and, perhaps more importantly, toward the specific patient in particular. Thus, a chemotherapy drug reported in the literature to be 80% effective in alleviating bone pain would appear to be a reasonable palliative intervention. However, in a heavily pretreated patient with multiple drug resistance, such an agent might be considerably less effective, with the risk of toxicity outweighing any potential benefit, particularly if pain relief is incomplete and of only brief duration. Radiotherapy or spinal decompression can be effective modalities for preventing spinal cord compression and lower extremity paralysis, but they are essentially useless interventions for that purpose in a patient who is already paraplegic.

HOW SIGNIFICANT ARE POTENTIAL TOXICITIES, SIDE EFFECTS, COMPLICATIONS, AND POSTINTERVENTION DISCOMFORT?

Clearly, adverse effects of treatment influence the patient's QOL. The assessment of benefit versus risk requires a full understanding of the potential for undesired, negative, and even life-threatening consequences. For example, what are the chances that a patient with extensive bone metastases who has been heavily pretreated with chemotherapy and external radiotherapy will develop severe pancytopenia with symptomatic anemia and thrombocytopenia following proposed treatment with radiostrontium? What is the likelihood of recurrent infection and sepsis following endoscopic stenting for biliary obstruction? In this regard, are metal stents better than plastic stents? What are the chances of perforating a viscus when performing a paracentesis to relieve discomfort caused by malignant ascites?

WHAT IS THE PATIENT'S BASELINE LEVEL OF FUNCTION?

This question recognizes that invasive procedures and interventions that have high efficacy and low-risk profiles may nonetheless be futile in improving the overall well-being and QOL of patients whose functionality is severely impaired and not likely to improve with the proposed intervention. Consequently, such procedures would seem to be of little palliative value, particularly when the symptoms at which they are directed can be adequately controlled by less invasive means. For example, will a patient with metastatic breast carcinoma and severe dyspnea secondary to lymphangitic pulmonary carcinomatosis benefit from testing to confirm suspected hypercalcemia even though hypercalcemia can be easily treated? Should sclerotherapy for bleeding esophageal varices be advised for a patient with terminal cirrhosis and irreversible hepatic encephalopathy? Should a patient with far-advanced, terminal dementia and pneumonia be treated with intravenous antibiotics?

WHAT IS THE LIFE EXPECTANCY OF THE PATIENT?

It would be illogical to initiate any therapeutic intervention unless there is a reasonable probability that the patient will survive for a sufficient time to realize a benefit from the procedure. Nonetheless, patients continue to be subjected to all kinds of aggressive therapies, even within a short time prior to death. In a study of 200 consecutive deaths at a large urban academic medical center, only 13% of the patients on mechanical ventilation and 19% of those on artificial nutrition and hydration underwent withdrawal of these interventions prior to death. In an Israeli ICU, no patient had antibiotics, nutrition, or fluids withheld. At a US Veterans' Administration hospital, 27% of patients received ventilatory support and 18% were restrained during the last 48 hours of life. On the other hand, other studies indicate that for patients with metastatic cancer, antibiotics are commonly withheld at the very end of life, and interventional surgery for abdominal emergencies (obstruction, bleeding, dehiscence) is quite rare. Nevertheless, even in this situation most patients continued to receive blood transfusions and intravenous fluids.

As discussed in detail in Chapter 1, predicting prognosis is never easy. However, with the judicious use of clinical guidelines and sound clinical judgment, physicians are getting more adept in predicting when life is coming to an end, especially when death approaches. By making these assessments, physicians can assist patients and families in making therapeutic decisions that will allow patients who have sufficiently long to live to benefit from indicated procedures, while avoiding such procedures in patients whose time is short.

Accurate prognostication is also critical in assessing the significance of potential delayed or late onset adverse effects attributable to prior aggressive intervention. For example, many radiation oncologists continue to prescribe protracted, low-fractionation radiotherapy for end-stage cancer patients for fear of causing radiation toxicity, even though this toxicity would have a predicted time of onset long after the death of the patient.

WHAT DOES THE PATIENT WANT?

The principle of autonomy allows competent patients to request or refuse any proposed intervention no matter how beneficial that treatment is likely, or not likely, to be. The physician is ethically obligated to provide sufficient information to allow the patient to reach an informed decision and professionally responsible to recommend and strongly espouse a course of action that is believed to be beneficial for the patient, while ensuring that the patient has had all appropriate options presented for consideration. Once the patient has made a decision, a mature and understanding physician will accept a patient's final decision, and, particularly in the context of end-of-life care, will be sure that the patient feels neither rejected nor abandoned even if the option chosen by the patient is not the one recommended by the physician. However, it must be remembered that a physician also has autonomous rights and professional integrity, and if a patient should make a choice that a physician believes is medically ineffective or detrimental, or morally inconsistent with the physician's values, he or she should feel no obligation to initiate or participate in patient-desired interventions, but should instead assist the patient in finding a physician who will be comfortable providing this intervention.

DIAGNOSTIC TESTS

Diagnostic laboratory and imaging studies are appropriate and indicated in end-of-life care when the information obtained will assist in decision making about therapeutic interventions to control symptoms. On the other hand, routine testing for the purpose of monitoring the patient is generally not advisable.

For example, consider an alert, ambulatory patient with an unresectable gastric carcinoma, but no overt evidence of gastrointestinal (GI) bleeding, who complains of anorexia, weight loss, and chronic fatigue. The physician orders weekly complete blood cell counts with the thought that should the hemoglobin concentration decrease to less than 8 g/dL, a blood transfusion will be necessary. This type of testing, which fosters therapeutic interventions on the basis of arbitrary laboratory values rather than on the patient's symptoms, makes little sense, particularly in the care of patients with end-stage disease. In contrast, should the same patient notice the passage of black stools, along with episodes of dizziness, palpitations, and increasing shortness of breath, measurement of hemoglobin concentration would be worthwhile to confirm the presence of severe anemia, provided, of course, that the patient would agree to interventions, such as a blood transfusion.

On occasion, patients thought to be at the end of life may need to undergo highly invasive procedures to clarify a suspected but previously unconfirmed diagnosis. Patients believed to have malignancies on the basis of abnormal imaging studies, suspicious needle aspirations, or other test results sometimes refuse to allow definitive biopsies or other procedures needed to obtain a tissue diagnosis, and elect a palliative approach to their care. Should their illness not follow the expected course, these patients may be amenable to a new diagnostic evaluation including new imaging studies and even tissue sampling.

Diagnostic testing may have the most utility when there has been a sudden or acute change in the patient's status from the usual condition or level of function. In these circumstances, testing, as an adjunct to historical and physical assessment, may clarify not only the etiology of the change, but also indicate the potential for reversibility and restoration of the *status quo ante*. The most common events that may require diagnostic studies in selected patients near the end of life are listed in Table 18–2 and discussed below.

MENTAL STATUS CHANGES

Acute and subacute changes in mental status of end-stage cancer patients as well as in patients with terminal noncancer diagnoses may be associated with metabolic disorders; infection and sepsis; toxic drug reactions and interactions; primary central nervous system events including thrombotic and embolic infarction, bleeding, and metastasis; delirium and psychiatric disorders.

Hypercalcemia

Hypercalcemia is the most common life-threatening, cancer-associated metabolic disorder. It occurs in 10% to 20% of all cancer patients and, when due to humoral mechanisms, may occur in the absence of bone metastases. When recognized, the symptoms of hypercalcemia are usually rapidly reversible with saline hydration and intravenous bisphosphonates such as pamidronate. Other active agents include calcitonin, corticosteroids, gallium nitrate, and plicamycin. With the exception of imminently dying patients, or patients with extremely poor performance status and refractory symptoms, serum calcium testing is reasonable for end-stage cancer patients with the new onset or exacerbation of fatigue, lethargy, confusion, stupor, muscle weakness, or seizures, particularly in association with constipation, nausea, vomiting, ileus, anorexia, thirst, polyuria, weight loss, and pruritus.

TABLE 18–2. Potentially Useful Diagnostic Interventions in Palliative Care

SYMPTOM	ETIOLOGY	DIAGNOSTIC INTERVENTION
Acute or subacute change in mental status	Hypercalcemia	Serum calcium and albumin levels
	Hyponatremia and other electrolyte abnormalities	Serum sodium and/or other electrolyte levels
	Hypothyroidism	Serum T4 and TSH levels
	Medication toxicity	Serum drug levels, if available
		Renal and liver function tests, as appropriate
	Brain metastases	CT scan of brain
New bone pain	Bone metastases and/or impending pathological fracture	X-rays
		Bone scan
Back pain with/without neurological symptoms	Spinal cord compression	MRI of spine
Dyspnea	Pleural effusion	Chest x-ray
	Anemia	Hemoglobin or hematocrit level

Hyponatremia

Similar symptoms may be associated with other correctable metabolic disorders such as severe hyponatremia sometimes associated with the syndrome of inappropriate antidiuretic hormone secretion (SIADH). Hyponatremia at the end of life may also be caused by salt-wasting states associated with adrenal insufficiency (as in some patients with advanced AIDS) and chronic renal failure, cirrhosis, and end-stage liver disease, hypothyroidism, and medications including diuretics, chlorpropamide, amitriptyline, thioridazine, vincristine, and cyclophosphamide. It should be remembered that when treating hyponatremia in end-stage patients, severe fluid restriction may not be accepted by the patient and family. In patients with SIADH, demeclocycline may ameliorate the symptoms associated with hyponatremia and allow more flexibility in fluid intake.

Hypoglycemia

Hypoglycemia is an all too often overlooked cause of confusion in altered mental status in patients near the end of life, who are being treated for diabetes mellitus, especially if the patients have been on a regular antidiabetic regimen for some time. As a patient's condition deteriorates, reduced oral intake or metabolic alterations may result in a reduced requirement for the routine insulin or oral hypoglycemic agent the patient had been receiving. If this goes unrecognized by the family or caregivers and appropriate dosage adjustments to the patient's regime are not made, hypoglycemia can result. Therefore, whenever a diabetic patient near the end of life becomes confused or unresponsive, a glucose bolus, either orally (if tolerated) or intravenously, should be administered and a blood sugar should be checked as part of the evaluation.

Other Metabolic Abnormalities

Additional, potentially reversible, symptomatic chemical abnormalities, which may manifest as altered consciousness or mental function include disorders of potassium and magnesium metabolism that are as likely to be iatrogenic in origin due to the primary terminal diagnosis or to coexistent morbidities. Testing for these, as well as for hypothyroidism, which is a fairly common late consequence of prior cancer treatment, azotemia caused by drug toxicity or obstructive uropathy, and hepatic encephalopathy, is indicated when therapeutic intervention is contemplated.

Medication Toxicities

Changes in mentation and level of consciousness that are attributable to medications occur frequently toward the end of life. The need to control a multiplicity of symptoms nearly always provokes a proliferative pharmaceutical response with a resulting enhanced probability of drug interactions. Declining hepatic and renal function may be associated with increasingly abnormal pharmacokinetics resulting in accumulation of a drug or its active metabolites to toxic levels. Empirical dose adjustments may sometimes be effective and adequate. This approach is commonly followed when titrating opioid analgesics. However, measurement of blood levels may sometimes be necessary to identify which of the multiple drugs is responsible for the toxic side effects. When in doubt, blood level determinations may be essential before and after adjusting medications such as anticonvulsants for which it is important to maintain a therapeutic range.

Neurological Abnormalities

The appearance or exacerbation of lethargy, weakness, confusion, headaches, memory loss, altered mental state, psychosis, focal neurological deficits, seizures, nausea, and vomiting may indicate brain metastases, infectious encephalopathy, or cerebral infarction or hemorrhage. As will be discussed in Chapter 19, radiotherapy and corticosteroids relieve clinical symptoms in 70% to 90% of patients with brain metastases, although the median survival is only 4 to 5 months from institution of treatment.

Because of the potential for meaningful palliative benefit and reversal of symptoms, imaging studies to confirm the diagnosis and to rule out cerebral infarction or hemorrhage can be considered even in an end-stage patient who has an otherwise reasonable performance status. On the other hand, when imaging studies suggest the likelihood of carcinomatous meningitis, or the clinical index of suspicion is high, a confirmatory lumbar puncture is probably unnecessary in an end-stage patient because the response to palliative intrathecal therapy is generally poor.

Imaging studies can also be significant in evaluating neuropsychiatric dysfunction in patients with end-stage AIDS. Symptoms attributable to cerebral toxoplasmosis may decrease with systemic therapy whereas the prognosis for even palliative improvement in patients with primary central nervous system lymphoma, progressive multifocal leukoencephalopathy, and AIDS dementia continues to be very poor.

Infections

Infections and sepsis are the common cause of altered mental status when patients are near the end of life. The issue of whether infections should be evaluated and treated is discussed in the following text (see the section entitled Antibiotics for Sepsis and Intercurrent Infection).

PAIN

Patients with advanced cancer and well-controlled symptoms who develop new onset of increasingly severe pain invariably have evidence for progressive parenchymal, soft tissue, or neuroinvasive disease, or pathologic fracture in a site of pre-existent osseous metastasis. Most often, careful physical assessment will suffice to establish the etiology (e.g., painful hepatomegaly associated with progressive liver metastases). Sometimes, however, radiographic or radionu-

clide imaging (i.e., bone scan) will be necessary to identify and treat new sites of skeletal metastasis, and impending or overt pathologic fracture.

Particular mention should be made of the ambulatory patient with refractory cancer who develops back pain which is often progressive, excruciating, and unrelenting. Such a patient, unless actively dying, requires immediate evaluation for spinal cord compression. If one waits for the patient to develop evidence of motor, sensory, or autonomic dysfunction, the patient will probably be paraplegic for the rest of his or her life. For those patients with spinal cord compression who are ambulatory at the time of diagnosis, 79% continue to be ambulatory on completion of radiotherapy. For those with weakness and who are unable to walk at the time of diagnosis, only 45% will be ambulatory on completion of treatment. (Treatment of spinal cord compression will be discussed in Chapter 19.) In addition to physical and neurological examination, patients with suspected spinal cord compression will usually also require some combination of plain spine radiographs, bone scan, magnetic resonance imaging, and, now less commonly, contrast myelography. Radiographic studies may also be indicated in patients with terminal noncancer diagnoses especially for the detection and treatment of painful fractures caused by falls or osteoporosis.

OTHER EVALUATIONS

Additional examples of diagnostic tests that may be apropos in selected patients at the end of life include chest radiographs for the diagnosis and treatment of symptomatic pleural effusions, echocardiography for constrictive pericardial effusions, electrocardiography for symptomatic supraventricular arrhythmias, Doppler venograms for deep vein thrombosis, prothrombin time/international normalized ratio (PT/INR) to monitor anticoagulation, and abdominal radiography for possible mechanical small bowel obstruction. In fact, no test or study should be excluded per se, provided that, in each individual circumstance, it meets the test of therapeutic applicability for palliation of symptoms on the basis of the questions discussed above, and is, of course, acceptable to the patient.

SURGICAL, ENDOSCOPIC, AND OTHER INVASIVE INTERVENTIONS

Although invasive interventions are generally thought upon as outside the scope of services that hospice and palliative care programs provide, carefully selected surgical, endoscopic, and other invasive interventions play a definite role in ensuring patients receive state-of-the-art end-of-life care. A list of potential invasive interventions can be found in Table 18–3 and are discussed below.

PALLIATIVE ORTHOPEDIC SURGERY

Apart from issues of pain management and potential neurological injury as discussed above, progressive osseous metastatic disease is oftentimes associated with ambulatory dysfunction, gait and postural instability, falling, and loss of functional independence, particularly when complicated by incipient or actual pathologic fracture. Moreover, the problem is not confined to advanced oncology patients. The incidence of severe osteopenia and osteomalacia is substantial in frail and elderly patients, particularly so in those with end-stage, chronic cardiovascular, pulmonary, renal, and neurological illnesses, especially when compounded by nutritional compromise or treatment with corticosteroids. The incidence of falling in such individuals approaches 80% on an annual basis. All too often, these falls result in fractures and other serious disabling injuries that accelerate dying, and materially detract from the quality of remaining life. Previously ambulatory patients often become bed-bound, and, in the absence of

a strong supportive service, such as a hospice team, patients who live independently in their own homes may be placed in nursing homes or other similar facilities for the remainder of their lives. In appropriate circumstances, palliative orthopedic surgery can avert some of these dire outcomes, even for patients with very limited life expectancies.

Hip and Other Long Bone Fractures

Hip fractures are either femoral or acetabular in nature. In the case of femoral fractures, underlying diagnosis, concurrent illnesses, mental status, performance status, anticipated life expectancy, prefracture ambulatory status, and patient/family goals and wishes are significant factors in the decision-making process. Patients with a short prognosis who were previously nonambulatory for reasons not directly attributable to pathology at the site of fracture probably should not be surgical candidates. Subsequent pain on turning or transferring may be managed with mechanical immobilization of the fractured limb and properly prescribed analgesics. A similar approach could be offered to formerly ambulatory patients, whose life expectancy is estimated to be less than a month, recognizing that some of these patients might prefer an orthopedic intervention, which could get them quickly back on their feet. These patients and families should be advised, however, that it is unusual for patients with such short life expectancies to be successfully discharged postoperatively.

Although cast immobilization is an excellent option in many cases for younger, nontumor patients with femoral fractures, who can afford to invest 8 to 10 weeks in the healing process, patients at the end of life rarely can afford that kind of time. Thus, for end-stage patients, regardless of the underlying diagnosis, internal medullary rod fixation for intertrochanteric and shaft fractures, and prosthetic reconstruction for fractures of the femoral head and neck, are often recommended. For patients with pathologic fractures, bone cement is commonly added for further

TABLE 18–3. Surgical, Endoscopic, and Other Invasive Palliative Interventions

CONDITION	PROCEDURE
Orthopedic conditions	
Hip fracture	Open reduction-internal fixation
Fracture of long bone	Open reduction-internal fixation
Vertebral compression fracture	Percutaneous vertebroplasty with or without balloon kyphoplasty
Extremity gangrene	Palliative amputation in select patients
Fungating extremity tumor mass with pain, bleeding, and infection	Palliative amputation in selected patients
Bowel obstruction	Laser photocoagulation
	Stent placement
	Laparoscopy
	Diverting enterostomy
	Gastrostomy tube for drainage
Malignant dysphagia	Stent placement
	Alcohol injection
	Laser therapy
	Photodynamic therapy
	Argon plasma coagulation
	Mechanical dilatation
Biliary obstruction	Endoscopic stent placement
	Percutaneous stent placement
Upper tract obstructive uropathy	Cystoscopic stent placement
	Percutaneous nephrostomy
Bronchial obstruction	Stent placement
	Photodynamic therapy
	Laser therapy
Vascular obstruction	Stent placement
Pleural effusion	Thoracentesis or chest tube with or without sclerotherapy (doxycycline, bleomycin, talc)
	Indwelling pleural catheter
	Chest tube with Heimlich valve
Ascites	Paracentesis
	Indwelling catheter
	Peritoneovenous shunts in selected patients
Pericardial effusion	Pericardiocentesis via echocardiographic guidance
	Sclerotherapy (doxycyline, bleomycin)
	Pericardial window

stabilization, and postoperative radiotherapy may be offered depending on the overall prognosis. Fixation of long bone fractures may be accomplished with minimal blood loss or morbidity, and patients can progress to immediate weight bearing the day after surgery. 96% of patients experience good or excellent relief of pain after internal fixation.

In contrast, patients with acetabular fractures require extensive joint reconstruction; this surgery has significant potential for morbidity and complications, and fewer patients experience good or excellent pain relief. Therefore, these extensive procedures are rarely applicable to patients receiving end-of-life care.

The most common site for long bone fractures other than the femur is the humerus. As with hip fractures, the decision to perform surgery and the surgical technique chosen for fracture of other long bones must be individualized on the basis of the individual patient's characteristics as discussed earlier, the area of fracture, and the particular qualities of the bone involved. Pain and discomfort caused by humeral fractures can often be managed by immobilizing the involved extremity, especially in patients who are nonambulatory and in whom overall performance status is poor.

Vertebral Fractures

Vertebral fractures in patients near the end of life may either be pathological due to malignancy or due to osteoporosis. Surgical repair of vertebral compression fractures is very unusual in patients who are terminally ill and would only be considered in patients who are experiencing impending spinal cord injury. In these situations, all the various factors that enter into decision making, including the patient's underlying illness, comorbid or concurrent illnesses, mental status, performance status, anticipated life expectancy, prefracture ambulatory status, and patient/family goals and wishes would have to be considered. In addition, if the etiology is pathologic, and the malignancy is sensitive to radiation therapy, this

might be considered as an alternative to surgical repair. (A full discussion of the treatment of spinal cord compression with radiation therapy can be found in Chapter 19.)

However, a newer, less invasive form of therapy for vertebral compression fracture has been in use for the past several years and is developing an increasing role in the palliative treatment of this condition. This technique is known as "percutaneous vertebroplasty," and it involves injecting acrylic cement into a collapsed vertebral body to stabilize and strengthen the fractured vertebra. As this technique alone does not restore the shape or height of the vertebral body, an adjunctive technique, known as "kyphoplasty" has been developed, in which a high pressure balloon is first placed in the bone and expanded to restore vertebral height, following which cement is injected to stabilize the bone.

In two series evaluating the effectiveness of balloon kyphoplasty to treat vertebral compression fractures due to both osteoporosis and malignancy (without accounting for patient prognosis), pain was significantly improved in an overwhelming majority of patients (>90% in one study) within a week of the procedure, and significant pain relief was maintained in one study for a duration of 2 years following the procedure. Although the role of percutaneous vertebroplasty with or without balloon kyphoplasty in end-of-life care has not been well defined, a recently published article presented three patients with advanced metastatic cancer who each underwent percutaneous vertebroplasty (without balloon kyphoplasty) for the treatment of refractory pain secondary to one or more vertebral compression fractures. All three patients had significant pain relief within 24 hours and significant reduction in the high-dose analgesia that they been previously receiving. The patients survived 3 weeks, 1 month, and 7 weeks. Although the authors appropriately point out that randomized trials regarding the use of percutaneous vertebroplasty in palliative care are lacking, they suggest that this technique may have a role in the palliative treatment of patients near the end of life who suffer from intractable pain secondary to vertebral compression fractures or who experience intolerable analgesic side effects due to the doses required to control their pain.

PALLIATIVE AMPUTATION

In caring for patients with terminal diseases, a recommendation to amputate an extremity is frequently a source of conflict for patients and family members, for patients/families and physicians, and among physicians with differing perceptions of how best to help the patient. This potential for disagreement is most pronounced in patients with end-stage, chronic, nonmalignant diseases, usually associated with multiple comorbidities; who develop vascular compromise and gangrene; and who were not perceived as imminently dying prior to the acute event. In these circumstances, many physicians believe that withholding surgical intervention in deference to a patient's wishes is a violation of their professional integrity as well the ethical principles of beneficence and nonmaleficence. There is also the belief that amputation may be the most effective palliative intervention for controlling pain and foul drainage even in patients with a relatively short prognosis, although delineated "dry gangrene" is not invariably associated with severe pain or infection. It should also be recognized that very few end-of-life patients will be candidates for postamputation prostheses or rehabilitation.

Despite the issues and concerns noted above, the medical literature has identified patients with "advanced limb ischemia" for whom a palliative nonsurgical treatment approach would be considered reasonable. These patients usually have one or more major comorbidities, including heart disease, cerebrovascular disease, advanced pulmonary disease, diabetes, or renal insufficiency. In one published series of 30 patients treated with a nonsurgical approach, half of the patients had three or more of the delineated comorbidities, with half having significant heart disease. Two-thirds of the patients were immobile, and almost half had a prior stroke. Patient survival in this population ranged from less than 24 hours (7 out of 30 patients) to 42 days following the decision to avoid surgery, and the median survival was 3.5 days.

As with all decision making, satisfactory conflict resolution depends on a careful and critical assessment of the patient's baseline physical, mental, and psychological function; rigorous definition of the goals after amputation in the context of the overall prognosis; and potential for restoration of function. There must also be a truthful informed consent process, and ultimately, respect for the patient's wishes as expressed either directly, with an advanced directive, or by a properly delegated health care surrogate. Consultation with an experienced ethics committee is often useful and advisable in these circumstances.

For patients with locally advanced malignancies, even in the presence of extensive metastatic disease, palliative amputation may be necessary to control local pain, fungation, bleeding, infection, gangrene, or severe lymphedema that has not been amenable to nonsurgical attempts at palliation. It is generally recommended in the literature that patients who are being considered for palliative amputation have at least a 3-month expected survival, should be in reasonable medical condition to tolerate the procedure, and have a performance status greater than 50%.

Although major amputations are often viewed as offering little to already compromised patients, significant improvements in performance status and pain control have been documented in the majority of small groups of carefully selected patients in the literature.

BOWEL OBSTRUCTION

Bowel obstruction most commonly occurs in patients with end-stage, refractory ovarian, colorectal, and gastric carcinoma, and less frequently in patients with metastatic breast cancer, lung cancer, and melanoma. Small bowel obstructions are more often the result of multiple intrabdominal implants, whereas large bowel obstructions more commonly occur at a single site. Symptoms of obstruction are often exacerbated by inflammatory edema, constipation, cancer or treatment-induced fibrosis, abnormalities in intestinal motility, decreased production of intestinal enzymes and secretions, change in the fecal flora, or adverse effects of medications. As some of these, such as inflammatory edema, constipation, and adverse medication effects may sometime be correctable, they should be managed medically prior to considering any surgical intervention.

In patients with extensive systemic cancer, bowel obstruction, which commonly fluctuates between partial and complete, is usually associated with multiple extraluminal metastatic implants. Consequently, surgery, even when technically feasible, rarely results in palliation of significant duration. In one series, only a bit more than half of the patients survived more than 60 days postoperatively, and nearly half of these individuals had intermittent symptoms of obstruction until death. Clinical features predicting a poor surgical outcome include diffuse intraperitoneal carcinomatosis, palpable abdominal masses, recurrent ascites, cachexia (especially in elderly patients), poor nutritional status, hypoalbuminemia, malignant pleural effusions, and extensive hepatic or pulmonary metastases. Therefore, medical management including the use of octreotide, opioids, anticholinergic drugs, corticosteroids, antiemetics such as haloperidol, and (in the absence of colicky pain) motility-enhancing agents, is generally the preferred approach near the end of life (See Chapter 8, Gastrointestinal Symptoms), with palliative surgery being considered primarily for those patients who are not high risk for poor outcomes and have a prognosis of at least several months.

If surgery is contemplated, the type of procedure considered would be dependent on the nature of the obstruction. If the obstruction is confined to a single site, as may be the case with large bowel disease, resection may be considered. When resection is not possible, or if the obstruction is multifocal due to carcinomatosis, then bypassing the obstruction with an enterostomy or intestinal stoma is usually the best option, with the placement of a large gastrostomy tube for drainage being reserved for patients for whom an ostomy is not feasible.

Recently, laparoscopic approaches to malignant bowel obstruction are being increasingly utilized, with potential advantages including reduced pain and shortening of the hospital stay. Unfortunately, laparoscopy is not appropriate for patients with carcinomatosis or dense adhesions, limiting its usefulness in many of the patients who present with bowel obstruction near the end of life and who either have extensive intra-abdominal disease or have had multiple prior surgeries making adhesions very likely. Studies to date are limited and the optimal role for laparoscopy has not yet been defined.

Endoscopic procedures can provide effective palliation with less complications. Endoscopic laser photocoagulation allows effective palliation in 85% to 95% of the patients, with negligible mortality and treatment complications in less than 10% of patients treated so. Photodynamic therapy (PDT) with porfimer sodium may further enhance the response.

The development of enteral self-expandable metal stents placed by fluoroscopic or endoscopic guidance has greatly improved the outcomes for patients with gastric outlet obstruction. Following stent placement, patients are reported to be able to begin eating more quickly, tolerate solids sooner and more often, and have shorter and more cost-effective hospital stays when compared with more traditional methods of obstruction relief. Early complications include stent malpositioning and perforation whereas late complications that have been reported include tumor ingrowth or overgrowth, stent migration, bleeding, and perforation.

Expandable stents have also been found to be effective in treating large bowel obstruction, with effective relief of obstructive symptoms 80% to 90% of the time. As with the upper GI tract, the stents are placed via fluoroscopic or endoscopic guidance. Clinical success, defined as colonic de-compression within 48 hours of stent placement, has been reported in about 90% of patients in several reported series. The most serious com-plication is perforation, which occurs in a little less than 4% of patients and usually requires sur-gical intervention. Other complications include mild rectal bleeding, abdominal pain, pseudo-obstructive episodes due to fecal impaction, and occlusive tumor ingrowth into the stent lumen. The duration of effective stent function has been reported to range from several weeks to more than 1 year and has almost always exceeded the pa-tient's lifespan. Stent placement requires less in-patient time and appears to be more cost-effective than a surgical colostomy. When appropriate, stent placement may be part of a multimodal pal-liative plan incorporating laser therapy and local radiotherapy and brachytherapy.

MALIGNANT DYSPHAGIA

As for bowel obstruction, palliation of malig-nant dysphagia by external radiotherapy and brachytherapy are most effective when used in conjunction with endoscopic interventions. A variety of techniques have proven effective in-cluding prosthetic stents, alcohol injection, laser therapy, PDT, argon plasma coagulation, and mechanical dilatation.

Treatment with self-expanding, membrane-coated metallic stents has a good and prompt ef-fect on dysphagia and has been perhaps the great-est recent advance in endoscopic palliation of malignant dysphagia and tracheoesophageal fis-tulas. Compared with radiotherapy and chemo-therapy, in which dysphagia is relieved in about 50% of treated patients, 80% to 90% of patients treated with stent insertion are free of dysphagia. The membrane coating prevents or retards tu-mor ingrowth into the stent. Complications are unusual but include chest pain, bleeding, perfo-ration, distal migration, and mediastinitis.

Injection of 100% alcohol under endoscopic guidance has been used to treat exophytic bulky lesions at all levels of the esophagus. Although dysphagia ultimately improved in 81% of pa-tients treated in one series, two treatments were needed on average to achieve success, and dif-ficulty swallowing recurred after a mean of 35 days in two-third of the patients. Complications included chest pain and fever for 12 to 24 hours following treatment, and a small percentage of patients develop mediastinitis or sepsis.

Endoscopic palliation with Nd-YAG laser therapy appears to have a complementary role to other techniques including dilatation, stent place-ment, and radiotherapy. As a solitary modality, laser therapy is usually administered at weekly in-tervals, with improvement in dysphagia observed after 3 to 4 weeks in 80% to 90% of patients. With the addition of external radiotherapy after initial laser treatment, the need for further endoscopy was substantially decreased.

PDT, in which the patient is given a hemato-porphyrin derivative, usually porfimer sodium, that accumulates in the malignant tissue and is then activated by passing light-delivery catheters through the endoscope, is useful for exophytic or flat lesions, especially those that are long and might be difficult to treat with a laser, and for tumor ingrowth or overgrowth of expandable metal stents. This technique produces somewhat longer responses to dysphagia than does laser therapy, and its complications include chest pain, odynophagia, fever, pleural effusion, and a 10% to 30% incidence of tracheoesophageal fistulas. In addition, there is a 60% to 70% incidence of skin injury secondary to sunlight exposure, other sources of radiant heat, or even strong flu-orescent lights, limiting patient activity for 30 to 45 days following treatment. In addition, the ex-pense of the photosensitizing agent makes this procedure less cost-effective when compared with other techniques.

Argon plasma coagulation is an ablative tech-nique that passes an electric "plasma arc" through the tumor, destroying the tissue. In one series of 83 patients with inoperable esophageal cancer, 58% of patients responded with only one treatment session, 26% of patients required a second treatment, and 16% of patients did not have a positive outcome. Two-thirds of patients required retreatment every 3 to 4 weeks until death, and one-third ultimately required a stent. The role of argon plasma coagulation is not yet well defined because of its similarity to laser therapy.

As a QOL issue, rapid restoration of the ability to swallow both food and secretions suggests that endoscopic stent placement may be the most appropriate palliative intervention for patients with even a very short life expectancy. On the other hand, mechanical dilatation, laser, photodynamic, and radiation therapy may have a complementary role for patients who are likely to survive long enough to benefit. These modalities also help in managing obstruction at the gastric cardia where stent placement may be technically difficult.

BILIARY OBSTRUCTION

Biliary stenosis or obstruction in patients with pancreatic carcinoma, cholangiocarcinoma, or extensive liver metastases is almost always accompanied by extremely distressing symptoms of jaundice, pruritus, anorexia, indigestion, nausea, vomiting, and wasting. With the exception of patients with a very short life expectancy, alleviation of these symptoms by endoscopic, percutaneous, or surgical bypass procedures often results in tangible improvement in both physical and psychological well-being. Currently, surgical bypass is generally performed only in those patients undergoing laparotomy with intention to cure who are subsequently found to have unresectable disease. Cholecystoenteric and choledocoenteric bypasses appear equally effective. Not surprisingly, for patients with advanced, end-stage disease, both are associated with considerable morbidity, and some patients never regain their preoperative performance status. Therefore, as endoscopic stenting provides at least an equivalent duration of survival with significantly less morbidity, obstructive jaundice in patients near

the end of life should almost always be treated either endoscopically or percutaneously. For patients with coexistent gastric outlet obstruction, laparoscopic gastrojejunostomy appears to be an excellent alternative to classical surgery, providing a good functional result with only minimal impairment of the QOL.

Endoscopic stenting involves retrograde cannulation of the common bile duct, performance of a sphincterotomy, and placement of either a plastic or metallic endoprosthesis. On occasion, the procedure may be technically difficult, time-consuming, and exhausting for the patient. Successful stent placement is considerably greater with this technique (95%) when the obstructing lesion involves the distal common bile duct, as typically seen in patients with pancreatic carcinoma. When the site of obstruction is more proximal and closer to the hilum of the liver, success rates decline to only 50%, and morbidity and mortality increase. For these lesions, percutaneous stent placement (with either internal or external drainage) may be more prudent, with a higher success rate, albeit a greater incidence of immediate serious complications.

The most common long-term complication of stent placement is clogging, which typically occurs after 3 to 4 months with plastic prostheses, and over a longer time period with metallic stents. Therefore, the choice of stent should depend on the anticipated life expectancy of the patient. The two most important independent risk factors for predicting prognosis are tumor size and presence of distant metastatic disease. For patients with tumors exceeding 3 cm in size, the median survival is 3.2 months, compared with 6.6 months for those with smaller tumors. The median survival for patients with metastatic disease is 2.5 months compared with 9 months for those without metastases.

Other than clogging, additional causes for recurrent jaundice include tumor overgrowth or ingrowth, duodenal obstruction due to tumor invasion, and stent impaction into the bile duct wall. Cholangitis occurs in 20% of the patients, sometimes with consequent sepsis. The responsible bacteria often have a high frequency of antibiotic resistance. As with all other end-of-life crises, a decision as to how aggressively to treat either clogging or infection depends on a careful appraisal of the patient's overall condition, prognosis, and desires.

UPPER TRACT OBSTRUCTIVE UROPATHY

The inevitable endpoint of bilateral ureteral obstruction is renal failure and uremia. The clinical manifestations of untreated uremia include increasing fatigue, anorexia, dulling of the sensorium, and eventual coma, presumably associated with decreasing perception of pain and suffering, culminating in a "peaceful" death, in a reported median time frame of 3 to 7 months. In as much as this clinical cascade has traditionally been regarded as a blessing for the patient with far advanced, symptomatic cancer, much as pneumonia was identified as the "friend" of the senile elderly, there has been little fervor for aggressive intervention for upper urinary tract obstruction in patients with end-stage disease. The older and largely outdated technique of open nephrostomy had a 50% rate of major, life-threatening complications, more than 40% of the patients never left the hospital, and 30% died within 52 days of surgery. The overall median survival was 3.3 months.

Studies suggest that in patients with end-stage malignancy, the results are little different using modern techniques of cystoscopic ureteral stenting and percutaneous nephrostomy. In a study of approximately 100 patients with advanced malignancy (mean age 68 years), the median survival after palliative endourologic urinary diversion was 3.5 months, of which 1.5 months was spent in the hospital.

Complications of percutaneous nephrostomies and stents include a very high risk (65%) of febrile urinary tract infections, dislodgement of the nephrostomy tube (10%), and perirenal abscesses (8%). There is a 3% risk of hemorrhage during the insertion of percutaneous catheters (3%), and these patients also run the risk of urinary leakage and skin excoriations, which have reportedly been associated with adverse QOL outcomes. In one study specifically evaluating QOL following percutaneous nephrostomy placement, only 11 out of 17 patients reported an acceptable outcome for 2 months or more.

A recent procedure that shows some promise is a subcutaneous nephrovesical bypass procedure, which has the advantage of eliminating the presence of percutaneous nephrostomy tubes. Early studies using this approach show improved results, with no dislodgement of the tubes reported, the ability of patients to void normally, and improved QOL reported by most patients. The role of this procedure, however, is not yet defined and additional studies will be required before it can be used routinely.

While this and other new approaches to ureteral bypass are being developed to help reduce complications, the high risk of complications and poor QOL outcomes reported to date suggest that the decision whether to bypass ureteral obstruction should be individualized on the basis of the patient's wishes, and that, in general, it is difficult to recommend these procedures as appropriate for most patients at the end of life.

BRONCHIAL OBSTRUCTION

In addition to radiotherapy (see Chapter 19), endoscopic management of symptomatic tracheobronchial airway stenosis can provide significant palliation for patients with malignant airway obstruction. Multimodality therapy including combinations of laser therapy, radiation therapy, and expandable metallic stent placement can improve survival and QOL for patients with complete malignant bronchial obstruction. Metallic stents can even alleviate obstruction in the area of the carinal bifurcation with little evidence of complications directly attributable to the stent. PDT with porfimer sodium was recently approved for palliation of symptoms for patients with completely or partially obstructing endobronchial non–small cell lung cancer. One month or later, PDT alleviated symptoms of dyspnea and cough in about 25% of treated patients and hemoptysis in nearly 80%. PDT appeared more effective than Nd:YAG laser therapy, particularly regarding hemoptysis. PDT cannot be used concurrently with radiotherapy but may be used sequentially. It is contraindicated in patients with respiratory–esophageal fistulas or with tumors eroding into major vessels. Patients will be photosensitive for at least 30 days and must avoid direct sunlight or even bright indoor light without skin and eye protection. Some patients may experience severe chest pain after PDT.

VASCULAR OBSTRUCTION

Aside from their established use in the management of occlusive coronary and peripheral vascular disease, expandable metallic stents are increasingly employed for the management of vascular occlusive disease associated with malignancy such as superior vena cava (SVC) syndrome. In a series of 12 patients with SVC syndrome, most of whom had advanced bronchogenic carcinoma, 11 patients had immediate relief of obstruction after radiologically controlled placement of self-expanding metal stents. There were no major complications. SVC obstruction recurred in only one patient after 3 months. The other patients survived without relapse for 1 to 10 months.

In a larger series of 76 patients with SVC syndrome in which stent insertion was compared with radiotherapy, stenting provided faster relief of symptoms and significantly greater improvement in symptoms than did radiation therapy. Significantly fewer patients developed recurrent symptoms after stent insertion than with radiotherapy, and there were three times as many complications in patients treated with radiation therapy alone compared with those who were stented. It was therefore suggested that percutaneous stent insertion should be the palliative procedure of first choice for malignant SVC obstruction.

Expandable stents can also alleviate symptoms caused by portal hypertension in patients with locally advanced biliary cancer or with liver metastases. With the transjugular intrahepatic portosystemic stent-shunt technique, symptoms of portal hypertension, including tense ascites, mesenteric congestion, and variceal bleeding disappeared after the procedure. There was a significant improvement of the patients' performance status allowing early ambulation.

PLEURAL EFFUSIONS

Compared with pericardial effusions (see in the following text), malignant pleural effusions are commonly encountered in patients with end-stage malignancy. Typical symptoms include progressive dyspnea, orthopnea, persistent coughing, and chest pain. In as much as these symptoms can materially compromise the quality of an even severely limited life, and treatment is generally successful in alleviating symptoms, palliative intervention is nearly always justified.

Classical treatment usually consists of sequential thoracenteses or large-bore tube thoracostomy, usually with sclerotherapy. For patients with an overall estimated life expectancy of very short duration, placement of a small, indwelling pleural catheter can be used successfully to drain the pleural space, even in a home setting. This procedure has considerably less morbidity than either repeated thoracentesis or tube thoracostomy, and an incidence of pneumothorax below 5%.

For patients with a somewhat longer life expectancy, tube thoracostomy and sclerotherapy are usually recommended. Traditional large-bore tube thoracostomy with chest tubes connected to continuous wall suction and underwater drainage requires inpatient care, limits patient mobility, often causes considerable patient discomfort, and is expensive. Studies suggest that ambulatory pleural drainage with a small-bore catheter connected to a closed gravity drainage bag system is a safe, effective, and more patient-friendly alternative. In one series, half of the patients treated with small-bore catheters and sclerotherapy had a complete response of at least 30 days duration. In a randomized study comparing large and small-bore catheters (18 patients), all patients found the large catheter somewhat or very unpleasant, whereas this was the case for only two patients with the small catheter. Regarding the need for subsequent thoracentesis, the small catheter was no less effective than the large one. Based on this admittedly preliminary evidence, increased use of small-bore catheters seems reasonable, particularly in the context of end-of-life care.

An ideal sclerosing agent is not yet available. Tetracycline has been studied most extensively, but it is no longer available in the United States for intrapleural administration. Doxycycline (500 mg) is highly effective, with 92% of patients in one trial free of recurrent pleural effusion for at least 3 months following instillation. Side effects include pain in the majority of patients, fever, and sometimes, troublesome cough. Patients should be pretreated with opioid analgesics prior to sclerotherapy with doxycycline. Intrapleural bleomycin (60 units) can also be used as a sclerosing agent. It is not painful, but can cause transient fever, and is expensive. Dose adjustments are advisable in elderly patients and in those with renal insufficiency to avoid systemic toxicity (alopecia, mucositis, and skin ulcers).

Talc powder, in the form of a slurry, may also be instilled via a chest tube, with a reported efficacy of 80% to 90%. Talc is inexpensive, but requires knowledge of special sterile technique by the pharmacist, and is associated with significant pain, fever, and, on occasions, with respiratory distress syndrome. Talc may solidify, especially in small-bore chest tubes, leading to residual loculated effusions. Talc may also be administered by insufflation (poudrage) via videothoracoscopy. This minimally invasive approach may be justified in end-stage patients with longer life expectancies who have failed to respond to conventional tube thoracostomy. This technique may also be valuable in patients with refractory chylous effusions.

Patients with persistent pleural drainage who cannot be sclerosed, or those with a persistent air leak, can be successfully managed as outpatients or at home via chest tube with a Heimlich valve.

ASCITES

Management of massive, tense ascites is a problem in end-of-life care in two types of patients with differing pathophysiology: (1) end-stage cancer patients (usually gynecologic, breast, or colorectal cancer); (2) end-stage liver disease (usually associated with cirrhosis). In nonmalignant ascites, sodium retention, mediated by neural and humoral mechanisms, causes an increase in total body sodium and water with ascitic fluid in equilibrium with total body fluid. In contrast, malignant ascites, usually caused by some combination of fluid secretion by tumor implants and interference with normal venous and lymphatic drainage, accumulates independently from total body volume. The clinical significance of this distinction is that although dietary water and salt restriction and judicious use of diuretics are integral to the management of nonmalignant ascites, they are of little value, and sometimes contraindicated, in a patient with malignant ascites.

The only goal in treating ascites at the end of life is to alleviate the typical symptoms of abdominal distension, early satiety, anorexia, indigestion, reflux, nausea, immobility, and respiratory distress. There is no advantage to treating asymptomatic patients.

Nonmalignant Ascites

For patients with nonmalignant, end-stage liver disease, the combination of salt and water restriction, and prescription of diuretics (usually spironolactone or amiloride) is effective in controlling fluid overload in 90% of the patients. It should be pointed out, however, that overly aggressive diuretic therapy can exacerbate fatigue due to electrolyte imbalance, lead to falls due to orthostatic hypotension, and add to patient discomfort by causing sleep deprivation due to frequent nocturia and embarrassing episodes of urinary incontinence. Recent reports in the literature have suggested that octreotide and midodrine (an alpha-1 adrenergic agonist) may have some benefit in patients with refractory ascites, but the data to date are anecdotal only, and more studies will be required before these agents could be considerable reasonable additions to the armamentarium for patients near the end of life.

For patients who continue to be symptomatic despite medical management, large volume paracentesis is generally safe and effective, with removal of up to 5 L of fluid at a single session. Nonedematous, hypoalbuminemic patients may sometimes require concurrent infusion of plasma volume expanders during paracentesis to avoid symptomatic hypotension. For patients whose life expectancy exceeds more than a few weeks, an indwelling catheter may promote greater comfort, although with some increased risk of infection. Radiologically placed port-a-cath devices or nephrostomy-type tubes may be a satisfactory alternative to surgical placement of a Tenckhoff peritoneal dialysis catheter. Peritoneovenous shunts are rarely indicated in end-of-life care, especially in patients with terminal liver disease in whom their use is sometimes complicated by an increased risk of sepsis, disseminated intravascular coagulation, shunt occlusion, and a significant incidence (10–20%) of perioperative death.

Malignant Ascites

As indicated above, fluid restriction and diuretics are rarely effective in controlling malignant ascites, and may promote symptomatic intravascular volume depletion. Paracentesis is the most commonly used means of managing malignant ascites and is recognized as being highly effective. The use of plasma volume expanders is generally not necessary after paracentesis for malignant ascites.

If fluid reaccumulation requires the patient to undergo frequent procedures, then, as with nonmalignant ascites, a radiologically implanted port-a-cath device may be a reasonable alternative to repeat paracentesis. Although sclerotherapy with bleomycin or doxycycline may retard fluid reaccumulation, it is only effective in about 30% of patients, and is of dubious value especially in patients with short life expectancies. Similarly, intraperitoneal infusion of radioisotopes or chemotherapy such as cisplatin is probably neither necessary nor warranted for symptom management near the end of life. Finally, a 1997 randomized trial evaluating the use of intraperitoneal tumor necrosis factor (TNF) as an adjunct to paracentesis did not confirm any benefit to the addition of TNF, despite preliminary positive results in some phase I and II trials.

Although peritoneovenous shunts are also ill-advised in patients in whom death is anticipated within several weeks, a beneficial effect was reported in 19 patients with malignant ascites in whom predicted life expectancy was several months. All had a prior unsatisfactory experience with repeated paracentesis and diuretics. The shunts were inserted under general anesthesia and were associated with an average hospital stay of 6 days. Sixteen patients had excellent shunt function with resolution of ascites and associated symptoms. Late shunt occlusion occurred in five patients with recurrence of ascites, but patency was reaccomplished in four out of the five. The median survival was 5.5 months, and 14 patients were free of ascites at the time of their deaths.

PERICARDIAL EFFUSIONS

Although pericardial metastasis and malignant effusions are not infrequent, especially for patients with cancers of the breast, lung, and with lymphoma, most patients never have signs and symptoms directly related to these complications. When symptomatic, patients most commonly complain of dyspnea with exertion or at rest, coughing, and chest pain or heaviness. The severity of the symptoms is related to the rate at which the effusion accumulates. Manifestations of pericardial tamponade may therefore occur early with a relatively small volume, rapidly accumulating infusion, or later in the course, when the volume of fluid relative to pericardial distensibility is so great as to increase intrapericardial pressure and impair diastolic ventricular filling. Signs and symptoms of tamponade include neck vein distension, hypotension, resting tachycardia, and pulsus paradoxus. Peripheral edema occurs less commonly, but, when present, can lead the physician to err in prescribing diuretics, which may worsen the underlying pathophysiology.

Patients with pericardial tamponade are usually critically ill at the time of presentation. However, even patients with refractory, end-stage disease who, at the onset of tamponade, are not so debilitated due to other cancer manifestations as to cause imminent death, are likely to have increased comfort and a better quality of remaining life as a result of therapeutic intervention. The procedure of choice is echocardiographically guided pericardiocentesis and attempted intrapericardial sclerosis with either doxycycline or bleomycin. Success in controlling recurrence is generally achieved 70% to 80% of the time with minimal toxicity. With doxycycline, multiple instillations may be necessary. The experience with bleomycin is still quite limited. There are also anecdotal reports of success with interleukin-2 and interferon alpha-2b, but there is no evidence that these agents are more advantageous than the traditional ones. For hemodynamically compromised patients with a better overall performance status and a life expectancy of more than 3 to 4 months, pericardiocentesis followed by subxiphoid pericardiectomy (pericardial "window") is a more durable palliative approach. This discussion, of course, presupposes refractoriness to chemotherapy. However, for patients with longer prognoses, radiosensitive malignancies, and no prior irradiation of the chest and mediastinum, radiation therapy may also be considered.

ANTIBIOTICS FOR SEPSIS AND INTERCURRENT INFECTION

Sepsis is a common sentinel event in both elderly and debilitated patients with end-stage disease. In addition to fever, symptoms of sepsis include altered mental status and delirium, dyspnea, pain, and lassitude.

Multiple studies indicate that, with the possible exception of patients with far-advanced metastatic cancer, even actively dying patients continue to receive intravenous antibiotics almost up to the moment of death. Regarding whether there is any benefit to treating such patients, the results are mixed. At one palliative care unit, although 72% of known infections were treated with antibiotics, most patients died nonetheless during the same admission. On the other hand, a study on the use of parenteral antibiotics in a different palliative care unit showed that they were considered helpful in 62% of patients treated for a variety of infections including the urinary tract, lower respiratory tract, and soft tissues/skin or wounds. Positive outcomes were most commonly observed for infections of the urinary tract and for patients who were either considered terminal (within a few days of death) or in a stable phase, as opposed to those who were considered to be deteriorating or in an acute phase.

Therefore, as with other palliative interventions, the decision regarding whether or not to treat a patient near the end of life with antibiotics for infection needs to be individualized. When sepsis is related to an infected or occluded catheter, central line device, or stent, or attributable to a drainable collection, or associated with painful cellulitis, antibiotics may be warranted, depending on the patient's premorbid condition and level of function. Intervention may also be appropriate when a patient develops an intercurrent localized infection, such as a urinary tract infection. Under these circumstances, appropriate cultures and imaging studies may be reasonable, even in the context of end-of-life care, for while one might argue that antibiotic treatment should be entirely empirical in terminal patients, the continuing and growing problem of antibiotic resistance suggests that the rules for proper selection of antibiotics should not be relaxed even at the end of life.

TRANSFUSIONS AND HEMATOPOIETIC GROWTH FACTOR

ANEMIA

Regardless of the terminal diagnosis, anemia that is sufficiently severe to cause symptoms can be a significant problem in end-of-life care. Contributing factors to anemia in the terminal patient can include concurrent debility and nutritional inadequacy, blood loss, renal or hepatic insufficiency, and bone marrow suppression associated with prior chemotherapy and radiotherapy or the anemia of "chronic disease." Current treatment options include transfusion of red blood cells and administration of subcutaneous erythropoietin.

Red blood cell transfusions are generally well tolerated and, with appropriate arrangements with a blood bank, can be safely administered in a home setting. This is supported by recent Swedish study demonstrating that 82 (58%) out of 141 patients on "advanced home care" were successfully transfused at home. In this same study, transfusions were of benefit to 117 (68%) out of 174 total patients who were transfused irrespective of location.

Despite the documented benefits, however, there are potential significant complications including severe allergic reactions and possible fluid overloading. Furthermore, in terminally ill patients, symptoms such as marked fatigue, breathlessness, palpitations, and dizziness may be due to multiple etiologies other than anemia and may not improve significantly even after transfusion.

Therefore, one must always keep in mind that a recommendation for red blood cell transfusion should never be triggered by some arbitrarily predetermined value of hemoglobin concentration or hematocrit. Rather, the decision should be based on a critical assessment of the symptoms, the patient's ambulatory and functional status, and the history of response to prior transfusions.

There are few indications for the use of erythropoietin in end-of-life care. The main virtue of erythropoietin is that, when effective, patients have fewer fluctuations in hemoglobin concentrations compared with those treated with intermittent transfusions, and the risk of transfusion reactions is obviated. In a 2004 Swedish study evaluating the potential benefits of erythropoietin in a group of unselected cancer patients with cachexia to prevent the appearance of anemia, biochemical benefits were noted, but they were not translatable into improvements perceived by the patients. More recently, studies showing a decrease in survival among cancer patients and an increase in the number of patients experiencing cardiovascular and thromboembolic events when treated with erythropoietin to maintain hemoglobin levels at 12 g/dL or above have significantly negatively impacted its use.

Therefore, with the exception of a few selected end-stage patients with refractory anemia already benefiting from treatment, erythropoietin would seem to have a very limited role to play in the treatment of patients near the end of life.

GRANULOCYTOPENIA AND THROMBOCYTOPENIA

Granulocytopenia and thrombocytopenia become issues in end-of-life care primarily in patients with end-stage hematologic illnesses or AIDS. Granulocytopenia may be a significant side effect of various antibiotics and antiviral agents used to treat or prevent opportunistic infections in AIDS. Although definitive antiretroviral treatment should not be within the purview of end-of-life programs, aggressive prophylaxis of QOL-threatening opportunistic infections in patients with refractory disease is a proper goal of palliative care. Granulocyte colony stimulating factor (G-CSF) is often prescribed in conjunction with these treatments to minimize the risk of concurrent granulocytopenia. However, it has not been clearly demonstrated that G-CSF reduces the rate of severe infection or mortality from infection when given prophylactically, and therefore, it should not represent "routine" care for end-stage patients.

Regarding severe thrombocytopenia, patients with terminal hematologic disease (leukemia or myelodysplasia) or bone marrow failure due to other causes are almost invariably refractory to transfused platelets by the time they are referred for end-of-life care. Consequently, except in unusual circumstances, platelet transfusions are unlikely to have significant palliative benefit and should be discouraged. Similarly, intravenous gamma globulin, which is sometimes indicated for the treatment of immune thrombocytopenia in patients with AIDS, is generally not applicable in patients with end-stage disease. Thrombopoietin has not yet been approved for use in the United States, and its role, if any, in end-of-life care, is yet to be defined.

FINAL WORDS

"You think it's beautiful to die for your country. The first bombardment taught us better. Actually, it's better not to have to die at all!"

from *All Quiet on the Western Front*

It seems paradoxical to depict techniques for alleviation of suffering as "invasive" or "aggressive," terms that evoke images of carnage and destruction. Although many people reluctantly come to accept the inevitability of death, everyone who has given the matter any thought wishes his death to be a "good" one. Few individuals

equate this desire with the experience of medical trench warfare, where they are cut off from the "home front" and subject to continual bombardment with ostensibly "friendly fire." As palliative soldiers, what attitude ensures that as we choose and deploy our weapons, we never forget the overall interests and aspirations of the population we are trying to liberate?

I chose the discussion of the palliative use of blood products as the concluding section of this chapter with that question in mind. On multiple occasions, the Bible identifies the blood as synonymous with *nefesh*, sometimes rendered as soul, but best translated as the "essence of life." If, we focus only on specific symptoms and lose sight of the global suffering of our patients, then, despite our most effective invasive interventions, we are likely to be regarded, as were our English predecessors of the 19th century, not as healers, but as no more than body snatchers. On the other hand, when we make the effort to penetrate the patient's *nefesh*, to recognize and alleviate not only physical, but also emotional and spiritual distress, the most aggressive palliative maneuvers will be accepted as life-restoring, even if not lifeprolonging. In the words of Maimonides: *"In the sufferer, let me see ever the human being."*

BIBLIOGRAPHY

General Introduction

Alpert HR, Emanuel L: Comparing utilization of lifesustaining treatments with patient and public preferences. *J Gen Intern Med* 13:175-181, 1998.

Altwein J, Ekman P, Barry M, et al: How is quality of life in prostate cancer patients influenced by modern treatment? The Wallenberg Symposium. *Urology* 49(4A Suppl):66-76, 1997.

Berger A, Portenoy RK, Weissman DE, eds: *Principles and Practice of Supportive Oncology.* Philadelphia, PA, Lippincott-Raven, 1998.

Berger JT, Majerovitz D: Stability of preferences for treatment among nursing home residents. *Gerontologist* 38:217-223, 1998.

Billings JA: Palliative care: Definitions and controversy. *Princ Prac Support Oncol* 1:1-10, 1998.

Bonnefoi H, A'Hern RP, Fisher C, et al: Natural history of stage IV epithelial ovarian cancer. *J Clin Oncol* 17:767-775, 1999.

Braddock CH III, Edwards KA, Hasenberg NM, et al: Informed decision making in outpatient practice: Time to get back to basics. *JAMA* 282:2313-2320, 1999.

Brown NK, Thompson DJ, Prentice RL: Nontreatment and aggressive narcotic therapy among hospitalized pancreatic cancer patients. *J Am Geriatr Soc* 46:839-848, 1998.

Council on Ethical and Judicial Affairs, AMA: Medical futility in end-of-life care. *JAMA* 281:937-941, 1999.

Covinsky KE, Wu AW, Landefeld S, et al: Health status versus quality of life in older patients: Does the distinction matter? *Am J Med* 106:435-440, 1999.

Doyle D, Hanks GWC, Macdonald N, eds: *Oxford Textbook of Palliative Medicine*, 2nd ed. Oxford, Oxford University Press, 1998.

Dunn GP. Surgery and palliative medicine: New horizons. *J Palliat Med* 1:215-219, 1998.

Eidelman LA, Jakobson DJ, Pizov R, et al: Foregoing life-sustaining treatment in an Israeli ICU. *Intensive Care Med* 24:162-166, 1998.

Emanuel EJ, Fairclough DL, Slutsman J, et al: Understanding economic and other burdens of terminal illness: The experience of patients and their caregivers. *Ann Intern Med* 132:451-459, 2000.

Fins JJ, Miller FG, Acres CA, et al: End-of-life-decision making in the hospital: Current practice and future prospects. *J Pain Symptom Manage* 17:6-15, 1999.

Goodlin SJ, Winzelberg GS, Teno JM, et al: Death in the hospital. *Arch Intern Med* 158:1570-1572, 1998.

Groeger JS, White P Jr, Nierman DM, et al: Outcome for cancer patients requiring mechanical ventilation. *J Clin Oncol* 17:991-997, 1999.

Hoffman K, Glimelius B: Evaluation of clinical benefit of chemotherapy in patients with upper gastrointestinal cancer. *Acto Oncol* 37:651-659, 1998.

Karlawish JHT, Quill T, Meier DE, for the ACP-ASIM End-of-Life Care Consensus Panel: A consensus-based approach to providing palliative care to patients who lack decision-making capacity. *Ann Intern Med* 130:835-840, 1999.

Kinzbrunner BM: The terminally ill patient. In: Abeloff MD, Armitage JO, Lichter AS, Niederhuber JE, (eds). *Clinical Oncology*, 2nd ed. New York, Churchill Livingstone, 2000.

Klastersky J: Supportive care in oncology. *Bull Mem Acad R Med Belg* 152:10-11, 371-378, 1997.

Leland JY, Schonwetter RS: Advances in hospice care. *Clin Geriatr Med* 13:381-401, 1997.

Maltoni M, Nanni O, Pirovano M, et al: Successful validation of the palliative prognostic score in terminally ill cancer patients. *J Pain Symptom Manage* 17:240-247, 1999.

Miner TJ, Jaques DP, Tavaf-Motamen H, Shriver CD: Decision making on surgical palliation based on patient outcome data. *Am J Surg* 177:150-154, 1999.

Patmaik A, Doyle C, Oza AM: Palliative therapy in advanced ovarian cancer: Balancing patient expectations, quality of life and cost. *Anticancer Drugs* 9:869-878, 1998.

Pirovano M, Maltoni M, Nanni O, et al: A new palliative prognostic score: A first step for the staging of terminally ill cancer patients. Italian Multicenter and Study Group on Palliative Care. *J Pain Symptom Manage* 17:231-239, 1999.

Razavi D: Quality of life: A new end point in patients treated with chemotherapy for advanced cancer. *Topics Support Care* 28:2-3, 1998.

Sabbatini P, Larson SM, Kremer A, et al: Prognostic significance of extent of disease in bone in patients with androgen-independent prostate cancer. *J Clin Oncol* 17:948-957, 1999.

Scott CB: Issues in quality of life assessment during cancer therapy. *Semin Radiat Oncol* 8(suppl 1): 5-9, 1998.

Stephens RJ, Hopwood P, Girling DJ: Defining and analysing symptom palliation in cancer clinical trials: A deceptively difficult exercise. *Br J Cancer* 79:538-544, 1999.

Weeks J: Evaluating palliative therapies for hormone-refractory prostate cancer: Clinical trials and clinical care. In: Perry MC, ed. *American Society of Clincal Oncology*. Fall Educational Book: 1998, pp. 157-158.

Surgery, Endoscopy, and Other Invasive Interventions

Abdel-Wahab M, Gad-Elhak N, Denewer A, et al: Endoscopic laser treatment of progressive dysphagia in patients with advanced esophageal carcinoma. *Hepatogastroenterology* 45:1509-1515, 1998.

Adler DG, Baron TH: Endoscopic palliation of malignant dysphagia. *Mayo Clin Proc* 76:731-738, 2001.

Arnell T, Stamos MJ, Takahashi P, et al: Colonic stents in colorectal obstruction. *Am Surg* 64:986-988, 1998.

Baron TH, Dean PA, Yates MR III, et al: Expandable metal stents for the treatment of colonic obstruction: Techniques and outcomes. *Gastrointest Endosc* 47:277-286, 1998.

Beattie GJ, Smyth JF: Phase I study of intraperitoneal metalloproteinase inhibitor BB94 in patients with malignant ascites. *Clin Cancer Res* 4:1899-1902, 1998.

Binkert CA, Ledermann H, Jost R, et al: Acute colonic obstruction: Clinical aspects and cost-effectiveness of preoperative and palliative treatment with self-expanding metallic stents—a preliminary report. *Radiology* 206:199-204, 1998.

Brune IB, Feussner H, Neuhaus H, et al: Laparoscopic gastrojejunostomy and endoscopic biliary stent placement for palliation of incurable gastric outlet obstruction with cholestasis. *Surg Endosc* 11:834-837, 1997.

Burger JA, Ochs A, Wirth K, et al: The transjugular stent implantation for the treatment of malignant portal and hepatic vein obstruction in cancer patients. *Ann Oncol* 8:200-202, 1997.

Burton AW, Reddy SK, Shah HN, et al: Percutaneous vertebroplasty—A technique to treat refractory spinal pain in the setting of advanced metastatic cancer: A case series. *J Pain Symptom Manage* 30:87-95, 2005.

Campbell WB, Verfaillie P, Ridler BMF, Thompson JF: Non-operative treatment of advanced limb ischemia: The decision for palliative care. *Eur J Vasc Endovasc Surg* 19:246-249, 2000.

Clementsen P, Evald T, Grode G, et al: Treatment of malignant pleural effusion: Pleurodesis using a small percutaneous catheter. A prospective randomized study. *Respir Med* 92:593-596, 1998.

Cwikiel M, Cwikiel W, Albertsson M: Palliation of dysphagia in patients with malignant esophageal strictures. Comparison of results of radiotherapy, chemotherapy and esophageal stent treatment. *Acta Oncol* 35:75-79, 1996.

De Gregorii MA, Mainar A, Tejero E, et al: Acute colorectal obstruction: Stent placement for palliative treatment—Results of a multicenter study. *Radiology* 209:117-120, 1998.

Dohmoto M, Hunerbein M, Schlag PM: Palliative endoscopic therapy of rectal carcinoma. *Eur J Cancer* 32A:25-29, 1996.

Doyle JJ, Hnatiuk OW, Torrington KG, et al: Necessity of routine chest roentgenography after thoracentesis. *Ann Intern Med* 124:816-820, 1996.

Feretis C, Benakis P, Dimopoulos C, et al: Palliation of large-bowel obstruction due to recurrent rectosigmoid tumor using self-expandable endoprostheses. *Endoscopy* 28:319-322, 1996.

Fiocco M, Krasna MJ: The management of malignant pleural and pericardial effusions. *Hematol Oncol Clin North Am* 11:253-265, 1997.

French EJ, Adler DG: Endoscopic therapy for malignant bowel obstruction. *J Support Oncol* 5:303-310, 319, 2007.

Galtanis IN, Hadjipavlou AG, Katonis PG, et al: Balloon kyphoplasty for the treatment of pathological vertebral compression fracture. *Eur Spine J* 14(3):250-260, 2005.

Greillier L, Barlesi F, Doddoli C, et al: Vascular stenting for palliation of superior vena cava obstruction in non-small cell lung cancer patients: A future standard procedure? *Respiration* 71:178-183, 2004.

Gross CM, Kramer J, Waigand J, et al: Stent implantation in patients with superior vena cava syndrome. *Am J Roentgenol* 169:429-432, 1997.

Hirte HW, Miller D, Tonkin D, et al: A randomized trial of paracentesis plus intraperitoneal tumor necrosis factor-α versus paracentesis alone in patients with ascites from recurrent ovarian carcinoma. *Gynecol Oncol* 64:80-87, 1997.

Katayama A, Konishi T, Hiraishi M, et al: A combination of laser therapy, radiation therapy, and stent placement for the palliation of complete malignant bronchial obstruction. *Surg Endosc* 12:1419-1423, 1998.

Kalambokis G, Fotopoulos A, Economou M, et al: Effects of a 7-day treatment with midodrine in non-azotemic cirrhotic patients with and without ascites. *J Hepatol* 46:213-221, 2007.

Kalambokis G, Fotopoulos A, Economou M, et al: Octreotide in the treatment of refractory ascites of cirrhosis. *Scand J Gastroenterol* 41:118-121, 2006.

Kouba E, Wallen EM, Pruthi RS: Management of ureteral obstruction due to advanced malignancy: Optimizing therapeutic and palliative outcomes. *J Urol* 180:444-450, 2008.

Krouse RS: Surgical palliation of bowel obstruction. *Gastroenterol Clin North Am* 35:143-151, 2006.

Ku JH, Lee SW, Jeon HG, et al: Percutaneous nephrostomy versus indwelling ureteral stents in the management of extrinsic ureteral obstruction in advanced malignancies: Are there differences? *Urology* 64:895, 2004.

Ledie JT, Renfroe MB: Kyphoplasty treatment of vertebral fractures: 2-year outcomes show sustained benefits. *Spine* 31(1):57-64, 2006.

Lee BH, Choe DH, Lee JH, et al: Metallic stents in malignant biliary obstruction: Prospective long-term clinical results. *AJR Am J Roentgenol* 168:741-745, 1997.

Lee CW, Bociek G, Faught W: A survey of practice in management of malignant ascites. *J Pain Symptom Manage* 16:96-101, 1998.

Malawer MM, Buch RG, Thompson WE, Sugarbaker PH: Major amputations done with palliative intent in the treatment of local bony complications associated with advanced cancer. *J Surg Oncol* 47:121-130, 1991.

Mares DC, Mathur PN: Medical thoracoscopic talc pleurodesis for chylothorax due to lymphoma: A case series. *Chest* 114:731-735, 1998.

McNamara P, Sharma K: Surgery or palliation for hip fractures in patients with advanced malignancy? *Age Ageing* 26:471-474, 1997.

Mentzer SJ: Surgical palliative care in thoracic disease. *Surg Clin North Am* 85:315-328, 2005.

Nicholson AA, Ettles DF, Arnold A, et al: Treatment of malignant superior vena cava obstruction: Metal stents or radiation therapy. *J Vasc Interv Radiol* 8:781-788, 1997.

Old JL, Calvert M: Vertebral compression fractures in the elderly. *Am Fam Physician* 69:111-116, 2004.

O'Sullivan GJ, Grundy A: Palliation of malignant dysphagia with expanding metallic stents. *J Vasc Interv Radiol* 10:346-351, 1999.

Patz EF Jr: Malignant pleural effusions: Recent advances and ambulatory sclerotherapy. *Chest* 113 (Suppl):74S-77S, 1998.

Paz IB: Major palliative amputations. *Surg Oncol Clin North Am* 13:543-547, 2004.

Pereira-Lima JC, Jakobs R, Maier M, et al: Endoscopic biliary stenting for the palliation of pancreatic cancer: Results, survival predictive factors, and comparison of 10-French with 11.5 French gauge stents. *Am J Gastroenterol* 91:2179-2184, 1996.

Ponec RJ, Kimmey MB: Endoscopic therapy of esophageal cancer. *Surg Clin North Am* 77:1197-1217, 1997.

Ponn RB, Silverman HJ, Federico JA: Outpatient chest tube management. *Ann Thorac Surg* 64:1437-1440, 1997.

Prat F, Chapat O, Ducot B, et al: A randomized trial of endoscopic drainage methods for inoperable malignant strictures of the common bile duct. *Gastrointest Endosc* 47:1-7, 1998.

Prat F, Chapat O, Ducot B, et al: Predictive factors for survival of patients with inoperable malignant distal biliary strictures: A practical management guideline. *Gut* 42:76-80, 1998.

Pulsiripunya C, Youngchaiyud P, Pushpakon R, et al: The efficacy of doxycycline as a pleural sclerosing agent in malignant pleural effusion: A prospective study. *Respirology* 1:69-72, 1996.

Raikar GV, Melin MM, Ress A, et al: Cost-effective analysis of surgical versus endoscopic stenting in the management of unresectable pancreatic cancer. *Ann Surg Oncol* 3:470-475, 1996.

Rogan M: *Porfimer Sodium Phototherapy for Obstructing Endobronchial Non-small Cell Lung Cancer. Photofrin Prescribing Information.* New York, Sanofi Pharmaceutical, Inc., 1999.

Runyon BA: Treatment of patients with cirrhosis and ascites. *Semin Liver Dis* 17:249-260, 1997.

Ryan JM, Hahn PF, Mueller PR: Performing radiologic gastrostomy or gastrojejunostomy in patients with malignant ascites. *Am J Roentgenol* 171:1003-1006, 1998.

Sargeant IR, Tobias JS, Blackman G, et al: Radiotherapy enhances laser palliation of malignant dysphagia: A randomised study. *Gut* 40:362-369, 1997.

Savin M, Kirsch MJ, Romano WJ, et al: Peritoneal ports for treatment of intractable ascites. *J Vasc Interv Radiol* 16:363-368, 2005.

Schmidbauer J, Kratzik C, Klingler HC, et al: Nephrovesical subcutaneous ureteric bypass: Long-term results in patients with advanced metastatic disease—improvement of renal function and quality of life. *Eur Urol* 50:1073, 2006.

Segreti EM, Morris M, Levenback C, et al: Transverse colon urinary diversion in gynecologic oncology. *Gynecol Oncol* 63:66-70, 1996.

Shah R, Sabanathan S, Lowe RA, Mearns AJ: Stenting in malignant obstruction of superior vena cava. *J Thorac Cardiovasc Surg* 112:335-340, 1996.

Shekarriz B, Shekarriz H, Upadhyay J, et al: Outcome of palliative urinary diversion in the treatment of advanced malignancies. *Cancer* 85:998-1003, 1999.

Shiraishi T, Kawahara K, Shirakusa T, et al: Stenting for airway obstruction in the carinal region. *Ann Thorac Surg* 66:1925-1929, 1998.

Shumate CR, Baron TH: Palliative procedures for pancreatic cancer: When and which one? *South Med J* 89:27-32, 1996.

Siersema PD, Dees, van Blankenstein M: Palliation of malignant dysphagia from oesophageal cancer. Rotterdam Oesophageal Tumor Study Group. *Scand J Gastroenterol Suppl* 225:75-84, 1998.

Smith GS, Barnard GF: Massive volume paracentesis (up to 41 liters) for the outpatient management of ascites. *J Clin Gastroenterol* 25:402-403, 1997.

Sonett JR: Endobronchial stents: Primary and adjuvant therapy for endobronchial airway obstruction. *Md Med J* 47:260-263, 1998.

Tham TC, Carr-Locke DL, Vandervoort J, et al: Management of occluded biliary Wallstents. *Gut* 42:703-707, 1998.

Tsang TS, Freeman WK, Sinak LJ, Seward JB: Echocardiographically guided pericardiocentesis: Evolution and state-of-the-art technique. *Mayo Clin Proc* 73:647-652, 1998.

Wickremesekera SK, Stubbs RS: Peritoneovenous shunting for malignant ascites. *N Z Med J* 110:33-35, 1997.

Wilkins HE III, Cacioppo J, Connolly MM, et al: Intrapericardial interferon in the management of malignant pericardial effusion. *Chest* 114:330-331, 1998.

Wilkinson SP: Treatment options for cirrhotic ascites. *Eur J Gastorenterol Hepatol* 10:1-3, 1998.

Antibiotics

Clayton J, Fardell B, Hutton-Potts J, et al: Parenteral antibiotics in a palliative care unit: Prospective analysis of current practice. *Pall Med* 17:44-48, 2003.

Grossman RF: The value of antibiotics and the outcomes of antibiotic therapy in exacerbations of COPD. *Chest* 113(suppl 4):249S-255S, 1998.

Pereira J, Watanabe S, Wolch G: A retrospective review of the frequency of infections and patterns of antibiotic utilization on a palliative care unit. *J Pain Symptom Manage* 16:374-381, 1998.

Robinson WM, Ravilly S, Berde C, Wohl ME: End-of-life care in cystic fibrosis. *Pediatrics* 100:205-209, 1997.

Transfusions and Hematopoietic Growth Factors

Adamson JW: Epoietin alfa: Into the new millennium. *Semin Oncol* 25(suppl 7):76-79, 1998.

Drüeke TB, Locatelli F, Clyne N, et al: Normalization of hemoglobin level in patients with chronic kidney disease and anemia. *N Engl J Med* 355:2071-2084, 2006.

Coyle TE: Hematologic complications of human immunodeficiency virus infection and the acquired immunodeficiency syndrome. *Med Clin North Am* 81:449-470, 1997.

Geissler RG, Schulte P, Ganser A: Clinical use of hematopoietic growth factors in patients with myelodysplastic syndromes. *Int J Hematol* 65:339-354, 1997.

Griggs JJ, Blumberg N: Recombinant erythropoietin and blood transfusions in cancer chemotherapy-induced anemia. *Anticancer Drugs* 9:925-932, 1998.

Harper SE, Tendler C: Important drug warning. Subject: Additional trials showing increased mortality and/or tumor progression with epogen, procrit, and aranesp. http://www.fda.gov/medwAtch/safety/2008/epo_DHCP_03102008.pdf, published 3/7/08. Accessed February 11, 2009.

Herter J: Hematopoietic supportive care. *Clin Cancer Res* 3:2666-2670, 1997.

Lindholm E, Daneryd P, Korner U, et al: Effects of recombinant erythropoietin in palliative treatment of unselected cancer patients. *Clin Cancer Res* 10:6855-6864, 2004.

Martinson U, Lundstrom S: The use of blood transfusions and erythropoietin-stimulating agents in Swedish palliative care. *Support Care Cancer* 17:19-203, 2009.

Osterweil N: Higher hemoglobin targets for chronic kidney disease linked to heart complications. MedPage Today, http://www.medpagetoday.com/ProductAlert/Prescriptions/4540, Published November 16, 2006. Accessed February 11, 2009.

Peck P: Black box warning ordered for aranesp, epogen, and procrit. MedPage Today, http://www.medpagetoday.com/ProductAlert/Prescriptions/5231, Published March 9, 2007. Accessed February 11, 2009.

Remuzzi G, Ingelfinger JR: Correction of anemia—payoffs and problems. *N Engl J Med* 355:2144-2146, 2006.

Singh AK, Szczech L,. Tang KL, et al: Correction of anemia with epoetin alfa in chronic kidney disease. *N Engl J Med* 355:2085-2098, 2006.

Stockelberg D, Lehtola P, Noren I: Palliative treatment at home for patients with haematological disorders. *Support Care Cancer* 5:506-508, 1997.

Thomas G, Ali S, Hoebers F, et al: Phase III trial to evaluate the efficacy of maintaining hemoglobin levels above 120 g/dL with erythropoietin vs above 100 g/dL without erythropoietin in anemic patients receiving concurrent radiation and cisplatin for cervical cancer. *Gynecol Oncol* 108:317-325, 2008.

SELF-ASSESSMENT QUESTIONS

1. When considering whether to treat a terminally ill patient with an invasive palliative intervention, which of the following characteristics is LEAST important factor to take into account?

    A. What does the patient want?

    B. Does the intervention have a high probability of efficacy?

    C. What does the physician want?

    D. What are the potential toxicities of the intervention?

    E. What is the life expectancy of the patient?

2. You are caring for a patient on your hospice program with a diagnosis of advanced dementia. She is 93 years old, unresponsive, bed bound, and receives her nourishment by a PEG feeding tube. She is lying in bed comfortably in the long-term care facility where she lives, with no evidence of shortness of breath or tachycardia. However, routine laboratory studies done by the facility shows that she has a hemoglobin level of 8 g/dL. What would be the most appropriate next step in the patient's management?

    A. Transfuse the patient with 2 units of packed red blood cells.

    B. Start the patient on erythropoietin to increase her hemoglobin to 10 g/dL.

    C. Check stools for occult blood, and do a GI work-up if positive.

    D. Request a consultation with a hematologist.

    E. Do not transfuse or work-up and discontinue the routine blood work.

3. You are caring for a 79-year-old male with end-stage cardiac disease on vasodilators and large doses of diuretics. He has been an insulin-dependent diabetic for many years and has a history of cirrhosis secondary to alcohol. His 78-year-old spouse, who is his primary caregiver, has reported that over the

last several days he has been having periods of mental confusion. In looking for potentially correctable causes of the patient's altered mental status, which of the following laboratory results would be LEAST likely in this patient?

    A. Elevated serum calcium

    B. Elevated BUN

    C. Elevated serum ammonia level

    D. Low blood glucose

    E. Low serum sodium

4. Which of the following end-of-life care patients would be LEAST likely to benefit from surgical repair of a femoral fracture?

    A. A 75-year-old female with refractory metastatic breast cancer to the bone who fell while shopping and has a life expectancy of 4 to 6 months.

    B. An 80-year-old female with far advanced dementia who has been bed bound for 2 years due to her neurological condition and has a life expectancy of 1 to 2 months.

    C. A 78-year-old female with advanced chronic obstructive lung disease on steroids who can ambulate only short distances due to her dyspnea and has a life expectancy of 6 to 8 months.

    D. A 74-year-old male with advanced Parkinson disease who can only ambulate with the assistance and the support of a walker and has a life expectancy of 3 to 4 months.

5. All of the following characteristics are associated with patients who should NOT be considered for palliative amputation EXCEPT:

    A. History of a prior stroke

    B. Significant heart disease

    C. The presence of dry gangrene

    D. Life expectancy of more than 3 months

    E. Performance status less than 50%

6. Which of the following is the most serious complication of expandable stents utilized to palliate large bowel obstruction?

A. Pseudo-obstruction due to fecal impaction
B. Occlusive tumor growth into the stent lumen
C. Perforation
D. Rectal bleeding
E. Abdominal pain

7. All of the following are true regarding the use of PDT to palliate an obstruction, EXCEPT:

A. The patient is treated with a hematoporphyrin derivative
B. The light source that the tumor is exposed to comes from an Nd-YAG laser.
C. It is most useful for the treatment of exophytic lesions
D. It may relieve obstruction caused by tumor ingrowth into expandable metal stents.
E. Patients must avoid sunlight exposure and fluorescent light for more than 1 month following treatment.

8. You are treating a 67-year-old male on your hospice program, who has terminal lung cancer. His major symptom is dyspnea, related to a large left pleural effusion for which a thoracentesis, without sclerotherapy, was done prior to hospice admission. He is being admitted to the hospice inpatient unit for repeat thoracentesis. He has expressed a desire to return home as soon as possible and does not want to have any more thoracenteses after this one, nor does he want to return to the hospice inpatient unit. All of the following statements regarding management options following thoracentesis for this patient are true EXCEPT:

A. If he has a short life expectancy, he could be sent home with a small, indwelling pleural catheter.
B. Doxycycline sclerotherapy has about 90% success rate for at least 3 months following instillation.

C. Side effects of doxycycline sclerotherapy include pain, fever, and cough.
D. Talc sclerotherapy is safe, effective, and easy to administer.
E. The dose of bleomycin used for sclerotherapy must be adjusted if patients have renal insufficiency.

9. You are treating a 73-year-old female with advanced colorectal carcinoma and liver metastases. She is complaining of abdominal distention secondary to progressive malignant ascites. All of the following statements regarding the treatment of her ascites are true EXCEPT:

A. Diuretics and fluid restriction have about a 90% chance of successfully controlling her ascites.
B. Plasma expanders are generally not needed following paracentesis.
C. An implanted port-a-cath device may be useful if she requires frequent paracenteses.
D. Sclerotherapy with doxycycline is effective in less than one-third of patients.
E. A peritoneovenous shunt may be beneficial if she requires frequent paracenteses and has a life expectancy of at least several months.

10. Based on a recently reported study regarding the use of antibiotics in a palliative care unit, which of the following groups were commonly observed to have positive outcomes from antibiotic therapy?

A. Patients who were actively deteriorating.
B. Patients with infections of the lower respiratory tract.
C. Patients with urinary tract infections.
D. Patients who were in an acute phase of illness.
E. Patients with infections of skin or soft tissue.

Palliative Chemotherapy and Radiation Therapy

James M. Sinclair, Gaurav Mathur, and Neal J. Weinreb

PART 1
PALLIATIVE CHEMOTHERAPY

INTRODUCTION

Currently, there are more than 100 individual chemotherapeutic drugs approved by the United States Food and Drug Administration for use in the "war on cancer." These include cytotoxins of multiple biochemical classes, hormonally active agents, cytokines, targeted agents, vaccines, and monoclonal antibodies, as well as cytoprotective drugs to prevent or reduce toxicity, and adjunctive medications intended to boost the efficacy of the primary chemotherapeutic agents. Unfortunately, despite continued improvements in screening, locoregional control, and adjuvant therapy, which have translated into higher cure rates and greater survival, recurrent metastatic disease still occurs commonly, and, when it does, it usually results in a fatal outcome.

Therefore, many patients with advanced cancer, especially when disease continues to progress in the face of standard therapies, are faced with the difficult decision as to whether they should choose to continue to receive cytotoxic chemotherapy to attempt to prolong the length of life and/or to try to preserve quality of life (QOL). As palliation of symptoms can often occur with aggressive supportive care, which has less toxicity than cytotoxic chemotherapy, prolongation of survival is usually the primary reason that most patients with advanced cancers decide to continue to receive cytotoxic treatment. In fact, studies have shown that, contrary to previous findings based on physicians' self-report data, health-related QOL considerations currently play a relatively minor role in decisions regarding modification or discontinuation of palliative chemotherapy. As counseling patients with incurable cancer about the risks and benefits of additional therapy is one of the most challenging tasks

in the practice of oncology, some oncologists, may present a subjective estimation of survival based on their personal experience, rather than on any specific scientific data resulting in both physicians and patients maintaining an overly optimistic belief in the value of palliative chemotherapy to avoid death anxiety and maintain a sense of control over cancer. That this is true is borne out by recent studies that suggest that patients with advanced cancer may be overtreated in their last months of life, likely due to this highly desirable, but usually unattainable goal of life prolongation.

Notwithstanding the extensive armamentarium described above, for most cancers, patients with metastatic disease are essentially incurable, with disease progression leading to symptomatic morbidity and inevitable death. Consequently, with a few notable exceptions such as testicular carcinoma, Hodgkin disease, some forms of non-Hodgkin lymphoma, and the acute leukemias, current treatments for metastatic cancer should be regarded as palliative therapy with some ability to prolong life in certain tumor types.

Patients with advanced metastatic malignancy usually experience multiple progressive symptoms including nociceptive and neuropathic pain, fatigue, anxiety, bowel irregularity, depression, malaise, anorexia, nausea, dysphagia, breathlessness, and cough. Curiously, however, as judged from the contents of most published reports, clinical trial design has traditionally ignored symptom relief as a therapeutic endpoint, concentrating instead on analyses of objective measurable tumor response or prolongation of life. In fact, although these latter endpoints are scientifically significant to physician investigators, they are less important to patients than the effect of treatment on symptoms and QOL. For example, in a study where patients with cancer were given the hypothetical choice between receiving supportive care or chemotherapy, 22% of the patients said they would opt for chemotherapy for a potential survival benefit of 3 months, whereas 68% of the patients said they would choose chemotherapy if it substantially reduced symptoms even if there was no potential prolongation of life.

In many randomized studies, the survival of patients in the treatment arm is compared with a matched cohort of patients who receive "best supportive care," a concept, which usually includes antibiotics, analgesics, transfusions, corticosteroids, or any other symptomatic therapy including psychotherapy. Few studies indicate how this supportive care is standardized as "best." One study, for example, defines "best supportive care" as "the best care available as judged by the attending physician, according to institutional standards for each center." In light of published surveys in which even medical oncologists acknowledge that pain and symptom management in patients with cancer continues to be suboptimal, it is disturbing to note how infrequently details of symptom management and response are provided for both treatment and "best supportive care" groups in published clinical trials. Furthermore, few trials, including those in which QOL is assessed, control for the effect of adjunctive treatments such as antiemetics, corticosteroids, and hematopoietic growth factors, which are commonly offered to chemotherapy patients. In addition, these studies often fail to control for the difference in patient/health care professional contacts between the treatment group, who may go to the doctor's office or outpatient department to receive a weekly injection or infusion, and the "best supportive care" patients, who may only see the professional at the time of the monthly data gathering visit common to both groups of patients. Lack of control for these factors, which could by themselves affect patient well-being and hence, patient survival, must raise serious questions as to the validity of these studies, which often demonstrate very modest, but statistically significant, survival advantages for the patients receiving chemotherapy.

The emphasis on objective tumor response and survival analysis rather than on symptom improvement has created another paradox. To detect small, but statistically significant differences in survival, and, in an effort to minimize the incidence of life-threatening toxicity, most clinical trials in advanced metastatic disease exclude patients with poor performance status, those who are sickest, most symptomatic, and therefore, in greatest need of palliative intervention. For example, a study of irinotecan in patients with far advanced colorectal carcinoma excluded patients with bulky liver or lung metastases, large abdominal masses, or unresolved bowel obstruction. Logically, one would anticipate that a truly effective palliative treatment would have the greatest effect on patients with the most severe symptoms. Obviously, the fear of causing toxic side effects that would negatively influence the quality of remaining life must be a valid and important concern in terminally ill patients, and analysis of toxicity is a vital component of any legitimate palliative study. It is possible that entering patients with poor performance status could interfere with response rate or survival benefits that could interfere with desired drug approval. However, arbitrary exclusion of patients with poor performance status and severe symptomatology creates the possibility that these patients will either be denied access to treatment, which may have palliative benefit and relatively low risk of toxicity, or, conversely, will be exposed to treatment that could cause undue toxicity without symptomatic benefit, as the therapy, while effective in a group of patients with relatively good performance and a low symptom burden, was never tested in this patient population.

Recently, outcomes related to symptom control and QOL assessment are being incorporated into oncology clinical trials. It is generally assumed that unrelieved and increasing patient discomfort and disability translates into an ever-worsening QOL. Conversely, symptom relief and functional improvement should logically be associated with higher QOL scores. However, as previously pointed out, the correlation between control of symptoms and QOL is frequently weak or, on occasions, nonexistent. Therefore, good study design should incorporate both elements of symptom outcomes and QOL measurement. One measure of symptomatic improvement is termed the "clinical benefit response" (see Table 19–1). This is defined as a significant, sustained

TABLE 19–1. "Clinical Benefit" Response to Chemotherapy

- Sustained improvement in pain
  - Decreased pain with no change in analgesia
  - Same level of pain with less analgesia
- Improvement in performance status
- Stabilization or improvement in weight

improvement in pain, performance status, weight, or other relevant symptom, with no deterioration in other symptoms. In assessing pain responses, for example, decreasing opioid usage or a step-down on the WHO analgesic ladder is often used as an important end point and scored as a significant success. However, although the correlation between decrease in analgesic use correlates with decreased pain and increased function and well-being may be a useful and significant outcome and a good proxy measure for improved pain control, the decrease in opioid use should not be the primary goal unless the patient has significant opioid side effects that are worse than the side effects of the palliative chemotherapy. Preoccupation with analgesic dose reduction as an independent end point may inadvertently contribute to fueling "opiophobia," the unwarranted fear of using opioids, which has proven to be such an obstacle in achieving good pain management, particularly at the end of life.

A number of reports have been published demonstrating a clinical benefit for chemotherapy for patients with a variety of advanced, end-stage malignancies. Nevertheless, surveys indicate that a significant proportion of physicians recommend only supportive care for patients with widespread metastatic disease, expecting that patients will have a short but peaceful end to their life, protected from the side effects of chemotherapy. Obviously, chemotherapy is not for every patient. Selection should be performed carefully to spare patients who have little chance to benefit from chemotherapy from exposure to side effects of ineffective treatments. However, as suggested in the studies below, palliative chemotherapy may sometimes add significantly to patient comfort, even at the end of life.

BRONCHOGENIC CARCINOMA

Many symptoms and manifestations of advanced lung cancer are directly attributable to defined anatomical metastases. Examples include somatic pain caused by discrete bone metastases or chest wall invasion, neuropathic pain associated with plexopathies, intractable coughing and hemoptysis attributable to endobronchial tumors, headache and changes in mentation caused by superior vena cava (SVC) syndrome or brain metastases, and dyspnea caused by malignant pleural effusions. Because locoregional interventions such as radiotherapy are the procedures of choice for palliating such symptoms, systemic chemotherapy is rarely reported in terms of its success in alleviating specific manifestations of metastatic disease. Rather, palliative chemotherapy is usually described in terms of the ability to improve QOL, a parameter that does not always reference specific symptoms such as generalized pain, fatigue, dyspnea, anorexia, wasting, anxiety, and depression.

SMALL CELL BRONCHOGENIC CARCINOMA

For patients with small cell bronchogenic carcinoma, however, even in those with extensive disease, systemic chemotherapy may be of significant palliative benefit. With first-line therapy, well-documented response rates of greater than 50% have been observed in most studies, with improvement in symptoms and QOL for most patients. Corresponding substantial increases in symptom-free survival suggest that most patients with small cell lung cancer who are started on de novo chemotherapy should not be thought of, or regard themselves, as recipients of end-of-life care. On the other hand, when patients with small cell lung cancer relapse after initial therapy, as, unfortunately, usually occurs, second-line chemotherapy is rarely of objective palliative benefit. However, when there has been an interval of at least several months between cessation of the primary treatment and relapse, reinstitution of the initial chemotherapy regimen, or treatment with oral etoposide and parenteral irinotecan sometimes is associated with temporary tumor regression and improvement in symptoms.

NON–SMALL CELL BRONCHOGENIC CARCINOMA

For the 75% of lung patients with cancer who have non–small cell histology, chemotherapy trials with newer regimens incorporating agents such as cisplatin, carboplatin, gemcitabine, paclitaxel, docetaxel, pemetrexed, erlotinib, bevacizumab, and vinorelbine, show 1-year survival rates of 35% to 40% in patients with stage IV disease. Most oncologists recommend a trial of doublet chemotherapy such as gemcitabine with cisplatin, carboplatin with paclitaxel, cisplatin with docetaxel, or cisplatin with vinorelbine for patients with good performance status. Unfortunately there is little to no palliative benefit data in trials using these doublets. Although these combinations are considered the standard of care, the question remains open whether the modest increase in survival is associated with sufficient clinical benefit to justify the side effects and toxicity of treatment. Therefore, there are a significant number of physicians, from a variety of specialties including primary care, pulmonary medicine, medical oncology, radiation oncology, and thoracic surgery, who recommend only supportive care for patients with advanced stage IV non–small cell lung cancer, especially if the patient has a poor performance status and/or suffers from a significant symptom burden.

Although the data are far from definitive, some studies have suggested that QOL may be improved for patients with metastatic disease as well as those with unresectable stage III disease who are treated with combination chemotherapy. However, a meta-analysis based on 11 randomized controlled trials involving 1,190 patients published in 1997 reported that not one trial successfully measured QOL using QOL assessment instruments. Several chemotherapy trials have documented relief of cancer-related symptoms such as pain, cough, and hemoptysis in most treated patients, although the outcomes of these trials must be taken with a grain of salt as, in all but one of these trials, patients with poor performance status were excluded to spare them treatment-related toxicity. In one study where elderly patients and those with poor performance status were included, a modest clinical benefit was reported in some patients.

Single-agent palliative chemotherapy with weekly vinorelbine has provided modest positive results, with about 25% to 40% of patients reporting improvements in either performance status or a variety of cancer-related symptoms such as cough, hemoptysis, dyspnea, and pain. In this study, more patients benefited from chemotherapy than was suggested by the objective response rate, suggesting that symptom palliation may not be dependent on demonstrated tumor regression. Erlotinib, an oral agent that targets epidermal growth factor receptor, has significant toxicity and little data supporting its palliative benefit in lung cancer.

In summary, as there is an increase in the attention being paid to symptom relief as a measured outcome in advanced bronchogenic non–small cell carcinoma, there may be a limited role for palliative chemotherapy in selected patients with a good performance status who are near the end of life.

BREAST AND PROSTATE CARCINOMA

These two very prevalent cancers share some characteristics that are of significance in end-of-life care. When patients with either of these malignancies present with advanced metastatic disease, many of them can achieve dramatic symptomatic relief, disease regression, and prolongation of life through the use of relatively nontoxic hormonal treatments.

Another shared characteristic is that patients with systemic breast and prostate carcinoma may have long, chronic courses, particularly when disease is restricted to osseous metastases. Effective palliative interventions, such as radiotherapy and bisphosphonates, are therefore frequently employed in both diseases even at a time well before the patient is close to the end of life, and their effects are well known and reliable for palliation of symptoms at the end stage of disease as well.

Breast and prostate carcinoma differ, of course, in their sensitivity to currently available cytotoxic agents, which are usually regarded primarily as life-prolonging tools, and, therefore, their role purely for the purpose of symptom palliation is rarely reported.

BREAST CANCER

Multiple chemotherapeutic drugs are active as single agents or in combination for the treatment of metastatic breast cancer. The most common "classic" combinations include cyclophosphamide, doxorubicin, and 5-FU (fluorouracil) (60% response rate), and cyclophosphamide, methotrexate, and 5-FU (40% response rate). Other chemotherapeutic drugs that have activity include docetaxel, vinorelbine, paclitaxel, gemcitabine, epirubicin, carboplatin, bevacizumab, ixabepilone, mitoxantrone, albumin-bound nanoparticle paclitaxel, liposomal doxorubicin, vincristine, vinblastine, infusional 5-FU, and an oral 5-FU analog, capecitabine. In 25% of breast cancer that is HER-2/neu positive trastuzumab, lapatinib, alone or in combination with chemotherapy offer an improved survival and/or tumor response. Although most patients with advanced metastatic breast cancer are treated with several sequential regimens before being judged to have chemotherapy-refractory disease, there is little information about how effective these treatments are in alleviating symptoms. There is a study, however, supporting a role for capecitabine as a palliative agent for patients with breast cancer who are refractory to anthracyclines and paclitaxel, reporting a positive clinical benefit in 20% of the patients treated, whereas an additional 30% of patients experienced stabilization of their clinical condition.

PROSTATE CANCER

In contrast to breast cancer, androgen-independent prostate carcinoma tends to be refractory to treatment. Second-line hormonal therapy, chemotherapy (single agent or combination), or various investigational therapies such as monoclonal antibodies have not produced durable remissions. However, some chemotherapy regimens have been described as having palliative benefit. In a randomized trial comparing mitoxantrone/prednisone combination (M + P) to prednisone alone, 29% of patients receiving M + P had a positive response, defined as a two-point or greater decrease in pain intensity on a six-point pain scale, lasting for a minimum of 6 weeks. Twelve percent of the patients treated with prednisone alone had a similar response ($P = 0.011$). Other patients had stable pain intensity but were able to reduce their analgesic consumption by at least 50%. Docetaxel has been compared to mitoxantrone in hormone refractory prostate cancer and demonstrates a better overall survival and better QOL. Unfortunately, these studies do not compare the palliative efficacy of the chemotherapeutic agents or prednisone to alternative interventions for bone pain, such as radiotherapy or radioisotopes. Other agents that have been shown to produce subjective improvements in symptoms (as well as reduction in prostate-specific antigen levels) include paclitaxel, estramustine, etoposide, vinblastine, and the combination of estramustine and paclitaxel.

PANCREATIC CARCINOMA

Until recently, chemotherapy was considered ineffective in pancreatic cancer. In recent years, however, there are data suggesting that various chemotherapeutic agents may improve physical symptoms of patients with advanced disease.

In a single comparative study of patients with advanced pancreatic cancer, gemcitabine was found to be more effective than fluorouracil with respect to survival duration and general clinical status. More significantly, this investigation fostered the development of the methodology for assessing clinical benefit as described earlier in this chapter and as illustrated in Table 19–1. The outcome of gemcitabine therapy in more than 3,000 patients with advanced pancreatic cancer (80% stage IV disease) demonstrated clinical benefit in 18.4% of treated patients after approximately 20 weeks of therapy, as compared with an objective tumor response rate of 12%. The median survival was 4.8 months and the 12-month survival was 15%. Treatment was discontinued in only 5% of patients because of adverse reactions. Although the study lacked a true control group, the investigators claimed that these results indicated notable disease-related symptom improvement, especially in light of the heretofore refractory nature of advanced pancreatic carcinoma to standard treatment. The study also did not address other symptoms or manifestations of pancreatic carcinoma such as obstruction, jaundice, and pruritus. Based on this study, gemcitabine was approved by the US Food and Drug Administration for the palliative treatment of advanced pancreatic carcinoma.

COLORECTAL CARCINOMA

Conventional palliative chemotherapy for advanced colorectal cancer has, by and large been restricted to fluorouracil and related agents, often in combination with leucovorin (folinic acid). This combination has been reported to lead to improved QOL in treated patients compared with those treated with "supportive care." Recent studies utilizing irinotecan and oxaliplatin in fluorouracil refractory patients have suggested that patients receiving either agent had a longer survival, fewer tumor-related symptoms, and a better QOL than those treated with supportive care alone. Hepatic intra-arterial chemotherapy with 5-FUDR may alleviate discomfort in some patients with extensive liver metastases.

Bevacizumab, cetuximab, and panitumumab have activity in metastatic colon cancer but no published palliative benefits.

OTHER MALIGNANCIES

In patients with advanced transitional cell carcinoma of the urinary tract who had previously received cisplatin, therapy with gemcitabine provided subjective symptomatic relief from pain, cystitis, dysuria, hematuria, and peripheral edema. Toxicity was reported as mild and consisted of influenza-like symptoms and myelosuppression. The median survival was 5 months.

Gemcitabine is also reported to have activity in patients with refractory germ cell tumors. However, the published reports have no information on symptom response or QOL.

Frail, elderly patients with refractory anemia with excess blasts in transformation or with overt acute myelocytic leukemia are extremely difficult to manage. Most of these patients do poorly with intensive induction chemotherapy. Aside from symptoms due to anemia, which can be managed with red blood cell transfusions, patients often suffer from recurrent infections and from bleeding complications. Life expectancy with supportive care only is usually 1 to 2 months. However, in one study, most patients who received a weekly regimen of low-dose cytosine arabinoside and thioguanine for at least 6 to 10 weeks became independent of platelet and red blood cell transfusions for periods up to 2 years. The treatment was well tolerated and suitable for outpatient palliation.

CONCLUSIONS ON THE ROLE OF PALLIATIVE CHEMOTHERAPY NEAR THE END OF LIFE

An objective assessment of the studies presented above is admittedly somewhat deflating. Not a single study revealed a truly dramatic reversal in symptoms, although such an expectation is undoubtedly unrealistic for patients with such advanced disease. There is now evidence that physicians and patients maintain overly optimistic beliefs in the value of palliative chemotherapy to avoid death anxiety and maintain a sense of control over cancer. Nevertheless, as increased attention is concentrated on the effects of chemotherapy on palliation of symptoms, a clearer picture should emerge as to those circumstances in which it will contribute to overall patient comfort at the end of life. Although one must remain cautious, the data suggest that chemotherapy may, at times, be an appropriate palliative intervention for specific patients

with specific malignancies. It is incumbent upon the hospice and palliative care teams who offer such palliative chemotherapy to ensure that the goals of therapy are clearly defined, for themselves as well as for the patient and family. Palliation of symptoms can often be accomplished with aggressive supportive care with less toxicity and greater efficacy than chemotherapy. All concerned must also have the ability, resources, and willingness to treat toxic side effects in a manner consistent with the overall needs and desires of the patient.

PART 2
PALLIATIVE RADIATION THERAPY

INTRODUCTION

Compared to chemotherapy, the role of radiation therapy in palliative care is well established. When pain, bleeding, or symptoms of obstruction are attributable to a localized malignant lesion, appropriately delivered radiation therapy can provide effective symptom control. When considering utilizing palliative radiation therapy for patients near the end of life, hospice and palliative clinicians should always be mindful of the principles of invasive therapies outlined in Chapter 18, as these factors can play a critical role in determining the efficacy of the intervention for the specific patient being treated.

OVERVIEW OF RADIATION THERAPY

Radiation therapy is used in a variety of tumor settings. Its major effect is through the destruction of tumor cell DNA. This occurs when ionizing radiation, such as a beam of photons, strikes the genetic material in the cell nucleus. This genetic damage causes cancer cells to reproduce more slowly, or not at all. If the genetic damage is sufficient, the cell may be killed by the radiation itself. Cancer cells are more susceptible to radiation because they are constantly reproducing (S-phase), and the DNA tends to be more vulnerable during this phase. In addition, cancer cells are often unable to repair the damage the way healthy cells can through polymerases and related enzymes.

Radiation has historically been delivered in one of two ways. Brachytherapy is a form of radiation therapy in which a radioactive source is placed inside or near an area requiring treatment. It is commonly used to treat head and neck cancers, prostate, and cervical cancers. In external beam radiotherapy (EBRT), a linear accelerator creates a high-energy beam of subatomic particles. The radiation beams are aimed from several angles of exposure to intersect at the tumor, providing a much larger absorbed dose than in the surrounding healthy tissue. Minimizing damage to the healthy tissue is important both in preventing side effects as well as preventing new tumor development. In addition to the traditional approach to delivering EBRT via a linear accelerator, there are newer techniques, which include stereotactic radiosurgery (or cyberknife radiosurgery) and gamma knife radiosurgery. What sets these technologies apart from traditional EBRT is a more precise target area through technologies such as magnetic resonance imaging (MRI) and computed tomography scanning. Gamma knife radiosurgery, for example, has been used with good results in brain tumors whose radiation field might be too large for traditional EBRT.

Radiation is measured in Gray (Gy), a standard international unit. A Gray is the absorption of one joule of ionizing radiation by 1 kg of matter. The total dose is the total amount of radiation to be delivered into the patient's body. A typical curative total dose for a solid tumor might be in the range of 60 to 80 Gy. Total doses in palliative radiotherapy are generally much less. In curative radiotherapy, the total dose cannot be administered

all at once, as such a dose would be extremely toxic, and in many cases lethal. Instead, the total dose is divided into fractions, smaller doses spread out over time. This is important for several reasons. It allows healthy cells time to repair cellular radiation damage, although tumor cells are often unable to do so, making them more susceptible to the next fraction. Fractionation also allows tumor cells that were in a radioresistant phase of the cell cycle during one treatment to cycle into a sensitive phase before the next fraction is given. Also, some tumor cells are chronically hypoxic due to lack of blood supply. These hypoxic tumor cells are more radioresistant but may reoxygenate between fractions, thus becoming susceptible to radiation by the next fraction.

Assessment, evaluation, and treatment is performed and supervised by a radiation oncologist, a physician with specialized training in radiation delivery. Generally, the patient is seen in the office for an evaluation and then scheduled for radiation therapy treatment planning or simulation. The patient lies in an appropriate position on the linear accelerator, and markings are made on the skin to identify the exact location where treatment is to be delivered. The patient's head may be immobilized using a special thermoplastic mask that molds to the shape of the patient's head and face. The treatment course is then planned, including the total dose and number of fractions to be given. The dose itself is invisible, silent, and without pain or any sensation.

SIDE EFFECTS OF RADIATION THERAPY

Side effects from radiation therapy are generally classified as acute and late-stage. Acute side effects (listed in Table 19–2) tend to occur within days of a treatment and are caused by damage to healthy tissue. They usually resolve shortly after the treatment course is completed without lasting impact. Acute effects are prolonged when the patient receives more fractions, even when the dose per fraction is low. Late or delayed side

TABLE 19–2. Acute Side Effects of Radiation Therapy

SIDE EFFECT	TREATMENT
Erythema and skin breakdown	Hydrocortisone/wound care
Alopecia	Reassurance, regrowth
Nausea and vomiting	Antiemetic therapy
Diarrhea	Prevention, antidiarrheals
Dysuria	Fluid intake, pyridium
Mucositis	Local anesthetic, treat thrush
Fatigue	Reassurance, emotional support

effects (listed in Table 19–3) generally do not present for 6 to 12 months, but when they do present they are often catastrophic, with the damage to the body often being irreversible. As these delayed complications of radiation therapy may be caused by a single high dose of radiation, it is primarily to avoid these significant toxicities that the total dose of radiation to be delivered is divided into fractions.

Thus, when patients are being treated for cure, long-term remission, or palliation in a situation where the patient's prognosis is more than

6 months, radiation oncologists have devised treatment schedules that call for a high total radiation dose divided into a number of fractions to avoid late toxicity.

RADIATION THERAPY IN END-OF-LIFE CARE

As already stated above, palliative radiotherapy clearly can play a significant role in providing patients with advanced cancer effective symptom control. However, as with any invasive palliative intervention, the clinician must carefully consider each patient for whom radiation therapy is being contemplated to maximize the chances that the treatment will be effective.

Patient performance status, for example, has been correlated with both the degree and duration of response. Patients with poor performance status often achieve less satisfactory and less durable pain relief than those with better performance scores. The level of ongoing patient fatigue is another critical variable to consider, as fatigue is a common, almost universal side effect of radiation. Therefore, when patients are already severely fatigued from their primary illness, the net effect of a course of radiotherapy may be

TABLE 19–3. Late Effects (6–12 months) of High-Dose Radiotherapy

ORGAN SYSTEM	POTENTIAL EFFECTS
Skin	Atrophy, fibrosis, telangiectasia, necrosis
GI tract	Stricture, telangiectasia, bleeding, perforation, malabsorption, enteritis, colitis, proctitis
Bladder	Oliguria, hematuria, stricture, fistula
Oropharynx	Mucosal atrophy, telangiectasia, bleeding, dental caries, osteonecrosis
Lung	Pneumonitis, fibrosis
CNS	Myelitis, necrosis
Eye	Cataract, dry eyes, entropion, ectropion

further deterioration of the patient's overall condition, as opposed to symptomatic improvement. Finally, one must keep in mind that studies show that it will take a course of radiation therapy between 2 and 4 weeks to be effective. Based on these variables, therefore, palliative radiation is generally only suitable for the patient who has at least a month to live.

Regarding treatment schemas, it is crucial to remember that patients receiving end-of-life care are often not expected to live past 6 months. Therefore, unlike patients being treated for cure or remission, end-of-life care patients are at much lower risk for delayed radiation toxicity. In many circumstances, a treatment schedule known as hypofractionation, which lowers the number of fractions and allows for a much higher dose per fraction, may be utilized. By reducing the number of treatments, the number of visits that the patient is required to make to the radiation therapy center is also reduced. The patient is exposed to less risk of fatigue from the daily trek by car or ambulance to the center, and instead can spend more time doing what he or she wants to do. With less frequent exposure to radiation therapy, there is a lower risk of acute side effects. Most importantly, since it takes the therapy 2 to 4 weeks to be effective, the sooner the treatment is completed, the more rapid the onset of symptom relief. This, of course, is crucial to all patients, but especially to those who do not have the luxury of spending the time to wait for a response.

A 2004 survey showed that most hospice professionals felt that radiotherapy is important in the palliative treatment of patients with advanced cancer. However, according to the data, less than 3% of patients served by those hospices actually received radiotherapy. The most common barriers to palliative radiotherapy included the short life expectancy of hospice patients, transportation difficulties, the cost of radiotherapy, and educational deficiencies between radiation oncologists and hospice/palliative medicine physicians. Hypofractionation and single-dose treatment schedules can potentially solve most of these issues, with the exception of the last. Radiation oncolo-

gists struggle with a dilemma: if the patient lives longer than expected, the high-dose radiation in a hypofractionated schedule could precipitate delayed toxicity, which could be devastating to the patient. Therefore, they are reluctant to utilize the hypofractionated schedules. This was borne out a number of years ago in a survey of 2,500 members of the American Society for Therapeutic Radiology and Oncology, which showed that traditional longer fractionation schemes were advocated by 90% of the physicians. Although the advocates of traditional fractionation was most pronounced among older radiation oncologists, and in nonacademic, private, community practice settings, it raises the issue that information sharing between radiation oncologists and hospice/palliative medicine physicians still has a fair way to go to achieve optimal utilization of radiation therapy for patients with cancer near the end of life.

With a basic understanding of radiation therapy and its overall role in end-of-life care, the specific indications for palliative radiotherapy, listed in Table 19–4 will be discussed.

TABLE 19–4. Indications for Palliative Radiotherapy

- Bone pain secondary to osseous metastases
- Back pain due to impending or progressing spinal cord compression
- Neurologic deficits associated with brain metastases
- Cough, hemoptysis, dyspnea, and pain due to primary or metastatic lung tumor
- Symptomatic superior vena cava (SVC) obstruction
- Malignant dysphagia due to obstructive tumor
- Painful hepatomegaly
- Pain, obstruction, or bleeding due to pelvic masses
- Symptoms due to massive splenomegaly
- Visual impairment from uveal metastases

BONE PAIN

External Beam Radiation Therapy

The pain from osseous metastases can be quite severe and is one of the most common indications for palliative radiotherapy. Between 50% and 80% of patients will experience improvement in their pain after radiation therapy, and up to 35% will have complete pain relief. Notably, pain relief generally begins about 2 weeks after treatment, and maximal pain relief is realized between 4 and 6 weeks after treatment.

Beginning as far back as the early 1980s, a significant number of large trials have been conducted comparing the efficacy of a single fraction of 8 or 10 Gy with the standard multiple fraction treatment, typically consisting of 30 to 35 Gy divided over 2 to 3 weeks. A review of a number of these studies showed that there was no significant difference in the duration of pain relief between the single-fraction and the multiple-fraction groups. Pain relief lasted for 3 months in 70% of patients, 6 months in 37% of patients, and 12 months in 20% of patients. Studies looking at single dose effectiveness have shown that a single 8-Gy dose provided significantly more pain relief than a single 4-Gy dose, suggesting that 8 Gy is the lowest optimal single fraction that should be recommended.

Most recently, an RTOG prospective randomized trial of more than 900 patients with breast or prostate cancer and bone metastases was conducted that compared treatment with 30 Gy in 10 fractions to a single 8-Gy fraction. Again, no significant differences in pain relief were observed at 3 months, with the rates of complete pain relief being 15% (8 Gy arm) and 18% (30 Gy arm), and the rates of partial pain relief being 50% (8 Gy) and 48% (30 Gy). At 3 months, one-third of patients no longer required analgesia, and of some interest was that there was significantly more toxicity in the 30-Gy arm (17%) as compared with the 8-Gy arm (10%) (Hartsell et al., 2005).

Based on these and other studies, the American College of Radiology (ACR) has recently recommended, as part of its "Therapeutic Guidelines for the Treatment of Bone Metastases," that "(a) shorter radiation schedule, like a single fraction, is advantageous for patients with poor prognostic factors" (which clearly applies to patients near the end of life). They cite four reasons for their recommendation: a single fraction is easier for a patient with a poor performance status to tolerate; response and survival are equal for single- and multiple-fraction treatment at 3 months, and median survival of patients with poor prognostic factors is less than 6 months; retreatment after a single fraction may be used as a means of periodically reducing tumor burden; and a single-fraction treatment is very cost-effective. They do note, however, that due to the risk of toxicity to adjacent structures such as the larynx, esophagus, and stomach, that, although single-fraction treatment should be utilized for nonvertebral metastases, it should be avoided when treating vertebral lesions (Janjan et al., 2009).

Systemic Radioisotopes

Systemic radioisotopes are also effective for the management of painful osseous metastases with effective palliation of pain from bone metastases being reported to last more than 6 months in 60% to 80% of patients with breast or prostate cancer. As they can be given by a single intravenous injection on an outpatient basis, they are also convenient to administer. One major advantage is that selective absorption limits the exposure of normal tissue, thus reducing toxicity and theoretically increasing the therapeutic ratio. Systemic radionuclide therapy may therefore be suitable for patients who have had even extensive EBRT. However, there is risk of significant myelosuppression, including severe thrombocytopenia, in patients who have been heavily treated with prior chemotherapy. Systemic radioisotopes are rarely effective for patients with predominantly lytic lesions and no radionuclide uptake on a bone scan. Therefore, a nuclear bone scan should be performed in assessing appropriateness of radionuclide therapy. Urinary incontinence, inability to follow radiation safety precautions, and severe renal insufficiency are also contraindications to radionuclide treatment as they have renal excretion.

The two most commonly utilized radioisotopes today are strontium-89 and samarium-153. One of the limitations of strontium is that pain relief may not occur for about 4 weeks following administration, whereas samarium has been reported to provide improvement in pain in about 2 weeks. Both agents have been associated with a flare reaction, with a resultant transient intensification of pain during first 24 to 48 hours following treatment. Patients should be warned about this possible effect and receive additional analgesics in sufficient dosage to control the increased level of pain. Because of the relatively long time period before pain control is achieved with strontium-89, and because most patients near the end of life who would be candidates for radiopharmaceuticals already have significant bone marrow suppression due to prior therapies, the role of radiopharmaceuticals for patients near the end of life is limited.

Bisphosphonates

Although bisphosphonates constitute medical therapy and are not a form of radiation therapy, their use in the treatment of bone pain suggests their inclusion in this discussion. There are number of medications currently available, including parenteral pamidronate, zoledronate, and ibandronate, and oral ibandronate and clodronate (with oral clodronate not being available in the United States as of 2009). They are primarily used to treat patients with diffuse skeletal metastases in breast cancer, multiple myeloma, and prostate cancer, and their primary indication in these patients with cancer is to reduce bone destruction secondary to metastatic disease by reducing osteoclast activity. This has been shown to reduce patient risk to various "skeletal-related events" secondary to bone metastases, including pathological fracture and hypercalcemia. These agents have also demonstrated modest activity in

the control of bone pain, although current guidelines for their use recommend that they should only be used for pain management in patients with bone pain that is refractory to appropriate analgesic management and radiation therapy.

Regarding the role of bisphosphonates in the treatment of patients near the end of life, most studies on these agents have been carried out on patients with prognoses well in excess of those generally expected by patients near the end of life. In a review of the role of bisphosphonates in the treatment of breast cancer (Gainford, 2005), it was noted that the benefits of bisphosphonates are time-dependent, and only begin to be identifiable 6 months after treatment is initiated. Therefore, with no formal studies having been conducted using these agents in patients with poor prognoses, it seems reasonable to conclude that starting one of these agents in an end-of-life care patient would make little, if any, sense. On the other hand, it is conceivable that patients already being treated with and benefiting from a bisphosphonate will be referred to a hospice or palliative care program and will want to continue to receive the agent to continue to reduce the risk of complications from their metastatic bone disease. Again, as no formal studies have been conducted to evaluate the optimal duration of bisphosphonate therapy or the potential benefits of bisphosphonates in patients with poor prognoses, the decision as to whether to continue the agent should be made on an individual patient basis, applying the general principles discussed in Chapter 18.

Back Pain and Spinal Cord Compression

The vertebral column is the most common site for skeletal metastases. Spinal cord compression due to extradural tumor growth occurs in 5% of patients with cancer, and affects an estimated 20,000 patients per year in the United States alone. The most common tumors to metastasize to spine are lymphoma and breast, lung, and prostate carcinoma.

Excruciating back pain is the most common symptom. It is typically progressive and unrelenting, and is usually worse with recumbency. It may awaken the patient from sleep, and often persists despite even properly prescribed opioid analgesics. The pain can usually be localized with vertebral palpation. Progression is sometimes dramatic and rapid. Patients may lose motor function and experience sensory dysfunction including numbness, paresthesias, or loss of tactile sensation. There may be autonomic dysfunction including urinary and fecal incontinence. A differential diagnosis includes epidural or subdural abscess, hematoma, herniated disk, carcinomatous meningitis, radiation- or chemotherapy-induced myelopathy, and intramedullary spinal cord metastases.

The diagnostic work-up should include a complete physical and neurological examination, plain spine radiographs, and MRI of the entire vertebral column, as there may be multiple levels of cord compression. When MRI is available, contrast myelography is rarely necessary.

With radiotherapy, nearly 80% of patients with spinal cord compression who are ambulatory at the time of diagnosis remain so on completion of treatment. Unfortunately, early intervention continues to be the exception rather than the rule. In one reported series, 78% of the patients were nonambulatory when initially seen by the radiation oncologist. For patients who are already paraplegic, neurological recovery is highly improbable, but they may nevertheless require treatment for pain relief. When spinal cord compression is first suspected, dexamethasone (10 mg IV initially followed by 4 mg orally every 6 hours) is usually initiated, and continued during the course of radiotherapy. Dexamethasone should be tapered and discontinued, if possible, to avoid corticosteroid toxicity after the radiation course is complete. Surgical decompression is generally not recommended, particularly in patients with refractory systemic disease who are near the end of life, except for extremely rare circumstances in which there is spinal instability, compression by bone, or failure of previous radiotherapy, and the patient's overall condition and prognosis justifies the morbidity of surgical intervention. Even then, it should be remembered that patients with poor performance status, as typically seen in hospice patients, have unfavorable outcomes and high surgical mortality.

The treatment volume should include 1 to 2 vertebrae above and below the level of the block. There is no data concerning the use of a single-fraction high-dose radiation in spinal cord compression, but as noted in the discussion on bone pain above, the ACR does not recommend the use of single-fraction high-dose radiation therapy to the vertebral column due to the risk of toxicity to adjacent structures such as the larynx, esophagus, and stomach.

Although cord compression is a neurologic emergency, the clinician must individualize treatment to the patient. Radiotherapy is not indicated for patients who are very near death. The consequences of inappropriate radiation can be worse than paralysis, including hastening death. Patients whose functional status is poor, especially those who were not ambulatory prior to the event, are unlikely to gain anything from radiation, despite the best intentions of the clinicians.

Impending Pathological Fracture

Regarding the prophylaxis and treatment of pathologic bone fractures, radiotherapy primarily plays an adjunctive role to surgical fixation (see Chapter 18). Painful lesions that measure at least 3 cm in size or destroy at least 50% of cortex of a tubular bone as seen in a single x-ray should be considered for surgical fixation prior to irradiation therapy. Postoperative radiotherapy is usually recommended to forestall additional tumor induced bone lysis, and to allow new bone synthesis. The usual dose is 20 Gy in five fractions, although single-dose radiotherapy may also be effective. In patients who are not surgical candidates because of poor performance status or short prognosis, single-fraction radiotherapy may alleviate pain, as described above, and the chance of fracture may be reduced through the use of weight supporting devices or immobilization of the affected extremity.

MALIGNANT BRAIN LESIONS

Because of the potentially dire ramifications for diminished mental status, functional abilities, and overall QOL, the development of brain metastases can be devastating for patients and their caregivers, even in the face of otherwise extensive and refractory metastatic cancer. Symptoms are attributable to tissue damage and increased intracranial pressure and may include anorexia, nausea, vomiting, fatigue, weakness, lethargy, confusion, headaches, memory loss, altered mental state, psychosis, focal deficits, seizures, and coma. In patients with end-stage disease, brain metastases are more commonly multiple than solitary. However, the degree of disability is often disproportionate to the bulk of tumor.

For patients with new or recurrent solitary brain metastases who have no evidence of active extracranial disease, surgical resection or stereotaxic radiosurgery are sometimes considered options of choice. However, as these conditions do not pertain to patients with refractory, end-stage disease, these modalities are, for all intents and purposes, inappropriate for end-of-life care. Indeed, it has been demonstrated that for patients with solitary brain metastasis and active extracranial disease, surgery plus radiotherapy offers no advantage over radiotherapy alone.

Whole brain radiotherapy does effectively palliate clinical symptoms in 70% to 90% of patients with solitary or multiple brain metastases, with 75% to 80% of remaining survival time spent in an improved or stable neurologic state. A course of 20 Gy in five fractions is as effective as a more protracted schedule. An ultrarapid schedule consisting of a single dose of 10 Gy was inferior in both the rate of complete disappearance of neurological symptoms as well as duration of symptom improvement.

Acute toxic effects of whole brain radiotherapy are usually confined to erythema of the scalp, dry desquamation, and alopecia, provided that the patient is simultaneously treated with corticosteroids, as is traditional. The late side effects of cranial radiotherapy, including dementia, are not of concern when treating patients near the end of life.

For some patients with brain metastases, manifestations of systemically advanced disease, and a brief anticipated life expectancy of only several weeks, the best palliative approach might be to avoid radiotherapy and use pharmacological supportive measures such as corticosteroids and anticonvulsants for symptom management. In fact, patients with brain metastases whose symptoms fail to improve in response to corticosteroids probably have irreversible damage and are unlikely to benefit from more aggressive measures such as radiotherapy.

MALIGNANT LUNG LESIONS

Patients with primary or metastatic intrathoracic tumors may suffer from a number of debilitating local symptoms including chest pain, cough, hemoptysis, dyspnea, dysphagia, hoarseness, fatigue, and anxiety. EBRT for symptom control is extensively used, and fortunately a number of recent studies support the use of hypofractionated treatment schedules. In particular, a dose of 16 or 17 Gy divided in two treatments appears to palliate symptoms just as well as traditional courses of 20 to 25 treatments without changing survival time. Moreover, there are fewer side effects. Symptoms that improve include dyspnea, hemoptysis, cough, and pain, and symptom control typically lasts for up to 50% of the remaining survival time. External radiation may be a useful adjunctive technique following endoscopic interventions such as laser therapy, photodynamic therapy, and/or stent placement, all of which can provide rapid symptomatic relief.

Patients with mass lesions in the chest may present with SVC compression. Symptoms related to the mass lesion include dyspnea, orthopnea, cough, hoarseness, vocal cord paralysis, dysphagia, chest pain, and syncope. Typical physical findings include tachypnea and tachycardia, fixed dilatation of the neck and arm veins, dilatation of the thoracic collateral circulation, cyanosis, facial plethora, conjunctival, facial, and upper extremity edema, and increased intracranial pressure. Although SVC syndrome is traditionally regarded as a medical emergency, the onset is usually gradual, and, only rarely is the presentation rapid and life-threatening. Rapid acuity of onset is, however, associated with a poorer response to treatment.

Immediate measures for the management of SVC syndrome include administration of oxygen, diuretics, and elevation of the head. Corticosteroids are often used. Traditional radiotherapy treatment is 20 to 30 Gy in 5 to 10 fractions, but there is evidence that 24 Gy in three fractions of 8 Gy weekly for 3 weeks is just as efficacious. Although radiotherapy has been the standard for the treatment of SVC, recent studies have suggested that vascular stenting may be a viable alternative (see Chapter 18).

MALIGNANT DYSPHAGIA

In addition to radiotherapy, potential palliative therapies for advanced esophageal cancer at the end of life include corticosteroids, chemotherapy, and endoscopic procedures, either alone or in combination. EBRT is effective and noninvasive, but relief occurs only over a period of 4 to 6 weeks. Therefore, radiation should probably not be considered in a patient whose life expectancy is significantly less than a month, or whose functional status is severely compromised.

Brachytherapy offers more rapid symptomatic relief and may be combined with EBRT for a more durable response in patients with better outlooks. For patients with a life expectancy of less than 3 months, brachytherapy alone is generally sufficient. EBRT also enhances the response to laser endoscopy for malignant dysphagia and reduces the necessity for subsequent therapeutic endoscopy to maintain lifelong palliation. However, although the optimal palliative approach for malignant dysphagia is yet to be determined, it appears that insertion of a self-expanding metal-

lic, membrane-coated stent (discussed in Chapter 18) may be the procedure of choice, with a prompt response and successful palliation of symptoms expected in more than 95% of cases.

PAINFUL HEPATOMEGALY, PELVIC SOFT TISSUE MASSES, AND OTHER INDICATIONS

Pain due to liver capsular distension from metastatic disease can be diminished in 75% to 90% of patients who complete a course of radiotherapy to the entire liver. Complete pain relief is achieved in about half of the patients within a median time of 10 to 12 days. Using a regimen of 10 fractions of 2 to 3 Gy, the median duration of response is approximately 3 months for patients with an expected survival of 4 to 6 months. Side effects are relatively minimal with about 20% of patients experiencing nausea and vomiting. Late hepatic toxicity, although theoretically possible, is not of concern for patients with a short life expectancy.

Recurrent gynecologic and colorectal tumors often result in pelvic pain, vaginal or rectal bleeding, and foul discharge. Single doses of 10 Gy to the pelvis can be effective in relieving symptoms of pain or bleeding. This approach is also effective for relief of pain and bleeding for patients with chemotherapy-refractory ovarian carcinoma. Side effects generally consist primarily of diarrhea. Evidence suggests that repeating the dose at monthly intervals two more times can substantially increase the response rate to treatment, but that those patients who do survive longer than expected are at greater risk for late-effect bowel toxicity, including severe diarrhea. This concern appears to manifest at approximately 9 months after treatment.

Patients with advanced, refractory myeloproliferative and lymphoproliferative disorders may suffer from massive splenomegaly. Symptoms include severe episodic abdominal pain, hypersplenism, portal hypertension, "crushed stomach" syndrome, and high output cardiac failure. Splenic irradiation in doses of more than 5 Gy delivered in multiple fractions was effective in relieving pain for several months in approximately 90% of treated patients, and in decreasing splenomegaly in about 60%. Prior splenic infarctions and subsequent fibrosis often limit the response in terms of reduction in splenic size.

Patients with disseminated breast, lung, and prostate cancer may suffer visual loss secondary to uveal metastases. Because preservation of vision is a significant QOL issue even at the end of life, uveal metastases should be treated with palliative radiotherapy. Most patients respond to a short, fractionated course of EBRT, administered with a technique that minimizes exposure of the lens, with improved or stabilized vision.

BIBLIOGRAPHY

Palliative Chemotherapy

Ajani JA: Chemotherapy for gastric carcinoma: New and old options. *Oncology* 12(suppl 7):44-47, 1998.

American Society of Clinical Oncology: Clinical practice guidelines for the treatment of unresectable non-small cell lung cancer: Adopted on May 16, 1997 by the American Society of Conical Oncology. *J Clin Oncol* 15:2996-3018, 1997.

Blum JL, Jones SE, Buzdar AU, et al: Multicenter phase II study of capecitabine in paclitaxel-refractory metastatic breast cancer. *J Clin Oncol* 17:485-493,1999.

Bunn PA Jr, Vokes EE, Langer CJ, Schiller JH: An update on North American randomized studies in non-small cell lung cancer. *Semin Oncol* 25(4 suppl 9):2-10, 1998.

Christakis NA, Lamont EB: Extent and determinants of error in doctors' prognoses in terminally ill patients: Prospective cohort study. *BMJ* 320:469-473, 2000.

Conroy T, Guillemin F: Quality of life in advanced colorectal cancer (Letter). *J Clin Oncol* 17:1644, 1999.

Cunningham D, Pyrhonen S, James RD, et al: Randomised trial of irinotecan plus supportive care versus supportive care alone after fluorouracil failure for patients with metastatic colorectal cancer. *Lancet* 352:1413-1418, 1998.

Detmar SB, Muller MJ, Schornagel, et al: Role of health-related quality of life in palliative chemotherapy decisions. *J Clin Orthod* 20:1056-1062, 2002.

Einhorn LH, Stender MJ, Williams SD: Phase II trial of gemcitabine in refractory germ cell tumors. *J Clin Oncol* 17:509-516, 1999.

Elderly Lung Cancer Vinorelbine Italian Study Group: Effects of vinorelbine on quality of life and survival of elderly patients with advanced non-small cell lung cancer. *J Natl Cancer Inst* 91:66-72, 1999.

Ellis PA, Smith IE, Hardy JR, et al; Symptom relief with MVP (mitomycin C, vinblastine and cisplatin) chemotherapy in advanced non-small cell lung cancer. *Br J Cancer* 71:366-370, 1995.

Emanuel EJ, Young-Xu Y, Levinsky NG, et al: Chemotherapy use among medicare beneficiaries at the end of life. *Ann Intern Med* 138:639-643, 2003.

Glare P, Virik K, Jones M, et al: A systematic review of physicians' survival predictions in terminally ill cancer patients. *BMJ* 327:195-201, 2003.

Glimelius B, Ekstrom K, Hoffman K, et al: Randomized comparison between chemotherapy plus best supportive care with best supportive care in advanced gastric cancer. *Ann Oncol* 8:163-168, 1997.

Graziano F, Cataano G, Cascinu S: Chemotherapy for advanced pancreatic cancer: The history is changing. *Tumori* 84:308-311, 1998.

Greenway BA: Effect of flutamide on survival in patients with pancreatic cancer: Results of a prospective, randomised, double-blind, placebo-controlled trial. *BMJ* 316:1935-1938, 1998.

Gridelli C, Perrone F, Gallo C, et al: Vinorelbine is well tolerated and active in the treatment of elderly patients with advanced non-small cell lung cancer. A two-stage phase II study. *Eur J Cancer* 33:392-397, 1997.

Hernandez-Boluda JC, Sierra J, Esteve J, et al: Treatment of elderly patients with AML: Results of an individualized approach. *Haematologica* 83:34-39, 1998.

Hickish TF, Smith IE, OBrien ME, et al: Clinical benefit from palliative chemotherapy in non-small cell lung cancer extends to the elderly and those with poor prognostic factors. *Br J Cancer* 78:28-33, 1998.

Lara PN JR, Meyers FJ: Treatment options in androgen-independent prostate cancer. *Cancer Invest* 17:137-144, 1999.

Lopez PG, Stewart DJ, Newman TE, Evans WK: Chemotherapy in stage IV (metastatic) non-small cell lung cancer. Provincial Lung Disease Site Group. *Cancer Prev Control* 1:18-27, 1997.

Lorusso V, Pollera CF, Antimi M, et al: A phase II study of gemcitabine in patients with transitional cell carcinoma of the urinary tract previously treated with platinum. *Eur J Cancer* 34:1208-1212, 1998.

Matsuyama R, Reddy S, Smith TJ: Why do patients choose chemotherapy near the end of life? A review of the perspective of those facing death from cancer. *J Clin Oncol* 24:3490-3496, 2006.

Millikan RE: Chemotherapy of advanced prostatic carcinoma. *Semin Oncol* 26(2):185-191, 1999.

Munshi NC, Tricot GJ: Single weekly cytosine arabinoside and oral 6-thioguanine in patients with myelodysplastic syndrome and acute myeloid leukemia. *Ann Hematol* 74:111-115, 1997.

Noble S, Goa KL: Gemcitabine. A review of its pharmacology and clinical potential in non-small cell lung cancer and pancreatic cancer. *Drugs* 54:447-472, 1997.

Otto T, Krege S, Otto B, et al: Therapy with mitomycin C, folic acid and 5-fluorouracil in treatment of metastatic, refractory urinary bladder carcinoma—Phase II study (In German). *Urologe A* 36:243-247, 1997.

Petrylak DP, Macarthur RB, O'Connor J, et al: Phase I trial of docetaxel with estramustine in androgen-independent prostate cancer. *J Clin Oncol* 17(3):958-967, 1999.

Scheithauer W, Rosen H, Kornek GV, et al: Randomised comparison of combination chemotherapy plus supportive care with supportive care alone in patients with metastatic colorectal cancer. *BMJ* 306:752-755, 1993.

Shanafelt TD, Loprinzi C, Marks R, Novotny P, Sloan J: Are chemotherapy response rates related to treatment induced survival prolongations in patients with advanced cancer. *J Clin Orthod* 22:1966-1974, 2004.

Shepherd FA: Chemotherapy for non-small cell lung cancer: Have we reached a new plateau? *Semin Oncol* 26(1 Suppl 4):3-11, 1999.

Silvestri G, Pritchard R, Welch HG: Preferences for chemotherapy in patients with advanced non-small cell lung cancer: Descriptive study based on scripted interviews. *BMJ* 317:771-775, 1889.

Slevin ML, Stubbs L, Plant HJ, et al: Attitudes to chemotherapy. Comparing views of patients with cancer with those of doctors, nurses, and general public. *BMJ* 300:1458-1460, 1999.

Small EJ, Marshall ME, Reyno L, et al: Superiority of suramin + hydrocortisone (S + H) over placebo + hydrocortisone (P + H): Results of a multi-center double-blind phase III study in patients with hormone refractory prostate cancer (Abstract). *Proc Am Soc Clin Oncol* 17:1187a, 1998.

Souhami RL, Spiro SG, Rudd RM, et al: Five-day oral etoposide treatment for advanced small-cell lung cancer: Randomized comparison with intravenous chemotherapy. *J Natl Cancer Inst* 89:577-580, 1997.

Storniolo AM, Enas NH, Brown CA, et al: An investigational new drug treatment program for patients with gemcitabine: Results for over 3000 patients with pancreatic carcinoma. *Cancer* 85:1261-1268, 1999.

Tannock IF, de Wit R, Berry WR, et al: Docetaxel plus prednisone or mitoxantrone plus prednisone for advanced prostate cancer. *N Engl J Med* 351(15):1502-1512, 2004.

Tannock IF, Osoba D, Stockler MR, et al: Chemotherapy with mitoxantrone plus prednisone or prednisone alone for symptomatic hormone-resistant prostate cancer: A Canadian randomized trial with palliative end points. *J Clin Oncol* 14:1756, 1996.

Thatcher N, Hopwood P, Anderson H: Improving quality of life in patients with non-small cell lung cancer: Research experience with gemcitabine. *Eur J Cancer* 33(suppl 1):S8-S13, 1997.

Thatcher N, Jayson G, Bradley B, et al: Gemcitabine: Symptomatic benefit in advanced non-small cell lung cancer. *Semin Oncol* 24(suppl 8):S8-S6-S8-S12, 1997.

Tsavaris N, Tentas K, Tzivras M, et al: Combined epirubicin, 5-fluorouracil and folinic acid vs no treatment for patients with advanced pancreatic cancer: A prospective comparative study. *J Chemother* 10:331-337, 1998.

Palliative Radiation Therapy

Abratt RP, Shepherd LJ, Salton DG: Palliative radiation for stage 3 non-small cell lung cancer—A prospective study of two moderately high dose regimens. *Lung Cancer* 13:137-143, 1995.

Anderson PM, Wiseman GA, Dispenzieri A, et al: High-dose samarium-153 ethylene diamine tetramethylene phosphonate: Low toxicity of skeletal irradiation in patients with osteosarcoma and bone metastases. *J Clin Oncol* 20:189-196, 2002.

Arcangeli G, Giovinazzo G, Saracino B, et al: Radiation therapy in the management of symptomatic bone metastases: The effect of total dose and histology on pain relief and response duration. *Int J Radiat Oncol Biol Phys* 42:1119-1126, 1998.

Ben Josef E, Shamsa F, Williams AO, Porter AT: Radiotherapeutic management of osseous metastases: A survey of current patterns of care. *Int J Radiat Oncol Biol Phys* 40:915-921, 1998.

Berenson JR, Hillner BE, Kyle RA, et al: American Society of Clinical Oncology clinical practice guidelines: The role of bisphosphonates in multiple myeloma. *J Clin Oncol* 20:3719-3736, 2002.

Bezjak A, Dixon P, Brundage M, et al: Randomized phase III trial of single versus fractionated thoracic radiation in the palliation of patients with lung cancer (NCIC CTG SC.15). *Cancer Treat Rev* 29:123-125, 2003.

Bhatt ML, Mohani BK, Kumar L, et al: Palliative treatment of advanced non small cell lung cancer with weekly fraction radiotherapy. *Indian J Cancer* 37:148-152, 2000.

Cole D: A randomized trial of a single treatment versus conventional fractionation in the palliative radiotherapy of painful bony metastases. *Clin Oncol (R Coll Radiol)* 1:59-62, 1989.

Cross CK, Berman S, Buswell L, et al: Prospective study of palliative hypofractionated radiotherapy (8.5 Gy 3 2) for patients with symptomatic non-small-cell lung cancer. *Int J Radiat Oncol Biol Phys* 58:1098-1105, 2004.

Donato V, Zurlo A, Bonfili P, et al: Hypofractionated radiation therapy for inoperable advanced non-small cell lung cancer. *Tumori* 85:174-176, 1999.

Gainford MC, Dranitsaris G, Clemons M: Recent developments in bisphosphonates for patients with metastatic breast cancer. *BMJ* 330:769-773, 2005.

Gava A, Bertossi L, Zorat PL, et al: Radiotherapy in the elderly with lung carcinoma: The experience of the Italian "Geriatric Radiation Oncology Group". *Rays* 22(suppl):61-65, 1989.

Gaze MN, Kelly CG, Kerr GR, et al: Pain relief and quality of life following radiotherapy for bone metastases: A randomised trial of two fractionation schedules. *Radiother Oncol* 45:109-116, 1997.

Gelblum D, Mychalczak B, Almadrones L, et al: Palliative benefit of external-beam radiation in the management of platinum refractory epithelial ovarian carcinoma. *Gynecol Oncol* 69:36-41, 1998.

Halle JS, Rosenman JG, Varia MA, Fowler WC, Walton LA, Currie JL: 1000 cGy single dose palliation for advanced carcinoma of the cervix or endometrium. *Int J Radiat Oncol Biol Phys* 12: 1947-1950, 1986.

Hartsell WF, Scott CB, Bruner DW, et al: Randomized trial of short- versus long-course radiotherapy for palliation of bone metastases. *J Natl Cancer Inst* 97:798-804, 2005.

Hillner BE, Ingle JN, Chlebowski RT, et al: American Society of Clinical Oncology 2003 update on the role of bisphosphonates and bone health issues in women with breast cancer. *J Clin Oncol* 21:4042-4057, 2003.

Hoegler D: Radiotherapy for palliation of symptoms in incurable cancer. *Curr Prob Cancer* 21:135-183, 1997.

Hoskin P, Price P, Easton D, et al: A prospective randomized trial of 4 Gy or 8 Gy single doses in the treatment of metastatic bone pain. *Radiother Oncol* 23(2):74-78, 1992.

Janjan NA: An emerging respect for palliative care in radiation oncology. *J Palliat Med* 1:83-88, 1988.

Janjan NA: Radiation for bone metastases. Conventional techniques and the role of systemic radiopharmaceuticals. *Cancer* 80(8 suppl):1628-1645, 1997.

Janjan N, Lutz ST, Bedwinek JM, et al: Therapeutic guidelines for the treatment of bone metastases: A report from the American College of Radiology appropriateness criteria expert panel on radiation. *J Pall Med* 12:427-431, 2009.

Jeremic B, Shibamoto Y, Acimovic L, et al: A randomized trial of three single-dose radiation therapy regimens in the treatment of metastatic bone pain. *Int J Radiat Oncol Biol Phys* 42:161-167, 1998.

Kirkbride P, Warde P, Panzarella A, Aslanidis J: A randomized trial comparing the efficacy of single fraction radiation therapy plus ondansetron with fractionated radiation therapy in the palliation of skeletal metastases. *Int J Radiat Oncol Biol Phys* 48:185, 2000. Abstract 147.

Kramer GW, Wanders SL, Noordijk EM, et al: Results of the Dutch national study of the palliative effects of irradiation using two different treatment schemes for non-small-cell lung cancer. *J Clin Oncol* 23:2962-2970, 2005.

Lingareddy V, Ahmad NR, Mohiuddin M: Palliative reirradiation for recurrent rectal cancer. *Int J Radiat Oncol Biol Phys* 38:785-790, 1997.

Lupattelli M, Maranzano E, Bellavita R, et al: Short-course palliative radiotherapy in non-small-cell lung cancer: Results of a prospective study. *Am J Clin Oncol* 23:83-93, 2000.

Lutz ST, Spence C, Chow E, et al: Survey on use of palliative radiotherapy in hospice care. *J Clin Oncol* 17:3581-3586, 2004.

Lutz ST, Huang DT, Ferguson CL, et al: A retrospective quality of life analysis using the lung cancer symptom scale in patients treated with palliative radiotherapy for advanced non-small cell lung cancer. *Int J Radiat Oncol Biol Phys* 37:117-122, 1997.

McFarland JT, Kuzma C, Millard FE, Johnstone PA: Palliative irradiation of the spleen. *Am J Clin Oncol* 26:178-183, 2003.

Macbeth FR, Bolger JJ, Bailey AJ, et al: Randomized trial of palliative two-fraction versus more intensive 13-fraction radiotherapy for patients with inoperable non-small cell lung cancer and good performance status. *Br J Cancer* 65:934-941, 1996.

Medical Research Council. Inoperable non-small cell lung cancer (NSCLC): A medical research council randomized trial of palliative radiotherapy with two fractions or ten fractions. Report to the medical research council by its lung cancer working party. *Br J Cancer* 63:265-270, 1991.

Medical Research Council: A medical research council randomized trial of palliative radiotherapy with two fractions or a single fraction in patients with inoperable nonsmall cell lung cancer and poor performance status. *Br J Cancer* 65:934-941, 1992.

Mercadante S: Malignant bone pain: Pathophysiology and treatment. *Pain* 69:1-18, 1997.

Mertens WC, Filipczak LA, Ben-Josef E, et al: Systemic bone-seeking radionuclides for palliation of painful osseous metastases: Current concepts. *CA Cancer J Clin* 48:361-374, 1998.

Nielson OS, Bentzen SM, Sandberg E, et al: Randomized trial of single dose versus fractionated palliative radiotherapy of bone metastases. *Radiother Oncol* 47:233-240, 1998.

Oneschuk D, Bruera E: Palliative management of brain metastases. *Support Care Cancer* 6:365-372, 1998.

Paulino AC, Reddy SP: Splenic irradiation in the palliation of patients with lymphoproliferative and myeloproliferative disorders. *Am J Hosp Palliat Care* 13:32-35, 1996.

Pignon T, Scalliet P: Radiotherapy in the elderly. *Eur J Surg Oncol* 24:407-411, 1998.

Plataniotis GA, Kouvaris JR, Vlahos L, et al: A short radiotherapy course for locally advanced non-small cell lung cancer (NSCLC): Effective palliation and patients' convenience. *Lung Cancer* 35:203-207, 2002.

Price P, Hoskin P, Easton D, et al: Prospective randomized trial of single and multifraction radiotherapy schedules in the treatment of painful bony metastases. *Radiother Oncol* 6:247-255, 1986.

Prie L, Lagarde P, Palussiere J, et al: Radiotherapy of spinal metastases in breast cancer. Apropos of a series of 108 patients. *Cancer Radiother* 1:234-239, 1997.

Rees FJ, Devrell CE, Newman HF, et al: Palliative radiotherapy for lung cancer: Two versus five fractions. *Clin Oncol (R Coll Radiol)* 9:90-95, 1997.

Rodrigues CI, Njo KH, Karim AB: Hypofractionated radiation therapy in the treatment of superior vena cava syndrome. *Lung Cancer* 10:221-228, 1993.

Roos D, Turner S, O'Brien P, et al: Randomized trial of 8 Gy in 1 versus 20 Gy in 5 fractions of radiotherapy for neuropathic pain due to bone metastases (Trans-Tasman Radiation Oncology Group, TROG 96.05). *Radiother Oncol* 75:54-63, 2005.

Sawyer EJ, Timothy AR: Low dose palliative radiotherapy in low grade non-Hodgkin's lymphoma. *Radiother Oncol* 42:49-51, 1997.

Senkus-Konefka E, Dziadziuszko R, Bednaruk-Mynski E, et al: A prospective, randomized study to compare two palliative radiotherapy schedules for non-small-cell lung cancer (NSCLC). *Br J Cancer* 92:1038-1045, 2005.

Simpson J, Francis M, Perez-Tamayo R, Marks RD, Rao DV: Palliative radiotherapy for inoperable carcinoma of the lung: Final report of the RTOG multi-institutional trial. *Int J Radiat Oncol Biol Phys* 11:751-758, 1985.

Spanos WJ, Wasserman T, Moez R, et al: Palliation of advanced pelvic malignant disease with large fraction pelvic radiation and misonidazole: Final report of RTOG phase I/II study. *Int J Radiat Oncol Biol Phys* 13:1479-1482, 1987.

Spanos W, Guse C, Perez C, et al: Phase II study of multiple daily fractionations in the palliation of advanced pelvic malignancies: Preliminary report of RTOG 8502. *Int J Radiat Oncol Biol Phys* 17:659-661, 1989.

Steenland E, Leer J, van Houwelingen H, et al: The effect of a single fraction compared to multiple fractions on painful bone metastases: A global analysis of the Dutch bone metastasis study. *Radiother Oncol* 52:101-109, 1999.

Stevens MJ, Beqbie SD: Hypofractionated radiation for inoperable non-small lung cancer. *Australas Radiol* 39:265-270, 1995.

Sundstrom S, Bremnes R, Aasebo U, et al: Hypofractionated palliative radiotherapy (17 Gy per two fractions) in advanced non-small-cell lung carcinoma is comparable to standard fractionation for symptom control and survival: A national phase III trial. *J Clin Oncol* 22:765-768, 2004.

Sykes AJ, Kiltie AE, Stewart AL: Ondansetron versus a chlorpromazine and dexamethasone combination for the prevention of nausea and vomiting: A prospective, randomised study to assess efficacy, cost effectiveness and quality of life following single-fraction radiotherapy. *Support Care Cancer* 5:500-503, 1997.

Tan R, Young A: The role of chemoradiotherapy in maintaining quality of life for advanced esophageal cancer. *Am J Hosp Palliat Care* 15:29-31, 1998.

Teo P, Tai PH, Choi D, et al: A randomized study on palliative radiation therapy for inoperable non-small cell carcinoma of the lung. *Int J Radiat Oncol Biol Phys* 14:867-871, 1988.

Vyas RK, Suryanarayana U, Dixit S, et al: Inoperable non-small cell lung cancer: Palliative radiotherapy with two weekly fractions. *Indian J Chest Dis Allied Sci* 40:171-174, 1998.

Wong R, Thomas G, Cummings B, et al: The role of radiotherapy in the management of pelvic recurrence of rectal cancer. *Can J Oncol* 6(suppl 1):39-47, 1996.

Wong RKS, Wiffen PJ: Bisphosphonates for the relief of pain secondary to bone metastates. *Cochrane Database Syst Rev* (2):CD002068, 2002.

Yarnold J: Eight-Gy single fraction radiotherapy for the treatment of metastatic skeletal pain: Randomized comparison with a multifraction schedule over 12 months of patient follow-up. On behalf of the Bone Pain Trial Working Party. *Radiother Oncol* 52:111-121, 1999.

Yuen KY, Shelley M, Sze WM, et al: Bisphosphonates for advanced prostate cancer. *Cochrane Database Syst Rev* (4):CD006250, 2006.

SELF-ASSESSMENT QUESTIONS

1. In a study which asked patients with cancer to choose between chemotherapy and supportive care in a hypothetical case scenario, what percentage of patients said they would opt for chemotherapy if it substantially reduced symptoms, even if there was no prolonged survival?

   A. 22%
   B. 36%
   C. 50%
   D. 68%
   E. 95%

2. Which of the following outcomes would NOT be included as part of a "clinical benefit response" to chemotherapy?

   A. Decreased pain with no change in analgesic dose
   B. Improvement in performance status
   C. Reduction in size of a palpable tumor mass
   D. Improvement in weight
   E. Decreased analgesic dose with the same level of pain

3. Which of the following best characterizes the "best supportive care" arms of trials comparing it with palliative chemotherapy in the treatment of advanced malignancies?

   A. "Best supportive care" is the best care available as judged by the attending physician, according to institutional standards.
   B. Most "best supportive care" trials control for the effects of adjunctive treatments such as antiemetics and corticosteroid.
   C. Most "best supportive care" trials provide detailed descriptions of patient responses to symptom management interventions.
   D. Most "best supportive care" trials control for the number of patient/health care provider contacts in the two study arms.
   E. "Best supportive care" is standardized in most of the studies in the literature.

4. In which of the following malignancies was the first chemotherapy trial utilizing the "clinical benefit response" reported?

   A. Small-cell bronchogenic carcinoma
   B. Pancreatic carcinoma
   C. Prostate carcinoma
   D. Colorectal carcinoma
   E. Non–small cell bronchogenic carcinoma

5. All of the following statements regarding patient performance status and its influence on the use of palliative chemotherapy or palliative radiation therapy are true EXCEPT:

   A. Patients with a poor performance status are not included in many palliative chemotherapy trials.
   B. A poor performance status is associated with less satisfactory pain relief to palliative radiation therapy.
   C. An improvement in performance status following palliative chemotherapy is considered a "clinical benefit response."
   D. A good performance status is associated with more durable pain relief to palliative radiation therapy.
   E. A poor performance status is associated with a reduced likelihood of a "clinical benefit response" to palliative chemotherapy.

6. Which of the following characteristics associated with a hypofractionation radiation therapy treatment schedule makes it a viable option for patients near the end of life?

   A. Decreased risk of acute toxicity due to smaller number of treatments
   B. Less frequent trips to the radiation therapy treatment center
   C. Decreased risk of delayed toxicity due to short patient life expectancy
   D. More rapid onset of symptom relief since treatment is completed sooner

7. All of the following statements regarding the use of EBRT for the treatment of bone pain are true EXCEPT:

A. The efficacy of single-fraction treatment is equal to that of standard multiple-fraction treatment.

B. Single-fraction treatment can be used to treat bone pain due to vertebral metastases.

C. In one study, toxicity was greater in the multiple-fraction treatment arm than in the single-fraction treatment arm.

D. Retreatment after a single fraction may be used to periodically reduce tumor burden.

E. A single dose of 8 Gy is more effective than a dose of 4 Gy.

8. All of the following statements regarding the management of spinal cord compression are true EXCEPT:

A. Excruciating back pain is the most common symptom.

B. MRI has replaced contrast myelography as the diagnostic study of choice.

C. Many patients who are nonambulatory will be able to ambulate following radiation therapy.

D. The treatment area should include at least 1 to 2 vertebrae above and below the level of the block.

E. Patients who are not expected to recover neurologically should be treated with radiation therapy for pain control.

9. All of the following statements regarding the management of SVC syndrome are true EXCEPT:

A. Although SVC is considered a medical emergency, its gradual onset, in most cases, gives one some time for evaluation and treatment.

B. Symptoms include dyspnea, hoarseness, chest pain, and syncope.

C. Medical management consists of oxygen, diuretics, elevation of the head of the bed, and corticosteroids.

D. Vascular stenting may be considered a viable alternative to radiation therapy in some patients.

E. Three once a week fractions of 8 Gy each has been shown to be less effective than the traditional treatment of 20 to 30 Gy in 5 to 10 fractions.

10. Which of the following statements regarding the use of palliative radiation therapy is TRUE?

A. EBRT is superior to stent placement in the treatment of malignant dysphagia secondary to esophageal carcinoma.

B. Treatment of pelvic pain or bleeding secondary to recurrent gynecological or colorectal tumors can be treated with a single dose of 10 Gy to the pelvis.

C. Painful hepatomegaly due to liver capsular distention can be treated with a single dose of 10 Gy to the liver.

D. Massive splenomegaly can be treated with a single dose of 10 Gy to the spleen.

E. The treatment of uveal metastases with radiation therapy should be avoided in patients near the end of life.

Invasive Cardiac Interventions

Barry M. Kinzbrunner

INTRODUCTION

In recent times, patients with advanced and end-stage cardiac disease are accessing hospice and palliative care programs in growing numbers. In 2007 alone, approximately 168,000 patients with end-stage heart disease were served by hospice programs. In addition, the American College of Cardiology/American Heart Association (ACC/AHA) 2005 Guidelines for the Diagnosis and Management of Chronic Heart Failure in the Adult has recommended hospice or palliative care as appropriate interventions when patients with refractory heart failure are approaching the end of life.

Among the challenges that end-of-life care providers face when caring for patients with end-stage cardiac disease is that many of these patients come with various interventions in place, initiated at an earlier stage of the disease, that they, and often-times their physicians, believe are of benefit either in reducing symptoms or in some cases, prolonging survival, even within a limited time frame. For example, it has become increasingly commonplace for patients with advanced cardiac disease to receive an automated implantable cardioverter-defibrillator device (AICD) long before their heart disease has reached the stage where hospice or palliative care would be considered. Many of these patients also have pacemakers either for primary rhythm disorders or for the purpose of cardiac resynchronization. In addition, when congestive heart failure reaches a truly refractory stage, patients are often treated with intravenous inotropic agents or, if not a transplant candidate, with implantable ventricular assist devices with the hope of ameliorating symptoms. Many patients awaiting cardiac transplantation also require the kind of supportive care that only hospice and palliative care programs are designed to provide either prior to transplant or in some cases, until the end of life since not all patients survive to transplantation.

Therefore, it is incumbent on hospice and palliative care providers to have a working knowledge of these "invasive" cardiac therapies and to know how to manage patients who present for care with one or more of these interventions already in place.

AUTOMATED IMPLANTABLE CARDIOVERTER-DEFIBRILLATORS

BACKGROUND

AICDs are surgically implanted, battery-powered devices that automatically resuscitate patients by recognizing and terminating fatal ventricular arrhythmias (such as ventricular tachycardia and ventricular fibrillation) and internally delivering an electric shock of up to 40 joules to the myocardium. These devices were originally approved by the FDA in 1985. The indications for which patients may receive an AICD include New York Heart Association (NYHA) Class II or III heart failure on optimal medical therapy, expected survival of greater than 1 year, and either ischemic or nonischemic cardiomyopathy with an ejection fraction below 35%, or a history of a hemodynamically significant ventricular arrhythmia or cardiac arrest. These devices may also be placed prophylactically in high-risk patients with a family history of sudden cardiac death.

Studies with AICDs have shown improved survival in patients suffering from left ventricular dysfunction and hemodynamically significant ventricular tachycardia or resuscitated from sudden cardiac death, whether or not the patients have coexisting coronary artery disease. In addition, survival was improved when AICDs were implanted prophylactically in patients 30 days or more following myocardial infarction who had an ejection fraction of 30% or less, irrespective of whether arrhythmias were present.

In a study comparing the quality of life of patients with AICDs with those receiving medical antiarrhythmic therapy with amiodarone or a placebo, psychological well-being was found to be significantly improved in the AICD group at 3 and 12 months, with the significance being lost at 30 months, leading to the conclusion that AICD therapy was not associated with any detectable adverse quality-of-life effects during 30 months of follow-up. Despite the increased survival associated with these devices, there are well-documented reports of significant pain and anxiety associated with an AICD shock. Therefore, it is not entirely surprising that when the patient experienced an AICD shock in the month preceding a scheduled quality-of-life assessment (3, 12, and 30 months), quality of life was found to be significantly decreased in multiple domains (Mark et al., 2008). This finding, as is discussed in the following text, is of great relevance to patients nearing the end of life who have an AICD in place.

AICD DEACTIVATION

Although it is highly unlikely that hospice and palliative care programs would ever have the request made to place an AICD into a patient, it is certainly likely that, with the widespread and increasing use of these devices, end-of-life care providers will be asked to care for patients who already have these devices implanted. The challenge for patients, families, and professional caregivers in this setting, given the pain, anxiety, and documented poor quality of life associated with an AICD shock, is whether to consider deactivating the device, and if so, at what point in the illness to do so. For if an AICD is not deactivated prior to the death of a terminally ill patient, there is a significant risk that the patient will receive one or more shocks during the active dying process, which can be exceedingly disturbing to the patient, if she or he is aware, and to the family.

Anecdotal reports on nursing blog sites on the Internet describe in great detail the extreme distress experienced by patients and families when the patient has been shocked prior to or at the time of death. These reports have been confirmed in a retrospective study published in 2004 that additionally documented that of 27 families who

had reported that loved ones received a shock in the last month of life, 8 reported that patients were shocked at least once only minutes before death (Goldstein et al., 2004).

The formal process of AICD deactivation itself is relatively straightforward. The first order of business is to contact a technician capable of deactivating the device. In some situations, the patient will have the necessary information, which includes the name of the manufacturer of the specific AICD implanted and the contact information for a representative of that organization. If the patient does not have the information, it can usually be obtained from the office of the physician who placed the device. In other circumstances, the necessary expertise and equipment to deactivate the device may be available directly from the cardiologist's office. Once this is accomplished, after obtaining a physician's order to deactivate the device, the technician would go to the patient's home with a reprogramming device and make the necessary changes to the AICD's programming. In the event that a patient does not want the device deactivated, but shocks are causing the patient distress, the parameters that trigger the device can be altered through reprogramming. The deactivation process is painless to the patient, and, as a ventricular arrhythmia which would trigger the device is unlikely at the moment of deactivation, concerns about causing immediate patient death are unfounded. It should also be noted that if the patient's AICD also functions as a pacemaker, the cardioverter-defibrillator can be deactivated without affecting the pacemaker. (See discussion below regarding deactivating pacemakers.)

Unfortunately, often times, as is discussed in the following text, deactivation is considered only after the patient has experienced a shock, and it is not always possible to have a technician come to the home immediately, especially if the need arises at night or on a weekend. In these situations, the device can be temporarily deactivated by using a magnet that will inhibit the AICD from sensing ventricular arrhythmias and, therefore, will prevent shocks from occurring. The magnets are medical in nature and made specifically for this purpose, and as the sensitivity to a magnetic field varies among AICDs, information about sensitivity of the specific AICD to magnetic interference, and the magnetic strength required, should be obtained from the manufacturer. The magnet can be taped to the chest wall over the device, and should remain in place until formal deactivation is accomplished.

Not surprisingly, the greatest challenge to obtaining patient agreement to deactivate an AICD device when end of life is near is the lack of communication on this issue between the patient and family, and the physician. In the 2004 study discussed earlier, only 27 (not the same as the group of 27 patients who were shocked) of the 100 families interviewed as part of the study had discussions about deactivating the device. Following these discussions, 21 of the 27 decided to deactivate the device, with most deactivations occurring days or hours prior to death. Only 9 of the 27 families who reported that patients received shocks prior to death had deactivation discussions following the patient receiving a shock and 6 of the 9 chose to have the AICD deactivated (Goldstein et al., 2004).

Further evidence regarding the lack of communication about the option of AICD deactivation near the end of life between patients and the physicians who care for them comes from two 2008 studies that reported on the attitudes, respectively, of patients and physicians to the deactivation of AICDs. Of 15 patients with AICDs, some of whom had the device for more than 1 year and some of whom had experienced at least one shock, it was reported that none of them ever had a deactivation discussion nor did any of them know that deactivation was an option. When informed that it was, most patients expressed the desire that their physicians make deactivation decisions, while one patient was quoted as saying that deactivation was "like an act of suicide." Although patients did express considerable anxiety over shocks and the desire for more information, all patients believed that the devices were exclusively beneficial (Goldstein et al., 2008, p. 7).

In the companion study, 12 physicians, 4 electrophysiologists, 4 cardiologists, and 4 internal medicine/geriatricians were interviewed. Although many of the doctors admitted that advance care planning should include discussions on the option of AICD deactivation, they acknowledged that they rarely, if ever, did so. They attributed this to differences in the intrinsic nature of AICDs as compared with other end-of-life care management decisions. Reasons for this that were provided during the interviews included the small internal nature of the AICD, with no visible reminder to trigger discussion; the absence of an established relationship with the patient (primarily relevant for the specialists); and their own concerns about withdrawing care (Goldstein et al., 2008, p. 2).

Another study exploring the ethical concerns of professional caregivers regarding deactivating AICDs showed that 52% of those surveyed believed that the devices were "life-sustaining while only 2% believed that deactivation was consistent with euthanasia or assisted suicide." Nevertheless, more than 89% of those surveyed believed that patient fears regarding inappropriate or poorly tolerated shocks were instrumental in granting requests for device activation (Kahn, 2006).

Although these studies are a good first step in understanding the issues and in increasing awareness in the medical community about the need for dialogue with patients and families about the option of AICD deactivation as part of advance care planning, the fact remains that at present, the responsibility to initiate discussions with patients and families regarding this issue more often than not devolves to the hospice and palliative care providers who care for these individuals during the final phase of life. Therefore, the National Hospice and Palliative Care Organization published a position statement on the care of hospice patients with AICDs. The statement includes guidelines (listed in Table 20–1) that, if adopted by hospice and palliative care providers, will help educate patients and families regarding the nature of AICD discharges, the implications

TABLE 20–1. NHPCO Guidelines for Patients with AICDs

- All patients with AICDs should be identified on admission and this should be documented properly
- The possibility of AICD discharge during the dying process should be thoroughly explained to patients and their designated caregivers as early as possible after admission to a hospice or palliative care program
- The option of deactivating AICDs should be thoroughly explored with patients and their caregivers as soon as possible after admission
- Patients, their designated caregivers, and health care team members should be educated that deactivating an AICD does not constitute euthanasia or physician-assisted suicide, nor is it likely to hasten death
- Patients, their designated caregivers, and health care teams should be informed about any decision to deactivate an AICD and about the methods to achieve deactivation.
- The process of AICD identification, education of the involved parties, discussions about goals of care, and possible device activation should be incorporated smoothly into current hospice and palliative care practices

Source: National Hospice and Palliative Care Organization: *Position Statement on the Care of Hospice Patients with Automatic Implantable Cardioverter-Defibrillators.* Alexandria, VA, NHPCO, 2008. http://www.nhpco.org/files/public/NHPCO_ICD_position_statement_May08.pdf. Accessed November 12, 2009.

of such discharges when close to or at the end of life, and the option of deactivation at whatever point in the course of illness that the patient/family deems appropriate, based on the patient's goals of care. These guidelines can also ensure that professional caregivers are prepared for either formal or emergent deactivation of an AICD if requested by a patient or family.

PACEMAKERS

BACKGROUND

Pacemakers have been in widespread use for many years, with estimates that more than 600,000 pacemakers are implanted yearly. They are indicated for a variety of cardiac brady-arrhythmias and may also be placed following radiofrequency ablation therapy for difficult to

control atrial fibrillation. More recently, in patients with NYHA class III or IV heart failure, an ejection fraction of 35% or less, and evidence of ventricular dysynchrony (QRS duration >120 ms and/or left bundle branch block), cardiac resynchronization therapy utilizing biventricular pacing to improve cardiac output has been utilized, with at least one study demonstrating improved quality of life, increased exercise tolerance, and reduction in symptoms.

PACEMAKER DEACTIVATION

As with AICDs, it would be unusual for a hospice or palliative care provider to be confronted with a patient who, at the time of or following admission to the program, would be considered a candidate for pacemaker placement. The one exception, perhaps, would be the rare patient with refractory heart failure whose cardiologist might see potential symptom benefit from cardiac resynchronization therapy, and this situation would have to be considered on its own merits based on the patient's short-term prognosis, chances for symptom improvement, and the patient's stated goals of care.

The most likely scenario for patients near the end of life is a request for deactivation of the pacemaker. This request stems, at least in part, from the mistaken belief by patients and their families that pacemakers may keep the heart beating after the patient would otherwise have died, prolonging the dying process and patient and family suffering. Although this belief is clearly untrue, it is unusual for deactivation of a pacemaker to result in immediate patient death, as patients are rarely, if ever, 100% pacemaker-dependent, especially during the dying process where tachycardias are the most common rhythm. However, deactivation of pacemakers, unlike AICDs, can result in immediate negative consequences to patients in the form of symptoms of fatigue, dizziness, or dyspnea from the bradycardia or progressive heart failure brought about by discontinuation of the device.

That these negative consequences are of concern has been demonstrated in the study cited earlier evaluating the ethical concerns of professionals regarding device deactivation. Sixty-three percent of the study participants thought there was an ethical distinction between deactivating a pacemaker and deactivating an AICD. Almost 90% of the respondents considered pacemakers to be life sustaining (AICDs: 52%), whereas 18.5% considered pacemaker deactivation equivalent to euthanasia or physician-assisted suicide (AICDs: 2%) (Kahn, 2006).

Regarding the techniques for deactivation, older pacemakers can be deactivated with magnets similar to what was described earlier for AICDs, while newer pacemakers, which are magnetically shielded, require the intervention of a cardiologist or other technician. As with all decisions of this type, patient/family education and communication as well as the patient's goals of care are key when considering a request for pacemaker deactivation.

BATTERY REPLACEMENT

All cardiac devices, including pacemakers and AICDs, are battery-powered self-contained units. At present, most pacemaker batteries generally last from 5 to 8 years, while those used to power AICDs may last 3 to 5 years. (This is, of course, subject to change as technology improves.) The leads that attach the power source to the heart are much more durable, and may last for 20 years or more. Replacing the battery is a minor surgical procedure during which the pacemaker case, which includes the battery, is removed from the leads, and a new case with a fresh battery is reattached to the same leads. This can usually be performed under local anesthesia with conscious sedation, except when there is an AICD involved, in which case the patient requires unconscious sedation to avoid feeling the test shock that ensures that the device is functioning.

For various reasons, patients near the end of life who have a cardiac device may decide not to have the battery replaced as its power is waning. Factors that are considered in this decision include the patient's current medical condition, short-term prognosis and the patient's ability to tolerate the procedure, the risk of progressive cardiac symptoms if the pacemaker ceases to function, and, of course, the patient's goals of care.

LEFT VENTRICULAR ASSIST DEVICE

The left ventricular assist device (LVAD) is a mechanical pump that is implanted between the left ventricle and the aorta to assist the failing heart. Its computer controller and power pack remain outside the body, with recharging required nightly. Its primary use has been to support cardiac function as a "bridge" to eventual cardiac transplantation. However, more recently it has found additional utilization in patients with refractory heart disease who are not transplant candidates, in what is described in the cardiac literature as "destination therapy."

In the one major study evaluating the LVAD in patients who were not transplant candidates, 1- and 2-year survival rates of patients randomized to receive an LVAD were significantly better than those of patients receiving "optimal medical management" (52% vs. 25% at 1 year, 23% vs. 8% at 2 years). However, the LVAD patients had twice the incidence of significant adverse effects including infection, bleeding, and stroke than patients receiving medical management.

Given the high morbidity and mortality rates associated with LVAD therapy, its role in the treatment of patients with refractory heart failure in a hospice or palliative care setting would seem to be extremely limited. However, as with all such treatment, end-of-life care providers should view the continuation of a device such as an LVAD on an individual patient basis, weighing such factors as the patient's current medical condition and needs and, most importantly, the patient's goals of care.

PARENTERAL INOTROPIC AGENTS

Inotropic agents are medications that increase cardiac contractility, resulting in beneficial hemodynamic effects in patients with acute and chronic heart failure. These medications have been utilized to temporarily improve cardiac function as a bridge to possible cardiac transplantation. In addition, although the evidence base is weak, infusion of inotropic agents has been shown to improve symptoms and functional status and possibly reduce hospitalizations in patients with advanced heart failure who are not transplant candidates, albeit with the trade off that there

is a high mortality, ranging from 40% to 95% in various reported series. As this latter group of patients, for the most part, are candidates for hospice and palliative care services, it would seem appropriate that, at least for those who are receiving symptomatic benefit from the parenteral inotropes, the medication should be continued.

The agents that are most commonly used are either dobutamine or milrinone. Dosage schedules vary, and despite the increased mortality risk, there has been a move toward intermittent infusion of these agents either in the home or at an outpatient center. A study evaluating intermittent parenteral inotropic therapy in patients with refractory heart failure demonstrated that 44 of the 73 patients in the study (44%) were able to have the therapy discontinued after a variable number of infusions, and remained without symptoms requiring repeat inotrope infusion, emergency department visit, or hospitalization for a period ranging from 201 to 489 days. Eighteen patients (25%) died, 4 patients (5%) required continuous infusion of an inotrope for symptom control, and 6 (8%) patients were withdrawn from the study program for various reasons (Lopez-Candales et al., 2004).

As long as patients are willing to recognize the increased risk of sudden death, it would appear that for at least some patients with refractory heart failure, there may be a palliative role for the intermittent infusion of inotropes on an outpatient basis. Hospice and palliative care programs who provide this intervention need to ensure that in addition to patient and family education and proper patient selection based on an individual patient's goals of care, that the staff is properly trained to manage these patients.

CARDIAC TRANSPLANTATION

There has always been a significant amount of debate about the role of hospice and palliative care providers in the care of patients awaiting cardiac transplantation. On the side in favor of caring for these patients is the notion that not all patients will survive long enough to receive a transplant. Since these patients need good symptom management and supportive care while awaiting transplant, as well as assistance coping with the possibility that they may die before a transplant is available, they should be cared for. On the other side of the argument are those who believe that patients who desire to receive a transplant want care that is incompatible with the philosophy of hospice and palliative care.

Stated another way, the question of whether a hospice or palliative care program is the appropriate care environment for patients awaiting transplant is best determined by each patient's stated goals of care. For patients who have goals of care primarily centered around palliation of symptoms, who, while willing to undergo a transplant should a heart become available but, for example, have expressed the desire not to be rehospitalized for recurrent heart failure or resuscitated should they experience cardiac arrest, it would seem reasonable to provide hospice or palliative care services pending transplant. However, for patients who desire all interventions necessary to maintain life, including hospitalization, cardiopulmonary resuscitation (CPR), and mechanical support pending availability of a transplant, it would seem that traditional care, rather than hospice and palliative care, would be the most appropriate environment.

When addressing questions of cardiac transplantation, parenteral inotropic therapy, cardiac assist devices, pacemakers, and/or AICDs, by centering the discussion around patient goals of care, decisions regarding how and when these interventions may be appropriately utilized in hospice and palliative care programs may be best determined.

BIBLIOGRAPHY

Allnurses.com. Implantable defibrillators/pacers. http://allnurses.com/hospice-nursing/implantable-defibri-llators-pacers-319889.html. Accessed August 21, 2008.

Arnsdorf MF, Knight BP: Patient information: Implantable cardioverter-defibrillators. http://www.uptodate.com/patients/content/topic.do?topicKey=~vYXPq02CRDHW. Accessed November 13, 2009.

Beattie J: *British Heart Foundation: Implantable Cardioverter Defibrillators in Patients Who Are Reaching the End of Life.* London, British Heart Foundation, 2007. http://www.bhf.org.uk/plugins/PublicationsSearchResults/DownloadFile.aspx?docid=decc6282-883c-4be8-9e35-7ef65556a9cc&version=-1&title=M105+Implantable+Cardioverter+Defibrillators+(Icds)+In+Patients+Who+Are+Reaching+The+End+Of+Life&resource=M105. Accessed August 21, 2008.

Boston Scientific LifeBeat Online: Cardiac device replacement: What to expect. http://www.bostonscientific.com/templatedata/imports/HTML/lifebeatonline/spring2006/recovery.shtml. Accessed November 13, 2009.

Christensen SA: Turning off your pacemaker. When terminal illness intervenes, a cardiac pacer can be deactivated. Suite101.com. http://medicalethics.suite101.com/article.cfm/turning_off_your_pacemaker. Accessed November 12, 2009.

Cleveland Clinic: Implantable ventricular assist device (VAD). http://my.clevelandclinic.org/heart/disorder/heartfailure/lvad.aspx. Accessed November 13, 2009.

Cleveland Clinic-Heart: 82 year old refusing pacemaker battery replacement. Heart disease (expert forum). Medhelp. http://www.medhelp.org/posts/Heart-Disease/82-Year-old-refusing-pacemaker-battery-replacement/show/917671. Created April 6, 2009. Accessed November 13, 2009.

Felker GM, O'Connor CM: Inotropic therapy for heart failure: An evidence-based approach. *Am Heart J* 142:393-401, 2001.

Fogoros RN: Pacemakers—What you should know. About.com. http://heartdisease.about.com/cs/arrhythmias/a/pacemakers.htm. Created November 27, 2003. Accessed November 13, 2009.

Goldstein NE, Lampert R, Bradley E, et al: Management of implantable cardioverter defibrillators in end-of-life care. *Ann Intern Med* 141:835-838, 2004.

Goldstein NE, Mehta D, Siddiqui S, et al: "That's like an act of suicide." Patients' attitudes toward deactivation of implantable defibrillators. *J Gen Intern Med* 23(suppl 1):7-12, 2008.

Goldstein NE, Mehta D, Teitelbaum E, et al: "It's like crossing a bridge." Complexities preventing physicians from discussing deactivation of implantable defibrillators at the end of life. *J Gen Intern Med* 23(suppl 1):2-6, 2008.

Goodlin SJ, Kutner JS, Connor SR, et al: Hospice care for heart failure patients. *J Pain Symptom Manage* 29:525-528, 2005.

Harrington MD, Luebke DL, Lewis WR, et al: Cardiac pacemakers at end-of-life. Fast Facts and Concepts. http://www.eperc.mcw.edu/fastfact/ff_111.htm. April, 2004. Accessed November 12, 2009.

Hunt SA, Abraham WT, Chin MH, et al: ACC/AHA 2005 guideline update for the diagnosis and management of chronic heart failure in the adult— Summary article: A report of the American College of Cardiology/American Heart Association Task Force on Practice Guidelines (Writing Committee to Update the 2001 Guidelines for the Evaluation and Management of Heart Failure). *Circulation* 112:1825-1852, 2005.

Kahn K: Ethical concerns identified regarding deactivating pacemakers, ICDs in terminally ill patients. Medscape Medical News, May 22, 2008. http://www.medscape.com/viewarticle/532903. Accessed November 12, 2006.

Lopez-Candales A, Carron C, Schwartz J: Need for hospice and palliative care services in patients with end-stage heart failure treated with intermittent infusion of inotropes. *Clin Cardiol* 27:23-28, 2004.

Mark DB, Anstrom KJ, Sun JL, et al: Quality of life with defibrillator therapy or amiodarone in heart failure. *New Engl J Med* 359:999-1008, 2008.

McCloskey WW: Use of intravenous inotropic therapy in the home. *Am J Health Syst Pharm* 55:930-935, 1998.

McDonagh TA: Challenges in advanced chronic heart failure: Drug therapy. http://www.medscape.com/viewarticle/580107. Accessed October 21, 2009.

National Hospice and Palliative Care Organization: *Position Statement on the Care of Hospice Patients with Automatic Implantable Cardioverter-Defibrillators.* Alexandria, VA, NHPCO, 2008. http://www.nhpco.org/files/public/NHPCO_ICD_position_statement_May08.pdf. Accessed November 12, 2009.

Otto CM, Weitz HH, Benitez RM, et al: Arrhythmias. In: *MKSAP 15: Cardiovascular Medicine.* In: Alguire PC, ed, Philadelphia, American College of Physicians, 2009a, pp. 49-61.

Otto CM, Weitz HH, Benitez RM, et al: Heart failure. In: *MKSAP 15: Cardiovascular Medicine.* In: Alguire PC, ed, Philadelphia, American College of Physicians, 2009b, pp. 29-41.

Otto CM, Weitz HH, Connolly HM, et al: Arrhythmias. In: *MKSAP 14: Cardiovascular Medicine.* In: Alguire PC, Epstein PE, eds, Philadelphia, American College of Physicians, 2006a, pp. 33-47.

Otto CM, Weitz HH, Connolly HM, et al: Heart failure. In: *MKSAP 14: Cardiovascular Medicine.* In: Alguire PC, Epstein PE, eds, Philadelphia, American College of Physicians, 2006b, pp. 23-33.

Quaglietti S, Pham M, Froelicher V: A palliative care approach to the advanced heart failure patient. *Curr Cardiol Rev* 1(1):45-52, 2005.

Stevenson LW: Clinical use of inotropic therapy for heart failure: Looking backward or forward? Part II: Chronic inotropic therapy. *Circulation* 108:492-497, 2003.

WebMD Heart Disease Health Center: Heart disease and the left ventricular assist device. http://www.webmd.com/heart-disease/treating-left-ventriculvar-device. Accessed November 13, 2009.

SELF-ASSESSMENT QUESTIONS

1. All of the following are indications for placement of an automated implantable cardioverter-defibrillator (AICD) EXCEPT:

    A. NYHA Class II or III heart failure on optimal medical therapy
    B. Expected survival of less than 1 year
    C. Cardiomyopathy with an ejection fraction of 35% or less
    D. Prior history of cardiac arrest
    E. Prophylactically in a high-risk patient with a family history of sudden cardiac death

2. All of the following statements regarding the efficacy of AICDs are true EXCEPT:

    A. Survival is improved in patients who had AICDs placed 30 days post myocardial infarction and had ejection fractions below 30%, whether they had arrhythmias or not.
    B. Quality of life of patients with AICDs has been reported to be superior to that of patients treated with amiodarone at 3 and 12 months following placement of the device.
    C. An AICD shock is associated with significant pain and anxiety.
    D. Quality of life within 1 month of a patient being shocked by an AICD is the same as for patients who have never been shocked.
    E. Survival is improved in patients with left ventricular dysfunction and a history of a resuscitated sudden cardiac death.

3. All of the following are true regarding the deactivation of an AICD EXCEPT:

    A. The deactivation process is painless to the patient.
    B. Formal deactivation requires the use of a reprogramming device that can be obtained from the manufacturer of the device.
    C. Emergency deactivation can be achieved with the use of a magnet.
    D. If the AICD has a pacemaker function, this function can be preserved when the cardioverter-defibrillator is deactivated.

    E. Deactivation preferably should occur prior to admitting the patient to the hospice program.

4. True statements regarding patient knowledge about AICD deactivation that were reported in a 2008 study by Goldstein et al. include all of the following EXCEPT:

    A. Patients are generally informed about the option of deactivation at the time the AICD device is placed.
    B. Most patients prefer that their physician play an active role in making deactivation decisions.
    C. One patient commented that deactivation "was like an act of suicide."
    D. Patients expressed considerable anxiety over the possibility of an AICD shock.
    E. Patients believed that the AICD device was exclusively beneficial.

5. True statements regarding physician attitudes toward AICD deactivation include all of the following EXCEPT:

    A. Physicians believe that the option of AICD deactivation should be discussed as part of advance care planning.
    B. Physicians rarely discuss AICD deactivation with patients.
    C. More than 50% of physicians believe that AICDs are "life-sustaining" in nature.
    D. More than 50% of physicians believe that AICD deactivation is consistent with euthanasia or physician-assisted suicide.
    E. Physicians cite their own concerns about withdrawing care as a reason why they avoid discussing AICD deactivation with patients.

6. All of the following statements concerning patient or family requests for deactivation of a pacemaker are true EXCEPT:

    A. Patients and families believe that the pacemaker will keep the heart beating after the patient would otherwise have died, prolonging the dying process.

B. It is common for deactivation of a pacemaker to result in immediate patient death.
C. Pacemaker deactivation may result in symptoms of fatigue, dizziness, or dyspnea.
D. More than 18% of physicians believe that pacemaker deactivation is consistent with euthanasia or assisted suicide.
E. Newer pacemaker models are shielded to prevent deactivation with a magnet.

7. All of the following statements regarding pacemaker and AICD battery replacement are true EXCEPT:

A. Pacemaker batteries generally last from 5 to 8 years.
B. Pacemaker leads may last for 20 years or more.
C. Pacemaker battery replacement is a minor surgical procedure that can generally be performed in the outpatient setting under local anesthesia with conscious sedation.
D. Patients having an AICD battery replaced must receive unconscious sedation to avoid feeling pain when the defibrillator is tested.
E. A patient decision to not have a pacemaker battery replaced is consistent with assisted suicide.

8. All of the following statements regarding left ventricular assist devices (LVADs) are true EXCEPT:

A. LVADs were originally designed as a "bridge" to support the cardiac function until eventual cardiac transplantation.
B. LVADs implanted in patients who were not candidates for transplantation had a 1-year survival over double that of patients treated with optimal medical management (52% vs. 25%).
C. Complications of infection, bleeding, stroke did not occur in LVAD patients with any greater frequency than in patients managed medically.
D. Patient mobility with an LVAD is limited because the power pack needs to be recharged nightly.

E. The role of LVADs in the treatment of patients with refractory heart failure receiving hospice services is extremely limited.

9. All of the following statements regarding the use of parenteral inotropic agents are true EXCEPT:

A. Inotropic agents may reduce hospitalization in some patients with advanced heart failure.
B. There is an increased risk of patient mortality associated with infusion of inotropic agents.
C. Intermittent infusion of inotropes may improve symptoms in some patients with refractory heart failure.
D. Intermittent infusion of inotropes may be accomplished in the home or outpatient setting.
E. Patients receiving intermittent infusion of inotropic agents require these infusions at least twice a week to maintain symptom control.

10. Which of the following statements regarding the role of hospice programs in the care of patients with advanced heart failure awaiting cardiac transplantation is TRUE?

A. Hospices should never care for patients awaiting cardiac transplantation because the care they want is incompatible with the principles of hospice care.
B. All patients awaiting cardiac transplantation should be admitted to hospice because if they do not receive a transplant, they will die within 6 months.
C. Patients who have goals of care focused on symptom palliation may be appropriate to receive hospice services while awaiting transplantation.
D. Patients who want to continue to receive care in the intensive care unit may be appropriate to receive hospice services while awaiting transplantation.

Invasive Respiratory Care

Freddie J. Negron and Joel S. Policzer

PART 1
INVASIVE RESPIRATORY INTERVENTIONS

Freddie J. Negron

The use of noninvasive ventilatory support devices in the management of pulmonary disorders has grown significantly since the mid-1990s for a number of reasons, including the treatment of sleep disordered breathing, the ability to allow for safer medical transport practices, and as an alternative to intubation in an emergency department.

This technology has found its way into palliative care, allowing patients and families, under the right circumstances, additional care options for the palliation of symptoms in the home setting in a safe and effective fashion. The issue, as always, remains the balance of the benefits of this technology versus its burdens, all in the context of the goals of care that the patient and family have established.

It is interesting to note that the American College of Chest Physicians in their position paper (Chest, 2005) regarding patient having acute and chronic cardiac and respiratory diseases stated that pulmonologists should "seek to prevent, relieve, reduce or soothe the symptoms of disease or disorder without affecting a cure.... Palliative care in this broad sense is not restricted to those who are dying or those enrolled in hospice programs." In this context, the role of noninvasive positive pressure devices in palliative care will be further explored.

OXYGEN THERAPY

Since virtually all palliative interventions for respiratory insufficiency will necessarily include oxygen supplementation, it is useful to briefly review oxygen therapy. For the vast majority of pa-

tients, the provision of oxygen is a comfort measure without any definitive positive physiological effects. Supplemental oxygen is commonly used to palliate dyspnea, although the evidence of benefit for this is mainly anecdotal. Head-to-head trials of oxygen versus room air are small and do not provide evidence that oxygen provides better relief of shortness of breath. However, this is not to deny that there can be a palliative effect from its use; even if the benefit is mainly psychological, the provision of oxygen, as with a concentrator, is safe and simple with few potential complications. This approach needs to be explained to patients and their caregivers as they may have expectations regarding the potential benefits of oxygen based on prior hospital experiences when patient recovery was possible.

As the provision of oxygen in the palliative care setting is primarily for comfort, the use of pulse oxymetry as a guide to titrate oxygen flow may not be warranted and may actually complicate decision making. If a patient is provided oxygen and feels less dyspneic, but the measured oxygen saturation has not changed, how has knowledge of the oxygen saturation added to the patient's comfort? Conversely, if the oxygen saturation is normalized by supplemental oxygen, but the patient has no change in symptoms, what has been accomplished? It would seem that best provision of care is to depend on careful observation and examination of the patient in order to determine the most appropriate flow rate, rather than depending on arbitrary measured pulse oxyimetry that does not correlate with symptoms and/or symptom relief.

Whenever possible, it is preferred that oxygen be provided via nasal cannula. Although the use of an oxygen mask can provide more accurate and higher flow rates of oxygen, the use of a mask may make the patient feel constrained or provide a feeling of "suffocation." If a patient finds the nasal cannula too restrictive, simply nicking the prongs will allow them to be more acceptable, as long as the flow is directly into the nostrils.

One should be aware that oxygen concentration through a nasal cannula is an approximation; however, this is not usually an issue for patients receiving palliative care near the end of life. If a patient requires a flow rate more than 2 L/min, the oxygen should be humidified to avoid the potential development of nasopharyngeal dryness, which can lead to bleeding.

NONINVASIVE POSITIVE PRESSURE VENTILATION

When the use of standard noninvasive palliative measures to treat respiratory distress, such as incentive-spirometry, chest physiotherapy, deep breathing exercises and/or positive airway pressure techniques (pursed-lip breathing), are unsuccessful, the patient may be a candidate for a form of noninvasive positive pressure ventilation.

Noninvasive positive pressure ventilation has been evolving since the mid-eighteenth century. Dräger and Barack used one such device for resuscitation of people who drowned and for the treatment of acute pulmonary edema, respectively. The iron lung became the mainstay of this therapy in the 1950s and 1960s during the polio epidemic and for the treatment of Da Nang lung and acute respiratory distress syndrome (ARDS) during the Vietnam conflict.

Noninvasive positive ventilation (NPPV) as a form of ventilatory support is more convenient and cost-effective than full mechanical ventilation. This can allow some patients with ventilatory dependence to be cared for either at home or in other nonhospital settings. In the past 10 years, there has been significant improvement in patient interfaces, such as nasal masks and nasal pillows, which have vastly improved patient adherence and long-term acceptance.

The objective of NPPV devices is to achieve larger lung volumes. They accomplish this by decreasing the work of breathing and thereby improving alveolar ventilation while simultaneously resting the respiratory musculature. In a group of patients with advanced cancer, a setting where the treatment of acute respiratory failure using ventilatory support is generally avoided, NPPV was studied. The Pavia group in Italy (Cuomo, 2004) treated 23 patients with advanced solid tumors and acute respiratory failure, a situation associated with an 87% mortality rate, with NPPV. The causes of the patients' respiratory failure were either an exacerbation of a pre-existing chronic airflow obstruction or acute pneumonia. Thirteen of 23 patients were discharged alive, while the other 10 died after an unsuccessful trial of NPPV. This study suggests that some patients with advanced cancer who develop reversible causes of respiratory failure may benefit from ventilatory support with NPPV.

This study shows that interventions that have not been considered to be appropriate for end-of-life patients may actually be of benefit in certain situations. The care of these vulnerable patients must be individualized and the expanded range of options carefully evaluated for their potential benefit and expected burdens on a case-by-case basis. As always, the care must not only be consistent with the medical status and expected survival of the patient, but most importantly with the goals of care that have been established by the patient for himself or by her decision makers.

There are various types of noninvasive positive pressure devices, including intermittent positive-pressure ventilators (IPPV), continuous positive airway pressure devices (CPAP), and bi-level positive airway pressure machines (BiPAP). The choice of device is often driven by local practice preferences and by the type of equipment that is most readily available, rather than any significant advantage of one type of device over another.

INTERMITTENT POSITIVE PRESSURE VENTILATION

Intermittent positive pressure ventilation (IPPV) is a mode of ventilation that was perfected and used in aviation medicine during the latter days of World War II and its aftermath. It stents open the airway of patients who are breathing on their own, thereby transiently improving lung volumes, decreasing the work of breathing, relieving refractory atelectasis, and, at least theoretically, improving ventilation–perfusion mismatch. It is driven by either bulk air pressure or by oxygen and is pressure-triggered to a variable maximum, with 3 to 5 cm H_2O being an example of an easily tolerated pressure. After intense debate regarding its efficacy in the early 1990s, IPPV's role today is limited to the administration of B-adrenergic agents and mucolytics.

CONTINUOUS POSITIVE AIRWAY PRESSURE

Continuous positive airway pressure (CPAP), first described in 1936 (Poultron), functions by continuously providing positive pressure throughout inspiration and expiration. The results of this are increases in vital capacity and functional residual capacity, with reduced minute ventilation. CPAP is provided via a mask, delivering 5 to 20 cm H_2O pressure. It can serve as an adjunct for bronchial hygiene therapy and can decrease breathlessness in cases of acute respiratory distress and severe pulmonary edema. It is considered the standard of care in the treatment of sleep-disordered breathing. Medications, such as bronchodilators, can be administered when a CPAP device is being utilized.

The main objection to CPAP is that patients are forced to exhale against resistance, which can promote and exacerbate diaphragmatic asthenia, as well as a sensation of general respiratory discomfort.

BI-LEVEL POSITIVE AIRWAY PRESSURE

Bi-level positive airway pressure (BiPAP) devices function by delivering a set inspiratory pressure against a lower expiratory pressure. A newer version of the BiPAP device allows the clinician to provide time-cycled and time-triggered breaths (spontaneous and timed ventilation). The BiPAP

device delivers air through either a nasal cannula or a face mask, making BiPAP much easier for users to adapt to and allowing patients with neuromuscular disease to successfully be supported by the device. As the BiPAP device allows different pressures to be set for inspiration and expiration, patients are able to get more air in and out of the lungs without needing a lot of natural muscular effort. The improvement in gas exchange with BIPAP is a result of an increase in alveolar ventilation. Externally applied positive end-expiratory pressure (PEEP) decreases the work of breathing; therefore, patients generate a lower negative inspiratory force, allowing them to more easily initiate a new breathing cycle.

In palliative care, BiPAP is utilized for hypercapnic hypoventilatory respiratory failure, pulmonary edema, chronic obstructive lung disease combined with sleep-disordered breathing, amyotrophic lateral sclerosis (ALS), and other motor neuron disease, especially those with bulbar symptoms. The indications are to palliate breathlessness, make breathing more comfortable, and improve oxygenation with hopes for improvement in comfort, while avoiding mechanical ventilation. As always, consideration of these interventions and their initiation should only occur when their potential utilization is consistent with the patient and family's goals.

OTHER ASSIST OR ADJUNCT DEVICES

There are several other devices that have found a firm niche in the care of chronic motor-neuron diseases, such as ALS, the muscular dystrophies, chest-wall deformities, and multiple sclerosis. Among these devices are incentive spirometers, handheld positive pressure devices, and the mechanical insuflattor–exsuflattor device.

Incentive spirometry is a lung expansive technique that mimics a yawn or a sigh. The spirometer device contains a ball that ascends as the patient inspires, providing the patient with visual feedback that serves as guidance as to the depth of a breath needed to achieve a predetermined volume. Some argue that similar results could be achieved with deep breathing exercises alone, without the visual guidance provided by the spirometer.

Small handheld positive airway pressure devices (e.g., Flutter® and Acapella®) work by creating "oscillations" in the pressures of the airway when the patient exhales through it, assisting in mucus clearance. Some of these devices are capable of working in conjunction with nebulizers to deliver bronchodilator medication.

The Mechanical Insufflator–Exsufflator is a portable electric device that uses a blower and a valve to apply a positive and then negative pressure to the airway, assisting in clearing retained secretions (e.g., Cough-Assist®).

care planning and for re-evaluation of their goals of care, especially if the patient's clinical condition is progressively declining (Moss et al., 1996).

There are a number of different portable volume ventilators available for home use, including the Puritan Bennett Companion 2801, Lifecare PLV-100/102, and the Intermed Bear 33. The Lifecare and Intermed models are capable of providing oxygen concentrations more than 0.21. The mode control allows the operator to select control, assist-control, or to synchronize intermittent mandatory ventilation. Some models are capable of providing PEEP. For a detailed description of current ventilators available at the time of this writing, please refer to Mosby's Respiratory Care Equipment, Mosby 2004.

PORTABLE VOLUME VENTILATORS

While the use of mechanical ventilators for resuscitation of acute hypoxic ventilatory failure has little, if any, role in hospice care, portable volume ventilators are finding an increased role as they can be used to provide ventilatory support in the home environment for patients receiving palliative care. Patients in a number of European countries, Canada, and, more recently, the United States have been treated with this modality, and reports have suggested higher patient satisfaction and an increase in patient quality of life; the use of these portable volume ventilators in the home setting is significantly cost-effective compared to long-term institutionalization.

Indications for the use of portable volume ventilators on a long-term basis include ineffectiveness or decreased effectiveness of noninvasive ventilation, intolerance to the side effects posed by noninvasive ventilation, or a desire by the patient to continue ventilatory support as part of their goals of care. Utilizing these ventilators in a palliative care setting can also allow patients and families additional time to refocus on advance

CONCLUSION

In summary, the use of ventilatory support devices has a limited but important role in the care of selected patients with respiratory insufficiency near the end of life, to allow patients to access the maximum palliative and end-of-life care options available to them. Therefore, interdisciplinary team physicians and nurses should become familiar with the techniques and equipment that enhance their ability to provide compassionate treatment of the multidimensional aspects of dyspnea that often plague patients as life is drawing to a close.

PART 2
REMOVAL OF MECHANICAL VENTILATORY SUPPORT

Joel Policzer

While caring for patients who remain on mechanical ventilators is highly unusual in a hospice setting, it is becoming increasingly common to provide end-of-life care either in a hospice or palliative care setting to patients who are on mechanical ventilators for the purpose of providing a safe environment for the discontinuation of the ventilatory support. The need for this has arisen because, as medical care has become more and more complex, there has been greater utilization of respiratory support on a mechanical ventilator to sustain a patient while other care is given in an attempt to reverse the other critical illnesses. If the associated illnesses do not improve, if the cause of respiratory failure cannot be reversed, or if the burden of continuation of ventilator support outweighs the benefits for the patient and family, then plans need to be made to remove this support in a humane and caring way so that the patient does not suffer from hypoxia or air hunger.

The protocol described below assumes that all conversations have already been held, that the medical caregivers have already helped the patient and family through the decision-making process, and everyone is agreed that removal of the ventilator is the appropriate path to follow in the patient's care at this time. (See Chapter 3 for a discussion of how to discuss this type of issue with the patient and/or family.) As well, the assumption is that all discussions have been documented in the patient record and all appropriate legal documents that are required have been reviewed and signed.

PREPARATORY STEPS

Once agreement is reached to discontinue the ventilator, then planning begins for its removal. The first decision is where this will happen. Often, the patient is in a critical care unit and the decision has to be made whether this is the best location for removal to occur. ICUs are busy places designed so that the staff has continual visual contact with patients; privacy is hard to achieve. Also, the noise of staff tending to other patients, monitors beeping, phones ringing, and the bright light levels increase the level of stress and it is nearly impossible to provide a calm, peaceful environment. If it is at all possible and compatible with the facility's policy, the patient, while remaining on the ventilator, should be moved to a private room on a medical floor, or to a hospice or palliative care unit if there is one within the facility, and the patient stabilized there before the procedure begins.

At times, a patient who has spent considerable time in a facility will request a transfer home prior to ventilator removal. In addition, there are, of course, patients that are being cared for at home who are on a mechanical ventilator. The special considerations for accommodating discontinuation of a mechanical ventilator outside a medical facility will be addressed separately below.

Once the proper location in the facility to remove the ventilator has been decided upon, the next decision is who should be present. If there is a request that many family and friends be present, the clinical staff in charge will have to determine how many people can be accommodated; crowding in the room should be avoided so that the atmosphere remains calm and the medical staff has easy access to the patient.

It should be specifically discussed whether family clergy should be present or should visit prior to discontinuing ventilatory support; if the family does not have personal clergy, the services of a chaplain should be offered. In addition, it should be strongly recommended that a clinical social worker be present for support; even if family members indicate that they will be fine, no one knows what their reactions will be until they occur.

Other decisions that need to be addressed are the timing of the procedure, who needs to make final visits with the patient, the visitation or presence of pets, whether special music will be played, and so on. The basic consideration here is that as this is likely the patient's final chance to interact with people close to him or her as well as experience things (i.e., music) that bring pleasure or enjoyment, every effort should be made to allow the patient to visit with whoever s/he needs to and to experience, within the realm of possibility, whatever is important, prior to discontinuing the ventilator.

REMOVAL PROTOCOL

The goals that guide the protocol of ventilator removal are based on the following principles: maximal comfort of the patient, maximal level of patient unawareness to achieve maximal comfort, and maximal symptom support to ease potential respiratory distress.

As the protocol is initiated, there should be a complete review of the decision with the patient and/or family to verify that the procedure will go forward. The protocol should be reviewed in detail with everyone who will be present so that all understand what symptoms and signs are expected and what will be done about them. There should be verification that all documentation is in place in the record, that a physician's order for this procedure has been obtained, and that a Do Not Resuscitate order and appropriate form are signed.

It is especially important to specifically discuss with the patient and family that possibility the patient's death may not occur immediately upon removal of the ventilator's support. Conventional wisdom would suggest that the ventilator has been needed because the patient was not able to "breathe on his own"; however, one has to consider that this often means that the patient was not able to breathe *optimally* on his own. Respiratory efforts may resume but without sufficient capacity to allow the patient to return to his or her previous life and usual activities. It needs to be reinforced that the fact that a patient resumes breathing after being taken off the ventilator does not mean that the ventilator was not needed in the first place, does not mean that it was the wrong decision to remove the ventilator, and does not mean that the patient will continue to improve. It is useful to remind families that the ventilator is a tool to support a patient that cannot breathe adequately on his own; since in the case of their loved one, the underlying medical problem did not improve, she will not be able to breathe well enough on her own without the ventilator, and they made the choice that they did not want her to always depend on the machine to help her breathe. And as always, the families must be told that whatever shortness of breath or dyspnea accompanies the postventilator state will be treated aggressively.

It is suggested that the minimum clinical staff that needs to be present includes a physician with experience in this process or a respiratory therapist, a nurse with similar experience, and a clinical social worker. If the patient's attending physician, pulmonologist, or intensivist will not be participating in the protocol and have transferred care to another physician, for example a physician working for a hospice or palliative care service, it should be policy that the physician now involved in the procedure personally examine the patient prior to orders being written for discontinuation of the ventilator.

A suggested protocol for discontinuation of a mechanical ventilator can be found in Table 21–1. Protocols vary by institution, with the major differences being the choice of medications for sedation and relief of symptoms. As already discussed earlier, what all protocols have in common is the provision of peaceful and comfortable environment, the presence of loved ones to the extent desired, and sufficient medication to ensure maximum patient comfort throughout the process.

POSTVENTILATOR CARE

In addition to the medical care that the patient will need to assure comfort during the postventilator period, the family will need strong support if

TABLE 21–1. Suggested Protocol for Discontinuation of Mechanical Ventilation

1. Remove all restraints and unnecessary medical equipment. Discontinue monitoring of vital signs and pulse oximetry; silence alarms on all equipment.
2. Prepare space at the bedside for family members who wish to be present.
3. Keep ventilator settings as they had been for the present.
4. IV access is the preferred route for medication administration. Keep any IV line patent either with KVO rate fluids or via saline lock. If IV access is compromised and patient/family decline to have it re-established, medications can be given via subcutaneous route. Oral or sublingual routes are not appropriate for this situation.
5. Assure that patient is unaware prior to any change of ventilator settings. The goal is a Ramsay Sedation Score of 5 (sluggish response to light glabellar tap or loud noise) or 6 (no response to same stimuli).
   a. Patient who is opioid naïve: administer morphine sulfate 10–20 mg IV bolus followed by morphine sulfate infusion at rate of 50% of initial bolus per hour.
   b. Patient who is truly allergic to morphine sulfate: hydromorphone 5 mg IV bolus followed by hydromorphone infusion at 0.5–1.0 mg per hour
   c. Patient receiving opioid analgesia: bolus dose should be basal dose of morphine increased by 50%.
   d. Titrate all doses to achieve appropriate Ramsay score and maintain with adjustments of infusion rate and bolus doses as needed
   e. Benzodiazepine medications can be used in the place of opioids or as a supplement to them. Midazolam or lorazepam can be given as a bolus of 0.04 mg/kg followed by infusion at 1–2 mg per hour.
6. Once the patient is properly sedated, set the FIO_2 on the ventilator to 21% and observe for signs of respiratory distress. If distress is observed, intervene with supplemental doses of morphine, nebulized bronchodilators, and/or steroids, as indicated.
7. Remove the patient from mechanical ventilation. Patients can either have the ventilator disconnected for "rapid weaning," or "slow weaning" can be achieved by decreasing assist control or IMV by intervals of two breaths every 2–4 minutes. In the latter, the goal is to achieve an IMV of 0 in 15–20 min.
8. Deflate cuff and remove tracheostomy or endotracheal tube and control any secretions as needed.
9. Postextubation assess carefully for signs of distress and treat as necessary.
   a. Respiratory distress: Administer bolus doses of morphine or hydromorphone every 10 min as needed.
   b. Anxiety: Administer bolus doses of a benzodiazepine every 10 min as needed.
   c. Excessive secretions: Occasional suctioning or use atropine ophthalmic solution 1%, one or two drops sublingual every hour as needed.
10. If the patient begins to breathe independently, administer humidified oxygen at 2 L/min for comfort and verify that orders are written for doses of opioids and/or benzodiazepines for respiratory distress and anxiety, acetaminophen for fever, anti-emetics, and atropine for excess secretions.

the patient has resumed independent breathing. It is expected that if the patient survives beyond 1 to 2 days, the family will begin to question the original decision to remove the ventilator; they will require education that resumption of breathing does not mean improvement of the underlying or associated illnesses and that prolonged survival is unlikely, with or without the ventilator.

In addition, there will need to be a discussion regarding whether to provide artificial hydration or nutrition. It is natural for family members to look at their loved one who has now survived for a few days, breathing without ventilatory support, and question whether they are now allowing him or her to "starve to death." If the patient has not improved clinically, has not spontaneously regained alertness, and is continuing to breathe shallowly, then it is unlikely that hydration or nutritional support will improve the situation. The family needs to review their goals of care and be guided toward the idea that the underlying disease is no better. In addition, in this situation, giving enteral or parenteral feedings or fluid may not be tolerated by their loved one, in which case s/he will experience increased shortness of breath that will worsen the clinical situation. Obviously, if a patient is showing signs that their underlying clinical situation may be improving, then aggressive measures need to be instituted to support the patient until the clinical course determines itself.

CONSIDERATIONS FOR VENTILATOR REMOVAL AT HOME

There are two scenarios that may result in a request for ventilator removal at home. One, of course, would be a patient who is on chronic mechanical ventilation already being cared for at home. The second would be a patient who is hospitalized or in another type of facility requesting ventilator removal and who wants to return home one final time before the ventilator is discontinued. These two situations create added logistical considerations that have to be planned for before the decision to remove the ventilator in the home setting can be made.

The prime consideration is personnel. Are there sufficient numbers of experienced clinical people available to participate in this intervention in the home? One needs to plan for the possibility that this procedure may take hours. Is there a physician willing and able to visit the patient, and to be present, if asked, during ventilator removal? Are there sufficient nurses to attend to the

patient during the entire period? If the patient begins to breathe independently, are there RNs who will be able to stay at the bedside continuously to manage the care?

Next, one has to consider the physical requirements. If the patient is not already at home, where will the temporary ventilator come from? Who will manage the ventilator settings? Which model needs to be supplied so that it will actually fit through the residence door? Compact, mobile ventilators now exist; is one of these available? Does the residence have grounded plugs so that the ventilator can actually be plugged in? If discontinuation of the ventilator is not going to be done immediately, what plans are in place for generator back-up in the case of power failure, or has the decision been made that in the event of power failure the patient will undergo rapid weaning?

Finally, there has to be planning to ensure that all medications, medical supplies, and equipment are available and in the home prior to the procedure. It is recommended that a checklist be created and that the responsible clinical team ensures that all necessary items, including oxygen, a suction device, tubing, catheters, and cannulas are in the home prior to the patient's arrival. An appropriate quantity of all medications that one might anticipate needing, including parenteral opioids and benzodiazepines, nebulized bronchodilators and steroids, and atropine eye drops, should also be obtained. It is recommended that the amount of each medication that should be procured is double what one would estimate requiring for a 24-hour period. While this may seem to be excessive, one has to remember that in a patient's residence, the ability to "call pharmacy or central supply and have them send STAT" does not exist.

All this is in addition to the planning noted earlier for ventilator withdrawal in a facility. One should not proceed with this in the home setting unless every single detail of staff, physical infrastructure, and medical equipment/medication is fully planned for and available. If not, there is a great risk that this procedure can deteriorate into one with a distressed patient aware and gasping for breath; this must be avoided at all costs.

BIBLIOGRAPHY

American Association for Respiratory Care: Use of positive airway pressure adjuncts to bronchial hygiene therapy. *Respir Care* 38:516, 1993.

Brochard L: Non-invasive ventilation for acute respiratory failure *JAMA* 288:932-935, 2002.

Cairo JM, Pilbeam SP: Lung expansion devices, Chapter 7. In: *Mosby's Respiratory Care Equipment*, 7th ed. St. Louis, MO, Mosby Publishing, 2004, pp. 191-210.

Cairo JM, Pilbeam SP: Noninvasive ventilation, Chapter 14. In: *Mosby's Respiratory Care Equipment*, 7th ed. St. Louis, MO, Mosby Publishing, 2004, pp. 773-786.

Cuomo A, Delmastro M, Ceriana P, et al: Non-invasive mechanical ventilation as a palliative treatment of acute respiratory failure in patients with end-stage solid cancer. *Pall Med* 18(7):602-610, 2004.

Deheny L, Berney S: The use of positive pressure devices by physiotherapists. *Eur Respir J* 17:821-829, 2001.

Gilani A, Hinn A, Jacobson PL: Fast Facts and Concepts #73: Respiratory Failure in ALS, 2nd ed. July 2006. End-of-Life/Palliative Education Resource Center: http://www.eperc.mcw.edu. Accessed November 10, 2008.

Leach R: Palliative medicine and non-malignant, end-stage respiratory disease, Chapter 10.4. In: Doyle D, Hanks G, Cherny NI, Calman K, eds. *Oxford Textbook of Palliative Medicine*, 3rd ed. Oxford, Oxford University Press, 2005, pp. 895-916.

Marrr L, Weissman DE: Withdrawal of ventilatory support from the dying adult patient. *J Support Oncol* 2:283-288, 2004.

Moss AH, Oppenheimer EA, Casey P, et al: Patients with amyotrophic lateral sclerosis receiving long-term mechanical ventilation. *Chest* 110:249-255, 1996.

Nava S, Cuomo A, Maugeri S, Selecky P: Non-invasive ventilation and dyspnea in palliative medicine (correspondence). *Chest* 129:1391-1392, 2006.

Policzer JS, Rapaport DK, O'Mahony S, McHugh M: Withdrawal of ventilatory support: cases from inpatient hospice, hospital-based palliative care service, and at home; practice protocols and guidelines. Program and Abstracts of the 15th Annual Assembly of the American Academy of Hospice and Palliative Medicine, Orlando, FL, February 6–9, Session 407, 2003.

Removal of Mechanical Ventilation in the Dying Patient; VITAS Standard; © VITAS Innovative Hospice Care; 2008.

Selecky PA, Eliasson CA, Hall RI, et al: Palliative and end-of-life care for patients with cardiopulmonary diseases: American College of Chest Physician Position Statement. *Chest* 128:3599-3610, 2005.

Sharma S: Non-Invasive Ventilation. http://www.emedicine.com May 15, 2006. Accessed November 10, 2008.

Szalados JE: Discontinuation of mechanical ventilation at end-of-life: the ethical and legal boundaries of physician conduct in termination of life support. *Crit Care Clin* 23(2):317-337, 2007.

SELF-ASSESSMENT QUESTIONS

1. Regarding oxygen use in end-of-life care, which of the following is TRUE?

   A. Pulse oximetry is a necessary guide to follow the use of supplemental oxygen treatment.
   B. Breathlessness is a subjective symptom and the patient will decide if use of oxygen makes their dyspnea less.
   C. Oxygen always needs to be administered under inspiratory pressure for benefit.
   D. The administration of oxygen will avoid the need for noninvasive ventilatory devices.
   E. Palliation of shortness of breath will require flow rates higher than 2 L/min

2. Which of the following interventions used to relieve dyspnea would be likely LEAST utilized in a patient on a hospice program?

   A. Oxygen
   B. CPAP
   C. BiPAP
   D. Positive pressure ventilators
   E. IPPV

3. Indications for the use of BiPAP to treat respiratory insufficiency include the following conditions EXCEPT

   A. Amyotrophic lateral sclerosis
   B. Muscular dystrophy
   C. Airway obstruction due to head and neck cancer
   D. Multiple sclerosis
   E. Chest wall deformities

4. All the following statements are true EXCEPT

   A. Pulmonary edema can create a situation of alveolar hypoventilation.
   B. A normal oxygen saturation will preclude the use of oxygen to palliate breathlessness.
   C. On a palliative care service, use of a ventilator can be beneficial to allow a patient time to decide on their goals of care.
   D. Bronchodilators can be administered to patients using BiPAP.
   E. Incentive spirometry devices have advantages over deep breathing exercises because the patient gains positive feedback from watching the ball rise with inspiration.

5. Which of the following interventions should NOT be tried before considering intervention with noninvasive positive pressure ventilation?

   A. Treadmill rehabilitation program
   B. Incentive spirometry
   C. Chest physiotherapy
   D. Deep breathing exercises
   E. Pursed-lip breathing

6. When planning for removal of a ventilator, which of the following people SHOULD be present?

   A. The administrator of the facility
   B. Relatives of the patient in the adjoining bed
   C. The patient's daughter who cannot stop crying and begging her mother not to do this
   D. The patient's son and grandchildren who are devastated at the loss of the patient but see this as supportive of their father's/grandfather's last wish
   E. The facility's code team

7. When planning withdrawal of a ventilator in a patient's residence, which of the following is TRUE?

   A. It requires no more planning than a procedure done in a facility.
   B. The electrical wiring of the house is not an issue.
   C. Experienced clinical staff is important.

D. Medications can be given by the oral/
sublingual route because IVs are not used
at home.
E. There is no need for psychosocial support because the patient is in his own
home.

8. Which of the following statements about
the role of physicians in the process of
discontinuing a mechanical ventilator is
TRUE?

A. The physician in charge of writing the
orders and managing the intervention
should have examined the patient and reviewed the medical record.
B. The physician of choice in this situation is
a pulmonologist or an intensivist.
C. It is the ordering physician's responsibility, not a respiratory therapist's, to remove
the patient's endotracheal tube.
D. The presence of a physician during ex-
tubation decreases the need for a social
worker.
E. Only a physician can counsel patient and
family on this intervention

9. All of the following should be part of the
preparation before withdrawal of ventilator
support EXCEPT

A. Assure IV access
B. Have the patient at a Ramsay sedation
score of 2
C. Have availability of sufficient supply of
opioids and benzodiazepines
D. Have suction in the room
E. Assure presence of all necessary clinical
support staff

10. Which of the following statements is TRUE
regarding discontinuation of a mechanical
ventilator?

A. Staff must be prepared to reintubate the
patient if respiratory distress occurs
B. Excess oral and tracheal secretions are
best palliated by an anticholinergic patch
C. Respiratory distress can be palliated by
benzodiazepines
D. It is not necessary to continue supplemental oxygen once the ventilator has been removed
E. The endotracheal tube should be left in
place to allow for ease of suctioning

Ethical Dilemmas

SECTION FOUR

CHAPTER

22

Advance Directives and CPR at the End of Life

Barry M. Kinzbrunner and Domingo Gomez

INTRODUCTION

Throughout the history of mankind, decisions about how to care for people who are approaching the end of life have been made according to the cultural mores of the times. In primitive societies, the "medicine man" and the chief of the tribe would make these decisions based on their religious and political power, and their decisions went essentially unquestioned. As civilization evolved, various deities, the "oracles," and religious figures were often consulted as to life and death issues, although the ancient Greeks and Chinese also pioneered the use of physicians to provide expert advice on health and disease. Throughout most of the Middle Ages, religious groups remained the most important advisors to people who had serious or terminal illness. However, toward the end of the Middle Ages, Mediterranean Jewish and Arab physicians increasingly became the repositories of medical knowledge and providers of medical advice to the point that even devout Christians called on them when faced with advanced illnesses. During the Renaissance, with medical knowledge advancing more slowly than the arts, religious leaders again took center stage away from physicians when it came to assisting patients and families in coping with serious illnesses and death.

The discovery of the nature of infectious diseases and isolation techniques during the latter half of the nineteenth and into the twentieth century had a significant influence on prolongation of life, shifting public attention back to the physician as the chief health care advisor. The introduction of antibiotics in the 1940s made diseases like syphilis, tuberculosis, pneumonia, and cholera no longer dreaded as harbingers of certain death. New anesthesia techniques in the 1950s allowed patients to receive mechanical ventilatory assistance, supporting them during difficult surgical procedures and postoperative recovery, with a high likelihood of full recovery. Mechanical ventilatory support was eventually extended to trauma victims and, ultimately, to support vital functions in decompensated patients with acute and chronic medical illnesses. The addition of cardiac defibrillators further enhanced the ability to support and prolong the lives of patients who were victims of cardiac as well as respiratory arrest.

With the increased use of mechanical ventilatory support and other forms of advanced life support, medical facilities developed the Intensive Care Unit (ICU) to ensure that patients received this care in the proper environment. During this same time period, improvement in nutritional support, both by enteral and parenteral methods, allowed physicians to also provide nutritional support to patients who were unable to eat on their own. The refinement and widespread application of these techniques allowed physicians to effectively support and prolong the lives of patients who had previously succumbed to advanced and life-threatening illnesses.

As with all new modalities of treatment, the widespread use of advanced life support and artificial nutritional support has not only had benefits, but adverse consequences as well. While some patients who would otherwise have died have been given a new lease on life, other patients who had no realistic hope for recovery had their lives extended artificially for weeks and months. As patients and families became more aware of the futility of advanced life support in certain clinical circumstances, some began to assert their wishes not to have the dying process prolonged by artificial means. This philosophy of care began as a grassroots movement, with landmark legal cases, such as Quinlan, Cruzan, and others, leading to legal precedents that gave patients the right to refuse life-prolonging treatment near the end of life. This ultimately led to the development of advance directives, documents that provide instructions to health care providers as to how individual patients choose to be treated near the end of life when they are unable to make independent health care decisions.

To encourage all patients to create advance directives while they are capable of making decisions about their care, the US Congress passed the "Patient Self-Determination Act" (PSDA) in

TABLE 22–1. Features of the Patient Self-determination Act (PSDA)
• Passed 11/1990; Effective 12/1/1991
• Requires Medicare and Medicaid providers to give adult individuals, at the time of inpatient admission or outpatient enrollment, certain information about their rights under the law of the state they are in, governing advance directives, including
• The right to participate in and direct their own health care decisions
• The right to accept or refuse medical or surgical treatment
• The right to prepare an advance directive
• The act also prohibits institutions from discriminating against a patient who does not have an advance directive or from denying care based on a patient's advance directive instructions.

November 1990. The primary features of this legislation, which became effective on December 1, 1991, are listed in Table 22–1. In essence, the PSDA mandates that Medicare and Medicaid providers inform patients, in writing, of their rights to execute an advance directive and to assist them in executing such a directive if they choose to do so. The PSDA also mandates that Medicare and Medicaid providers may not deny patients access to health care services based upon their advance directive instructions.

It is the primary goal of this chapter to review the subject of advance directives, defining what they are, exploring the principles behind their development, and gaining an understanding of how they function. This chapter will then evaluate the historical driving force behind the development of advance directives, such as choices regarding cardiopulmonary resuscitation (CPR) at the end of life. A second major issue addressed by advance directives, choices regarding artificial nutritional support and hydration at the end of life, is covered in Chapter 24.

ADVANCE DIRECTIVES

Advance directives are specific instructions, prepared in advance of serious illness, that are intended to direct the medical care for specific individuals if they become unable to express their health care choices at a future date. This allows patients to participate in making their own decisions regarding the care they would prefer to receive if they are unable to make their wishes known. There are several different types of advance directives in use today in the United States, listed in Table 22–2 and discussed below.

LIVING WILL

The living will is a legal document, written and signed by an individual in the presence of witnesses, that conveys the instructions of the individual regarding health care interventions desired or not desired in the event the person suffers from a terminal illness or certain other irreversible illnesses (defined differently by different

TABLE 22–2. Types of Advance Directives
• Living will
• Durable (or special) health care power of attorney
• Combined living will/health care power of attorney document
• Verbal advance directive

TABLE 22–3. Interventions Addressed by Living Wills

- Cardiopulmonary resuscitation
- Nutritional support by other than oral means
- Hydration by other than oral means
- Antibiotics
- Transfusion of blood products
- Invasive procedures and diagnostic studies including, but not limited to
  - Blood tests
  - Spinal taps
  - X-rays and scans
- Desire to be hospitalized or remain at home

role. A critical responsibility for the health care proxy is that when called upon to make a surrogate decision, the decision must be based, not on what the proxy would choose, but on what the surrogate believes that the incapacitated individual would choose if the person were able to express his or her own wishes. Unlike the living will, which only comes into play when the person suffers from a terminal illness or certain other irreversible illnesses, the durable power of attorney allows the health care surrogate to make decisions for the incapacitated individual whenever the person is incapable of making a choice, whether the incapacitating illness is terminal, irreversible, or ultimately correctable.

states, see section "Advance Directives and State Law") and is incapable of verbally communicating wishes regarding health care. (This document should not be confused with a last will and testament, the purpose of which is to distribute assets after a person's death.) While living wills have been traditionally thought of as addressing choices primarily limited to interventions such as CPR, nutrition, and hydration, they may, in fact, address a wide variety of other interventions, as delineated in Table 22–3.

DURABLE (OR SPECIAL) HEALTH CARE POWER OF ATTORNEY

The durable (or special) health care power of attorney is a legal document that allows an individual to appoint a responsible person (usually called a health care surrogate or proxy) who is empowered to make health care decisions in the event the individual becomes unable to make and communicate such decisions personally. This document provides for power to make medically related decisions only, and does not give the surrogate the authority to make legal or financial decisions. While health care proxies are usually family members, any individual, such as a close friend, a member of clergy, or even a physician, may, with their permission, be designated for this

COMBINED LIVING WILL/HEALTH CARE POWER OF ATTORNEY

The major challenge with the durable health care power of attorney is to ensure that the surrogate actually knows (or has a pretty good idea of) what the individual would have chosen had the person been capable of expressing his or her own wishes. Hopefully, this was accomplished through conversation or written instructions when the person gave the decision-making responsibility to the health care proxy. One way to ensure that this happens is for an individual to execute what, for lack of a better term, is a combined living will/ health care power of attorney. The health care surrogate could then rely on the living will section of the document to guide the decisions that he or she makes for the incapacitated person.

VERBAL ADVANCE DIRECTIVES

Many individuals have, in the course of conversation with loved ones, expressed their desires around care at the end of life, but did not have the foresight to execute a written advance directive prior to becoming unable to make a health care decision. Alternatively, for psychological reasons, some individuals just cannot bring themselves to sign a document that addresses issues revolving around the end of life. For these people, the documentation of their verbal instructions by their physician or health care provider (i.e., hospice) may be sufficient to constitute a legitimate advance directive. In fact, nowadays these are the most common kind of advance care directives.

Verbal advance directives may be provided by patients, or, in many states, by next of kin in a similar fashion to the health care power of attorney. The ability of next of kin to make proxy decisions for patients varies from state to state. (This will be discussed in the section Advance Directives and State Law).

The key to the verbal advance directive is documentation. It is crucial that, whether the source of the information is the patient or the appropriate legal next of kin, the medical record should clearly document the nature of the conversation held regarding the patient's condition, offered options of care, and the decisions made around the various potential interventions discussed.

DO-NOT-RESUSCITATE (DNR) ORDER

A "Do-Not-Resuscitate" (DNR) order is a physician's order that states that CPR is not to be initiated if a cardiac or respiratory arrest occurs. Technically, it is not an advance directive, but is the order given by a physician honoring the advance directive (written or verbal) of a patient or the patient's health care proxy that the patient does not desire CPR. It should be noted that while a physician can theoretically give a DNR order on any patient for whom s/he deems it be appropriate, it has become common practice, (as well as policy in many institutions and law in many states) for physicians not to give such an order in the absence of a verbal or written advance directive or the health care proxy's permission.

Another DNR document that has become increasingly common and is in use in many states is termed the "Out-of-Hospital DNR." When this document, signed by the patient or health care surrogate (if the patient is incompetent), witnesses, and a physician, is present in an individual's home, then emergency medical services (EMS) paramedics, who are generally instructed to provide CPR to any person that has experienced a cardiopulmonary arrest, are not compelled to start CPR.

ADVANCE DIRECTIVES AND STATE LAW

While the "Patient Self-Determination Act" (PSDA) is a federal statute, the nature of advance directives and the laws that govern them are state specific, with the laws of each state varying considerably regarding terminology, the scope of decision-making, restrictions, and the formalities required for executing an advance directive. For example, different states will have different definitions of what constitutes a terminal illness for purposes of a living will (which may also differ from the hospice definition of 6 months or less as defined by the Medicare Hospice Benefit and discussed extensively in Chapter 1 of this book). States will also differ as to what other medical conditions (i.e., irreversible neurological condition, persistent vegetative state, end-stage condition), if any, would permit medical decision making based on a living will. States also define the requirements for appointing a durable health care power of attorney and may differ regarding the degree of evidence required (i.e., verbal or written) to establish that the decision being made by the surrogate is what the person would have chosen. The states differ in their legal definitions of substituted decision makers. For example, Florida defines a "surrogate" as the person legally appointed by the patient to act "in the place of" that patient when capacity is impaired. A "proxy" is a volunteer, picked from a hierarchy of people, who acts "in the best interest of" the patient. As has been said, not all states concur with these definitions; for the purposes of this discussion, the terms will be used fairly interchangeably. Therefore, when advising patients on executing these documents, it is important to ensure that they meet the specifications of the state in which the patient resides. Information specific to individual states may be obtained from such organizations as the State Medical Association, the State Nursing Association, or the State Bar Association. Most hospitals, medical centers, and hospices will also be able to provide the appropriate information. Another excellent source for state-specific advance directives on the Internet is the Web site "Caring Connections," sponsored by the National Hospice and Palliative Care Organization (NHPCO), which has links to sample advance directive documents for each of the 50 states (http://www.caringinfo.org).

Regarding interstate validity of advance directives, many states recognize out-of-state advance directives if the directive meets either the legal requirements of the state where executed or the state where the treatment decision arises, while several states are silent on this question. However, even if an advance directive fails to meet the technicalities of state law, health care providers are encouraged to value the directive as important, if not controlling, evidence of the patient's wishes.

In the absence of written advance directives, many states have provisions that will allow documented verbal instructions to be followed regarding care or the oral designation of a health care surrogate. In some states, this can be established based on the word of the treating physician, while in others, there are varied requirements, which may include the testimony of one or more witnesses, the confirmed terminal diagnosis for the patient, or the restriction of the designation to the current hospitalization or course of treatment.

For patients who are unable to make their own decisions and for whom no written or verbal advance directive exists, most states have established provisions for substitute decision making within their advance directive statutes. This usually includes the establishment of a hierarchy of relatives that have precedence in health care decision making for incapacitated patients (in varying order state to state and including health care professionals in some states) and often also includes provision for a court-appointed guardian to make health care decisions for patients who have no relatives and have not left any written advance directive instructions. There remain a small number of states that do not allow health care proxy decisions to be made for patients in the absence of written advance directives.

ADVANTAGES OF ADVANCE DIRECTIVES

There are a number of potential advantages to the use of advanced directives, listed in Table 22–4, the key advantage being the respect of patient autonomy.

Autonomy derives from the deontological school of thought, which emphasizes duty and acting from the right intentions. One of those right intentions involves treating people with respect, which leads directly to the concept of autonomy, or respecting the capacity and the right of rational agents to self-determination. In a clinical setting, autonomy is defined as the right of patients to have self-determination when it comes to choosing between different therapeutic

TABLE 22–4. Potential Advantages of Advanced Directives

PATIENT ADVANTAGES	HEALTH CARE PROVIDER ADVANTAGES
Expression of autonomy	Knowledge of patient's wishes
Decreased personal worry	Decrease in unnecessary therapeutic and diagnostic interventions
Decrease in family anxiety and guilt	Decrease in health care costs
	Decrease in medicolegal concerns

alternatives. By choosing to execute an advance directive (an expression of autonomy unto itself), patients provide family caregivers and professional health care providers with the information necessary to ensure that their choices regarding care at the end of life are respected and followed. In the form of a living will, autonomy is expressed in writing, while in the form of a durable power of attorney, the assumption is made that the health care proxies are making health care choices for patients based on the knowledge of what the patients would have chosen.

Patients who execute advance directives may have the advantage of worrying less about the prospects of receiving therapy that they would otherwise not desire. Families are often appreciative of the fact that, especially when living wills are used, they do not have the anxiety and guilt associated with being forced to make life and death decisions for a loved one. Providers benefit by knowing what therapeutic interventions patients do and do not desire near the end of life. The providers can then care for patients in an appropriate, beneficial, and cost-effective manner, respecting patient autonomy and reducing the risk of medicolegal repercussions.

sations until the patient is nearing a time of crisis, when the need to make decisions about interventions such as CPR at the end of life are a virtual reality. As covered in depth in Chapter 3, many practitioners still have significant difficulty speaking with patients and families and "breaking the bad news" that the end of life is approaching. The additional burden of the discussion and decision making around advance directive issues is often too overwhelming for patients and families to comprehend and digest at the same time that the "bad news" is confronted. Therefore, it is recommended that advance directive conversations between physicians and patients be held at a time before "bad news" needs to be discussed, such as while the patient may be chronically ill, but not yet approaching the terminal phase. This will reduce the potential for overwhelming the patient and family during a time of great crisis and allow for more thoughtful decision making to occur.

The content of the discussion is of great importance. Table 22–5 lists some of the issues that need to be reviewed by the physician. Patients should be offered the option of executing a living will, a durable power of attorney, or both, based upon individual and family preference. A thorough explanation of the structure and function of each

HOW TO ASSIST PATIENTS IN EXECUTING ADVANCE DIRECTIVES

Physicians own a great deal of the responsibility to empower and encourage patients to execute advance directives. Physicians should have advance directive discussion with all patients under their care. It is especially important for physicians to discuss these issues with patients who suffer from chronic illnesses that have a high risk of progressive mental and physical debility and to do this before the patients become incapable of making health care decisions.

The timing of the discussion is important. Most often, physicians, as well as patients and families, tend to avoid advance directive conver-

TABLE 22–5. Content of Advanced Directive Discussions

- Types of advanced directives
  - Living will
  - Durable power of attorney
  - Verbal instructions
- State regulations regarding advanced directives
- Pros and cons of specific interventions (see Table 22–3)
- For living wills, use specific language to describe therapeutic choices
- Review patient preferences and update frequently
- Advance directives are not irrevocable

of these documents, including state specific requirements, should be provided to the patient and family. It is suggested that for many patients, it is desirable to execute a combined living will/health care power of attorney. As discussed earlier, living wills are only effective when a patient suffers from a terminal illness or suffers from certain other irreversible illnesses (that, as discussed earlier, may differ from state to state). If a patient's condition falls short of the state's specific legal definition that allows for activation of a living will at a time when the capacity to make a health care decision is absent, having identified a health care surrogate will allow the necessary decisions to be made based upon the patient's expressed wishes.

While it is better to have a written advance directive, verbal instructions remain important as supplements to written instructions as well as serving as advance directives on their own. Patients may be physically unable to execute an advance directive or may be unwilling to commit their wishes to paper for psychological reasons. In either event, in the absence of written advance directives, oral instructions that are reduced to writing by the patient's physician or another health care provider may adequately provide information on how a patient wants to be cared for near the end of life.

Therapeutic decisions that are commonly articulated in advance directives related to the interventions listed in Table 22–3 should be thoroughly discussed. The physician should present the potential benefits and potential harms of each intervention to the patient and family so that informed decisions on each item can be made. It is urged that all patient decisions around specific therapeutic options be clearly spelled out both in the patient's medical record as well as in the advance directive documents.

It is very important for the physician to emphasize to patients and families that advance directives, once executed, are not irrevocable documents. They are, instead, evolving documents, reflective of the continuing conversations between physicians and their patients and families regarding patient wishes for care at the end of

life, and, therefore, should be reviewed and updated with patient and family on a frequent basis.

MYTHS ABOUT ADVANCE DIRECTIVES

There are a number of misconceptions about advance directives that present barriers to their effective use. These are listed in Table 22–6 and discussed below. It is important for physicians to become familiar with these issues and be prepared to discuss or defuse them when they are raised as concerns by patients and families.

ADVANCE DIRECTIVES MEAN "DON'T TREAT"

There is a mistaken notion that when patients execute advance directives, especially when the directives include instructions not to provide CPR, that no treatment will be provided. Nothing could be further from the truth. The content of an advance directive is entirely dependent upon the patient's specific wishes and values. Questions regarding whether a patient chooses to receive any specific treatment modality can and should be clearly delineated in the advance directive

---

TABLE 22–6. Myths about Advance Directives

- Advance directives mean "Don't Treat"
- Appointing a health care proxy means giving up control
- Lawyers are necessary to execute advance directives
- Physicians and health care providers do not have to honor advance directives
- Families can freely make decisions in the absence of advance directives
- Advance directives are only for old or sick people

discussion and documented as discussed earlier. Even in the circumstance in which a patient has left advance directive instructions not to receive any form of life-sustaining treatment, standards of end-of-life care mandate appropriate interventions that provide pain and symptom control, comfort care, and respect for one's dignity.

APPOINTING A HEALTH CARE PROXY MEANS GIVING UP CONTROL

Another misperception about advance directives, specifically durable health care power of attorney documents, is that when individuals designate health care proxies, they relinquish their own authority to make health care decisions. In fact, as long as individuals remain able to make decisions, their consent must be obtained for medical treatment. The health care surrogate only becomes directly responsible for decision making when the patient becomes incapacitated. Health care providers cannot legally ignore patients in favor of health care proxies when patients are competent and choose to make their own decisions. Indeed, in most states, advance directives have no legal effect unless and until the patient lacks the capacity to make a health care decision. A minority of states does allow patients to defer to proxies when still able to make their own decisions; however, patients always retain the right to override their proxies or revoke already existing advance directives.

LAWYERS ARE NECESSARY TO EXECUTE ADVANCE DIRECTIVES

An attorney is not necessary in order for an individual to complete an advance directive, although some persons may find a legal opinion helpful. To assist patients and families in executing advance directives in as easy a manner as possible, physicians' offices and other health care provider agencies should make the appropriate advance directive forms available. In states that have advance directive statutes, "official" versions of living will or health care power of attorney documents should be readily available. Sample advance directive documents specific to each state can be found on numerous websites, with Caring Connections, sponsored by the National Hospice and Palliative Care Organization (http://www.caringinfo.org), being just one example.

PHYSICIANS AND HEALTH CARE PROVIDERS DO NOT HAVE TO HONOR ADVANCE DIRECTIVES

This statement is false. Health care providers are required to honor advance directives. The law is clear that medical providers cannot treat an individual against his or her wishes. If a physician acts contrary to a patient's advance directive or contrary to the decision of patient's authorized proxy, the physicians would risk the same liability as if they were to ignore the verbal instructions of a fully competent patient. Treatment could then be construed as constituting battery. However, there is a caveat that the written advance directive be clear regarding the specific circumstances being addressed. In the absence of a clear directive, physicians, in many instances, will use their best judgement, which could result in a patient receiving care contrary to his or her wishes expressed in advance directives.

Unfortunately, there are a number of circumstances in which, despite the existence of advance directives, patients received care that they documented they did not want to receive. For example, there are times when the physician or health facility is unaware of the existence of an advance directive. To try and avoid this, the PSDA requires that whenever a patient is admitted to a hospital, nursing home, home health agency, or hospice, the provider must inquire whether or not the patient has an advance directive (as well as giving the patient the opportunity to execute one). If an advance directive exists, the facility or service has the responsibility to ensure that the advance directive is made part of the medical record. Unfortunately, this does not always happen. Therefore, the patient or health care proxy should make sure that any advance directives are available to the facility or service, and that copies of all appropriate documents are placed on the medical record.

Another important challenge to the proper execution of advance directives, as noted earlier, relates to the lack of detailed instructions in the documents. Simply using general language that rejects "heroic measures" or "treatment that only prolongs the dying process" does not give much guidance and leaves treatment decisions open to interpretation bias. Therefore, living wills should be detailed in defining what treatments a patient does and does not want. Likewise, when a patient designates a surrogate via a health care power of attorney, the patient should have provided the health care proxy with specific instructions on how they desire to be cared for.

Conscientious objection to advance directive instructions is another important reason why these documents are not always followed. In most states, if a health care provider (whether a physician, a facility, or a service provider) objects to an advance directive based on reasons of conscience, state law permits the physician or the facility to refuse to honor it. However, providers are obligated to notify patients or families of their objections to the advance directive instructions at the time of admission or, in the case of the physician, when the issue arises. In circumstances where a provider cannot accept a patient's or health care proxy's advance directive choices, the patient's care should be transferred to another provider who is willing to comply with the patient's or proxy's instructions.

Finally, persons who are dying, but living at home, may receive unwanted efforts at cardiopulmonary resuscitation, despite having advance directives to the contrary, if a crisis occurs, EMS is called and there is no "Out of hospital DNR" document in the home. Therefore, it is important that physicians and other health care providers ensure that patients complete this form when it is determined that the patient is near the end of life, and the patient has expressed, through an advance directive or via health care proxy, that CPR is not desired.

FAMILIES CAN FREELY MAKE DECISIONS IN THE ABSENCE OF ADVANCE DIRECTIVES

Many individuals believe that advance directives really are not necessary, relying instead on next of kin to make decisions for them when they become incapable themselves. Unfortunately, this is only partly true, and families may not always be able to freely assume the role of decision-maker when the situation demands. In many states, if there is no advance directive, state law designates default "proxies," typically family members, who are permitted to make some health care decisions. The hierarchy of health care proxy among next of kin varies from state to state, which contribute to internal family conflicts at a time when family members need to be supportive of each other and their terminally ill family member. In the absence of family, a few states allow a health care professional (i.e., a social worker) or a "close friend" to make proxy health care decisions, while in other states, the lack of family forces a court-appointed guardian to be designated to make decisions. The end result in these circumstances is that individuals who have little or no contact with patients or knowledge of their wishes will be making health care decisions for them, seriously increasing the risk that patients will receive care that they would not have wanted to receive.

ADVANCE DIRECTIVES ARE ONLY FOR OLD OR SICK PEOPLE

Advance directives are not only for the old and infirm. While it may be natural to link death and dying issues with old age, younger patients and families may also be faced with making difficult decisions about end-of-life care. Consider that perhaps the most well-known landmark court cases addressing patient rights at the end of life (Nancy Cruzan, Karen Ann Quinlan, and, most recently, Terri Schiavo) involved relatively young adults. The stakes may actually be higher for younger persons in that, if tragedy strikes, their lives might be prolonged for years or even decades in an undesired condition. Therefore, advance directives are for all adults to execute and make available to their next of kin as well as their physicians and other health care providers.

HOW WELL DO ADVANCE DIRECTIVES WORK?

In 2003, with the PSDA being in effect for over a decade at that time, the US Agency for Health care Research and Quality (AHRQ) reviewed the medical literature to that time in order to determine what effects the statute had regarding improving advance care planning and ensuring that patient preferences regarding health care near the end were honored. A summary of the key findings are listed in Table 22–7.

Unfortunately, what AHQR found was that there is still a long way to go. While the number of patients who had executed some form of advance directive had improved from the 7% to 8% reported in the first edition of this chapter, several reviewed studies showed that less than 50% of all severely or terminally ill patients had an advance directive in the medical record. More disconcerting was that only 12% of patients with an advance directive had received physician input,

TABLE 22–7. AHQR Findings on the Effectiveness of Advance Directives

- Less than 50% of the severely or terminally ill patients studied had an advance directive in their medical record
- Only 12% of patients with an advance directive had received input from their physician in its development.
- Between 65% and 76% of physicians whose patients had an advance directive were not aware that it existed.
- Having an advance directive did not increase documentation in the medical chart regarding patient preferences.
- Advance directives helped make end-of-life decisions in less than half of the cases where a directive existed.
- Advance directives usually were not applicable until the patient became incapacitated and "absolutely, hopelessly ill."
- Providers and patient surrogates had difficulty knowing when to stop treatment and often waited until the patient had crossed the threshold to actively dying before the advance directive was invoked.
- Language in advance directives was usually too nonspecific and general to provide clear instruction.
- Surrogates named in the advance directive often were not present to make decisions or were too emotionally overwrought to offer guidance.
- Physicians were only approximately 65% accurate in predicting patient preferences and tended to make errors of under-treatment, even after reviewing the patient's advance directive.
- Surrogates who were family members tended to make prediction errors of over-treatment, even if they had reviewed or discussed the advance directive with the patient or assisted in its development.
- Care at the end of life sometimes appears to be inconsistent with the patients' preferences to forgo life-sustaining treatment and patients may receive care they do not want.

Source: Kass-Bartelmes BL, Hughes R, Rutherford MK. *Advance care planning: Preferences for care at the end of life.* Rockville, MD, Agency for Healthcare Research and Quality, 2003. Research in Action Issue #12. AHRQ Pub No. 03-0018.

and that between 65% and 76% of the physicians of patients who had advance directives were not aware that the documents existed. Advance directives were helpful in making end-of-life decisions in less than half of the patients where a directive existed, and they were often not applied until the patient had become "incapacitated," "hopelessly ill," or "actively dying," in part because providers and surrogates had difficulty knowing when it was best to stop treatment, and therefore, often waited to invoke the advance directive until a fatal outcome was clearly apparent. Language contained in many advance directives was not specific enough to provide clear instructions, and surrogates were often either not present or too emotionally distraught to make decisions. Surrogates who were family members also often requested more treatment for their loved ones than desired, even when the patients had discussed their wishes with the surrogates before the medical crisis occurred.

These findings led to the conclusion that care at the end of life sometimes appears to be inconsistent with the patients' preferences to forgo life-sustaining treatment and patients may receive care they do not want. To remedy this and ensure that patients receive more effective advance care planning, the AHQR has recommended that physicians take the responsibility to initiate and guide advance care planning discussions in a structured five-step process, listed in Table 22–8, which encompasses many of the ideas discussed earlier in the section "How to Assist Patients in Executing Advance Directives."

TABLE 22–8. AHQR Recommendations for Physicians for Improving Effectiveness of Advance Directives

- Initiate a guided discussion before the patient is terminally ill
- Introduce the subject of advance care planning and offer information
- Prepare and complete advance care planning documents
- Review the patient's preferences on a regular basis and update documentation
- Apply the patient's desires to actual circumstances

SOURCE: Kass-Bartelmes BL, Hughes R, Rutherford MK. *Advance care planning: preferences for care at the end of life.* Rockville, MD, Agency for Healthcare Research and Quality, 2003. Research in Action Issue #12. AHRQ Pub No. 03-0018.

CPR AT THE END OF LIFE

As already noted, the PSDA requires that all Medicare and Medicaid providers inform patients in writing when the patient is admitted to the facility or service of their right to create an advance directive and to assist them in executing such a directive if they choose to do so. The

PSDA also mandates that Medicare and Medicaid providers may not deny patients access to health care services based upon their advance directive instructions.

This latter statutory requirement potentially raises major issues for patients receiving hospice care or other forms of end-of-life care when death is near. After all, it is generally assumed that a patient who elects hospice care has also agreed not to receive CPR when life comes to an end. However, the PSDA has been interpreted to require that a hospice provider (as well as any other provider of palliative care) must take a patient under care if s/he meets prognosis eligibility requirements, even in the face of an advance directive that states that the patient desires CPR. Needless to say, this interpretation of the PSDA has caused significant ethical dilemmas for end-of-life care providers regarding how to care for these patients in an appropriate and responsible fashion.

To more fully understand the scope of the ethical challenges confronted by end-of-life care providers when caring for patients who desire CPR at the end of life, the issue will be examined in the context of the four cardinal ethical values:

autonomy, beneficence, nonmaleficence, and two forms of justice, distributive justice (availability of resources) and social justice (what is good for the society as a whole). (See *Introduction* of this book for a definition of each of these ethical values.) In view of the fact that patient autonomy is currently the overriding ethical value, and the driving force behind the PSDA, it will be addressed last.

CPR AND BENEFICENCE

The basic procedure referred to as cardiopulmonary resuscitation was developed in the late 1950s and 1960s, primarily to revive patients who experienced cardiac or respiratory arrest (e.g., acute arrhythmia or drowning). As resuscitative techniques have been refined over the years, the use of CPR has been extended to patients with virtually any acute or chronic illnesses. In fact, CPR has become a "default" procedure, assumed to be desired by all individuals unless they specifically request that they do not want CPR performed.

Overall, survival rates for patients who require CPR is approximately 15%, with considerable variability in survival rates reported depending upon the specific patient population studied. Table 22–9 lists reported survival rates, stratified by several key variables, for elderly patients (generally defined as ≥70) receiving CPR. These variables include the location where the arrest occurred, whether or not the arrest was witnessed, whether or not vital signs were initially detected, and the presence of chronic illness. While 39% of a selected group of elderly cardiac patients have been reported to survive CPR, the outcome of CPR in all other reported studies is fairly dismal. Ambulatory elderly patients and patients who still had detectable vital signs are reported to have approximately 10% survival, while those patients who arrest while in the hospital or have witnessed arrest survive approximately 5% to 7% of the time. Survival of patients following an unwitnessed cardiorespiratory arrest, an arrest outside the hospital, and/or without vital signs when CPR was initiated was reported as 1% or less. While no studies

TABLE 22–9. Survival to Hospital Discharge for Elderly Patients Requiring CPR for Cardiopulmonary Arrest

CHARACTERISTIC	SURVIVED TO DISCHARGE (%)
Out of hospital arrest	0.8
In-hospital arrest	6.5
Witnessed arrest	5.2
Unwitnessed arrest	0.9
Vital signs present	10.2
Vital signs absent	1.1
Ambulatory elderly	10
Selected cardiac patients-in hospital	39
Chronically ill elderly	<5

have been on the terminally ill elderly, chronically ill elderly patients, including those with malignancies, neurologic disease, renal failure, respiratory disease, and sepsis (some of whom at least would potentially be receiving hospice or end-of-life care) have a less than 5% probability of leaving the hospital alive with survival of such patients approximating zero in many studies.

CPR AND NONMALEFICENCE

The performance of CPR is not without the potential for harm, irrespective of whether the ultimate outcome is patient survival or death. Autopsy studies following CPR have demonstrated fractures of ribs and sternum, bone marrow emboli, epicardial hemorrhage, mediastinal hematomas, aspiration pneumonia, and hemorrhage into various other cardiac and respiratory structures. Surviving patients may experience many of these same complications, as well as chest wall burns secondary to ventricular defibrillation. They also have the added risk of having permanent neurological sequelae including, but not limited to, brain death, persistent vegetative state, seizures, and impairment of higher intellectual functions.

CPR AND JUSTICE

Examining distributive justice, one can intuitively conclude that performing CPR at the end of life is more costly than avoiding the procedure. While hard data specific to CPR is lacking, it has been demonstrated that hospitalized patients who had advance directives in place prior to death spent less than one-third the resources of hospitalized patients who had no documented advance directive.

Social justice suggests that the society considers the ready availability of CPR to be in its best interest, based on the fact that, as already mentioned earlier, CPR is considered a default condition. The question that needs to be asked, however, is whether having CPR as a default condition is in the best interest of society as a whole. This is a far more complex question than one might surmise, especially in view of the facts related to beneficence and nonmaleficence presented earlier. While it is beyond the scope of this chapter to answer the question as it affects the society as a whole, one must seriously question whether the societal good is met by having CPR be the default situation in patients who are near the end of life.

CPR AND AUTONOMY

That autonomy is the preeminent value regarding the question of CPR at the end of life has been made abundantly clear by the passage of the PSDA. Autonomy in this area is further emphasized by the fact that hospice and end-of-life care providers must serve eligible patients who request CPR. Hospice and end-of-life care providers are respectful of patient autonomy in this area, and most hospice providers, in compliance with the PSDA, will admit patients who are eligible for care and have requested CPR. Physicians are generally supportive of allowing patient preference to dictate whether or not CPR is performed at the end of life, although it is suggested that patient autonomy is more often respected when CPR is desired than when it is not.

For autonomy to properly function in this setting, however, there needs to be a caveat that patients possess the necessary information that allows them to make appropriate choices. Herein is the major challenge, as the literature suggests that, at least to date, patients as a whole are not well-informed when making decisions about matters such as CPR at the end of life.

There is a great deal of public misperception about the nature of CPR. While 94% of people who participated in a study evaluating their knowledge of CPR knew that CPR included chest compressions, only 43% recognized that CPR might entail needing "paddles on the chest" (although perhaps a higher percentage are aware of this now due to the advent and widespread availability of "automated external defibrillators") and only 36% knew that it could include placing a "tube in the windpipe." The mass media has seriously affected the public's perception of the successfulness of CPR, with television shows and movies often depicting a much higher degree of successful resuscitation than has been demonstrated in the medical literature.

That proper information is vital to helping patients express autonomy in this area is underscored by a study evaluating the influence of patient knowledge regarding the probability of survival following CPR and patient preferences. When patients were questioned about CPR preferences during an acute illness or a chronic illness, the percentage of patients desiring CPR significantly decreased (acute: 41–22%; chronic: 11–5%) after they were informed of the probability of survival following the procedure. By demonstrating that most patients do not want to undergo CPR when they are informed of the probability of survival after the procedure, this study affirms the importance of physicians providing their patients with the information necessary to help them express their autonomy in this area.

Unfortunately, despite the fact that patients are capable of synthesizing the information necessary to make informed and autonomous decisions about CPR at the end of life, only approximately 25% of patients are having such discussions with their physicians. (A full discussion on the subject of physician/patient communications at the end of life can be found in Chapter 3.) More importantly, more than 50% of patients who have not had a discussion with their physicians about CPR at the end of life do not want to have the discussion in the first place. This serious lack of communication between patients and physicians has

led, not surprisingly, to many patients receiving CPR in support of their autonomy, where, if they had been properly informed, their expressions of autonomy might have been very different.

CPR AT THE END OF LIFE: SYNTHESIS OF ETHICAL VALUES AND FINAL THOUGHTS

Table 22–10 summarizes the salient issues regarding CPR in relationship to each of the cardinal ethical values. Analysis of this information suggests that, with little if any medical benefit

TABLE 22–10. Ethical Issues Related to CPR at the End of Life

ETHICAL VALUE	PROS	CONS
Autonomy	1. Legislated by the PSDA 2. Respected by hospices and other end-of-life care providers 3. Physician support—more so when choice is for CPR 4. Patients would make appropriate CPR choices if properly informed	Lack of patient information to make an informed autonomous decision, as indicated by 1. Public misperception of nature of CPR 2. Public misperception of successful CPR 3. Only 25% of patients speak with physicians about CPR preferences 4. More than 50% of patients do not want to speak with physicians about CPR preferences
Beneficence	None in patients with chronic or terminal illness	1. Overall survival rate approximately 15% 2. Unwitnessed arrest, out of hospital, or no vital signs, survival 1% or less 3. Chronically ill elderly, survival rate <5%
Nonmaleficence	None reported	1. Autopsy studies indicate risk of fractures, hemotomas, and aspiration 2. Survivors also risk chest wall burns and permanent neurological sequelae
Justice distributive	None reported	Fold increased in average cost of final hospitalization in patients without advance directive vs. patients with advance directive
Social	CPR is default situation	No clear evidence that providing CPR to patients at the end of life is in the best interests of the society

and the potential for significant medical harm, the ethical values of beneficence and nonmaleficence would clearly be violated if one were to provide CPR to patients at the end of life. Distributive justice would also dictate that CPR at the end of life be avoided. The ethical position of social justice in relationship to CPR is less clear and remains the subject of continued debate. Finally, autonomy clearly dictates that if desired, CPR should be provided to patients who request this procedure.

Weighing all this together, with three of the four major ethical values suggesting CPR should be avoided at the end of life, one could certainly make the ethical case, autonomy not withstanding, that to provide CPR to patients at the end of life would be in violation of the principles of medical ethics. Reality is quite different, however. Autonomy is clearly the dominant ethical value in our society today, to the point that on the issue of CPR, it actually supercedes all the other values. Therefore, and reinforced by federal law, patients who desire CPR at the end of life are entitled to receive it, despite the medical evidence that it is ineffective at the end of life and despite the violation of most other medical ethical values.

While awaiting shifts in societal values or changes in legislation, how is the provider of end-of-life care to proceed? Clearly, good autonomous decision-making needs to be accompanied by information. Physicians need to meet with patients and families and discuss their CPR preferences with them, disclosing to them all the medical facts related to the benefits, risks, and outcomes of CPR at the end of life. Likewise, hospice providers and other providers of end-of-life care should discuss these issues carefully and thoroughly with patients and families when patients are referred and admitted for palliative care. If these conversations are held thoughtfully, it is likely that most patients and families will choose, either verbally or with a written advance directive, to avoid CPR at the end of life.

The dilemma is how to properly care for patients who continue to express the desire to receive CPR at the end of life. Physicians will usually address this issue by simply acquiescing to the patients or families wishes while keeping the lines of communication open. Hospices and other end-of-life care providers confronted with patients who desire CPR, recognize a challenge and an opportunity. Being respectful of both patient autonomy and the PSDA, hospice providers will admit these patients. Integral to the hospice palliative plan of care for these patients and families is appropriate education, with the goal being to have these patients or health care surrogates evaluate their decisions for CPR on an on-going basis, and to continually reassess their goals of care in view of the patient's changing clinical status. Often the patient or surrogate will come to the decision that CPR no longer matches their goals. For the patient or family where such education does not result in the choice that the patient forgoes CPR, there is always the option to leave the hospice program at any time to receive the desired care.

When dealing with human beings, especially as life is drawing to an end, there are no circumstances that are perfect or ideal. There will always be specific situations where, despite the best efforts of all concerned, individual patients or families will opt to receive CPR when it will be clearly ineffective. Physicians, hospices, and other providers of end of life can all be instrumental in reducing these situations to a minimum by better understanding how to help their patients provide advance directive instructions that are legal and binding, by properly documenting these instructions, and, most importantly, by educating their patients and families about the medical facts of procedures such as cardiopulmonary resuscitation at the end of life.

BIBLIOGRAPHY

Bedell SE, Delbanco TL, Cook EF, Epstein FH: Survival after cardiopulmonary resuscitation in the hospital. *N Engl J Med* 309:569-576, 1983.

Bradley EH, Rizzo JA: Public information and private search: Evaluating the Patient Self-Determination Act. *J Health Polit Policy Law* 24(2):239-273, 1999.

Caring Connections: National Hospice and Palliative Care Organization. http://www.caringinfo.org. Accessed February 23, 2009.

Chambers CV, Diamond JJ, Perkel RL, Lasch LA: Relationship of advance directives to hospital charges in a Medicare population. *Arch Int Med* 154:541-547, 1994.

Curtin LL: DNR in the OR: Ethical concerns and hospital policies. *Nurs Manage* 25:29, 1994.

Curtis JR, Park DR, Krone MR, Pearlman RA: Use of the medical futility rationale in do-not-attempt-resuscitation orders. *J Am Med Assoc* 273:124-128, 1995.

Danis M, Mutran E, Garrett JM, et al: A prospective study of the impact of patient preferences on life-sustaining treatment and hospital costs. *Crit Care Med* 24:1811-1817, 1996.

Ditto PH, Danks JH, Smucker WD, et al: Advance directives as acts of communication. *Arch Intern Med* 161:421-430, 2001.

Emanuel LL, Danis M, Pearlman RA, et al: Advance care planning as a process: Structuring discussion in practice. *J Am Geriatr Soc* 43(4):440-446, 1995.

Fischer GS, Tulsky JA, Rose MR, et al: Patient knowledge and physician predictions of treatment preferences after discussion of advance directives. *J Gen Intern Med* 13:447-454, 1998.

Gordon M, Cheung M: Poor outcome of on-site CPR in a multi-level geriatric facility: Three and a half years experience at the Baycrest Centre for Geriatric Care. *J Am Geriatr Soc* 41(2):163-166, 1993.

Hoffmann JC, Wenger NS, et al: Patient preferences for communication with physicians about end-of-life decisions. *Ann Intern Med* 127,1-12, 1997.

Kass-Bartelmes BL, Hughes R, Rutherford MK: *Advance Care Planning: Preferences for Care at the End of Life*. Rockville, MD, Agency for Healthcare Research and Quality, 2003. Research in Action Issue #12. AHRQ Pub No. 03-0018.

Members of the 1991 NHO Ethics Committee: *Do-Not-Resuscitate (DNR) Decisions in the Context of Hospice Care*. Arlington, TX, National Hospice Organization, 1992.

Moss AH: Informing the patient about cardiopulmonary resuscitation. *J Gen Intern Med* 4:349-354, 1989.

Murphy DJ, Murray AM, Robinson BE, Campion EW: Outcomes of cardiopulmonary resuscitation in the elderly. *Ann Intern Med* 111:199-205, 1989.

Murphy DJ, Burrows D, Santilli S, et al: The influence of the probability of survival on patient preferences regarding cardiopulmonary resuscitation. *N Engl J Med* 330:545-549, 1994.

Schonwetter RS, Teasdale, Taffet G, Robinson BE, Luchi RJ: Educating the elderly: Cardiopulmonary resuscitation decisions before and after intervention. *J Am Geriatr Soc* 39:372-377, 1991.

Scofield GR: Is consent useful when resuscitation isn't? *Hastings Cent Rep* 21:28-36, 1991.

Singer GR: Do-not-resuscitate orders. *J Florida Med Assoc* 8(1):30-34, 1994.

State in end-of-life care: Focus: Oregon's POLST Program. A Publication of the National Program Office for Community–State Partnerships to Improve End-of-Life Care. Midwest Bioethics Center. 1021-1025 Jefferson Street, Kansas City, MO 64105-1329. April 1999, issue 3.

Steinbrook R, Low B: Resuscitating advance directives. *Arch Int Med* 164:1501-1506, 2004.

Teno JM, Licks S, Lynn J, et al: Do advance directives provide instructions that direct care? *J Am Geriatr Soc* 45:508-512, 1997.

Teno JM, Lynn J, Phillips RS, et al: Do formal advance directives affect resuscitation decisions and the use of resources for seriously ill patients? *J Clin Ethics* 5(1):23-30, 1994.

Teno JM, Lynn J, Wenger N, et al: Advance directives for seriously-ill hospitalized patients: effectiveness with the Patient Self-Determination Act and the SUPPORT intervention. *J Am Geriatr Soc* 45:500-507, 1997.

Virmani J, Schneiderman LF, Kaplan RM: Relationship of advance directives to physician–patient communication. *Arch Intern Med* 154:909-913, 1994.

SELF-ASSESSMENT QUESTIONS

1. All of the following are forms of advance directive EXCEPT
   A. Living will
   B. DNR order
   C. Health care power of attorney
   D. Combined living will/health care power of attorney
   E. Verbal advance directive

2. When a health care surrogate or proxy is asked to make a decision for a patient who is incapable of making a medical decision, on which of the following does the surrogate primarily base the decision?
   A. What the surrogate would do in the same situation.
   B. What the physician recommends
   C. What the patient would want done
   D. What a health care attorney recommends
   E. Input from the physician and a health care attorney

3. All of the following are regulated by individual state laws EXCEPT:
   A. Patient Self-Determination Act
   B. Definitions for activation of living will
   C. Requirements for appointing a durable health care power of attorney
   D. Hierarchy of decision makers if there is no advance directive
   E. Level of proof that surrogate's decision is consistent with patient wishes

4. While all of the following are advantages to use of advance directives, which of these is the most important advantage?
   A. Physician knowledge of patient wishes
   B. Decrease in family anxiety and guilt
   C. Decrease in unnecessary health care interventions
   D. Respect of patient autonomy.
   E. Decrease in health care costs

5. Which of the following statements about advance directives is true?
   A. Advance directives are not irrevocable.
   B. Advance directives mean "don't treat"
   C. Appointing a health care proxy means giving up control
   D. Advance directives are only for old or sick people
   E. Health care providers do not have to honor advance directives

6. The Patient Self-Determination Act, implemented in December 1991, mandated that all providers receiving federal funding through Medicare and Medicaid give all patients admitted to their care the opportunity to create an advance directive. Which of the following outcomes regarding research on the impact of the PSDA on the use of advance directives is true?
   A. More than 50% of the severely or terminally ill patients studied had an advance directive in their medical record.
   B. Having an advance directive increased documentation in the medical chart regarding patient preferences.
   C. The majority of patients with an advance directive had received input from their physician in its development.
   D. Advance directives helped make end-of-life decisions in less than half of the cases where a directive existed.
   E. Care at the end of life is usually consistent with the patients' preferences to forgo life-sustaining treatment.

7. Which of the following statements regarding the role of the physician in assisting patients with creating an advance directive is true?
   A. The best time to have the conversation is at the same time the physician informs the patient of a terminal prognosis.
   B. The physician should emphasize to the patient the importance of making advance

directive choices right the first time, since once the document is written, it cannot be changed in the future.

C. The pros and cons of both living wills and durable health care power of attorney documents should be clearly spelled out for the patient.

D. As long as the physician knows what the patient means, the language in the advance directive can be left vague.

E. If the patient is unwilling to write an advance directive, verbal instructions to the physician are acceptable, even if they are not documented.

8. Which of the following groups of patients has the best chance of surviving until hospital discharge following CPR for cardiopulmonary arrest?

A. Witnessed arrest
B. Selected cardiac patients in-hospital
C. Chronically ill elderly
D. Ambulatory elderly
E. Arrest with vital signs initially present

9. All of the following statements regarding the public's view of CPR are true EXCEPT

A. Most people know that CPR may include placing a "tube in the windpipe."
B. The public overestimates the percentage of successful CPR outcomes.
C. More people would choose to forgo CPR during an acute or chronic illness if they were better informed of the outcomes.

D. More than half of people do not want to speak to their physicians about CPR.
E. Only about 25% of people speak with their physicians about CPR.

10. As medical director of your local hospice you are asked to meet with a 62 year-old man with terminal metastatic lung cancer. He also has a history of heart disease. He was about to be admitted to your hospice program, but when the nurse spoke with him about his advance directive, he made it very clear that he wanted CPR if his heart should stop or he should stop breathing. The purpose of your visit is to discuss his advance directive wishes with him further. At the end of your conversation, he is firm that he still wants CPR. Which of the following would be your most appropriate plan going forward?

A. Discharge him from the hospice since he still wants "aggressive care."
B. Tell him you will honor his request, but write a DNR order on his chart.
C. Document your conversation, take no further action, and when the time comes, provide CPR as this is what the patient wants.
D. Tell him that you will not provide CPR even if he wants it.
E. Continue to visit him and provide ongoing education as to the poor outcomes of CPR in patients with his illnesses.

CHAPTER

23

Physician-Assisted Suicide, Euthanasia, and Palliative Sedation

Joel S. Policzer, Richard Fife, Richard A. Shapiro, and Neal J. Weinreb

INTRODUCTION

The development and routine application of advanced, life-prolonging technology, especially in chronic, irreversible, incapacitating illnesses, has raised difficult clinical, ethical, legal, and political issues for the practice of medicine. With attention increasingly directed at the quality, rather than merely the duration of life, and with a shift in the physician–patient relationship away from professional paternalism and toward absolute patient self-determination, the question "whose life is it anyway?" has been extended to include ending life on patient demand. Consequently, physician-assisted suicide (PAS) and euthanasia have been in the forefront of medical-ethical issues, and continue to be the focus of intense public debate in the United States. A number of authors and organizations have also begun to use the term "physician-assisted death" (PAD) as a less judgmental substitute for PAS, although the original name is still commonly used, as it will be here.

Within the medical community, interest and controversy about physician-assisted suicide were sparked by the anonymous article "It's Over, Debbie" (*JAMA*, 1988) and by the thoughtful case presentations and subsequent writings by proponents such as Dr. Timothy Quill. The participation by Dr. Jack Kevorkian in assisted suicides in Michigan graphically brought the subject before the public and the courts. Although Kevorkian's actions appeared to violate statutory law, jurors repeatedly refused to convict him to the extent that he claimed his participation was restricted to assisting in suicide. However, when he carried his activity to the point of videotaping and publicizing a "mercy killing," a Michigan jury found him guilty of murder. This suggested that, at least at that time, the public continued to maintain a clear distinction between euthanasia, still considered unacceptable, and assisted suicide, for which there appears to be an increasing amount of popular support, albeit to varying degrees, in various areas of the country.

The organized medical community, as represented by national organizations such as the AMA, regards PAS with disfavor. The American Academy of Hospice and Palliative Medicine, the professional organization for physicians and other clinicians caring for patients at end of life, has a Position Statement dated 2007, which says, in part,

> Despite all potential alternatives, some patients may persist in their request specifically for PAD. The AAHPM recognizes that deep disagreement persists regarding the morality of PAD. Sincere, compassionate, morally conscientious individuals stand on either side of this debate. AAHPM takes a position of "studied neutrality" on the subject of whether PAD should be legally regulated or prohibited, believing its members should instead continue to strive to find the proper response to those patients whose suffering becomes intolerable despite the best possible palliative care. Whether or not legalization occurs, AAHPM supports intense efforts to alleviate suffering and to reduce any perceived need for PAD."

Surveys suggest that there is a difference between the public's attitude toward PAS and euthanasia and the attitudes of physicians. One-third of the public support these interventions regardless of the medical situation described; one-third oppose these interventions in all circumstances; and one-third would support an intervention in certain circumstances, usually a patient in intractable pain. It also appears that the public may no longer distinguish between assisted suicide and euthanasia, at least in the context of this study. The majority of physicians, however, do not view either intervention as ethical. Only 40% of physicians would support PAS, but most support it if forced to choose between legalization of it or an outright ban. Yet, even among those physicians who might support the intervention, few would personally participate. Physicians do distinguish between these interventions and do not support euthanasia.

Although the justices of the United States Supreme Court ruled unanimously in 1997 that there is no constitutional right to assistance in committing suicide, the court clearly indicated that state legislatures were empowered to address the issue and that the individual states would be appropriate "laboratories" in which the ramifications of PAS might be explored. Nonetheless, proposed legislation to allow PAS was defeated in 26 states in 1997 to 1998, and voters rejected state ballot initiatives to legalize PAS in California, Michigan, and Washington State; yet a significant minority (30–40%) favored these proposals. Oregon voters, however, approved the "Oregon Death with Dignity Act" in 1996 by a 60% majority. Opponents of the Oregon legalization of PAS sought to circumvent the state law by threatening physician participants with penalties specified in the federal Controlled Substance Act. This approach was ultimately rejected by the United States Supreme Court in 2006.

As of the time of this writing, Washington State passed its own Death with Dignity Act in 2008, modeled on the Oregon act, with a 58% majority. In addition, the Supreme Court of the state of Montana, in a ruling issued on December 31, 2009, supported a 2008 lower court decision that the state's constitutional privacy and human dignity rights allow a terminally ill patient to "die with dignity," making Montana the third US state to legalize PAS. However, 38 states still treat PAS as a crime whereas only a few (NC, UT, WY, OH) do not consider this a criminal act but do not condone or sanction it.

Regardless of judicial, legislative, and political positions, physicians still have a significant part to play in individual decisions of life extension and termination. They will continue to be asked to make judgments and recommendations regarding the extension of the length of life, assessment of the quality of life, and defining options for the relief of pain and suffering. The possibility of further legalization of PAS will place an even greater responsibility and burden on health care professionals, and be a challenge to the traditional concepts of the physician's mission.

The purpose of this chapter is to assist physicians with an interest in end-of-life care in grappling with the issue as to whether, and under what circumstances, assisted suicide might be considered as a therapeutic option in the management of patients with terminal disease.

DEFINITIONS

PHYSICIAN-ASSISTED SUICIDE (PAS) OR PHYSICIAN-ASSISTED DEATH (PAD)

Following a patient-initiated request, a physician provides the means for the patient to end his or her life. Typically, the physician offers counseling, information, and instruction, prescribes (and sometimes delivers) the requisite medication, but does not otherwise participate in the final act. The presence of the physician during the suicide process is sometimes encouraged, but remains a matter of patient and physician preference. (Guidelines and legal requirements in Oregon, Washington State, and the Netherlands, where PAS is either legal or legally tolerated, will be discussed later.)

EUTHANASIA

The term is derived from the Greek *Eu* (good) and *Thanatos* (death). Although helping a terminally ill patient achieve a "good death" is the goal of everyone involved in hospice medicine and end-of-life care, in modern usage euthanasia is a direct action taken by a physician or other third party with the intention of ending a patient's life as a response to unmitigated pain and suffering.

The term "voluntary euthanasia" refers to the action of a physician and a competent patient who jointly agree, via a process of informed consent, to terminate the patient's life. Involuntary euthanasia is a commonly practiced veterinary procedure ("putting an animal down"), but could be conceivably applied (with trepidation) to the act of ending the life of a terminally ill, suffering patient lacking decision-making capacity at the request of a legally authorized health care surrogate. Rare episodes reported in the Netherlands notwithstanding, independent action by the physician or other third party (e.g., a husband shooting his severely demented wife), even if felt to be in the patient's best interest, is not euthanasia, and could legally be considered murder. Euthanasia implies an active role for the physician. "Passive euthanasia," which has been used synonymously with withholding or withdrawing treatment on the patient's instruction tends to blur the distinction between these separate end-of-life issues, and is a term best avoided (see below).

PALLIATIVE SEDATION

For some terminally ill patients near the natural end of life, alleviation of discomfort due to pain, dyspnea, bleeding, or other symptoms may not be achieved with conventional means. Because such patients experience not only marked physical but also severe emotional and spiritual distress often associated with agitation, the physician, with appropriate consent from the patient or family, may prescribe doses of medication sufficient to sedate and keep the patient unconscious until death occurs. This is commonly termed "terminal or palliative sedation." See below for a full discussion. (The actual medical indications and techniques for using terminal sedation as a therapeutic intervention at the end of life are discussed in Chapter 12.)

DOUBLE EFFECT

In as much as death from PAS as commonly practiced by administration of barbiturates is not instantaneous and occasionally may not ensue for as much as 24 hours, there is a legitimate question as to the difference between PAS and palliative sedation. It is classically argued that with PAS, the intent of the physician is to help to bring death for the purpose of relieving pain and suffering. With palliative sedation, the intention of the physician, as reflected in the choice and dosage of medication, is to alleviate pain and suffering rather than to hasten death, although the latter outcome frequently occurs and may often be welcomed by the patient's family and the physician. The ethi-

cal justification for this distinction is the principle of *double effect*.

The principle of *double effect* refers to an action that may have two distinct effects, one planned and desired, and another anticipated but unwanted or unneeded. An example is the administration of chemotherapy to a patient with cancer. The desired effect is tumor regression and prolongation of life. The potential undesired side effects include neutropenia and fatal septicemia. The principle of *double effect* teaches that if the primary goal of the action is to cause a certain desired effect, and the patient is informed and aware of the potential adverse consequences or undesired effects, assuming there is no negligence in the provision of the medical intervention, then no moral culpability is attached should the unfavorable outcome occur.

Although the formulation of the principle of double effect is often attributed to medieval scholastics, its origins date to late antiquity, as it is repeatedly applied in Talmudic reasoning and jurisprudence. The proper application of the principle depends not only on the actor's intent, but also on the proximate inevitability of the undesired effect, and on an assessment as to whether the action chosen is proportionate to the severity of the problem to be addressed and is the best or only alternative. For example, one cannot cut off the head of a squawking chicken in an attempt at noise abatement and then deny accountability for the chicken's death on the basis of double effect!

The application of the doctrine of double effect to end-of-life care has been criticized by some medical ethicists who argue that "at best, it is often claimed disingenuously or, at worst, it has become a [shallow] meaningless mantra recited by . . . surreptitious practitioners of euthanasia cloaked as palliative care clinicians."

INTENT

Human intentions are usually complex, sometimes ambiguous, frequently inconstant, often difficult to pin down, and easily subject to manipulation. For this reason, it has been suggested that "appeal to intention offers no basis for a clear moral distinction between [such closely similar actions as] withdrawing life-sustaining treatment and PAS." Dr. Marcia Angell has argued that intent is important in criminal law (e.g., differentiating murder from manslaughter), whereas "the situation is different for compassionate physicians caring for the terminally ill, [who] want to relieve their patients' suffering, . . . sometimes in whatever way possible." Others would argue, however, that assessment of intent is not only a linchpin of all legal and justice systems, but is critical for even the most rudimentary social interactions (e.g., is the lion out for a postprandial stroll or on a preprandial prowl, and might its intention change unpredictably, and is it worth trying to know?).

Because virtually all human action can be invested with moral significance, and because ends do not necessarily justify means, intent, although often difficult to evaluate, should not be easily dismissed. Even nonverbalized intent may sometimes have ethical and even legal significance. It stands to reason, therefore, that when dealing with emotionally charged end-of-life issues, the prudent physician will document with even greater care than usual, the full details of physician–patient interactions, so as to leave the least possible doubt about the intentions of all parties involved.

PROFESSIONAL INTEGRITY

Just as the patient's autonomy and right to self-determination must be respected, the physician is entitled to take "professional actions that are consistent with one's ethical and moral beliefs, and [to avoid] actions that are contrary to one's beliefs" (Oregon Death and Dignity Act). This right, also referred to as conscientious practice or conscientious objection, allows a clinician to withdraw from a patient relationship when the patient's wishes conflict with the clinician's own moral beliefs. The application of this principle is contingent on nonabandonment of the patient's

continuing needs and sufficient notice to effect the transfer of care to another physician.

IS THE DEBATE REGARDING PAS SIMPLY A MATTER OF SEMANTICS?

Among both proponents and opponents of legalized PAS, there are those who contend that the debate is nothing more than a question of semantics. Some argue that there is no essential ethical difference between withholding life-prolonging treatment at the instruction of an informed, competent patient and honoring the request of that patient for a supply of medication sufficient for a successful suicide. In the case of an incompetent patient with a properly executed advanced directive, why distinguish between withdrawal of life-sustaining equipment on instruction of a designated health care surrogate and the request of that same surrogate that the physician administer a lethal injection? Is a living will that abjures aggressive, life-prolonging treatment anything other than a predated, highly contingent, promissory suicide note? What about the competent patient who determines to hasten death by refusing food and drink, or the physician whose prescription of heavy sedation to alleviate pain, dyspnea, or other symptoms inevitably, although allegedly without intention, accelerates the end of life?

Although seemingly irrational, our society currently sanctions all of the above activities except PAS and euthanasia. The justices of the Second Circuit United States Court of Appeals advanced this very argument when overturning New York State legislation prohibiting PAS. However, the thinking of the Second Circuit was rejected by the United States Supreme Court, which firmly espoused a strong legal distinction between refusing unwanted treatment and PAS. Although nuance of language is subject to the same logical criticism as assessment of intention, it is similarly essential to a functional legal system and indeed to all social intercourse. The formulation of arbitrary distinctions may sometimes be the sole mechanism to achieve compromise and consensus in a diverse, pluralistic community.

General support for patient self-determination, including refusal of undesired treatment, which is not easily accepted by all ethnic and religious groups, might be jeopardized if the distinction from suicide is blurred or removed. Furthermore, the distinction between withholding/withdrawal of treatment and PAS may not necessarily be totally arbitrary. Refusal of food, drink, and treatment can constitute the autonomous actions of patients or their representatives and are subject only to a physician's advice, but not to his consent. Although a physician who disagrees with the patient's decision may withdraw and transfer care to a colleague, if there were no alternative physician available, the physician would have no choice but to comply with the patient's wishes.

Assisted suicide, on the other hand, presupposes the *voluntary* compliance of the physician, who, based on the principle of professional integrity and conscientious practice, has no ethical or legal obligation to participate. Even if the physician's involvement is not there, the patient still has recourse to other means of committing suicide. All these might be seen as sufficient grounds to argue that the distinction between refusal of treatment and PAS/euthanasia is substantive and not merely semantic.

HISTORY AND BACKGROUND OF ASSISTED SUICIDE AND EUTHANASIA

ANCIENT GREECE AND ROME

Episodes of assisted suicide and euthanasia are recorded in the classical literary and historical sources of antiquity. There is abundant evidence that these actions were in common use in ancient Greece and Rome. Antiquity, of course, does not automatically confer moral legitimacy on these procedures, as abhorrent practices such as human sacrifice and infanticide for population control were also practiced in ancient civilizations. Consider the following examples: "There must be a law that no imperfect or maimed child shall be brought up, and to avoid an excess of population, some children must be exposed, for a limit must be fixed to the population of the state" (Aristotle, Politics VII). "Children also, if weak and deformed we drown, not through anger, but through the wisdom of preferring the sound to the useless" (Seneca, Concerning Anger).

THE BIBLE

Of greater relevance to the current debate are case reports describing withdrawal of treatment, assisted suicide, and euthanasia in texts such as the Bible and Talmud, which are the basis of the Judeo-Christian-Islamic life-affirming traditions that have largely shaped the American ethos. Saul, the first king of Israel, defeated in battle, surrounded by the enemy, and anticipating capture, humiliation, and a tortured death, asked his armor-bearer to kill him with his own sword. The armor-bearer conscientiously objected and refused, whereupon Saul, as soldiers have done even in modern times, fell on his sword and died. Whether this suicide was condemnable or laudatory to avoid desecration of God's name has been debated by Biblical commentators, but it has been emulated by generations of martyrs who chose suicide rather than being forced to violate cardinal principles of faith.

The epilogue of the Saul story is also relevant to this chapter. A messenger, looking to curry favor with David, Saul's rival and successor, brought news of the king's death. Possibly embellishing the details, he related how he had found Saul dying of his self-inflicted wounds, and, in the spirit of mercy killing, finished him off. To his undoubted dismay, David did not take kindly to the deed and ordered the messenger's execution, although it is not clear whether this represented a rejection of the concept of euthanasia or merely concern about *lese majesté*.

THE TALMUD

The Talmud relates a number of episodes suggesting that natural death is preferable to prolonged physical or emotional suffering. Furthermore, there is a suggestion that life-prolonging maneuvers may be withheld or withdrawn from dying, suffering patients in the story of Rabbi Judah the Prince, whose maid was praised for interrupting the prayers of his colleagues and students, which she perceived as an impediment to a beneficent death.

Euthanasia is mentioned and endorsed in association with the martyrdom of Rabbi Hananiah ben Tradyon, who was burned at the stake by Romans. One of the guards, knowing that death was inevitable, and wishing to prevent further cruelty, removed a sponge that was tortuously damping the flames, thus mercifully hastening the Rabbi's death and gaining himself a guaranteed ticket to paradise.

Finally, there is an episode of euthanasia by proxy that may be of relevance to assisted suicide. Rabbi Ulla, on a journey from Babylon to Israel, camped with two men who quarreled. The situation turned violent and one man slit the throat of the other. With the victim exsanguinating on the ground, the perpetrator asked Ulla whether he had done the right thing. Ulla, fearing for his own life, assented, and secretly hoping to spare the dying victim prolonged agony, suggested that the incision be extended to transect the trachea, thus causing immediate death. Troubled as to whether he might be an accessory to murder, he later reviewed the case with his teacher, Rabbi Yochanan, who justified Ulla's action as necessary for self-preservation. Because it was not condemned as unnecessary or excessive, one might presume that the "assisted euthanasia" was approved, or even expected, behavior.

Of course, these anecdotes relate to unusual circumstances and may not necessarily be applicable to everyday life. As a general rule, western religious tradition emphasizes the sanctity of life, and, despite a strong belief in an afterlife, with few exceptions, emphasizes the importance of prolonging life in this world. Consequently, suicide and euthanasia are anathema to these major world religions. Furthermore, from a religious viewpoint, the physician is conceived of as a divinely authorized healer and a restorer of life. Therefore, physician participation in suicide or euthanasia is doubly problematic. Secularists, on the other hand, also regard "life" as one of the inalienable rights of humankind, but coupled to "liberty" (autonomy) and conceivably modified by "the pursuit of happiness." The position that these three basic rights are coequal in importance, as contrasted with the religious outlook, which regards the latter two as not absolute, creates the philosophical gradient that moves the controversy about euthanasia and PAS.

THE UNITED STATES AND THE UNITED KINGDOM

In 1994, Ezekiel Emmanuel reviewed the history of euthanasia in the United States and in the United Kingdom. The first reference to euthanasia in the English language is found in Sir Thomas More's Utopia (1516): "They console the incurably ill by sitting and talking with them and by alleviating whatever pain they can. Should life become unbearable for these incurables, the magistrates and priests do not hesitate to prescribe euthanasia. . . ."

In the late eighteenth century, the framers of the United States Constitution rejected the age-old concept that inflicting painful suffering had instructive, deterrent, or redemptive value by prohibiting cruel and unusual punishment. Although the morality and social utility of capital punishment continues to be hotly debated, there has been an inexorable movement toward that even the most reprehensible criminal is entitled to protection from physical pain and suffering. The trend to medicalize executions by using lethal injection has parenthetically focused attention on why we appear to treat condemned criminals with greater compassion than we treat victims of the ravages of terminal illness.

After 1846, as anesthesia with ether and chloroform was increasingly applied to surgical procedures, suggestions were offered that these agents might also be useful in alleviating terminal suffering. In 1870, Samuel Williams proposed using morphine in conjunction with general anesthetics to intentionally end a patient's life. Debates about the ethics of euthanasia continued for the next 35 years, further fueled by controversy linked to emerging Darwinian theories such as "survival of the fittest" as applied to social utilitarianism. In 1906, a bill to legalize euthanasia was introduced and eventually defeated in the Ohio legislature. For much of the twentieth century, euthanasia and PAS continued to be illegal throughout the United States and in most of the rest of the world.

NAZI GERMANY

A notable exception was Nazi Germany where state-sanctioned euthanasia was promoted to advance that regime's perverted concepts of racism, eugenics, and purification of society. Even today, it seems easy to be taken in by the diabolically upbeat Nazi propaganda films designed to convince the German people that culling the physically and mentally disabled was not only crucial for the protection and development of the Fatherland, but was also a humane benefit and favor for the victims themselves. The moral depravity of this approach, and its indelible association with the Nazi program of barbarous medical experimentation and mass genocide, continues to influence the current debate over PAS and euthanasia for patients with devastating terminal illness.

TODAY

Public awareness and interest in PAS and euthanasia appear to have paradoxically increased in direct proportion to advances in medical knowledge and the resultant substantial gains in expected longevity over the past 50 years. The routine application of technologically advanced, artificial, life-prolonging devices and techniques regardless of clinical appropriateness has supplanted the experience of a natural death, shifted the process of dying away from home and family to the hospital and health care professionals, and altered the definition of death itself.

Increased longevity has seen a shift in terminal disease states away from infectious illnesses and toward malignancies and chronic, irreversible degenerative organ failure disorders. Many physicians, sometimes under pressure from patients and their families, continue to over-emphasize ephemeral hopes for curative success and ignore or minimize existent symptoms and side effects of life-prolonging treatment.

On the other hand, the public, although increasingly conditioned to expect medical miracles, is well aware that, with the progression of chronic illness, the level of independent function and quality of life inexorably decrease, and the symptoms of disease become ever more distressing. The heightened emphasis on quality, and not only quantity, of life is reflected in a growing sentiment the management of terminal illness needs to be recaptured from the health care profession and asserted by individual patients and their loved ones. This change in the public attitude toward end-of-life care has contributed to both the development and growth of hospice and palliative medicine and also increased pressure to consider the ending of an undesired life as a therapeutic option.

The debate over PAS and euthanasia has intensified during the previous decades, particularly after the publication of two articles in which physicians described personal participation in hastening a patient's death in response to perceived pain and suffering. The first paper entitled "It's Over, Debbie" was published anonymously in *JAMA*, and purportedly related the clinical relationship between a young resident on call and a 20-year-old woman with terminal ovarian carcinoma. The patient, who weighed only 80 pounds and appeared much older than her

20 years, was cachectic and suffering relentless pain and intractable vomiting. The resident described the situation as a "gallows scene" and stated that her only words to him were "let's get this over with." He proceeded to administer a lethal dose of morphine with the clear intention of causing a death that quickly ensued.

The second paper, in the New England Journal of Medicine, was written by Dr. Timothy Quill, an internist and hospice medical director. It described the story of his long-time patient, Diane, who presented with acute myelomonocytic leukemia. Although Diane was young and good candidate for aggressive induction chemotherapy with a 25% chance for long-term survival, after discussing her options with her family and physician, she decided to forego an attempt at curative treatment in favor of a palliative approach. She availed herself of hospice services, but increasingly stated neither her family nor the hospice seemed to be able to deal adequately with the emotional pain and suffering, as well as the growing bone pain, and sense of dependence and isolation. She requested help from her physician to end her pain and suffering, and, after considerable soul-searching and detailed discussions with Diane, Quill prescribed medication and helped Diane understand how to take a lethal dose.

The response of the medical community to "It's All Over, Debbie" was generally unfavorable. The resident had a brief and apparently shallow professional relationship with his patient, appeared to have had no contact or input from her family, and left no indication he had considered or proposed other options such hospice, or sought additional consultation before acting unilaterally. Indeed, there was even speculation that the entire story was fictional and written for the purpose of stimulating discussion. In contrast, Quill, whose candid disclosure potentially jeopardized his medical career, had a deep and professionally intimate knowledge of his patient's mind-set and family situation. After many detailed and emotionally charged discussions with the patient, he could in good conscience conclude that he had

come to know, respect, and admire Diane's desire for independence and her decision to stay in control of her own life. Nevertheless, although there has been widespread recognition of Quill's personal and professional integrity and intellectual acumen, his assertion that PAS is a constitutional right and his advocacy of the legalization of PAS are not currently supported by a majority of physicians in the United States.

PAS/EUTHANASIA IN THE NETHERLANDS

The Netherlands has a population of approximately 16 million, of which 14% are older than 65 years. With a death rate of 8.69/1,000 population, there are an estimated 139,000 total annual deaths. In 2001, physician-assisted suicide (PAS) accounted for 2.6% of all deaths, an increase from 2.1% in 1990. More recent surveys have shown a decrease to 1.2% of deaths, for reasons that will be discussed below.

In contrast to attitudes of American physicians, PAS is supported by a majority of Dutch physicians. Most Dutch pharmacists are also supportive of euthanasia and PAS and are prepared to fill prescriptions written for these purposes.

In 2002, the Netherlands legalized euthanasia. While euthanasia is still technically considered a criminal offence, the law codified a 20-year-old convention of not prosecuting physicians who have committed euthanasia in specific circumstances. The *Dutch Euthanasia Act* states that euthanasia and physician-assisted suicide are not punishable if the attending physician acts in accordance with criteria of due care. These criteria concern the patient's request, the patient's suffering (unbearable and hopeless), the information provided to the patient, the presence of reasonable alternatives, consultation of another physician, and the applied method of ending life. To demonstrate their compliance, the Act requires physicians to report euthanasia to a review committee. The law allows a medical review board to suspend prosecution of physicians who performed euthanasia when each of the following conditions is fulfilled:

- The patient's suffering is unbearable with no prospect of improvement.
- The patient's request for euthanasia must be voluntary and persist over time (the request cannot be granted when under the influence of others, psychological illness, or drugs).
- The patient must be fully aware of his/her condition, prospects, and options.
- There must be consultation with at least one other independent physician, who needs to confirm the conditions mentioned above.
- The death must be carried out in a medically appropriate fashion by the physician or patient, in which case the physician must be present.
- The patient is at least 12 years old (patients between 12 and 16 years of age require the consent of their parents)

In a survey of Dutch physicians published in 2006, most cases of euthanasia were reported by general practitioners. Because of the way medicine is practiced in the Netherlands, this means that the majority of euthanasia cases were performed at home, rather than in a hospital. The mean age of patients was 63 years, and 88% had cancer as a diagnosis. The most important reasons for requesting euthanasia were suffering without improvement (82%), loss of dignity (63%), weakness and fatigue (43%), meaningless suffering (37%), pain (36%), and dependency (33%). Of note, depression was a reason in only 1% of patients.

In 2005, the Royal Dutch Medical Association (RDMA) published a national guideline for palliative sedation, and since that time there has been a steady increase in cases treated with this modality, with a concurrent fall in the number of euthanasia cases. The RDMA guidelines require that sedation be given for a refractory symptom with mostly a somatic nature, that the patient be involved as much as possible in decision making before sedation, that symptom management continue during sedation, that artificial hydration during sedation is not recommended, and that life expectancy from the terminal condition not exceed 1 or 2 weeks. When a physician survey was done in 2007, it was reported that Dutch physicians distinguish palliative or continuous sedation from euthanasia, patient requests for euthanasia decreased by 50%, and patient involvement in decision making increased significantly. There was an increase in the reported symptom of exhaustion as a reason for the request; this symptom can be physical due to deterioration brought on by the terminal illness as well as have a psychoexistential dimension due to social interactions and fear of the future.

PAS IN THE UNITED STATES: THE OREGON EXPERIENCE

PAS was legalized in Oregon in October 1997 with the passage of the Death with Dignity Act. Under this statute, eligibility for PAS is restricted to patients older than 18 years of age who are residents of Oregon and who are terminally ill (i.e., life expectancy of less than 6 months), are mentally "capable" of making and communicating decisions about their health care and, on their own volition, make two oral requests for PAS separated by an interval of 15 days and one written, witnessed request. (See Table 23–1, which compares the guidelines for PAS in the Netherlands and Oregon.) The patient's primary physician and a consultant are required to confirm the terminal diagnosis and prognosis and determine that the patient has capacity. If either physician believes the patient's judgment is impaired due to depression or some other psychiatric or psychological disorder, the patient must be referred for counseling. The physician must inform the patient of all feasible alternative options, including pain control and hospice and palliative

TABLE 23–1. Guidelines for PAS/Euthanasia: Comparison of the Netherlands and Oregon

GUIDELINE	NETHERLANDS	OREGON
Physician action	Euthanasia/PAS	PAS only
Conscientious objection	Yes	Yes
Age requirement	Adult	Adult
Legal residency	None stated	Prior waiting period required
Mentally capable	Yes	Yes (physician certified)
Voluntary only	Yes	Yes
Multiple requests	Yes (repeated, consistent, and documented)	Yes (oral × 2; 15 d interval) + witnessed written)
Indication	Intolerable suffering	Terminal disease
Mandatory consultation	Yes	No
Coexistent "psych" illness	Counseling optional	Counseling mandatory
Psychiatric illness	Yes	No
Offer alternative options	Not required	Mandatory
Mandatory reporting	Yes	Yes
Legality	Technically illegal	Legal
Immunity from prosecution	Highly probable	Yes

care, and review the risks and results of ingesting the lethal dose of medication. Physicians must report all prescriptions for lethal medications that are actually given to the patient. Physicians are not compelled to participate in PAS in violation of their own moral convictions and are protected from criminal prosecution when they adhere to the requirements of the legislation.

During 1998, the first year of legalized PAS, 23 patients received prescriptions for lethal medications and 15 died after taking the prescribed medications (barbiturates in all cases, usually with anti-emetics). Of the eight patients not choosing to take their own lives, seven died of their terminal illnesses, and one committed suicide during 1999. Thirteen of the 15 patients had cancer, and eight were older than 69 years of age. (Although not so stated, one has the impression that death was not as imminent in these patients as in the Dutch patients described above.) The time from medication ingestion to unconsciousness ranged

from 3 to 20 minutes, and the time from ingestion to death ranged from 15 minutes to 11.5 hours. No vomiting or seizures were reported. Eight patients who received prescriptions did not use them, with six having died of their underlying illnesses. Of the two who remained alive in January 1999, one subsequently died of the underlying illness and the second committed suicide during 1999. The frequency with which physicians were present during the act of suicide was not reported.

Updated statistics in 2008 show that from 1998 to 2007, physicians wrote a total of 541 prescriptions for lethal doses of barbiturates, either secobarbital or phenobarbital, and 341 patients died as a result of taking these medications. Of the other 200 patients, 13 were still alive at the end of 2007 and the rest had died of their underlying diseases. The median age of patients who took the barbiturates was 69 years, almost all were white (although this may be more a reflection of the racial demographics of Oregon), and they were well-educated. Approximately 86% were enrolled in hospice programs and almost all died at home.

Although nearly 82% of patients had a cancer diagnosis, the rates of assisted suicide were higher among people with amyotrophic lateral sclerosis (25 per 1,000) and HIV-AIDS (23 per 1,000) than among people with cancer (4 per 1,000). The most frequent reasons for choosing assisted suicide, mentioned by more than 80% of people, were loss of autonomy, loss of dignity, and the inability to enjoy life. Only 1 in 5 cited poor pain control and a tiny minority cited financial concerns.

Regarding physician involvement, most Oregon physicians have never written a prescription for a lethal dose of medication. The 85 prescriptions written in 2007 were issued by only 45 physicians.

Concern has been raised as to whether depression was under-recognized or under-reported among Oregonians requesting PAS with the result that patients with potentially treatable depression were instead allowed to end their own lives. In prior studies of terminally ill patients, the rates of depression have ranged from 59% to 100%, yet between 1998 and 2006 only 12.6% of people who requested a lethal prescription were referred for psychiatric evaluation. In 2007, no patients were referred. Nevertheless, it is conceded that the potential magnitude of the role of depression in requests for PAS requires further investigation, and there is debate whether, pending further evidence, all patients requesting assistance with suicide should undergo a mental health consultation.

Rather than taking the state down a slippery slope of unintended consequences with assisted death being an important cause of demise, it is clear that the passage of the Oregon Death with Dignity Act has resulted in PAS being an option for only a small number of people. The side benefits of this Act have been a substantial improvement in palliative care in Oregon, an improvement in palliative care training of physicians, better communication of patients for their end-of-life treatment, and an increase in rates of hospice referrals.

The experience in Washington State will be watched with interest as the population there is larger and less homogeneous than in Oregon; it is too soon as of this writing to see what impact, if any, the court decision in Montana will have on the issue. Similar initiatives have been introduced in the legislatures of Vermont, Hawaii, and California, but, at least at present, they remain unsuccessful.

THE DISPUTATION: ARGUMENTS PRO AND CON

In the United States, legitimization and legalization of physician-assisted suicide as a therapeutic option remains a controversial issue in end-of-life care. Profound differences over fundamental ethical questions and societal values have resulted in seemingly irreconcilable positions with little evidence for the existence of any middle ground. There is little disagreement about the clinical concerns that have motivated those who have put the issue of PAS "into play" in the arena of public opinion. The controversy swirls around the issue as to whether PAS violates professional and societal ground rules sufficiently so as to make it totally inadmissible.

IN FAVOR OF PAS

The proponents of PAS as a therapeutic option in end-of-life care have offered four major reasons as compelling justifications for their position (Table 23–2). A clearer understanding of the relative significance of each, from the perspective of the patient and family, has emerged from the experience with PAS in Oregon (see above).

Inadequate or Unavailable Pain and Symptom Management

One of the most haunting and disturbing images in American literature is Thomas Wolfe's

TABLE 23–2. Conditions Promoting Consideration of Physician-Assisted Suicide

CONDITION	MANIFESTATION
Physical suffering	Inadequate or unavailable pain and symptom management
Emotional suffering	Irreversible loss of control and independence
Social suffering	Intractable socioeconomic burdens of terminal illness
Existential suffering	Hopelessly worsening quality of life

description of the death of his own brother as depicted by Ben Gant in the novel *Look Homeward Angel*: "Ben's thin lips were lifted in a constant grimace of torture and strangulation, [and the] sound of his gasping—loud, hoarse, unbelievable, filling the room and orchestrating every moment of it—gave to the scene its final note of horror." Although written 70 years ago, this could be a contemporaneous description of a dying, undertreated patient with AIDS, COPD, or cancer. A number of studies indicate a high prevalence of uncontrolled pain and dyspnea, among other symptoms in dying patients. It is hardly surprising that some patients would elect to accelerate their own death rather than undergo protracted, unrelenting physical suffering, even if only contemplated and not yet experienced. Under such circumstances, if a rational person chooses to die rather than to live miserably, should society have the right to say no?

Autonomy and Privacy: The Patient's Right to Choose

Even when adequate symptom palliation is achieved, the Oregon experience indicates that dying patients assign particular importance to control over their body and the right to self-determination. Autonomy is a hallmark principle of clinical ethics. The right to refuse unwanted treatment and the constitutional right to privacy were key elements in the precedent-setting 1976 Quinlan decision regarding unwanted artificial ventilation and in the Cruzan decision involving the right to remove a feeding tube from a patient in a persistent vegetative state. The courts have extended the right to refuse treatment even to

patients with nonterminal conditions. The 1986 opinion in Bouvia v. Superior Court (CA) stated "The right to die is an integral part of our right to control our own destinies so long as the rights of others are not affected." Today, a patient can refuse any life-sustaining procedure or treatment, and unassisted suicide is not generally illegal. That being so, why should a person not be free to choose any mode of "final exit" that does not endanger others, even if the cooperation of another party such as a physician is necessary?

Perception of Being a Burden

As patients with terminal illnesses progressively lose physical independence, they often suffer from erosion of their self-image and a loss of self-worth. They are also usually aware of the invariably onerous financial burden imposed on others by their deteriorating condition, not only in terms of medical expenses, but also in terms of the investment of time, effort, and money by family and friends. One study of attitudes toward euthanasia and PAS in the United States indicated that 60% of the respondents chose "economic burden" as a reason for PAS as opposed to only 20% who chose "avoiding pain." Although the Oregon results indicated that patients who requested PAS were not at greater economic disadvantage than those who did not, it is uncertain that this finding is applicable to other areas of the country or the world in general in which economic disparity may be more pronounced. In any event, does society have the right to refuse PAS to those terminally ill patients who regard it as the best option for alleviating what has been termed "social suffering"?

Existential Suffering

Even if the patient is not suffering physically and is not a financial burden, emotional pain and distress cannot be ignored. Is it possible that the patient's perceived quality of life can be so low that it is unethical to force the individual to continue that life? Is such an emotional state necessarily synonymous with a syndrome of pathological depression that would render the patient incompetent to make life decisions? Consider the case of a 42-year-old psychologist whose disability and weakness progressed to complete quadriplegia and total dependence on others. "She was imposing on her family as they were forced to watch her dying slowly. . . her pain was adequately controlled, but this existential suffering remained profound." She requested assistance in dying, but was told that was illegal. Rather, she was offered total sedation. "In the physician's mind, this approach was justified by the inability to relieve her psychological and existential distress while maintaining a wakeful state." Is this approach truly different or better from an ethical viewpoint than PAS?

IN OPPOSITION TO PAS

The counter arguments to legalization of PAS are summarized in Table 23–3 and also should be examined with reference to the published reports from Oregon that were described earlier.

Improved Access to Adequate Hospice and Palliative Care Obviates Need for PAS

PAS need not be and ought not to be a subject for controversy because a model for quality end-of-life care for the terminally ill is already available. The real debate should be about improved access to hospice and palliative care programs. Although there are more than 4,500 hospice providers in the United States, the quality of hospice care is variable, and there are millions of people in this country who do not have access to hospice services. Funding restrictions

TABLE 23–3. Arguments Against Legalization of Physician-Assisted Suicide

1. Improved access to hospice and palliative care obviates need for PAS
2. Individual patient autonomy rights must yield to the overall societal concern for the sanctity of human life
3. PAS is a "slippery slope" leading to social injustice and depravity
4. PAS is incompatible with the role of the physician as healer and protector of life

and overly restrictive and rigid interpretation of the Medicare rule mandating a life expectancy of 6 months or less have placed restraints on the ability of many hospices to respond appropriately to need and have resulted in a majority of patients being referred to hospice less than two weeks before death. With education and legislative changes, hospice and palliative care could markedly reduce suffering in almost all terminally ill patients, rendering PAS unnecessary. Of course, there would still be the rare, exceptional case where suffering was intractable and resistant. And, it should also be noted that 86% of the Oregon patients who elected PAS were enrolled on hospice programs!

Patient Autonomy Is Not Limitless

The Bouvia decision (see above) emphasized the right to control one's destiny, provided that the rights of others are not affected. Daniel Callahan reasons that because PAS requires assistance by another person, it is no longer a private act, but a form of communal action. Although the individual physician who opposes PAS may abstain on the basis of conscientious objection, it is argued that PAS threatens the very fabric of society by cheapening and denigrating the perceived value of human life. There is a solid core of opinion, usually but not always religiously based, that life is sacred and infinitely precious no matter its "quality" and that this belief is key to preserving our moral status. Because society has an overriding responsibility to protect the sanctity of life, individual freedom of action, such as to allow PAS, should be abrogated in favor of the overall good.

PAS Is a "Slippery Slope" Leading Inevitably to Social Depravity

Some advocates for PAS also support euthanasia for sick patients who cannot kill themselves. "This comes as no surprise to opponents of PAS [who] predicted long ago that if assisted suicide is permitted, euthanasia would not be far behind." Reacting in part to an older Dutch experience, opponents of PAS foresee euthanasia without consent, euthanasia for mental illness, and eventually, euthanasia for the physically handicapped, the elderly, the demented, the homeless, and anyone else deemed socially useless or undesirable. For those who are skeptical that highly cultured societies would never countenance such behavior, "slippery slope" debaters justifiably introduce Adolph Hitler, Joseph Goebbels, Joseph Mengele, and their followers into evidence. Closer to home, there is already sufficient concern in this country about abusive, self-serving managed care practices that have caused politicians of all stripes to recognize the need for some type of "patient bill of rights." Can we be truly sure that were PAS to be broadly legalized, patients might not come under subtle pressure to make the request? There seems to be no evidence for this in Oregon to date, but can we afford to be complacent?

PAS Is a Violation of the Hippocratic Oath

PAS is antithetical to the role of the physician as a healer and protector of life whose most basic obligation is *primum non nocere,* "first, do no harm." As deliberately killing a patient is regarded as harm *par excellence,* this maxim would appear to clearly apply to any action by a physician that serves to hasten death. Advocates for PAS such as Dr. Sherwin Nuland prefer to treat the Hippocratic Oath and similar formulations as ancient, perhaps occasionally relevant guidelines, which should be interpreted and modified as necessary in accordance with the physician's appraisal of a patient's needs and desires, and in accordance with the physician's individual conscience. "To seek refuge in ancient aphorisms is to turn away from the unique needs of each of our patients who have entrusted themselves to our care." The observation that a strong majority of American physicians oppose legalization of PAS and would refuse to participate even if legally able suggests that *primum non nocere* continues as a significant component of the professional psyche of most physicians.

RESPONDING TO A PATIENT'S REQUEST FOR PAS

The ultimate resolution of this debate is unclear. It seems likely that, given the undercurrent of public support, assisting terminally ill patients in ending their own lives will become more of a reality in our society in the years to come. In addition to guidance from an individual's conscience and religious beliefs, if present, what advice should a physician seek in responding to a legal request for PAS? The Assisted Suicide Consensus Panel of the University of Pennsylvania Center for Bioethics offered the following paraphrased suggestions in a paper in Annals of Internal Medicine, which are also listed in Table 23–4.

IDENTIFY, ACKNOWLEDGE, AND CLARIFY THE REQUEST

Using open-ended questions (see chapter on communication skills) encourage patients to feel comfortable in sharing their ideas and feelings. If it is evident that a patient is seeking PAS, address the issue head on. If the patient appears

TABLE 23–4. Suggested Physician Responses to a Request for Physician-Assisted Suicide

1. Identify, acknowledge, and clarify the request.
2. Explore the patient's concerns and address total suffering.
3. Achieve a shared understanding of the goals of treatment.
4. If treatment goals cannot be achieved, search for acceptable alternatives to PAS.
5. If the patient insists on suicide, clarify the level of participation expected and conscientiously acceptable to the physician.
6. Offer all information relevant to informed consent, including realistic options.
7. Do not hesitate to seek emotional support from colleagues.

SOURCE: Adapted from Tulsky JA, Ciampa R, Rosen EJ: Responding to legal requests for physician-assisted suicide. *Ann Intern Med* 132:494-499, 2000.

to be skirting the issue, probe cautiously to find out whether PAS is indeed under consideration. In the absence of some patient initiative, do not recommend PAS as a therapeutic option.

EXPLORE THE PATIENT'S CONCERNS AND ADDRESS TOTAL SUFFERING

Try to identify the elements of suffering that are fueling the patient's desire to hasten death. As indicated above, these most often involve concern about loss of independence, loss of control of bodily functions, worsening and unrelenting symptoms, and fear of being a burden to family and friends. After an in-depth discussion, the patient may agree to consider alternate approaches other than suicide.

ACHIEVE A SHARED UNDERSTANDING OF THE GOALS OF TREATMENT

When palliative treatment is proposed, the physician and patient should agree on realistic goals and endpoints of response. A key component of all palliative care is restoration of hope that continued living will be meaningful. Oftentimes, by focusing attention on particularly significant life events or milestones, even a short-term treatment

plan may assure the patient that he is back in control of his life.

IF TREATMENT GOALS CANNOT BE ACHIEVED, SEARCH FOR ACCEPTABLE ALTERNATIVES TO PAS

Seek additional expert consultation if treatment outcomes are sub-optimal. In the rare circumstance, when all standard and nonconventional options for palliation of suffering are exhausted, and the patient reasserts an interest in PAS, discuss other relevant and more universally acceptable options. These may include withdrawal of life-sustaining treatment such as dialysis, terminal sedation, or voluntary cessation of eating and drinking.

IF THE PATIENT INSISTS ON SUICIDE, CLARIFY THE LEVEL OF PARTICIPATION EXPECTED AND THAT IS CONSCIENTIOUSLY ACCEPTABLE FOR THE PHYSICIAN

Despite the best efforts of the attending physician and consultant experts, some patients will persist in requesting PAS. This is the time when the issue can no longer be avoided and each physician must decide how to respond based on personal belief and conviction. The principle of conscientious practice guarantees the physician's right to withdraw from the care of a patient who chooses a treatment that is morally objectionable for the clinician. It would seem that right would extend even to abstaining from a direct referral to a colleague who would be prepared to participate in PAS. However, the physician should be most careful not to abandon other necessary and appropriate care of the patient, unless specifically asked to withdraw.

OFFER ALL INFORMATION RELEVANT TO INFORMED CONSENT INCLUDING REALISTIC OPTIONS

Patients must be fully informed about their legal options as well as all the details of the PAS procedure, including potential complications. There should be agreement as to the physician's attendance during the suicide and the physician's role if events do not go smoothly. The patient and family need to be aware that the time from ingestion of lethal medication to death may be variable, occasionally extending for many hours. There should be a plan as to what to do if the attempted suicide fails or if patients change their minds mid-stream. Family members should be integrated into the discussion as they are likely to play an active role in assisting the suicide and must face the emotional consequences thereafter.

DO NOT HESITATE TO SEEK EMOTIONAL SUPPORT FROM COLLEAGUES

Many physicians will experience feelings of frustration, failure, emptiness, and abandonment when receiving a request for assisted dying, and more so should a patient actually commit suicide. Physicians and other health care professionals need to take care of each other, and the support of colleagues can be critical in affirming the physician's own sense of self-worth and continued mission as a healer.

FINAL THOUGHTS ON PAS

The debate about PAS is more subtle and sensitive than committed proponents and opponents are sometimes willing to acknowledge. Competent physicians caring for terminal patients have always been positioned somewhere on that notorious ethical slippery slope. The real conundrum is to define where on that slope we are willing to take a stand—a muddy and ambiguous task that subjects us to high levels of stress and to potential abuse.

Ultimately, what has to inform the physician's decision making, whether as regards PAS or any other aspect of the physician–patient relationship, is nothing more than as much wisdom and kindness as his education, character, and faith will permit. The challenge is well-described in the words of Dr. Walter J. Kade, the pseudonym of a physician who himself participated in PAS: "Although we have accepted our roles as comforters in end-of-life care, we have not struggled with or found solutions to active roles in accomplishing their deaths. I am grateful for the great disruption in my emotional stability that this experience precipitated. This act should never be easy, never routine. It should be among the most difficult and disquieting acts we embark upon." The question is: Will Dr. Kade pen those same words after PAS number 2, or number 5, or number 20? Writing in January 2010, we must, at this time, leave this question hanging and unanswered.

PALLIATIVE SEDATION

Despite aggressive and skilled attempts at palliation of symptoms in terminally ill patients, some patients will experience distress from symptoms that cannot be adequately relieved. In this situation, it may be necessary to consider sedating the patient to the point where he or she becomes unaware of their symptoms. As with all other interventions, this has to be considered in the context of the patient's goals of care, the intervention's potential benefits and burdens, and the ethical issues that surround it.

DEFINITIONS

A number of names have been attributed to this intervention. The original name of "terminal sedation" has fallen from favor because of the implication that the sedation is being used to "terminate" the patient, rather than the true source of the name, using sedation in a patient who is terminally ill and imminently dying. Quill et al. have proposed a three-level classification of sedation. *Ordinary sedaton* is used to relieve anxiety or depression, and if there is a decrease in the level of consciousness during waking hours, there would be a decrease in the dose of the sedating medication. *Proportionate palliative sedation* occurs when sedating medications are progressively increased along with the use of other measures to control symptoms; the result is a variable level of sedation during both waking and sleeping hours that relieves the intractable suffering of physical symptoms, such as pain or delirium. The goal is to use the minimal amount of sedation needed to achieve the relief of symptoms that is acceptable to the patient. *Palliative sedation to unconsciousness* is when the goal of the intervention is unconsciousness because the continued perception of symptoms is unacceptable to the imminently dying patient. Usually, patients are sedated rapidly and there is often no administration of artificial hydration or nutrition; sedation is continued until the patient's death. This form of sedation is much more ethically controversial, as will be discussed. This last form of sedation has now been referred to as *continuous deep sedation* in the European literature. Finally, Rousseau has described an intervention called *respite sedation* where a pa-

tient is sedated for a predetermined interval, say 24 to 48 hours, and then brought back to consciousness. This may often break a cycle of anxiety, agitation, or insomnia, and the patient may not require further alteration of the level of consciousness afterward.

Lo has pointed out the three characteristics that make use of sedation justified:

1. Alternate means of relieving symptoms have been ineffective or the side effects of these treatments are unacceptable. Most clinicians can bring to mind patients they have cared for whose pain was simply uncontrollable despite maximal use of opioids and other medications, or the opioids relieved the pain but the nausea was intolerable; patients who were so dyspneic from lung disease that they had the sensation of ongoing suffocation; intractable nausea and emesis; and so on. In these patients, most people would agree that decreasing the patient's awareness of the symptoms would be preferable, if not merciful and humane, treatment of the suffering.
2. The goal of sedation is to relieve the symptom, not to shorten the patient's life. The ethical issues that surround this concept will be discussed below.
3. The patient is near to, or at the point of, death, which makes it unlikely that the patient's life will be shortened. A study in the *Annals of Oncology* in 2009 looked at survival of patients in a cancer center who did and did not receive sedation for their symptoms. Survival in both groups was a median of 10 days. One can therefore surmise that this intervention was used in patients who were actively dying, yet sufficiently alert to be distressed by their symptoms, and their already short life expectancy was not compromised.

HOW PREVALENT IS THIS INTERVENTION?

Most studies on palliative sedation/continuous deep sedation come from Europe; this is not surprising given the fact that physician-assisted suicide and euthanasia are more acceptable in Europe and are legal in a number of countries.

In 2007–2008, 16.5% of the deaths in the United Kingdom were preceded by this form of sedation. The demographics of the patients included a relatively younger age and cancer as a diagnosis. When British physicians answered a questionnaire, nearly 20% of those responding indicated that they had attended a case of continuous deep sedation (CDS). They also indicated that 12% of these patients had requested a hastening of their death, and the sedation was requested in many of the others as a way to control intractable symptoms, or as an adjunct to withdrawal of life-sustaining measures such as ventilators or dialysis. The demographics of the physicians who voluntarily reported their experiences was also looked at and it was found that those physicians who participated in CDS supported euthanasia and were nonreligious.

In the Netherlands, the practice of sedation is used in approximately 10% of dying patients, as reported by Dutch physicians. Again, the symptoms that are most often palliated with this intervention are pain (51%), delirium (38%), and dyspnea (38%). In 60% of cases, the sedation was discussed with the patient, and in the other patients, the reason for not involving them in the discussion was the perception that the patient was incompetent or semi-conscious already. Most often hydration and nutrition were not offered to patients, as the physicians felt that withholding these interventions was a given in this situation.

ETHICAL ISSUES

The main ethical issue that arises in palliative sedation is whether, regardless of what it is called and how it is done, this is a form of active euthanasia. This can certainly be inferred from the Dutch experience where a sizable minority of physicians has reportedly advised this intervention with the intent of hastening the demise of the patient. In addition, in a minority of the patients, no discussion of this intervention was done with either patient or family before it was started, suggesting

that sedation may be used as a more "acceptable" means to the patient's end than direct euthanasia.

In the United States, physicians make a definite distinction between the two interventions, with the intent of the sedation being the main differentiating factor. Sedation is acceptable when symptoms are intractable and the patient's life expectancy is short; it is not acceptable and perceived as euthanasia, when the patient is not imminently dying and there is a stated request by the patient to hasten death.

An ethical dilemma that arises is whether to continue artificial hydration and nutrition in patients who are receiving any level of sedation for symptom relief. Does withholding of these not accelerate dying? Yet, if one considers that most of these patients are already far advanced in their dying process, then these patients have already stopped eating and drinking normal amounts on their own; so how is withholding these artificially when the patient has altered consciousness different from what was occurring when they were fully conscious?

It is also interesting to note that the majority of patients for whom palliative sedation is recommended have pain as their predominant symptom. It is generally accepted that pain can be controlled in greater than 90% of cases, so one has to raise the question: how aggressive and rigorous was pain management in these patients? If palliative sedation has become an accepted intervention for "intractable" symptoms, is there any concern that the definition of "intractable" may become increasingly lax? Is it possible that one can think of turning to sedation prior to exhaustive interventions to control pain in a dying patient?

The stated ethical basis of this intervention is the Rule of Double Effect where the sedation would be seen to be ethical because the intent of the action is not to end the patient's life. Yet, in a number of studies it has been shown that physicians often have more than one intent. Not only European physicians, but U.S. physicians as well have said that a significant minority would offer sedation not only as a means to control intractable symptoms but additionally as a means of hastening death. And focusing on "intent" can take away responsibility for the outcome of the action, as in "I didn't *mean* to do that."

It would seem to be better to focus on the proportionality of the dose versus the symptom. That way one can focus on what the clinician *does*, rather than what she *says*. In this way, the initial dose of sedation would be the lowest dose appropriate to control the symptom, and the increments in dose should be stated explicitly and be reasonable to other clinicians.

The final concern that needs to be addressed is under what circumstances is sedation not appropriate? As has been stated, clinicians may agree that sedation is an alternative for the imminently dying patient who is having intractable physical symptoms. However, as one moves back from the phase of imminent death, is this intervention still appropriate? How close to death must the patient be? What about the patient who is terminally ill, but not actively dying, with psychologic, existential, or spiritual suffering? Sedation likely will shorten that patient's life. The questions that remain to be answered are: is this at all acceptable and ethical? How much shortening of life can be ethically accommodated? How much suffering needs to be demonstrated? These are questions that beg for guidelines that may well be developed in the future. For the present, however, it is up to each clinician to use his or her clinical judgment to best meet the needs of each patient and family under care, and to utilize palliative sedation in an appropriate manner based on the indications and ethical considerations that have been discussed.

BIBLIOGRAPHY

Abramson N, Stokes J, Weinreb N, Clark WS: Euthanasia and doctor-assisted suicide: Responses by oncologists and non-oncologists. *South Med J* 91: 637-642, 1998.

American Academy of Hospice and Palliative Medicine: *Position Paper: Physician-Assisted Death.* Glenview, IL, AAHPM, 2007.

Angell M: Euthanasia in the Netherlands—Good news or bad? (Editorial). *New Eng J Med* 335:1676–1678, 1996.

Angell M: The Supreme Court and physician-assisted suicide—The ultimate right (Editorial). *New Engl J Med* 336:50-53, 1997.

Angell M: Caring for the dying—Congressional mischief (Editorial). *New Engl J Med* 341:1923–1925, 1999. (See correspondence *New Engl J Med* 342: 1049-1050, 2000.)

Anonymous: A piece of my mind. It's over, Debbie. *JAMA* 259:272, 1998.

Binstock RH: Long-term care for older people: Moral and political challenges of access. In: Monagle JF, Thomasma DC, eds. *Health Care Ethics: Critical Issues.* Maryland, Aspen Publishers, 1994.

Blendon RJ, Szalay US, Knox RA: Should physicians aid their patients in dying? The public perspective. *JAMA* 267:2658-2662, 1992.

Burt RA. The Supreme Court speaks: Not assisted suicide but a constitutional right of palliative care. *N Engl J Med* 337:1234-1236, 1997.

Caplan AL, Snyder L, Faber-Langendoen K: The role of guidelines in the practice of physician-assisted suicide. *Ann Intern Med* 132:476-481, 2000.

Cherny NI: The use of sedation in the management of refractory pain. *Principles Pract Support Oncol* 3:1-11, 2000.

Chin AE, Hedberg K, Higginson GK, Fleming DW: Legalized physician-assisted suicide in Oregon—the first year's experience. *New Engl J Med* 340:577-583, 1999.

Churchill LR, King NM: Physician-assisted suicide, euthanasia and withdrawal of treatment. *BMJ* 315: 137-138, 1997.

Dworkin G, Frey RG, Bok S: *Euthanasia and Physician-Assisted Suicide (For and Against).* New York, Cambridge University Press, 1998.

Emmanuel EJ: The history of euthanasia debates in the United States and Britain. *Ann Intern Med* 121:793-802, 1994.

Emanuel EJ, Daniels ER, Fairclough DL, Clarridge BR: The practice of euthanasia and physician-assisted suicide in the United States: Adherence to proposed safeguards and effects on physicians. *JAMA* 280:507-513, 1998.

Emanuel EJ, Fairclough DL, Slutsman J, Emanuel LL: Understanding economic and other burdens of terminal illness: The experience of patients and their caregivers. *Ann Intern Med* 132:451-459, 2000.

Faber-Langendoen K, Karlawish JHT: Should assisted suicide be only physician assisted? *Ann Intern Med* 132:482-487, 2000.

Field MJ, Cassel CK, eds: *Approaching Death: Improving Care at the End of Life.* Washington, DC, National Academy Press, 1997.

Fohr SA: The double effect of pain medication: Separating myth from reality. *J Palliat Med* 1:315-328, 1998.

Ganzini L, Nelson HD, Schmidt TA, et al: Physicians' experiences with the Oregon death with dignity act. *New Engl J Med* 342:557-563, 2000. (See correspondence *New Engl J Med* 343:150-153, 2000.)

Gordijn B, Janssens R: The prevention of euthanasia through palliative care: New developments in The Netherlands. *Patient Educ Couns* 41:35-46, 2000.

Groenewoud JH, van der Maas PJ, van der Wal G, et al: Physician-assisted death in psychiatric practice in the Netherlands. *New Engl J Med* 336:1795-1801, 1997.

Groenewoud JH, van der Heide A, Onwuteaka-Philipsen BD, et al: Clinical problems with the performance of euthanasia and physician-assisted suicide in the Netherlands. *New Eng J Med* 342:551-556, 2000.

Haley K, Lee MA, eds. *The Oregon Death with Dignity Act—A Guidebook for Health Care Providers*, 1st ed. Portland, OR, The Center for Ethics in Health Care, 1998.

Hendin H: *Seduced by Death: Doctors, Patients, and Assisted Suicide.* New York, WW Norton, 1998.

Hasselaar JGJ, Verhagen SCAHHVM, Wolff AP, et al: Changed patterns in Dutch palliative sedation practices after the introduction of a national guideline. *Arch Intern Med* 169:430-437, 2009.

Haverkate I, Muller MT, Cappetti M, et al: Prevalence and content analysis of guidelines on handling requests for euthanasia or assisted suicide in Dutch nursing homes. *Arch Intern Med* 160:317-322, 2000.

Jecker NS: Physician-assisted death in the Netherlands and in the United States: Ethical and cultural aspects of health policy development. *J Am Geriatr Soc* 42:672-678, 1994.

Kade WJ: On being a doctor. Death with dignity: Case study. *Ann Intern Med* 132:504-506, 2000.

Kissane DW, Kelly BJ: Demoralisation, depression and desire for death: problems with the Dutch guidelines for euthanasia of the mentally ill. *Aust N Z J Psychiatry* 34:325-333, 2000.

Lau HS, Riezebos J, Abas V, et al: A nation-wide study on the practice of euthanasia and physician-assisted suicide in community and hospital pharmacies in the Netherlands. *Pharm World Sci* 22:3-9, 2000.

Lo B, Rubenfeld G: Palliative sedation in dying patients: "We turn to it when everything else hasn't worked." *JAMA* 294:1810-1816, 2005.

Maltoni M, Pittureri C, Scarpi E, et al: Palliative sedation therapy does not hasten death: Results from a prospective multicenter study. *Ann Oncol* 20:1163-1169, 2009.

Meier DE, Emmons C, Litke A, et al: Characteristics of patients requesting and receiving physician-assisted death. *Arch Intern Med* 163:1537-1542, 2003.

Miller FG, Fins JJ, Snyder L: Assisted suicide compared with refusal of treatment: A valid distinction? *Ann Intern Med* 132:470-475, 2000.

More T: *Utopia and Other Writings.* New York, New American Library, 1984.

Muller MT, Van der Wal G, Van Eijk JT, Ribbe MW: Voluntary active euthanasia and physician-assisted suicide in Dutch nursing homes: are the requirements for prudent practice properly met? *J Am Geriatr Soc* 42:624-629, 1994.

Nuland SB: Physician-assisted suicide and euthanasia in practice (Editorial). *New Engl J Med* 342:583-584, 2000. (See correspondence *New Engl J Med* 343:150-153, 2000.)

Okie S: Physician-assisted suicide—Oregon and beyond. *N Engl J Med* 352(16):1627-1630, 2005.

Onwuteaka-Philipsen BD, van der Wal G, Kostense PJ, van der Maas PJ: Consultation with another physician on euthanasia and assisted suicide in the Netherlands. *Soc Sci Med* 51:429-438, 2000.

Peck MS: *Denial of the Soul.* New York, Random House, 1997.

Quill TE: Death and dignity: A case of individualized decision making. *New Engl J Med* 324:691-694, 1991.

Quill TE: Doctor, I want to die. Will you help me? *JAMA* 270:870-873, 1993.

Quill TE: *Death and Dignity: Making Choices and Taking Charge.* New York, WW Norton, 1993.

Quill TE, Lo B, Brock DW: Palliative options of last resort: A comparison of voluntarily stopping eating and drinking, terminal sedation, physician-assisted suicide, and voluntary active euthanasia. *JAMA* 278:2099-2104, 1997.

Quill TE, Dresser R, Brock DW: The rule of double effect—A critique of its role in end-of-life decision making. *N Engl J Med* 337:1768-1771, 1997.

Quill TE, Coombs Lee B, Nunn S: Palliative treatments of last resort: Choosing the least harmful alternative. *Ann Intern Med* 132:488-493, 2000.

Quill TE: Legal regulation of physician-assisted death—The latest report cards. *N Engl J Med* 356(19): 1911-1913, 2007.

Quill TE, Lo B, Brock DW, Meisel A: Last-resort options for palliative sedation. *Ann Intern Med* 151: 421-424, 2009.

Rietjens JAC, van Delden JJM, van der Heide A, et al: Terminal sedation and euthanasia. *Arch Intern Med* 166:749-753, 2006.

Rietjens JAC, van Delden JJM, Onwuteaka-Philipsen B, Buiting H, van der Maas P, van der Heide A: Continuous deep sedation for patients nearing death in the Netherlands: Descriptive study. *BMJ* 336:810-813, 2008.

Rosenblatt J: Montana becomes third state to legalize doctor-assisted suicide. Bloomberg.com, 1/1/2010. http://www.bloomberg.com/apps/news?pid=20601103&sid=axsJmWgpz0dE. Accessed February 23, 2010.

Rousseau P: Palliative sedation in the management of refractory symptoms. *J Support Oncol* 2:181-186, 2004.

Seale C: Continuous deep sedation in medical practice: A descriptive study. *J Pain Symptom Manage.* 39(1):44-53, 2010.

Shaiova L: Case presentation: Terminal sedation and existential distress. *J Pain Symptom Manage* 16:403-404, 1998.

Snyder L, Caplan AL: Assisted suicide: Finding common ground. *Ann Intern Med* 132:468-469, 2000.

Steinbrook R: Physician-assisted death—From Oregon to Washington State. *N Engl J Med* 359(24): 2513-2515, 2008.

Sullivan AD, Hedberg K, Fleming DW: Legalized physician-assisted suicide in Oregon—The second year. *New Engl J Med* 342:598-604, 2000. (See correspondence *New Engl J Med* 343:150-153, 2000.)

Swarte NB, Heintz AP: Euthanasia and physician–assisted suicide. *Ann Med* 31:364-371, 1999.

Tulsky JA, Ciampa R, Rosen EJ: Responding to legal requests for physician-assisted suicide. *Ann Intern Med* 132:494-499, 2000.

Van der Heide A, Onwuteaka-Philipsen BD, Rurup ML, et al: End-of-life practices in the Netherlands under the euthanasia act. *New Engl J Med* 356: 1957-1965, 2007.

Van der Maas PJ, van der Wal G, Haverkate I, et al: Euthanasia, physician-assisted suicide, and other medical practices involving the end of life in the Netherlands, 1990-1995. *New Eng J Med* 335: 1699-1705, 1996.

Willems DL, Daniels ER, van der Wal G, et al: Attitudes and practices concerning the end of life: A comparison between physicians from the United States and from the Netherlands. *Arch Intern Med* 160:63-68, 2000.

Wolfe J, Fairclough DL, Clarridge BR, et al: Stability of attitudes regarding physicin-assisted suicide and euthanasia among oncology patients, physicians, and the general public. *J Clin Oncol* 17:1274, 1999.

Wolfe T: Look *Homeward, Angel.* New York, Charles Scribner's Sons, 1947, p. 574.

SELF-ASSESSMENT QUESTIONS

1. Which of the following statements regarding attitudes toward physician-assisted suicide is TRUE?

   A. Physician-assisted suicide is universally endorsed by national medical organizations.
   B. Physician-assisted suicide is supported by the majority of the American public.
   C. The American public makes the distinction between physician-assisted suicide and euthanasia.
   D. American physicians make the distinction between physician-assisted suicide and euthanasia.
   E. The majority of American physicians would participate in assisted suicide.

2. All of the following statements are true EXCEPT

   A. Physician-assisted suicide is defined as the patient ending his own life, but another person may administer the lethal medication if the patient is too weak to do so on his own.
   B. Voluntary euthanasia means a physician and a competent patient agree to life termination.
   C. Euthanasia always implies that the physician plays an active role.
   D. Involuntary euthanasia means that the physician acts at the request of a surrogate for an incompetent patient.
   E. A physician acting alone to hasten a patient's death, without consent of the patient or her surrogate, could be seen as murder.

3. Regarding the Rule of Double Effect, if an action has two possible effects, one can proceed with the action if all of the following are true, EXCEPT

   A. If the benefit of the positive effect outweighs the burdens of the negative effect.
   B. If the negative effect is not the means to the positive effect.
   C. If the patient is aware of the two competing effects.
   D. If the intent of the action is the positive effect.
   E. If the negative effect occurs, the physician accepts liability even if the there was no negligence in performing the intervention.

4. All of the following are true regarding the practice of euthanasia in the Netherlands EXCEPT

   A. The Dutch Euthanasia Act protects practitioners if due care is taken in the performance of euthanasia and assisted suicide.
   B. The Act allows euthanasia if the patient has unbearable suffering without hope of recovery.
   C. Most interventions of euthanasia are done in the patient's home.
   D. Since guidelines were published in 2005, the rate of palliative sedation has increased and euthanasia has decreased.
   E. Depression is one of the major reasons for patients to request hastening of death.

5. Regarding the Oregon Death with Dignity Act, all of the following statements are true, EXCEPT

   A. From 1998 to 2008, less than 400 patients have ended their own lives under this Act.
   B. There has been a significant and continuous increase in the number of patients requesting lethal prescriptions year over year.
   C. Approximately 60% of the patients who were given prescriptions used them to end their lives.
   D. The majority of patients requesting prescriptions had a cancer diagnosis.
   E. The most common reason for the request was loss of autonomy.

6. All of the following are unintended consequences of the Oregon Death with Dignity
   Act, EXCEPT

   A. Physician-assisted suicide has become a
      major cause of death in Oregon
   B. Knowledge and sophistication of pallia-
      tive care have increased
   C. Hospice referrals in Oregon have in-
      creased
   D. Physician training in palliative care has in-
      creased
   E. Patients and physicians communicate bet-
      ter regarding end-of-life choices

7. All of the statements regarding the establishment and exercising of the right of autonomy
   are true, EXCEPT

   A. The Quinlan case established the right to
      refuse unwanted therapies.
   B. The Cruzan case established that artifi-
      cial nutrition and hydration can be re-
      fused.
   C. The Bouvia case (CA) established the
      right to control one's destiny.
   D. The request for physician-assisted suicide
      in Oregon and Washington State derive
      from the principle of autonomy.
   E. In Oregon and Washington State, if a pa-
      tient with capacity and autonomy requests
      a lethal prescription, the physician must
      write it.

8. All of the following are considered legal
   and acceptable forms of palliative sedation,
   EXCEPT

   A. Proportionate sedation
   B. Palliative sedation to unconsciousness
   C. Respite sedation
   D. Rapid sedation to respiratory suppression
   E. Ordinary sedation

9. Which of the following intractable symptoms, for which palliative sedation may be
   indicated, causes the most ethical challenges
   for end-of-life care providers?

   A. Pain
   B. Dyspnea
   C. Existential suffering
   D. Delirium
   E. Nausea

10. Regarding the concept of intent, all of the
    following are true, EXCEPT

    A. Intent allows physicians to use interven-
       tions with serious or lethal side effects as
       long as these were not the primary goals.
    B. Physicians always have only one intention
       when deciding on an intervention.
    C. Intent is better defined by what the clini-
       cian does, rather than by what s/he says.
    D. Focusing on intent can allow clinicians to
       think about the consequences of their acts.
    E. Intent is clearly seen in actions that seem
       reasonable to other clinicians.

Artificial Nutrition and Hydration

Lyra Sihra and Barry M. Kinzbrunner

INTRODUCTION

There are very few areas of Hospice and Palliative Medicine that are as medically, ethically, and culturally complex as the administration of nutrition and hydration at the end of life. This issue was magnified by the most publicized death in recent history, that of Theresa (Terri) Marie Schiavo. Her case painfully demonstrated the extreme polarization of opinions relating to this topic and illustrates the complexity that surrounds decisions regarding the use of nutrition and hydration at the end of life.

THE CASE OF TERRI SCHIAVO

Terri Schiavo suffererd a respiratory and cardiac arrest on February 25, 1990. She was subsequently diagnosed with persistent vegetative state. Despite an initially amicable relationship, Terri's husband, Michael Schiavo, and Terri's parents eventually disagreed over whether her tube feedings should be continued. As Terri's legal surrogate, Michael Schiavo petitioned the courts for discontinuation of her feedings in 1998. Her parents were opposed to the decision and filed multiple motions with the courts to prevent cessation of feedings. As media attention grew, diverging parties gathered allies on either side of the issue.

On November 2, 2003, then Florida Governor Jeb Bush sponsored a bill called "Terri's Law," which sought to continue tube feedings that had been ordered stopped by the judge hearing her case. The Florida Supreme Court struck down this legislation as unconstitutional and a breach of the separation of powers. Further appeals ensued, during which time Terri's feedings were continued.

After the third removal of her feeding tube, and for the first time in the history of the United States, the U.S. Congress passed a special law specifically for Terri on March 20, 2005, entitled "For the relief of the parents of Theresa Marie Schiavo." This legislation required a federal judicial review of her case. The president interrupted his vacation to return and sign the bill. The U.S. Supreme Court refused to hear the case.

TERRI DIED ON MARCH 31, 2005

This is the only time that a bioethical issue has activated the legislative, judicial, and executive branches of government. The case drew public protests from multiple interest groups, caused bewilderment among bioethicists (as this issue had been dealt with in prior court cases), and even caused the California Medical Association to adopt a resolution, also on March 20, 2005, entitled "Resolved: that the California Medical Association expresses its outrage at Congress' interference with these medical decisions."

Our society remains divided into segments of the population that believe nutrition and hydration at the end of life in incompetent patients is necessary and beneficial. Others view the same treatment as burdensome, not beneficial and even abusive. There are strong ethnic and cultural beliefs that food is essential for maintaining life and a sense of well-being. In addition, weight loss in many patients results in dramatic physical changes during the course of their terminal illness. These alterations in appearance may create significant anxiety for the patient and family by serving as a constant reminder of deteriorating health.

Case law does not consider the withholding or withdrawing of nutrition and hydration to be euthanasia, suicide, or physician-assisted suicide. The courts, based on the principle of autonomy, have affirmed the right of a competent patient to decline food or fluid. Our challenge is to provide guidance to a patient and family in making this decision in the face of differing cultural, societal, and religious values.

ETHICAL ISSUES

Advance Directives

While the topic of advance directives is discussed in depth in Chapter 22, a discussion as to how ethical decision making and advance directives relate directly to the issue of nutrition and hydration at the end of life is warranted. The ethical debate surrounding nutrition and hydration at the end-of-life centers around the question of whether such care is considered "medical treatment" versus "ordinary and proportionate." In the 1990 case of Nancy Cruzan, the Supreme Court stated that administration of nutrition and hydration without consent is "an intrusion on personal liberty." However, the case really centered on what kind of evidence is required to support the contention that a now-incapacitated patient did not desire artificial nutrition and hydration. The outcome of Nancy Cruzan's case and others is this: the withholding or withdrawal of nutrition and hydration from cognitively incapacitated patients requires a higher level of evidence (clear and convincing evidence) than other life-sustaining measures.

To that end, many states now have statutory provisions that require separate standards and "clear and convincing evidence" as justification for withholding or discontinuing nutrition and hydration from an incompetent person. In fact, Illinois excludes refusal of "artificial nutrition and hydration" as it would "result in death solely from dehydration or starvation rather than from the existing terminal illness." Instructions on completing an Illinois advanced directive states "if you wish to have artificial nutrition and hydration removed from your treatment plan, you must state this as a special instruction."

The fact remains that very few patients complete advance directives and the harsh reality is that a verbal request or preference is often ignored. A recent study examined the use of life-sustaining treatments in hospitalized patients aged 80 and older. It showed that although 70% wanted comfort care rather than life-prolonging care, still 18% of them received feeding tubes. A separate study of 154 hospitalized adults that underwent gastrostomy tube placement demonstrated that in 92% of cases, the consents were signed by surrogate decision makers (22% of consents were obtained over the telephone). However, the study indicated that 33 (21%) of those patients were judged to be competent to make their own decision. Only one of the 154 medical records had any documentation of a discussion regarding the procedure and its risks and benefits. On the basis of this data, it is not surprising that 70% of people who die in American hospitals die as a consequence of someone's decision to withhold or withdraw life-sustaining medical treatment.

When advance directives concerning nutrition and hydration are discussed, the ethical principles of beneficence and nonmaleficence, providing benefit and avoiding harm, are often overshadowed by cultural and social beliefs that food and fluids are essential to sustain life and provide for increased well being and recovery in illness, even in the face of a terminal prognosis. Unfortunately, clinicians often leave the decision to the patient or family without providing necessary guidance, resulting, in many instances, in patients, families, surrogates, and health care providers not being able to come to fully informed, thoughtful, and objective decisions on these most important issues. Although it may appear as if this approach empowers patients and families in their decision making, it also assumes that the patient or surrogate understands the treatments available, and their risks and benefits; knowledge remains the most crucial component of decision making. In situations of uncertainty, the evidence shows that people choose options that extend life. When these decisions are made in the absence of support from the clinician, suffering, regret, guilt, and anxiety will increase.

Model for Decision Making (Dr. David Fleming)

The question then becomes, how can we best help our patients and their families come to a decision regarding nutrition and hydration in the context of their beliefs, religion, and culture. This question becomes significantly more complex when the patient is incompetent to make decisions. The model proposed by David Fleming consists of five steps that clinicians can use to guide this decision making:

1. Clarify the facts—take into account the medical facts, patient wishes, and beneficence for the patient in general
2. Identify ethical concerns—autonomy versus paternalism, futility, withholding/withdrawing, identify who the surrogate decision maker is, and how are they making their decision (substituted judgement vs. best interest standard).
3. Frame the issue—use lay language, who will decide and by what criteria, and what is possible vs. what is best for the patient
4. Identify and resolve conflict—what is rational?
5. Make a decision

Using this model or other similar models can help guide us in these often painful conversations.

PATHOPHYSIOLOGY OF ANOREXIA/CACHEXIA

There is no other syndrome that outwardly typifies the terminal state like the anorexia and cachexia syndrome (the word cachexia is derived from the Greek words "kakos" and "hexis," meaning poor condition or bad health). Although strides have been made to correct the underlying disorders, the fatigue and unintentional weight loss that accompany this syndrome play a major role in end-of-life suffering. In fact, a recent survey study of terminally ill patients showed that anorexia, cachexia, and fatigue caused more suffering than pain or dyspnea. Anorexia and cachexia are characterized by insufficient intake of calories and protein, and hypercatabolism. The salient feature of the syndrome is systemic inflam-

TABLE 24–1. Diagnostic Criteria of Cachexia

Unintentional weight loss (5% of baseline weight)
BMI <20 in those aged <65 yrs and <22 in those aged 65 or more
Albumin <3.5 g/dL
Low fat-free mass (lowest 10%)
Evidence of cytokine excess (e.g., elevated C-reactive protein)
Increased resting energy expenditure
Resistance to refeeding

mation, which leads to muscle loss with or without loss of fat mass. It is associated with poor performance status and often precedes death.

The diagnostic criteria of cachexia are listed in Table 24–1 and include unintentional weight loss resulting in a lowering of the BMI, serum albumin levels, and fat-free mass. Accompanying these changes are an increased resting energy expenditure (REE) and a resistance to refeeding, further exacerbating the already existing weight loss. These changes are believed to be mediated, at least in part, by an increase in proinflammatory cytokines such as tumor necrosis factor or TNF alpha; interleukins 1, 2, and 6; C-reactive protein; and interferon. These substances cause a number of metabolic abnormalities, listed in Table 24–2, which include increased protein catabolism, decreased protein synthesis,

TABLE 24–2. Metabolic Abnormalities in Cachexia

Increased protein catabolism
Decreased protein synthesis
Impaired lipoprotein lipase
Increased lipolysis from adipose tissue
Decreased fat synthesis
Decreased total lipids

TABLE 24–3. Diagnosis Specific Features of Cachexia

Cancer	Release of cytokines, which induce systemic inflammation
	Increased resting energy expenditure
AIDS	Decreased oral intake, systemic inflammation, endocrine dysfunction
End-stage renal disease	Decreased ability to clear inflammatory cytokines, uremic toxicity, decreased gastric emptying, dietary restrictions
Congestive heart failure	Disruption of neuroendocrine balance, bowel wall edema causing nutrient malabsorption, poor tissue perfusion Increased resting energy expenditure
Chronic obstructive pulmonary disease	Increased resting energy expenditure, systemic inflammation
Aging	Systemic inflammation, decreased resting energy expenditure

altered lipid metabolism with impaired lipoprotein lipase, increased lipolysis from adipose tissue, decreased total lipids, and decreased fat synthesis. TNF alpha, produced from monocytes and tissue macrophages, causes release of nitrogen and amino acids from skeletal muscle in addition to loss of body fat. Significantly, TNF alpha also crosses the blood-brain barrier and produces an anorectic effect.

Clinically, the effects of cachexia are profound. Terminal diseases including various cancers, HIV/AIDS, end-stage congestive heart failure (CHF), end-stage renal disease (ESRD), advanced chronic obstructive pulmonary disease (COPD), and aging are all associated with different features of the anorexia/cachexia syndrome. Up to 80% of cancer and AIDS patients, 40% of ESRD patients, and 20% of COPD, CHF, and nursing home patients meet criteria for this syndrome. The pathophysiological features of anorexia/cachexia for each of the aforementioned terminal illnesses are listed in Table 24–3 and will be discussed in depth below.

ANOREXIA/CACHEXIA IN CANCER

Cancer-related cachexia (also termed cancer anorexia/cachexia syndrome or CACS) has been the most extensively studied of all of the diseases in which cachexia is found. Cachexia in cancer is associated with shorter median survival, poor response to chemotherapy, and increased risk of toxicity from treatment. The incidence of weight loss in cancer differs according to tumor type with pancreatic and gastric having the greatest incidence (83%), followed by head and neck (72%), lung (55–60%), and breast (10–35%). Systemic inflammation is the most pronounced process responsible for the anorexia and cachexia observed in cancer patients. The tumor itself (in part through tumor-derived proteolysis inducing factor or PIF) is responsible for the release of cytokines that help to initiate the expression of genes that are involved in the process of muscle proteolysis.

Symptoms of malignant diseases that may also directly contribute to anorexia and weight loss include abdominal fullness and early satiety, taste change, nausea, emesis, and mouth dryness. Uncontrolled pain is often associated with decreased oral intake, as are changes in smell, mucositis secondary to opportunistic infection, and a learned aversion to specific foods. In patients with head and neck or gastrointestinal malignancies, mechanical obstruction may contribute to malnutrition, especially late in the course of the illness. Malabsorption is only rarely implicated in the

CACS, occurring in some patients with gastrointestinal or hepatobiliary carcinomas, and in other patients already severely anorectic and cachectic secondary to enzymatic deficiencies from atrophy of small intestinal villi. Various therapeutic interventions aimed at the malignant disease, specifically surgery and its accompanying postoperative period, chemotherapy, and radiotherapy, with side effects including gastrointestinal mucositis and ulceration, nausea, and emesis, may also contribute to poor nutritional status.

ANOREXIA/CACHEXIA IN HIV/AIDS

Another disease that is classically associated with cachexia is AIDS. Prior to Highly Active Anti-Retroviral Therapy (HAART), weight loss occurred in 50% to 84% of all HIV+ patients. Still, today, 80% of patients who die of AIDS have weight loss and malnutrition as a concurrent cause of death. Cachexia in HIV/AIDS (HIV wasting syndrome) is defined as weight loss of greater than 10% of baseline weight associated with chronic diarrhea or chronic weakness and documented fever in absence of concurrent illness. The weight loss is more a result of decreased oral intake (which may be due to involvement of the GI tract due to infections) than to increased resting energy expenditure. Muscle wasting is associated with systemic inflammation and endocrine dysfunction. Since HAART, the most common endocrine manifestation has become the lipodystrophy syndrome in which fat is lost from the face, arms and legs and accumulates in the trunk and abdomen. It is associated with insulin resistance and increased cardiovascular risk.

ANOREXIA/CACHEXIA IN END-STAGE RENAL DISEASE (ESRD)

Two-thirds of patients on hemodialysis (HD) die within 5 years of initiation of HD, and cachexia in ESRD is prognostically significant in this population. Decreased serum albumin is a stronger predictor of death in ESRD than hypertension or hypercholesterolemia. Half of all patients on HD have an albumin level in the range that meets diagnostic criteria for cachexia. Interestingly, an increase in body mass is associated with decreased mortality. Features characteristic of cachexia in ESRD include a decreased ability to clear proinflammatory cytokines, uremic toxicity, decreased gastric emptying (which leads to anorexia), dietary restrictions, and an increased prevalence of comorbid illnesses that limits possible therapeutic interventions.

ANOREXIA/CACHEXIA IN END-STAGE CHF AND COPD

The incidence of cachexia in end-stage CHF is up to 20% of patients, while patients with cardiac cachexia have a mortality of 50% in 18 months. In CHF, cachexia is defined as a greater than 6% loss of dry weight over a period of greater than 6 months and a 10% loss of lean body tissue. Unique features attributed to CHF cachexia include a disruption of the neuroendocrine balance, bowel wall edema leading to nutrient malabsorption, poor perfusion of tissues, and an increased resting energy expenditure.

In end-stage COPD, malnutrition and protein loss compound the problem of dyspnea due to the loss of mass in the respiratory muscles. Prognostically, COPD patients with a BMI of less than 25 have an increased mortality. The central process responsible for cachexia in COPD patients is an increase in resting energy expenditure.

ANOREXIA/CACHEXIA IN AGING

Weight loss in elderly persons is generally incompletely explained by underlying chronic illness, and systemic inflammation has been found to play a contributing role. Indeed, 30% to 40% of persons aged >75 years are 10% or more underweight. Unlike most other types of cachexia where REE is increased, in the elderly, REE is actually diminished.

Elderly debilitated patients who suffer from a nonmalignant terminal illness will generally experience anorexia and weight loss primarily due to the functional loss of the ability to independently eat rather than to metabolic or humoral factors. It should be noted that patients with terminal malignant disease may experience anorexia and weight loss from this as well, compounding the changes that occur secondary to the CACS. The loss of functional independence in eating has been associated with impaired mobility, impaired cognition, modified consistency diets, upper extremity dysfunction, abnormal oral–motor examinations, absence of teeth and dentures, xerostomia, and behavioral indicators suggestive of abnormalities in the oral and pharyngeal stages of swallowing. Consistent with these problems, the vast majority of elderly patients who require nutritional support suffer from various forms of chronic neurological debilitation, including severe cerebrovascular disease, Parkinson's disease, Alzheimer's disease, and other forms of dementia. A number of patients will have the concurrent effects of anorexia/cachexia due to CHF and COPD, as previously described. A few patients will experience dysphagia secondary to a nonmalignant obstructive processes such as Zenker's diverticulum, Schatski's rings, esophageal webs, peptic strictures, and thoracic aortic aneurysms.

ASSESSMENT OF ANOREXIA/CACHEXIA

Table 24–4 highlights the information crucial to a proper assessment of a patient having anorexia and cachexia. Initial assessment involves a detailed history and physical exam. The history

TABLE 24–4. Assessment of Anorexia/ Cachexia

Detailed history and physical exam
Laboratory studies
    CBC, electrolytes, BUN/Cr, TSH, albumin, testosterone, cortisol
    Inflammatory markers (CRP and ESR)
Indirect calorimetry (measure resting energy expenditure)
Bioelectric impedance (BEI) to measure body composition

should focus not only on the aspects of the terminal disease itself, but also on psychosocial issues as well. Pertinent information to be obtained in the history is listed in Table 24–5. Psychosocial factors that need to be explored include the level of poverty, the adequacy or inadequacy of the caregiver to provide the patient with nutrition, and whether the diet provided to the patient may be inedible, spoiled, of poor quality, or of inadequate quantity. Psychiatric factors that contribute to anorexia and cachexia may include depression, psychosis, dementia, and delirium. Uncontrolled or poorly controlled pain, dyspnea, nausea, vomiting, diarrhea, anosmia, altered taste perception, fatigue, or malaise may contribute

TABLE 24–5. Historical Factors that Contribute to Weight Loss

TYPE	EXAMPLE
Psychosocial factors	Poverty, inadequate caregiver support
Psychiatric factors	Depression, dementia
Mechanical factors	Poor oral health, obstruction
Physical symptom factors	Pain, dyspnea, nausea, emesis

TABLE 24–6. Important Physical Findings in Evaluating Anorexia/Cachexia

Weight
Anthropomorphic measures
Muscle strength and mobility of extremities
Interosseous and temporal muscle mass, looking
    for wasting
Oral and dental exam
Abdominal exam

to loss of appetite and weight. Finally, various physical and mechanical problems that should be looked for include poor oral hygiene or oral disease, odynophagia, dysphagia (due to neurological or gastrointestinal disease), difficulty chewing (either mechanical, such as temporo-mandibular joint dysfunction or neurological disease), delayed gastric emptying, and bowel obstruction.

The areas of focus of the physical examination are listed in Table 24–6. Current weight should be sought and compared to prior weights. If weight cannot be obtained, then the degree of muscle wasting and subcutaneous fat loss should be estimated, and mid-arm circumference and triceps skinfold measurement should be obtained in order to determine the mid-arm muscle area (MMA). Wasting of peripheral tissues, such as the interosseous and temporal muscles, should be noted, and the examiner should look for the loose-fitting clothes that often are symbolic of anorexia and weight loss in this setting.

An oral and dental examination should be performed to assess for quality of dentition, tongue strength and mobility, symmetry of palatal elevation, and masses or the oral cavity (possibly previously undiagnosed). An abdominal examination will detect potential masses that may be causing partial or complete obstruction, hepatomegaly, or splenomegaly, which are often present in protein calorie malnutrition, and areas of tenderness. A rectal examination to rule out the possibility of severe constipation as a contributing factor to a pa-

tient's lack of appetite may also be crucial. In addition to looking for muscle wasting as discussed earlier, an assessment of muscle strength and mobility of extremities may provide additional clues to possible reasons for a patient's inability to eat. This will also help in the fall risk assessment.

Laboratory testing and other diagnostic studies are usually reserved for situations when the information may be useful in properly treating the patient. When indicated, these studies may include measurement of body composition using bioelectric impedance (BEI), CBC, electrolytes, BUN/Cr, TSH, albumin, testosterone, cortisol and inflammatory markers (CRP and ESR), and indirect calorimetry. If the history suggests difficulty swallowing on a mechanical basis or another gastrointestinal etiology, then appropriate studies such as barium swallow may be done. REE (determined by indirect calorimetry) can be measured, and if it is greater than the calculated REE, then a hypermetabolic state is present. The body mass index (BMI) is less useful as it does not assess body composition. It is also misleading since obese patients with severe cachexia may still have a "normal" BMI.

TREATMENT OF ANOREXIA/CACHEXIA

With an understanding of the underlying pathophysiologic mechanisms responsible for anorexia and cachexia in various end-stage diseases and with the knowledge of how to assess patients to determine the specific causes for the syndrome in individuals with advanced illnesses, interventions can be prescribed that will hopefully improve the nutritional status of patients near the end of life. While it must be remembered that in many situations improvement in caloric intake will be of limited usefulness, as it cannot alter the underlying pathophysiologic mechanisms of anorexia and cachexia, the symbolic importance to families of providing nutritional support and attempting to improve the nutritional status of loved ones who are ill cannot be sufficiently underscored.

Many interventions have been studied for the treatment of the anorexia/cachexia syndrome. They include various pharmacologic and non-pharmacologic interventions designed to improve oral intake and also include providing direct nutritional support by either enteral or parenteral means.

PHARMACOLGIC INTERVENTIONS

The most significant advancement in treatment of the anorexia/cachexia syndrome has been the elucidation of the physiologic changes that take place, leading toward the potential for more targeted approaches to treatment.

While this has led to the study of many pharmacological interventions that are used to treat anorexia and cachexia, all of which are listed in Table 24–7, only megestrol acetate, corticosteroids, and to a lesser extent, metoclopramide, have a high level of evidence supporting their use. These important agents will be discussed below,

followed by a more limited discussion of some other agents that have been or are currently being investigated.

Recommended Medications for the Treatment of Anorexia/Cachexia

MEGESTROL ACETATE   Megestrol acetate, a synthetic progestin, has principally been studied in patients with cancer and AIDS, and also been explored as an appetite stimulant in patients with COPD. Its primary mechanism of action is to cause an increase in appetite, possibly by inhibiting the release of cytokines and acting directly on the hypothalamus. Actual weight gain may take several weeks and occurs in only approximately 20% of patients. The weight gain observed is primarily due to an increase in body fat mass. Subsequently, there is no significant improvement in fat-free mid-arm muscle area, nutritional laboratory parameters (albumin, prealbumin) do not show improvement, and there are no significant reductions in markers of systemic inflammation (i.e., CRP). However, studies performed within the last 10 years do indicate an improvement in quality-of-life measures, with symptomatic improvement in appetite and overall

TABLE 24–7. Pharmacological Treatment of Anorexia/Cachexiq		
Proven therapies		Megestrol acetate: 480–800 mg daily; Corticosteroids: dexamethasone: 4–8 mg daily, prednisone: 20–40 mg daily; Metoclopramide: 10 mg tid ac and hs
Therapies with limited benefit	NSAID	Anabolic steroids
	Melatonin	Onandrolone
	Thalidomide	Testoserone
Therapies not recommended	Dronabinol	Cyproheptadine
Therapies currently under investigation	Pentaoxifylline	Human growth hormone
	ACEI/ARB	Eicosapentanoic acid (EPA)
	Statins	Macrolide antibiotics
	Beta blockers	Insulin

well-being being observed in approximately 50% of patients with anorexia/cachexia syndrome after as little as 1 to 2 weeks of treatment. As the goals of therapy in palliative care should be focused on improvement in appetite, which is much more clearly demonstrable and correlates well with quality of life, rather than absolute weight gain and significant improvement in objective measures, megestrol acetate is an acceptable option in these patients.

In a comparison study between megestrol acetate and dexamethasone, megestrol was found to have fewer side effects than dexamethasone and demonstrated a trend toward better weight gain. Although megestrol is significantly more expensive (up to 20 times the cost of dexamethasone) and has a higher risk for deep vein thrombosis, because of its relative effectiveness and lower side effect profile when compared to dexamethasone, it should be considered first line for anorexia/cachexia if the patient has an appropriate life expectancy to consider long-term use (weeks to months).

The optimal dose is between 480 to 800 mg daily. No significant benefit has been demonstrated at doses less than 480 mg per day. However, since the most significant side effects, including hypertension, hyperglycemia, and adrenal suppression, are dose dependent, starting at doses of 160 mg per day is still recommended, with upward titration as tolerated.

CORTICOSTEROIDS There are multiple randomized controlled trials that demonstrate the effectiveness of corticosteroids (usually, dexamethasone) in improving appetite and decreasing fatigue in patients with the anorexia/cachexia syndrome, most typically when they suffer from advanced malignancies. In these patients, steroids are thought to act, in part, by suppression of release of tumor necrosis factor and other metabolic products from the tumor itself. They may also improve appetite indirectly through their antiemetic and analgesic effects.

Steroids have been shown to improve appetite in 50% to 75% of patients with advanced cancer. The improvement generally occurs within several days of initiation of the medication, with maximum appetite stimulation achieved within 4 weeks. Unfortunately, the improvement in appetite tends to be short-lived, and most patients experience recurrent anorexia over the next several weeks. The recommended dose of steroids for the treatment of anorexia usually range from 4 to 8 mg per day for dexamethasone and from 20 to 40 mg per day for prednisone.

Reported toxicity to steroids includes oral candidiasis in approximately 1/3 of patients, the development of edema and cushingoid features in up to 20%, while 5% to 10% of patients develop dyspepsia, weight gain, behavioral changes, or ecchymoses. Other gastrointestinal complications, occurring in less than 10% of treated patients, include esophagitis, gastrointestinal bleeding, and perforation. Thus, although steroids may have some efficacy as an appetite stimulant in the terminally ill, the lack of durability of this effect and concerns over toxicity may limit the utility of this class of medication to those patients with a very short life expectancy, usually less than 6 weeks.

METOCLOPRAMIDE One of the causes of anorexia in patients with advanced illness may be early satiety, often due to delayed gastric emptying. Metoclopramide, an agent that increases lower esophageal sphincter pressure and increases gastric emptying, has been demonstrated to be effective in the treatment of this form of anorexia, as well as for symptoms of bloating, belching, and nausea, in patients who suffer from the previously mentioned Cancer-Associated Dyspepsia Syndrome (CADS). Improvement in similar symptoms in diabetics with gastroparesis suggests that in some patients who would otherwise require gastrointestinal intubation, metoclopramide may be beneficial in improving their symptoms without resorting to mechanical intervention. The recommended dose of metaclopramide is 10 mg three times a day before meals with a fourth dose at bedtime.

Medications with Limited Benefit in the Treatment of Anorexia/Cachexia

OXANDROLONE The anabolic steroid oxandrolone is FDA approved to promote weight gain and has demonstrated increases in muscle mass in several studies. In a study of patients with weight loss due to COPD, oxandrolone showed an increase in lean body mass after 2 months of treatment. Importantly, these patients also had an improvement in their functional status during the study. As it has been studied in AIDS and COPD, it may have utility in these patients. It may also be reasonable to give testosterone in cases in which hypogonadism complicates anorexia/cachexia.

NONSTEROIDAL ANTI-INFLAMMATORY DRUGS Most of the abnormalities involved in the pathogenesis of anorexia/cachexia are related to mediators of inflammation. Ibuprofen alone has been shown to reduce resting energy expenditure and acute phase reactants in cancer patients. In a trial comparing megestrol acetate plus ibuprofen with megestrol plus placebo, there was significant weight gain and improvement in quality-of-life scores in the megestrol/ibuprofen group.

This study would suggest that the combination of megestrol and ibuprofen may be very reasonable approach to the treatment of anorexia/cachexia syndrome in patients with life-limiting diseases, especially if the patient requires an NSAID for analgesia as well. However, as the toxicities of NSAIDs are well known and can be formidable in this patient population, careful patient selection is important.

MELATONIN Melatonin appears to suppress cytokine activity by reducing levels of TNF. In several studies of cancer patients, melatonin has been shown to decrease cachexia and asthenia in patients at a dose of 20 mg at night. Additionally, it decreases chemotherapy-related side effects. As its main side effect is sedation, it would be a good choice if treatment for insomnia were needed as well.

THALIDOMIDE Thalidomide has been studied in cancer and noncancer-related anorexia/cachexia syndrome. The trials suggest an improvement in appetite, nausea, and general well-being. One study showed a reversal in loss of lean body mass in patients with esophageal cancer. In patients with HIV, thalidomide treatment resulted in significant weight gain, half being fat-free mass.

Thalidomide inhibits TNF alpha and has effects on other cytokines. It is unknown whether these effects also contribute to its efficacy in management of insomnia, sweating, nausea, and neuropathic pain. Although the studies to date appear promising, there is not sufficient evidence to recommend its use for the routine treatment of anorexia/cachexia syndrome in patients with advanced life-limiting illnesses. However, it may be of utility in patients having advanced multiple myeloma, where the agent has some limited direct antineoplastic effects as well.

Agents Not Recommended for the Treatment of Anorexia/Cachexia

CYPROHEPTADINE Cyproheptadine is an antihistamine and serotonin antagonist that had been attributed with causing weight gain in a number of clinical conditions including childhood asthma, anorexia nervosa, and in patients with tuberculosis, prompting its use as a potential appetite stimulant. Unfortunately, multiple studies have failed to demonstrate any appreciable improvement in appetite or weight gain, suggesting that original positive results were due to placebo effect. Therefore, especially due to the significant side effects of dizziness and increased sedation, the use of this agent in terminally ill patients should be avoided.

CANNABINOIDS Cannabinoids (delta-9-tetrahydrocannabinol, THC, and cannabidiol, CBD) have been studied for effectiveness in anorexia/cachexia, with dronabinol, a synthetic cannabinoid, already FDA approved as an appetite stimulant in patients with AIDS-related cachexia and for chemotherapy-induced nausea and emesis. Recent studies however, including a randomized, double blind, placebo-controlled phase III trial comparing cannabis extract, dronabinol (THC), and placebo, found no differences between the three groups for the primary end points of appetite and quality of life after 6 weeks of treatment, suggesting that the positive results previously reported may have been secondary to a significant placebo effect. In addition, these agents have significant neurotoxicity, including dizziness, somnolence, and disassociation, severely limiting their use in the elderly and those patients with already impaired cognitive abilities. Therefore, because of the high risk and lack of demonstrated benefit, there is insufficient evidence to recommend cannabinoids for routine treatment of anorexia/cachexia syndrome for patients near the end of life.

Other agents currently being studied include growth hormone, pentoxifylline, beta blockers, statins, the atypical antipsychotic medications (mirtazipine and olanzipine), and macrolide antibiotics, but to date, none of these can be recommended for the primary treatment of anorexia/cachexia.

NONPHARMACOLOGIC INTERVENTIONS

There are many other simple and often overlooked treatments that can be recommended to patients in dealing with anorexia. These measures are listed in Table 24–8. It is important to recognize that stomatitis, mouth ulcers, or other oral lesions may present a significant impediment to food consumption and can generally be treated with topical antimicrobials if there is an infectious etiology, topical anesthetics, and meticulous mouth care. Patients who complain of chronic nausea and other gastrointestinal symptoms need to be promptly assessed and aggressively treated.

Be creative in suggesting modification of eating habits. Patients with early satiety can be given more frequent smaller meals rather than insisting that they follow the traditional pattern of three meals per day. Consider serving the smaller meals on smaller plates which may provide patients with a psychological boost, a sense of accomplishment by being able to finish a meal. Most importantly, allow patients to eat what they want and when

TABLE 24–8. Nonpharmacologic Treatments for Anorexia

Assess for treatable causes	Oral thrust
	Nausea, emesis, constipation,
	Metabolic disturbances
Dietary counseling to help patient adjust eating habits	Increase attractiveness of meals
	Smaller portions
	Smaller plates
	Allow patient to eat whenever desired
	Lift dietary restrictions, i.e., low salt, ADA
	Allow favorite foods
	Avoid strong smells, spices
	Avoid hot foods
Dietary counseling to explain changing dietary needs to patient and family	Need for less food
	Lifting of dietary restrictions

they want. Many patients are on dietary restrictions for other chronic medical conditions and would like nothing better than to eat what has been, in the past, a forbidden food. In the palliative care setting, encourage this, and compensate by adding an additional dose of a medication if needed. These maneuvers are relatively simple and may add significantly to the quality of a patient's remaining life.

DIRECT NUTRITIONAL SUPPORT

ORAL NUTRITIONAL SUPPORT

Interest in providing oral nutritional support to patients with malignant diseases dates back at least to 1956, when nine patients with progressive cancer were force fed on a metabolic ward, in an attempt to document any alterations in nutritional status. While positive findings included weight gain and nitrogen retention for some patients early in the course of treatment, the weight gain was primarily due to intracellular fluid accumulation, and the nitrogen balance reequilibrated from positive to the baseline negative state in short order. More importantly, in about half the patients, there was clinical evidence to suggest that the supplemental feedings caused the malignant process to accelerate.

A randomized controlled study performed in the 1990s, studying the effects of oral nutritional support on patients with various malignancies being treated with chemotherapy, demonstrated that neither aggressive dietary counseling nor specific dietary instructions significantly improved patient response to chemotherapy, quality of life, or survival. In addition, dietary interventions such as macrobiotic diets, hyper-vitamin therapy, and shark cartilage, that were popular during the last two decades of the twentieth century have never been demonstrated to be effective in treating the anorexia/cachexia syndrome. Despite the negative historical data regarding oral nutritional sup-

plementation in patients with advanced illness, there have been some recently reported options that may show some promise.

Supplementation of amino acids, such as arginine and glutamine, has been shown to block mediators of cachexia with resultant gain in weight and increase in skeletal muscle mass. In view of these findings, an oral supplement containing β-hydroxy-β-methyl butyrate, arginine, and glutamine is occasionally used as an adjunct in patients with cancer-related anorexia/cachexia syndrome. Another popular supplement is eicosapentanoic acid (EPA), which has been shown to inhibit the production of various inflammatory mediators, including cytokines and PIF. Unfortunately, despite its continued popularity, recent studies have not demonstrated any nutritional or symptomatic benefit to date.

Generally, attempts to reverse weight loss with oral supplementation, as in patients with COPD, are extremely difficult and short lived, as has been demonstrated in studies. Patients who are given a high-energy diet gain small amounts of weight and have concurrent improvement in respiratory muscle strength. These gains, however, quickly disappear once the diet returns to the preintervention diet.

NON-ORAL NUTRITIONAL SUPPORT

For patients who are unable to swallow, whether due to obstructing malignant lesions in the oropharynx or esophagus, or chronic neurological disorders, enteral nutrition via intubation of the gastrointestinal tract has been the method of choice for providing nutritional support. The most common method of non-oral enteral nutrition is through a percutaneous endoscopic placed gastrostomy tube (PEG). While the nasogastric (NG) tube was historically considered the least complex way to provide nourishment to these patients (as no invasive procedure is required), the high incidence of pulmonary aspiration and self-extubation, the latter resulting in subsequent trauma to patient, family, and health care staff when replacing the tube, led to the development and subsequent popularity of the PEG tube as the vehicle of choice. Today, most patients at the end of life who receive PEG tubes are cognitively impaired elderly patients and many live in nursing homes.

Many studies evaluating the efficacy of PEG tubes have been performed to date, and, unfortunately, have not yielded the results that most expect or desire to see. While PEG tubes are placed for a number of indications, including weight loss, aspiration pneumonia, prevention of decubitus ulcers and improvement in the healing of existing lesions, improvement in nutritional parameters, and reduction in infection risk, studies to date have not supported benefit for any of these indications. Even patient survival, which one would intuitively think would improve with PEG tube feedings, has not been demonstrated when compared to oral feedings with proper aspiration precautions. These outcomes continue to remain controversial, as no prospective RCTs have been done nor are any likely to be performed due to the ethical complexities that this type of research would present.

Despite the lack of demonstrated benefit to PEG tube placement, there are significant risks that are well documented. By far, the most common adverse consequence is aspiration of gastric contents. Yet, it is the avoidance of aspiration that is the very reason most commonly given to families as a rationale for PEG tube placement. Other complications include local infection, leaking, and tissue trauma; abdominal pain and bloating; diarrhea; pulmonary edema; and increased respiratory tract secretions. It should be pointed out that overfeeding of patients is an all too common reason for aspiration pneumonia and other complications. This is especially true when patients are bed-bound and inactive and, therefore, are not expending the calories that one might expect would be used by a healthier, more active patient of the same height and weight. In such circumstances, counseling regarding reducing the feedings to more appropriate rates that reflect true patient caloric needs would be a rea-

sonable approach to help avoid PEG tube complications in this patient population.

Finally, studies evaluating patient mortality following PEG tube placement have shown that up to one-half of all patients who receive a PEG tube for nutritional support succumb to their primary illness within one year of PEG placement. This raises serious questions regarding the need for better patient selection.

Yet, despite the risks and lack of benefit, the rates of PEG tube placement continue to increase. Multiple factors may play a role. Patients may choose PEG tube feedings or families may desire loved ones to be fed as expressions of their cultural or religious values. Segments of the general public perceive that PEG tube feedings are of benefit and serve to respect and maintain the value of life. Providers may perceive financial advantages to the use of PEG tubes, as services related to the placement are usually covered by health insurance while paying for an attendant to spoon feed a patient who is physically unable to eat is labor-intensive and is generally not a covered service. Finally, liability concerns regarding the failure to have it inserted may influence the decision to place a PEG tube.

Support for the observation that PEG tube placement is increasing comes from recent study done in hospitalized patients with advanced dementia which showed that out of 192 patients, 62% of the patients that did not have a PEG tube at the time of admission had one placed during the index hospitalization. Importantly, admissions specifically for PEG placement were excluded from the study. Nursing home residents and persons of African-American ethnicity were more likely to receive PEG tubes. This study, like others, showed high short-term mortality for these patients and lack of a survival advantage.

The use of PEG tubes in the nursing home has been specifically studied and these studies have yielded a number of important trends and observations. Approximately, one-third of cognitively-impaired residents in nursing homes have PEGs, with the requests for these tubes most commonly coming from the nursing home staff. Those nursing homes that have speech therapists on staff have higher rates of PEG tube placement, and there is a higher rate of PEG placement in non-Caucasian patients (60% African-American vs. 28% Caucasian). There are geographic differences in PEG tube placement rates, with higher rates in seen the southern United States, 40% in North Carolina and 64% in Washington, DC as opposed to only a 9% rate in Maine. Finally, nursing home survey studies demonstrate that there is the perception that a tube-fed patient is being well cared for and that everything is being done to assure nutritional status. This helps the facility avoid deficiencies and citations related to weight loss as evidence of abuse and neglect.

Despite the overwhelming negative evidence regarding PEG tube placement in the population of patients with advanced illness, there are circumstances under which a PEG is clearly indicated, including selected patients who are unable to swallow due to tumor obstruction of the oropharynx or esophagus and who still sense hunger. In addition, one must be cognizant of the important cultural and religious issues that often influence the decisions that patients and families make regarding the desire for enteral nutritional support when medical indications are either very weak or absent. However, with the preponderance of medical evidence to date demonstrating that there is significant morbidity and mortality associated with PEG tube placement, it is imperative that patients who are provided nutritional support via gastrointestinal intubation be carefully selected and be provided with the appropriate caloric intake that is sufficient to meet their needs without undue risk of toxicity. In this way, patient dignity and quality of life can be maintained in a safe and effective manner.

TOTAL PARENTERAL NUTRITION

Total parenteral nutrition (TPN) has historically not been considered beneficial in terminally ill patients at the end of life. It is associated with significant morbidity, primarily infection and fluid overload, and until recently, there has not been good evidence for its use. Recent studies have shown that a very specific population of cancer patients, those with malignant bowel obstruction (and other related GI dysfunction such as short owel syndrome and malabsorption), can derive some benefit from TPN. Patient selection usually depends upon a prognosis of greater than 2 to 3 months and a Karnofsky Performance Score of greater than 50%. These are patients in whom death by starvation would occur earlier than if death had been due to disease progression.

Other than in the specific situations aforementioned, the overwhelming majority of the evidence shows that, in patients with advanced cancer receiving TPN, there is no survival benefit (with several studies showing decreased survival) and an increased susceptibility to infection and other complications. Therefore, with very few exceptions, TPN is not indicated for patients with advanced illnesses near the end of life.

HYDRATION AT THE END OF LIFE

A majority of hospitalized patients receive intravenous fluids in the period just prior to death, despite evidence that hydration is of negligible benefit to these patients, and, in fact, may be accompanied by significant adverse effects. There often are emotional and cultural imperatives that compel patients and families to insist that parenteral hydration is provided, regardless of whether it is beneficial or harmful to the patient. In addition, physicians and other health care professionals are concerned about patient discomfort caused by symptoms of dehydration near the end of life.

SYMPTOMS OF DEHYDRATION AT THE END OF LIFE

Symptoms of dehydration and potential interventions to treat these symptoms are listed in

TABLE 24–9. Symptoms of Dehydration of Patients Near the End of Life

SYMPTOM	OCCURRENCE	TREATMENT
Thirst	Common	Small amount of oral fluid or ice chips
Dry mouth	Common	Meticulous mouth care
		Small amounts of artificial saliva
Nausea and emesis	Rarely reported	Symptomatic medications
		Parenteral hydration may be indicated in selected patients
Headache		
Cramps		
Postural hypotension	Occasional in ambulatory patients	Parenteral hydration may be indicated
Lethargy	Common	May not be indicated as it may protect against pain and other discomforting symptoms in bed bound patients
Drowsiness		
Fatigue		

Table 24–9. They include thirst, dry mouth, nausea, headaches, cramps, postural hypotension, and central nervous effects including lethargy, drowsiness, and fatigue. Thirst is the symptom of overriding concern to families and physicians, although for some patients, the loss of the pleasure in drinking may be more important.

In fact, thirst may be less of a problem than most perceive, as it has been shown that healthy elderly males, who were deprived of fluid for 24 hours, experienced a reduction in thirst compared to normal younger males treated in the same fashion. Furthermore, it may even be that dehydration at this last stage of life is beneficial for most patients because may accelerate in the development of starvation ketosis, which reduces sensations of thirst and hunger and may additionally provide some relief from pain due to its anesthetic effects.

Metabolic abnormalities resulting from dehydration that are of concern to clinicians may include azotemia, hyperosmolality, hypernatremia, hyperkalemia, and hypercalcemia. While these conditions should be appropriately treated with parenteral fluids and other measures when the patient still has significant quality time remaining, concerns that these abnormalities cause discomfort in the last days of life are greatly exaggerated. Studies have demonstrated that, despite lack of parenteral hydration, patients near the end of life do not experience significant changes in serum sodium, osmolality, or blood urea nitrogen.

TREATMENT OF DEHYDRATION AT THE END OF LIFE

Interventions to treat symptoms of dehydration near the end of life are listed in Table 24–9. Most symptoms can be treated without resorting to parenteral fluids. Thirst, the symptom about which families worry most, may be managed in the majority of patients by providing them with small amounts of oral fluid or ice chips. While clearly insufficient to alter any of the metabolic abnormalities associated with decreased fluid intake, the small amount of oral intake provided will usually satisfy the patient's desire to drink fluids as well as ameliorate any thirst the patient may be experiencing. Dry mouth may be successfully managed with meticulous mouth care. Symptoms of lethargy, drowsiness, and fatigue are not uncommon, but in most cases are not believed to be harmful, especially when patients are close to death.

Nevertheless, recent studies have begun to suggest that there may be more of a role for parenteral fluids than previously thought. Although randomized trials have not been published to date, observational studies suggest that symptoms of delirium (particularly opioid-induced, as renal clearance of opioid metabolites will be improved), sedation, or fatigue, postural hypotension, and treatment of opioid-induced myoclonus might improve in some terminally ill patients who receive a limited amount of parenteral fluid (typically, 1 L per day or less).

Caution must be applied to avoid the many significant risks associated with parenteral hydration which include increased peripheral edema, respiratory tract secretions, gastrointestinal secretions that may cause nausea, vomiting, or aspiration, worsening ascites and pleural effusions, and possible prolongation of the dying process. One should be aware that these negative consequences of parenteral hydration are often overlooked by family members caring for terminally ill patients who are actively approaching death. Near the end of life, fluid needs decrease and it is more difficult for the body to properly mobilize and incorporate the fluids that are provided. Significant third-spacing of fluid can often be the result. In addition, hydration does not alleviate the sensation of thirst.

To minimize the potential risks associated with parenteral hydration, and in order to minimize patient discomfort, hydration in the end-of-life setting is typically given using hypodermoclysis, often simply referred to as 'clysis'. Derived from the Greek meaning to irrigate or wash, lysis is defined by the administration of fluid not given by mouth. Hypodermoclysis uses a butterfly needle (23–25 gauge), which is inserted into the subcutaneous tissue of the upper chest, abdomen, or extremities. Approximately 1 L of fluid (usually,

normal saline) can be administered daily by this technique. Although hyaluronidase to breakdown interstitial barriers has been studied in an attempt to improve fluid absorption, hypodermoclysis is quite effective on its own. The advantages to subcutaneously administered fluids are a decreased incidence of trauma and bleeding, lack of need for an infusion pump, and the ease by which it can be done in the home setting. If needed, medications can also be given subcutaneously. Medications that may be administered in this fashion are listed in Table 24–10.

There have been attempts at developing guidelines for the administration of hydration at the end of life. A recent study suggested that hydration should be limited to 1,000 mL per day in patients with peripheral edema, ascites, and pleural effusions due to the potential for exacerbation of these conditions. In addition, hydration should be limited to 500 mL or less, or avoided completely, when patients have distress related to respiratory tract secretions.

What is most important, however, is to be sure that one is providing parenteral hydration to treat a specific symptom. The key is to have a

TABLE 24–10. Medications That May Be Administered by Hypodermoclysis	
SYMPTOM	**MEDICATION**
Pain	Morphine
	Hydromorphone
	Fentanyl
	Methadone
	Ketorolac
Delirium and other CNS symptoms	Midazolam
	Phenobarbital
Gastrointestinal	Metoclopramide
	Octreotide
	Ondansetron
	Promethazine
Respiratory secretions	Glycopyrrolate

conversation with the patient or decision-makers to determine what the expected outcome of hydration is. Once this has been established, negotiate a time period for a trial of hydration and then reassess what has happened. If the goals are not met and the hoped for outcome does not occur, then hydration can be discontinued. And one has to remember that there will occasionally be families who need the visual assurance of a fluid bag to know that they have fulfilled their psychologic and/or cultural duties to their loved one. As long as the patient will tolerate a slow infusion of fluid, and is not harmed by it, this type of "doing something" will provide comfort to and ease the grieving of the family once the patient has died. Obviously, if the patient begins any signs of distress with this hydration, it must be interrupted immediately. Therefore, use of parenteral fluids in the patients in the terminally ill, preferably by hypodermoclysis, should be used judiciously for symptomatic patients who have a distressing symptom that will improve with fluid administration, or when medication cannot be administered by a noninvasive route. For the overwhelming majority of patients who are near the end of life, however, symptoms of decreased fluid intake will respond just as effectively to palliative interventions such as small amounts of fluids, ice chips, and good oral care.

VOLUNTARILY STOPPING EATING AND DRINKING (VSED)

An ethical dilemma that does not receive much media attention is the issue of VSED, which, one can argue, is an ultimate expression of a person's sense of autonomy and self-determination. VSED is a decision made by a competent patient who is able to eat and drink and who intentionally chooses to hasten death by refusing food and fluid. Survey studies show that patients who choose VSED are ready to die, sense a poor quality of life, and want to control the manner of their

death. Death usually occurs within 1 to 3 weeks after food and fluid is stopped.

VSED is a difficult issue because forcing food and fluid on a competent patient who refuses them violates the bioethical principle of autonomy and could be considered assault and battery. Indeed, the court cases of Cantor and Thomas describes two cases in New York filed by nursing homes who requested permission to forcibly administer nutrition and hydration to competent residents who resisted feeding. The nursing homes argued on the basis of a New York statute that authorizes prevention of suicide. In both cases, the judge refused to intervene.

The real question for physicians is how to respond to a patient who desires VSED. Controversy exists on whether a physician has the moral obligation to inform the patient that the option for VSED exists as a way to hasten death. Some say that providing this option would be akin to advising that a patient commit suicide. Others say that not giving the patient this option would be negligent omission of describing all the possible legal end-of-life options. In final analysis, the physician does have the duty to actively listen to a patient and their desire for VSED.

Finally, the issue of dehydration and discomfort is addressed in a recent study in nursing home residents in whom a decision was made to forgo nutrition and hydration. More than half of patients who made this decision died within one week. Symptom scores were highest at the time the decision was made to stop nutrition and hydration. In patients who died within two weeks, the symptom scores decreased progressively until death. In patients who survived longer than two weeks, the discomfort decreased in the first five days but then increased again but did not reach baseline levels. In the end, 85% of patients died within 2 weeks of stopping food and fluids.

Other studies have found that patients who forgo nutrition and hydration had lower levels of discomfort than (1) patients in the nursing home with dementia and pneumonia and (2) patients with dementia in long-term care facilities in the United States who had no intercurrent disease.

A study of nurse experience with patients who stopped eating and drinking was the perception that the overall quality of death was good.

CONCLUSION

The challenge to palliative medicine health professionals is to determine the goals of care set by the patient and family, to understand the options available to meet those goals and to be able to explain the options in an understandable way to patients and families. It is one's responsibility to strike a balance between the respect for patient autonomy, culture, and religious beliefs and the obligation to recommend what is medically sound and for the benefit of the patient.

In the majority of cases, a detailed medical and psychosocial history combined with a careful physical examination can provide most of the information needed to formulate an approach to treatment of anorexia/cachexia. Non-pharmacologic treatments should always be applied while reserving pharmacologic approaches for specific patients who still have a reasonable life expectancy (more than 2 weeks). While the future may bring more pharmacologic options, the choice of interventions will continue to depend on the diagnosis, pathogenesis of the illness, and careful patient selection.

Parenteral and non-oral enteral nutrition are rarely indicated and are associated with significant adverse effects. Even with the lack of evidence of benefit of these therapies, they are commonly recommended by physicians and other health care professionals, while highly effective interventions, such as mouth care, ice chips, and the modification of dietary intake to allow the patient to eat whatever they desire, on their own schedule, are often overlooked.

Even more distressing is the fact that patients who either choose, or are required by cultural or ethic values, to elect artificial nutrition or hydration at the end of life are not managed to avoid complications. While it may be very reasonable to provide artificial nutritional support or hydration to these patients based upon their individual needs, too often this therapy is administered based on fixed quantities without consideration of the patient's limited ability to incorporate the nutrition or hydration, resulting in increased morbidity or premature mortality from fluid overload or aspiration.

In conclusion, the provision of artificial nutritional support and hydration to terminally ill patients, as with any other intervention, must be considered for each patient on an individual basis, taking into account the ethical principles of autonomy, beneficence, and nonmaleficence. Noninvasive interventions, such as allowing ad lib oral intake, providing spoon feedings and providing sips of fluid and ice chips, should be considered therapeutically on par with invasive interventions. Paying attention to detail, considering correctable causes of decreased oral intake, and if artificial support is indicated, avoiding toxicity are all vital to providing patients with high quality end-of-life care, which should be the hope and goal of all therapy provided to patients who suffer from illnesses that limit life expectancy.

BIBLIOGRAPHY

Andrew I, Hawkins C, Waterfield K, Kirkpatrick G: Anorexia–cachexia syndrome—Pharmacological management. *Hosp Pharm* 14:257, 2007.

Annas GJ: "Culture of life" politics at the bedside—The case of Terri Schiavo. *N Engl J Med* 352:1710, 2005.

Boyd KJ, Beeken L: Tube feeding in palliative care: Benfits and problems. *Palliat Med* 8:156, 1994.

Bozzetti F, Cozzaglio L, biganzoli E, et al: Quality of life and length of survival in advanced cancer patients on home parenteral nutrition. *Clin Nutr* 21:281, 2002.

Brett AS, Rosenberg JC: The adequacy of informed consent for placement of gastrostomy tubes. *Arch Int Med* 161:745, 2001.

Bruera E: ABC of palliative care: Anorexia, cachexia, and nutrition. *BMJ* 315:1219, 1997.

Bruera E, Ernst S, Hagen N, et al: Effectiveness of megestrol acetate in patients with advanced cancer: A randomized, double-blind, crossover study. *Cancer Prev Control* 2:74, 1998.

Bruera E, Legirs MA, Kuehn N, Miller MJ: Hypodermoclysis for the administration of fluids and narcotic analgesics in patients with advanced cancer. *J Pain Symptom Manage* 5:218, 1990.

Bruera E, Macmillan K, Kuehn N, et al: A controlled trial of megestrol acetate on appetite, caloric intake, nutritional status, and other symptoms in patients with advanced cancer. *Cancer* 66:1279, 1990.

Bruera E, Sala R, Rico MA, et al: Effects of parenteral hydration in terminally ill cancer patients: A preliminary study. *J Clin Oncol* 23:2366, 2005.

Burge FI: Dehydration symptoms of palliative care cancer patients. *J Pain Symptom Manage* 8:454, 1993.

Callahan CM, Haag KM, Buchanan NN, Nisi R: Decision-making for percutaneous endoscopic gastrostomy among older adults in a community setting. *J Am Geriatr Soc* 47:1105, 1999.

Caplan AL, McCartney JJ, Sisti DA: *The Case of Terri Schiavo: Ethics at the End of Life.* Amherst, NY, Prometheus Books, 2006.

Casarett D, Kapo J, Caplan A: Appropriate use of artificial nutrition and hydration—fundamental principles and recommendations. *N Engl J Med* 353:2607, 2005.

Cerchietti L, Navigante A, Sauri A, Pallazzo F: Hypodermoclysis for control of dehydration in terminal stage cancer. *Int J Palliat Nurs* 6:370, 2000.

Congleton J: The pulmonary cachexia syndrome: Aspects of energy balance. *Proc Nutr Soc* 58:321, 1999.

Del Fabbro E, Dalal S, Bruera E: Symptom control in palliative care, part II: Cachexia/anorexia and fatigue. *Palliat Med* 9:409, 2006.

Deutsch J, Kolouse JF: Assessment of gastrointestinal function and response to megesterol acetate in subjects with gastrointestinal cancers and weight loss. *Supp Care Cancer* 12:503, 2004.

Duerksen DR, Ting E, Thomson P, et al: Is there a role for TPN in terminally ill patients with bowel obstruction? *Nutrition* 20:760, 2004.

Dy SM: Enteral and parenteral nutrition in terminally ill cancer patients: A review of the literature. *Am J Hosp Palliat Med* 23:369, 2006.

Finucane TE, Bynum JP: Use of tube feeding to prevent aspiration pneumonia. *Lancet* 348:1421, 1996.

Finucane TE, Christmas C, Travis K: Tube feeding in patients with advanced dementia. A review of the evidence. *JAMA* 282:1365, 1999.

Finucane TE, Christmas C, Leff BA: Tube feeding in dementia: How incentives undermine health care quality and patient safety. *J Am Med Dir Assoc* 8:205, 2007.

Ganzini L, Goy ER, Miller LL, harvath TA, Jackson A, Delorit M: Nurses' experiences with hospice patients who refuse food and fluids to hasten death. *N Engl J Med* 349:359, 2003.

Gillick MR: Rethinking the role of tube feeding in patients with advanced dementia. *N Engl J Med* 342:206, 2000.

Grauer PA: Appetite stimulants in terminal care: Treatment of anorexia. *Hosp J* 9:73, 1993.

Huang Z, Ahronheim JC: Nutrition and hydration in terminally ill patients: An update. *Clin Geriatr Med* 16:313, 2000.

Johnson KS, Elbert-Avila KI, Tulsky JA: The influence of spiritual beliefs and practices on the treatment preferences of African Americans: A review of the literature. *J Am Geriatr Soc* 53:711, 2005.

Lacey D: Tube feeding, antibiotics, and hospitalization of nursing home residents with end-stage dementia: Perceptions of key medical decision makers. *Am J Alzheimers Dis Other Demen* 20:211, 2005.

Lawlor PG, Gagnon B, Mancini IL, et al: Occurrence, causes, and outcome of delirium in patients with advanced cancer: A prospective study. *Arch Intern Med* 160:786, 2000.

Loprinzi CL: Management of cancer anorexia/cachexia. *Support Care Cancer* 3:120, 1995.

Loprinzi CL, Michalak JC, Schaid DJ, et al: Phase III evaluation of four doses of megestrol acetate therapy for patients with cancer anorexia and/or cachexia. *J Clin Oncol* 11:762, 1993.

MacDonald N, Easson AM, Mazurak VC, Dunn GP, Baracos VE: Understanding and managing cancer cachexia. *J Am Coll Surg* 197:143, 2003.

McCann RM, Hall WJ, Groth-Juncker A: Comfort care for terminally ill patients. The appropriate use of nutrition and hydration. *JAMA* 272:1263, 1994.

Meier DE, Ahronheim JC, Morris J, Baskin-Lyons S, Morrison S: High short term mortality in hospitalized patients with advanced dementia. *Arch Int Med* 161:594, 2001.

Mercadante S, Ferrera P, Girelli D, Casuccio A: Patients' and relatives' perceptions about intravenous and subcutaneous hydration. *J Pain Symptom Manage* 30:354, 2005.

Miller MG, McCarthy N, O'Boyle CA, Kearney MA: Continuous subcutaneous infusion of morphine vs. hydromorphone: A controlled trial. *J Pain Symptom Manage* 18:9, 1999.

Mirhosseini N, Fainsinger RL, Baracos V: Parenteral nutrition in advanced cancer: Indications and clinical practice guidelines. *J Palliat Med* 8:914, 2005.

Mitchell SL: Financial incentives for placing feeding tubes in nursing home residents with advanced dementia. *J Am Geriatr Soc* 51:129, 2003.

Mitchell SL, Buchanan JL, Littlehale S, Hamel MB: Tube feeding versus hand feeding nursing home residents with advanced dementia: A cost comparison. *J Am Med Dir Assoc* 4:27, 2003.

Mitchell SL, Kiely DK, Gillick MR: Nursing home characteristics associated with tube feeding in advanced cognitive impairment. *J Am Geriatr Soc* 51:75, 2003.

Mitchell SL, Kiely DK, Lipsitz LA: The risk factors and impact on survival of feeding tube placement in nursing home residents with severe cognitive impairment. *Arch Intern Med* 157:327, 1997.

Mitchell SL, Kiely DK, Lipsitz LA: Does artificial enteral nutrition prolong the survival of institutionalized elders with chewing and swallowing problems? *J Gerontol A Biol Sci Med Sci* 53:M207, 1998.

Mitchell SL, Lawson FM: Decision making for long-term tube-feeding in cognitively impaired elderly people. *CMAJ* 160:1705, 1999.

Mitchell SL, Teno J, Roy J, Kabumoto G, Mor V: Clinical and organizational factors associated with feeding tube use among nursing home residents with advanced cognitive impairment. *JAMA* 290:73, 2003.

Modi SC, Whetsone LM, Cummings DM: Influence of patient and physician characteristics of percutaneous endoscopic gastrostomy tube decision making. *Palliat Med* 10:359, 2007.

Morita T, Shima Y, Miyashita M, Kimura R, Adachi I: Japan palliative oncology study group: Physician and nurse reported effects of intravenous hydration therapy on symptoms of terminally ill patients with cancer. *J Palliat Med* 7:683, 2004.

Morita T, Tei Y, Tsunoda J, Inoue S, Chihara S: Determinants of the sensation of thirst in terminally ill cancer patients. *Support Care Cancer* 9:177, 2001.

Morley JE, Thomas DR, Wilson MM: Cachexia: Pathophysiology and clinical relevance. *Am J Clin Nutr* 83:735, 2006.

Nelson KA, Walsh TD: Metoclopramide in anorexia caused by cancer-associated dyspepsia syndrome (CADS). *J Palliat Care* 9:14, 1993.

Nelson KA, Walsh D, Sheehan FA: The cancer anorexia–cachexia syndrome. *J Clin Oncol* 12:213, 1994.

Oh DY, Kim JH, Lee SH, et al: Artificial nutrition and hydration in terminal cancer patients: The real and the ideal. *Support Care Cancer* 15:631, 2007.

Oster MH, Enders SR, Samuels SJ, et al: Megestrol acetate in patients with AIDS and cachexia. *Ann Int Med* 121:400, 1994.

Pasman HRW, Onwuteaka-Philipsen BD, Kriegsman DMW, Ooms ME, Ribbe MW, Van Der Wal G: Discomfort in nursing home patients with severe dementia in whom artificial nutrition and hydration is forgone. *Arch Int Med* 165:1729, 2005.

Pasman HRW, Onwuteaka-Philipsen BD, Ooms ME, van Wigcheren PT, van der Wal G, Ribbe MW: Forgoing artificial nutrition and hydration in nursing home patients with dementia. *Alzheimer Dis Assoc Disord* 18:154, 2004.

Pirrello RD, Chen CT, Thomas SH: Initial experiences with subcutaneous recombinant human hyaluronidase. *J Palliat Med* 10:861, 2007.

Plonk WM, Arnold RM: Terminal care: The last weeks of life. *J Palliat Med* 8:1042, 2005.

Quill TE, Byock IR: Responding to intractable terminal suffering: The role of terminal sedation and voluntary refusal of food and fluids. *Ann Intern Med* 132:408, 2000.

Quill TE, Lo B, Brock DW: Palliative options of last resort: A comparison of voluntarily stopping eating and drinking, terminal sedation, physician-assisted suicide, and voluntary active euthanasia. *JAMA* 278:2099, 1997.

Ritchie C, Kvale E, Bruera E: Cachexia in advanced illness: When to treat and how to treat. AAHPM Annual Assembly, Tampa, FL, February, 2008.

Schmoll E: Risks and benefits of various therapies for cancer anorexia. *Oncology* 15:436, 1992.

Schwarz J: Exploring the option of voluntarily stopping eating and drinking within the context of a suffering patient's request for a hastened death. *Pallliat Med* 10:1288, 2007.

Shega JW, Hougham GW, Stocking CB, et al: Barriers to limiting the practice of feeding tube placement in advanced dementia. *J Palliat Med* 6:885, 2003.

Sieger CE, Arnold, JF, Ahronheim JC: Refusing artificial nutrition and hydration: Does statutory law send the wrong message? *J Am Geriatr Soc* 50:544, 2002.

Somogyi-Zalud E, Zhong Z, Hamel MB, Lynn J: The use of life-sustaining treatments in hospitalized persons aged 80 and older. *J Am Geriatr Soc* 50:930, 2002.

Steiner N, Bruera E: Methods of hydration in palliative care patients. *J Palliat Care* 14:6, 1998.

Strasser F, Luftner D, Possinger K, et al: Comparison of orally administered cannabis extract and delta-9-tetrahydrocannabinol in treatment patients with cancer related anorexia–cachexia syndrome: A multicenter, phase III, randomized, double-blind, placebo-controlled clinical trial from the cannabis in cachexia study group. *J Clin Oncol* 24:3394, 2006.

Tatsuya M, Bito S, Koyama H, et al: Development of a national clinical guideline for artificial hydration therapy for terminally ill patients with cancer. *Palliat Med* 10:770, 2007.

Tsai JS, Wu CH, Chiu TY: Symptom patterns of advanced cancer patients in a palliative care unit. *Palliat Med* 20:617, 2006.

van der Steen JT, Ooms ME, van der Wal G, Ribbe MW: Penumonia: The patient's best friend? Discomfort after starting or withholding antibiotic treatment. *J Am Geriatr Soc* 50:1681, 2002.

van Rosendaal GM, Verhoef MJ, Kinsella TD: How are decisions made about the use of percutaneous endoscopic gastrostomy for long-term nutritional support:*Am J Gastroenterol* 94:3225, 1999.

Viola RA, Wells GA, Peterson J: The effects of fluid status and fluid therapy on the dying: A systemic review. *J Palliat Care* 13:41, 1997.

Warden V, Hurley AC, Volicer L: Development and psychometric evaluation of the pain assessment in advanced dementia (PAINAD) scale. *J Am Med Dir Assoc* 4:9, 2003.

Wolfson J: Defined by her dying, not her death: The guardian ad litem's view of schiavo. *Death Stud* 30:113, 2006.

SELF-ASSESSMENT QUESTIONS

1. What percentage of patients 80 and older would want their care focused on comfort rather than prolonging life?

   A. 10%
   B. 30%
   C. 50%
   D. 70%

2. On which bioethical principle have the courts affirmed the rights of a competent patient to decline food or fluid?

   A. Autonomy
   B. Beneficence
   C. Nonmaleficence
   D. Justice

3. In the model for decision making proposed by David Fleming, the first step that should be taken is

   A. Identify ethical concerns
   B. Frame the issue
   C. Clarify the facts
   D. Identify and resolve conflict

4. The salient feature of anorexia and cachexia is

   A. Unintentional weight loss
   B. Protein calorie malnutrition
   C. Systemic inflammation
   D. Loss of fat mass

5. Resting energy expenditure (REE) in COPD is

   A. Increased
   B. Decreased
   C. Unchanged
   D. Varies based on the individual patient

6. What percentage of patients with anorexia/cachexia who are treated with megestrol acetate experience an increase in appetite and overall well-being?

   A. 10%
   B. 30%
   C. 50%
   D. 70%

7. The use of cannabinoids has been shown to

   A. Cause increase in muscle mass
   B. Have a significant placebo effect
   C. Improve cognitive abilities
   D. Have few side effects

8. Which of the following is true when patients receive artificial nutritional support via feeding tubes?

   A. They have a lower incidence of aspiration
   B. They have improved rates of wound healing
   C. They have a reduced risk of infection
   D. One-year mortality rates up to 50% have been reported.

9. What is the approximate percentage of nursing home patients in the United States with severe cognitive impairment that have feeding tubes?

   A. 20%
   B. 30%
   C. 40%
   D. 50%

10. Observational studies in terminal cancer patients suggests that small amounts of parenteral fluid may do all the following, EXCEPT

    A. Decrease sedation
    B. Decrease opioid induced myoclonus
    C. Decrease delirium
    D. Decrease blood pressure

Specific Populations

End-of-Life Care in Patients with AIDS

Alen Voskanian and Michael Wohlfeiler

INTRODUCTION

In the era of highly active antiretroviral therapy (HAART), AIDS does not have a uniformly terminal prognosis and for the most part has become a chronic disease. However, despite the improvements in treatment, the estimated number of deaths among persons with AIDS in the United States still remains high at 14,016 for 2006 based on the National Center for HIV/AIDS. Therefore, patients with AIDS still need hospice and end-of-life care and they represent a unique population for several reasons. First, precise prognostic determinations can be difficult because most of the deaths that used to occur from opportunistic infections are, at least to some extent, treatable. Second, continual improvements in antiretroviral therapy and opportunistic disease prophylaxis and treatment have continually increased the interval between AIDS diagnosis and death which in turn has led to the increased incidence of death from non–AIDS-related conditions. Third, patients with AIDS also present significant psychosocial and socioeconomic challenges that health care providers must pay close attention to and address appropriately.

Those infected with the AIDS virus are mostly younger people in their second through fourth decades of life. Increased life expectancy has led to an increase in the number of HIV-infected patients who are in their 50s and beyond. Since people dying with AIDS tend to be younger, end-of-life care providers have had to learn to deal with psychosocial problems that are substantially different from those seen in the more typical, predominantly elderly, patient population. Further complicating the psychosocial care of terminal AIDS patients is the fact that there is still fear and stigmatization accompanying a diagnosis of HIV, as many persons infected with the disease tend to be from groups already marginalized by the society and often suffer from depression and other mental illnesses that need further evaluation and treatment.

DETERMINING PROGNOSIS IN AIDS

One of the greatest challenges in providing end-of-life care for AIDS patients has always been the difficulty in determining which patients are appropriate for hospice and end-of-life care. The very nature of HIV disease has made these determinations very difficult. Since most of the morbidity and mortality of AIDS, which used to result from opportunistic infections are now usually treatable, patients do not follow an inexorably progressive and fatal course. Additionally, as treatment modalities have improved, the interval between diagnosis with AIDS and death has lengthened. Less than a decade ago, the average survival after a first episode of *Pneumocystis carinii* pneumonia (PCP) was approximately 10 months. However with the development of antiretroviral therapy, followed later by HAART, and improvement in opportunistic infection prophylaxis, that period has steadily increased and may now conceivably be indefinite. This constantly changing prognosis in AIDS makes it difficult for clinicians to determine which AIDS patients have progressed to a stage of disease that makes it appropriate for them to receive end-of-life care.

Despite these challenges, the National Hospice and Palliative Care Organization (NHPCO) Medical Guidelines Task Force, in 1996, published medical guidelines for determining prognosis in selected non-cancer diseases, including AIDS. These guidelines are discussed in Chapter 1 (Table 1–14) and, for completeness, are reprinted here as Table 25–1.

It is important to note that the factors delineated by the Task Force represent guidelines rather than absolute criteria for determining

TABLE 25–1. Guidelines for Determining a Prognosis of 6 Months or Less for Patients with Acquired Immunodeficiency Syndrome (AIDS)

CD4+ count <25 cells/μL in periods free of acute illness
or
HIV RNA (viral load) >100,000 copies on a persistent basis

HIV RNA (viral load) <100,000 copies in the presence of:
    Patient refusal to receive antiretroviral or prophylactic medications
    Declining functional status
    One or more "other factors" listed below

HIV-related opportunistic illnesses	Prognosis for survival
Disease	
CNS lymphoma	2.5 mo
Progressive multifocal leukoencephalopathy	4 mo
Cryptosporidiosis	5 mo
AIDS wasting syndrome (loss of 1/3 lean body mass)	<6 mo
MAC bacteremia, untreated	<6 mo
Visceral Kaposi's sarcoma, unresponsive to treatment	50% 6 mo mortality
Renal failure, refuses dialysis	<6 mo
Advanced AIDS dementia complex	6 mo
Toxoplasmosis	6 mo

Other factors associated with a poor prognosis for patients with AIDS
    Chronic persistent diarrhea for 1 yr
    Persistent serum albumin <2.5 g/dL
    Concomitant substance abuse
    Age >50
    Decision to forego antiretroviral therapy, chemotherapy, and prophylactic drug
       therapy related to HIV disease and related illnesses
    Congestive heart failure, symptomatic at rest

Reprinted, with permission, from Stuart B, Connor S, Kinzbrunner BM, et al: *Medical Guidelines for Determining Prognosis in Selected Non-Cancer Diseases.* Arlington, VA, National Hospice Organization, 1st ed. 1995, 2nd ed. 1996.

prognosis. The Task Force acknowledged that HIV mortality is a dynamic variable that is affected by a number of factors: new and changing therapies, the practitioner's skill and experience in management of HIV disease, and the individual patient's ability to tolerate treatment. Because of the waxing and waning clinical course that can be so characteristic of AIDS, it was suggested that the clinical course over the previous months might be more reflective of the patient's prognosis. For example, a patient whose clinical condition is consistent with the guidelines established by the NHPCO and continues to progressively get weaker and have a decline in functional status despite optimal treatment should be considered for end-of-life care.

The following AIDS-defining conditions were more likely to be diagnosed during the last 12 months of life based on a study of the clinical profile of end-stage AIDS in the era of HAART (Welsh and Morse, 2002):

- HIV dementia
- Progressive multifocal leukoencephalopathy (PML)
- Wasting
- Mycobacterium avium complex
- Lymphoma
- Cytomegalovirus infection

Another study on predictors of mortality for patients with advanced disease in an HIV palliative care program found that age and markers of functional status were more predictive of mortality than traditional HIV prognostic variables (Shen et al., 2005).

On the basis of the most recent analysis of data from the HIV Outpatient Study, which is a prospective, multicenter, observational cohort study among 6,945 HIV-infected patients followed from January 1996 to December 2004, deaths that included AIDS-related causes decreased from 3.79/100 person-years in 1996 to 0.32/100 person-years in 2004. There was an increase in deaths involving liver disease, bacteremia/sepsis, gastrointestinal disease, non-AIDS malignancies, and renal disease. The percentage of deaths due exclusively to non–AIDS-defining illnesses increased from 13.1% in 1996 to 42.5% in 2004.

ANTIRETROVIRAL THERAPY NEAR THE END OF LIFE

The NHPCO Medicare Guidelines Task Force noted that patients receiving antiretrovial therapy may have a greatly lengthened prognosis and, therefore, may generally not be appropriate to receive hospice or end-of-life care. There is controversy regarding the benefits of HAART near the end of life in patients who have developed resistance to their current regimen. Continuing HAART can cause selective pressure on the HIV virus and render the HIV virus less fit, which can potentially lead to less constitutional symptoms. Since most of the benefits of HAART are long term, one could conclude that by the time a patient with AIDS transitions to palliative care, there is probably little if any benefit to continuing antiretroviral therapy. The fact that the patient is now in the terminal stages of the disease can be considered evidence that antiretroviral therapy is no longer effective, most likely due to the development of antiretroviral resistance. Because of the toxicities and inability of patients to tolerate antiretroviral medications many hospice and palliative care programs discontinue antiretroviral medications. Despite that, it may be psychologically very difficult for the patient to give up the only therapy that is directed at the underlying HIV infection.

PALLIATIVE CARE OF PATIENTS WITH AIDS

Palliative care in AIDS can be conceptualized as a continuum consisting of specific therapy directed at AIDS-related illnesses such as infection and malignancy, as well as treatments focused primarily on providing comfort and symptom control at the very end of life.

Specific treatments directed at AIDS-related infection or malignancy are not generally perceived as part and parcel of end-of-life care. However, efforts to have patients access hospice and palliative care services earlier in the course of AIDS dictates that end-of-life care providers be willing to provide such care when indicated, based on the patient's overall clinical condition and quality-of-life concerns. For example, a terminally ill AIDS patient with cytomegalovirus (CMV) retinitis who is still well enough to read or interact with family and friends may be treated with ganciclovir while on a hospice program, as quality of life concerns would dictate that this patient should not be allowed to go blind. If, however, the patient's underlying AIDS has progressed to the point that he or she is comatose or severely encephalopathic, then continuing intravenous therapies for CMV is unlikely to enhance quality of life. At that stage it is more likely that the discomfort and toxicities associated with drug treatment would outweigh benefit for the patient's quality of life.

Likewise, with regard to primary or secondary prophylaxis against opportunistic infections, each prophylactic regimen should be evaluated by weighing the likely benefit of that regimen on the patient's quality of life against the toxicities and discomfort likely to be associated with it. As the patient's clinical status declines, a point will inevitably be reached at which the balance shifts away from continuing such therapies and warrants discontinuation of all opportunistic prophylaxis.

Therefore, as treatment and prophylaxis of common AIDS-related opportunistic infections and malignancies seen near the end of life are discussed below, it is important to keep these principles in mind.

OPPORTUNISTIC INFECTION TREATMENT AND PROPHYLAXIS NEAR THE END OF LIFE

Symptoms in AIDS are often a direct consequence of specific opportunistic infections (OIs). Since most OIs respond partially or completely to appropriate therapy, symptoms may, at times, be palliated most effectively by prevention or treatment of the underlying infection. Therefore, in an end-of-life care setting, the primary purpose of prophylaxis and treatment of OIs must be relief of symptoms rather than restorative or curative care. The most common OIs that are seen in AIDS patients near the end of life are PCP, CMV retinitis, and Mycobacterium avium intracellulare (MAC). Table 25–2 details a summary of each of the OIs symptoms and recommended treatments for AIDS patients near the end of life.

Pneumocystis Carinii Pneumonia

PCP is the most common of all OIs. The primary symptoms of PCP are typically fever, cough, and dyspnea on exertion. The cough is usually dry and nonproductive. In the palliative care setting, treatment of acute PCP should be considered for patients who, though terminal, are not imminently dying and still have an acceptable quality of life. It is preferable to administer PCP treatment as oral therapy using any of the following medications:

- Trimethoprim sulfamethoxazole (TMP-SMX)
- Clindamycin plus primaquine
- Trimethoprim plus dapsone
- Atovaquone suspension
- Trimetrexate with leucovorin

If a patient refuses therapy or cannot tolerate the toxicities associated with therapy, management should be based purely on symptom control. The patient should receive supplemental oxygen and morphine to relieve dyspnea. Corticosteroids are often a useful adjunctive therapy to improve dyspnea and hypoxemia. (See Chapter 7 for a full discussion of the treatment of dyspnea at the end of life.) Corticosteroids or nonsteroidal anti-inflammatory drugs (NSAIDs) may also be effective in reducing the fever and generalized discomfort of PCP.

PCP occurs in approximately 80% of patients who do not receive prophylaxis. Therefore, it is reasonable, even near the end of life, to treat all patients who tolerate oral TMP-SMX with a dose of one double-strength tablet daily or one double-strength tablet three times per week as primary or secondary prophylaxis for PCP infection. The PCP prophylaxis should be considered in all HIV-infected patients who have a CD4 count less than 200 cells/mm^3.

Cytomegalovirus Retinitis

CMV can cause disease in a wide variety of sites, though by far the most common is the

TABLE 25–2. Common Opportunistic Infections in Patients Near the End of Life with AIDS

INFECTION	COMMON SYMPTOMS	TREATMENT	DOSE
PCP	Fever	Prophylaxis: TMP − SMX	1 DS tablet daily or 3 times a week
	Cough	Treatment: TMP + SMX	2 DS tablets q 8 h × 21 d
	Dyspnea	TMP + Dapsone	TMP: 5 mg/kg PO tid +
			Dap: 100 mg PO qd for 21 d
		Clindamycin + Primaquine	Clindamycin 600 mg IV or
			300–450 mg PO q 8 h +
			primaquine 15 mg base PO
			q 24 h × 21 d
CMV retinitis	Blindness	Primary prophylaxis:	
		Not recommended near	
		the end of life	
		Treatment:	Valganciclovir 900 mg PO q 24 h
		Valganciclovir and	
		ganciclovir intraocular	
		implant	
MAC complex	Fever	Treatment should be	NSAIDs
	Night sweats	symptomatic only near	Steroids (dexamethasone 2 mg
	Weight loss	the end of life	PO qd)
	Diarrhea	Toxicity of prophylaxis and	Analgesics
	Fatigue	primary treatment of	Antidiarrheals
	Cytopenias	infection outweigh	
		potential benefits in	
		terminally ill patients	

retina of the eye. If left untreated, CMV retinitis can progress rapidly to blindness. Preservation of sight is an obvious quality of life issue and, as such, treatment of active CMV disease or secondary prophylaxis for previous infections should be considered appropriate palliative care.

The choice of therapies for treatment and suppression of CMV retinitis includes oral valganciclovir, intravenous ganciclovir, foscarnet, and cidofovir. Intravenous ganciclovir is used for the treatment of active CMV while either the oral form or an intravitreal implant can be used for maintenance therapy. However, it should be noted that the oral form is associated with a risk of more rapid rate of CMV progression. Both the intravenous and oral forms of ganciclovir can cause significant bone marrow suppression (primarily

neutropenia) that can be problematic and should be monitored.

Cidofovir is only administered every 2 weeks (after the induction dosing of weekly for 2 weeks) that would seem to make it ideal for a hospice setting. Unfortunately, it has significant nephrotoxicity, making it a difficult agent to use near the end of life. Foscarnet has nephrotoxicity similar to cidofovir and maintenance therapy requires daily infusions, making it even more problematic.

Regarding prophylaxis, whereas PCP will occur in almost 80% of AIDS patients who are not receiving prophylactic therapy, CMV retinitis occurs in only approximately 25% of patients not treated prophylactically. Suspicion of CMV retinitis is usually raised by the patient's report of symptoms and is then readily detectable by ophthalmologic examination. Once diagnosed, CMV retinitis generally responds rapidly to treatment. Therefore, primary prophylaxis to prevent CMV retinitis is generally not indicated in the palliative care setting.

Mycobacterium Avium Complex

Mycobacterium avium complex (MAC) can develop in AIDS patients with CD4 counts of less than 50 cells/mm^3. Disseminated disease causes multiple nonspecific symptoms that include fever, night sweats, weight loss, diarrhea, fatigue, and cytopenias. Treatment of disseminated MAC disease requires the administration of two to three antibiotics, with a combination of clarithromycin and ethambutol being most commonly utilized. Azithromycin is sometimes substituted for clarithromycin and rifabutin can be added as a third agent. Side effects of the above antibiotics might outweigh their benefits in end-stage AIDS patients; therefore, in those circumstances, MAC treatment may be discontinued in patients who are near the end of life.

When antibiotics are discontinued due to undue toxicity, the focus of care should shift to pure symptom management. Symptoms such as diarrhea and fever should be treated with standard symptom management approaches (see below). One study has found that for patients who were unable to tolerate MAC therapy or who were symptomatic despite therapy, dexamethasone at a dose of 2 mg daily will significantly alleviate a number of symptoms.

Primary prophylaxis is usually initiated in patients with CD4 count below 50 cells/mm^3. Azithromycin at a dose of 1,200 mg per week is the preferred agent.

TREATMENT OF HIV-ASSOCIATED MALIGNANCIES AT THE END OF LIFE

Assessment of the efficacy of palliative care for HIV-associated malignancies should take into account medication side effects, ease of drug administration, and effectiveness of symptom relief and patient acceptability. The two most common cancers seen in AIDS patients are Kaposi's sarcoma (KS) and lymphoma, though the prevalence of other neoplasms such as rectal carcinoma is increasing.

Kaposi's Sarcoma

KS in patients with HIV is a different entity than the classic form of the disease that is seen predominantly in older white males of Mediterranean and northern and eastern European extraction. In the setting of HIV infection, KS affects primarily homosexual and bisexual men and is a much more aggressive neoplasm. KS is caused by human herpes virus 8. KS manifests as mucocutaneous and visceral lesions. The incidence of KS has declined dramatically in North America, Europe, and Australia since the advent of HAART.

Mucocutaneous KS may cause pain due to the location and size of the lesions. It also often causes edema secondary to lymphatic obstruction. Visceral lesions will cause pain and other symptoms that vary with the organ or organs involved. For example, KS of the gastrointestinal tract (the most common extracutaneous site) will often cause abdominal pain, melena, hematochezia, anemia, diarrhea, or weight loss. Pulmonary involvement may present with dyspnea and/or hemoptysis.

Palliation of symptoms may be best achieved by using standard KS treatments, such as chemotherapy and radiation therapy, to reduce the size of the lesions. As with all therapies, an appropriate risk–benefit assessment must be made and the therapy should be continued only as long as the palliative benefit outweighs the side effects. Patients for whom chemotherapy or radiation therapy is not appropriate, standard symptom management principles apply.

Lymphoma

The two types of lymphoma most commonly seen in AIDS patients are non-Hodgkin's lymphoma and primary central nervous system lymphoma

(PCNSL). Either form of lymphoma is generally aggressive and poorly responsive to treatment. In addition, the very substantial toxicities of the available treatments generally preclude their use in a palliative care setting. As such, lymphomas should be palliated with traditional measures such as corticosteroids, analgesics, and other symptom management interventions.

SYMPTOM MANAGEMENT OF PATIENTS WITH AIDS NEAR THE END OF LIFE

AIDS patients near the end of life have unique symptoms that require direct management. As with all patients, it should be stressed that symptom management must be individualized. All decisions regarding the appropriateness of interventions should be made by weighing of benefits and toxicities of the proposed treatment as discussed earlier.

Fever

The evaluation of fever in patients with advanced AIDS is presented in Table 25–3. The first step is to assess the patient for obvious sources of infection such as infected intravenous lines, catheters, and decubiti. The clinician should consider the possibility that previous infections for which the patient has been receiving secondary prophylaxis

(e.g., MAC, CMV, or PCP) have reactivated. If that seems probable, appropriate empiric therapy should be initiated if such therapy is likely to maintain or improve the patient's quality of life. The possibility of noninfectious causes of fever such as drug or tumor fever should also be considered. If those are thought to be likely, the offending drug should be withdrawn or, for tumor fever, nonsteroidal anti-inflammatory medications should be administered. If the etiology of the fever remains unclear and the patient has a good performance status, it may be appropriate to initiate a limited work-up aimed at detecting readily reversible conditions. This may include such diagnostic procedures as a chest radiograph, routine laboratory studies, and urinalysis. A trial of empiric broad-spectrum antibiotic therapy can be initiated but should be discontinued after 3 to 5 days if there is no response. If the fever persists despite antibiotics and the etiology remains unknown or if a patient's poor performance status precludes a work-up and an empiric trial of antibiotics, the fever should be treated symptomatically with antipyretics or with steroids such as dexamethasone (2–4 mg/d).

Gastrointestinal Symptoms

Patients with AIDS suffer from a variety of gastrointestinal disorders, most commonly related to

TABLE 25–3. Evaluation of Fever in Patients with Advanced AIDS

POTENTIAL SOURCE	RECOMMENDED INTERVENTION
IV line or indwelling catheter	Remove or replace
Decubiti	Treat (see Chapter 11)
Reactivation of opportunistic infection PCP, CMV, MAC	Empiric treatment if appropriate (see Table 25–2)
Medication	Discontinue potentially offending agent
Tumor fever	NSAID
If above ruled out:	
Patient with good performance status	Limited evaluation followed by 3–5 d of empiric antibiotics
Patient with poor performance status or no response to empiric antibiotic	Symptomatic treatment with NSAID or Dexamethasone 2–4 mg/d

OIs or medications. Although a full discussion of gastrointestinal symptoms and treatments near the end of life is covered in Chapter 8, information unique to patients with HIV will be discussed below.

DYSPHAGIA, ODYNOPHAGIA, HICCUPS, AND DRY MOUTH Dysphagia, odynophagia (painful swallowing), and hiccups can be relatively common in late stage AIDS and are usually the result of esophagitis. The most frequent cause of esophagitis is Candida infection. Other etiologies include CMV, herpes simplex infection, and aphthous ulcerations. Dysphagia and odynophagia can also occur as a result of neoplastic processes such as KS and lymphoma. Even if the patient has a preserved appetite, esophageal symptoms can prevent the patient from eating or drinking. If the pain or obstruction is severe enough, the patient may not even be able to swallow normal oral secretions.

Esophageal symptoms should be evaluated by first obtaining a good history. Most patients will complain of odynophagia or dysphagia with both liquids and solids. Physical examination will frequently, but not always, reveal oropharyngeal candidiasis. The three types of oral candidiasis most commonly associated with HIV infection are thrush or the pseudomembranous type, the erythematous (atrophic) type, and angular cheilitis. Mild to moderate oral candidiasis should be treated with application of topical antifungal agents such as nystatin suspension or clotrimazole troches four to five times per day. Severe disease may be treated with systemic azoles such as fluconazole or itraconazole. The antifungal drug of choice is fluconazole given as a 200 mg loading dose followed by 100 mg daily for at least 14 days. The treatment options for angular cheilitis include clotrimazole, nystatin or miconazole ointment, ketoconazole cream, and triamcinolone ointment or cream.

If the symptoms do not improve with antifungal therapy, other causes such as ulcerative disease should be considered. Unfortunately a definitive diagnosis of ulcerative disease and its etiology requires invasive diagnostic procedures such as endoscopy with biopsy. If CMV or herpes is thought to be likely, it is reasonable to consider an empiric trial of ganciclovir or other anti-herpes treatment. If there is no improvement in symptoms after 7 to 10 days, therapy should be discontinued and other diagnoses considered. For aphthous ulcerations, topical treatment with oral steroid preparations or tetracycline oral suspensions can be used. In severe or refractory cases, oral corticosteroids (e.g., prednisone 40–60 mg daily) can be effective. Alternatively, thalidomide (100–300 mg daily) can be used. Although the FDA approved thalidomide in 1998 for treatment of erythema nodosum leprosum, numerous studies have demonstrated its effectiveness in treating oral and esophageal aphthous ulcerations.

Hiccups can have a variety of causes including central nervous system lesions or infections, diaphragmatic irritation due to tumor invasion or inflammation, metabolic derangement, or systemic infection. In HIV-infected patients, however, esophagitis is usually the most common predisposing condition. When esophagitis results from gastroesophageal reflux disease, treatment with H_2-antagonists like ranitidine or proton pump inhibitors such as omeprazole is indicated. For symptomatic treatment, chlorpromazine is most commonly used. Although this is the only drug FDA approved for the treatment of hiccups, there are anecdotal reports of successful treatment with other medications such as baclofen.

Xerostomia, or dry mouth, can develop in 10% to 25% of HIV-infected patients. Decreased salivary flow can be secondary to infections, medications, or crystal methamphetamine use. Management of xerostomia includes hydration techniques such as use of ice chips and toothettes, sugarless and sour gum or candy, and artificial saliva. Systemic management of xerostomia includes the use of pilocarpine tablets or solution.

NAUSEA AND VOMITING The patient's current medications should be evaluated to assess possible causes of the nausea and vomiting and any nonessential medications should be eliminated or changed. Conditions such as pancreatitis, gastritis, peptic ulcer disease, and gastroparesis are frequent causes of nausea and vomiting in patients with AIDS and these causes should be considered.

Pharmacologic therapy should be directed both at specific suspected diseases (e.g., H_2-antagonists for gastritis, metoclopramide for gastroparesis) and at symptom control with anti-emetics. The most commonly used anti-emetics are the phenothiazines and include prochlorperazine and promethazine. The use of adjunctive medications such as steroids (dexamethasone), benzodiazepines, anti-histamines (diphenhydramine, hydroxyzine), or anticholinergics may enhance the effectiveness of anti-emetics. Other interventions that can be tried include changing the patient's diet or giving the patient smaller, more frequent meals until symptoms are under adequate control. If the vomiting is so severe that the patient is unable to take oral medications, the anti-emetics should be administered parenterally or by suppository. Chronic nausea may respond to dronabinol, 2.5 to 5 mg twice a day. Finally, appropriate precautions, such as elevation of the head of the bed, must always be taken to minimize the patient's risk of aspiration during episodes of vomiting.

DIARRHEA   An attempt should first be made to determine the etiology of the diarrhea and whether the onset is acute or whether this is a chronic problem. If acute, one must consider whether it may be due to infection, such as cryptosporidiosis or giardiasis, or whether it is secondary to medication side effects, as may occur with anti-retroviral agents or antibiotics. Therefore, medications should be carefully reviewed as a possible cause of the diarrhea and suspect medications should be discontinued.

In some patients, a brief trial of an antiparasitic agent such as metronidazole or paromomycin may be indicated. Anti-motility agents such as loperamide or diphenoxylate or bulk supplements like psyllium should be tried initially for symptom control. Severe, chronic diarrhea, which may be secondary to changes in the intestinal wall due to the HIV virus itself, may respond only to opioids

such as oral tincture of opium. The usual starting dose is six drops (0.6 cc) in 2 ounces of water every 4 hours. The dose should then be titrated until symptom control is achieved. There is no maximum dose for tincture of opium. With any of these agents, the patient must always be monitored for the development of constipation or fecal impaction, especially when fluid intake is inadequate.

Octreotide is a synthetic somatostatin analog that is approved for treatment of profuse water diarrhea caused by vasoactive intestinal peptide tumors and carcinoid tumors. It has shown variable effectiveness in treating diarrhea in AIDS patients. Its major disadvantages are its high cost and the fact that it needs to be administered subcutaneously on a regular basis.

Dyspnea and Respiratory Distress

A full discussion of dyspnea and respiratory distress can be found in Chapter 7. Causes of dyspnea in end-stage AIDS patients include pneumonia and acute pneumothorax from either community-acquired or opportunistic pathogens. The etiology of dyspnea may become apparent via a thorough physical examination and history. Simple blood tests such as a CBC may be necessary to rule out conditions such as anemia. Diagnostic procedures such as chest radiograph and oxygen saturation can be obtained but only if data are likely to be of benefit in managing the patient's condition. Initiation of empiric therapy such as antibiotics for suspected bacterial pneumonia or PCP may be appropriate. Supplemental oxygen, opioids, and anxiolytics can be used to decrease respiratory distress and increase patient comfort.

Alteration in Mental Status, Seizures

A full discussion of neurological symptoms near the end of life can be found in Chapter 9. Alterations in mental status can occur due to a variety of reasons. Evaluation to determine the etiology of the change in mental status or the new onset of seizures should be limited to patients whose quality of life and prognosis have previously been of an acceptable degree and who have now undergone an acute change. Focused laboratory studies may, for example, rule out potentially correctable electrolyte abnormalities or other metabolic disturbances. Nuclear or radiographic diagnostic imaging may be helpful in selected circumstances when there is a high index of suspicion that the patient suffers from an easily treatable condition that will restore the person's quality of life (e.g., cerebral toxoplasmosis). However, it would be equally acceptable to avoid the imaging study and treat such patients with a limited course of empiric therapy for the suspected reversible condition (e.g., toxoplasmosis) and monitor the patient for a response to the treatment.

With regard to therapies focused purely on symptom management, antiepilectics such as phenytoin and carbamazepine are generally used as seizure prophylaxis. Active seizures can be treated with benzodiazepines such as lorazepam and diazepam. For HIV encephalopathy (also known as AIDS dementia complex), the patient can be considered for a trial of psychostimulants such as methylphenidate. If the patient develops agitation or psychosis, phenothiazines such as haloperidol or chlorpromazine may be beneficial.

Asthenia

A full discussion of asthenia can be found in Chapter 13. Asthenia, or chronic debilitating fatigue, is a common symptom in AIDS patients that is often associated with impaired physical functioning. Although fatigue may be considered by some to be an unavoidable sequella of advanced HIV disease, its significant effect on quality of life makes it a particularly distressing symptom for many patients. Estimates of the prevalence of fatigue among patients with AIDS range from 40% to 50%. Some studies have shown a higher prevalence of fatigue among HIV-infected women compared with HIV-infected men. Other variables that appear to be correlated with fatigue include more advanced disease (as indicated by greater numbers of phys-

ical symptoms and treatment for AIDS-related medical conditions) and high levels of psychological distress. Hypogonadism in men is one of the main causes of fatigue. Other symptoms that suggest hypogonadism are sexual dysfunction, loss of muscle mass, and osteoporosis. It is important to keep in mind that fatigue is often a symptom of depression. Differentiating between medical and psychological etiologies of fatigue can be very difficult in clinical practice. Further complicating the assessment is the fact that the medical and psychological factors are often multifactorial and frequently coexist. Treatment of asthenia in patients with end-stage AIDS may include steroids (prednisone 20 mg once or twice a day, or dexamethasone 2–4 mg two to four times a day), as well as heavy doses of reassurance and support.

Depression

A full discussion of depression can be found in Chapter 9. Not surprisingly, depression is a common comorbid condition in end-stage AIDS. Depression not only negatively affects the patient's quality of life, but may also exaggerate pain and other symptoms. As such, it is exceedingly important to recognize and treat depression. The class of antidepressants known as selective serotonin reuptake inhibitors (SSRIs) should be the first choice in treating depression. The SSRIs are taken only once daily, have generally mild and manageable side effects, and tend to be very effective. There are multiple SSRIs available and the choice of a particular one should be individualized to the patient.

Pain Management

A full discussion of the treatment of pain near the end of life can be found in Chapter 6. Pain is extremely common in late-stage AIDS. Several studies have shown it to be the most common symptom, affecting 75% to 80% of patients. Studies have also shown pain to be underreported and undertreated.

Neuropathic pain is the major challenge in managing the pain of patients with AIDS. It may result from a toxic peripheral neuropathy secondary to drugs such as the nucleoside analogs d4T (Zerit®), ddI (Videx®), or ddC (Hivid®), or it may be due to HIV infection itself. Neuropathic pain can be disabling if severe. It usually presents first in the feet and may progress up the legs or to other parts of the body.

Neuropathic pain unfortunately does not respond well to opioids alone. Traditionally, tricyclic antidepressants such as amitriptyline have been the drugs of choice for first-line treatment of peripheral neuropathy. These drugs are of limited benefit in reducing neuropathic pain in AIDS patients, however, and dose-related side effects such as somnolence and orthostatic hypotension further limit their usefulness. Anticonvulsants such as gabapentin are also used to treat neuropathic pain.

When patients develop difficulty with swallowing, alternate routes of pain medication delivery such as transdermal patches or subcutaneous infusion of pain medication should be considered.

Weight Loss

A weight loss of at least 10%, with diarrhea or chronic weakness and documented fever for at least 30 days not attributable to a condition other than the HIV infection itself, is defined as Wasting syndrome. Malnutrition and weight loss can reflect malabsorption or high energy expenditure secondary to OIs, malignancy or HIV itself. Hypogonadism in men has also been associated with weight loss. Palliative treatments for weight loss and anorexia include corticosteroids, dronabinol, megestrol acetate, oxandrolone, and testosterone replacement.

Pruritus

Pruritus is very prevalent in patients with advanced HIV disease. Eosinophilic folliculitis (EF) is one of the main causes of pruritus in AIDS patients. EF lesions consist of small follicular papules and pustules that measure 2 to 3 mm in diameter. EF is associated with low CD4 counts and low nadir counts. The exact cause of this rash is not known but it appears that a hypersensitivity to the *Demodex folliculorum* mite can be the culprit. EF is very resistant to treatment and topical steroids rarely provide relief. Topical permethrin (Elimite) has been shown to provide some relief. Other oral treatments include itraconazole and metronidazole tablets.

CONCLUSIONS

The care of patients with AIDS has changed markedly since the disease was initially described in the early 1980s. Primarily affecting younger people, and once a rapidly fatal disease, AIDS has now become a chronic and controllable illness, with the inevitability of death postponed for significant and meaningful periods of time. Unfortunately, all patients with AIDS still face the prospect of a premature death, challenging those who provide hospice and palliative care to patients near the end of life to meet their unique needs. It is hoped that the information presented earlier will assist in that process.

BIBLIOGRAPHY

Breitbart W, McDonald MV, Rosenfeld B, et al: Fatigue in ambulatory AIDS patients. *J Pain Symptom Manage* 15(3):159-167, 1998.

Broder S, Merigan TC, Bolognesi D: *Textbook of AIDS Medicine.* Baltimore, MD, Williams & Wilkins, 1994.

CDC HIV/AIDS Media Facts: HIV and AIDS in the United States: A picture of today's epidemic. http://www.cdc.gov/hiv/topics/surveillance/

Chaisson RE, Benson CA, Dube MP, et al: Clarithromycin therapy for bacteremic Mycobacterium avium complex disease. A randomized, double-blind dose-ranging study in patients with AIDS. AIDS Clinical Trials Group Protocol 17 Study Team. *Ann Intern Med* 121(12):905-911, 1994.

Chin DP, Reingold AL, Stone EN, et al: The impact of mycobacterium avium complex bacteremia and its treatment on survival of AIDS patients: A prospective study. *J Infect Dis* 170:578-584, 1994.

Crum NF, Riffenburgh RH, Wegner S, et al: Comparisons of causes of death and mortality rates among HIV-infected persons: analysis of the pre-, early, and late HAART (highly active antiretroviral therapy) eras. *J Acquir Immune Defic Syndr* 41:194-200, 2006.

DenOuden P: *AAHIVM Fundamentals of HIV Medicine, 2007 edition*. Washington, DC, AAHIVM, 2007, pp. 335-346.

Hogg RS, Strathdee SA, Craib KJ, et al: Lower socioeconomic status and shorter survival following HIV infection. *Lancet* 344:1120-1124, 1994.

Kinzbrunner BM: *Vitas Pain Management Guidelines*. Miami, FL, Vitas Healthcare Corporation, 1999.

Krentz HB, Kliewer G, Gill MJ, et al: Changing mortality rates and causes of death for HIV-infected individuals living in Southern Alberta, Canada from 1984 to 2003. *HIV Med* 6(2):99-106, 2005.

Mellors JW, Rinaldo CR Jr, Gupta P, et al: Prognosis in HIV-1 infection predicted by the quantity of virus in plasma. *Science* 272:1167, 1996.

Mills GD, Jones PD: Relationship between CD4 lymphocyte count and AIDS Mortality, 1986–1991. *AIDS* 7:1383-1386, 1993.

Moore J, Schuman, P, Schoenbaum E, et al: Severe adverse life events and depressive symptoms among women with, or at risk for, HIV infection in four cities in the United States of America. *AIDS* 13:2459-68, 1999.

Moore RD, Chaisson, RE: Natural history of opportunistic disease in an HIV-infected urban clinical cohort. *Ann Int Med* 124(7):633-642, 1996.

Neaton JD, Wentworth DN, Rhame F, et al: Considerations in choice of a clinical endpoint for AIDS clinical trials. Terry Beirn Community Programs for Clinical Research on AIDS (CPCRA). *Stat Med* 13(19-20): 2107-2125, 1994.

Nicholas P: Self-care for peripheral neuropathy in HIV disease. In: XIIIth International AIDS Conference; July 9-14, 2000; Durban, South Africa. Abstract ThPeB5250.

Palella FJ Jr, Baker RK, Moorman AC, Chmiel J, Wook K, Homberg SD; HIV outpatient Study investigators. Mortality in the highly active antiretroviral therapy era: Changing causes of death and disease in the HIV outpatient study. *J Acquir Immune Defic Syndr* 44(3):364, 2007.

Reiter GS: Palliative Care and HIV, Part I: OIs and Cancers. *AIDS Clin Care* 8(3):21-22, 1996.

Saag MS, Holodniy M, Kuritzkes DR, et al: HIV viral load markers in clinical practice. *Nat Med* 2:625, 1996.

Sansone GR, Frengley JD: Impact of HAART on causes of death or persons with late-stage AIDS. *J Urban Health* 77:166-175, 2000.

Schofferman J, Brody R: Pain in far advanced AIDS. In: Foley KM, Bonica JJ, Ventafridda V, et al., eds. *Advances in Pain Research and Therapy*, Vol. 16. New York, Raven Press, 1990, pp. 379-386.

Selwyn P, Rivard M: Palliative care for AIDS: Challenges and opportunities in the era of highly active anti-retroviral therapy. *J Palliat Med* 6(3):475-487, 2003.

Shen JM, Blank A, Selwyn PA: Predictors of mortality for patients with advanced disease in an HIV palliative care program. *J Acquir Immune Defic Syndr* 40(4):445-447, 2005.

Spector SA, McKinley G, Lalezari JP, et al: For the Roche Cooperative Ganciclovir Study Group. Oral ganciclovir for the prevention of cytomegalovirus disease in persons with AIDS. *N Engl J Med* 334:1491-1497, 1996.

Stuart B, Connor S, Kinzbrunner BM, et al: *Medical Guidelines for Determining Prognosis in Selected Non-Cancer Diseases*, 2nd ed. Arlington, VA, National Hospice Organization, 1996.

Welsh K, Morse A; and the Adult Spectrum of Disease Project in New Orleans: The clinical profile of end-stage AIDS in the era of highly active antiretroviral therapy. *AIDS Patient Care STDS* 16:75-81, 2002.

Wormser GP, Horowitz H, Dworkin B: Low-dose dexamethasone as adjunctive therapy for disseminated Mycobacterium avium complex infections in AIDS patients. *Antimicrob Agents Chemother* 38(9):2215-2217, 1994.

SELF-ASSESSMENT QUESTIONS

1. Which of the following AIDS-related illnesses is more likely to be diagnosed earlier than the last 12 months of life?

   A. Mycobacterium avium complex (MAC)
   B. Pneumocystis carinii pneumonia (PCP)
   C. Cytomegalovirus infection (CMV)
   D. Progressive multifocal leukoencephalopathy (PML)
   E. Lymphoma

2. You have just admitted a 27-year-old male with far advanced AIDS to your hospice program. The patient is on antibiotic prophylaxis for PCP, CMV, and MAC. Which of the following would be the most appropriate recommended course of action regarding whether or not continue the prophylactic antibiotic therapy?

   A. Discontinue all the prophylactic antibiotics
   B. Continue prophylaxis for PCP only
   C. Continue prophylaxis for PCP and CMV
   D. Continue all the prophylactic antibiotics
   E. Continue prophylaxis for PCP and MAC

3. As the medical director of the local hospice, you are consulted on a 25-year-old male with advanced AIDS who has developed visual difficulties consistent with CMV retinitis. He is still active, and very concerned about losing his vision. His attending physician would like to start him on therapy and has contacted you to discuss various therapeutic options. Which of the following would be the best therapeutic option for this patient?

   A. Intravenous ganciclovir
   B. An intravitreal ganciclovir implant
   C. Intravenous cidofovir
   D. Intravenous foscarnet
   E. No antibiotics, as this is a hospice patient

4. Regarding AIDS-associated malignancies, all of the following statements are true EXCEPT:

   A. AIDS-related Kaposi's sarcoma (KS) is a much more aggressive neoplasm than the classic form of KS.
   B. The most common extracutaneous site of KS is the gastrointestinal tract.
   C. Primary central nervous system lymphoma (PCNSL) is one type of AIDS-related lymphoma.
   D. AIDS-related lymphomas are generally very aggressive but respond well to antineoplastic therapy.
   E. When antineoplastic therapy is not indicated, patients should be treated symptomatically with steroids, analgesics, and other palliative measures.

5. You are caring for a 26-year-old female, who is on your hospice program with advanced AIDS. She is bed bound and has a Palliative Performance Score (PPS) of 30. She has been having recurrent fever for the last several days. She has no evidence of an AIDS-related malignancy, no indwelling catheters, no decubiti or other sites of possible infection on physical examination, no evidence to suggest reactivation of any opportunistic infections, and medications as a possible etiology of her fever has been ruled out. Which of the following would be the best next step in her management?

   A. Chest x-ray, laboratory studies, and urinalysis, followed by a trial of broad-spectrum antibiotics.
   B. A trial of broad-spectrum antibiotics without doing the chest x-ray, laboratory studies, and urinalysis.
   C. Symptomatic therapy of the fever with dexamethasone.
   D. Full work-up for fever, including cultures and diagnostic scans, followed by a trial of broad-spectrum antibiotics.

E. Full work-up for fever, including cultures and diagnostic scans. Await culture results prior to starting antibiotics.

6. A 32-year-old male with advanced AIDS is being seen in palliative care consultation with complains of dysphagia and odynophagia. What is the most common cause of his symptoms?

A. Aphthous ulcerations
B. Candidal esophagitis
C. CMV esophagitis
D. Herpes simplex esophagitis
E. KS

7. A 38-year-old female with advanced AIDS is complaining of severe debilitating fatigue. Which of the following statements regarding her fatigue is TRUE?

A. The prevalence of fatigue in AIDS ranges from 60% to 70%.
B. There may be a higher prevalence of fatigue in HIV-infected men compared with women.
C. Fatigue in AIDS may be associated with high levels of psychological distress.
D. Fatigue in AIDS does not correlate with the number of physical symptoms experienced by the patient.
E. Steroids should be avoided in patients with advanced AIDS who experience fatigue.

8. A 28-year-old male with advanced AIDS is complaining of severe hyperesthesia in both legs, from the feet to the mid-calf, consistent with peripheral neuropathy. All of the following statements regarding this patient's complaints are true EXCEPT:

A. The prevalence of pain in advanced AIDS ranges between 75% and 80%.

B. His pain may be secondary to medications used to treat the HIV virus.
C. His pain may be secondary to the HIV infection itself.
D. Tricyclic antidepressants are of great benefit in reducing neuropathic pain in AIDS patients.
E. Gabapentin may be an effective agent in the treatment of this patient's neuropathic pain.

9. Which of the following best describes AIDS Wasting Syndrome?

A. Weight loss of 5%, diarrhea, chronic weakness, and fever for 30 days.
B. Weight loss of 10%, diarrhea, chronic weakness, and fever for 30 days.
C. Weight loss of 10%, diarrhea, and chronic weakness without fever for 30 days.
D. Weight loss of 5%, diarrhea, and chronic weakness without fever for 30 days.
E. Weight loss of 10% and chronic weakness, with or without diarrhea or fever for 30 days.

10. You are treating a 33-year-old male with advanced AIDS who has developed severe pruritis. A diagnosis of eosinophilic folliculitis (EF) is made. All of the following regarding EF are true EXCEPT:

A. EF lesions consist of small follicular papules and pustules.
B. EF is associated with low CD4 counts and low nadir counts.
C. The rash may be secondary to hypersensitivity to the *Demodex folliculorum* mite.
D. EF responds well to topical steroids.
E. Metronidazole tablets may be given to treat EF.

CHAPTER

26

Care of the Pediatric Patient at the End of Life

Lynn Ann Meister and Judith Ann Haythorne Macurda

INTRODUCTION

Children receiving hospice care can be compared to snowflakes. No two snowflakes are alike, and we can only enjoy their beauty for a short time.
Diane Majeski, hospice nurse

The death of a child is a life-changing experience for all involved. Children with life-threatening conditions present multiple challenges to providers of medical care who generally focus on life and conquering disease. These providers may feel a sense of failure when they cannot "save" a child. Children with terminal illnesses also present challenges to their parents and family members. These individuals may feel powerless that they cannot do more to improve the quality or the length of their child's life. Dying children present challenges to all affected by their eventual death, including classmates, friends, and neighbors. Dying children also present challenges to the health care system in general as their needs have not always been met within the existing structure of our health care system. In addition, children who die can present challenges even after their death, for the ongoing life of the family and others may be affected by prolonged and unresolved grief.

Improvement in end-of-life care for adults has occurred over the past 30 plus years since the institution of hospice care in the United States. Although close to one-half of all adults who die each year receive some hospice services, only 1 in 10 of the more than 50,000 children who die each year benefit from formal end-of-life care. Similarly, palliative care services for children have been lacking in our country. Although over 50,000 infants and children die each year in the United States, there are also 500,000 children living with life-threatening illnesses and 12 million children living with special health care needs. Many of these children and their families could benefit from palliative care services.

Palliative care is a concept of care that arose from hospice care to meet the needs of people with life-threatening illnesses and is a practice that may be instituted from the time of diagnosis, in some instances, to improve quality of life. Chapter 2 defines and provides a full discussion of the principles of palliative care. As with hospice care, control of pain and other physical symptoms, as well appropriate management of psychologic, social, and spiritual problems is vital. The goal of palliative care is achievement of the best possible quality of life for patients and their families. Palliative care and hospice programs offer a support system to help families cope during the patient's illness as well as during their own bereavement. Although these statements have defined palliative care for the terminally ill adult patient for more than 30 years, the needs of dying children and their families have only been actively recognized to any great degree in the past decade.

In 2005, 28,000 infants younger than 1 year of age and 25,000 children and adolescents aged 1 to 19 years died in the United States. Accidents accounted for 42.4% of the deaths in children and adolescents and assault accounted for 10.9%. Most of these children died while undergoing acute care therapy and would not be appropriate for palliative or hospice care. The remaining 46.7% of children and the infants succumbed to disorders related to premature birth and low birth weight, congenital malformations, genetic syndromes, chromosomal abnormalities, and other anomalies, malignancies, heart disease, neurodegenerative disorders, and HIV infection. Many of these children are appropriate candidates for palliative or end-of-life care from the time of diagnosis.

For the more than 12,000 children diagnosed with cancer each year in the United States, 20% will die. Improvement in symptom management associated with end-of-life care in children with malignancies has not advanced at the same rate as curative and disease-modifying therapies; however, the palliative care needs of dying children and their families gained significantly greater attention in 2000 when, in the New England

Journal of Medicine, Wolfe and colleagues reported the results of interviews with the parents of children who had died of cancer at Boston Children's Hospital/Dana Farber Cancer Institute. Eighty-nine percent of the parents stated that their children "suffered a lot" in their last month of life. The children's primary symptoms were not only pain, fatigue, dyspnea, and constipation, but there were also complaints of depression, sadness, and other symptoms that could have been ameliorated by the presence of a palliative care team. As stated in a responding editorial:

> Children are not just "little adults," and caregivers skilled in the care of dying adults generally lack the expertise to deal with the unique medical and psychosocial needs of children. The overwhelming success of programs for the treatment of childhood cancer and the tremendous stakes involved in saving the life of a child make both parents and caregivers reluctant to abandon a curative approach. Thus, the continuation of the aggressive care is encouraged even if there is little or no realistic hope of a favorable outcome. The push for a cure means that less attention is often given to controlling symptoms. Commonly, aggressive treatments are not abandoned until shortly before death. Thus, there is little or no time for patients, family members or caregivers to address emotions, anticipatory grieving or to participate in decisions about care.
>
> Morgan ER, Murphy SB.
> [Editorial] *N Engl J Med* 342:347-348, 2000.

These sentiments attracted international attention to the substantial suffering at the end-of-life experienced by children with cancer and prompted the development of interdisciplinary pediatric palliative care teams across our nation and others. Through educational programs for oncologists and formalized training programs in hospice care and palliative medicine, changes are being seen. Nearly a decade later, in 2008, Wolfe published a follow-up study interviewing parents of children who died of cancer at the same institution between 1997 (the year their pediatric palliative care service was formed) and 2004. The parents reported that their children suffered less

and their care was more consistent with the principles of palliative care.

COMPARISON OF ADULT AND PEDIATRIC HOSPICE CARE

Although conceptually similar, some of the needs of children and their families under hospice or palliative care are markedly different from those of adults, and these needs can be barriers which prevent children from receiving the care they deserve. Some of the differences are shown in Table 26-1. One basic difference is that the child has not achieved a "full and complete life" and consequently the family and caregivers want to do everything possible to treat the child and thus prolong his life. Palliative care is about providing quality of life for whatever time the child has left, so interventions aimed at prolonging life can be pursued as long as their goal is to also provide comfort, but when these interventions become burdensome the plan must be modified. The family must be helped to realize at this stage that they are not "giving up," but rather "letting go."

Another major difference is that the child is in a developmental process and is not considered legally competent. This is in sharp contrast to adults who can make their own decisions regarding disease-modifying and life-prolonging therapies and may have delineated advance directives that instruct and bind their families and medical care providers to follow their wishes about health care. Advance directives written by children younger than 18 years do not currently have legal standing.

Yet another difference is attitudinal. Medical caregivers, especially those who care primarily for adults, may not be adequately trained in assessing and treating pain and symptoms occurring in children. In addition, medical caregivers who are focused on curative modalities may not

TABLE 26–1. Differences Between Hospice Care for Children and Adults

CHILDREN	ADULTS
Patient Issues	
• Not legally competent	• Mentally competent, possible advance directives
• Child in a developmental process which affects understanding of life and death, sickness and health, God, etc.	• Understanding more complete
• Has not achieved a "full and complete life"	• Often advanced in age
• Lack of verbal skills to describe needs, feelings, etc.	• Verbal skills may be good
• Child protects parents and significant others at own expense	
• Child often in a highly technical medical environment	• Frequently at home
Family Issues	
• Protection of the child from information about his or/her health	• Diagnosis known
• Desire to do everything possible to save the child	• Realistic expectations
• Potential difficulty dealing with siblings	
• Financial stress	• Financial stress
• Fear that care at home is not as good as in the hospital	• Home care frequently chosen
• Grandparents feel helpless in dealing with their children and grandchildren	
• Family needs relief from burden of care	• Respite may be necessary
Caregiver Issues	
• Desire to protect children, parents, siblings	
• Feeling a sense of failure in not saving the child	• Prognosis accepted
• Lack understanding of children's cognitive level	
• Feeling sense of "ownership" of children, even at the expense of parents	
• Out-of-date ideas about pain in children, especially infants	
• Lack of knowledge about children's disease processes	
• Influence of "unfinished business" on style of care	
Institutional/Agency Issues	
• Less reimbursement or none for children's hospice/home care	• Medicare, Medicaid, private insurance
• High staff intensity caring for children at home	
• Ongoing staff support necessary	
• Children's services have immediate appeal to public	
• Special competencies are needed in pediatric care	
• No established admission criteria	• Established admission policies
• Unusual bereavement needs for family members.	

SOURCE: Adapted, with permission, from Children's Hospice International 2000 Informational Overview.

pay adequate attention to symptom control or focus on important psychospiritual aspects of care. Parents as well are often poorly prepared for the death of their child because the focus has been only on curative approaches.

PEDIATRIC AND ADULT HOSPICE CARE IN THE UNITED STATES

Since the passage of the Medicare Hospice Benefit legislation in the United States, hospice care has been functionally defined as appropriate for people with 6 months or less to live and who are seeking palliative (comfort) care. Medicaid and most private insurance providers have adopted a similar scope for their benefits. Many children, especially those with malignancies, may continue to receive disease-modifying therapies aimed at cure or life prolongation until the very end of their lives. Consequently, they are not considered eligible for hospice care under the traditional definition. Further, because the disease-modifying treatment might be successful, it is also difficult to firmly establish a terminal prognosis. Therefore, the Institute of Medicine and others have recommended that Medicaid and private insurers restructure their hospice benefits for children and modify policies restricting benefits for other palliative services to increase patient/family access to these much needed services.

Pediatric hospices in the United States have generally developed programs that are not as restrictive as the traditionally defined hospice. Their funding is more "creative," often depending heavily on fund raising and charity, and their admission criteria are more lenient to better meet the needs of the children and their families. Pediatric hospitals have also become more sensitive to the psychosocial needs of their patients and families and have improved their attention to symptom management. Partnerships between hospice care and pediatric oncologists are developing since research has shown that when hospice care is introduced earlier, children are more likely to be described as calm and peaceful at the end of their lives.

Finally, terminally ill children served within the traditional hospice system in the United States have a different diagnosis mix when compared with their adult counterparts. Although cancer remains the dominant terminal illness in all age groups, adults served by hospice care also suffer from chronic debilitating illnesses such as dementia, end-stage cardiac disease, and degenerative diseases like amyotrophic lateral sclerosis. In contrast, children in hospice care with diagnoses other than cancer tend to have congenital malformations and chromosomal anomalies, progressive neurodegenerative diseases, neuromuscular disorders, disorders of mucopolysaccharide metabolism, and congenital cardiac conditions.

THE TEAM APPROACH

Once a child has been identified as being an appropriate candidate for palliative care, a referral should be made to either a hospital-based program or the local homecare organization. The responding team should consist of a well-trained primary physician, a care coordinator, a child psychologist, child-life specialists, pediatric-trained nurses, and a bereavement specialist, as well as a chaplain. The focus should be upon the medical and psychosocial issues of the child with the life-threatening condition and his family, as illustrated in Figure 26–1. Once the team is established, the first step to quality patient and family care involves assessment and planning. Physical concerns, such as pain and nonpain symptoms should be addressed first with both pharmacologic and nonpharmacologic treatment plans. Next, psychosocial concerns, including fears, coping mechanisms, communication, previous experiences with death, and resources for bereavement should be investigated. The family's religious beliefs should be reviewed and respected. Advanced care planning, including the identification of the decision makers and

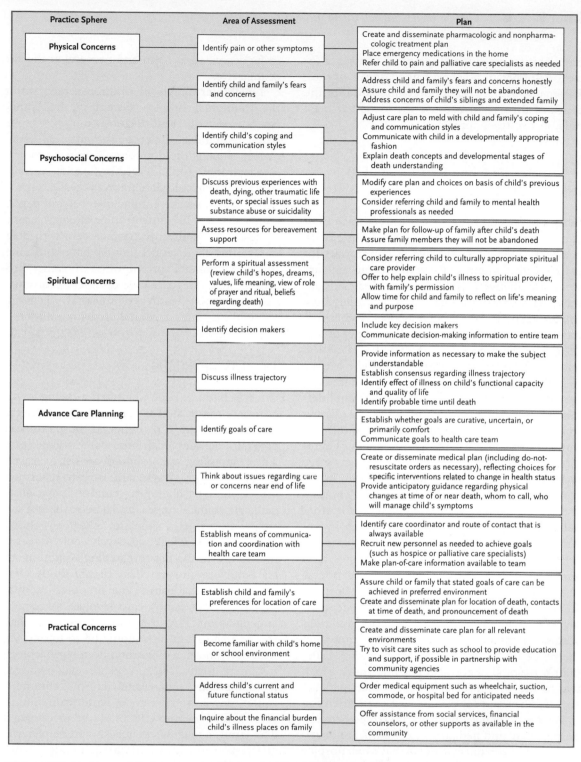

Figure 26–1. Essential elements in the approach to pediatric palliative care algorithm.

SOURCE: Reproduced, with permission, from Himelstein B: Pediatric palliative care. *NEJM* 350: 1754, 2004.

establishment of goals of care, are important. One must assess the patient's and family's knowledge of the illness, provide information and make end-of-life plans. Practical concerns also must be addressed such as location of care, home and school environment, procurement of medical equipment, and finances.

PEDIATRIC PAIN MANAGEMENT

Pain and symptom evaluation should be given first priority in the initial assessment of the child with a life-threatening condition. Pain is the most important barrier to quality care at the end of life. Historically, pain has been undertreated in children, even to the point where neonates have undergone surgery without anesthesia. This has occurred in spite of the fact that newborns have been shown to experience decreased morbidity and mortality when given appropriate pain medication. Although pain management has greatly improved in recent years, children are still frequently inadequately medicated for pain. This undermedication results from physician lack of knowledge about pharmacologic and nonpharmacologic practices as applied to children and from misconceptions and myths suggesting that young children do not perceive pain in the same way as adults.

In response to the widespread under treatment of children with pain, many medical institutions and organizations, including the World Health Organization, have made pain control and palliative care in children a priority over the past two decades. This has resulted in an increase in awareness of the problem and improvement in the treatment of pain in children. A recently published study found that based on parental report on a group of terminally ill children, pain was the most commonly treated symptom. However, of the 76% of the study children treated for pain, the treatment was successful in less than 30% of

the children. Thus, there is still a great need for improvement.

A thorough discussion of the management of pain at the end of life can be found in Chapter 6, and the reader is referred to this chapter for a detailed review of the principles of pain management of patients near the end of life. The following discussion is confined to pain management issues unique to terminally ill children.

PHYSIOLOGY OF PAIN

There are two main types of physical pain: nociceptive and neuropathic. Nociceptive pain includes somatic pain and visceral pain. Somatic pain is a direct result of peripheral tissue damage in bones, joints, muscle, skin, or connective tissue. It is usually described as aching or throbbing and is well-localized. This type of pain responds to both opioids and, especially in the case of bone pain, to nonsteroidal anti-inflammatory agents (NSAIDs). Visceral pain arises from organs such as the stomach, gall bladder, and pancreas. The two main mechanisms of visceral pain arise from either tumor invasion of the organ capsule that results in aching and fairly well-localized pain, or obstruction of a hollow viscus, which results in cramping and poorly localized pain. Both types of nociceptive pain usually respond to nonopioids and opioids.

Neuropathic pain is caused by stimulation of either the peripheral or the central nervous system. It is generally described as burning or stabbing in nature. Neuropathic pain generally responds to adjuvant analgesics such as anticonvulsants or tricyclic antidepressants, with or without the addition of opioids.

Nociceptive systems in children have been described as "plastic," in that they can perceive pain from a given amount of tissue damage in various ways. The amount of pain perceived by the child can be influenced by emotional factors such as anxiety and fear, behavioral factors such as social activities and physical restraint, and cognitive factors such as expectations and understanding.

Consequently, to adequately control children's pain requires not only the pharmacologic administration of appropriate analgesics, but also non-pharmacologic techniques.

MISCONCEPTIONS AND FEARS REGARDING PAIN CONTROL IN CHILDREN

Multiple barriers to adequate pain management exist in children as well as adults. Some of these barriers are similar, including but not limited to the fear of addiction, the fear that the need for analgesia means the illness is progressing, and the fear of respiratory depression due to opioid toxicity. There are also several myths about pain and pain management that are unique to children. These are listed in Table 26–2 and are discussed below.

Infants Do not Feel Pain

Historically it was believed that young infants do not feel pain. It has been shown, however, that the central nervous system of a 26-week old fetus has the structural and neurochemical ability to experience pain. Newborns, even those born prematurely, and children show elevated stress responses as measured by biochemical parameters, as well as increased morbidity and mortality when receiving inadequate analgesia perioperatively as compared with those who receive proper

---

TABLE 26–2. Myths that Create Barriers to Effective Pain Management Specific to Children

Infants do not feel pain
Children tolerate pain better than adults
Children are unable to communicate appropriately about their pain
Children will tell caregivers when they are having pain

---

pain control. Neonates may experience increased sensitivity to pain because their inhibitory pain tracts are underdeveloped.

Children Tolerate Pain Better Than Adults

There is a serious misconception that children have a higher tolerance to pain than adults. In fact, children's ability to tolerate pain increases with age. Older children experience less pain with procedures than younger children. Children do not become accustomed to pain or painful procedures. Rather, they often experience increased anxiety and perception of pain with repeated procedures. The child's first experience with a procedure will determine how he handles future procedures, making adequate pain control essential.

Children Are Unable to Communicate Appropriately about Their Pain

Children are, in fact, able to communicate where and how much they hurt. Children as young as 3 years have been taught to use appropriate pain scales (Fig. 26–2, Table 26–5, see discussion below) such as a "faces" pain scale, and can localize pain by pointing to an area of their body. What is true is that special assessment skills are necessary to properly evaluate children's pain. These must be tailored to the child's developmental stage, remembering that the child may have regressed due to illness or matured beyond his years.

Children Will Tell Caregivers When They Are Having Pain

Although children can usually share information about their pain, they may not always do so. Younger children may have inadequate communication skills and older children may not report pain because they may fear the treatment, for example, injections. Others may have adjusted to chronic pain. The level of activity of a child may or may not reflect the pain level. A child may elect to watch television or sleep rather than play

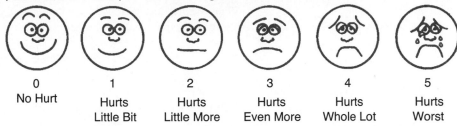

MY PAIN RATING SCALE*

Please keep a record of how well your child's pain medicines are working. Rate your child's pain before and after pain medicine is given.

| 0 | 1 | 2 | 3 | 4 | 5 |
| No Hurt | Hurts Little Bit | Hurts Little More | Hurts Even More | Hurts Whole Lot | Hurts Worst |

Explain to your child that each face is for a person who has no hurt (pain) or some or a lot of hurt (pain). Point to each face and say the words under the face. Ask the child to pick the face that best describes how much hurt he (or she) has. Record the number of that face in the Pain Rating column. If your child's pain is above 2, or if you have other concerns with pain, let your nurse or physician know.

Date and time	Pain rating	Medicine I took	Side effects, such as drowsiness or upset stomach

Figure 26–2. Wong-Baker FACES Pain Rating Scale.

SOURCE: Reproduced, with permission, from Hockenbury MJ, Wilson D: *Wong's Essentials of Pediatric Nursing*, 8th ed. St. Louis, MO, Mosby, 2009.

outside, and may use distracting activity such as playing with puzzles to cope with pain.

PAIN ASSESSMENT

The evaluation of pain in a child who may be non-communicative by virtue of his age or behavior is difficult and a number of different approaches or pain assessment tools must be employed. Pain in children can be consistently and objectively assessed by the use of pediatric assessment tools and pain-rating scales. The assessment should include not only physical factors, but also social and emotional factors as well. One useful acronym is the QUEST approach to pediatric pain assessment (Table 26–3). It promotes the use of mul-

tiple sources for a systematic and complete pain assessment.

The healthcare team should empower parents and family members by requesting and trusting

TABLE 26–3. QUEST: Assessment of Pain in the Pediatric Patient

Question the child
Use pain-rating scales
Evaluate behavior and physiologic changes
Secure parents' involvement
Take action and evaluate the results

SOURCE: Reproduced, with permission, from Baker CM, Wong DL: QUEST: a process of pain assessment in children, *Orthop Nurse* 6(1):11-21, 1987.

TABLE 26–4. Pain Experience History	
CHILD FORM	**PARENT FORM**
Tell me what pain is	What word(s) does your child use in regard to pain?
Tell me about the hurt you have had before.	Describe the pain experiences your child has had before.
Do you tell others when you hurt? If yes, who?	Does your child tell you or others when he or she is hurting?
What do you do for yourself when you are hurting?	How do you know when your child is in pain?
What do you want others to do for you when you hurt?	How does your child usually react to pain?
What don't you want others to do for you when you hurt?	What do you do for your child when he or she is hurting?
What helps the most to take your hurt away?	What does your child do for himself or herself when he or she is hurting?
Is there anything special that you want me to know about you when you hurt? (If yes, have the child describe).	What works best to decrease or take away your child's pain?
	Is there anything special that you would like me to know about your child and pain? (If yes, describe.)

SOURCE: BA Joyce, JG Schade, JF Keck, et al: From reliability and validity of preverbal pain assessment tools. *Issues Comp Pediatr Nurse* 17(3), 121-135, 1994. Copyright 1994 Hemisphire Pub. Corp., Adapted with permission.

their input regarding pain levels and effective treatments. A complete pain assessment includes a report based on the patient's and the parents' description of the pain. The most valuable information is received from the children themselves, but the parents' input should also be sought because they know their child best (Table 26–4). Specific words used by the child to describe pain should be used (e.g., hurt, "owie," and "boo-boo,") to establish proper lines of communication. As with adults, physical examination, behavioral observations, and physiologic measures are the other components of a pain assessment.

Multiple behavioral pain assessment scales for young children have been developed (Fig. 26–2 and Table 26–5). To obtain reliability and validity in assessing pain, the same observer should reevaluate the child whenever possible. Therefore, especially in patients being cared for at home, parents should be trained in the use of the chosen scale so they can report to hospice nurses or other clinical personnel in a common language.

The pain assessment scale that is being used for a child should be clearly recorded in the chart. It should be used, and the results recorded, on routine visits, during exacerbation of pain, and within an hour following new interventions. It is important for the child to become familiar with the scale as early in the disease process as possible for best results. The Faces scale has been successfully used by children as young as 3 years. Another useful method for determining pain is with the use of five red poker chips. The chips are placed on a table in front of the child who is instructed to take away chips to the level pain he is experiencing. In addition to the type of scales use, goals for pain control should be delineated and discussed with the family and with the patient when appropriate.

TABLE 26–5. Behavioral Pain Assessment Scales for Young Children

FLACC SCALE SCORING

CATEGORIES	0	1	2
Face	No particular expression or smile	Occasional grimace or frown, withdrawn, disinterested	Frequent to constant quivering chin, clenched jaw
Legs	Normal position or relaxed	Uneasy, restless, tense	Kicking or legs drawn up
Activity	Lying quietly, normal position, moves easily	Squirming, shifting back and forth, tense	Arched, rigid, or jerking
Cry	No cry (awake or asleep)	Moans or whimpers; occasional complaint	Crying steadily, screams or sobs, frequent complaints
Consolability	Content, relaxed	Reassured by occasional touching, hugging, or being talked to, distractible	Difficult to console or comfort

RILEY INFANT PAIN SCALE ASSESSMENT TOOL

	0	1	2	3
Facial	Neutral/smiling	Frowning grimacing	Clenched teeth	Full cry expression
Body movement	Calm, relaxed	Restless/fidgeting	Moderate agitation or moderate mobility	Thrashing, flailing, incessant agitation, or strong voluntary immobility
Sleep	Sleeping quietly with easy respiration	Restless while asleep	Sleeps intermittently (sleep/awake)	Sleeping for prolonged periods of time interrupted by jerky movements or unable to sleep
Verbal/voice	No cry	Whimpering, complaining	Pain crying	Screaming, high-pitched cry
Consolability	Neutral	Easy to console	Not easy to console	Inconsolable
Response to movement/ touch	Moves easily	Winces when touched/moved	Cries out when moved/touched	High-pitched cry or scream when touched or moved

Each of the five categories (F)face; (L) Legs; (A) Activity; (C) Cry; (C) Consolability is scored from 0–2, which results in a total score between 0 and 10.

SOURCE: Merkeland S, et al: The FLACC: a behavioral scale for scoring postoperative pain in young children. *Pediatr Nurse* 23(3), 293-297, 1957. Copyright 1997 by Jannetti Co. University of Michigan Medical Center. Reprinted with permission.

Slade JG, Joyce BA, Gerkensmeyer J, and Keck JF: Comparison of three preverbal scales for post operative pain assessment in a diverse pediatric sample. *J Pain Symptom Manage* 12(6), 348-359, 1996. Copyright 1996 Elsevier Science Inc. Reprinted with permission.

NONPHARMACOLOGIC PAIN INTERVENTIONS

Nonpharmacologic interventions are frequently effective in the pediatric population for improving pain control. They have been categorized primarily as physical, behavioral, or cognitive. Physical interventions include thermal stimulation, massage, and touch in general. Examples of behavioral interventions include relaxation therapy and behavioral modification. Cognitive interventions include distraction, such as looking at books or blowing bubbles, and guided imagery. When a child's attention is completely absorbed by one of these techniques, the neuronal responses caused by tissue damage are actually reduced, the child is not simply ignoring his or her pain.

PHARMACOLOGIC MANAGEMENT OF PAIN IN CHILDREN

Use of appropriate analgesic medications will relieve pain in most children. As in adults, and as expressed by the World Health Organization

(WHO), the four main concepts behind adequate pain control are the following:

By the ladder
By the clock
By the appropriate route
By the child

By the Ladder

The basis of pharmacologic pain management in children, as in adults, is the WHO's analgesic ladder (Fig. 26–3). It presents a three-step approach to pain management on the basis of mild, moderate, or severe pain with appropriate analgesic choices for each step. The first step for controlling mild pain is a nonopioid analgesic. Acetaminophen or an NSAID agent is the drug of choice if the child can take oral medication. If the pain is not controlled with these alone, a mild opioid, usually codeine, is added and the acetaminophen or NSAID is continued. If the pain persists, then a strong opioid, preferably morphine, should be added. At this point,

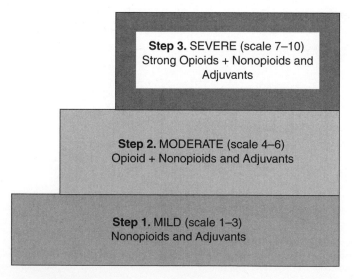

Figure 26–3. The World Health Organization (WHO) analgesic ladder.

SOURCE: WHO's pain ladder. World Health Organization. http://www.who.int/cancer/palliative/painladder/en/. Accessed March 16, 2010.

TABLE 26–6. Starting Oral Doses for Nonopioid Drugs

MEDICATION	ADMINISTRATION	COMMENTS
Acetaminophen	10–15 mg/kg/dose PO/PR q 4–6 h Max dose 4,000 mg/24 h	Administer q 6–8 h in neonates Does not inhibit platelet function Not anti-inflammatory
Ibuprofen	10 mg/kg/dose PO q 6–8 h Max dose 40 mg/kg/24 h	Anti-inflammatory May cause platelet dysfunction and bleeding gastrointestinal and renal toxicity

the acetaminophen or NSAID should be continued but the weak opioid discontinued. Tables 26–6 and 26–7 show commonly used nonopioid and opioid drugs and the recommended doses in pediatric patients.

By the Clock

Medication should be administered "by the clock" on a regular schedule to prevent pain rather than on an as-needed basis to treat recurrent pain. This relieves the caregiver of continually having to assess the child for routine pain medication and leads to better pain control. Additional "rescue" doses of a short-acting medication should be available for intermittent or breakthrough pain.

By the Appropriate Route

Medications should be taken "by the appropriate route," that is, the route that is the simplest, most effective, and least painful for the child. If the child can tolerate oral medications, either liquids or pills, this is the preferred route. At times, subcutaneous (SC) or the intravenous (IV) route may be necessary for rapid pain control or titration or if the child is unable to tolerate oral medications. Both of these methods are compatible with patient-controlled analgesia pumps, which can be controlled by either the child or the primary caregiver if the child is too young or otherwise not able to self-medicate. The SC route is especially useful in the home setting as it avoids the need for an IV line.

Intramuscular injections are to be avoided since they are painful and drug absorption is irregular. The rectal route is generally disliked by children and also results in inconsistent absorption. However, if there is transient vomiting or if the child is comatose, it may be necessary to use the rectal route.

By the Child

All medications should be adjusted "by the child" based on what the needs are at any given time. There is no single dose that should be appropriate for all children. Strong opioids do not have a ceiling dose and must be titrated to the patient's comfort. Although most of the common opioid side effects such as fatigue or pruritus resolve within a few days of initiation, if unacceptable side effects develop such as persistent severe myoclonus or uncontrollable vomiting, an alternative opioid should be selected.

Pediatric Use of Specific Opioids

MORPHINE Morphine is the recommended strong opioid of choice for controlling severe pain in children. It is the "gold standard" to which other opioids are compared. The recommended starting dose is 0.2–0.4 mg/kg orally, every 4 hours, and it can be titrated until the pain is relieved.

TABLE 26–7. Starting Doses for Opioid Drugs

MEDICATION	ORAL ADMINISTRATION	COMMENTS	IV ADMINISTRATION
Codeine	0.5–1.0 mg/kg/dose PO q 4–6 h Max dose 60 mg/dose	Tablets: 30 mg Liquid: 3 mg/mL	
Acetaminophen and Codeine	0.5–1.0 mg codeine/kg/dose PO q 4–6 h	Tablets: #3: acetaminophen 300 mg and codeine 30 mg Tablets: #4: acetaminophen 300 mg and codeine 60 mg Elixir: acetaminophen 120 mg/5 mL and codeine 12 mg/5 mL (tsp)	
Oxycodone	0.05–0.2 mg/kg/dose PO/SL q 4 h Sustained release: 10 mg PO q 12 h	Tablets: 5, 15, 30 mg Immediate release Solution: 1 mg/mL, 20 mg/mL Sustained-release tablets (Oxycontin): 10, 20, 40, 80, 160 mg	
Morphine	Infants and children: Immediate release (IR): 0.15–0.3 mg/kg/dose PO/SL q 3–4 h Sustained release (SR): 0.3–0.6 mg/kg/dose PO q 12 h	Tablets (IR): 15 mg Tablets (SR): 15, 30, 60, 100 mg Solution: 10 mg/5 mL, 20 mg/mL	Neonates: 0.05–0.1 mg/ kg/dose IV/SQ q 3–4 h Infants and children: 0.05–0.1 mg/kg/dose q 3–4 h
Fentanyl	Transdermal patch (>12 yr): 25 μg/h q 72 h Lozenge (>2 yr and 15–40 kg): 5–15 μg/kg (max 400 μg) >40 kg: 5 μ/kg (max 400 μg)	Patches: 12.5, 25, 50, 75, 100 μg/h	1 μg/kg/dose
Hydromorphone	0.03–0.06 mg/kg/dose q 3–4 h PO/SL Adults: 1–4 mg q 3–4 h PO/SL	Tablets: 2, 4, 8 mg	0.003 mg/kg/dose q 3–4 h IV/SQ
Methadone	0.1 mg/kg/dose q 4 h for first 2–3 doses then q 6–12 h Max dose: 10 mg/dose	Tablets: 5, 10 mg Solution: 1 mg/mL Concentrate: 10 mg/mL	0.1 mg/kg q 4 h to 12 h Max dose 10 mg

In infants younger than 6 months, the pharmacokinetics of morphine are different. The starting dose of morphine in infants should be between one-quarter and one-third of the initial dose for older children, based on mg/kg. Morphine should be administered to infants where observation and interventions are available in the case of respiratory depression. If oral administration is not possible, SC or IV infusion starting at 0.03 mg/kg/h should be initiated, or, if the child has been on oral morphine an appropriate conversion should be made.

HYDROMORPHONE   Hydromorphone is similar to morphine in its pharmacokinetics and effectiveness. It may produce less sedation, nausea, and pruritus than morphine. At the time of this writing there is no long-acting oral form of hydromorphone. Hydromorphone can be useful if morphine causes intolerable side effects. The starting dose of hydromorphone is 0.03 to 0.08 mg/kg/dose every 4 to 6 hours as necessary. Hydromorphone should be used with caution in infants and young children, and should not be used in neonates due to potential central nervous system (CNS) effects.

OXYCODONE   Oxycodone is considered a strong opioid and is available in immediate- and sustained-release forms in addition to combination products with acetaminophen. At this time there are no parenteral preparations available. The initial dose is 0.05 to 0.15 mg/kg/dose every 4 to 6 hours. Oxycodone can be titrated in the same way as morphine and does not have a ceiling dose.

METHADONE   Methadone is recommended for children who are unable to tolerate morphine or hydromorphone due to side effects of nausea or sedation. It is a synthetic long-acting opioid analgesic with a prolonged and unpredictable half-life (averaging 19 hours in children and 35 hours in adults, but ranging from 6 to 200 hours) that requires careful dosage adjustments. The duration

of analgesia is shorter than the half-life that requires the dosing to be more frequent initially. Due to its long half-life, methadone accumulates slowly and may lead to symptoms of overdosage over several days even in a child that appears to be doing well initially. Methadone may cause respiratory depression, sedation, increased intracranial pressure, hypotension, and bradycardia. The respiratoy effects last longer than the analgesia and lower dosages should by used in children with renal or hepatic impairment. Oral duration of action is 6 to 8 hours initially and 24–48 hours after repeated doses. Not until after 48 hours or more of methadone administration should a routine schedule can be initiated. Methadone is particularly useful in the management of neuropathic pain.

FENTANYL   Fentanyl is available in a patch form for transdermal absorption and in the form of oral lozenges for short-acting, immediate-release medication. The patches are recommended only in children older than 12 years, or greater than 50 kg, and the safety and efficacy are still being established in pediatrics. They are not recommended for acute pain because 12 to 16 hours are required from application of the patch to achieve steady blood levels. Due to delay in onset, difficulty in titration for changing pain, and absorption issues, transdermal fentanyl patches are not routinely recommended in pediatric patients. They may be useful in older patients with stable chronic pain where analgesic requirements have already been determined.

The doses for fentanyl lozenges for children older than 2 years are listed in Table 26–7. They are not recommended in children younger than 2 years or who weigh less than 15 kg.

Neonatal Dosing Considerations

Special dosing consideration should be given to neonates and infants due to differences in their pharmacokinetics and pharmacodynamics. Only acetaminophen can be administered at the regular recommended dose (10–15 mg/kg) for short periods of time without danger of hepatotoxicity. Because the rate of absorption is slower and the half-life of acetaminophen is prolonged in infants, the dosage schedule should be every 6 hours rather than every 4 hours.

In spite of these differences, opioids should be used for severe pain in neonates. The starting doses in infants younger than 6 months should be one-quarter to one-third of the suggested doses. Generally, the pharmacokinetics of opioids in infants older than 6 months and children are similar to those in adults; however, neonates show reduced clearance of most opioids. This increased sensitivity to morphine and other opioids is probably the result of a combination of factors including immature liver function, decreased clearance by the kidney, smaller volume of distribution, and possibly increased permeability into the brain. These factors in combination with the newborn's immature responses to hypoxia and hypercarbia may result in respiratory depression at relatively low doses of morphine. This depression can be reversed with naloxone. The recommended dose of naloxone is 1 to 2 μg/kg given at frequent intervals (every 2–3 minutes) to reverse hypoventilartion without reversing analgesia. Monitoring of infants for respiratory depression should continue for at least 24 hours after morphine is discontinued.

Opioid Side Effects

Although all opioids have similar side effects in both adults and children, recommended medications for their management are slightly different for children than those frequently used for adults. Some of the side effects such as nausea and sedation may improve over the first few days, whereas others will need to be treated. Assessment of possible side effects should be performed with both the parent and the child because children may not spontaneously volunteer information. As most common opioid side effects may also occur as stand-alone symptoms, the treatments of these side effects are discussed in the section on Symptom Management.

Adjuvant Medications

Adjuvant medications are drugs that are often necessary to treat specific types of pain, either alone or in combination with opioid analgesics (see Chapter 6 for a full discussion). The most common reason for the use of adjuvant analgesics is the treatment of neuropathic pain. Direct involvement of the nerves by tumor invasion or as a side effect of chemotherapy may result in neuropathic pain. This type of pain is frequently described as shooting, burning, or stabbing. It often responds well to tricyclic antidepressants and anticonvulsants, but high doses of strong opioids may be necessary when it does not. Tricyclic antidepressants are classically used for burning type of pain; however, many clinicians use them as first-line medications for all neuropathic pain.

Amitriptyline and nortriptyline are the most commonly used medications. Amitriptyline should be started at 0.1 to 0.2 mg/kg at bedtime. The primary side effect is sedation, thus the preferred bedtime dosing. Dry mouth, blurred vision, constipation, and urinary retention may also occur. An EKG should be performed before initiation of therapy as arrhythmias have been reported. The dose may be increased by 50% every 2 to 3 days up to 0.5 to 2.0 mg/kg at bedtime although many patients will not tolerate the larger doses. The analgesic effect is usually seen in 3 to 5 days.

Anticonvulsants are useful for the treatment of neuropathic pain that is described as shooting or stabbing. Gabapentin is increasingly being used for neuropathic pain; the dose of gabapentin is 5 mg/kg PO at bedtime. It may be increased to twice daily on day 2 and three times per day on day 3. The maximum dose is 10 to 20 mg/kg three times per day or 1,800 mg/day, although some patients require as much as 3,600 mg/day. Side effects include nystagmus, thought disorder, and hallucinations, along with headaches, weight gain, and myalgias. When stopping treatment, patients should be weaned off gradually, rather than discontinuing the agent abruptly. Adjuvant analgesic drugs and the dosages recommended for children are listed in Table 26–8.

TABLE 26–8. Adjuvant Drugs for Pain and Other Symptoms

DRUG CATEGORY	DRUG DOSE	INDICATIONS	COMMENTS
Antidepressants	Amitriptyline—start at 0.2 mg/kg and escalate by 25% q 2–3 d to max 1–2 mg/kg if needed	Neuropathic pain insomnia	Beneficial effects seen within 3–5 d Anticholinergic side effects, dysrhythmias (pre-rx EKG)
Anticonvulsants	Gabapentin—start at 2–5 mg/kg/dose qhs and increase to bid then tid to max 20 mg/kg tid slowly	Neuropathic pain	
Neuroleptics	Haloperidol—0.01 mg/kg/dose PO q 8 h or 0.02 mg/kg/dose q 8 h IV/SC	Anxiety	Can cause dystonic reactions—treat with diphenhydramine 1 mg/kg or use concurrently
Sedatives, hypnotics, anxiolytics	Lorazepam—0.02–0.05 mg/kg/ dose PO/SL/PR/IV q 4–6 h Diazepam—0.05–0.1 mg/kg PO/PR/IV q 4–6 h	Anxiety Muscle spasm	
Antihistamines	Diphenhydramine—1 mg/kg/ dose PO/IV q 4–6 h PRN Hydroxyzine—0.05–1 mg/kg/ dose PO q 4–6 h	Opioid-induced pruritus/nausea Anxiety Insomnia	
Psychostimulants	Methylphenidate—start at 0.1–0.2 mg/kg bid and escalate to 0.3–0.5 as tolerated, give q AM and noon	Opiod-induced sedation	Can exacerbate dysphoria or agitation
Corticosteroids	Dexamethasone-dose depends on clinical situation—usually 6–12 mg/m²/d	Increased intracranial pressure Spinal cord compression Bone metastasis Bowel obstruction	Side effects: edema, gastrointestinal upset and bleeding, increased appetite, mood swings Try to use lowest effective dose

SYMPTOM MANAGEMENT

CONSTIPATION

Constipation (see Chapter 8 for a full discussion) is an expected side effect of opioid analgesic use. Opioids cause constipation by reducing bowel motility and secretions. Unlike other opioid side effects, constipation does not improve with time. Neurologic conditions, spinal cord compression by tumor, and abdominal tumors may also cause constipation. In addition, children at the end of life often do not drink or eat well and are immobile, thus exacerbating their constipation. Although increased fiber, fluid, and bulk in

TABLE 26–9. Treatment of Constipation in Children

MEDICATION	AGE	DOSE
Docusate Sodium	<3 yr	10–40 mg/24 h
	3–6 yr	20–60 mg/24 h
	6–12 yr	50–500 mg/24 h
Senna	All ages	10–20 mg/kg/dose
Lactulose	1 month to 1 yr	55–109 mg qhs (max 218 mg/24 h)
	1–5 yr	109–218 mg qhs (max 436 mg/24 h)
	5–15 yr	218–436 mg qhs (max 872 mg/24 h)
	or	or
	<2 yr	2.5–7.5 mL bid
	>10 yr	2.5 mL bid
	2–10 yr	15–30 mL bid

Consider combination of docusate and senna or lactulose and senna.

the diet may help treat constipation, medications are often necessary. Medications used to treat constipation in children include osmotic agents (lactulose or magnesium sulfate), stool softeners (docusate), and stimulants (senna or bisacodyl). Osmotic agents such as Lactulose come in liquid form, are well tolerated and do not cause cramping. When using a stool softener such as docusate sodium, it should be administered in combination with a stimulant such as senna. The stimulants may cause cramping; however, they are usually well tolerated when started prophylactically on a once daily basis at the same time that the child is started on opioids. Recommended dosages based on age are presented in Table 26–9.

NAUSEA AND EMESIS

The etiology of the nausea or emesis (See Chapter 8 for full discussion) should first be determined to permit institution of effective therapy. The vomiting reflex may be in response to irritation of the chemoreceptor trigger zone (CTZ) in the area postrema in the brainstem by toxins or drugs, irritation of the cortex by increased intracranial pressure or emotional stimuli, or the gastrointestinal tract by mechanical obstruction, toxins, or drugs. Opioid analgesics and other medications frequently induce nausea and emesis by irritating the CTZ as well as by decreasing gastrointestinal motility. Opioid-induced nausea is usually not very severe and will improve after 3–4 days on a stable dose. In refractory cases, changing or rotating the offending agent is generally preferred, but if the suspect medication is medically indicated and necessary, antiemetics will be required. Metoclopramide, an agent that regulates gastrointestinal motility in low doses, may be beneficial.

Phenothiazines are among the most commonly used agents for nausea in adults, and they work by depressing emetogenic activity at the CTZ. However, phenothiazines may cause extrapyramidal symptoms (EPS), which can be particularly troublesome complications in children. Therefore, despite the overall wide usage of phenothiazines, some pediatric experts recommend that these agents should only be used after other antiemetic agents have proven unsuccessful in controlling a child's symptoms. Prochlorperazine, promethazine, or chlorpromazine are the most commonly used phenothiazines, although the first two medications are contraindicated in children younger than 2 years.

Other medications used to treat nausea and emesis include metaclopramide, antihistamines, and agents that reduce gastric acid secretion. Metaclopramide works both centrally by inhibiting the CTZ and peripherally by accelerating gastric emptying. It too can cause EPS, which can be prevented or reversed by the use of the antihistamine diphenhydramine. Antihistamines also work on the CTZ, possibly by blocking labyrinthine impulses. Vomiting due to gastritis should be treated by a combination of antacids and a histamine (H2) blocker or an acid-pump inhibitor.

Vomiting may be due to intermittent or partial bowel obstruction. Surgery to bypass the obstruction or a gastrostomy may be considered, but these procedures may not be appropriate in some situations. The obstruction may be relieved by the use of steroids. Anticholinergic agents such as glycopyrrolate reduce secretions and contractility. Octreotide may also decrease gastrointestinal secretions, thus decreasing nausea and vomiting. Some children may need a nasogastric tube placed for decompression. If vomiting is refractory, two or more classes of medications may be combined to increase effectiveness. Although benzodiazepines such as lorazepam do not have specific antiemetic effects, they are frequently given in combination with the above-mentioned medications.

Projectile emesis, usually accompanied by little or no nausea, is often associated with increased intracranial pressure from primary or secondary malignant lesions in the CNS. Projectile emesis may be effectively treated with high doses of steroids, such as dexamethasone.

Nausea and vomiting from certain chemotherapeutic agents may respond well to ondansetron or granisetron. Although these agents are most effective for this application, they are also effective in treating opioid-induced nausea and vomiting. For refractory cases, benzodiazepines, such as lorazepam, and antipsychotics, such as haloperidol, can be tried. A list of antiemetics, and their dosage schedules in pediatric patients, are presented in Table 26–10.

Nonpharmacologic interventions that may help with nausea and vomiting include changing the child's diet to include foods such as clear liquids (ginger ale and other sodas, apple juice, and Jello). Popsicles, sherbet, ice chips, yogurt, and other cold foods may also appeal to children. Room temperature foods are frequently better tolerated than hot foods. Generally, foods that are greasy, spicy hot, or characterized by a strong odor should be avoided. Multiple small meals or snacks are better tolerated than larger servings. Distraction with television or games may also help.

DYSPNEA AND RESPIRATORY DEPRESSION

Shortness of breath may be seen in the child with pulmonary metastases, ascites, heart or lung disease, or pneumonia. Oxygen may provide symptomatic relief along with bronchodilators and inhaled or oral steroids. Systemic opioids such as morphine cause a decrease in the respiratory drive and a subsequent decrease in the feeling of shortness of breath. Benzodiazepines such as lorazepam, or in severe cases, haloperidol, may help with associated anxiety.

Respiratory depression (see Chapter 7 for full discussion) from opioid therapy is very rare. Pain stimulates the respiratory drive. A reduction in opioid dose can be considered with titration to maintain pain relief without respiratory depression. In the rare instance of respiratory arrest, naloxone can be given in small frequent doses of 1 to 2 μg/kg every 2 to 3 minutes to avoid acute severe, painful withdrawal symptoms.

EXCESS SECRETIONS

Excess oral secretions are frequently apparent in the dying child who can no longer swallow. The noisy sounds made as the child breathes can be extremely upsetting to family members. These

TABLE 26–10. Medications to Treat Nausea and Vomiting

MEDICATION	DOSE	COMMENTS
Promethazine	0.25–1 mg/kg/dose PO q 4–6 h	Only for ages >2 yr May cause EPS, reverse with diphenhydramine
Chlorpromazine	0.5–1 mg/kg/dose PO q 6 h 1 mg/kg/dose PR q 6 h	Only for age >6 months Side effects: similar to above
Prochlorperazine	0.1 mg/kg/dose PO/PR/IM q 6 h	Only for age >2 yr or >10 kg Side effects: similar to above
Dexamethesone	10 mg/m^2 PO/IV	
Diphenhydramine	1.0 mg/kg/dose PO/IV q 6 h	
Hydroxyzine	0.5 mg/kg/dose PO/IM q 6 h	
Lorazepam	0.025 mg/kg/dose PO/IV q 6 h	
Metoclopramide	0.5–1.0 mg/kg/dose PO/IV q 6 h GI motility dose: 0.1 mg/kg/dose PO q 6 h	Use with diphenhydramine to prevent dystonic reactions
Ondansetron	0.15 mg/kg/dose PO/IV q 6 h or 0.45 mg/kg daily	
Granisetron	10 mcg/kg/IV 30 minutes prior to chemotherapy or radiation therapy	Max dose 2 mg Only for age >2 yr

are caused by a thin layer of secretions over the glottis. The child is usually not in distress. Excess secretions are best treated by anticholinergics such as sublingual hyoscyamine or oral glycopyrrolate. Atropine is effective, but the side effects are often intolerable. Scopolamine patches placed behind the ear can be used for children over 15 kg.

AGITATION

Hypoxia frequently causes agitation and restlessness in addition to apparent shortness of breath. Opioids and oxygen are the treatments of choice. Morphine may be used at the rate of 0.3 mg/kg/dose by mouth every 3 to 4 hours and titrated as necessary. Benzodiazepines such lorazepam given 0.05 to 0.1 mg/kg/dose every 4–6 hours orally as needed may also be useful. Haloperidol 0.025 to 0.05 mg/kg per 24 hours divided two to three times daily by mouth as an initial dosing regimen may also be useful for controlling agitation and hallucinations. It may also be useful in controlling nightmares that frequently occur in the preterminal child.

SEIZURES

Because the occurrence of a seizure (see Chapter 9 for full discussion) may be extremely distressing to the family and caregivers, the possibility of a seizure occurring and the appropriate management should be discussed in advance. It should be emphasized that seizures are usually self-limiting, and appropriate first-aid measures should be reviewed. Maintenance anticonvulsant therapy should be continued as long as possible. If seizures, especially status epilepticus, are anticipated appropriate medications and dosages should be available in the home. Phenobarbital suppositories are helpful for anticonvulsant therapy after the child can no longer swallow. Diazepam rectal gel is also useful for the management of acute seizures and status epilepticus.

SLEEP DISTURBANCES

Sleep disturbances are common in pediatric patients who are near death. Often, such children will sleep on and off during the day and be awake at night. This sleep pattern creates difficulty for caregivers, who generally need to sleep at night. If a child's insomnia has an identifiable cause, such as pain, depression, anxiety, or medication side effect, appropriate treatment should be initiated. If the insomnia is related to depression, amitriptyline 0.5 to 2 mg/kg at bedtime or nortriptyline 1 to 3 mg/kg may be helpful. If chronic opioid administration results in excessive sleepiness that is not due to disease progression and lowering opioid doses is not possible, then a psychostimulant like methylphenidate may be helpful. The initial dose is 0.1 mg/kg/dose every 4 hours as needed or twice daily at 8 AM and noon. Nonpharmacologic interventions such as guided imagery, distraction, and relaxation techniques may also be helpful.

ANXIETY

Anxiety is a common occurrence in terminally ill children. In younger children it may be difficult to differentiate pain from anxiety or fear. Nonpharmacologic measures such as emotional and spiritual support and strong family relationships, in addition to support from the hospice team, may help to allay a child's anxiety. If pharmacologic interventions are necessary, the benzodiazepines are the preferred agents. If these medications are not successful, the phenothiazines may be useful.

END-OF-LIFE CARE FOR CHILDREN AT HOME

End-of-life care for children in the United States, whether provided by a hospice or a nonhospice palliative care program, is generally provided in the child's home. There are many issues to consider when choosing to have end-of-life care provided in the home. First, although children overwhelmingly prefer to be cared for at home, the family needs to make the commitment to having the child at home, coping with the associated stress, and sharing tasks.

Parents are actually able to provide more attention and support to the siblings when the child is cared for at home. When the terminally ill child is cared for in the hospital, the parents are with the ill child to the detriment of the siblings who may know little of their sibling's status.

With the child at home, his brothers and sisters can assist in his care and entertainment to the best of their abilities. This can lead to enhanced communication between the family and the child. It increases the feeling of control for the parents and decreases the isolation of the dying child. Studies have shown that, with this "normalization" of family life, children are more peaceful in death, and that bereavement is less complicated for the surviving parents and siblings.

STAFFING ISSUES

Due to the complex issues associated with terminally ill children, the entire end-of-life care team must be actively involved in the care plan. The team should consist of, at minimum, a physician, a nurse, a social worker, and a chaplain, who all have experience in caring for terminally ill children. Although home health aid services may be offered, the parent or primary caregiver frequently prefers to provide the child's personal care.

If possible, the physician who cared for the child in the acute care setting should continue to care for the child during hospice care. Although this may be difficult at times, especially if the primary care physician or pediatrician is unfamiliar with the principles of hospice and palliative care, studies have shown that maintaining the relationship between the child, the family, and the primary physician aids in a smooth transition to appropriate end-of-life care. In the event that the primary physician or pediatrician is unfamiliar with pain and symptom management principles in terminally ill children, the hospice or palliative care medical director should provide consultative support to assure that the child and his family receives the most effective pain and symptom management possible.

The child and his family will frequently form a relationship with one particular member of the hospice team—often a nurse. If this individual is not available to make a home visit, usually a telephone call from that individual will often be more effective than a home visit from a substitute nurse. Such a "broken" relationship may have lasting negative effects on the acceptance of care and the quality of life of the dying child.

FAMILY COMMUNICATION REGARDING THE TERMINALLY ILL CHILD

One of the most sensitive issues in pediatric end-of-life care relates to how family members communicate with the dying child about his or her condition. Children, even young ones, generally are aware of the fact they are dying. However, because parents frequently want to protect their children from information about their health, and children want to protect their parents from worry that they may die, the result is a lack of meaningful communication about the eventual death. When this occurs, a dying child may become increasingly isolated at the very time when love and support is most needed. Such children may end up feeling guilty and alone, while the parents

and siblings often experience significant psychologic stress. This situation may be illustrated by the following case:

> Timmy was a ten-year old boy who was dying from a cancer. His family had felt strongly that he should not be told of his terminal status and continually avoided discussing the issue with him. Because he had some difficulty with nausea, Timmy was on a bland diet. One day Timmy decided he really wanted a taco to eat. His mother told him this was not possible due to his diet, to which Timmy replied: "For heaven's sake, I'm dying! Let me have the taco!" At last the subject was broached and meaningful communication followed.

When discussing death with children, adults need to follow the child's lead regarding the timing and extent of the conversation. Communication may be brief and the conversation should be specific and literal. Expressions comparing death to a trip or a long sleep can be confusing to a child and should be avoided. Sometimes, nonverbal communication through art, music, and puppets is the easiest way for both adults and children to communicate.

It is important to acknowledge the completeness of the child's life and to give him or her a sense of accomplishment by acknowledging the impact his or her life will continue to have on the family and community. Both children and adults need to know it is normal to experience a wide range of emotions when facing death. Older children need to be part of the discussions and decision making regarding their own death, and their wishes should be respected as much as possible. All children need to be reassured of continuing love and physical closeness in addition to adequate symptom control. Lastly, it is necessary to realize that there are times when children need to be alone, such as when they withdraw or are noncommunicative. Caregivers should give children the space they need during this time, while making should children know that the caregivers will be there when called.

TABLE 26–11. Children's Understanding of Death Related to Age

AGE	LEVEL OF UNDERSTANDING OF INTERVENTIONS
Birth to 3 yr (infant–toddler)	Unable to differentiate temporary separation from abandonment. Death may be understood as separation from parents. Natural fears about being left alone, strangers, pain. Provide maximum physical comfort through exposure to familiar persons, consistency, favorite toys/objects.
3–6 yr (preschool)	Recognizes death, but not its irreversibility. Expansion of death concept to include loss of loving and protective object. Death is a temporary departure, reversible. Concrete and magical thinking. Fears separation. Issues of guilt. Minimize separation from parents, correct perceptions of illness as punishment, assuage guilt, use precise language.
6–12 yr (school age)	Develops concrete understanding of death and its concepts. Appreciation of removal from one kind of physical existence to another. Beginning to understand that death is permanent. Death associated with fear of separation and guilt. Evaluate fears of abandonment, be truthful, provide details if asked, allow child to participate in decision making
12–19 yr (Adolescent)	Death is recognized as a final, irrevocable act, yet accompanied by disbelief in the possibility of one's personal death. Issues of independence versus dependence, sexuality, isolation, anger, withdrawal and body image arise. Decision making requires honesty, trust, and respect.

CHILDREN'S UNDERSTANDING OF DEATH

As children grow and develop they assimilate the concepts relating to death (see Chapter 27 for a more in-depth discussion) of irreversibility, universality, nonfunctionality, and causality. Irreversibility refers to the understanding that dead things do not become alive again. With universality it is understood that all living things will die at some time. Nonfunctionality refers to the ending of all life functions. Causality relates to why people die. These concepts must be integrated with the child's developmental level and age, and are listed in Table 26–11.

Children from birth to age 3 years are unable to differentiate temporary separation from abandonment but by the age of 3 years are able to recognize death as an entity. Children from

3 to 6 years may recognize death but not that it is irreversible. Children in this age group may use fantasy and "magical thinking." Using "magical thinking" the child may think he can cause death by his thoughts, and consequently may suffer from misplaced guilt. By age 7 years, most children understand all the death concepts of irreversibility, universality, nonfunctionality, and causality.

BEREAVEMENT

A full discussion on bereavement related specifically to the loss of a child can be found in Chapter 27.

CONCLUSION

Pediatric hospice care as we know it can and does make a difference. Hospice facilitates the inclusion of the patient and family in the decision-making process. It allows the child to remain at home in familiar surroundings with loving caregivers. In addition to preventing suffering by providing good pain and symptom relief and leading to a more peaceful death for the child, hospice also facilitates bereavement for the parents and siblings.

Although nothing can eliminate the pain associated with a child's death, hospice care can facilitate bereavement for parents and siblings. Unfortunately, only a small percentage of the families that could benefit from hospice services actually receive them, but this is changing in the United States. In the year 2000, the American Academy of Pediatrics issued their recommendations for pediatric end-of-life care (Table 20–12). In response to the continuing challenges involved in pediatric palliative and end-of-life care, the Institute of Medicine of the National Academies interdisciplinary panel of pediatric experts issued a consensus report entitled "When Children Die" in 2003 stating that "children with fatal and potentially fatal conditions and their families fail to receive competent and compassionate and consistent care to meet their physical, emotional, and spiritual needs." They called for professional education, policy reform, increased public awareness, and research focused on pediatric palliative care all of which are finally being addressed by organizations such as the American Academy of Pediatrics, The National Hospice and Palliative Care Organization, The American Academy of

TABLE 26–12. American Academy of Pediatrics' Committee on Bioethics: Recommendations for Pediatric End-of-Life Care

1. Palliative care and respite programs need to be developed and be widely available to provide intensive symptom management and promote the welfare of children living with a life-threatening or terminal conditions.
2. At the diagnosis of a life-threatening or terminal condition, it is important to offer an integrated model of palliative care that continues throughout the course of the illness, regardless of the outcome.
3. Changes in the regulation and reimbursement of palliative care and hospice services are necessary to improve access for children and families in need of these services. Modifications in current regulations should include (1) broader eligibility criteria concerning the length of expected survival; (2) the provision of respite care and other therapies beyond those allowed by a narrow definition of "medically indicated." Adequate reimbursement should accompany these regulatory changes.
4. All general and subspecialty pediatricians, family physicians, pain specialists and pediatric surgeons need to become familiar and comfortable with the provision of palliative care to children. Residency, fellowship training and continuing education programs should include topics such as palliative medicine, communication skills, grief and loss, managing prognostic uncertainty, and decisions to forgo life-sustaining medical treatment, spiritual dimensions of life and illness, and alternative medicine. Pediatric board and sub-board certifying examinations should include questions on palliative care.
5. An increase in support for research into effective pediatric palliative care programming, regulation and reimbursement, pain and symptom management, and grief and bereavement counseling is necessary.

SOURCE: Policy statement: Palliative care for children (RE0007). *Am Acad Pediatr* 106(2):351-357, 2000.

Hospice and Palliative Medicine, The Center to Advance Palliative Care, the Hospice and Palliative Nurses Association, and others. *The National Consensus Project for Quality Palliative Care: Clinical Practice Guidelines for Quality Palliative Care* published by a consortium of these organizations in 2004 are meant to be clinical guidelines that promote patient- and family-centered care of consistent and high quality for patients of all ages. What remains now is to enlarge upon the hospice and palliative care model so more children and their families can be served and achieve optimal end-of-life care.

BIBLIOGRAPHY

Anand KJ: Clinical importance of pain and stress in preterm neonates. *Biol Neonate* 73(1):1-9, 1998.

Baker CM, Wong DL: QUEST: A process of pain assessment in children. *Orthop Nurse* 6(1):11-21, 1987.

Brenner P: *2000 Overview*. Alexandria VA, Children's Hospice International, 2000.

Brenner PR: The Volunteer component. In: Armstrong-Dailey A, Zarbock S, eds. *Hospice Care for Children*. Oxford, UK, Oxford University Press, 2001, pp. 213-231.

Carter BS, Levetown M, eds: *Palliative Care for Infants, Children, and Adolescents: A Practical Handbook*. Baltimore, MD, The Johns Hopkins University Press, 2004.

Davies B, Dorninica, F, Stevens M, Faulkner KW, Pollard B: The development of peadiatric palliative care. In: Doyle D, Goeffrey WCH, MacDonald N, eds. *Oxford Text Book of Palliative Medicine*. Oxford, UK, Oxford University Press, 1996, pp. 1087-1106.

Davies B, Eng B: Special issues in bereavement and staff support. In: Doyle D, Goeffrey WCH, MacDonald N, eds. *Oxford Text Book of Palliative Medicine*. Oxford, UK, Oxford University Press, 1996, pp. 1085-1095.

Davies B, Howell D: Special services for children. In: Doyle D, Goeffrey WCH, MacDonald N, eds. *Oxford Text Book of Palliative Medicine*. Oxford, UK, Oxford University Press, 1996, pp. 1077-1084.

Davies B: After a child dies: Helping the sibling. In: Armstrong-Dailey A, Zarbock S, eds. *Hospice Care for Children*. Oxford, UK, Oxford University Press, 2001, pp. 157-171.

Dussel V, Kreicbergs U, Hilden JM, etal. Looking beyond where children die: Determinants and effects of planning a child's location of death. *J Pain Symptom Manage* 37(1):33-43, 2009.

Faulkner KW: Children's understanding of death. In: Armstrong-Dailey A, Goltzer SZ, eds. *Hospice Care for Children*. New York, Oxford University Press, pp. 9-21,1993.

Field MJ, Behrman R, eds: When children die: improving palliative and end of life care for children and their families. *Institute of Medicine of The National Academies,* Report. Washington DC, The National Academies Press, 2003.

Foley KM: Controlling the pain of cancer. *Sci Am* 275(3):164-165, 1996.

Friedrichsdorf S, Kang T: The management of pain in children with life-limiting illnesses. *Pediatr Clin North Am* 54(5):645-672, 2007.

Gemke RJ, Zwaan, CM, Revesz T. Letter to the editor.*N Eng J Med* 342(26):1997-1999, 2000.

Gibbons MB: Psychosocial aspects of serious illness in childhood and adolescence. In: Armstrong-Dailey A, Zarbock S, eds. *Hospice Care for Children* Oxford, UK, Oxford University Press, 2001, pp. 49-67.

Goldman A (ed.) *Care of the Dying Child*. Oxford, UK, Oxford University Press, 1994.

Goldman A: Life threatening illnesses and symptom control in children. Doyle D, Goeffrey WCH, MacDonald N, eds. *Oxford Text Book of Palliative Medicine*. Oxford, UK, Oxford University Press, 1996, pp. 1033-1043.

Goldman A, Hain R, Liben S, eds. *Oxford Textbook of Palliative Care for Children*. Oxford, Oxford University Press, 2006.

Goldman A: Letter to the editor. *N Eng J Med* 342(26): 1997-1999, 2000.

Gortler E: Lessons in grief: A practical look at school programs. In: Armstrong-Dailey A, Zarbock S, eds. *Hospice Care for Children*. Oxford, UK, Oxford University Press, 2001, pp. 232-249.

Harper BC: Staff support. In: Armstrong-Dailey A, Goltzer SZ, eds. *Hospice Care for Children*. New York, Oxford University Press, 1993, pp. 184-197.

Himelstein B, Hilden J, Morstad Boldt A, et al: Pediatric palliative care. *N Eng J Med* 350:1752-1762, 2004.

Hirshfeld AB, Getachew A, Sesions J: Drug Doses, Sibery GK, Iannone R, eds. *The Harriet Lane*

Handbook, 15th ed. St Louis, MO, Mosby 2000, pp. 599-892.

Hockenberry-Eaton M, Barrera P, Brown M, Bottomley SJ, O'Neill JB: *Pain Management in Children with Cancer.* Houston, Texas Cancer Council, 1999.

Huff S, Joshi P: Pain and symptom management. In: Armstrong-Dailey A, Zarbock S, eds. *Hospice Care for Children.* Oxford, UK, Oxford University Press, 2001, pp. 23-48.

Levetown M, Carter MA: Child-centered care in terminal illness: An ethical framework. In: Doyle D, Goeffrey WCH, MacDonald N, eds. *Oxford Text Book of Palliative Medicine.* Oxford, UK, Oxford university Press, 1996, pp. 1108-1117.

Levetown M, Frager G: UNIPAC eight: The hospice/palliative medicine approach to caring for pediatric patients. In: Storey P, Knight CF, eds. *Hospice/ Palliative Care Training for Physicians.* New York, Mary Ann Liebert, Inc. Publishers, 2003.

Martin J, Kung H, Mathews T, et al: Annual summary of vital statistics: 2006. *Pediatrics* 121(4):788-801, 2007.

Martinson I: A home care program. In: Armstrong-Dailey A, Goltzer SZ, eds. *Hospice Care for Children.* New York, Oxford University Press, 1993, pp. 219-230.

McGrath PA: Pain control. In: Doyle D, Goeffrey WCH, MacDonald N, eds. *Oxford Text Book of Palliative Medicine.* Oxford, Oxford University Press, 1996, pp. 1013-1031.

Milch RA, Freeman A, Clark E, *Palliative Pain and Symptom Management for Children and Adolescents.* Washington DC, Division of Maternal and Child Health, US Department of Health and Human Services, 1989.

Miles MS, Demi AS: Toward the development of a theory of bereavement guilt: Sources of guilt in bereaved parents. *Omega* 12:299-314, 1984.

Miser JS, Miser AW: Pain and symptom control. In: Armstrong-Dailey A, Goltzer SZ, eds. *Hospice Care for Children.* New York, Oxford University Press, 1993, pp. 22-59.

Morgan ER, Murphy SB: Care of children who are dying of cancer. *N Eng J Med* 342(5):347-348, 2000.

Policy Document: National consensus project for quality palliative care: Clinical practice guidelines for quality palliative care, executive summary. *J Palliat Med* 7(5):611-626, 2004.

Policy Statement: Palliative care for children (RE0007). *Am Acad Pediat* 106(2):351-357, 2000.

Robin B: Analgesia and sedation. In: Sibery GK, Iannone R, eds. *The Harriet Lane Handbook,* 15th ed., St Louis, MO, Mosby 2000, 893-902.

Sahler OJZ, Frager G, Levetown M, Cohn FG, Lipson MA: Medical education about end-of-life care in the pediatric setting: Principles, challenges, and opportunities. *Pediatrics* 105(3):575, 2000.

Santucci G, Mack J: Common gastrointestinal symptoms in pediatric palliative care: nausea, vomiting, constipation, anorexia, cachexia. *Pediatr Clin North Am* 54(5):673-689, 2007.

Sligh JS: An early model of care. In: Armstrong-Dailey A, Goltzer SZ, eds. *Hospice Care for Children.* New York, Oxford University Press, 1993, pp. 219-230.

Stevens MM: Care of the dying child and adolescent: family adjustment and support. In: Doyle D, Goeffrey WCH, MacDonald N, eds. *Oxford Text Book of Palliative Medicine.* Oxford, Oxford university Press, 1996, pp. 1057-1075.

Stevens MM: Psychological adaptation of the dying child. In: Doyle D, Goeffrey WCH, MacDonald N, eds. *Oxford Text Book of Palliative Medicine.* Oxford, Oxford University Press, 1996, pp. 1145-1155.

Wolfe J, Hammel J, Edwards K, et al: Easing of suffering in children with cancer at the end of life: is care changing? *J Clin Oncol* 26(10):1717-1723, 2008.

Wolfe J, Grier HE, Klar N, et al: Symptoms and suffering at the end of life in children with cancer. *N Eng J Med* 342(5):326-333, 2000.

Wong DL, Backer C: Pain in children: Comparison of assessment scales. *Pediatr Nurs* 14(1):9-17, 1988.

Worden JW: *Grief Counseling and Grief Therapy: A Handbook for the Mental Health Practitioner,* 2nd ed. New York, Springer, 1991.

Worden JW, Monahan JR: Caring for bereaved parents. In: Armstrong-Dailey A, Zarbock S, eds. *Hospice Care for Children.* Oxford, UK, Oxford University Press, 2001, pp. 137-156.

World Health Organization Monograph: *Cancer Pain Relief and Palliative Care in Children.* England, World Health Organization, 1998.

SELF-ASSESSMENT QUESTIONS

1. As executive director of the hospice, you have decided to develop pediatric hospice services. In planning staff education, you realize that there are a number of significant differences between the care you provide to adults and what will be required to properly care for children. All of the following are differences that you will need to educate your staff about EXCEPT:

   A. As a child has not had a "full and complete life" the family more commonly desires life-prolonging treatment than is typical for adult hospice patients.
   B. Bereavement needs of the family are often much more complex.
   C. There is a special dispensation allowing terminally ill children to execute legally valid advance directives.
   D. Hospice admission criteria for pediatric hospice are much less well defined than those for adult hospice.
   E. Children of different ages will have different levels of understanding regarding what is happening to them.

2. Which of the following statements regarding the treatment of pain in children is TRUE?

   A. Neonates may be more sensitive to pain due to underdeveloped inhibitory pain tracts.
   B. The central nervous system of a 26-week-old fetus does not have the structural or neurochemical ability to experience pain.
   C. Children have a higher tolerance to pain than adults.
   D. Children are unable to communicate appropriately about their pain.
   E. Children will usually tell parents or caregivers when they are in pain.

3. You are evaluating a 10-year-old boy with advanced osteogenic sarcoma for pain. All of the following are important principles to remember during the regarding the assessment EXCEPT:

   A. Ask questions to the child in way he can understand them.
   B. Use pain rating scales such as the Wong/Baker faces or a 0 to 10 numeric scale.
   C. Observe and evaluate the child's behavior and how he reacts to the pain.
   D. Avoid involving the parents so as not to bias the evaluation.
   E. After intervening, reevaluate to assess the effectiveness of the intervention.

4. You are asked to evaluate a 3-month-old female infant with severe pain secondary to a congential neuroblastoma. On examination, the infant is constantly crying and her jaw is clenched. Her legs appear tense and restless, and she is continuously squirming back and forth. You try to calm her down with soothing sounds but she cannot be consoled. Based on the FLACC scale, you would document that this infant has a pain severity score of:

   A. 6
   B. 7
   C. 8
   D. 9
   E. 10

5. Regarding the same infant as in question # 4, you decide to start her on an opioid and acetaminophen in combination. Which of the following statements regarding the use of these agents in infants is TRUE?

   A. Acetaminophen can be administered at the same dose and frequency as in older children.
   B. Acetaminophen can be administered for prolonged periods without increased risk of hepatotoxicity.
   C. Morphine should be given at one-fourth to one-third the dose recommended in older children.

D. The risk of respiratory depression as a side effect is the same as in older children.

6. Of the following antiemetics, which can be administered to children under 2 years of age?

A. Chlorpromazine
B. Prochlorperazine
C. Promethazine
D. Granisetron

7. Your patient is a 13-year-old boy with a diagnosis of acute lymphoblastic leukemia who you have taken care of for many years. He has been the hospital numerous times, and has currently been in the hospital for several weeks for treatment of complications of chemotherapy. Posttreatment evaluation has unfortunately shown that his disease is progressive and resistant to further chemotherapy. You have discussed his terminal prognosis with his parents, and they would like to consider taking him home for his last days. They are concerned, however, what impacts this would have on their family life in general, and especially how this would affect the patient's two siblings, an 11-year-old sister, and an 8-year-old brother. All of the following are true statements regarding the potential impact of caring for the patient at home EXCEPT:

A. Parents can pay more attention and provide more support to their other children.
B. Siblings can participate in the care and entertainment of their brother.
C. The dying child will feel less isolated and have a more peaceful death.
D. Bereavement issues for the siblings are likely to be more complicated.

8. During what development age group do children begin to understand that death is permanent?

A. Infancy to 3 years (infant/toddler)
B. 3 years to 6 years (preschool)
C. 6 years to 12 years (school age)
D. 12 years to 19 years (adolescent teenager)

9. When an adult is discussing death with a child, which of the following regarding the nature of the conversation is TRUE?

A. The child should dictate the timing and extent of the conversation.
B. Expressions comparing death to a trip or a long sleep are encouraged.
C. The nature of the conversation should be general and nonspecific.
D. Nonverbal communication through art and music should be avoided.

10. You are the medical director of a hospice with a pediatric hospice program. A 12-year-old girl with a terminal clear cell sarcoma of the kidney tumor has been referred to your hospice by her family pediatrician, who has cared for her and her three siblings since birth. The pediatrician calls you to discuss the patient, and wants to know what the hospice's position would be regarding his continued involvement with the patient, especially as he has virtually no experience in the principles of hospice and palliative care. Which of the following would be reasonable to include in your discussion?

A. You should not stay involved as it is not important to maintain the relationship between the primary pediatrician, the patient, and family.
B. You can stay involved and you will be responsible to give all orders regarding the patient's palliative care.
C. You can stay involved and the hospice physician will consult with you regarding the patient's palliative care.
D. You should not be involved as you have no experience in the principles of hospice and palliative care.

Grief and Bereavement in Children

Robin Fiorelli

INTRODUCTION

Both mental health practitioners and parents alike have been misguided about how children and teens experience the loss of someone significant to them and about the most effective ways to assist a grieving child. In a systematic review of the prevailing misperceptions, Charles A. Corr listed most centrally the belief that children do not really grieve because they are too young to understand death. The reality is that children's grief may look different than that of adults, but it shares fundamental similarities as a physical and emotional reaction to the loss of a significant loved one.

The most compelling myth is that it is best to protect a child from death and also from grief. It is natural for adults to want to protect children from painful experiences. However fanciful this wish may be, children will grieve in their own unique ways and it is imperative that caring adults do not dictate or impede that process, instead, allow and even facilitate children's expression of grief.

Another myth is that funerals and memorial services are not age appropriate and children may be traumatized by the acute emotional experience at such an event. As will be discussed, current research suggests that a child should receive information about what the event will be like and then should be allowed to make up his or her own mind about participating, a decision adults should honor.

Another common myth is that children are "naturally resilient" and should just "bounce back" after a loss. This is not always the case and depends on contingencies such as concurrent stressful events, the child's understanding of the death, the child's developmental age, and the support received by adults in their life. On the other hand, John Bolby in his work on attachment and loss concluded that children are more susceptible to profound emotional scarring after experiencing a significant loss. Supposing this potential exists, its realization still depends on the factors already listed, most importantly the attitudes and behaviors of adults important in their lives.

Children tend to attribute physical symptoms to emotional experiences more than do adults. Many parents are familiar with the headache that appears when a child is overwhelmed with emotion or with the stomach ache that appears the morning before a school test. There is much debate about whether children really experience emotions more as a physical sensation than do adults or whether they know that adults in their lives are more apt to heed physical rather than emotional symptoms.

This chapter begins by outlining children's concepts of death and grief responses, differentiated by developmental level and chronologic age, through adolescence. The most common physical, emotional, social, and spiritual grief reactions of children and teens will be explored in depth, following which, complicated grief reactions in children and teens will be outlined. The chapter then shifts to a discussion on how to prepare a child for the impending death of a loved one, what to tell them when the death actually occurs, and the questions one might expect children to ask during this difficult time. The chapter then turns to the topic of how to assist bereaved children and teens in expressing and coping with their grief as well as where to find additional sources of support for the grieving child and teen. Suggestions for grieving parents in caring for their own grief needs are also included. How children may attend and participate in funerals and memorial services, including guidance for how to discuss burial and cremation with children, and how to help grieving children participate in memorial activities, including those on anniversaries or birthdays, are shared. Finally, two of the most significant losses for a child will be examined closely, that of a parent and that of a sibling.

CHILDREN'S CONCEPTS OF DEATH AND RESPONSES TO GRIEF

Each child is unique in his or her understanding of death and response to grief. This understanding is largely influenced by the child's developmental level and chronologic age. There can be tremendous overlap, however, between the age groups because children and adolescents move from one developmental level to another at very different rates.

INFANCY (TO AGE 2)

Babies do not have the cognitive capability to understand an abstract concept like death. They function very much in the present, so when someone significant dies, babies become more acutely aware of loss and separation. They also react to the emotions and behaviors of significant adults in their environment and also to any disruptions in their nurturing routine and schedule. If there is a sudden change, they feel tremendous discomfort.

Therefore, in response to a loss, babies may search for the deceased and become anxious as a result of the separation. Common reactions include: irritability and protest, constant crying, a change in sleeping and eating habits, decreased activity, and weight loss.

PRESCHOOL (AGE 2–4)

When will my mommy be home?

How does (the deceased) eat or breathe?

Preschool children do not comprehend the concept of "forever." For this age group, death is seen as temporary and reversible. Even when a preschooler is told that mommy is not coming back, for example, she or he may ask the same question again an hour later. These children often have difficulty visualizing death as separate from life, and not as something that can happen to them. Preschool children love to play "peek-a-boo" games where adults in their life disappear and then reappear again. It is through these games that they slowly begin to understand the concept of "gone for good."

Because preschoolers tend to be present-oriented, their grief reactions are brief although often very intense. As these children are going through the developmental stage where they are learning to trust and form basic attachments, when a significant adult in their life dies, they become very concerned about separation and altered patterns of care. Children this age typically have a heightened sense of anxiety concerning separations and rejections because they do not have the capacity yet to use fantasy to gain control over what is happening.

They also respond to the emotional reactions of adults in their life. If they sense their parents are worried or sad, they may cry or throw tantrums either because they are concerned or as a way to distract their parents from difficult emotions. Typical grief responses of the preschool child include confusion, frightening dreams and night agitation, and regressive behaviors such as clinging, bedwetting, thumb sucking, inconsolable crying, temper tantrums, and even withdrawal from others. They may search intensely for the deceased despite assurance they will not return. They also may exhibit anxiety toward strangers.

EARLY CHILDHOOD (4–7)

It's my fault. I was mad at my mother once and I told her I wish she would die and then she died.

The roadrunner in the cartoon always comes back to life, so I know Daddy will too

As with preschoolers, children in the 4 to 7 age group tend to view death as temporary and reversible. They sometimes feel responsible for the death because they believe that negative thoughts or feelings they have had about the deceased caused their demise. This "magical thinking" stems from the belief that everything in their environment revolves around them and that they can control what happens. Even when children at this age are exposed to death through the media or at school, they still may believe that if you are careful enough you can avoid death.

Children at this age may also connect occurrences that do not have anything to do with each other. For example, if a child bought a certain toy the day that her sister died, she may attribute the toy to causing the sister's death, especially if the real cause of the death is not fully explained to her.

Not surprisingly, therefore, children of this age group, much like their younger counterparts, may repeatedly search for the deceased or ask where they are. Repetitive questioning about the death process, such as "What happens when you die?" "How do dead people eat?" is often common. They will often express their grief feelings through play instead of verbally. Themes of family loss and death may surface as they play with dolls or action figures. They may play act the death itself or the funeral.

Sometimes, children at this age appear unaffected by the death and act as if nothing happened, but this doesn't mean that they are oblivious *or* that they have accepted the death. It may just signify their inability in the moment to acknowledge very painful reality. They also may model their grief reaction after the adults in their lives, feeling uncertain how to express grief feelings. Other typical responses include anger, sadness, confusion, and difficulty eating and sleeping.

As with preschoolers, this age group may regress as a way to receive more nurturance and attention during this difficult time. Children who have experienced a loss at this age tend to be fearful that other loved ones will leave them as well. Sometimes they form attachments to people who resemble the deceased in some way.

MIDDLE YEARS (AGES 7–10)

Do your fingernails and hair keep growing when you die?

If I smoked cigarettes, would I die?

Although children between the ages of 7 and 10 often still want to see death as reversible, they begin to see it as both final and universal. Children in this age group sometimes visualize death in the form of a tangible being such as a ghost or boogeyman. They are very curious about the details of death, cremation, and burial and may ask candid questions

Even though they know death can happen to anyone and that there are many things that cause death, they still do not typically think of death as something that can happen to them or their family members, instead, to only old or very sick people. They may believe that they can escape from death through their own efforts. They also might view death as a punishment, particularly before age 9. Sometimes they are unable to comprehend how the death will affect their lives, which can become a source of anxiety.

Children in the middle years often become concerned with how others are responding to the death as they become less focused on themselves and more on others. They may fear that other loved ones will die as well. Sometimes they may become overly concerned about their own health and may fear bodily harm and death.

Some children in this age group may act out their anger and sadness and experience difficulties in school due to a lack of concentration. On the other hand, they may have a jocular attitude about the death, appearing indifferent, or they may withdraw and hide their feelings. Other typical responses include shock, denial, depression, changes in eating and sleeping patterns, and regression to an earlier developmental stage.

This age group tends to have more coping strategies available than younger children and may fantasize how they would prevent the death from happening again as a way to gain control over the situation. Death is also play-acted in children at this age, for example, through war games, especially for those children who have difficulty expressing feelings verbally.

Children in this age group may assume the role of the deceased in the family or the mannerisms of the deceased. They may also take on tasks or chores normally performed by the deceased, such as care for their siblings. They may idealize the deceased as a way of maintaining a bond with them.

PREADOLESCENT (AGES 10–12)

> None of my friends could ever relate to what it's like losing their Dad.

> While I know that Grandma is not coming back and I will miss her, I don't understand why my Mom is so upset about it

Preadolescents conceive of death in much the same way as children in the middle years with a few additions. Preadolescents are in the process of establishing their own identity, increasing their independence from their parents and other adults and increasing their dependence on their peer group. In understanding death, preadolescents attempt to understand both the biologic *and* emotional process of death. They are, however, more able to understand the facts surrounding the death of someone than they are the feelings surrounding the death.

It is common for preadolescents to want to cover up their feelings about their loss so as not to appear "different" from their peer group. They fear that expressing sad feelings may be seen as a sign of weakness (particularly for boys). For this reason, they may appear removed and indifferent. Preadolescents may also express their grief feelings in uncharacteristic ways such as through anger outbursts, irritability, and bullying behavior. Feelings may also be exhibited through physical complaints, moodiness, changes in sleeping and eating patterns, indifference toward schoolwork, or isolation from their peers. They may show concern for practical issues after the death such as how the household will survive without the deceased or how they personally will be taken care of. They also might have questions regarding religious and cultural beliefs related to death.

ADOLESCENT (AGES 13–15)

These years are often marked by stressful physical changes. Boys are usually a little slower to mature than girls in this age range, but the stress of change is ever-present—from radical growth spurts to facial skin problems. Teens in this age range are seeking to establish their unique identity, often separate from parents and family. They are beginning to think about spiritual and philosophical ideas for the first time in truly abstract ways. And, they generally experience powerful and deep emotions that they may feel no one can understand.

One of the difficult tasks a grieving teenager faces is integrating loss into his or her current emotional life. This integration can be compounded by physical and hormonal changes. Grief may be expressed by frequent headaches or stomach aches, or through feeling sad and depressed. Another common reaction is for middle teens to manifest their grief in mood swings and outbursts of anger. Some teens withdraw to a safe place, such as a bedroom, where the anger may be acted out by pounding on a wall or beating a pillow. Some may act out the anger through inappropriate social behavior, pouting, or aggression toward others. Grades may decline in part due to sleep disturbances, which are often combined with depression and a general feeling of meaninglessness.

It is not unusual for middle teens, both girls and boys, to want a special "friend," such as a teddy bear to hug and sleep with during this time. It may be important for a caregiver to protect this information from other family members and friends, especially in the case of a boy. The teenager also may want to wear a special article of clothing that belonged to the deceased. He or she may adopt certain mannerisms or behaviors associated with the deceased loved one, or idealize his or her relationship with the deceased. Being tolerant of what may be seen as "childish" or immature behavior allows middle teenagers to process the loss in their own, personal and important ways.

ADOLESCENT (AGES 15–18)

Adolescents in the 15 to 18-year-old age group are in the process of becoming young adults. They want to be treated with respect and collegiality. Providing assistance to grieving adolescents, therefore, can be complicated by the fact that although they may be young adults, they do not have the full experience of adulthood. They are also in the process of differentiating and distancing themselves from the parental figures in their lives. The peer group is their major authority—and how they are seen and judged by their peers is of primary importance to them.

These older teens often become sullen and noncommunicative. Their anger may be expressed through exaggerated conflict with parental figures, pushing hard to overturn formerly understood limits. They may become insecure about the future, question the meaning of life, and question or abandon the family's belief system. They may have sleep problems, such as recurrent or disturbing dreams and insomnia. Sometimes they regress and become immature and childish, or they mask their fears with jokes and sarcastic remarks.

Sometimes, older adolescents who suffer a loss may idealize the deceased loved one. They may adopt mannerisms, habits, and preferences of the deceased. They may want to wear certain items of clothing, especially a hat, shirt, or jacket that belonged to their special loved one. Or they may react by feeling abandoned and angry at unfulfilled expectations in their relationship with the deceased.

NORMAL GRIEF REACTIONS IN CHILDREN

We now examine more in detail the typical and normal grief reactions that children and adolescents experience during the grief process. Some grief reactions with children occur immediately and others may occur at a later point. In general, children's grief tends to manifest in physical and behavioral expression rather than verbal expression.

In addition to developmental level and chronologic age, the main factors that influence how a child grieves are the relationship with the person that has died, the nature of the death (when, how, and where the person died), the child's own personality, previous experiences with death, religious, and cultural beliefs, input from the media, and above all, what they are taught about death and grief from adults and the availability of family, social, and community support. The more common physical, cognitive, and behavioral reactions that may occur to children during the normal grief process are listed in Table 27–1 and are discussed below.

PHYSICAL SYMPTOMS

I don't feel good. I feel sick to my stomach.

Last night I dreamed that Johnny came back to visit me. He was all grown up, though, and he had a mean look and wanted to hurt me.

Chief somatic complaints of a grieving child include headaches, stomach aches, fatigue, lack of energy, muscle aches, tightness in the throat, difficulty breathing (especially when they first learn about the death), skin rashes, change in eating patterns (lack of appetite or excessive appetite), change in sleeping patterns (both falling asleep, staying asleep, and sometimes prolonged sleeping), odd and frightening dreams, hyperactivity and hypersensitivity (especially if

TABLE 27–1. Normal Grief Reactions in Children

REACTION	EXAMPLES		
Physical symptoms	Headache	Muscle aches	Changes in eating habits
	Stomach ache	Throat tightness	Difficulty breathing
	Fatigue	Skin rashes	Changes in sleep habits
	Lack of energy	Hyperactivity	Odd and frightening dreams
		Hypersensitivity	
Cognitive symptoms	Inability to concentrate		
	Obsessed with or preoccupied with deceased		
	Preoccupation with the death, or the meaning of death		
	Carrying objects owned by the deceased		
	Repetitively looking at photos of the deceased		
	Visual hallucinations of the deceased		
	Adopting deceased's roles or physical mannerisms		
Behavioral changes	Emotional shock		Anger and acting out
	Denial		Regressive behavior
	Sadness, despair		Fear, anxiety, panic
	Depression		Jealousy
	Guilt, shame, self-blame		Acceptance

the loss was traumatic). Most of these physical symptoms are temporary and go away with time when the child begins to receive adequate grief support. Some children develop physical symptoms that resemble the symptoms of the illness that they observed in the deceased. This may be a child's attempt to stay connected in some way with the deceased or a way to express his or her own fear about getting sick. When children receive a great deal of attention for their physical symptoms, they may exaggerate the "sick role" as a means to obtain socially acceptable attention for their grief feelings.

COGNITIVE SYMPTOMS

I couldn't focus on my school work today. I don't remember one thing that I learned.

My Dad was the best father in the world. He never even once got mad at me

When I went to sleep last night, my Mom came and sat in the chair by my bed.

Many bereaved children describe an inability to concentrate for any length of time after a significant loss. Their thoughts seem to be taken up with the death and loss of their loved one. Rabbi Earl A. Grollman discusses how children idealize the deceased as a way of coping with their loss. In an attempt to counter unhappy thoughts, the child may become obsessed with only the positive qualities of the deceased. Some older children become preoccupied with "why" the death happened, may want to know all the facts surrounding the death, and may search for the "meaning" of the death. Some children search for their lost loved ones with the hope of finding them. They may seek out places they used to go together. Other children become temporarily preoccupied with memories of the deceased, asking other adults to tell stories about the deceased over and over again, carrying objects of the deceased around with them, and looking at photos repetitively.

Visual hallucinations of the deceased are also common and are experienced as very real to the child. Sometimes they can be comforting and other times terrifying. Identification with the deceased by incorporating mannerisms or taking on the deceased's roles such as disciplining the other children are also common. All these behaviors are an attempt by the bereaved child to reconnect and relate to his or her deceased loved one. They should all be viewed as a normal part of the grief process unless they persist unnaturally long or cause a great deal of distress for the child.

EMOTIONAL SHOCK AND DENIAL

> I don't believe you. My mother will come back. You are wrong.

> Even though it's a year later, I still can't believe that Grandma is gone.

Usually, when the realization of the death is too overwhelming, the child temporarily denies that it happened. Denial of the death is not unusual, but it can be difficult for adults to endure. It should be viewed as a protective mechanism; a way for the child to comprehend painful information at the speed with which they are ready. Denial is most common in the first few months following the death, but may reappear at different times throughout the grief process.

SADNESS, DESPAIR, AND DEPRESSION

> I don't want to live without my Dad.

> I miss my Mommy and I want her back.

There are many different ways that children exhibit feelings of sadness and despair following a loss. They may express it verbally, nonverbally through a depressed demeanor, through tears, or by becoming withdrawn, isolated, and quiet. Children sometimes react in total despair and are inconsolable when they first learn the news of the death. The full realization of the loss does not happen all at once, but as it does, sadness, loneliness, and depression can follow.

ANGER AND ACTING-OUT BEHAVIOR

> I hate you and wish you had died instead of Dad.

> I hate school. I hate my friends. I hate my family. I hate my life. I hate everything.

It is often easier for children to feel mad, then to feel sad and children typically strike out with anger at the people with whom they feel closest and most safe. There are many reasons why grieving children feel angry. They may feel angry at the person who died for leaving them, angry at God, at others in their family, and at the doctor for not doing more to save their loved one. They may be angry at themselves because they believe they caused the death (magical thinking) or that they did not do enough to prevent the death. Anger often originates from feelings of helplessness and lack of control.

There are some bereaved children that channel their anger by defying authority, rebelling against everything and by displaying somewhat antisocial tendencies. Antisocial behavior in a bereaved child is often an attempt to keep themselves away from any close relationships and the possibility of being "abandoned" again. It is important to note that anger expression generally is more socially acceptable among boys than girls. Younger children are often more physically expressive and direct when they are angry. They throw things, hit and kick, and have tantrums. Anger outbursts are often set off by seemingly unimportant triggers in bereaved children.

REGRESSIVE BEHAVIORS

It is very common for bereaved children to regress in some way to an earlier developmental or chronologic age. Death of a loved one can cause complete disruption in their routine and in their sense of safety, and regression to a time in their life where they felt more secure and familiar should be seen as a healthy adaptation to a traumatic situation. Usually, regressive behaviors are temporary and subside with time as the child receives appropriate grief support. It is important that adults in a grieving child's life find a balance between allowing the regression and gently expecting the child to return to his or her former level of functioning.

Examples of regressive behaviors include bedwetting and thumb sucking, difficulty separating from significant others, demanding attention, regressing from prior advances toward independence, difficulty with developmentally appropriate tasks, needing to sleep in parent's bed, needing to be held or rocked, reverting to fantasies of an earlier age, talking in baby language, giggling inappropriately, and inability to function with peers.

FEAR, ANXIETY, AND PANIC

Are you going to die when you go to sleep tonight like Grandma did?

Who is going to take me to school now that Daddy died?

I think I'm going to get cancer too.

Children often react with fear and panic when they lose someone significant to them and may be afraid of the intensity of their own feelings. They become concerned about how other grieving adults will fare. They worry as well about the changes in care-giving and nurturance that come with the loss. Some grieving children become concerned that someone else close to them will die and that they will have to feel that pain again. In some cases, these children withdraw from other important adults so as not to repeat the hurt.

Bereaved children often feel afraid of becoming sick or of dying themselves. They may become afraid of the dark, of sleeping alone and of being separated from or abandoned by other significant adults. Unfortunately, this is especially true if a parent has died and the other parent is somewhat detached from the child because of the parent's own grief reaction.

GUILT, SHAME, AND SELF-BLAME

It's all my fault that Janey died. I told her I wished she was dead when she broke my doll and now she is dead.

I never liked my brother. He always teased me. Now I feel so guilty because he died.

Bereaved children sometimes believe they are responsible for the death, especially if they had ever wished the deceased dead. Some children feel guilty if they experience relief that the person has died, even though this is very normal reaction, especially if their loved one had been suffering. Other children feel guilty because they had a difficult relationship with the deceased. Frequently interrelated to self-blame is a sense of helplessness and worthlessness. If grieving children feel helpless, they may try to gain some control by thinking what they would have done differently to change the situation.

JEALOUSY

I can't go to the Father/Daughter dance because I don't have a father.

I hate when all the kids at school talk badly about their parents. They should feel lucky they HAVE parents.

It is very common for bereaved children to feel like they have been short-changed in some way, especially if the loss is that of a parent. It becomes particularly difficult for them during holidays such as Mother's or Father's Day, at their birthdays or graduations, and when they receive awards, because all these events serve as continual reminders to them of their loss. Feeling jealous that other children have parents is very common.

ACCEPTANCE

When Dad first died I thought my life was over. Now I feel like I'm starting to look forward to things again.

J. William Worden, a leading expert in grief and loss, describes the process by which a child begins to accept a significant loss. Acceptance of the loss comes gradually as does the understanding that the death is final. Most children describe a kind of "new normal" as they begin to adjust to the loss. They still think about their loved one that died and understand that their life has been changed, but they begin to reconstruct a life without their loved one in it. In the case of the death of a parent, they begin to feel secure that they will be taken care of and will have their needs met. They realize there are other significant adults available for support. Older children sometime state that going through a grief experience allowed then to learn to feel more compassion toward others and more tolerance for other problems and challenges in their own lives.

Alan Wolfelt, another leading expert on children's grief, calls the healing process that grieving children go through "reconciliation." He says that reconciliation happens when a whole and healthy person emerges from grief. The person recognizes that life will be different without the presence of the significant person who has died. Reconciliation is a process not an event, and it does not occur all at once—it is a slow, painful process. The most notable changes during the child's "reconciliation" process include a return to stable eating and sleeping patterns, a renewed sense of energy and well-being, a subjective sense of release from the person who has died, increased thinking and judgment capabilities, the capacity to enjoy life experiences, a recognition of the reality and finality of the death, and the establishment of new and healthy relationships.

NORMAL GRIEF EXPERIENCE FOR A TEENAGER

By the end of high school, 20% of today's students will have lost one of their parents; 90% will have experienced the death of a close relative or loved one. Add to this that 1 in every 1,500 secondary school students dies each year, and we can see that death and the resulting grief following death is a part of everyday life for many teenagers. Recognizing and providing constructive ways for teenagers to express their grief will help prevent prolonged or unresolved grief and depression.

Grief is as unique as the people who experience it, but there are some reactions to grief that we all feel and that are considered *normal or typical* grief reactions. For teens who experience the death of a loved one, these typical grief reactions, listed in Table 27–2, often resemble those described

TABLE 27–2. Normal Grief Experiences for Teenagers
Assuming mannerisms, traits, or wearing clothes of the deceased. Emotional regression and even bed-wetting, which can be most upsetting for teenagers. Needing to repeat again and again stories of their loved one Saying nothing at all Becoming overly responsible (the "new" man or woman of the house), which distracts them from their own feelings by taking care of everyone else. The need to integrate the loss into their budding identity Anger and lashing out at others that can happen at any time for no real reason Intense anger at the deceased for dying, and later feelings of guilt for being angry. Mood changes over the slightest things; unexpected outbursts or crying. A feeling that the loss is not real and did not happen at all

earlier for children, albeit in a somewhat older age context.

Teenagers experience their loss at different times in their development and the first and second year may be the most difficult. Part of normal development for a teenager is to reintegrate what they have learned about their loss into their current developmental stage. Special days and important times may serve as reminders of their absent loved one. The process of integrating the loss may resurface on these special days. For example, a high school senior wore his deceased father's shirt to his graduation exercises. A 19-year-old bride proposed her first toast to her deceased grandmother, a most significant figure in her life.

COMPLICATED GRIEF REACTIONS IN CHILDREN AND TEENAGERS

Prior to her mother's death from liver cancer, Sarah had been doing well in school, was captain of the gymnastic team and had several close friends. As Sarah and her Mom were very close, it was expected that Sarah would have a difficult time adjusting to her Mom's death, although everyone remarked how "well" Sarah was coping as her mother was dying. Her father explained, "She seemed to hold it all together so well." Even after the death, Sarah returned to school and to her normal routine fairly quickly. "Then all at once everything started to fall apart. It was as if she finally understood that her mother was really gone." Sarah started missing school and her grades began to slip. She lost interest in gymnastics and quit the gymnastic team. She had trouble getting out of bed and began saying that she wished she were dead. She rejected her peers' attempts at helping her and stopped answering the phone. Her Dad noticed that she stopped caring about her appearance and that she even looked disheveled. At first, her Dad was patient and thought it would pass. He was so involved in his own mourning that he didn't seem to notice just how serious her depression had become. He finally called the school

counselor who referred him to a grief specialist who worked with children. Sarah was reluctant at first, not believing that anything would help. Finally, she agreed to go, began to express her anger and sadness, and over the course of several months began to resume her normal activities and functioning.

Thus far, the emotional, physical, and behavioral grief responses that have been described are **normal** expressions of grief in children and adolescents. A child may experience some or all of these reactions or may show no overt reaction at all. However, if any of these typical responses to grief are **prolonged, extreme, pervasive, affecting the child's ability to function normally** in school or with their peers, or in providing self-care, like in the case with Sarah, the grief would now be considered "complicated." Examples of complicated grief reactions are listed in Table 27–3. When a bereaved child exhibits any of these behaviors, immediate professional advice and assistance should be sought. There are many community sources that provide support for grieving children including school guidance counselors, pediatricians, clergy, mental health practitioners, and hospice bereavement personnel. Further discussion of how to manage complicated grief reactions in children and teenagers can be found below.

PREPARING A CHILD FOR THE DEATH OF A LOVED ONE

PREDEATH SUPPORT

If an adult can prepare a child or teen for the death of a loved one, it is important to do so as soon as possible before the death occurs. First, asking a child what he or she knows about a loved one's illness allows the adult to discover any misperceptions that the child may have, and assists the adult in knowing where to start from in educating

TABLE 27–3. Complicated Grief Reactions in Children and Teenagers

BEHAVIOR	EXAMPLES
Suicidal thoughts and behaviors	"I just want to kill myself"
	Giving away valued possessions
	Preoccupation with suicidal themes in media
	Desire to be with deceased loved one
	Self-punishment ideation or behaviors
Prolonged sleep disturbances	Insomnia
	Nightmares
Persistent personality changes	Neat, well-groomed child abandons bathing, grooming, and dressing habits
	Eating habits change: too much or too little
	Extrovert turns into introvert
	Optimist becomes pessimist
	Pleasant child becomes a bully
	Secure child becomes anxious and afraid
Aggressive behavior	Dangerous risk-taking behaviors
	Behavior dangerous to others
Excessive or inappropriate guilt	Child ruminates how she or he caused death of loved one
Extreme fatigue or loss of energy on a prolonged daily basis	Inability to get out of bed that lasts more than 10 d
Extreme withdrawal or isolation	Inability to socialize with others
	Despair
	Depressed affect
Pervasive fantasies that interfere with normal functioning	Belief that loved one will return, especially if she or he is good
Phobias that interfere with functioning	Fear of getting sick
	Fear of dying
	Avoiding anything having to do with death
Hypervigilance	Checking on other parent constantly
	Checking themselves and others for symptoms that mirror those experienced by the deceased
	Hyperalertness in a car if loved one died in a car accident
Persistent assumption of mannerisms of the deceased	Assumption of chores and responsibilities of deceased that are not developmentally appropriate
Preoccupation with the deceased to the point that it interferes with normal function	
Drug and/or alcohol use	

the child about the illness and prognosis. It is imperative that the adult presents the information in a gentle and calm manner, allowing the child to voice questions and concerns. Children can usually absorb only a little information at a time.

It is important to look for "teachable moments"—moments when the child seems open to learning. It should be explained that all living things must die. The adult could show the child plants and insects that have died and tell them that because people are living things, they die too. Explain that the changing seasons are another example of the cycle of life and death. The child should be told that the images they see of death in television cartoons are not always authentic and that death is irreversible. The adult can explain to the child that people usually live a long life, but that sometimes when someone develops a very serious illness, he or she dies before becoming old. The adult can also explain that doctors usually help people live long healthy lives, but that sometimes even doctors cannot stop some people's bodies from malfunctioning. Using several adjectives like "very, very sick" or "very, very old" helps the child distinguish between someone with a common cold versus someone with a terminal illness and between their parents, who may seem old to them, and elderly people. The child should be reassured that this is not a punishment, or God's fault or anyone's fault, but that sometimes it just happens. She or he can also be reassured that death is usually not painful and that it is almost always quiet.

When a loved one is dying, if a child is old enough to understand what is happening and both the child and the dying person would like to see each other, the child should be allowed to visit the loved one. The child should be prepared beforehand about what she or he might see or hear and what feelings might be experienced. The child should be told what the loved one might look like, and the setting, including medical equipment if applicable, should be described. Depending on the age of the child, it may be advisable to keep the visit short. Visiting with a dying loved one might be a way for a child to understand the reality of the death, and a way for important communication to take place between the child and the loved one. The key is that the visit must be the child's choice. If the child does not want to visit, a supportive adult should attempt to elicit why the child is resistant, but the child's wishes should be honored.

Throughout the illness, a child should be told about changes in a loved one's condition as they arise. A child should be allowed to care for a loved one in a way that he or she chooses, be it through writing cards or bringing a glass of water or tissues. Sometimes, caring for a dying loved one allows a child to feel less helpless.

HOW TO TALK TO A CHILD WHEN THE DEATH OCCURS

Ideally, a child or teen should be told in a gentle and caring way about the death as soon as it occurs, by someone they trust and feel close to. It might be helpful to prepare the child for the news by saying, "I'm afraid I have some bad news." The explanation should be kept simple, avoiding euphemisms such as, "passed away," "expired," "went away," or "went to sleep." These euphemisms may cause the child to believe the person will come back or wake up, or conversely, may cause the child to be afraid to go to sleep at night. A suggested approach might be, "Daddy has died. He was very, very sick. Daddy had a disease that made him very weak and he was not able to get better. Daddy is now unable to move, feel, talk, eat, or hurt anymore." By being direct, the child's confusion and fantasies about what happened are usually diminished.

When a child is told about the death of a loved one, she or he needs to be allowed a lot of time for expressing reactions and feelings, as well as for raising questions and concerns. By sharing their own feelings with a child, adults can help normalize what the child might be feeling. The child should also be made aware of what others in their environment may be feeling and thinking and should be reminded that sadness, anger, and fear are all normal feelings when someone dies. It is also important that the child is told what funeral arrangements or rituals will happen next, so they know what to expect. They should be reassured by being told specifically what will happen to them and how they will be taken care of.

TYPICAL QUESTIONS THAT CHILDREN HAVE ABOUT DEATH

It is important that the questions posed by children and adolescents are answered in a specific, straightforward, and brief fashion, and reflect the developmental level of the child. Children can usually absorb only bits of information at a time so it is important to pay attention to their cues. Checking to see if a child has understood what has been said is also critical. Adults unsure of the meaning behind a child's question should probe further by asking what the child meant or knows about the topic. Children often repeat the same questions merely as a way to assimilate the answers. It is also okay for adults to tell the child they do not know the answer to a specific question.

Some of the most common questions children ask are the following:

Why did daddy die?: It is important to probe further to assess whether they are asking this question because they feel sad, angry, or guilty about the death. If so, it is imperative to allow the child to express those thoughts and feelings. The child should be reassured that death does not seem fair. It may also be that they are asking about the physical process of death.

When is mommy coming back?: It is okay to tell a child in a gentle loving way that people who die do not come back; that as much as she or he may want mommy to come back, she can't because she is dead. Sometimes, it is reassuring for a child to know that she or he can always hold onto feelings and memories about a loved one and that in that way, the loved one will always be with him or her. It may also be reassuring for a child to know that the feelings of sadness that he or she is experiencing about a loved one being gone will go away over time.

Where is daddy now?: Before answering this question, it is helpful to know where the child thinks daddy is. The adult's response would then be based on that belief. If the child believes daddy is in heaven, because that is the family's spiritual belief, than that belief should be validated. Also, to minimize confusion, it might be helpful to remind the child about the burial, for example, that the loved one was placed in a casket underground.

Will you die too?: It is important when answering this question to give reassurance and support and also to answer honestly. An example would be: "I will die sometime but I hope to be here a long time yet. I do not have any serious illnesses." Sometimes when a child asks this question, she or he is afraid of losing another loved one. A clarifying question might be," Are you worried that I won't be here to care for you?"

How long will I live?: A response might be that no one knows how long they will live, but that no one lives forever. The child should be reassured that *most* people live until they are old and that many old people are not worried about death.

GUIDELINES FOR HELPING BEREAVED CHILDREN EXPRESS THEIR GRIEF

A hundred years ago death was much more a natural part of a child's experience. Grandparents often lived with families, so children witnessed them growing older and dying. Modern medicine has made strides in reducing infant and child mortality and has prolonged life expectancy for the elderly, so children witness fewer deaths. More and more elderly die in nursing homes and hospitals, outside the home environment. The exclusion of death from children's lives requires us to teach them explicitly about death and grief.

In *Mourning and Melancholia*, Sigmund Freud outlined his belief that young children did not have the capacity to mourn. He believed that only as a child developed into an adolescent did they acquire the ego capacity to grieve. More contemporary research has concluded that children do in fact have the capacity to experience and express grief, but it is often more intermittent and drawn out over a longer period of time than with adult grief. General guidelines for helping children express their grief are presented in Table 27–4, whereas guidelines that address some of the most common specific feelings that children experience are listed in Table 27–5.

TABLE 27–4. General Guidelines for Helping Grieving Children Express Grief

---

Allow children to express grief in their own ways.

Do not pressure children to resume normal activities before they are ready.

Allow children to feel that it is OK to talk about death and grief.

Be available to listen.

Let children know that having and expressing feelings are normal.

Avoid expressions that suppress grief.

Gently intervene if the child is taking on the role of a bereaved adult.

Grieving adults should not hide feelings from children.

Allow children to express religious and spiritual concerns.

Allow children to remain in familiar surroundings. Avoid sending children away.

The grieving process helps people heal from their pain. Pain is a natural reaction when we lose someone close and children are capable of accepting pain of loss directly and openly. When adults try to protect children from such pain, they are usually, in reality, trying to protect themselves. The most important thing to remember in helping children cope with the death of a loved one is to allow them to express their grief in their own way and in their own time. It is important not to pressure children to resume their normal activities if they are not ready.

Children tend to have "grief bursts" followed by play and normal activities. Children may not be able to succinctly verbalize what they are feeling and instead may demonstrate their feelings through their behavior and play. They may laugh or play at a time that feels inappropriate to an adult.

Children need to feel that it is okay to talk about death and grief. However, if a child does not want to talk about grief, adults also need to respect that desire. Adults should let the grieving child know that they are available to listen and help and that any feelings they have, such as anger, sadness, fear or regret, are normal. Hugging and touching helps the grieving child feel secure in expressing emotions and also reassures the child that he or she is loved and will be cared for. Alan Wolfelt feels that if grieving children are ignored, they may suffer more from the sense of isolation that from the loss itself.

Messages relayed to a grieving child such as "Don't cry. You need to be strong," "You're the man in the family now," or "Be a good girl. Your mommy needs your help now more than ever," suppress grief expression in children and set up unfair expectations of them. Adults should gently intervene if they observe a child taking on the roles and tasks of a bereaved adult. Grieving children should not be allowed to take on the role of the "confidante" or partner of one parent if the other has died.

It is important that adults not hide their own feelings of grief from a bereaved child. If they do, they teach them that experiencing these

TABLE 27–5. Guidelines for Managing Specific Expressions of Grief

EXPRESSION	SUGGESTED ACTIONS
Sadness/depression	Draw memories of the deceased and show to others
	Show photographs and describe keepsakes to others
	Develop a memory scrapbook
	Engage in physical activity
Anger	Allow child to dissipate anger with various activities
	Ask children about their anger
	Ask the child to suggest ways of responding to anger
	Maintain household rules and chores
Guilt and regret	Write a letter or draw a picture describing "unfinished business" with the deceased
	Write a note about feelings of guilt and tie it to a helium balloon in order to "let it go"
	Create puppets so that child puppet can talk to puppet of the deceased
Fear	Help child identify fears
	Provide repetitive reassurance that all will be OK
	Spend time alone with child and reassure that s/he is special and loved
Physical complaints	Ask about other possible feelings, symptoms, or emotions
	Remind the child why the death occurred
	Pediatrician visit to reassure child

feelings are *not* okay, that they are something to be ashamed of or to be kept to oneself. It is also true that grieving adults should not grieve profusely and at length in front of a child as it might frighten and worry the child.

Religion is an important source of strength for many adults and children during the grief process. Children takes things literally, so explanations such as "It is God's will" or "Bonnie is happy in heaven" could be frightening or confusing rather than comforting, particularly if religion has not played an important role in the child's life. It's important to inquire how the child perceives what is explained about the death. It is also important that children be allowed to express their religious and spiritual concerns.

Parents may be tempted to "send children away" when there is a loss—either to protect them from painful feelings or because it is difficult to care for them while grieving themselves. During the grieving period, children are often most comforted by familiar surroundings and routines, and separation may increase their fears about abandonment.

SADNESS/DEPRESSION

Grieving children that are sad or depressed require a lot of support and attention so that they can express their sad feelings and work them through. Helen Fitzgerald, a well-known children's grief therapist, recommends several techniques for helping a depressed grieving child. She suggests having the child draw good and bad memories of the deceased and share them with others. The child could also could show photographs and describe keepsakes to others and develop a memory scrapbook. For a child that feels so despaired about a loss, it might be helpful to ask the child to fantasize how life might be different if she or he was not so sad. Encouraging the child to engage in physical activity is another useful technique with a depressed child.

> Johnny was very withdrawn and depressed for several months after the death of his mother. Finally, his grief counselor suggested he make a "God box" where he could write down all his sad feelings and put them in the box and God would help him feel better. He wrote a new note almost every day and soon his father noticed that he seemed more cheerful.

ANGER

It is sometimes easier for a child to feel mad rather than sad or guilty. Anger is not always rational and it can escalate by feeding upon itself. Anger does need to be expressed, however, and adults can be helpful in teaching grieving children how to express anger in constructive ways. Unexpressed anger can turn into depression or into anger that is out of control.

Children generally tend to express their anger physiologically. Instead of asking an angry child to "calm down" it may be more useful to allow them to dissipate their anger in other ways such as running, exercising, scribbling on paper, ripping paper, singing, and sculpting play dough. It is important to not try to deal with the cause of anger until the intensity has decreased. Adults can ask children questions about their anger at a time when they are not angry. It might be helpful to ask questions like, "What usually leads to your feeling angry?" or "How does your body tell you that you are becoming angry?" Examining these precipitating factors usually diminishes the intensity if the anger and gives the child a sense of control by learning what triggers an angry response.

It is helpful to ask the child what he or she thinks are more appropriate ways to respond to angry feelings. It is also appropriate for an adult to set a limit with an angry bereaved child who is acting out. "It's not okay to hit me but you can hit this pillow." Maintaining household rules and chores actually increases the sense of normalcy and security for a grieving child.

> Stephen had been very close to his grandfather and when he died, his parents noticed he began bullying his younger siblings and picking fights at school. They called his football coach who suggested that Stephen might "work out" some of his aggression by staying after practice and "ramming" the dummy players. After two weeks of "extra" practices, Stephen was much less aggressive with other children.

GUILT AND REGRETS

Some children have regrets about negative aspects of the relationship with the deceased or regrets about things that did not happen or were not said prior to the death. Examples might be: "I never told my mother I loved her," "I lied to my father and never told him the truth," "I was mad at my Mom the day she died," or "I didn't have a chance to say goodbye."

Helen Fitzgerald describes some techniques that are useful with children in helping them work through feelings of guilt and regret. One suggestion is to write a letter to or draw a picture for the deceased describing their "unfinished business." Another suggestion is to have the child write a note about what she or he feels guilty about, tie the note to a helium balloon, and then release the balloon into the sky. For younger children, she suggests making two puppets and drawing one puppet face as the child and the other as the deceased person. The child puppet could tell the puppet of the deceased what they feel guilty about or what they regret about the relationship.

> After her mother's death, Emily's father noticed that she seemed very preoccupied and unable to focus on her schoolwork. After several months, he referred her to the school counselor who had

experience in working with bereaved children. When she suggested Emily write letters to her mother, Emily seemed relieved to be able to "communicate" with her mother in this way. Emily then asked the counselor to read the letters. They were full of ways that Emily believed she could have prevented her mother's death. After several of these letters and the counselor's educating Emily on the nature of her mother's serious illness, Emily began to relax and was able to focus on her school work again.

FEARS

It is important to help fearful children identify what they are afraid of specifically and then to address each fear individually. Children who are fearful generally need repetitive reassurance that they will be OK. It is also important that a parent or other significant adult spend time alone with and focused on the grieving child, reassuring the child that they are special and loved.

> Both of Anwar's siblings had been killed in an automobile accident. Anwar was terrified of riding in a car for months after their death and was also afraid that someone else close to him would die. His parents and family provided a great deal of love and support during this time. His father decided to help him confront his fear of riding in the car by taking incremental steps. First they sat in the car for a long time as Anwar expressed sorrow about his loss and his anger at the driver that hit the car. Later, his father backed out of the driveway reassuring Anwar that he was safe. The next day he drove down the street assuring Anwar about how accomplished a driver he was. Soon Anwar was able to ride in a car again without fear.

PHYSICAL COMPLAINTS

When grieving children routinely have physical complaints like headaches and stomach aches, it is sometimes helpful to ask what other feelings they may be having as well. They may not disclose their emotions right away, but they may begin to make their own connection between their physical and emotional concerns.

If the physical complaints mirror those of the deceased, it is helpful to remind a child why the death happened. A visit to the pediatrician may also be advised, so the child can hear reassurance from the doctor that nothing is wrong with them.

> Jose complained of headaches for weeks after his father's death. He was the oldest son and felt he had to be "strong" for his other siblings and for his mother, so he expressed very little emotion. Two months after his father's death, his uncle asked Jose if he wanted to visit the cemetery. When they arrived, Jose began to cry when they came to the grave. He and his uncle spent several hours while Jose talked to his father and reminisced with his uncle. After that, Jose no longer complained about headaches.

BEREAVEMENT SUPPORT GROUPS FOR GRIEVING CHILDREN

Child bereavement support groups are among the most successful ways to provide support to a grieving child, particularly for older children. Donna L. Schuurman, Executive Director of the Doughy Center, an agency that specializes in the grief and loss issues of children, suggests that children should be grouped by age and developmental level in grief groups. She also suggests that mixing death types and relationships to the deceased are acceptable but that children experiencing different losses (i.e., divorce, death) should not be mixed in the same group. Children support groups are typically less structured than adult groups and usually incorporate play time.

One of the most important reasons that bereavement groups are helpful is that grieving children discover in the group that there are other children whose experiences are similar to theirs. Being in a peer group with other bereaved children helps normalize their experience and reactions, helps then to understand that their feelings are important, and allows them to feel hopeful by listening to other children who are coping successfully. In bereavement support groups, children learn that they can express themselves in healthy ways and also learn tips from one another about how to deal with similar emotions and circumstances.

SUPPORT FROM SCHOOLS FOR GRIEVING CHILDREN

Children spend a great deal of time in school and both teachers and peers can be an important source of support for a grieving child. Teachers and school counselors should be told about the progress of the illness while the child's loved one is still alive *and* of the death when it happens. The teacher should be aware of what the child knows about the illness and could be given advice on how best to support the child. Teachers can also help by monitoring the child's emotional state and behaviors in the time following the death. The school may need to alter assignments or provide extra instructional assistance for a grieving child.

The teacher should share with the child's classmates' information about the death and also provide guidance on what they can do and say and how they might be helpful when the grieving child returns to the classroom. Children could be prompted to say, "I was sorry to hear about your sister," or "I felt sad when I heard about your father dying." Welcome back posters or sympathy cards are very appropriate.

It is important to remember that some children spend more time processing their loss with peers than with other adults. On the other hand, some children, especially older children, do not want to feel different than their peers and may be hesitant to share their loss as it might single them out as different from others.

PLAY THERAPY FOR GRIEVING CHILDREN

A child's play is often the main avenue through which a grieving child expresses his or her grief, particularly younger children. When young children are trying to comprehend death, one can often observe rituals where they bury animals and insects in the ground or use dolls and action figures to play out the both the dying and grief processes. Through play, children can take apart traumatic experiences and replay them in a way that is comforting to them, and they can do this in relative safety, one step removed from reality. If parents or teachers find that a child's play has taken on a rigid, sad, or repetitive character, they should talk openly with the child about what is being experienced.

Many grief therapists who work with young grieving children use play therapy to assist the child in coming to terms with their loss. The advantages of play therapy are that young children tend to have a limited verbal ability for describing their feelings, they tend to have a limited emotional capacity to tolerate stress and the pain of loss, they have a shorter attention span, and finally, young children communicate their feelings, wishes, fears and attempted resolutions to their problems through play. The goals of therapy for the bereaved child are to help facilitate the mourning process and to help clarify any cognitive confusion the child may have about the death.

GUIDELINES FOR HELPING GRIEVING TEENS

Table 27–6 presents the "Bill of Rights for Grieving Teens." Written by a grieving teenager, this document, is, in essence, guidelines for how to assist teens who are bereaved.

The most important thing an adult caregiver can do for grieving teens is to be available to them. Availability means being approachable, nonjudgmental, caring, and appropriate. Letting them know you are there to talk at any time and letting them know you will hear what they are saying, no matter what it is, will make all the difference in your ability to be a helpful presence for teenagers who have suffered a loss.

Do not assume they will come to you to talk. You will need to ask if they want to talk. And, if a grieving teen asks, "What do you want to talk

---

TABLE 27–6. Bill of Rights for Grieving Teens

A grieving teen has the right . . . .

- To know the truth about the death, the deceased, and the circumstances
- To have questions answered honestly
- To be heard with dignity and respect
- To be silent and not tell you her or his grief emotions and thoughts
- To not agree with your perceptions and conclusions
- To see the person who died and the place of death
- To grieve any way he or she wants without hurting self or others
- To feel all the feelings and to think all the thoughts of his or her own unique grief
- To not have to follow the "Stages of Grief" as outlined in a high school health book
- To grieve in one's own unique, individual way without censorship
- To be angry at death, at the person who died, at God, at self, and at others
- To have his or her own theologic and philosophic beliefs about life and death
- To be involved in the decisions about rituals related to the death
- To not be taken advantage of in this vulnerable mourning condition
- To have irrational guilt about how he or she could have intervened to stop the death

Written by teenagers at the Dougy Center (http://www.dougy.org/grief-resources/bill-of-rights/); Reprinted with permission of the Doughy Center, Portland, OR.

---

about?" tell him or her. Be open and address your own feelings or difficulties regarding your loved one's death. Be honest. Avoid euphemisms such as, "passed on" or "left us." Use the deceased person's name or family role (like mother, grandmother, etc.). It's also OK to say, "I don't know" if she or he asks you a difficult question. Don't pretend to understand something that you don't; your teenager likely will learn that you don't, if he or she doesn't pick up on it immediately. Then be open to just *listening*. Ask leading questions that invite your teenager to talk to you. Review the conversation, asking your teenager to summarize what you discussed. This provides opportunities to clarify if there are misconceptions or misunderstandings.

If you are unable to talk about death with your teenager, find someone else who feels comfortable talking about it, like another relative, another bereaved teen, or a professional, such as a social worker, faith practitioner, or school counselor.

Share your own thoughts, concerns, and feelings. Acceptable expressions of grief will be demonstrated by your example. Give your teenagers permission to grieve by allowing them to see you grieve. Telling stories, reading, and writing poetry and journaling are all useful means of expressing one's grief. These things could be shared with others or not.

Share and discuss religious beliefs with your teenager. If your teenager has spiritual questions you can't answer, admit it and seek the assistance of your faith professional (minister, priest, rabbi, imam). Try not to react negatively if your teenager is expressing faith or beliefs that are different from the accepted family practice. Older teens especially will be developing their own faith practices to prepare for future losses. This may require some religious "experimentation" on the older teen's part. Refer him or her to your local faith professional.

Being an adult companion to a bereaved teen, especially if you are a parental figure, may make you the focal point of anger and, perhaps, cruel remarks. This can be especially difficult to tolerate if you are experiencing your own grief. Try not to engage the teenager in a way that will result in building barriers, but shift the focus to the underlying pain the teenager is trying to mask with these remarks. The bereaved teen may not be approachable at the moment that the remarks are made; you may want to establish a time to talk in the future and describe what you want to talk about when making your "appointment."

Times before, during and immediately after a death are disruptive. Try to re-establish a routine, with appropriate expectations and limits, as soon as possible. Teenagers as well as younger children need the reassurance and sense of security that comes from structure, rules and limits. The main difference in an older teen is that you should be open to negotiate the rules and limits appropriate to the teen's age. Remembering your own fears and anxieties during this period of your life may help you be less rigid and more reasonable in negotiating rules and limits.

Teens need to be allowed to mourn intermittently. Two teenagers who were present for the home death of their father were seen playing video games within an hour of his death. Some family members wondered if this was "appropriate" behavior. It was fortunate that a hospice professional was present to reassure the family that this was normal, and that teenagers need to be given room to mourn in their own ways. Sometimes the overwhelming nature of the loss requires teenagers to "take a break" from their mourning and engage in whatever may distract them from the loss. Also be ready for mood swings and emotional expressions at unexpected times. Be prepared for resurfacing of emotions on special days or anniversaries, such as birthdays, holidays, and the anniversary of the death.

The secure presence of some understanding, caring and appropriately affectionate adult role models can make all the difference to a teenager's experience of and ability to cope with his or her grief. Remember that each teenager's grief is unique. Let him or her teach you what the loss means and then help the teenager to his or her own meaning as he or she grows up with this loss.

In most cases, teenagers who have experienced the death of a loved one will not need professional help. Continuing to live a routine life in a loving caring environment of friends, family and community will provide the support and refuge they need to learn to live with their loss and prepare for future losses life undoubtedly will put in their way.

However, in some situations, professional help is needed. After any experience of violent death, whether that violence is manmade (such as murder, an act of war or mob violence) or natural (such as flood, tornado, earthquake, or hurricane), the evaluation of a caring family-oriented healthcare professional may be appropriate. In these situations, the possibility of long-term complications, such as posttraumatic stress disorders, should be addressed.

Always seek professional help and evaluation if the teen has developed symptoms that are of a concern to you. Grief is often expressed through behavior. Your teenager needs to hear that you care about him or her even if the teen is acting out. If grief is severe or prolonged, don't hesitate to seek grief counseling for your teenager. Family and friends can provide a wealth of support, when relationships are established that are trusting and appropriate. Individual counseling can help address personal issues. Child and family counselors are a primary source of assistance to the whole family in grief. Support groups can help your teenager feel less isolated and different from other teens. Peer groups are usually more authoritative than parents during the teen years. A well-facilitated youth group can help immensely with teenagers' grief.

When seeking grief counseling for a bereaved teen, the first place to go to obtain appropriate help should be the teenager's primary healthcare provider. The family healthcare provider can make appropriate referrals to mental health providers or recommend other interventions that may be necessary. The provider may also help access any insurance benefits that may be available, or make referrals to public health resources.

The teenager's school may be another important resource, as a large part of a teenager's time is spent at school. If a teenager is having a difficult time with his or her grief, the school staff, such as teachers and the guidance counselor should be involved. They can be invaluable allies in helping a teenager with his or her grief. In addition, guidance counselors often know about community resources. Inform the teenager's school guidance counselor and teachers of the death, and how close your teenager was to the deceased. Ask teachers and guidance counselors to provide you with feedback if they see any changes—good or bad—in your teenager's behavior or performance at school. Watch for academic decline. Grieving teenagers may not be well-rested due to insomnia or interrupted sleep patterns. They may have trouble concentrating in class or completing homework. Offer assistance and, if necessary, see if the school can recommend a tutor.

There are also many resources in the general community. A growing number of communities have bereavement centers with programs for children and teenagers. Also, many communities have self-help phone numbers or help hotlines that may list bereavement services available in your community for children and teenagers. Some communities will have a public mental health center, and these centers often will help to evaluate and refer teenagers who are having a difficult time with bereavement, especially when they are depressed, despondent, or unusually angry. Another source of community help for bereavement care is your local hospice provider—even when the deceased was not a hospice patient. Hospices generally provide resources and referrals for bereavement care at no cost.

Youth groups that are either recreational, such as the YMCA or Scouts, or religious youth groups, may be a useful resource to assist the grieving teen, as participating teenagers receive nurture and distraction from their routine in a wholesome environment. Some of these youth groups may even provide direct access to counselors who can address and assist with grief recovery. One's local temple, church, or mosque, and the local minister, rabbi, pastor, imam, or other spiritual counselor is another important resource to consider if you are looking for help with bereavement. Many local faith groups provide bereavement groups and pastoral counseling that address issues of bereavement from a spiritual point of view.

The internet can provide a wealth of information and support for grieving teenagers. Keep in mind that while there is also a lot of inappropriate information on the internet, there are reputable sites that provide an opportunity to read information and write or start your own blog (a web site with short entries and links to personal or other websites on a particular subject, i.e., bulletin boards). Libraries and book stores offer reading in the area of grief and grief recovery.

GRIEVING PARENTS NEED TO TAKE CARE OF THEMSELVES

Although this chapter focuses on the care of bereaved children, one would be remiss in not at least touching on the need for grieving parents to care for themselves while caring for bereaved children. Many parents find this particularly challenging, which is why it is imperative that adults make a special effort to get the support and assistance they need so that in turn they can attend to the grief needs of their children. Some adults, however, do find it particularly therapeutic to give to a grieving child, because it can be healing to provide assistance to someone else. To ensure the best possible interactions can occur between grieving parents and children, several suggestions are provided in Table 27–7. A full discussion of bereavement care for adults can be found in Chapter 17.

TABLE 27–7. Suggestions for Grieving Parents

- Take time for themselves to sort out their own concerns, doubts, and fears. It is hard for an adult to be reassuring to a child when they have their own unresolved fears.
- Take care of their physical health—rest, eat right, exercise moderately, and avoid alcohol and drugs.
- Keep a grief journal, read books about grief, and join a bereavement support group. Many grief experts also suggest waiting on making any major life decisions.
- Take people up on their offer to help and support. Relatives and friends can run errands, take care of the children, or assist with the final arrangements. It is very important not to become isolated.
- Allow the child to care about them as well as long as the child doesn't become consumed with care.
- Have someone they can share the responsibility of providing emotional grief support to the child.

GUIDELINES FOR CHILDREN ATTENDING FUNERALS AND MEMORIAL SERVICES

Therese Rando, a well-known grief and loss expert, explains that rituals allow structure for important events that happen throughout our lives, including death. A funeral offers a controlled time where individuals can emotionally and physically ventilate their feelings. Funeral rituals generate social support and offer opportunities to find meaning, by applying spiritual and philosophical understandings to loss. Funeral rituals are most effective when they are personal and involve participation from friends and family.

When the death of a loved one occurs, adults are faced with difficult choices about whether to include children and teenagers in death rituals such as funerals and memorial services. As a general guideline, children should be allowed to attend a wake, funeral, and burial if they want to. Children can also be involved in the funeral planning. Joining family members for these rituals gives them a chance to receive grief support from others and a chance to say goodbye in their own way to the deceased.

Children should never be forced to attend a funeral or memorial service. It is important, however, to understand the children's reasons for not wanting to attend, so any fears or questions can be addressed. Questions that might assist adults in understanding a child's fears or concerns might include: "What is the thing you are most afraid of about the funeral?" or "What do you think you might feel if you were to go to the memorial service?"

Always prepare children for what will happen at any death ritual. Describing the funeral process step by step (what they will see, how other people might react, how they might feel) can help allay children's anxieties about the event. It is important to reiterate that crying or not crying are both OK. Extra attention and affection from adults may be necessary so children do not feel forgotten or neglected, remembering not to embarrass a teenager in front of his or her peer group. It is helpful to make arrangements with a trusted adult so a child could leave the funeral or memorial service early if he or she wishes.

Children should *never* be forced to view or touch the body; they need to be given a choice that will be respected. If they are going to view the body, it is helpful to remind them that death is final and to describe how the body might look. An explanation could go like this: "Sally will be lying in a wooden box called a casket. She will look like she is sleeping, but she is not. She is dead. Her chest will not rise and fall because she is not breathing." For some children, touching the body may satisfy their curiosity, be a way of saying goodbye, or be an expression of love. If a child decides to touch the body, he or she should be told that the body will feel cold and hard. Some children, however, do not need to touch or see the body to know that the death is real. If a child does not want to see or touch the body, an adult could relay that the body was seen and that the deceased was not living or breathing.

Children should be asked if there is anything they would like buried with their loved one. It is often comforting for the child to place a small gift, a drawing, a letter, or a picture of themselves in the casket.

EXPLAINING BURIAL AND CREMATION TO A CHILD

If the deceased will be buried, it is helpful to explain to children in detail what that means so they will not develop fantasies about where their loved one was put to rest. An explanation may go like this: "The casket will be sealed shut and then taken to a cemetery where there are several other bodies buried under the ground (or placed in a hole in the wall of a building called a mausoleum). They have to be placed there because, like with a dead squirrel, their body will begin to decompose because it is no longer living."

It is sometimes difficult for a child to understand cremation. When describing it, it is important to remind the child that the dead person no longer feels anything, so it is not painful. If the child wants to view the body before a cremation, most mortuaries can arrange for this. When de-scribing cremation to a child, it might be helpful to say: "Cremation happens at a place called a crematory. There they use heat to change the body into ashes. These ashes are usually placed in a special box and the family decides what they want to do with the ashes."

WAYS TO COMMEMORATE THE LOSS WITH A GRIEVING CHILD

During the grieving process, there comes a time to bring emotions into perspective, modify patterns of thinking, develop a new awareness of the loss and the importance of life, and start to free oneself from the profound pain of grief. This change, and it can be a significant one, is facilitated by the act of commemoration. Commemorating a loss can be a public or private event, elaborate or simple. The important thing with a grieving child is that the ritual should be planned with the child's consent and is not imposed. The child could be asked to actively participate by sharing ideas for commemorating the deceased.

A helpful way to commemorate a loss is to visit the cemetery or final resting place of the deceased. It may be a means for the child to say goodbye or to satisfy natural curiosity. As with funerals, it is important to describe to children beforehand what they will see and how they may feel at the cemetery, and allow them to ask questions. Often families take flowers, pictures, small gifts, or notes to place on the grave. It is helpful if adults share their feelings while visiting the grave to give permission to the children to share as well. It is also helpful to process afterwards any thoughts and feelings about the visit.

Phyllis Silverman, William Worden, and others have described how bereaved youngsters often maintain a connection of some type to the deceased person who they loved, such as a parent. They may believe the parent is somehow with them when they are awake. There are many rituals and activities that children enjoy doing that enhance a positive connection to the deceased. Adults should allow grieving children ample opportunity to share their memories of their loved one and adults should talk about the deceased person as often as possible. Viewing photo albums, telling stories, visiting special places where they went with their deceased loved one, having memorable possessions of their loved one are all important commemorative activities.

There are many creative ways to commemorate the loss as well. One is to write letters to the deceased. The letters could be kept in a special place, could be shared, or could be burned in a ceremony. The burning of letters is especially significant if there was unfinished business in the relationship, particularly with older children. Artwork can be very therapeutic for grieving children as it allows them a nonverbal channel to express themselves. It is important to allow children the choice about whether or not to share their artwork with others. Some children may choose to write about their emotions and memories in a poem, story, or journal. Other creative ideas include making a scrapbook or photo album, making a treasure box where mementos of the deceased can be stored, planting memorial trees or plants, and donating money to charity in their loved one's name.

HOLIDAYS AND SPECIAL ANNIVERSARIES

Holidays and special anniversaries can be very difficult for grieving children and adolescents, especially during the first year. Holidays and anniversaries serve both as a reminder of the loss and of pleasant memories of the deceased. It is sometimes difficult for children to watch others enjoy the holiday, when for them it just brings up the void they feel. Often, the anticipation of the holiday can be worse than the holiday itself.

It is important to let bereaved children know in advance that they might experience some painful feelings during the holiday or anniversary. It is also helpful to plan with them in advance ways to make these events more tolerable. Holiday rituals that included their loved ones could be altered and new rituals developed.

Mother's and Father's Day can be particularly difficult for children that have lost a parent. They may choose to commemorate their loss by visiting the cemetery or visiting a special place where they have positive memories of their parent. If they are supposed to participate in an activity with the parent, for example, a Mother's Day celebration, they may choose to take a "substitute mother" to the event.

As the first anniversary of the death approaches, children often find themselves reliving very intensely the last days of their loved one's life. Children often need extra reassurance and support during this anniversary. It is also important that the adults in their life share their own feelings about the anniversary and memories about the deceased.

Children often choose to celebrate the birthday of their deceased loved one. They might make a birthday gift for their deceased loved one, or bake a cake and light birthday candles. The celebration could include sharing memories about past birthdays with their loved one. A visit to the cemetery might be a special way to allow a child to say "happy birthday" to their deceased loved one. Other holidays may be commemorated in a similar fashion, by giving gifts, sharing memories of the deceased, and developing special rituals.

DEATH OF A PARENT OR SIGNIFICANT ADULT

Parents naturally love their children and children depend upon parents for survival and stability. Silverman believes that what a child experiences as lost along with the death, how they talk about their deceased parent or significant adult, and how they understand his or her place in their lives, can be even more critical than age-specific understanding of death. The death of a parent or significant adult seems to be more difficult if the death was sudden *or* if the child lacks a solid replacement figure.

Some children fantasize that their parent will return, and others have the wish to die so they can be reunited with their deceased parent. Usually, this is a fleeting desire rather than true suicidal ideation. Children expressing these wishes, however, should be questioned more deeply, and an investigation made as to whether they do have a specific plan and means available to carry out their wishes.

Silverman describes the accommodation and adaptation to the loss of a parent or significant adult that a bereaved child experiences throughout his or her life. These children tend to revisit the meaning of their parent's death over and over again at different developmental stages. They also re-experience the loss at events such as graduation, marriage, and the birth of a child.

Some bereaved children idealize their parent or significant adult as a way to keep their pleasant, comforting memories of them alive. This can be adaptive unless it gets in the way of a child expressing angry feelings toward the parent for "leaving" or for any "unfinished business" in the relationship. It is important that surviving parents allow the idealization of the deceased parent, but also stress with children how much they love them and reassure them of their care and support.

DEATH OF A SIBLING

When a sibling dies, the surviving child reacts to both the loss of the sibling *and* to the change in behavior and grief process of his or her parents. The grief response of siblings may be longer or shorter than parents and they may have a different understanding of the death. Siblings are often asked numerous questions about their brother's or sister's death from their peers and from other adults. This can feel overwhelming to a child.

An ill child often receives more attention from parents than their siblings who are well. The surviving children often believe they will get more attention from their parents after the death of their sibling and then are disappointed when those expectations are not met. Surviving children may also grapple with identity and role issues after the loss. "Am I still a little brother?" or "Who's going to take out the garbage now?"

Sometimes, grieving parents are overprotective of the remaining siblings, concerned that they may die or become ill as well. Other parents place unreasonable expectations or demands on the remaining siblings, for example, asking them to take on the responsibilities and roles of or to have the same attributes as the deceased sibling. It is important that parents avoid being either overprotective or overpermissive with grieving siblings, despite the temptation. Care should be taken to not make comparisons between the deceased child and any siblings, as it may lead the surviving children to feel inadequate. Care should also be taken not to assign inappropriate responsibilities to a child that the deceased sibling used to have, especially responsibilities that are not developmentally appropriate.

For all these reasons, grieving siblings need a lot of reassurance from their parents that they are loved for who they are and that they will be cared for and supported. They need to be reminded that they did not cause their brother's or sister's death. They also should be encouraged to share memories and hold keepsakes of their deceased sibling and to participate in family rituals related to the deceased child.

CONCLUSION

Bereaved children and adolescents are unique in that they experience the pain of loss earlier than other people, earlier than they are expected to. Bereaved children are also unique in that they may not completely comprehend the meaning of "gone for good," instead, may hold onto an inner representation of the deceased. Children who are grieving the loss of a parent or significant adult differ from other children in that they lose the innocent belief that their parents will be there to care for them forever. Surviving siblings or children whose young friends have died are forced to face the fact that young people sometimes die earlier than they are supposed to.

This chapter outlines the typical emotional, physical and behavioral manifestations of children and adolescent grief and offers guidelines for interventions that adults can provide to grieving children. When adults really listen to grieving children and take their cues for action from them, adults learn that what grieving children most need is unconditional love, reassurance that they will be cared for, inclusion in the mourning process, and availability to work through their grief. Adults also can be comfortable that the community at large can play a significant role in the positive outcome of a grieving child.

When adults talk openly and honestly with children about death, especially before the child ever faces a loss and if children are given the straight facts about death, they begin to understand death as a natural part of life, instead of something to be feared or something that happens to others and never to them or their families. This affords children the time necessary to be able to face the reality of death and to properly mourn, and as a result, attain a positive outcome to their grief process.

BIBLIOGRAPHY

Bolby J: *Attachment and Loss: Loss, Sadness and Depression-Volume III.* New York, Basic Books, 1980.

Cline, KD: *A Family Guide to Helping Children Cope.* California, American Cancer Society, 1988.

Corr CA: Eight myths about children, adolescents and loss. In: Doka KJ, ed. *Living With Grief,* Washington, DC, Hospice Foundation of America, 2000, p. 33.

Corr CA: What do we know about grieving children and adolescents?. In: Doka KJ, ed. *Children, Adolescents and Loss: Living With Grief.* Washington, DC, Hospice Foundation of America, 2000, p. 28.

Doka KJ, ed: *Children, Adolescents and Loss: Living with Grief.* Washington, DC, Hospice Foundation of America 2000.

Doka KJ: Using ritual with children and adolescents. In: Doka KJ, ed. *Children, Adolescents and Loss: Liv-*

ing with Grief. Washington, DC, Hospice Foundation of America, 2000, p. 154.

Doka KJ, ed: *Children Mourning, Mourning Children.* Washington, DC, Hospice Foundation of America, 1995.

Dyregrov Atle: *Grief in Children: A Handbook for Adults.* London, Jessica Kingsley Publishers, 1990.

Fitzgerald H: *The Grieving Child.* New York, Simon & Schuster, 1992.

Grollman Earl: *Bereaved Children and Teens: A Support Guide for Parents and Professionals.* Boston, Beacon Press, 1985.

Grollman EA: Grieving children: Can we answer their questions?. In: Doka KJ, ed. *Children Mourning, Mourning Children.* Washington, DC, Hospice Foundation of America, 1995, p. 21.

Huntley T: *Helping Children Grieve.* Augsburg, Augsburg Fortress, 1991.

Kroen WC: *Helping Children Cope with the Loss of a Loved One.* Minneapolis, MN Free Spirit Publishing, Inc, 1996.

Osterweis M, Solomon F, Green M, eds: *Bereavement: Reactions, Consequences and Cure.* Washington, DC, National Academy Press, 1984.

Pennells Sr., M, Smith, SC: *The Forgotten Mourners: Guidelines for Working with Bereaved Children.* London, Jessica Kingsley Publishers, 1995.

Seibert D, Drolet JK, Fedro JV: *Helping Children Live with Death and Loss.* Carbondale, IL, Southern Illinois University Press, 2003.

Schuurman DL: The use of groups with grieving children. In: Doka KJ, ed. *Children, Adolescents and Loss: Living with Grief.* Washington, DC, Hospice Foundation of America, 2000, p. 175.

Silverman P: When parents die. In: Doka KJ, ed. *Children, Adolescents and Loss: Living with Grief.* Washington, DC, Hospice Foundation of America, 2000, p. 221.

Silverman P, Nickman S, Worden W: Detachment revisited: The child's reconstruction of a dead parent. In: Doka KJ, ed. *Children, Adolescents and Loss: Living with Grief.* Washington, DC, Hospice Foundation of America, 2000, p. 131.

Walsh, F, McGoldrick, M: *Living Beyond Loss: Death in the Family,* 2nd ed. New York, W.W. Norton, 2004.

Webb NB: Play therapy to help bereaved children. In: Doka KJ, ed. *Children, Adolescents and Loss: Living with Grief.* Washington, DC, Hospice Foundation of America, 2000, p. 78.

Wolfelt A: *Helping Children Cope with Grief*. Bristol, Accelerated Development, 1983.

Wolfelt A: *A Child's View of Grief: A Guide for Caring Adults*. Houston, TX, Service Corporation International, 1990.

Worden, JW: *Children and Grief: When a Parent Dies*. New York, Guilford Publications, 2001.

RESOURCES FOR GRIEVING CHILDREN
Books for Children

Aliki: *The Two of The*. New York, Harper Publisihers, 1987.

Blackburn LB: *The Class In Room 44-When A Classmate Dies*. Omaha, NE, Centering Corporation, 1991.

Boulden JJ: *Saying Goodbye*. Weaverville, CA, Boulden Publishing, 1992.

Brown, LK, Brown MT: *When Dinosaurs Die: A Guide to Understanding Death*. Boston, Little, Brown Books, 1996.

Brown MW: *Dead Bird*. New York, Harper Collins, 1995.

Buchanan-Smith D: *A Taste of Blackberries*. New York, Harper Collins, 1992.

Buscaliglia L: *The Fall of Freddie the Leaf*. Austin, TX, Holt, Rinehart and Winston, 1982.

Clifton L: *Everett Anderson's Goodbye*. Austin, TX, Henry Holt & Company, Inc., 1988.

DePaola T: *Nana Upstairs, and Nana Downstairs*. New York, Penguin Young Readers, 2000.

Douglas R: *Rachel and the Upside Down Heart*. New York, Penguin Group, 2006.

Fassler J: *My Grandpa Died Today*. New York, Behavioral Publications Co., 1971.

Harris RH: *Goodbye Mousie*. New York, Margaret K. McElderry Books, 2001.

Hazen, Barbara Shook: *Why Did Grandpa Die?* New York, Random House Children's Books, 1985.

Heegaard M: *When Someone Very Special Dies*. Minneapolis, Woodland Press, 1998.

Johnson J, Johnson M: *Tell Me, Papa*. Brooklyn, Center for Thanatology, 1980.

Krementz J: *How it Feels when a Parent Dies*. New York, Knopf, 1991.

Levine Jennifer: *Forever in My Heart*. Burnsville, NC, Compassion Books, 1992.

McNamara Jill: *My Mom is Dying*. Minneapolis, Augsburg Fortress, 1994.

Parker MB: *Jasper's Day*. Tonawanda, NY, Kids Can Press, 2002.

Romain T: *What on Earth Do You Do When Someone Dies?*. Minneapolis, Free Spirit Publishing, 1999.

Schwiebert P, DeKlyen C: *Tear Soup*. Portland, OR, Grief Watch, 1999.

Shavatt D, Shavatt E: *My Grieving Journey Book*. Mahwah, NJ, Paulist Press, 2001.

Simon N: *The Saddest Time*. Park Ridge, IL, Albert Whitman, 1986.

Van-Si L, Powers L: *Helping Children Heal From Loss*. Portland, OR, Portland State University, 1994.

Viorst J: *The Tenth Good Thing About Barney*. New York, Atheneum, 1972.

Wilhelm H. *I'll Always Love You*. New York, Dragonfly Books, 1988.

Winsch JL: *After the Funeral*. Mahwah, NJ, Paulist Press, 1995.

Wolfelt A: *Healing Your Grieving Heart: 100 Practical Ideas for Kids*. Ft. Collins, CO, Companion Press, 2000.

Yolen Jane: *Granddad Bill's Song*. New York, Penguin Young Readers, 1998.

Zalben Jane: *Pearl's Marigolds for Grandpa*. New York, Simon & Schuster, 1997.

Books for Teens:

Blume J: *Tiger Eyes*. New York, Random House, 1982.

Fitzgerald H: *The Grieving Teen: A Guide for Teenagers and Their Friends*. Wichita, KS, Fireside (also available in downloadable digital edition), 2000.

Fry VL: *Part of Me Died, Too: Stories of Creative Survival among Bereaved Children and Teenagers*. New York, NY, Dutton Books, 1995.

Gootman M: *When a Friend Dies: A Book for Teens About Grieving and Healing*. Minneapolis, Free Spirit Publishing, 2005.

Gravelle K: *Teenagers Face to Face with Bereavement*. Englewood Cliffs, NJ, Silver Burdett Press, 1989.

Grollman EA: *Straight Talk about Death for Teenagers: How to Cope with Losing Someone You Love*. Boston, MA, Beacon Press, 1993.

Grosshandler-Smith J: *Coping when a Parent Dies*. New York, Rosen Publishing Group, Inc, 1995.

Hughes L: *You Are Not Alone: Teens Talk About Life After The Loss of a Parent*. New York, Scholastic, Inc., 2005.

Kolf JC: *Teenagers Talk about Grief*. Grand Rapids, MI, Baker. Publishing Group, 1990.

Krementz J: *How it Feels When a Parent Dies*. New York, Knopf, 1988.

Myers E, Adams K: *When Will I Stop Hurting? Teens, Loss, and Grief.* Lanham, MD, Rowman & Littlefield Publishers, Inc., 2004.

Meyers K: *Truth about Death and Dying.* New York, Facts on File, Inc., 2005.

Samuel-Traisman E: *Fire in My Heart, Ice in My Veins: A Journal for Teenagers Experiencing a Loss.* Omaha, NE, Centering Corporation, 1992.

Wolfeldt A: *Healing Your Grieving Heart for Teens: 100 Practical Ideas.* Fort Collins, CO, Companion Press, 2001.

Internet Resources:

http://www.centerforloss.com/.
http://kidsaid.com/.
http://www.newhope-grief.org/teengrief/.
http://www.wnyafn.com/teengrief/.
http://www.dougy.org/.
http://www.centeringcorp.com/catalog/index.php.
http://www.compassionbooks.com/store/.
http://santaclaracountylib.org/kids/lists/death_dying_grieving.html.

SELF-ASSESSMENT QUESTIONS

1. All of the following are myths associated with children and grief in this culture EXCEPT?

    A. It is best to protect a child from experiencing grief
    B. Children should only be allowed to attend funerals and memorials if they choose to
    C. Children do not have the capacity to really understand death and grief
    D. Children are more resilient than adults and quickly "bounce back" after a loss

2. All of the following are considered typical grief reactions for infants and toddlers (until about age 4) EXCEPT:

    A. Anxiety related to the separation from a major attachment figure
    B. Understanding that death is final and irreversible.
    C. Irritability, protest, and crying
    D. Changes in eating and sleeping patterns
    E. Do not envision that death is something that can happen to them

3. All of the following are considered the important factors that influence how a child and teenager respond to grief and loss EXCEPT:

    A. Developmental level and chronologic age
    B. Nature of the relationship with the person that has died
    C. Child's own personality
    D. What they are taught about death and grief from adults
    E. Whether they know how to read or not

4. Which of the following behaviors exhibited by a child to the loss of a significant loved one is most likely to require trained, professional help to resolve?

    A. Memory difficulties
    B. Searching behavior
    C. Difficulty concentrating

    D. Preoccupation with memories of the deceased
    E. Idealization of the deceased

5. According to Alan Wolfelt, all of the following characteristics indicate that a child is beginning to adjust to the loss of a significant loved one EXCEPT:

    A. Return to stable eating and sleeping patterns
    B. Decision to forget their loved one and move on
    C. Increased thinking and judgment capabilities
    D. Establishment of new and healthy relationships.

6. Which of the following is considered a complicated grief reaction in a teenager?

    A. Assuming mannerisms, traits or wearing clothes of the deceased.
    B. Emotional regression and even bed-wetting, which can be most upsetting for teenagers.
    C. Becoming overly responsible (the "new" man or woman of the house)
    D. Prolonged sleep disturbances, including insomnia and nightmares
    E. Needing to repeat again and again stories of their loved one

7. All of the following are considered behaviors associated with complicated grief in a child or teenager EXCEPT:

    A. Excessive rumination about having caused the death
    B. Extreme withdrawal, isolation, and inability to socialize with others
    C. Pervasive fantasies that get in the way of normal functioning
    D. Anger and lashing out seemingly for no reason
    E. Persistent assumption of the mannerisms of the deceased, including those not developmentally appropriate

8. All of the following are considered appropriate interventions in preparing a child for the death of a loved one EXCEPT:

   A. It is important to wait to tell the child until just before the loved one dies so the child does not carry unnecessary anxiety prior to the death.
   B. The child should be told that the images they see of death in television cartoons are not always authentic and that death is irreversible
   C. The adult should use adjectives like "very very old" or "very very sick" to help the child distinguish between getting a cold and someone with a terminal illness
   D. If the child is old enough to understand what is happening and both the child and the dying person would like the visit, the child should be allowed to visit.
   E. If the child does not want to visit, a supportive adult should attempt to elicit why the child is resistant, but the child's wishes should be honored.

9. All of the following are helpful interventions by an adult who is trying to help a grieving child EXCEPT:

   A. Assure the child with specifics about how his or her care giving needs will be met.
   B. Keep the child in their environment and continue their routine as much as possible
   C. Tell the child that God wanted their loved one and that is why he or she died can be comforting to a child.
   D. Adults should not use children as their sole support during their grief.
   E. Respect a child's desire to not talk about their grief

10. All of the following are helpful interventions that an adult can use with a grieving child who is angry EXCEPT:

    A. Be direct and ask the child to "calm down."
    B. Help the child dissipate the anger by running or exercising
    C. Involve the child in art work such as scribbling, ripping paper, sculpting dough, etc.
    D. Ask questions like, "What usually leads to your feeling angry?" "How does your body tell you that you are becoming angry?"
    E. Ask the child what he or she thinks are more appropriate ways of responding to angry feelings.

End-of-Life Care and Critical Care: The Emergency Department and the Intensive Care Unit

Joel S. Policzer and Forrest O. Beaty

END-OF-LIFE CARE AND THE EMERGENCY DEPARTMENT

The emergency department (ED) in a hospital plays many roles. As its very basic role, it has been designed to be a place in the health care system for transition and triage, the point of entry to health care for people who require unexpected, unplanned life-saving or life-protecting treatments. It has become, in addition, the center to provide care for people with acute illnesses, exacerbation of longstanding chronic illness and trauma. Secondarily, it can provide care for people with a terminal illness who have no other support in the health care system. And, finally, it is a place of transition from one health care setting to another.

THE CAPACITY ISSUE

Most hospital EDs perceive that they are operating "at" capacity or are "over" capacity, especially EDs in urban areas, in hospitals with Level 1 trauma centers, and in hospitals with greater than 300 beds. There are many factors that contribute to this, and they are the same factors that contribute to the stresses on other parts of the health care system. The aging population, with an aggregate of multiple chronic health problems will, of necessity, require more visits to the ED when there is an exacerbation of any one or more of these health problems. The decreasing length of stay of patients in hospitals results in patients being moved out while still requiring the care of skilled nurses or while not fully healed; if posthospital follow-up is not scrupulously planned for, the patient will return to the ED at the first sign of any perceived complication. The shortage of registered nurses affects this care setting as it does all others; fewer nurses mean longer wait times for patients to be assessed and to enter the system. There is now pressure on the ED staff for productivity and the need for them to move growing numbers of increasingly complex patients through the system in a shorter period of time, resulting in decreased time for the staff to actually spend with patients. In addition, as of this writing, there are large numbers of patients who have no payment source for health care and who use the ED as their primary care clinic. Finally, the increasing fragmentation of the health care system, where clinics and physicians refer patients who appear to have acute problems to the ED after-hours, or sometimes even during working hours, results in overload of this care area.

PATIENT DEMOGRAPHICS

In 2002, Sanders already noted the disproportionate use of ED services by the elderly, reporting that while people 65 years of age or older made up 12% of the population, they represented 43% of ED visits and a similar percentage of admissions to the ICU from the ED. The primary diagnosis for ED utilization was congestive heart failure, and, not surprisingly, a large percentage of these visits occurred at night or on weekends, often as transfers from extended-care facilities. One can only imagine that this situation has worsened in the years since that study was published.

These elderly, compromised patients with multiple illnesses do not fit the "ideal" portrait of an ED patient: a patient whose illness has an unambiguous treatment and prognosis, whose illness is easily treated or triaged, and who is cooperative and compliant. They are best off not being treated in an ED, yet they are, as highlighted by the following, somewhat typical, patient example.

A.S., an 84-year-old man with chronic obstructive lung disease and congestive heart failure as his main illnesses, presents for the third time in 2 months to the ED for increasing shortness of breath. The patient admits to noncompliance with using his supplemental oxygen, cannot clearly remember taking his oral medications, but does recall using his nebulizer treatments multiple times. During his last crisis a few weeks ago, the patient required intubation but was successfully weaned after 72 hours. He was then briefly transferred to a skilled facility for pulmonary rehabilitation and teaching and then he returned home. The patient's primary physician is semiretired and does not take any calls; the patient relies on ED physicians, hospitalists, and pulmonary consultants for his care; however, he no longer drives and is unable to follow-up with posthospital visits. The patient's wife has dementia of increasing severity and it is the patient's responsibility to watch over her and keep her safe. She interferes with his care because she dislikes the noise of the oxygen concentrator and disconnects it when it is in use. The couple has two children who live close by but neither is able to assume responsibility for the care of their parents due to their own medical and social issues; the children are concerned that their parents are not being able to obtain their medication and may not even be able to get and prepare food. The patient is treated with diuretics in the ED and is responding well; it is not clear whether he will require acute hospitalization or not.

As one can see, this patient has many needs which are not currently being adequately met. The patient requires more structure to his situation. His needs include: more support and supervision to make certain that he has a supply of medications and is taking them appropriately; assistance in caring for his wife for whom he has become the primary caretaker despite his own worsening medical problems; adequate access to sustenance; and access to medical care in a setting that would prevent basic medical problems from escalating to the level of requiring a visit to the ED. In addition, there is the need for someone to sit with the patient and his family and assist them in developing goals of care so that future options for care are clarified and in accordance with what the patient wants for himself.

THE CULTURE OF ED CARE

Our medical culture is one of "rescue" and EDs are set up so that the priority of care for the emergency clinician is based on the severity of the illness or injury; the most severely ill or injured receive the most care and attention. The person at highest risk of unanticipated or unwanted death immediately goes to the top of the priority list. And it is precisely this culture of "rescue" that throws into relief the tension points between ED care and traditional end-of-life care.

First, end-of-life care assumes that there has been acceptance by the patient and family unit of the fact that the patient's death is inevitable and that adequate advance care planning has been done. It is nearly impossible for adequate advance planning to be done in the ED at the time of exacerbation of a chronic illness. The ED staff does not have sufficient clinical knowledge about the patient, nor a long-term relationship, to advise the patient and family about their options in an appropriate and compassionate manner.

Second, end-of-life care assumes that the trajectory of the patient's illness is known and fits into one of the known models of deterioration of a chronic illness. The ED is a place where illnesses are acute, visits are unexpected, and death often occurs without a trajectory.

Third, end-of-life care rests on the fact that there is sufficient time for a patient's needs to be palliated as they proceed through the trajectory of the terminal illness. However, time is clearly not a commodity in large supply in an ED.

Finally, end-of-life care incorporates the concept that care does not end with the patient's death; at that point the focus of care shifts from the patient to the family in the form of bereavement care. However, the ED is traditionally structured to see the patient alone as the focus of care, rather than viewing the patient and family as the unit of care, as is done by end-of-life (EOL) providers. This inability to provide care to a family after a patient's death may lead to more complicated grief and bereavement for families who have suffered the loss of a loved one in the ED, and can also result in increased distress in members of the ED staff.

COLLABORATION BETWEEN THE ED AND END-OF-LIFE CARE PROVIDERS

How can EOL care models that are available in the community assist the ED and its staff in caring for these patients?

The ED staff is often faced with "frequent flyers" in their department, patients who, lacking other options or resources, use the ED as their primary care provider. Therefore, the staff is often able to recognize the transitions that are occurring in these patients as they progressively deteriorate and require more care and structure in their lives.

Palliative care services have developed many facilities that can serve patients in these situations well. As these patients present to the ED for care of their various illnesses and attendant exacerbations, palliative care professionals can be asked to see the patients and their families to assist in care and decision making. Often, patients will continue to pursue aggressive interventions, perceived to be disease modifying, because they are unaware either of the lack of benefit of these interventions or of the existence of alternatives. When patients are informed that their current pattern of care, always returning to the hospital ED for any change in status or worsening of their symptoms, need not occur, they may well choose to pursue other options. These options either are referral to community, home-based palliative care services, if they exist, or referral to a hospice, if the patient is terminally ill. Although there is little data available, it is believed that the majority of patients who are referred to a palliative care service for evaluation and consultation are actually terminally ill and hospice-appropriate at the time of referral.

Of course, patients do not need to be frequent visitors to the ED for benefit to be derived from hospice or palliative care interventions. Any patient who is assessed to be in a life-threatening situation where aggressive care would not be warranted can access this type of care. Consider the following case:

Ms. R.D. is a 67-year-old woman with advanced amyotrophic lateral sclerosis. She is a widow and has no children, but does have a personal caregiver who is now with her 24 hours per day. She has been deteriorating steadily over the past few months and has an advance health care directive which specifies that she is not to be resuscitated and does not wish to have artificial feedings initiated. She has been using a BiPAP device that was started to maximize ventilation during sleep, but she is now using it during the day as well.

Family members have been advised of her deterioration, and they have come from a distance to say their goodbyes. Among them is a brother, with whom she has not been close for a number of years and his wife, a registered nurse. As Ms. D's respiratory status begins to worsen, the anxiety of her family members increases as well and the sister-in-law impulsively calls 911; the paramedics arrive and take her to the ED, without the documentation contained in her advance directive. Once the family members arrive in the ED as well, they began to lobby for aggressive interventions including endotracheal intubation and mechanical ventilatory support. However, when her caregiver arrived she informed the family and staff that this is exactly *not* what the patient wanted for herself. She takes it upon herself to return to the patient's residence to retrieve the advance directive.

Faced with competing interests and goals, a nonrelated caregiver who knows exactly what the patient wants and has documentation to prove it, and a family, who may have been peripheral for years, but are now present and vocal, the ED staff is able to obtain a rapid evaluation by the palliative care service. These professionals are able to quickly arrange a family meeting with family members, an ED representative, and the caregiver to discuss goals of care and immediate care planning. Fortunately, the family is able to verbalize that their desire for aggressive care is due to guilt over their lack of involvement in Ms. D's life and they are able to defer to the patient's wishes. A referral is arranged to a hospice and the patient is taken under care in their inpatient unit to stabilize her respiratory status as best as possible.

Values of Hospice Intervention

Hospice services have a number of roles to play in collaborating care with the ED. A primary role is the ability of a hospice provider to assist with the transfer of patients out of the ED itself. If a patient, for example, requires greater structure to the home environment so that it becomes a safe environment in which to provide care long term, the patient may initially be admitted directly from the ED to a hospice inpatient level of care where the patient's condition will be stabilized, while at the same time, changes in the patient's home environment can be addressed. If the patient's clinical condition does not warrant hospice inpatient care, the hospice can immediately begin to provide services in the patient's place of residence.

A question that is often asked is why should patients be referred to hospice if it is clear that they will survive only a few days or hours, or are actively dying on evaluation? One important answer to this query is that, irrespective of how long or short a time a patient spends on a hospice program, the patient's family will receive bereavement services for a full 12 months after the patient's death. As already mentioned above, bereavement care is a crucial component of EOL care, as it recognizes the needs of the family unit that requires support in order to adjust to the new reality of life without their loved one. Prior to the death of the patient, attention had been focused on the patient and bearing witness to the end of his or her physical life; now to be effective in beginning an appropriate grieving process, there must be a shift in context for bereaved family members to understand the meaning of changes in their lives brought about by their loss. Contin-

ued compassionate contact with the family is one way of assisting in this process. (See Chapter 17 for a full discussion of Grief and Bereavement.)

Hospice services are also of benefit to the ED staff, who routinely move from one stressful situation to another, one disaster to another, one recurring situation to another, and one death to another, without any time to debrief or deal with emotions. Whether termed death overload, grief overload, or compassion overload, the inability of staff to address their emotions will quickly take its toll resulting in job dissatisfaction, dissociation from patients and from their own families, and job burnout. In a worst-case scenario, it may also lead professionals to the abuse of alcohol or other substances to palliate their own distress. Ongoing debriefings with hospice social workers and chaplains will facilitate stress release and healthier behaviors in the staff.

END-OF-LIFE CARE IN THE ICU

Conventional wisdom would seem to hold that palliative EOL care and critical care are complete polar opposites. Critical care does appear to be the pinnacle of modern medical care, fueled by advances in technology starting in the 1950s. Hospice and Palliative Medicine started as counter-cultural movements in the 1970s in response to medicine's perceived nonstop battle against disease, with cure as the only acceptable goal, and with the dying patient seen as the victim of this system. At first glance the basic goals of these care systems also seem to be diametrically opposite: critical care focuses maximal efforts on the saving of life at all costs; palliative care is a care system that accepts death as a natural event.

But on closer inspection, one can see that there is truly a concordance of goals of the two "opposites." Both care models involve the sickest patients in the health care system, who consume large quantities of medical care and resources, not only including provider time and effort, but also interventions and pharmaceuticals as well. For example, it is not unusual for either an ICU patient or a hospice patient to have 8 to 15 medications as part of the plan of care. As Byock has described, the primary goal of each care model is the secondary goal of the other. Critical care has saving or extending life as its primary goal, and decreasing suffering and increasing quality of life as a secondary goal. Hospice and palliative medicine have the mirror image goals: decreasing suffering and increasing quality of life become primary, while saving or extending life assumes secondary roles.

Rather than pushing the models further apart, this situation can actually lead to significant overlap in how these two seemingly disparate models of care are practiced at the bedside. It is well known that ICU patients who have their pain, dyspnea, and other symptoms well-controlled have better outcomes due to more rapid mobilization which decreases their risk of pneumonia and deep vein thrombosis. In a similar fashion, patients cared for by a hospice or palliative care service, whose symptoms are scrupulously controlled, whose treatments and interventions are matched to their goals of care, and who receive ongoing, regular contact from their EOL providers, actually do live longer.

So, is there a role for palliative care in the ICU setting? In the last decade, it was estimated that approximately 20% of Americans died in an intensive care unit, that most ICU deaths involve patients older than 65 years, and that the care consumes almost 80% of all terminal hospitalization costs. As the American population ages and the Boomer generation ages, it is expected that these percentages will rise significantly, resulting in increased demands on an already stressed health care system. Therefore, it is becoming ever more important that patients cared for in the ICU setting receive care that optimally matches their clinical situation and goals: aggressive, disease-modifying care when there is good expectation of return to their previous function, and optimal supportive care when the underlying medical conditions cannot be improved.

Although common sense would dictate that matching care delivery in the ICU with patients' clinical situations and goals should be commonplace and fairly straightforward to accomplish, the fact is that there are several barriers that impede this from occurring: the increasing lack of continuity of care between the community and acute care hospitals, the culture of the ICU, and the difficulties inherent in determining the prognosis of critically ill patients. These barriers are discussed below, following which the vital role of palliative care services in overcoming these challenges will be explored.

CONTINUITY OF CARE

It is an accepted concept that the provider who knows the person best, whether physician, advance practice nurse, or physician assistant, will deliver optimal care to the patient based on the knowledge acquired from the close, ongoing provider–patient relationship: the clinician who knows the patient will know what the patient's goals are and how he or she wants care delivered in various situations. In addition, by knowing the clinician, the patient will have a higher level of confidence that the care being provided include the best and most appropriate interventions for the specific clinical situation. Confirming this, it has been shown that when there is continuity of care across care settings, there are positive outcomes: ED visits decrease, hospitalizations decrease, and health care expenditures decrease.

On the other hand, if a physician cares for a patient who is not well known to him, and where goals of care are not well established, it is not unusual for extra tests to be done and extra care to be given, resulting in outcomes that are often less than optimal. Consider the following scenario:

A patient develops a chronic cough. Is the patient's cough due to side effects of angiotensin-converting enzyme (ACE) inhibitor treatment of hypertension or a sign of significant lung disease? Although the patient's usual provider will likely know the answer to this, if the patient sees another provider and does not relate the cough to the initiation of the antihypertensive therapy, it is much more likely that the clinician will order a chest x-ray. When the x-ray is reported to show a small density in the right lower lobe which the patient's usual provider knows has been present and unchanged for years, and which the patient may have forgotten, the new provider, not knowing that this is an old lesion will recommend a biopsy. The patient has the biopsy, and suffers a pneumothorax as a complication.

Clearly, better continuity of care would have avoided the x-ray, the biopsy, and the pneumothorax.

Care delivery in our health care system continues to fragment. When patients are not clear who their physician or practitioner is, or when they are being shuffled from one primary care provider to another, they are much more likely to go to the ED or urgent care clinic rather than their provider's office when they become ill. As physicians are more often practicing in group settings and confining their activities to the outpatient setting, hospital care is increasingly being left in the hands of hospitalists who are not familiar with the acutely ill patients under their care. Aggravating the situation further is that upon discharge, if the patient is unable to return home, care is likely to be rendered by another group of providers in skilled and long-term care facilities, who again, are unfamiliar with the patient or the patient's health care goals and wishes. Even if the patient returns to outpatient care, there is a better than even chance that they will return to a different physician or provider. Each transition breaks down the continuity of care further, increasing the chances that patients will receive care that they do not desire and the likelihood of a poor and/or undesired outcome. Sadly, it is now estimated that over 60% of patients experience one or more such care transitions during the last 3 months of life.

The effect of the presence or lack of continuity of care on critical care has been explored by Sharma et al. In a retrospective review of the care of advanced lung cancer patients, they found that while nearly three-quarters of the study patients had care given continuously by one provider in an outpatient setting, the percentage of patients followed by that provider on transition to an inpatient setting, decreased during the study period, from 60% in 1992 to 51% in 2002. Further investigation showed that of the patients who had a continuous usual provider, 18% received ICU care during their final hospitalization while more than 22% of patients spent time in the ICU if they were not being cared for by their usual provider in the inpatient setting.

Needless to say, the lack of continuity of care in the inpatient setting (or any other health care setting for that matter) results in a lack of provider knowledge regarding health care choices and goals of care and increases provider reluctance to discuss these issues with patients and families.

ICU CULTURE

Baggs has noted that critical care units are places where the "culture" of the unit has a significant impact on the way care is given. Because of their origins in the technological advances of the last century, it is not surprising that critical care units are technology-intensive areas. Ventilators, hemodynamic monitoring devices, bedside dialysis, and so on are common. Nor should it be surprising that the assumption is made that patients who access this type of aggressive care do so because this is what they desire. If a patient does not want to be hooked up to machines and lines, why is this patient here in the first place?

In addition to the general philosophy of the ICU being one of invasive, high-tech care aimed at cure, the approach to ICU care can also be affected by the physicians in charge of and/or providing care to patients. For example, surgical ICUs generally adopt the personal philosophy of surgeons, who, by the nature of their chosen field, tend to focus on cure. Therefore, they are much more likely to be of the view that in the ICU the goal of the patient is to survive, resulting in the continuation of disease-directed care until all treatment options have been exhausted. In such ICUs, EOL care decisions usually revolve around the withdrawal of life-sustaining interventions at a time when death appears imminent, often times only hours before a patient's expected demise. Under these circumstances, patients often receive care that, if they or their families had been able to make their wishes known through earlier goals of care discussions, might have been avoided.

Medical specialists, especially in the critical care specialty fields such as cardiology and pulmonology, often view the goals of ICU in a similar way. However, they, as well as many primary care physicians involved in caring for patients in the ICU, have more recently been able to shift their focus in a more utilitarian direction when encountering patients who are destined not to do well. Under these circumstances, they are becoming more able to adopt a perspective that considers optimal utilization of resources, and a "hope for the best, but prepare for the worst" attitude. Therefore, they are becoming increasingly comfortable moving away from disease-driven care earlier in the ICU course, usually when it is apparent that the patient is ventilator-dependent and will require a tracheostomy, or when a percutaneous endoscopic gastrostomy (PEG) tube is required for artificial nutritional support. The need for these interventions often open the door that allows the physicians caring for the patient, or the palliative medicine specialist asked to consult, to discuss goals of care with the patient and/or the family earlier than would be the case in the surgical ICU setting.

PROGNOSTIC UNCERTAINTY

On admission to an ICU setting, there is usually congruence between patient and physician goals: the attempt to cure or significantly ameliorate a life-threatening medical problem and restore the patient to the optimum achievable level of health.

However, as care progresses, if patient's clinical condition does not rapidly resolve, it becomes increasingly less certain whether the patient will or will not recover from the acute situation. This prognostic uncertainty makes it difficult to know when to consider the option of shifting care from a disease-directed life-saving focus to a palliative one, and when to have goals of care conversations to consider the various options. Making such discussions even more complicated is that only approximately 5% of patients in an ICU can participate in their own decision-making, so these discussions are usually held with family members who are usually under tremendous stress due to their loved one's illness, and may not always have knowledge of what interventions the patient would desire in the current critical care situation.

There are tools available that, in theory, are designed to assist clinicians in prospectively predicting which patients being cared for in an ICU setting are likely to continue benefiting from critical care and which are not, allowing physicians to identify with which patients and families to have goals of care and EOL care conversations. However, in practice, these tools have not been found to be reliable enough to utilize on a routine basis. In a review of ICU outcome predictive models by Barnato and Angus, they reported that currently existing tools, even if they are well-calibrated for a specific population, do not appear to have predictive ability; the models are always retrospective, not prospective. For example, one can determine that a population of patients in a defined age group, with specific circulatory and vascular function, when treated with a specific intervention, will have a certain outcome when viewed retrospectively. However, one cannot prospectively predict that this outcome will occur in other patients, and one can certainly not generalize from these findings.

A major flaw in these models is that they do not factor in the quality-of-life issues, which for many patients play a major role in their decisions regarding the various interventions and options of care presented to them. It has been shown that people will choose an intervention with a high symptom burden if the chance of survival is worth the effort for them. Conversely, more than 75% of people will avoid a treatment of even low burden if the outcome includes significant functional or cognitive impairment, which they perceive as a reduction in quality of life. It is not survival alone, but the quality of continued survival, that significantly affects patient and family decision making regarding whether or not to initiate or continue specific interventions.

Another barrier to the utilization of these models is physician resistance. Often times, physicians caring for patients have more information on the patients than can be entered into a model, and such information may be relevant in the decision making for that particular individual. In addition, physicians may perceive a loss of professional authority when using one of these models to predict patient outcomes as opposed to relying on their clinical judgment. They may also fear legal reprisal if they follow the recommendations of the predictive model, and the outcome is not consistent with what was predicted.

PALLIATIVE CARE CONSULTATIONS IN THE ICU

Many ICU deaths today involve withholding or withdrawing life-sustaining treatments. Therefore, goals of care discussions leading to decisions involving EOL care are frequently held in these settings. During these conversations, it has been observed that physicians spend 70% of this "discussion" time speaking and telling, and only 30% actually listening. Families consider these discussions to be of crucial importance, actually ranking the importance of physicians' communication skills as high or even higher than the physicians' clinical skills. Communication involves receiving information as well as transmitting it, and the more time a family spends talking the more satisfied the family feels with the care.

Unfortunately, many physicians working in the critical care areas have neither the time nor the specific training to have meaningful goals of care and decision-making conversations with the families of patients being cared for. Therefore, in an effort to improve communication efforts with these families (and, of course, those patients who can participate in the conversations themselves), palliative care consultations provided by physicians and/or nurse practitioners with specialty level training in palliative care, sometimes with the support of other members (i.e., social workers and/or chaplains) of the interdisciplinary palliative care team, are being offered in many institutions in order to facilitate this process. Although at present, these consults are most often called when it is already apparent that a patient is not going to have positive outcome, they may also be requested earlier in the course of illness, when a patient's clinical course and outcome are still uncertain, allowing families to make the patient's wishes known to the physician(s) before a crisis ensues, reducing the risk that the patient will receive care that is not desired.

Although palliative care consultations have only been provided in the ICU setting during the last several years, studies looking at the effectiveness of improving communication between patients/families and critical care staff are available. One study evaluating the outcomes of mandated ICU conferences between clinical staff, physicians and nurses, and family within 72 hours of ICU admission demonstrated a decreased length of stay in the critical care unit for patients who ultimately die.

Another study on this topic evaluated the effectiveness of proactive ethics consultations (a precursor to palliative care consultations) that were mandated for patients in the ICU who had been on a ventilator for more than 96 hours. The stated goals of the consultation were to determine if an advance directive was in place; if so did the patient still have capacity to make health care decisions or if not, who, if anyone, was the designated health care surrogate; were there barriers to recovery; and were there any other unresolved issues. An additional purpose of the consultation was to facilitate discussion between the family and clinicians. Patients who had these consultations performed were more likely not to choose to life-sustaining treatment and the length of stay in the ICU decreased by 6 days.

These findings were then confirmed in randomized controlled studies in both a single-institution and a multicenter trial. When there were "values-based conflicts" between providers and families, or within families, palliative care consultations resulted in an average decrease of 9 days length of stay in the ICU, a decrease in life-sustaining treatments, but no decrease in overall mortality. In other words, palliative care consultations in an ICU setting does not result in an increase mortality of patients, rather they allow patients to receive the type of care they want in the setting where it is wanted.

In summary, it can be seen that critical care and palliative care are not mutually exclusive in their goals and each has the ability to enhance the care given in the alternative setting. As physicians and other providers recognize this, it will be possible to begin the most critical intervention early in the ICU stay: goals of care communication between the critical care physicians and staff, and the patient's family. Families have the burden of making the majority of decisions for ICU patients, often with little prior guidance from their loved one, and most of these revolve around whether or not to continue life-sustaining treatments. Optimal outcome for the critically ill patient involves solid, ongoing communication between the family and all of the health care team, regardless of discipline or specialty, and with the family knowing that they were listened to and their viewpoints were valued.

BIBLIOGRAPHY

Arnold RM, Kellum J: Moral justifications for surrogate decision making in the intensive care unit: Implications and limitations. *Crit Care Med* 31: S347-S353, 2003.

Aulisio MP, Chaitin E, Arnold RM: Ethics and palliative care consultation in the intensive care unit. *Crit Care Clin* 20:505-523, 2004.

Baggs JG, Norton AS, Schmitt MH, et al: Intensive care unit cultures and end-of-life decision making. *J Crit Care* 22:159-168, 2007.

Barnato AE, Angus DC: Value and role of intensive care unit outcome prediction models in end-of-life decision making. *Crit Care Clin* 20:345-362, 2004.

Byock I: Improving palliative care in intensive care units: Identifying strategies and interventions that work. *Crit Care Med* 34:S302-S305, 2006.

Buchman TG, Cassell J, Ray SE, et al: Who should manage the dying patient? Rescue, shame, and the surgical ICU dilemma. *J Am Coll Surg* 194:665-673, 2002.

Chan CK: End-of-life models and emergency department care. *Acad Emerg Med* 11:78-86, 2004.

Curtis JR: Communicating about end-of-life care with patients and families in the intensive care unit. *Crit Care Clin* 20:363-380, 2004.

Mosenthal AC: Palliative care in the surgical ICU. *Surg Clin N Am* 85:303-313, 2005.

Pawlik TM, Curley SA: Ethical issues in surgical palliative care: Am I killing the patient by "letting him go"? *Surg Clin N Am* 85(2):2753-2786, vii, 2005.

Schneiderman LJ, Gilmer T, Teetzel HD, et al: Effect of ethics consultations on nonbeneficial life-sustaining treatments in the intensive care setting: A randomized controlled trial. *JAMA* 290:1166-1172, 2003.

Sharma G, Freeman J, Zhang D, Goodwin JS: Continuity of care and ICU utilization during end of life. *Arch Intern Med* 169:81-86, 2009.

SELF-ASSESSMENT QUESTIONS

1. Which of the following statements about care delivered in a hospital Emergency Department (ED) is true:

   A. Elderly patients with chronic medical problems are best evaluated in the ED when they experience exacerbation of symptoms.

   B. Decreasing length of stay in hospitals is a reason for increased use of ED services.

   C. There are sufficient nurses in the ED to allow for the smooth flow of patients.

   D. Being a Level 1 trauma center does not put added stress on the ED because staffing levels are sufficient to account for this status.

   E. Patients' ability to pay has no effect on their utilization of ED services.

2. All of the following statements regarding the utilization of the ED by elderly patients are true EXCEPT:

   A. They represent more than 40% of ED visits.

   B. They represent more than 40% of admissions to the ICU from the ED.

   C. The most common diagnosis for an ED visit is dehydration.

   D. Most of these visits are at night or on weekends.

   E. Most of these visits represent transfers from long-term care facilities.

3. Which of the following characteristics, commonly seen in elderly patients, is the main reason why the ED is not an ideal environment for the chronically ill elderly to receive care?

   A. The patient has a straightforward medical problem with a defined treatment.

   B. The patient has a straightforward medical problem with a defined prognosis.

   C. The patient's problem is easily treated.

   D. The patient requires complex triage management.

   E. The patient is cooperative and compliant.

4. Which of the following statements regarding end-of-life care and the ED is true?

   A. Advance care planning is appropriate in the ED because the problem being treated is straightforward.

   B. The ED staff should have sufficient knowledge of the patient and family wishes to adequately counsel them on end-of-life (EOL) issues.

   C. The ED is able to quickly and appropriately palliate all the patient's needs.

   D. Care does not end with the patient's death and the ED staff should play a role in follow-up with the family for bereavement.

   E. The ED staff should be able to recognize the declining status of patients who return frequently and refer them for hospice/palliative care evaluation.

5. Collaboration between ED and hospice/palliative care (EOL) providers includes the following EXCEPT:

   A. EOL providers can consult with patients and families in the ED to assist in goals of care and advance care planning conversations.

   B. EOL providers can assist in the transfer of patients out of the ED while planning for their needs is underway.

   C. EOL providers can intervene with patients already under hospice care who are inappropriately transferred to the ED.

   D. EOL providers may provide support and counseling to the ED staff.

   E. EOL providers may provide bereavement services to family members providing that the patient receives EOL care for at least 24 hours prior to death.

6. All of the following statements regarding concordance between critical care and EOL life care are true EXCEPT:

    A. Both view patient death as an expected outcome of care.
    B. Both care for the sickest patients in the system.
    C. Both care for patients who consume large quantities of provider time.
    D. Both improve patient outcomes by aggressively controlling patient symptoms.
    E. Palliative care in the ICU improves patient and family satisfaction with care.

7. All of the following statements regarding care in ICU are true, EXCEPT:

    A. Twenty percent of Americans die in an ICU.
    B. Most ICU deaths are in patients older than 65 years.
    C. ICU care consumes approximately 80% of the total costs of terminal hospital care.
    D. A longstanding relationship between the patient and physician results in increased ICU costs.
    E. An increase in ICU utilization both in terms of cost and days of care is due to the fragmentation of the health care system.

8. All of the following statements about the culture of critical care units are true EXCEPT:

    A. ICUs are high-tech, interventional environments.
    B. Surgeons often adopt a "hope for the best, plan for the worst" attitude with patients in the ICU as they deteriorate.
    C. Patients admitted or transferred to the ICU are assumed to have agreed to this type of treatment.
    D. Medical specialists are more comfortable moving away from disease-driven care when patients require interventions such as a tracheostomy for chronic ventilator support.
    E. In surgical ICUs, EOL care decisions usually revolve around withdrawal of life-sustaining in the last days or hours of life.

9. Which of the following statements regarding the ability to predict the prognosis and outcome of ICU patients is true?

    A. Patients and clinicians usually have different goals when the patient is transferred to the ICU and these goals coalesce as care continues.
    B. The majority of patients in the ICU can participate in their own decision making.
    C. Prognostic tools are derived retrospectively and are poor tools to use prospectively to determine the prognosis of an individual patient.
    D. Quality of life is taken into consideration as a factor in prognostic tools.
    E. Physicians are very comfortable using prognostic tools to assist in their decision making on ICU patients.

10. Regarding palliative care consultations and other forms of provider/family communications in the ICU, which of the following statements is true?

    A. When speaking with families, physicians typically spend most of the encounter time listening.
    B. Family meetings increase the length of stay of ICU patients because families come to understand the need for intensive interventions.
    C. Palliative care interventions increase the mortality rate.
    D. Palliative care consultations result in longer ICU stays.
    E. Ethics consultations have been shown to result in an increased number of cases where the patient/family decides to forgo ventilator support.

Hospice in Long-Term Care

Jeffrey M. Kagan and Barry M. Kinzbrunner

INTRODUCTION

As briefly discussed in Chapter 2, it was recognized in the early years of the Medicare Hospice Benefit (MHB) that there was a group of elderly, terminally ill patients who were not able to be served by hospice programs under the terms of the MHB. These were patients that resided in long-term care facilities (LTCFs). At the time the MHB was first crafted, no provision was made to allow hospice to go into these facilities to care for patients living there. Often they had moved from their homes to these facilities due to custodial care needs that could not be met where they had been residing; they now had become terminally ill and had needs requiring care greater than what could be provided by the facility alone, therefore needing the added assistance of a hospice. This led to a modification of the MHB in the late 1980s that recognized the LTCF as the patient's new primary residence and on that basis permitted a hospice, under contractual agreement with an LTCF, to serve terminally patients who resided in the facility.

On the basis of data compiled by the National Hospice and Palliative Care Organization (NHPCO), 28.3% of hospice patients who were cared for and died in 2007 were residents in a LTCF (nursing home 22.8%, residential facility 4.5%), representing a significant percentage of the hospice population and a modest increase from the 27.1% who were cared for and died in 2006. As the general population continues to age and more elderly individuals are expected to reside in LTCFs during the coming years, the percentage of patients receiving end-of-life care in LTCFs is expected to continue to increase at an even more rapid pace. Therefore, it is incumbent upon end-of-life care providers to have a better understanding of how hospice and palliative care can be effectively delivered in a facility setting.

LONG-TERM CARE

WHAT IS LONG-TERM CARE AND WHERE IS IT PROVIDED?

Long-term care is formally defined as "a combination of medical, nursing, custodial, social, and community services designed to help people who have disabilities or chronic care needs, including dementia" (Family Caregiver Alliance, 2009). Less formally, it is about patients, most of them elderly and usually referred to as "residents" or "clients" by the facilities where they reside, who receive services that include but are not limited to those that are health related, that are intended to make their everyday lives easier and safer. Some of the more typical services patients may receive via long-term care include assistance with various activities of daily living (ADLs) such as bathing and dressing, nutritional support, recreation, transportation, medications, and personal fiscal management.

Long-term care may be provided in a wide variety of locations, based on the physical, medical, and emotional needs of the individual. These locations may run the gamut from assistance in an individual's private home all the way to hospitalization in a subacute, rehabilitative, or chronic care hospital. For the purposes of this discussion, however, the definition will be focused primarily on two key types of LTCFs where hospice and palliative care services are traditionally offered today: the skilled nursing facility (SNF) and the assisted-living facility (ALF).

The skilled nursing facility is a place of residence for people who have significant deficits in multiple ADLs and require some degree of around-the-clock care. Although the majority of the patients in SNFs require predominantly custodial care provided by certified nursing assistants under nursing supervision, available services in SNFs include nurses for skilled care (see below), physical, occupational and speech therapists, and social workers and recreational assistants.

For patients who need assistance in ADLs but are independent enough not to require around-the-clock care, long-term care may be provided in an ALF. In addition to receiving supervision or assistance with ADLs, ALF residents will have their activities monitored to help ensure their health, safety, and well-being, and may receive assistance in the coordination of outside health care services and administration or supervision of medications.

A modern approach to providing long-term care that combines the ALF and the SNF is the continuing care retirement community (CCRC), which provides a wide range of facilities and services usually on the same campus. The common theme of the CCRC concept is to allow elders to "Age in Place." A CCRC will usually offer residents the options of living in Independent Senior Apartments if they are relatively independent, an ALF is there if there are some care needs, and an SNF if their needs are around-the-clock. There is the flexibility within the community to allow residents to change levels of care as their needs change. For example, a resident in the ALF who is hospitalized may be temporarily transferred posthospitalization to the SNF for short-term rehabilitation and then later returned to the ALF when his or her condition improves. Individuals also move progressively along the continuum from more to less independent living as their chronic diseases progress, all the while being maintained in familiar surroundings and not requiring relocation to an entirely new and unknown facility.

HOW IS LONG-TERM CARE PAID FOR?

The majority of individuals who reside in assisted living facilities and CCRCs, and a lesser number of persons living in SNFs utilize private funds or long-term care insurance to pay for room and board and their other basic care needs. In addition, some CCRCs have an "entrance fee" to guarantee access to assisted or skilled care as required, while others have the cost of the higher levels of care built into the lease or purchase price of the initial unit occupied by the resident. For patients who are not insured and do not have sufficient assets to pay for long-term care, most states have room and board funds when patients require around-the-clock custodial care in an SNF available through the Medicaid program (Title XIX).

For patients who have skilled nursing needs, there is a limited amount of coverage through Medicare under the Part A "Skilled Nursing Facility Care Benefit." Key features of the Skilled Benefit are listed in Table 29–1. In order to qualify to receive services under the skilled nursing care benefit, a Medicare Part A beneficiary must have been hospitalized for a minimum of 3 consecutive days (including the day of admission but not the day of discharge), be admitted to the facility within 30 days of discharge from the hospital, and have skilled professional care needs either related to the reason for the hospitalization or that developed while already receiving SNF care for

---

TABLE 29–1. Features of Medicare "Skilled Nursing Care Facility Benefit"

- 3-d qualifying hospitalization
- Admission to skilled nursing facility (SNF) within 30 d of the qualifying hospitalization
- Medically necessary skilled care required for the medical condition treated during the hospitalization
- Care only be provided in an SNF inpatient environment
- Maximum coverage for 100 d
  - Reimbursed at 100% for first 20 d
  - Reimbursed at 80% for days 21–100

another reason. The required skilled care must be needed daily (with an exception for skilled rehabilitation therapy services that may only be scheduled 5 or 6 days a week) and can only be provided effectively in an SNF inpatient setting. (For patients receiving care under a Medicare Advantage program, the managed care organization may, in certain cases, choose to waive the 3-day qualifying hospitalization requirement providing they are paying for the skilled care as part of their overall coverage of the patient.)

The maximum number of days that a patient may receive care under the "Skilled Nursing Facility Care Benefit" following a qualifying 3-day hospital is 100 days. The first 20 days of care are fully paid for (including room and board) while days 21 to 100 are covered at 80% of the Medicare rate, with the patient or coinsurance responsible for a 20% copayment. If a patient is discharged from skilled care prior to using the full 100 days, and requires further skilled care within 30 days, they may resume skilled care without needing another qualifying hospitalization. If the 100 days have been used, or more than 30 days lapsed following completion of a skilled episode, then another 3-day qualifying hospitalization would be necessary in order for the patient to access the skilled benefit again.

HOSPICE AND LONG-TERM CARE

HOW IS HOSPICE CARE PAID FOR IN LONG-TERM CARE?

For the purposes of the MHB, LTCFs, including nursing homes and assisted-living facilities, are considered a patient's primary residence. Therefore, when Medicare beneficiaries live in either of these types of facility and are not receiving care under the Skilled Nursing Facility Care Benefit, they are eligible to receive hospice services un-

der the MHB. The basic level of care is identical to the "routine home care" provided to patients living in their own private residences. Higher levels of care may be provided to hospice patients living in a LTCF as well. Continuous care is provided in much the same fashion as it is in patients' homes. General inpatient care for patients living in LTCFs may take one of several forms. If the hospice has a free-standing or hospital-based inpatient facility, the patient may be moved to that facility for the period during which inpatient care is required. However, some hospices may have contracts with LTCFs to provide general inpatient care, in which case, patients living in such a facility will not have to leave the building to receive the higher level of hospice care. Sometimes, the patients will be relocated within the facility, if it has a dedicated hospice inpatient unit or a skilled nursing wing, while in other situations, patients will receive the higher level of services while remaining in their own bed. (For a more thorough discussion of hospice levels of care, see Chapter 2.)

Room and board payments for hospice patients residing in LTCFs and receiving services at either the routine home care or continuous care levels are not covered by the hospice. (For periods where a hospice patient is receiving general inpatient care, the room and board payment is paid for by the hospice if the patient stays in the facility.) For patients who either pay privately or have long-term care insurance to cover room and board, the arrangement with the facility remains the same. For patients who have their room and board paid by the Medicaid program, the payment schema changes somewhat. Rather than the Medicaid program continuing to pay the facility while the Medicare program pays the hospice, the payments for both the hospice services and the room and board are combined, with the room and board rate discounted to 95% of the full amount. This payment, known as the "unified rate," is paid to the hospice provider, who is then responsible to pay the room and board to the facility. The hospice and facility may agree contractually to a different room and board rate than the 95% paid by Medicaid, as long as the agreed upon payment does not exceed 100% of the actual room and board rate the facility would have been paid had the patient not enrolled in the hospice program. This payment schema operates in most states with few exceptions, when patients are dually Medicare and Medicaid eligible.

As mentioned earlier, patients residing in LTCFs can access hospice providing they are not receiving care under the Medicare Skilled Nursing Facility Care Benefit. The reason that both benefits cannot generally be accessed together is because they are both Part A benefits and are considered mutually exclusive. However, there is an exception. If a patient receiving hospice services under the MHB had a qualifying hospitalization for a particular medical condition that required skilled care under the Medicare skilled benefit following hospital discharge and that condition was clearly unrelated to the terminal illness, such a patient could receive services under both benefits.

As an example, suppose that a patient with lung cancer falls and breaks a hip and is hospitalized. If it is determined that the hip fracture is pathologic secondary to metastatic lung cancer, the patient would be unable to access both the hospice benefit and the skilled nursing benefit, and if both services were offered, the patient would have to make a choice as to which service would be best for posthospital care. On the other hand, if the hip fracture was found to be traumatic in nature and not related to the lung cancer, the patient could conceivably access both benefits if eligible, although if the fall were secondary to the debilitating effects of the lung cancer or there was osteoporosis found in the hip secondary to steroids that were being used to treat the lung cancer, one could still make the argument that the conditions were actually related even without evidence of metastatic cancer in the bone. Therefore, as there are no firm guidelines as to what constitutes a related or an unrelated medical condition for the purpose of accessing these two benefits in tandem, and due to the complexity illustrated by the example just discussed, one must be extremely cautious when considering whether this can be done.

It is highly recommended that if it is believed that a patient, such as the one described above, has two unrelated medical problems and is eligible for both hospice and skilled nursing benefits under Medicare, that the patient's attending physician or nursing home medical director, and the hospice medical director, document in the patient's medical record why they believe that the two medical problems are unrelated and that the patient, therefore, is entitled to both benefits.

COLLABORATION BETWEEN THE HOSPICE AND THE LONG-TERM CARE FACILITY

As is always the case when two somewhat disparate organization attempt to work together, hospice and LTCFs need to collaborate effectively in order to meet their common goal, the needs of the patients that they share. Their ability to collaborate with one another is complicated by the fact that both organizations are governed by sets of rules and regulations defined by the federal government and state governments where they operate, and like with many things of governmental origin, the two sets of regulations have not always been interpreted in ways that make them compatible with one another.

To help address this situation, the Hospice Conditions of Participation, revised in 2009, includes a specific section, §418.112, devoted specifically to standards that must be met by hospices that provide care to residents of LTCFs. These standards are listed in Table 29–2 and clearly state that even though the patient resides in the LTCF, it is the hospice that has responsibility for the professional management of the patient's hospice services, including making arrangements for hospice-related inpatient care when necessary, leaving the LTCF responsible for those issues not related to the patient's hospice care. The standards also require that the hospice properly orient and train the LTCF staff that will care for hospice patients, include the LTCF

TABLE 29–2. Features of Hospice Condition of Participation §418.112

- Resident eligibility, election, and duration of benefits same as for all other hospice patients
- Hospice assumes responsibility for professional management of resident's hospice services in accordance with hospice plan of care, including hospice-related inpatient care
- Written agreement between hospice and long-term care facility (LTCF)
- Hospice resident must have a written hospice plan of care, maintained in consultation with the LTCF staff
- Services must be coordinated
- Hospice staff must orient and train LTCF staff caring for hospice patients in hospice policies, procedures, and pain and symptom management

staff in the care planning of hospice residents, and establish documentation and communication requirements to ensure that the care provided to LTCF residents receiving hospice services is coordinated between the two organizations.

Crucial to the success of these standards is the establishment of specific requirements that must be detailed in the written agreement executed between a hospice and LTCF in which the hospice desires to serve patients. These requirements are listed in Table 29–3. By precisely detailing the responsibilities of the hospice staff and the LTCF staff in caring for patients and communicating with each other, it is anticipated that these standards will significantly improve the collaboration between the hospice and LTCFs in caring for patients that they have in common.

Nursing homes, one of the predominant types of LTCFs, have federally mandated requirements that must be adhered to as well, even when patients that they care for are also being cared for by a hospice program. Following admission of a patient, a comprehensive assessment must be performed, using a specific tool called the "Resident Assessment Instrument" (RAI). Incorporated into the RAI is the Minimum Data Set (MDS), which is a comprehensive assessment of a resident's functional capabilities that is utilized to help identify patient problems. Elements of the

MDS are reported to Center for Medicare and Medicaid services (CMS) on a regular basis and are used to assess the quality of care provided in nursing homes. When a problem is identified, the RAI process triggers the nurse caring for the patient to utilize the appropriate "Resident Assessment Protocol" (RAP) to further assess and care plan for the specific problem. A detailed discussion of the RAPs is beyond the scope of this chapter. However, a significant proportion of them, including those for problems such as delirium, cognitive loss, dehydration and fluid maintenance, pressure ulcers, and ADLs, to name a few, may be related to a hospice patient's terminal diagnosis. A major challenge lies in the divergence of goals: nursing home goals of care are generally rehabilitative in nature with a focus on improvement of the condition, while the expected outcomes of many of the aforementioned problems for hospice patients are for gradual deterioration without significant improvement.

In order to avoid conflict, therefore, it is crucial for nursing home and hospice staff to work together to coordinate the plans of care generated by both teams, and to ensure that all interventions and expected outcomes related to hospice problems, including those where improvement is not an expectation, are well documented. To do this, some hospices have adapted their care planning

TABLE 29–3. Requirements for the Written Agreement Between a Hospice and LTCF

- The manner in which the LTCF and hospice will communicate to ensure 24-h per day coverage to meet patient's needs
- The LTCF staff will notify the hospice immediately for the following:
  - A significant change in a patient's physical, mental, social, or emotional state
  - Clinical complications that suggest a need to modify the hospice plan of care
  - A need to transfer the patient to a higher level of care, such as general inpatient care or continuous care for a hospice-related condition
  - The death of a patient
- A provision that it is the hospice's responsibility to determine the appropriate course of hospice care, including determining the need for a change in level of care
- An agreement that the LTCF is responsible to continue to furnish 24-hour room and board care, and meet personal care and nursing needs that would have been provided by a primary caregiver at home
- An agreement that the hospice is responsible to provide services at the same level and extent that would have been provided had the patient been living at home.
- A delineation of the hospices responsibilities to provide all services as defined by the Medicare Hospice Benefit for the care of the patient's terminal illness and related conditions
- A provision that the hospice may use LTCF nursing personnel to assist in the administration of prescribed therapies in the hospice plan of care only to the extent that the hospice would use a patient's primary caregiver or other family members if the patient were living at home.
- A delineation of the responsibilities of the hospice and LTCF staff regarding the provision of bereavement services to the LTCF staff
- A provision that the hospice report to the LTCF administrator all alleged violations involving mistreatment, neglect, injuries of unknown source, or abuse within 24 h of becoming aware of the alleged violation

process and documentation for nursing home patients to be consistent with those found in the RAPs so that the nursing home staff and the hospice staff are on the same page. The hospice will, in adapting their care plans, follow the RAP problem list, use language similar to that used in the RAPs, and update their care plans in a fashion consistent with the RAP process. Goals and interventions will also be similar when appropriate, and because of these similarities, when goals for a hospice patient do not reflect the expected improvement that might be sought for a nursing home patient with a better prognosis, these similarities will lead to the nursing home staff to appropriately document the expected outcome for the terminally ill patient, avoiding both patient care and regulatory challenges. In this way, the facility staff is comfortable with the care provided by the hospice staff, and vice versa, and the patients being cared for by both the hospice and nursing home are the beneficiaries of the combined effort.

THE IMPACT OF HOSPICE CARE IN LONG-TERM CARE

Although it has been documented that LTCF staff perceive that the patients under their care receive good end-of-life care, published data prior to the widespread incorporation of hospice services into long-term care suggest that the reality does not support this perception. These studies have documented a high prevalence of unrelieved pain in facility patients, with such pain resulting in impaired mobility, increased depression, and a decrease in quality of life. Control of dyspnea in this patient population has also been shown to be poor. There were significant deficits reported in advance care planning, resulting in lower rate of documented "do-not-resuscitate" orders and continued widespread and increased use of feeding tubes despite growing evidence that these interventions are of limited or no benefit in patients with advanced dementia and other end-stage neurodegenerative diseases (see Chapters 22 and 24 for further discussion of these issues). Family members also felt that care of their dying loved ones left something to be desired. Studies have shown that families with relatives being cared for in facilities had very low expectations regarding the quality of care their loved ones received, that symptoms and other needs of the patients often went unrecognized and untreated, and that opportunities for advanced care planning and decision making were often missed.

This has all begun to change with the increased presence of hospices, working in collaboration with LTCFs to care for terminally ill patients who reside there. These patients have been reported to receive pain management that is consistent with accepted guidelines. They also have fewer hospitalizations and receive enteral tube feedings and parenteral fluid less often than similar patients not receiving hospice care. In addition, family members have perceived improvement in the care of their terminally ill loved ones following hospice admission.

As an added bonus, likely due to an increase in facility staff education and awareness of pain and symptom management and other aspects of the hospice philosophy of care, nonhospice patients living in facilities that have a significant number of hospice patients benefit as well. When compared with nonhospice facility patients with little or no hospice presence, those in facilities with a large hospice presence have fewer hospitalizations, have pain assessed and treated more frequently, and have dyspnea better managed.

NONHOSPICE PALLIATIVE CARE IN LONG-TERM CARE

As palliative care continues to evolve, and needs are identified for patients who are either not eligible for the MHB or who do not desire to access the benefit, some LTCFs, albeit to date on a limited basis, have attempted to provide such patients with access to palliative care. Some of these efforts have been educational in nature, while others have taken the form of formal consult services, with the primary consultation being provided either by a palliative medicine physician or nurse practitioner. In studies evaluating the success of such efforts, reduction of pain and other symptoms leading to improved quality of life for dying patients have been documented.

CONCLUSIONS

As our population continues to age, it is likely that increasing numbers of elderly individuals will spend their last years of life in a LTCF of some type. As these facilities will become the primary residences for these individuals, and are the likely places where most of their lives will end, it is incumbent upon these facilities to have the skill and compassion to provide appropriate palliative interventions to ensure that their patients receive quality end-of-life care. What better way to accomplish this than for the facilities to develop partnerships with hospice providers. As discussed and demonstrated earlier, by mutual education, open lines of communication on a frequent basis, and clearly delineating the responsibilities of both agencies to the patients and families under their care, LTCFs in partnership with hospices can successfully provide quality hospice and palliative care to patients living in these facilities, so that they live fully until their lives come to a peaceful conclusion.

BIBLIOGRAPHY

Assisted Living. Wikipedia, the free encyclopedia. http://en.wikipedia.org/wiki/Assisted-Living_Facility. Accessed March 24, 2009.

Baer WM, Hanson LC: Families' perception of the added value of hospice in the nursing home. *J Am Geriatr Soc* 48:879-882, 2000.

Bernabei R, Gambassi G, Lapane K, et al: Management of pain in elderly patients with cancer. SAGE study group. *JAMA* 279:1877-1882, 1998.

Buchanan RJ, Chol M, Wang S, Huang C: Analyses of nursing home residents in hospice care using the Minimum Data Set. *Palliat Med* 16:465-480, 2002.

Centers for Medicare and Medicaid Services: *Medicare Coverage of Skilled Nursing Facility Care.* Baltimore, MD, U.S. Department of Health and Human Services, Centers for Medicare & Medicaid Services, 2007.

Family Caregiver Alliance, National Center on Caregiving: Definitions, long-term care. http://www.caregiver.org/caregiver/jsp/content_node.jsp?nodeid=1703. Accessed March 24, 2009.

Ferrell BA: Pain evaluation and management in nursing homes. *Ann Intern Med* 123:681-687, 1995.

Keay TJ, Alexander C, McNally K, et al: Nursing home physician education intervention improves end-of-life outcomes. *J Palliat Med* 6:205-213, 2003.

McKinnon S: *Vitas Coordinated Plan of Care.* Presentation. Miami, FL, Vitas Innovative Hospice Care, 2004.

Miller SC, Gozolo P, Mor V: Hospice enrollment and hospitalization of dying nursing home patients. *Am J Med* 111:38-44, 2001.

Miller SC, Mor V, Teno JM: Hospice enrollment and pain assessment and management in nursing homes. *J Pain Symptom Manage* 26:791-799, 2003.

Miller SC, Teno JM, Mor V: Hospice and palliative care in nursing homes. *Clin Geriatr Med* 20:717-754, 2004.

Mitchell SL, Teno JM, Roy J, et al: Clinical and organizational factors associated with feeding tube use among nursing home residents with advanced cognitive impairment. *JAMA* 290:73-80, 2003.

NHPCO Facts and Figures: *Hospice Care in America.* Alexandria, VA, National Hospice and Palliative Care Organization, 2008.

Nursing home. Wikipedia, the free encyclopedia. http://en.wikipedia.org/wiki/Skilled_nursing_facility. Accessed March 24, 2009.

Reynolds K, Henderson M, Schulman A, Hanson LC: Needs of the dying in nursing homes. *J Palliat Med* 5:895-901, 2002.

Teno JM, Claridge BR, Casey V, et al: Family perspectives on end-of-life care at the last place of care. *JAMA* 291:88-93, 2004.

Teno JM, Weitzen S, Wetle T, Mor V: Persistent pain in nursing home residents. *JAMA* 285:2081, 2001.

Travis SS, Loving G, McClanahan L, Bernard M: Hospitalization patterns and palliation in the last year of life among residents in long-term-care. *Gerontologist* 41:153-160, 2001.

Tuch H, Strumpf N, Stillman D, et al: Developing and integrating palliative care programs in community nursing homes. *J Palliat Med* 6:297-309, 2003.

Weissman DE, Griffin J, Muchka S, Matson S: Improving pain management in long-term care facilities. *J Palliat Med* 4:567-573, 2001.

Wu N, Miller SC, Shield R, et al: The problem of assessment bias when measuring hospice effect on nursing home residents' pain, care in nursing home. *J Pain Symptom Manage* 26:998-1009, 2003.

SELF-ASSESSMENT QUESTIONS

1. On the basis of 2007 data compiled by the National Hospice and Palliative Care Organization (NHPCO), approximately what percentage of hospice patients were residents of a long-term care facility (LTCF)?

   A. 14%
   B. 28%
   C. 42%
   D. 56%
   E. 70%

2. All of the following are features of the Medicare Part A "Skilled Nursing Facility Care Benefit" EXCEPT:

   A. A hospital stay of at least 3 consecutive days within 30 days of admission to the facility.
   B. Skilled care that related to the reason for the hospitalization.
   C. Skilled care that can only be effectively provided in a skilled nursing facility.
   D. Skilled care that must be provided on a daily basis.
   E. Concurrent access to the Medicare Hospice Benefit if the skilled care is related to the patient's terminal diagnosis.

3. All of the following statements regarding care provided to LTCF residents under the Medicare Hospice Benefit are true EXCEPT:

   A. Room and board payments are covered for all patients.
   B. Patients can receive continuous care in the facility.
   C. For Medicaid patients, the "unified rate" payment scheme discounts room and board payments by 5%.
   D. The facility is considered the patient's primary residence.
   E. Patients can receive general inpatient care in the facility.

4. All of the following are standards set by the Hospice Conditions of Participation regarding hospice care provided in LTCFs EXCEPT:

   A. The need for a written agreement between the hospice and the LTCF.
   B. The hospice assumes professional management responsibility for all hospice services in accordance with the hospice plan of care.
   C. The hospice must provide orientation and training to the LTCF staff about hospice care.
   D. Residents living in LTCFs may be eligible for hospice under the Medicare benefit with a prognosis of 1 year or less.
   E. All hospice patients must have a written plan of care that is maintained in consultation with the LTCF staff.

5. According to the written agreement between a hospice and a LTCF, it is required to delineate that in all of the following situations EXCEPT which one must the LTCF staff immediately notify the hospice?

   A. A significant change in the patient's physical or emotional condition.
   B. A visiting family member who demands to speak to the hospice nurse immediately.
   C. Clinical complications that likely require modification of the plan of care.
   D. A need to transfer the patient to a higher level of care for a hospice-related condition.
   E. The death of a patient.

6. All of the following responsibilities must be included in the written agreement between the hospice and the LTCF EXCEPT:

   A. As the patient is living in a facility, the hospice may provide less nursing and nurses aide visits than would be required if the patient were living at home.

B. The hospice is responsible to determine whether the patient requires a change in the level of hospice care.

C. The hospice may use LTCF nursing personnel to assist in the administration of prescribed medications only to the extent that the primary caregiver would provide at home.

D. The LTCF is responsible to meet the personal care and nursing needs that would have been provided by the primary caregiver at home.

E. The hospice is responsible to provide bereavement services and support to LTCF staff.

7. Which of the following is the name of the required nursing home document that is used to assess and care plan for specific problems identified during the comprehensive assessment following admission?

A. RAI

B. MDS

C. RAP

D. CMS

E. ALF

8. All of the following are ways that hospices can coordinate the plan of care with the LTCF staff EXCEPT:

A. Have hospice care plans follow the RAP problem list.

B. Use language in the hospice care plans similar to that used in the RAPs.

C. Update hospice care plans in a fashion consistent with the RAP process.

D. Utilize interventions in hospice care plans similar to those used in RAPs.

E. Set goals for patient improvement as used in RAPs, even when patient improvement is not expected.

9. Prior to the widespread incorporation of hospice services into LTCF, studies regarding the state of end-of-life care in these facilities demonstrated all of the following EXCEPT:

A. A high prevalence of unrelieved pain

B. Poor control of dyspnea

C. A decrease in the use of feeding tubes

D. Low expectations by family members regarding the quality of care of their loved ones

E. A lower rate of "do-not-resuscitate" orders

10. Studies of the impact of hospice services on the care received by LTCF residents have shown all the following EXCEPT:

A. More hospitalizations

B. Less use of feeding tubes

C. Management of pain consistent with accepted guidelines

D. Family perceptions that care is improved

E. Improved dyspnea management in nonhospice LTCFs residents with a large hospice presence

The Geriatric Patient: Pain Management

Jeffrey M. Behrens

INTRODUCTION

The geriatric patient presents a unique challenge when it comes to pain management. Although the basic principles of pain management are the same, regardless of age, the geriatric patients represent a subset of patients with their own set of challenges. Over the years, hospice care has evolved from primarily caring for patients with malignancies to additionally caring for patients with advanced nonmalignant end-stage diseases such as congestive heart failure, COPD, end-stage renal disease, end-stage cerebrovascular disease, and general debility (aka "adult failure to thrive"), to name a few. The majority of these patients are elderly, and as a result, the majority of patients receiving end-of-life care will also be geriatric patients. As there is an entire chapter devoted to the basic principles of pain management (see Chapter 6), this chapter will be devoted to the unique challenges the clinician will face when dealing with the geriatric patient. Therefore, in addition to addressing issues related to patient's specific disease process and following the rules of basic pain management, the clinician will need to know how to adjust those rules in order to take into account the patient's advanced age.

BASIC PRINCIPLES

The key factors that affect how pain is managed in the geriatric population as compared to a younger patient population can be divided into three broad categories: metabolic changes that affect drug absorption and metabolism (i.e., pharmacokinetics and pharmacodynamics), the multifactorial nature of pain in the elderly, and differences in the way pain is reported due to, at least in part, a host of psychosocial factors unique to the older population. Each of these categories is discussed below.

DIFFERENCES IN METABOLISM (PHARMACOKINETICS AND PHARMACODYNAMICS)

Pharmacokinetics refers to the rates of absorption of medications into the body, their distribution through the body, and their metabolism and clearance from the body, while pharmacodynamics refers to the different effects of the same dose of a particular medication on different individuals. As a person ages, changes in pharmacokinetics and pharmacodynamics, listed in Table 30–1, must be accounted for when prescribing analgesia for the management of pain.

Geriatric patients have altered rates of absorption of orally administered pain medications due to changes in gastric pH, gastrointestinal motility, and altered blood flow to the gastrointestinal tract. As a person ages, gastric acid production falls, as does gastric motility. Absorption of drugs across membranes decreases and reduced blood flow results in decreased absorption as well. Therefore, one would expect lower concentrations of drug passed into the blood stream. However, this potential decrease in absorption is counterbalanced to varying degrees by reduced gastric motility, which allows more time for absorption to take place. These complexities require clinicians to carefully titrate medication doses on an individual basis.

TABLE 30–1. Differences in Pharmacokinetics and Pharmacodynamics in Geriatric Patients

Altered rate of drug absorption
Altered protein and fat binding of medications
Altered hepatic clearance of medications
Altered renal clearance of medications
Number of potential drug–drug interactions due to presence of comorbid medical conditions

The distribution of the drug throughout the body is also very dependent on the fat and water contents of the various tissues as well as the lipid and water solubility of the drugs.

In the geriatric patient, there is a decline in the lean body muscle mass, a reduction in the amount of total body water available and an increase in body fat. This affects the water/lipid ratios and, as a result, alters the active concentration of many drugs. The amount of active medication available is also affected by alterations in blood flow to the various organs, changing the amount of drug delivered to various parts of the body, and by the decrease in albumin levels seen in the elderly.

Clearance of the drug from the body is dependant on both the liver and the kidneys. Both of these organs undergo change as the body ages. The kidneys clear drugs based upon glomerular filtration, tubular secretion, and tubular reabsorption. Glomerular filtration is dependent on renal perfusion and renal mass. It is estimated that 25% of the total cardiac output is delivered to the kidneys and approximately 10% of this blood flow is filtered at the glomeruli. Because of a decrease in cardiac output, a decrease in blood flow secondary to vascular factors and age-related loss of renal mass, there is a creatinine clearance loss of 10% per decade after the age of 20.

In addition, comorbid conditions that are commonly seen in geriatric patients further decrease renal function. These include hypertension, diabetes, and atherosclerosis. Not only is renal function diminished by the direct effects of these comorbid conditions, but medications used to treat them also take their toll. For example, ACE inhibitors adversely affect glomerular filtration by decreasing renal perfusion pressures and altering the balance between the afferent and efferent renal arteriole pressures. This effect may exacerbated by the presence of renal artery stenosis, which is also commonly seen in the geriatric patient. Medication used to treat pain, such as the nonsteroidal anti-inflammatory agents (NSAIDs) also alters renal perfusion due to the alteration of prostaglandins that are necessary to dilate the intrarenal arteri-

oles. These alterations in intrarenal blood flow and prostaglandin-mediated vasodilatation also affect the pH within the renal cortex, alter the Na^+ concentrations in the loop of Henle and alter the tubular secretion and reabsorption properties of the kidney.

In the liver, drug metabolism is affected by the amount of drug delivered to it, as well as by changes in the function and effectiveness of various hepatic enzymes. Alterations in circulation commonly seen in the geriatric patient due to congestive heart failure and/or arteriosclerosis also affects delivery of drug to the liver. It has been estimated that there is a 24% to 47% reduction in the blood flow to the liver between the ages of 25 and 90, resulting in a progressive decrease in the hepatic clearance of various medications.

While age-related loss of hepatocytes compounded by comorbid conditions, such as hepatitis or cirrhosis, may also alter the liver's ability to metabolize drugs, the effect of age on hepatic enzyme activity is extremely variable. Some studies have shown decrease in hepatic enzyme activity, while others have shown none. Many of these changes are genetically determined and are not solely dependent on age. However, most studies have shown some decline in phase I and phase II oxidative metabolism but little change in conjugation.

Hepatic enzyme activity may also be affected by other medications that are commonly used in the geriatric population. Phenobarbital and rifampin, for example, are inducers of hepatic microsomal oxidase activity. Cimetidine, on the other hand, inhibits hepatic enzyme activity, as well as decreases hepatic blood flow, both of which will result in significantly lowered drug clearance.

While, as discussed earlier, there is a fair amount of pharmacokinetics data comparing older to younger individuals, there is much less pharmacodynamics data available, and what data does exist has primarily been collected from non-pain drug studies. For example, beta-blockers demonstrate a blunted response in the elderly vs. younger patients while benzodiazepines have been shown to have greater effects on elderly patients. Therefore, although there is no firm data available, one should always be cognizant of the possible enhanced effect of a given dose of a pain medication on a geriatric patient compared to a younger individual, which only serves to emphasize a key principle of pain management: titrating the dose to the needs of the individual patient.

To summarize this section, one should always take into consideration the effects that age will have on the potency and duration of activity of the various pain medications that one may wish to administer. Although one may experience a great deal of variation in analgesic dosages between individuals, the basic premise that should be followed is to "start low and go slow." One should start with the lowest possible effective dose and titrate the dose slowly, depending on the response obtained.

THE MULTIFACTORIAL NATURE OF PAIN IN THE GERIATRIC POPULATION

Unlike their younger counterparts, geriatric patients frequently suffer from pain from multiple sources concurrently. The presence of chronic pain is also more common.

Some studies have shown that between 25% and 50% of all community dwelling people over the age of 60 commonly experience pain. In one study involving interviews of surviving close contacts of deceased patients, 66% of the now-deceased patients had reported pain frequently, or all the time, one month before their death compared to a matched group of surviving patients of whom only 24% had pain. In a study involving 97 nursing home residents in a 311-bed facility, 71% reported between one and four different pain complaints, and out of those, 34% described their pain as constant or continuous and 66% reported their pain as intermittent. Of the 43 subjects with intermittent pain, 51% reported the pain daily. Another study of nursing home residents published in 1996 and reported

TABLE 30–2. Common Causes of Pain in the Geriatric Population

TYPE OF PAIN	FREQUENCY REPORTED (%)
Low back pain	40
Arthritis (RA, OA)	24–37
Cancer	33–75
Previous fracture sites	14
Neuropathic pain (DM, postherpetic)	11
Leg cramps	9
Claudication	8
Headaches (migraine, cluster, temp. art.)	6
Generalized	5

in 2007 gave similar results with 45% to 80% reporting pain. These residents reported daily pain 24% to 38% of the time. A study of 21,380 nursing home residents aged 65 and older, published in 2004 and reported in 2007, identified persistent pain in 49% of the residents with an average age of 83. Table 30–2 lists the most common causes of pain in the geriatric population with an approximation of the reported frequency, while Table 30–3 lists other causes of pain in the elderly for which frequency has not been reported.

DIFFERENCES IN THE REPORTING OF PAIN

There are innumerable reasons why geriatric patients report pain with different frequencies and to different degrees of severity than the younger population. Older patients fear that reporting pain will lead to their loss of independence. Frequently they, as well as their treating physicians, believe that pain is part of the normal aging process. There is also a concern among both elderly patients and their physicians that the treatment of pain with the various analgesics available will lead to untoward side effects that will create

TABLE 30–3. Less Frequent Causes of Pain in the Elderly

Improper positioning/use of restraints	Gastritis, diverticulosis(litis), hiatal hernia
Gout, pseudogout	Chronic pancreatitis, cholilithiasis
PMR	Urinary retention, cystitis
Spinal stenosis (cervical, lumbar)	Chest pain, angina
Osteoporosis (w or w/o fx)	Phantom limb pain
Phlebitis	Myofacial pain
Dental pain	Reflex sympathetic dystrophy
Constipation, fecal impaction, IBS	Post CVA pain

more difficulties than the pain itself. For patients residing in nursing homes, there is a legitimate concern that reporting pain will result in a diagnostic evaluation that will include the burden of having to be transported to outside offices or uncomfortable diagnostic facilities and the need to remain confined for several hours, which will exacerbate their discomfort. In addition, they may suffer the indignity of needing assistance to use the bathroom, potentially miss meals, and risk the side effects of various radiopaque dyes that are often used as part of the diagnostic evaluation. Some studies have reported that facility patients have a perception that the staff is "too busy" or fear they will be regarded as a "nuisance" if they complain of pain. These patients also suffer a higher degree of anxiety and depression about their declining health, which may result in either over- or under-reporting of pain.

This group of patients also has additional challenges, which make reporting of pain more difficult. Delirium and dementia affect their ability to accurately describe and report pain. Visual impairments due to cataracts, glaucoma, macular degeneration, and other common maladies will adversely affect their ability to answer written questions on a pain assessment questionnaire or respond to a visual pain scale. In the same manner, significant hearing impairments, which are very common in this age group, will hamper their ability to hear the questions posed by the examiner and may lead to incorrect answers, making the pain assessment inaccurate. Lastly, speech impediments due to prior strokes may frustrate the patient to the point where they will either be unwilling or unable to accurately report their degree of pain.

One study reported that older patients wish to be more involved in treatment decisions regarding management of pain; however, because of the various limitations listed above as well as the attitudes of many clinicians, the patients are not encouraged to actively participate, and as a result, may not accurately report their pain. The same study demonstrated that clinicians become frustrated and irritated when older patients request more analgesics than the staff believes is indicated. In reaction to the emotions expressed by the staff, the patients feel powerless and as a result tend to under-report their pain.

A pain panel assembled by the American Geriatrics Society in 1998 and reported in an article in 2003 stated that older patients will often under-report their pain when the word "pain" is used. This is no different than the well-known phenomenon of patients denying anginal chest pain, unless they are asked if the have "pressure, or heaviness" in their chest. The panel suggested that while doing a pain assessment, the questions "Are you feeling hurt?", "Are you uncomfortable?", or "Do you hurt anywhere?" should be used.

There are a number of recommendations as to how to address many of these barriers that negatively influence how geriatric patients report pain. These solutions have been proposed by various researchers as well as the experts from the American Geriatric Society (AGS) and the American Medical Directors Association (AMDA). They

TABLE 30–4. Barriers to Accurate Reporting of Pain in Elderly Patients and Recommended Solutions

BARRIER	SUGGESTED SOLUTIONS
Fear of loss of independence	Reassurance that treatment of pain will increase independence
Part of the "normal aging process"	Education
Fear of the analgesic medications	Education and reassurance
Transportation barriers for nursing home residents	Arrange for testing in the facility
Reluctance of nursing home residents to leave facility	Arrange for in-house testing
	More efficient scheduling
	Send a CNA to meet personal needs of patient. Send a box lunch
Fear that the testing will exacerbate other chronic conditions	Assure patient comfort during testing
Delirium/dementia	Use pediatric assessment tools (Pain thermometer) (Faces Pain Scale)
	Watch for nonverbal cues
	Give extra time to respond to questions
	Possible empiric trial of analgesics
Visual impairments	Large bold print. Visual cues
	Stronger lighting
	Magnifying glasses
	Nonglare paper
	Verbal Descriptor Scale (VDS)
Hearing impairments	Hearing aids
	Portable amplifiers
	Visual cues
Speech impairments	Visual cues
	Simple "yes/no" answers

are summarized in Table 30–4 and discussed below.

Education is first and foremost. Patients, families, caregivers, and clinicians need to be taught that although the presence of pain during aging is a common occurrence, it is NOT part of the "normal" aging process. It can be and should be relieved. In addition, all these parties need to know that proper pain control should *increase* a patient's independence rather than decrease it and that the proper and judicious use of analgesic medications will relieve pain without the undue risk of uncomfortable side effects, which can be effectively ameliorated if they do occur.

For patients residing in nursing homes, every effort should be made to minimize the inconvenience and discomfort that a pain work-up might entail. Diagnostic studies should be kept to a minimum, and whenever possible, portable diagnostic equipment should be brought to the facility to minimize the need to transport the patient. If it does become necessary to transport the patient to a diagnostic center or a consultant's office, every effort should be made to arrange an appointment time which would cause the least disruption of the patient's daily routine, including the consideration for meals and planned activities. Whenever possible, a facility CNA should accompany the patient to ensure their comfort, repositioning on the gurney, provision of toileting, and a boxed meal if necessary and appropriate.

Patients with delirium or dementia present a challenge when it comes to performing an adequate pain assessment. The usual tools used in the evaluation of younger adults may not be appropriate in these situations. In certain circumstances, the tools used in pediatric pain assessments may be used. These include the Pain Thermometer Scale and the Faces Pain Scale. If the patient is also visually impaired, these scales should be magnified. The patients with alteration in their cognitive status should also be evaluated by the use of nonverbal cues such as the observation of facial grimacing, body movements and postures (rubbing, bracing, guarding, touching), vocalizations (moans, groans, yelling, shouting, crying), or by observations in changes in behavior such as poor appetite, depressive symptoms, excessive anxiety, sleep disturbances, resistance to care, aggressive/agitated behavior, or withdrawal. For patients who have severe enough dementia to be nonverbal, there are several validated scales that have been published that the clinician may find useful. (Bjora and Herr) When nonverbal patients exhibit behaviors that are compatible with uncontrolled pain, a therapeutic trial of an appropriate analgesic agent, depending on the severity of the pain as indicated by the nonverbal pain scale, would be warranted.

For visually impaired patients, assessment tools should be printed in large bold type on nonglare paper. Lighting should be adequate and the use of magnifying devices should be considered. If the patient cannot see or cannot understand the 1–10 numerical descriptor scale or the Pain Thermometer or Faces Pain Scale, the Verbal Descriptor Scale (VDS) (Herr and Garand) may be used instead. This scale describes pain as

"slight pain," "mild pain," "moderate pain," "severe pain," "extreme pain," or "pain as bad as it could be." In two studies of community dwelling elders, this scale was preferred and more easily understood. In addition, in another study, it was understood by 73% of cognitively impaired hospitalized elders.

For hearing impaired patients, every attempt should be made to ensure their hearing aid is in good working order. If for some reason they do not have one, portable amplification devices should be used. The clinician should also attempt to sit closer to the patient or lean over to assist in communication. Extra time should also be devoted to performing the pain assessment. The clinician should speak slowly, in a clear loud voice facing the patient so as allow for visual cues and facial expressions and written cues can also be used. Extraneous noises should be eliminated whenever possible.

When evaluating the speech-impaired patient, the various visual assessment devices described earlier should be employed, together with the use of nonverbal observational clues, simple "yes/no" questions, head nodding, or any other appropriate communication technique.

TREATMENT OF PAIN IN THE ELDERLY

After the pain assessment is completed using the aforementioned recommendations, a treatment plan can be initiated. As with younger patients, the clinician has innumerable treatment options to choose from. These include administration of medications by various routes, injections of specific body parts, the use of nondrug modalities such as TENS units, acupuncture, physiotherapy, psychosocial, and surgical treatments. These modalities are discussed in great detail in the chapter on pain management. Although, by necessity, some of the material presented here will be repetitious, the emphasis will be on specific issues related to the management of geriatric patients. Unfortunately, there are very few randomized clinical trials that specifically have examined elderly patients. Therefore, much of the information presented is based on available data from the younger aged patients combined with consensus guidelines from the various geriatric societies including the AGS and AMDA. All of these guidelines take into consideration the high prevalence of altered renal and hepatic function as well as the alteration in body fat and water composition and loss of muscle mass seen in the geriatric population, which renders these patients, in most cases, more sensitive to the positive effects of these medications and more susceptible to their potential side effects. By the nature of having multiple comorbid conditions, these patients are generally receiving a fair number of additional medications as well, increasing the likelihood of adverse drug–drug interactions.

PHARMACOLOLGIC THERAPY

As with the younger population, the pain management guidelines for the geriatric patient follow the suggestions of the World Health Organization (WHO) stepladder approach. Therefore, for mild pain, it is recommended that patients be treated with nonopioid analgesics (with adjuvants as indicated), for moderate pain, combination opioid/nonopioid medications (with adjuvants), and for severe pain, opioid analgesics. As these guidelines and the various analgesics were discussed extensively in Chapter 6, the comments will be confined to issues specific to the geriatric population. Table 30–5 lists the more commonly available nonopioid analgesics with recommended starting doses in the elderly and any special precautions that need to be taken. Table 30–6 does the same for the opioid analgesics. The combination products are not listed individually, and the reader should look at their specific components to evaluate any concerns. More information on the combination agents can be found in Chapter 20.

Nonopioids

ACETAMINOPHEN   Although it does not possess anti-inflammatory properties, acetaminophen is still considered the drug of choice as first-line therapy for pain due to musculoskeletal causes, including rheumatoid arthritis and osteoarthritis. It may be given alone for mild pain (step 1), in combination with codeine, hydrocodone, or oxycodone for moderate pain (step 2), and it can be given as an adjunctive agent with morphine or other opioids when pain is severe (step 3). If administered along with morphine or another opioid, the opioid dosage requirement may be lessened.

The major side effect of acetaminophen is hepatotoxicity. Therefore, it should be avoided when patients suffer from chronic liver disease. Doses should not exceed 3 to 4 g per day, and in patients with compromised liver function, one should be alert to the possibility that worsening liver function may be a sign of early acetaminophen toxicity rather than progressive liver failure due to the patient's underlying illness. When evaluating the acetaminophen dose of a patient, therefore, one must take into account not only the dose of acetaminophen prescribed but also any over-the-counter combination medications that the patient is taking, since many of these products contain acetaminophen. Recent reports indicate acetaminophen may also increase the anticoagulant effect of warfarin.

Nonsteroidal Anti-Inflammatory Drugs (NSAIDs)

As their name implies, these agents possess anti-inflammatory properties, making them suitable for the treatment of a variety of pain syndromes, including musculoskeletal pain, dental pain, postfracture pain, various arthritic pains, as well being effective in the treatment of pain secondary to bone metastases. Despite their usefulness, and, hence their popularity, these agents must be used with caution in the geriatric population due to the risk of significant toxicity. These agents act to reduce inflammation and relieve pain by inhibiting

TABLE 30–5. Nonopioid Analgesics in the Geriatric Population

MEDICATION	RECOMMENDED STARTING DOSE IN GERIATRIC PATIENTS	ADVERSE EFFECTS	SPECIAL PRECAUTIONS IN THE ELDERLY
Acetaminophen	325 mg po q 4 h	Liver toxicity	Do not exceed 3–4 g/24 h (including combination products and OTCs). May increase anticoagulant effects of warfarin.
Nonsteroidal anti-inflammatory drugs (NSAID)	Varies by product	GI bleeding Renal failure Edema Hypertension Constipation Headache Altered mental status	Use short-term only Give with food Use PPIs to protect GI tract Do not use if history of GI disease, ethanol abuse, diuretic use, bleeding tendencies, renal insufficiency, CHF, ascites, dehydration
Tramadol	50 mg PO daily Maximum dose 300 mg/d	Nausea, vomiting, seizures	Avoid if patient has Liver disease Renal disease Seizure disorder Use of antidepressants Dose reduction for patients >75 y of age
Nonopioids to be avoided in the elderly			
Aspirin and Salicylates	Varies by product	GI distress GI bleeding	Not advised for use in the geriatric population
COX-2 inhibitors	200–400 mg PO q 12–24 h	Cardiovascular GI bleed	Not recommended for use in geriatric population.
Propoxyphene	65–100 mg PO q 4 h	CNS, cardiac, hepatic toxicity, respiratory depression	Not recommended for use in geriatric population

prostaglandin synthesis, which, especially in the geriatric population, can lead to increased secretion of gastric acid, resulting in the risk of upper GI toxicity, and may adversely affect intrarenal arterioles, which may worsen renal function and potentially lead to edema, hypertension, and possibly, renal failure. The renal effects may be exacerbated by a number of pre-existing conditions that are common in the elderly, including renal insufficiency, congestive heart failure, ascites, or, conversely, the concomitant use of diuretics, and/or dehydration. Other side effects that have been reported in the geriatric population have included cognitive impairment, constipation, and

TABLE 30–6. Opioid Analgesics in the Geriatric Population

MEDICATION	RECOMMENDED STARTING DOSE IN GERIATRIC PATIENTS	ADVERSE EFFECTS	SPECIAL PRECAUTIONS IN THE ELDERLY
Morphine Immediate release Sustained release	 2.5–10 mg q 4 h 10–30 mg q 12 h or 20 mg 24 h Titrate to effect	Constipation Nausea and vomiting Respiratory depression in opioid naïve patients	Start bowel program empirically, consider alternative in renal failure Chewing or crushing sustained-release preparations can be fatal
Methadone	5–10 mg q 8 h No maximum dose	Same as morphine, however less confusion, myoclonus, dry mouth	Long half-life, so dose should be escalated slowly Useful in patients with renal insufficiency Multiple drug–drug interactions Cardiac arrhythmias if hypokalemia Dosage conversion variable
Oxycodone Immediate release Sustained release	 5–10 mg q 4–6 h 10–20 mg q 12 h Titrate to effect	Same as morphine	Crushing or chewing sustained-release products can be fatal
Fentanyl Transdermal patch Oralet Buccal tabs	 25 mcg/24 h 200 mcg 100 mcg	Nausea and vomiting Dizziness Fatigue Headache Altered mental status Respiratory depression Urinary retention Constipation	Absorption of transdermal medication, increasing risk of toxicity, affected by body fat composition Monitor hydration status Fever and exposure to heat increase absorption Oralet and buccal tabs for breakthrough only and dose not related to baseline dose Possibly less constipating than morphine
Hydromorphone		Same as morphine	Same as morphine
Oxymorphone Immediate release Sustained release	2 mg q 3 h 5–10 mg q 4 h 10 mg q 12 h Titrate to effect	Same as morphine	Alcohol consumption increases serum concentrations

(continued)

TABLE 30–6. Opioid Analgesics in the Geriatric Population (*Continued*)

MEDICATION	RECOMMENDED STARTING DOSE IN GERIATRIC PATIENTS	ADVERSE EFFECTS	SPECIAL PRECAUTIONS IN THE ELDERLY
Codeine	15 mg q 4 h Max 60 mg q 4 h (ceiling effect)	Constipation, nausea, and vomiting Pruritis	High incident of side effects Dose limited
Hydrocodone (in combination with acetaminophen or NSAID)	5 mg q 4 h	Same as morphine	Same as morphine Dose-limited by acetaminophen or NSAID
Ketamine	0.1–0.3 mg/kg/h	Minimal	Limited to parenteral use only
Opioids to be avoided in the Elderly			
Meperidine	300 mg PO 75 mg IM q 3–4 h	Tremors, myoclonus, seizures Tissue irritation Muscle fibrosis	Should *never* be used in geriatric patients
Levoraphanol	2 mg q 4 h	Confusion	Not recommended for use in geriatrics
Opioid agonist–antagonists			
Pentazocine	50 mg q 4 h 2 IM (all q 4–6 h)	Psycho-mimetic effects	Not recommended for use in geriatrics
Nalbuphine	10 mg IM q 4 h	Psycho-mimetic effects	Not recommended for use in geriatrics
Butorphanol	2 mg IM q 4 h	Psycho-mimetic effects	Not recommended for use in geriatrics

The author would like to thank Susan Stanish, from the JFK Medical Center Library, who assisted with the literature search performed in preparation for this chapter.

headaches, although one study has suggested that long-term use of NSAIDs has been reported to lessen cognitive decline in Alzheimer's disease.

Some recommended strategies to minimize NSAIDs GI toxicity by the use of gastric protective agents such as proton-pump inhibitors or misoprostol and by recommending that the medication be taken with food. Misoprostol, unfortunately, has been associated with dose-related diarrhea in the geriatric population, limiting its use for this purpose. Prescribing lower doses of shorter-acting NSAIDs, such as ibuprofen, rather than the longer-acting preparations may also be helpful in reducing potential side effects. These medications should not be given to patients who are already being treated with steroids or anticoagulants. It must also be noted that some geriatric organizations have recommended these agents not be used at all in the geriatric population.

Drugs in this class include ibuprofen, naproxen, diclofenac, etodolac, flurbiprofen, ketoprofen, mefenamic acid, meloxicam, indomethacin, and nabumetone. Ketorolac is a NSAID that is useful for the management of acute pain and is available parenterally as well as orally. Its use discouraged in the elderly, as it may cause renal failure if administered for more than five consecutive days and is contraindicated in conditions commonly seen in the geriatric population, including dehydration, renal insufficiency, cirrhosis, or heart failure. In addition, mefenamic acid and naproxen should also be avoided in the elderly, due to their longer half-lives and increased risk of toxicity. Case reports have documented that ibuprofen is associated with cognitive dysfunction, which improved when the drug was discontinued. Indomethacin crosses the blood–brain barrier and is the most neurotoxic of the NSAIDs and as a result is considered to be an inappropriate drug to be used in the geriatric population.

TRAMADOL   Tramadol is a useful nonopioid alternative that may be useful in the geriatric population. It is indicated for the treatment of moderate to severe pain and has also been shown to be effective in the treatment of neuropathic pain. Unlike the medications discussed earlier, this drug does not cause GI bleeding, hypertension, or congestive heart failure. It does have some opioid-like effects, with the starting dose of 50 mg being equianalgesic to a dose of 60 mg of codeine without opioid side effects such as constipation or the risk of respiratory depression. It does, however, have a high incidence of nausea and vomiting, and must be used with caution in patients with hepatic or renal disease and in patients over the age of 75. It also must be used with caution in patients with a history of a seizure disorder as it lowers the seizure threshold, and it increases the risk of seizures in patients who are receiving antidepressants or MAO inhibitors.

SALICYLATES   The salicylates, of which aspirin is the prototype, should be avoided in the management of pain in the elderly, due to their increased toxicity. For, although they offer the advantage of anti-inflammatory activity over acetaminophen like the NSAIDs discussed earlier, they have an even higher risk of gastric side effects and bleeding than the NSAIDs, making them unsuitable

agents for use in the geriatric population. In addition to aspirin, medications in this class include choline magnesium trisalicylate and diflunisal, with the former offering the theoretical advantage of less gastropathy and platelet inhibition, although not enough to suggest that it would be safe to use in the geriatric population for pain control.

COX-2 INHIBITORS   These actually belong to the NSAID classification of medications, but unlike the nonselective NSAIDs discussed earlier, which also block COX-1 prostaglandin synthesis (gastric mucosa protection), these agents selectively block COX-2 prostaglandin synthesis (responsible for side-effects). In theory, therefore, it was hoped that these medications would be better tolerated, with less GI and renal side effects than their less-specific cousins. However, reports of adverse cardiovascular events associated with these medications resulted in the withdrawal of rofecoxib and valdecoxib from the market. Celecoxib is the only drug in this class remaining on the market. In addition to the increased risk of cardiovascular disease, significant reports of GI bleeding have led to the recommendation by most authorities that this class of medication be avoided in the elderly population.

PROPOXYPHENE   This drug is not recommended for use in the geriatric population. Available either plain or combined with acetaminophen or aspirin, it is estimated to be between 33% and 50% as potent as codeine, with 65 mg of propoxyphne being equianalgesic to 1,000 mg of acetaminophen. Its toxic metabolite, norpropoxyphene, may accumulate and produce hepatic and cardiac toxicity as well as increase the risk of respiratory depression. CNS toxicity in the form of seizures has also been reported. It has been demonstrated to increase the incidence of hospitalizations, emergency department visits, and deaths in nursing home residents and has been classified as an "inappropriate drug" for use in nursing home residents. Yet, despite this, it is still commonly prescribed.

Opioids

As in the younger population, opioid analgesics are the mainstay of treatment for moderate to severe pain in the geriatric population. As already noted earlier, opioids may be available as single agents, or, for the treatment of moderate pain, may be combined with acetaminophen or another nonopioid analgesic. There is a fair amount of discussion in the literature questioning whether there is any advantage to the use of the opioid/nonopioid combination products in the elderly. On the one hand, the small dose of opioid renders their effectiveness limited while at the same time reducing the risk of opioid toxicity. On the other hand, the dose limitations of these agents, often due to potential toxicity of the nonopioid, reduce their flexibility when the persistence of pain requires opioid dose escalation.

Opioids must be used with a high degree of care in the elderly due to the risk of toxic side effects including constipation, nausea, vomiting, confusion, and over-sedation, and the potential for respiratory depression. However, when used according to well-accepted treatment guidelines, these medications result in excellent pain control without untoward side effects. For the geriatric patients, guidelines recommend starting at the lowest effective dose and raising the dose slowly as needed to achieve pain control. All geriatric practitioners abide by the adage of "start low and go slow." Because of the alterations in metabolism that were previously discussed, many guidelines recommend a starting dose of 25% to 50% of the usual adult starting dose with dosage titrations in 25% increments as needed. The guidelines also recommend initially starting with the immediate-release, short-acting preparations, titrating to effect, and once an effective dose has been established, the patient may be converted to a sustained-release product, while continuing to have the immediate release product available for the treatment of breakthrough or incident pain. These guidelines are discussed in more detail in Chapter 20.

MORPHINE   While morphine is considered the treatment of choice for treating pain in the geriatric population, studies have demonstrated decreased morphine clearance and reduced volumes of distribution as compared to younger patients, resulting in higher and more prolonged drug levels. This means that elderly patients will generally be more sensitive to both the analgesic effects and potential toxic effects of any specific dose of morphine. Morphine metabolism by the liver produces an active compound, morphine-6-glucuronide (M6G), which may be responsible for up to 60% of its analgesic effects. This same compound, as well another hepatic metabolite, morphine-3-glucuronide (M3G) may also be the agents responsible for the myoclonus, hyperalgesia, nausea, vomiting, and sedation that may be seen when morphine doses are excessive. As these metabolites are cleared by the kidneys and accumulate in patients with renal insufficiency, it has been recommended, due to the reduced renal function generally present in geriatric patients, that starting morphine doses be approximately 50% of what is typically recommended for younger adult patients. Hydromorphone, fentanyl, hydrocodone, oxycodone and codeine all have similar renal excretion; only methadone metabolism is relatively independent of renal function.

The importance of preventing the common side effect of constipation cannot be understated. Therefore, as a rule of thumb, any time morphine is prescribed, a stool softener with or without a stimulant laxative should empirically be prescribed as well. This is discussed in more detail both in Chapter 20 on pain management and Chapter 8, which discusses the management of GI symptoms.

Two of the newer sustained release morphine products, Kadian® and Avinza®, may be useful for patients with dementia who are on restricted diets or are being fed via a PEG tube. These 24-hour sustained release products consists of capsules, which contain small beads from which morphine is slowly released into the GI tract during the digestive process. As such, the capsule can be opened and the beads can either be sprinkled on foods such as applesauce or flushed down a PEG tube of an appropriate size, allowing the patient to be easily medicated for pain once daily. As alcohol will increase the rate of GI absorption of morphine from the beads and increase the patient's risk of toxicity, alcohol products should be avoided when these medications are used.

METHADONE   This is a synthetic opioid that is chemically unrelated to morphine, and, therefore, may be used in "morphine-allergic" patients. It is available in oral and parenteral forms and can be administered by suppository as well. It has several unique properties; in addition to acting at the μ receptor, as does morphine, it also acts as an *N*-methyl-D-aspartate (NMDA) receptor antagonist, which makes it extremely useful in the treatment of neuropathic pain. Because of its efficacy against both nociceptive and neuropathic pain, as well as its cost effectiveness, it is now frequently prescribed by hospice and palliative care physicians. As it is metabolized by the liver to inactive metabolites, this drug causes much less in the way of the usual opioid side effects of confusion, hallucinations, myoclonus, dry mouth, and constipation, and it can be safely used in geriatric patients with renal insufficiency. Conversely, its very long half-life and the high incidence of multiple drug–drug interactions dictate that methadone be titrated extremely slowly and carefully to the desired analgesic effect over several days. It has also been shown to increase the likelihood of fatal cardiac arrhythmias in patients with low serum potassium levels.

This use of this drug does require finesse since the dosage conversions from morphine to methadone are variable and complex. For further discussion of how to properly use methadone, please see the discussion in Chapter 20.

OXYCODONE   This opioid is a semisynthetic derivative of morphine and is approximately 1.5 times as potent as morphine. It is available orally as an immediate release and as a sustained release product and is also available in combination with aspirin, acetaminophen, or ibuprofen. While it has no ceiling effect, its dose is limited when used in combination a nonopioid due to the dose limitations of the nonopioid moiety. The sustained-release preparations should not be used in opioid-naïve patients. This medication is as effective as morphine in reducing pain, and some geriatricians prefer this agent in the elderly due to reports in drug company-sponsored studies that oxycodone may cause confusion in a smaller percentage of patients than morphine. However, the inability to predict which patients may benefit from oxycodone over morphine, as well as its lack of cost-effectiveness compared to morphine, suggest that oxycodone may be efficiently used as a second-line agent for patients who have difficulty tolerating morphine.

FENTANYL   This is a synthetic phenyl piperidine derivative and a chemical congener of the reverse ester of meperidine (an analgesic to be avoided, see later). Despite its meperidine heritage, it does not share all of the same adverse properties. It is a pure μ agonist and has a very short duration of action. It also has the advantage of being lipophilic, allowing it to cross the skin and mucus membranes. Hence, its most popular dosage form, the transdermal delivery system, is extremely popular, including in the elderly, due to its ease of administration. It is also popular in the elderly due to the results of several drug company sponsored studies, which have suggested that fentanyl through the transdermal delivery system causes less constipation than oral opioids.

Despite its popularity in the geriatric population, one must be cautious when using the fentanyl transdermal delivery system in these patients. As many of the elderly are cachectic and have little to no body fat, and since body fat is critical to proper absorption of the medication, these patients run the risk of not being adequately medicated. In addition, as an elevated body temperature can significantly increase drug absorption, elderly patients who are prone to febrile illnesses can be put at greater risk for opioid toxicity when receiving analgesia in this fashion. Therefore, it is recommended that utilization of fentanyl by the transdermal delivery system be limited to patients who are unable to swallow or otherwise tolerate oral analgesics or who are at high risk for non-compliance.

Its ability to cross mucus membranes has also led to the development of a transmucosal lozenge and a buccal tablet. While these products seem attractive, especially as a noninvasive breakthrough alternative for patients who do not have an intact gastrointestinal tract, this is, unfortunately, not the case. 50% (buccal tablet) to 75% (transmucosal lozenge) of the medication given is actually absorbed through the GI tract and not directly through the buccal mucosa.

The major side effects of fentanyl are nausea, vomiting, dizziness, fatigue, headaches, and respiratory depression. Depending on the delivery system, in 10% of patients there can also be local pain and irritation at the site of the patch or oral ulcerations. Fentanyl may also be administered parenterally via subcutaneous or intravenous infusion, or via the intraspinal or intrathecal routes, although when administered, the risk of sedation and respiratory depression are significant.

HYDROMORPHONE This is a semisynthetic opioid produced by hydrogenating morphine. As of this writing, it is available only in a short-acting oral form (tablets or solution), although its short half-life and the need to administer the medication every 3 hours makes it somewhat less practical to use as a primary agent.

Its significantly greater potency as compared to morphine has made it a very useful agent when patients require subcutaneous analgesic administration due to the smaller fluid volume required.

OXYMORPHONE This is a metabolite of oxycodone and, unlike its parent, is also available in a parenteral and rectal formulation. It was recently introduced in the United States in both a short-acting and a long-acting formulation. It has no particular advantages in the elderly population, although patients must be cautioned not to consume alcohol, which will cause substantially increased serum concentrations and significantly increase toxic side effects.

CODEINE This is a "weak" form of morphine with approximately 1/7 its potency. It is only available in the oral form and is generally prescribed in combination with acetaminophen or an NSAID, although it is available on its own. Despite its popularity in the elderly when prescribed in combination, it should really be avoided, as it has a very high incidence of constipation, nausea, vomiting, and, due to its histamine-like properties, pruritis. For the drug to become metabolically active, it needs to be converted to morphine, and 10% of the population lacks the enzyme responsible for this conversion. The dose of the parent compound is limited by its side effects and the combination products are dose-limited by the nonopioid.

HYDROCODONE This opioid is only available in the oral form in combination with acetaminophen or an NSAID. It has the same side effect profile as morphine, and the combination product is dose limited due to the nonopioid. It has no special advantages or disadvantages in the elderly and seems to be a favorite of orthopedists for the treatment of postfracture and musculoskeletal complaints.

KETAMINE Ketamine is a dissociative anesthetic, but is included here because in subanesthetic doses, it may serve as a potent analgesic with minimal side effects. It interacts with many opioid receptors including μ, δ, and κ as well as monoaminergic and muscarinic receptors, calcium and sodium channels, and possibly the γ-aminobutyric acid (GABA) receptors. Like methadone, its NMDA receptor antagonistic activity makes it an ideal drug for the management of neuropathic pain. Unlike methadone, however, which may be given in the oral form, ketamine is only available in the intravenous or subcutaneous form, which limits its usefulness to the in-patient unit setting. Here, however, it may be the preferable drug since it is the most potent NMDA receptor antagonist presently available for clinical use.

MEPERIDINE   As stated in Chapter 6, meperidine is a medication that should be avoided in all patients and, therefore, certainly should not be used in the geriatric population. In fact, it is listed on the Beer's list of "inappropriate" medications for the elderly. To reiterate some of the challenges with meperidine, it has a more rapid onset of action than morphine and is much less potent than morphine, with a 50 mg tablet being equianalgesic to 650 mg of aspirin. When given subcutaneously, it is very irritating to tissues and when given IM, it cause muscle fibrosis. It is metabolized in the liver to a toxic substance, normeperidine, which causes dysphoria, irritability, tremors, myoclonus, and seizures. In patients who are also taking MAO inhibitors, meperidine can cause severe encephalopathy and death.

LEVORPHANOL   This drug is available both in the oral and subcutaneous form. Although it is a potent analgesic for treating chronic pain, it does accumulate due to a long half-life of 16 to 18 hours and it also commonly causes confusion. Therefore, it is not recommended for use in the elderly.

Opioid Agonist–Antagonist Agents

Pentazocine, nalbuphine, and butorphanol are all agonist–antagonist drugs. The idea behind these agents was that they would be able to provide analgesic effects while reducing the possibility of physical dependence. Unfortunately, this has not been seen on a practical level. They all possess analgesic ceiling effects and have a significant risk of psychotomimetic side effects. In addition, if patients are already receiving opioid agonists, they can precipitate opioid withdrawal symptoms. Pentazocine is available orally, while the other two agents are only available in the parenteral form. With all of these challenges, the use

of these agents is not recommended in the geriatric population.

Adjuvant Medications

As discussed in Chapter 6, there are certain pain syndromes for which opioids alone may not be sufficient to control pain, or, by themselves, require such high doses to control pain that the toxicity of the opioid is more distressing to the patient than the pain itself. In these circumstances, adjuvant medications may be helpful in combination with an opioid to control pain.

This principle certainly holds true in the elderly, where the risk of opioid toxicity is high, and where opioid side effects often are a deterrent to good pain control. For example, NSAIDs may be useful for the treatment of bone pain, providing the patient can tolerate them. Steroids may also be effective in treating bone pain, although here the more formidable side effects, which include salt and fluid retention, development of exacerbation of hypertension, diabetes, glaucoma, or osteoporosis, and possible steroid psychosis are of great concern. In these situations, a benefit-versus-risk decision needs to be made taking into account the severity of the pain, the potential for a positive response to the steroid medication, the patient's expected longevity, and the seriousness of any pre-existing co-morbid conditions.

Another important role for adjuvant medications in the geriatric population is the ability to counteract the untoward side effects of the primary drug. For example, the addition of a stool softener or laxative to an opioid regimen is virtually mandatory to prevent the troubling side effect of constipation, while many practitioners will prescribe a PPI to reduce the risk of gastrointestinal toxicity in a patient being treated with an NSAID.

One must be cautious, however, not to cause additional toxicity. For example, while adding hydroxyzine to morphine may reduce the risk of opioid-induced nausea, there is an increase of patient sedation. Similarly, when treating opioid-induced sedation with dexedrine, methylphenidate, or modafinil, one needs to take into account whether the patient has any pre-existing cardiac disease, a condition commonly found in the geriatric population. As already mentioned, one must weigh the benefits vs. the potential risk whenever considering whether or not to add one of these medications, and, perhaps more importantly, one must be careful to avoid polypharmacy due to the tendency to always add a medication when an untoward effect occurs. Sometimes, the more prudent approach is to discontinue a medication, or, in the case where an opioid analgesia is required and the toxicity cannot be effectively managed with an adjuvant, switching to an alternative opioid.

Adjuvants to Treat Neuropathic Pain

As one of the more common causes of poorly treated pain, the management of neuropathic pain deserves a separate discussion. The nonopioid tramadol, and the opioid methadone may be very useful in the treatment of neuropathic pain. For certain types of neuropathic pain, such as postherpetic neuralgia, topical medications are initially employed, followed sequentially by anticonvulsant and/or antidepressant medications. If these are ineffective, then methadone or tramadol is added. In other situations, when the patient has a pain of a more malignant nature, the anticonvulsants or antidepressants may be added to whatever opioid the patient is currently receiving, or, if side effects make this a challenge, methadone may be substituted for the primary opioid the patient is receiving. If this is ineffective, more invasive therapies need to be employed, such as intrathecal or epidural administration of drugs or even surgical intervention.

Anticonvulsants

Gabapentin has become the treatment of choice for neuropathic pain, with doses ranging from 100 to 3,600 mg/d. More recently, pregabalin, intended to be a more potent congener of gabapentin, has been approved. The challenge for the elderly is that these agents produce a number of troublesome side effects, including dizziness, unsteadiness of gait, and somulence, as well as weight gain and peripheral edema. Pregabalin also has been reported to induce euphoria. Therefore, extra caution needs to be exercised when using these drugs. Other anticonvulsants that may be used for the treatment of various neuropathic pain syndromes include carbamazepine (specific for trigeminal neuralgia), oxcarbazepine (which may have fewer side effects than carbamazepine), phenytoin, valproate, clonazepam, and topiramate. In several small clinical trials, lamotrigine has shown some promise for the treatment central poststroke pain and HIV-associated painful neuropathy. However larger trials have been inconclusive and this drug can cause a rash that has sometimes progressed to Stevens–Johnson syndrome, severely limiting its utility at present.

Antidepressants

The tricyclic antidepressants, which act by blocking the reuptake of serotonin and norepinephrine, were among the first agents to be shown to be effective in the treatment of neuropathic pain and have been a mainstay for its treatment for many years. However, the anticholinergic and antihistaminic effects of these agents, of which amitriptyline has been the most extensively studied, are usually very poorly tolerated by the elderly, and hence, these drugs may be found on the Beer's list of "inappropriate" medications to use in the geriatric population. It should be noted, however, that as the therapeutic dose of these agents to treat neuropathic pain may be significantly lower than that required for their antidepressant effects, they may sometimes be used with caution at low doses in the elderly population. Some of the tricyclics better tolerated in the elderly include nortriptyline and desipramine. All these agents have the increased risk of cardiac arrhythmias, orthostatic hypotension, delirium, and precipitation of an acute glaucoma attack, toxicities which are seen with increased frequency in the geriatric population.

Unfortunately, the newer selective serotonin reuptake inhibitors (SSRIs) have not been shown to be effective for the treatment of neuropathic pain. Some of the newer serotonin norepinephrine reuptake inhibitors (SNRIs) such as venlafaxine and duloxetine have shown some activity in treating some forms of neuropathic pain, with the added benefit of fewer side effects. However, their role has yet to be determined.

Antiarrythmics

Mexiletine (Mexitil®) has also been tried with questionable success; however, due its proarrythmic, GI, and other side effects, it is not recommended in the geriatric population.

Intravenous lidocaine has been used to reduce the pain induced by the injection of angiography contrast agents, embolization therapy for tumors, and administration of propofol prior to induction of anesthesia. In 2006, there was a case report of a 45-year-old woman who was given an infusion of lidocaine for severe opioid-refractory pain due to infarct of the thalamus; a condition known as central poststroke syndrome. She had complete relief of her pain and died two weeks later from her hemorrhagic stroke with midline shift. In reports such as this, the patients were 45 years old or less. Geriatric patients, however, are at increased risk of delirium, seizures, respiratory depression, and hemodynamic instability if this therapy is used, so it is most likely prudent to avoid this in the geriatric population.

Baclofen

Baclofen, which is actually indicated for the treatment of muscle spasticity due to multiple sclerosis and other spinal cord diseases including injury, has proven effective in the treatment of trigeminal neuralgia and may be tried in neuropathic pain not responding to the other therapies described earlier. It acts as a GABA-receptor agonist and has a wide dosage range of 20 to 200 mg/d. Unfortunately, however, it has a myriad of side effects, which include drowsiness, dizziness, weakness, fatigue, confusion, daytime sedation, headache, insomnia, visual hallucinations, hypotension, nausea, constipation, and urinary frequency. Therefore, it should be started in low doses and only gradually escalated to either effectiveness or intolerance. In addition to its impressive side effect profile, it may potentiate the action of antihypertensive medications, and patients receiving carbidopa and levodopa for Parkinson's disease are prone to mental confusion, hallucinations, and agitation. It may also increase blood glucose and can raise the liver enzymes. As these are all common pre-existing conditions in the elderly, this medication should only be used with extreme caution and at very low doses in the geriatric population.

Topical Preparations for the Management of Pain

5% lidocaine patches have commonly been used for the treatment of neuropathic pain arising from radicular arthritic sources or postherpetic neuralgia. The use of these patches has demonstrated no significant plasma levels even with the application of up to three patches per day. In addition, lidocaine is available in a topical formulation in various concentrations up to 10%. Another alternative is EMLA, which is a mixture of lidocaine and prilocaine. This preparation can only be applied to small areas, however, due to its high cost.

Clonidine patches have also sometimes been used off-label for the same indication. Unlike the lidocaine patches, which exert their effect locally, the Clonidine needs to be absorbed systemically. This results in centrally-mediated reduction of blood pressure. Side effects include hypotension with resulting syncope, dry mouth, and local skin sensitivity to the drug or the adhesive backing. Rapid discontinuation may result in a hypertensive crisis, hypertensive encephalopathy, stroke, or death. The manufacturer warns the prescriber to use extreme caution in patients with severe coronary insufficiency, conduction disturbances, recent myocardial infarction, cerebrovascular disease, or chronic renal failure. For all of these reasons, this drug should probably not be used in the geriatric population for pain control.

Capsaicin cream has been frequently used in the treatment of postherpetic neuralgia and diabetic neuropathy as well as the non-neuropathic pain from osteoarthric joints. Capsaicin is a naturally occurring neuropeptide found in capsicum fruit and is the active ingredient that makes chili peppers hot. It depletes substance P, which acts as a neurotransmitter from the peripheral nociceptive nerve endings in the skin and joints. After an initial period of heat and a burning sensation, it reduces the pain. It remains effective with chronic use. It is a desirable treatment in elderly patients due to its relative lack of side effects, ease of use, and lack of interaction with other medications. The 0.075% preparation is recommended for postherpetic neuralgia and the 0.025% preparation is used for diabetic neuropathy and osteoarthritic pain. It may take up to 2 to 3 weeks to obtain maximum effectiveness.

Recently, a patch containing 1.3% diclofenac epolamine (the NSAID Voltaren®) was released in the United States for topical treatment of minor strains, sprains, and contusions. It had previously been available in Europe since 1993. The 1% gel preparation of diclofenac sodium is also available for topical treatment of osteoarthritis. The most common side effects are skin irritation, pruritis, dermatitis, and burning. GI side effects do not occur. The patches need to be applied twice daily and are expensive.

A 1% naltrexone topical preparation has been demonstrated to relieve chronic pruritis. Morphine (4 g powder) has been mixed with various topical preparations, including 5% Lidocaine cream, Silvadene® cream, Eucerine® cream, Aloe Vera®, Hydrogel®, saline solution, and metronidazole gel for treatments of painful wounds. The morphine works locally (studies demonstrate virtually no systemic absorption) by decreasing substance P release and there may be some evidence to suggest that this may actually accelerate the healing process. A mixture of 20 mg of ketamine mixed with 1.5 cc of normal saline has been sprayed on infiltrating skin tumors and been reported to reduce pain.

Invasive Pain Management in the Elderly

As discussed in Chapter 6, one of the important principles of pain management is to use the least invasive route possible to achieve the maximum therapeutic benefit. Therefore, even in the elderly, if oral, topical, rectal, or parenteral opioids and adjuvant medications are ineffective, invasive interventions may sometimes be required. As with all patients, the decision to use an invasive intervention must take into account the benefits vs. risk, the life expectancy of the patient, and the potential for a positive outcome.

Because of the higher incidence of musculoskeletal and arthritic symptoms in the elderly, there may be a need for, for example, trigger-point injections for myofacial pain, joint capsule injections for inflammatory joint pain, or nerve blocks for intercostal neuralgia, postherpetic neuralgia, or painful ischemic peripheral vascular disease. Reflex sympathetic dystrophy, ischemic peripheral vascular disease, and various arthritic-induced radiculopathies may require the use of autonomic nerve blocks. Trigeminal neuralgia, which is not uncommonly seen in the geriatric population, may require the use of radiofrequency neuroablative techniques. For a further discussion of these and other invasive pain management interventions, please see the discussion in Chapter 20.

NONPHARMACOLOGICAL TREATMENTS FOR PAIN

Although this section was placed last in the discussion, these techniques are extremely important and should be employed early on in the course of treatment and should be initiated either prior to or in conjunction with the pharmacological therapies already discussed. This is especially important in the geriatric population, as these interventions are generally easy to administer and often lack the many side effects that pharmacological therapies entail.

Nonpharmacological interventions for the management of pain in the elderly may include, but are not limited to, physiotherapy, application of heat or cold, massage, TENS units, vibration therapy, acupuncture/acupressure, Tai Chi, psychosocial/spiritual interventions, and guided imagery/relaxation/distraction. All of these aforementioned techniques have been shown to relieve the pain from osteoarthritis, fibromyalgia, muscle spasms, and peripheral vascular disease. One study actually demonstrated improved collateral circulation after these activities. Repositioning of specific body parts and the application of pressure-relieving devices and/or splints are extremely beneficial for relief of various painful musculoskeletal conditions.

Application of cold has been demonstrated to minimize edema and reduce chronic back pain. Application of heat, taking care to avoid burns, is very beneficial to relieve arthritic pains and muscle aches although special care must be used when employing heat in cognitively impaired patients.

Massage therapy has been demonstrated to relieve muscle spasms, increase joint mobility, improve circulation, and relieve anxiety by decreasing the accumulation of irritants and inflammatory substances. It has also been shown to release endorphins and enkephalins that improve the sense of well-being, reduce anxiety, and relieve pain.

Some small studies have demonstrated the efficacy of acupuncture and acupressure to relieve pain, but due to poor study design, the results have been inconclusive. The Chinese have used acupuncture for centuries and have demonstrated excellent anesthetic properties. The theory behind this treatment is that the stimulation of the nerve fibers in the muscles releases endogenous endorphins. In addition, the pain stimulus generated by the insertion of the acupuncture needle is thought to modulate subsequent pain via the dorsal horn of the spinal cord. However, one meta-analysis of randomized trials of acupuncture used for the treatment of back pain found that 57% of the patients improved, although the benefits were short-lived. In 2000, the British Medical Association determined that acupuncture was an effective therapy for chronic back and neck pain as well as migraine headaches.

A meta-analysis evaluating the effectiveness of transcutaneous electrical nerve stimulation (TENS) demonstrated an effect beyond what was achieved with opioids alone; however, there were multiple variables including placebo effect and sampling error, rendering the results less than conclusive. TENS has been used for the treatment of chronic back pain, osteoporotic pain, and phantom limb pain. Because of loss of manual dexterity needed to operate the units and the higher frequency of cognitive impairment in the geriatric population, TENS unit therapy may be more difficult in the older population as compared to younger individuals.

By way of the pain modulation pathways, vibration therapy may relieve pain by inducing paresthesias and/or local anesthesia. One study demonstrated that, when using vibrations for 20 to 30 minutes two to three times per day, sharp pain was changed to a dull sensation and shown to eliminate the need for the use of TENS units in the subject patients. Pain relief was demonstrated for muscle pain and spasm, itching, neuropathic pain, phantom limb pain, oro-facial pain, and tendonitis. They also demonstrated added benefit by combining heat therapy and vibration therapy concurrently with superior results to either therapy alone. The article describes commercially available vibration devices that deliver 100 to 200 Hz vibrations.

Published studies have demonstrated the effectiveness of guided imagery, relaxation, and distraction techniques including watching TV, playing cards, arts and crafts, listening to music, visits from friends and family, and interacting with pets. Published studies have also shown the advantage of prayer and meditation. The psychosocial staff should be actively involved in the pain therapy treatment plan.

CONCLUSIONS

As was stated in the beginning of this chapter, the geriatric patients represent the vast majority of the patients one will encounter in the hospice and palliative care setting. Although the basic principles of pain management still apply, certain adjustments need to be made in light of the special challenges that these patients present. There are multiple pharmacological options available including nonopioids, opioids, adjuvants, and topical agents. There are also invasive and nonpharmacological techniques to further complement the armentarium. Each presents its own unique set of advantages and disadvantages. The clinician must weigh several factors when deciding which therapy or therapies to employ, including the etiology or etiologies of the pain, the potential benefits, and toxicities of the various medications available, taking into account the patient's pre-existing illnesses and comorbid conditions, the patient's potential functionality, and the patient's life expectancy, to name but a few. Only after considering all of these factors, which are unique to the geriatric population, will one be able to tailor a treatment plan that results in optimal pain relief with a minimum of adverse consequences.

BIBLIOGRAPHY

A diclofenac patch (Flector) for pain. *Med Lett* 50 (1277):1-2, 2008.

American Geriatrics Society: *Geriatrics Review Syllabus.*

American Geriatrics Society Panel on Chronic Pain in Older Persons: The management of chronic pain in older persons. *J Am Geriatr Soc* 46(5):635-651, 1998.

American Medical Directors Association: Clinical Practice Guidelines: Pain Management in the LTC Setting. Columbia, MD, 2003.

Ardery G, Herr K, Titler M, et al: Assessing and managing acute pain in older adults: A research base to guide practice. *Med Surg Nurs* 12(1):7-18, 2003.

Bernstein AL, Werlin A: Pseudodementia associated with the use of ibuprofen. *Ann Pharmacother* 37(1):80-82, 2003.

Bjoro K, Herr K: Assessment of pain in the nonverbal or congitively impaired older adult. *Clin Geriatr Med* 24(2):237-262, 2008.

Bharadwaj P, Danilychev M: Central post-stroke syndrome treated with parenteral lidocaine. *J Pain Symptom Manage* 32(5):400-401, 2006.

Brown D, McCormack B: Determining factors that have an impact upon effective evidence-based pain management with older people, following colorectal surgery: An ethnographic study. *J Clin Nurs* 15(10): 1287-1298, 2006.

Bruera E, Higginson I, Ripamonti C, von Gunten C: *Textbook of Palliative Medicine.* Oxford, Hodder Arnold Publications, 2006.

Cleary J: The pharmacological management of cancer pain. *J Palliat Med* 10(6):1369-1394, 2007.

Drugs for pain: treatment guidelines. *Med Lett* 5(56): 23-33, 2007.

Fentanyl buccal tablet (Fentora) for breakthrough pain. *Med Lett* 49(1270):78-79, 2007.

Fentanyl Transdermal System—Updated Information On Appropriate Prescribing, Dose Selection, and Safe Use. Rockville, MD, FDA Med Watch, 2007.

Feldt KS: Pain in the elderly. *Adv Nurse Pract* 13(6):51-52, 54, 2005.

Fitzgibbon EJ, Viola R: Parenteral ketamine as an analgesic adjuvant for severe pain: Development and retrospective audit of a protocol for a palliative care unit. *J Palliat Med* 8(1):49-57, 2005.

Fujii Y, Nakayama M: Prevention of pain due to injection of propofol with IV administration of lidocaine 40 mg + metoclopramide 2.5, 5, or 10 mg or saline: a randomized, double-blind study in Japanese adult surgical patients. *Clin Ther* 29(5):856-861, 2007.

Hanks-Bell M, Halvey K, Paice JA: Pain assessment and management in aging. *Online J Issues Nurs* 9(3):8, 2004.

Hazard Wm, Bierman E, Blass J, et al: *Principles of Geriatric Medicine and Gerontology*, 3rd ed. New York, McGraw-Hill, 1994.

Herr KA, Garand L: Assessment and measurement of pain in older adults. *Clin Geriatr Med* 17(3):457-478, 2001.

Hollenack K, Cranmer K, Zarowitz B, O'Shea T: The application of evidence-based principles of care in older persons (Issue 4): Pain management. *J Am Med Dir Assoc* 8(3 Suppl 2):E.77-E.85, 2007.

Keyounf JA, Levy EB, Roth AR, et al: Intraarterial lidocaine for pain control after uterine artery embolization for leiomyomata. *J Vasc Interv Radiol* 12 (9):1065-1069, 2001.

Manfredi P, Houde R: Prescribing methadone, a unique analgesic. *J Support Oncol* 1:216-220, 2003.

Mitchell C: Assessment and management of chronic pain in elderly people. *Br J Nurs* 10(5):296-304, 2001.

Slatkin N, Rhiner M: *Topical Approaches to Pain Management in Patients Having Refractory Skin and Mucosal Pain.* Presented at the Annual Assembly of the American Academy of Hospice & Palliative Medicine, Tampa, FL, 2008.

Stein WM: Pain in the nursing home. *Clin Geriatr Med* 17:575, 2001.

Stein WM, Ferrell BA: Pain in the nursing home. *Clin Geriatr Med* 12(3):601-613, 1996.

Wilcox SM, Himmelstein DU, Woolhandler S: Inappropriate drug prescribing for the community-dwelling elderly. *JAMA* 272(4):292-296, 1994.

SELF-ASSESSMENT QUESTIONS

1. In regards to pain and pain management, geriatric patients differ from younger patients in all of the following ways EXCEPT
   A. Geriatric patients metabolize drugs at a different rate
   B. Geriatric patients absorb drugs at a different rate
   C. The volume of distribution in elderly patients changes due to differences in fat content
   D. Geriatric patients are more likely to have pain from multiple sources
   E. Geriatric patients tend to under-report pain when compared to younger patients.

2. The most common cause for pain in the geriatric population is
   A. Chest pain
   B. Phlebitis
   C. Constipation
   D. Cancer
   E. Low back pain

3. Geriatric patients under-report pain for all of the following reasons EXCEPT
   A. Fear of loss of independence
   B. The belief that pain is a normal part of aging
   C. They are a stoic group
   D. They don't want to be regarded as a "nuisance"
   E. Fear of addiction

4. The first-line agent to be used for the treatment of mild to moderate pain in the elderly, regardless of cause is
   A. NSAIDs
   B. Aspirin
   C. COX-2 inhibitors
   D. Acetaminophen
   E. Propoxyphene

5. An opioid which should NEVER be used in the geriatric population is
   A. Morphine
   B. Meperidine
   C. Fentanyl
   D. Codeine
   E. Hydrocodone

6. In order for this drug to become active, it must be converted to morphine. Ten percent of the population lacks the necessary enzyme. This drug is
   A. Hydrocodone
   B. Oxycodone
   C. Codeine
   D. Oxymorphone
   E. Hydromorphone

7. This drug is commonly used in geriatrics; however, its use should be limited due to its dependence on degree of body fat, hydration status, and temperature:
   A. Fentanyl patch
   B. Lidocaine patch
   C. Methadone patch
   D. Capsaicin cream
   E. Diclofenac patch

8. Because of its high potency, this is the preferred parenteral drug to be used, especially when infused fluid volumes are an issue:
   A. Morphine
   B. Codeine
   C. Hydrocodone
   D. Methadone
   E. Hydromorphone

9. Of all the following, the best oral medication for the treatment of neuropathic pain in the geriatric population is
   A. Morphine
   B. Tramadol
   C. Gabapentin

D. Amitriptyline
E. Fluoxetine

10. This nonpharmacological therapy has been demonstrated to release endorphins:

A. Application of cold
B. Application of heat
C. TENS
D. Vibration therapy
E. Massage therapy

Diversity

Cultural Diversity and End-of-Life Care

Barry M. Kinzbrunner, Michele Grant Ervin, Freddie J. Negron,
Teresita Mesa, and Yolanda Castillo

INTRODUCTION

Barry M. Kinzbrunner

Growing up in the United States in the 1950s and 1960s, one would be frequently exposed in school to the idea that America was a "melting pot society." The idea was that as immigrants arrived on the shores of the United States, they would, over time, shed their historic identities and acculturate themselves within American society. In other words, the immigrants would assimilate and culturally become "Americans."

The idea of immigrant assimilation continued until sometime in the late 1970s or early 1980s when the desire to assimilate and join the "melting pot" was rejected by a significant number of Americans in favor of multiculturalism, in which individuals would continue to identify with their culture of origin. The catalyst for this change may have been the 1976 best-selling novel "Roots," authored by Alex Haley and subsequently turned into a widely viewed television mini series. "Roots" traced the author's ancestry all the way back to the Africa, where the first of his family to arrive on American soil by being kidnapped into slavery was born. Alex Haley's journey to trace his "roots" caught the imagination of a large part of the American public, many of whom also had "roots" outside of the American continent. So, rather than shed their immigrant culture and identify in favor of assimilating into the "melting pot," immigrants to America, and even first- and second-generation (or earlier) descendants of immigrants, have chosen to identify with their or their ancestor's ethnicity, culture, or religion of origin, and to incorporate the various values and rituals of their ancestral group into their everyday lives.

As the hospice movement developed in the United States during the 1970s (see Chapter 2 for further discussion), in a sense it adopted the "melting pot" concept that was prevalent from the perspective that it was generally believed that the vast majority of patients and families wanted the same things at the end of life. On a medical level, hospices often had specific policies about what interventions they would or would not provide, whereas on the spiritual side, it was generally believed that the "generic" chaplain would be able to meet the needs of virtually all end-of-life patients irrespective of whether the religious beliefs of the chaplain and patients he or she served were the same or vastly different (see Chapter 4 for further discussion of the role of the hospice chaplain).

Despite hospice's significant growth during the 1980s and 1990s, its leaders noted that only approximately one-third of all patients who died in the United States received hospice services, and that most of those who did received care for relatively short periods of time, and began to explore why the service was underutilized. This led to the identification of a number of barriers that deterred patients and families from choosing hospice care as the patient's life was approaching its end. Some of the identified barriers were medical in nature and are discussed more fully in Chapter 2. Other barriers, however, such as mistrust of the health care system, the mandate to "preserve life" at all costs, the idea that informing someone that they are terminally ill may hasten death, and the proscription to the concept of "giving up," were found to be deeply rooted in the ethnic, cultural, or religious beliefs of many patients and families who were in need end-of-life care and choosing not to access hospice services to provide that care. Underscoring these specific barriers, a recent report published as part of the larger "Coping with Cancer" study demonstrated that although 80% of white patients had participated in advance care planning, this was true of only 47% of black patients and the same percentage of Hispanic patients. Black (45%) and Hispanic (34%) patients were much more likely to request life prolonging care in the last few days of life than white (14%) patients, and also considered religion to be much important (black patients 88%; Hispanic patients 73%) than their white counterparts (44%) (Smith et al., 2008).

Recognizing the increased diversity of the population of patients requiring end-of-life care, hospices and nonhospice palliative care providers have been reaching out in a number of ways. "Generic" chaplains are being replaced by chaplains from multiple religions and multiple denominations within those specific faith groups to provide spiritual counseling to patients who share the same belief system. End-of-life care staff is being actively trained in the specific issues and needs of the diverse patient populations they care for, and in some instances, entire hospice teams have been formed to address the needs of a specific group who might speak a language other than English or come from a specific ethnic, cultural, or religious perspective.

With this in mind, this chapter and the one that follows explore the end-of-life needs and issues of a number of the more common ethnic, cultural, or religious groups that hospices and other end-of-life care providers are serving in the United States today. It must be pointed out that the information provided for any group is superficial at best, and readers are encouraged to access the references provided at the end of the each chapter if they are interested in more detail about any specific group.

CULTURAL ASSESSMENT

Before exploring some of the more common cultural, ethnic, and religious groups that are commonly encountered by end-of-life care providers, it is prudent to say a few words about the cultural assessment. The cultural assessment, of course, is the part of the comprehensive assessment in which caregivers elicit relevant information about a patient's and family's cultural, ethnic, or religious traditions. Table 31–1 is a list of some of the important pieces of information that caregivers should gather from patients or families to better

TABLE 31–1. Suggested Items for a Cultural Assessment
• Country of birth or immigrant status
• Patient's ethnic or cultural identity, if any
• Primary and secondary language
• Religious affiliation
• Importance of religious belief or faith
• Membership in formal religious organization
• Identification with community clergy
• Religious practices
• Food and dietary preferences or prohibition
• Socioeconomic status: level of education, occupation
• Health and illness beliefs and practices
• Customs and rituals around the dying process and death

understand any cultural, ethnic, or religious issues they have.

The cultural assessment can be done as a separate part of the assessment, or these questions about issues and preferences may be interspersed into other part of the assessment. A good example of the latter would be the incorporation of questions regarding religious preferences and practices into the spiritual assessment (see Chapter 16).

Eliciting information from each patient and family about their specific cultural, ethnic, and religious preferences is crucial to providing culturally sensitive care to the diverse population that end-of-life care providers serve. For, even though individual patients and families may identify with one or more cultural, ethnic, or religious group, the level at which they follow the traditions and practices of the group can be extremely variable. So, although one can learn about the diverse rituals, traditions, and end-of-life care needs of different ethnic, cultural, or religious groups, one cannot take that knowledge and apply or impose it on any specific patient and family who identifies with any specific group. It is only by doing a good cultural assessment that one can learn what aspects, if any, of a group's practices are relevant and important to the specific patient and family being cared for, and then tailor the care to meet those individual needs.

AFRICAN AMERICANS

Michele Grant Irvin

INTRODUCTION

Today, black Americans are the second largest minority group in the United States (13.5%), with an estimated population of approximately 40.7 million. Of these, the vast majority are African American, defined by Ronald Barrett as referring to the descendants of those blacks who were enslaved and transported to America between the seventeenth and nineteenth centuries and who have been socialized primarily through values inculcated in the United States (2009). (As it is recognized that there is an increasing population of blacks of Caribbean descent or more recently emigrated from Africa who may have significantly different cultural values and norms, this discussion will primarily confine itself to African Americans as defined above.)

African American culture in the United States has been significantly shaped by the long history of discrimination and prejudice that has continued long past the days of slavery into the present. With a disproportionately high percentage of African Americans falling below the poverty line (33%), and with less physicians per capita caring for patients in African American communities than in white ones, there is less access to health care services in general, leading to poorer overall health and to the highest morbidity and mortality rates of any ethnic group in the United States for multiple illnesses including heart disease, cancer, cerebrovascular disease, and HIV/AIDS. In ad-

dition, despite the increased mortality rate, and what would clearly be a high need for end-of-life care services, African Americans have had disproportionately low utilization of hospice, with only 7.2% of all hospice patients served in the United States in 2008 being African American. Therefore, as the culturally diverse needs of African Americans are explored in the context of end-of-life care, it is necessary to understand how these needs are affected by the overt health care disparities that exist in this community.

HISTORY AND CULTURE OF MISTRUST

Health care disparities affecting minority populations, including African Americans, have most recently been chronicled in the Institute of Medicine's 2003 published report entitled: "Unequal Treatment: Confronting Racial and Ethnic Disparities in Health Care." Among the disparities that were reported that affect the African American include the belief that they receive less attention than white patients, that they are patronized in the doctor's office, that physicians do not communicate properly with them, and that they more often than not leave their doctor's office unclear as to the diagnosis and options for treatment.

At the root of these and other health care disparities that exist within the African American community is an innate mistrust of the U.S. health care system by African Americans. This culture of mistrust is well earned, with the Tuskegee Syphillis Study, during which treatment was withheld from several hundred black sharecroppers to study the natural history of the disease, being the most infamous example. But certainly that was not the only cause of mistrust.

Lack of trust in the health care system was shown to be one of the main reasons why, in a study evaluating the utilization of advance directives among African Americans, 75% of the 102 persons studied refused to complete an advance directive, even after receiving education on the benefits of advance care planning (Bullock,

2006). In addition, it may be, at least in part, responsible for the findings of a study discussed in the general introduction to this chapter, that a lower percentage of black patients (47%) had participated in advance care planning as compared to white patients (80%) and that black patients (45%) were much more likely to request life-prolonging care in the last few days of life than white (14%) patients (Smith et al., 2008). Caregiver recognition of this mistrust and a willingness to discuss and acknowledge this with African American patients may often be the initial step in building a positive relationship between the parties that will be able to continue throughout the patients' care.

AFRICAN AMERICAN ATTITUDES TOWARD DEATH AND DYING

It must be recognized that when interacting with African Americans, there is an unconscious tendency to see the color of the skin and make assumptions about the person's culture. Therefore, it is important to realize that African Americans exhibit significant diversity regarding religion, socioeconomic status, status of origin, sexuality, language, and life experiences. Nevertheless, there is a body of research which suggests that most African Americans share some common attitudes toward death and dying as well as funeral rites.

As many African Americans share certain African traditions blended with the Western culture they have been living in for several generations, they tend to be accepting of death, viewing it as part of the continuum of life. They believe in life after death, and the idea that a person transitions from the physical world to the spiritual world. This has also led to the notion that the physical and spiritual world overlap rather than being distinctly separate, and that the spirits of deceased ancestors may be present in the community.

African Americans regard the process of death and dying and the treatment of the deceased with great reverence and respect. This has led to the importance of the funeral as a primary ritual with great social significance. African Americans tend to spend more discretionary income on funerals than whites, and highly value attendance at and participation in funerals as a significant social obligation, with lack of attendance often being perceived as a sign of disrespect (see later for a more thorough discussion of African American funeral customs).

Spirituality and Religion

There is a diverse spectrum of religious and spiritual practices in the African American community (Christian, Muslim, Buddhist, etc.) and patients' beliefs, whether based on religion alone, spirituality alone, or a mixture of the two, provide important coping and survival resources, especially during critical end-of-life periods. Studies, in fact, suggest that health care decisions and views on death and dying among African Americans may have more to do with the religious or spiritual orientation of the individual rather than to race alone. It is important to be aware that religion and spirituality permeate the daily lives of many African American patients. This explains a common phrase that may be heard while caring for patients, "it's in God's hands now." Awareness of this belief and demonstration of respect for the patient's beliefs during development of goals of care will enhance and build a trusting provider/patient relationship.

The centrality of religion in the African American community is also manifest in the role of the African American church and the church community (as well as other faith-based organizations and their communities) in providing comfort to families that have experienced loss, irrespective of whether a patient and family have strong ties to a church or are "unchurched" (without strong church affiliation).

Clergy, as representatives of the faith community, also play a central role in providing care and support to patients and families, again, primarily due to the strong reverence for death held by

African Americans as well as their beliefs in the spiritual transition of the deceased. Clergy are expected to visit the sick and dying to offer prayers and support, as well as encourage others in the faith community to do the same. When a death occurs, the clergyperson should visit the family as soon as possible to offer condolences and assist with funeral arrangements. Clergy are expected to be present and supportive during the wake or other prefuneral service, officiate at the funeral, deliver a personalized eulogy, support the bereaved family members, and participate in the committal service or other appropriate postfuneral rituals based on the patient's and family's faith and wishes. They should also participate in postfuneral gatherings held for the family.

Role of the African American Families

African Americans have very close-knit family structures, although they may not take the form of what is considered in Western society as the "traditional" family. Often referred to as "kin networks," these extended families may include grandparents, noncustodial parents, and other nonblood relatives who are given the honorific title "aunt" or "uncle." These kin networks may be crucially important during times of illness, especially terminal illness, as they are a significant source of care and support. Elder members of the kin network may be looked upon for advice and counsel regarding end-of-life care decision making (see below) and bereavement support needs to be extended to all members of a kin network following a death.

End-of-Life Care Decision Making

Due to a combination of the close-knit nature of the African American family as well as the innate mistrust of the health care system already discussed, African Americans traditionally "take of their own." They also have a low expectation of the services they are likely to receive from outside health care providers, including hospice and palliative care programs, as they have been chronically underserved by virtually all aspects of the health care system.

End-of-life decision making may pose challenges for African American patients and families as well. Many believe that choosing not to be resuscitated or refusing or withdrawing a feeding tube only gives the health care system license to provide substandard care or give up on them prematurely. Electing to execute an advance directive often increases feelings of hopelessness and patients and families may often feel conflicted when considering discontinuing life-prolonging therapy as there may some perception that they are giving up the hope that God will heal them. Discussion of these issues, therefore, has to be undertaken with a great deal of care, knowledge of the patient's and family's health care concerns, and an understanding of their cultural, spiritual, and religious values. Oftentimes, spiritual counselors or kin network elders can be of great assistance in facilitating these conversations.

AFRICAN AMERICAN FUNERAL CUSTOMS

As already mentioned, due to their reverence for death as a critical moment in life, African Americans view the funeral, and the active participation of family and community in the activities and rituals surrounding it, as an event of tremendous importance. Tying back to the African view that the funeral reflects the value of the individual to the community, many African Americans join funeral societies or have burial policies to ensure that they have a decent and proper funeral. Cremation is not widely accepted, although it is being used more in some communities in the last decade or so as the costs of burial continue to rise significantly.

Specific funeral customs vary considerable among African Americans on the basis of their specific religious affiliations. A prototype of an African American funeral, however, is often characterized as a traditional, emotional, "homegoing" service, consistent with the concept discussed earlier that the person is transitioning to the spiritual world. It often takes significant time to plan, and may not take place until approximately a week following the death. This time delay allows family members who live a distance from where the deceased will be interred to be able to travel to the funeral, which is extremely important, as family relationships can be significantly damaged if a family member is not present or does not properly participate at the funeral of a loved one. The more respected and esteemed the deceased, the greater is the time and resources spent on the service, so the added time also allows for the necessary resources to be gathered.

The funeral service itself may last for several hours and there is a great deal of emotional expression, often with a great deal spontaneity as well as by musical participation, and if there are postfuneral services (such as a committal followed by a family gathering and repast), the activities may last an entire day. As African Americans have become more acculturated into Western society, some, especially those who have moved into the middle or upper socioeconomic classes, have chosen to have funeral services more in keeping with white America, which tend to be less emotional, more formal, and more stoic.

Common to all African American funerals is the importance of the community participation. There is an implicit social obligation to gather and express support and condolences to the bereaved as well as to honor the deceased and one's presence at all aspects of the process (i.e., visiting the family when learning of the death, attending the funeral as well as all pre- and postfuneral activities) is considered the greatest expression of support one can provide.

In addition to one's presence, it is the norm for African Americans to provide the bereaved with support in the form of money, resources, and food. Here, again, the more personal one's involvement in this, the more highly valued is the expression of support. For example, although both are appreciated, the individual who prepares food for the family is regarded more highly than the individual who buys already prepared items.

CONCLUSIONS

With the understanding that African Americans should not be stereotyped and that there are significant cultural, spiritual, and religious differences, they share certain common issues that hospice and palliative care providers need to understand to help provide care to this significantly underserved population. Central to this is the recognition that many African Americans significantly mistrust the health care system, and that they often make decisions based on this mistrust and the idea that unless they advocate for themselves they will be undertreated by physicians and other service providers.

To assist end-of-life care providers in overcoming this significant barrier to access, Burrs et al. (2009) have made a number of recommendations, which include the following:

- Address the mistrust issue directly.
- Promote cultural proficiency in your practice and organization.
- Educate health care providers (all disciplines), the African American community, and major stakeholders (financing, health care systems) regarding hospice and palliative care referral and use.
- Acknowledge and continue to monitor for unequal care/access.
- Level the reimbursement field to provide better access to hospice and palliative care.
- Empower the African American community by identifying its leaders and resources and involving them in promoting hospice and palliative care.
- Develop policies/guidelines for health care providers that are evidence based and decrease likelihood of disparities in care.

By establishing a relationship of trust, which is often very challenging and rarely ideal, more African American patients who are approaching the end of life will have access to appropriate pain and symptom management, and will be more comfortable having conversations about goals of care and advance care planning.

HISPANIC PATIENTS

Freddie J. Negron, Teresita Mesa, and Yolanda Castillo

INTRODUCTION

Hispanic, derived and anglicized from the Spanish word *hispanos,* was a term originally used by people of Latin American descent living in New Mexico to refer to themselves. Its official use as an ethnic label was promoted in the 1970s by New Mexico Senator Joseph Montoya and others to be able to better identify and quantify people of Latin American descent in the U.S. census. Another term used to define this same group of people is Latino, likely derived from a shortening of these individuals region of origin, Latin America. From these beginnings, the terms Hispanic and Latino have been formally defined by the U.S. Office of Management and Budget as "persons of Mexican, Puerto Rican, Cuban, South or Central American, or other Spanish culture or origin, regardless of race."

Hispanics represent the single largest minority group in the United States, with a population estimated at 45.5 million (15.5% of the U.S. population). In addition, it is the fastest growing segment of the United States population with recent statistics from the Census Bureau demonstrating that Hispanics born as American citizens accounted for more than a third of the population increase in 2005. A significant number of U.S. cities, including Miami, New York, Los Angeles, San Antonio, and Chicago boast sizable Latino populations. With the continued growth of the Hispanic population, it is expected that they may become the majority in California as early as 2018 and it is anticipated that Texas may have a sufficiently large Latino population to elect a Hispanic Governor around the same time (Texas Monthly, 2008).

As the Hispanic population in the United States grows, the need for health care services, including services for patients near the end of life, will significantly increase. In fact, according to statistics published by the National Hospice and Palliative Care Organization, Hispanic patients accounted for 5.1% of those who accessed the hospice benefit in 2007. What makes this significant is not a dramatic increase from the prior year (4.9% in 2006), but the fact that in prior years the impact of Hispanic patients on hospice utilization was not deemed great enough to warrant measuring them as a separate group.

With expectations that hospice will be accessed by increasing numbers of Hispanic patients in the future, it is incumbent upon us to be better prepared to serve these patients by enhancing our understanding of the dynamics and the diversity of the Latino culture. Therefore, we address a number of issues that significantly impact the care of Hispanic patients near the end of life and their families. It should be noted that although Hispanics living in the United States originate from a number of different nations which have specific cultural distinctions, they also share a common heritage and have a great deal in common. Rather than focus on the differences, this discussion will concentrate on the similarities found within Hispanic culture as it pertains to caring for patients at the end of life.

DEATH AND DYING WITHIN THE HISPANIC CULTURE

As already noted, there is considerable variability among Hispanic patients regarding the approach to care and decision making at the end of life, based on factors such as race, country of origin, and country of birth, with those born in the United States and further removed from their country of origin tending to be more acculturated to "Western" customs typical of the United States. Irrespective of these differences, there are three common factors that significantly affect all

Hispanic patients when facing end-of-life issues: their religious beliefs, their respect for their physicians, and the overriding sense of family.

Role of Religion

The Hispanic community in the United States is, for the most part, fervently religious, with approximately 68% of all Latinos identifying themselves as Roman Catholic, the majority of them being immigrants. Of the remaining 32%, approximately 20% identify themselves as Protestants, 3% are of other Christian faiths, 1% are from non-Christian religions, and only approximately 8% of Hispanics do not identify with any religious group.

Irrespective of religious affiliation, the great majority of Hispanics incorporate God actively into their everyday lives. Many pray every day, most have a religious object in the home, and most attend a religious service at least monthly. At least one national survey also suggests that many Latinos who identify with a religion believe that miracles are performed today just as they were in ancient times. This religious intensity, not surprisingly, significantly influences how Hispanic patients and their families react when faced with end-of-life situations. Therefore, end-of-life caregivers, as part of their routine evaluation of Hispanic patients, must learn about their specific religious beliefs and practices to properly care for them.

Role of the Primary Care Physician

Latinos view their physicians with great respect and see them as major authority figures. Therefore, they will generally seek their physicians out for advice regarding health care choices and follow the physicians' instructions. This can have significant impacts on the end-of-life care that Hispanics patients receive, especially when physicians and end-of-life care providers are not in agreement about any aspect of a patient's plan of care, in which case the patient is more often than not, going to follow the advice of the physician. Therefore, it is incumbent upon professional caregivers who are providing end-of-life care to Hispanic patients to develop strong lines of communication with their patients' primary physicians, to avoid any potential conflict and ensure that the patients receive optimal symptom management.

Role of Family

Hispanics are extremely family-centered. It is very common for multiple generations to live together in an extended family household or, if they do not reside in the same household, they will often live in close residential proximity to one another. Life cycle events, such as births, birthdays, anniversaries, and holidays are occasions for extended Latino families to gather together to celebrate and provide support. Illnesses are viewed in a similar light, so it not unusual that, when a family member is approaching death, all members of the extended family who live in the household or in the proximity have an opportunity to participate in the care and anticipatory grieving of their loved one.

Many Hispanic families are patriarchal, whereas some families from Central or South America may be matriarchal. Whatever the case, it is the head of the family that is often looked upon as the ultimate decision maker. Nevertheless, when a family member is approaching the end of life, it is not unusual to have many members of the extended family involved in decision making, either providing input to the family head or legal health care surrogate or directly participating as a surrogate. Therefore, it is important to involve all concerned family members that have a relevant relationship with the patient, along with the patient and the primary physician, in establishing the goals of care.

When a loved one is nearing the end of life, Hispanic families often assume a protective role by not allowing any discussion of the ill family member's terminal prognosis. The assumption that is generally made is that if the patient was aware that life was coming to an end, the person would not be able to tolerate the information and would become extremely depressed or even consider taking his or own life. This "conspiracy of silence" may even extend to hospice caregivers, who are often requested by the family to avoid the use of the word "hospice" or similar terms that connote end-of-life care, and to not to wear a name badge in the home if it has the word hospice on it. What is more tragic is that the patient is often on the other side of this "conspiracy of silence" as he or she actually knows what is happening but does not want well-meaning family members to know that he or she knows. It is important for caregivers to not only recognize and respect this "conspiracy of silence" as a cultural norm, but to work within it to maintain the trust of the patient and family. However, when caregivers see the opportunity, they should take the time to facilitate communication between the patient and family members, so that, if agreed to by all concerned, the "conspiracy" can be broken, and patients and families can enjoy the remaining time they have without watching everything they say.

Nutrition and Hydration

For many Hispanic families, food is considered a powerful symbol of wellness, and in face of illness, it represents the hope of improvement and cure. For some, providing nutritional support to loved ones is so important, that they perceive a direct correlation between nutritional support or hydration and the amount of care that the loved one is receiving. For others, religious considerations dictate the provision of food and fluids. Many also believe that not providing patients with food or fluid is tantamount to allowing the patients to die of starvation or dehydration, which is considered emotionally to be a "painful and cruel" treatment. Therefore, when Hispanic patients nearing the end of life either refuse food or fluids or are unable to take them orally, families often request artificial nutritional support or hydration.

In this type of situation, the role of the end-of-life caregiver is one of empathy and respect for the family's request and point of view. Once one understands the cultural and, in many cases, religious motivations for the request, these con-

cerns can be addressed with appropriate education around the pros and cons of providing food and fluid to patients who are approaching the end of life. Creative solutions, such as providing small amounts of food via spoon-feeding or syringe, or small amounts of fluid by hypodermoclysis, can often reassure families that their loved ones are being properly cared for, not in pain or discomfort, and not being "starved to death," while avoiding the discomfort and potential unpleasant effects that often result when terminally patients are either tube fed or overhydrated (see Chapter 24 for a full discussion of nutrition and hydration at the end of life).

Morphine for the Management of Pain and Dyspnea

The word "morphine" evokes strong negative reactions in many Hispanics, likely related to the recollection of inappropriate uses of the drug in their countries of origin. Some equate "morphine" directly with euthanasia or physician-assisted suicide. These negative feelings about "morphine," not surprisingly, often create challenges for end-of-life physicians and other caregivers when morphine is necessary to control symptoms such as pain or dyspnea, as patients and their family members are often reluctant to allow morphine (and sometimes related opioids) to be prescribed and will refuse to take the medication. Complicating these challenges are that these same negative reactions can be found among many Hispanic physicians and nurses who are not well acquainted with the principles of palliative medicine, and they will often discourage patients under their care from taking morphine as well.

As discussed earlier, empathy, respect, and understanding why patients and families do not want to use "morphine" are the first step to finding a solution. Education remains the key, and often, a caring physician can explain how morphine will help the patient in a way that will allay any fears and preconceived ideas that a patient or family might have. If this is not successful, a creative solution, such as substituting an opioid with a name other than "morphine," such as oxycodone, might resolve the situation to the patient's benefit while respecting the family's concerns.

"SAYING GOODBYE"

When Hispanic patients enter the final phase of life, it is important for professional cargivers to visit with the patient on a daily basis. Hispanics generally choose to die at home, and multiple family members will usually be present at the bedside of their dying loved one around the clock. At the time of death, the reactions of family members vary across the entire spectrum, from quiet acceptance to loud aggressive behavior and expressions of denial.

Once the patient has died, the care of the body and funeral customs are dictated by the religious affiliation of the patient and family. As approximately 90% of Hispanics in the United States identify themselves as Christian (with more than two-thirds being Roman Catholic), a wake is usual prior to burial, with variable timing based on the religious practices of the specific church that the patient belonged to. Some will start the viewing of the body within 24 hours of death, continue the viewing throughout the night so that the body remains attended at all times, and have the burial occur the following morning. Others may have the body viewed for only a couple of hours and immediately proceed to the burial.

CONCLUSION

Hispanics in the United States, although often thought of as a single population due to a common language, actually consist of widely diverse subgroups of people from different countries with varying cultural norms. Of common importance to all, however, especially as one's life is nearing its end, are religious and cultural tradition, family, honor of the elderly, and respect for the physician. Each of these has a significant impact on how patients and families face end-of-life issues. Caregivers must remember that while virtu-

ally all Hispanic patients and their families view these factors with great importance, how they express them varies greatly, not only among different Hispanic religious and cultural subgroups, but among individuals within each particular subgroup as well. It is only by focusing on the individual patient and family, and knowing what is important to them, that one can provide true culturally sensitive care.

ASIAN AMERICAN PATIENTS

Barry M. Kinzbrunner

INTRODUCTION

Asian Americans are a heterogenous group of individuals that have migrated to the United States from the myriad of nations in the Far East and Pacific Rim, including China, Japan, Korea, Vietnam, the Philippines, and India, to name a few. Based on data from the 2000 U.S. census, there are approximately 12 million people who identify themselves as Asian American, representing 4.3% of the total U.S. population. They are also among the fast growing ethnic groups in the United States, with a documented population increase of 63% between the 1990 and 2000 census.

Religious practices vary among Asian Americans almost as much as country of origin. Based on Pew Research Institute Study from 2008, 45% identify themselves as Christian (17% Catholic, 27% Protestant), 14% Hindu, 9% Buddhist, and 4% Muslim, and 5% identify with a variety of other religions. Twenty-three percent of Asian Americans consider themselves to be unaffiliated with any specific faith. It should be noted that even with the more prevalent faiths, such as the various forms of Christianity, Asian Americans have brought their own unique traditions, rituals, and observances to these well-established religions and these unique traits may become apparent when end-of-life care issues arise.

As a whole, the Asian American community values family, and hence, it is not unusual for patients near the end of life to be cared for in the home, rather than in a facility. In addition, as Asian cultures tend to avoid airing personal problems, family is often where individuals go to seek guidance when things are not going well. Many Asian Americans, influenced by the value of self-control, do not tend to react emotionally to stress or show feelings very readily. In addition, the core values of guilt and shame play a significant role in the behaviors exhibited by Asian Americans in the public arena.

Language barriers, especially for more recent immigrants, may be a significant challenge, and both family and professional translators are often required to foster proper communication with patients.

With this background, the specific cultures and traditions of some of the more prominent Asian American groups will be explored, with an eye toward how they affect issues related to the care of these individuals as end-of-life approaches.

CHINESE AMERICAN

Chinese Americans are the largest Asian American group, with a population of over 2.7 million (22.6% of American Asians). Traditional Chinese religion is a mixture of Buddhist, Confucian, and Taoism, although many Chinese American families have converted to Christianity. Nevertheless, elements of their prior faiths may significantly influence behavior and beliefs. Chinese culture, for example, is heavily influenced by the Taoist philosophy of yin–yang, and in health care this translates into the belief that the harmony and balance of the mind, body, and spirit are the keys to maintaining good health.

Chinese Americans maintain a very closely knit family structure. Families are tightly bound, divorce is relatively uncommon, and children remain heavily involved with their parents throughout their lives. The significance of family loyalty transcends one's individual wishes, and there is an expectation that all emotional and financial support will come from within the family unit.

Respect for elders is an essential part of the familial culture, and there is a clear hierarchy among family members, with the oldest male member of the family usually serving as the spokesperson and decision maker. Direct eye contact with authority figures is frowned upon. Questioning of the family elder may be seen as a sign of disrespect as is referring to an elder by his or her first name.

Chinese Americans are often extremely modest and shy. Touching is generally reserved for close family and friends, and female patients may be uncomfortable when confronted with a male caregiver, so this situation should be avoided when possible.

With the high degree of family unity displayed by Chinese Americans, most elderly family members who are infirm or ill are cared for at home rather than in an institution. However, near the end of life, this may change as some Chinese Americans believe that dying in the home will bring bad luck and for these patients and families, when death is approaching, relocation of the patient to a hospice or palliative care inpatient facility may be required. Conversely, others believe that if one dies in an institution, the spirit may get lost, and in this situation, the patient will be best served by continuing to receive care in the home setting.

Although Chinese Americans make use of Western medicine, they still may choose to rely on traditional Chinese remedies for certain ailments, including medicinal teas and soups, as well as acupuncture for certain ailments. Many believe that the proper combination of yin and yang foods may prevent illness, although when one becomes ill, one may avoid certain types of food to try and restore the balance that is believed to have been lost. As illness is perceived to be, at least in part, a result of a loss of balance in one's life, Chinese American patients are often reluctant to discuss health issues or complain of pain and other symptoms to "save face."

Chinese American patients and families have a variety of views on the topic of terminal prognosis and death. Some patients are willing to discuss the issue, whereas others are not. In a similar vein, there will be families who are comfortable with the caregiver discussing this with their loved one, families who will want to the have the conversation with their loved ones themselves, whereas others do not want the patient told about the terminal illness. Professional caregivers, therefore, have to be aware of each specific patient's and family's wishes on this subject.

Funerals for Chinese Americans, especially those who were born in the United States, are more than likely consistent with the traditions and customs of whatever religious community they belong. However, immigrants, even if they have converted to Christianity, will often have funerals that are colored with traditions brought with them from China. These customs, which any individual person will desire to have followed to various degrees or not at all, vary based on the Chinese village that the person originally came from and as many believe that funerals are filled with bad omens, many of the rituals are designed to ward off bad spirits.

These rituals start in the home prior to the funeral, where at the time the family leaves for the funeral service, all the lights may be turned on to help the deceased's spirit find his or her way out. Looking back at the house is considered bad luck, as is returning to the house before the funeral service has been concluded, or the deceased's spirit may follow one back and become trapped.

During the funeral, the patriarch of the family sits closest to coffin with the rest of family seated based on their hierarchical importance in the family: spouse, children, grandchildren, siblings, and siblings' children. The eldest son is responsible to lead a period of wailing, which is considered a sign of respect and honor for the deceased. In traditional funerals, the bereaved wear white. In addition, men wear black armbands, whereas women wear green bows or flowers in their hair. These are then thrown into the grave before it is closed. Women will then wear red bows for the next 3 days.

The deceased is buried with the head pointing to the north, and it is preferable that the gravesite be on a hill with a water source nearby. It is considered bad luck to watch the casket as it is lowered, although a family member may be assigned the task of watching this to ensure that the casket remains closed for fear of bad spirits getting inside.

There is a tradition among some to give mourners small white envelopes with a coin and a piece of candy, termed *bak gim* or "white gold." This symbolizes money or a gift from the deceased. The candy is to be eaten immediately after the funeral to "sweeten" the solemn event, whereas the coin is to be spent on something that brings joy after the funeral's sadness. Another custom is to give a red envelope with a dollar bill. Red is considered good luck and, combined with the money, the envelope is supposed to restore any good fortune that was lost at the funeral.

After the services, the family returns home and upon entering the house, each member jumps over a small fire to cleanse themselves of bad spirits. They are then each given three grains of rice with a small amount of water to swallow, representative of the staples needed to sustain life: earth, wind, fire, and water. A funeral banquet is then sometimes held to help the bereaved "swallow their pain."

Three days after the funeral, the family returns to the grave to visit the deceased. Some Buddhist families will bring food and burn incense at the grave. Others burn paper objects, including money, clothes, and even cars, as offerings for the deceased to use in the afterlife.

FILIPINO AMERICANS

The second largest group of Asian Americans living in the United States are Filipinos, roughly 2.4 million (18.3%). Many have come to assist their families who remain in the Philippines economically. In Filipino American culture, the family is of utmost importance, and this includes the extended family. Elders are highly respected, and are shown respect by kissing the hand, forehead, or cheek. They place a high priority on cultural traditions to keep the family close. The extended family also benefits from emotional ties, family loyalty, and economic exchange, and is valued as a source of emotional sustenance and mutual support.

Religion is central to Filipino life. The majority of Filipinos in the United States are of the Roman Catholic faith, with small minorities identifying as Protestant or Muslim. Filipino Catholic ritual and tradition is colored by belief and customs brought from the Philipine Islands that were previously home. Most Filipino Americans speak and understand English, and many speak Spanish as well. In fact, as many Filipinos have Spanish surnames, one must not make the mistake of confusing a Filipino for someone of Hispanic origin.

Filipino Americans tend to appear shy and are very polite, avoiding direct eye contact, especially with superiors and authority figures. They tend to smile as sign of greeting or acknowledgment, and will often use facial expressions instead of verbally responding to questions. Filipinos use respect for all as the basis for social interaction. In addition, they place a high value on proper social conduct to avoid shame or "save face."

Many Filipino Americans believe that good health is achieved by maintaining balance, and that illness is the result of losing that balance. Illness is also associated with bad behavior and punishment, with the accompanying belief that one must correct the evil deed in order for health to be restored. Others believe that all physical ailments have supernatural causes. Patients may seek traditional Western health care, but many will also use folk medicine concurrently. Some who are ill will postpone seeking medical attention until they have attempted treatment with herbal remedies.

Prior to discussing advance care planning or a hospice or palliative medicine referral with a patient, the family elder and spokesperson, usually the father or eldest son, should be consulted. Most often, the family will want the responsibility to discuss the terminal illness and prognosis with the patient, and will often opt to make advance care planning decisions related to cardiopulmonary resuscitation (CPR) or nutrition and hydration.

Many Filipino Americans, even when elderly, place a high emphasis on youthfulness, and see death as occurring in the far future. However, once they lose physical dependence, they usually prefer to remain at home and be cared for by family members until death. However, when the family members responsible for care have other commitments, such as work or school, patients may sometimes, albeit reluctantly, be placed in a facility. Filipino American patients tend to be stoic when experiencing pain. For some, this may be due to a higher pain threshold than otherwise might be anticipated, whereas for others, the fear of addiction to analgesics may make them reluctant to agree to be medicated. They believe that death is "an act of God," that strong faith can thwart death, and when faith does not work to ward off the death, there may be guilt that one's faith was not strong enough to save the loved one who passed on.

Funeral customs, designed to assist the soul in its survival and passage into the next world, are quite elaborate as carried out in the Philippines. Public grieving is considered a sign of respect. Therefore, women are expected to grieve very openly and demonstrably, often fainting, swooning, or hugging the casket whereas men are more reserved. People also tend to grieve in groups rather than privately.

Once a death has occurred, the deceased should be blessed by a priest to ensure entry into heaven, following which the body is prepared for burial and laid out for visitation in the home. Word of mouth is the main method of communicating informaton about the death and funeral plans. During the time between death and burial, which may be from 3 to 7 days depending on logistics, the family ceases all personal and normal activities, and instead focuses on cooking and making preparations for the ongoing visitations prior to burial. Family and friends are expected to surround the body of the deceased 24 hours a day and the deceased is surrounded by lit candles and fresh flowers. Nightly prayers are recited in the home of the deceased family for an extended period of time (9 days in one report, 30 days in another) to aid the deceased in getting to heaven. Nightly prayers are again recited on the 40th day when it is believed that the soul is making its ascent to heaven.

The funeral itself is very elaborate, with the type of casket and flower arrangements being viewed as reflective of the deceased's life. Therefore, no expense is spared. The funeral is punctuated by a long procession on foot through the town. The procession takes an indirect route to the cemetery to allow people to pay their last respects to the deceased, and participants sing prayers during the procession.

Filipino culture believes in the idea that the "longer the grief, the better." Therefore, for up to a year, and often beyond, men will wear a black ribbon and women will dress in black to signify that they are in mourning. Masses for a specific deceased person may be held in several churches in the locale during the weeks following the death, at which family and friends of the deceased are expected. Families visit the grave of the deceased on multiple occasions during the months following burial, and a special mass is held on the first anniversary of the death.

In the United States, these rituals are not carried out to the same extent, and for Filipino immigrants, this has led to the wish of many to return to Philipines either prior to death (to reunite the family in life) or at death for a proper funeral and burial.

ASIAN INDIAN AMERICANS

Asian Indians are the third largest group of Asians to settle in the United States. Their population is approximately 1.9 million, which represents approximately 16.4% of the Asian American population. Like immigrants from other Asian nations, family is central. In the traditional Indian family,

in fact, the members of the extended family often live together as a single family unit. The elderly are often dependent on their children for support, and it is not uncommon for a husband's parents to join the family (as families in many parts of Indian society are matriarchal in nature) when they retire or need financial assistance. Grandparents play a significant role in child rearing, as they form a link to the Indian culture, religion, and heritage.

The vast majority of Asian Indian Americans are Hindu. Other religions practiced by members of this population include Sikhism, Buddhism, Christianity, and Islam. Although Indians have a national language, Hindi, which is spoken by over 40% of the population, there are actually over 300 languages and dialects spoken by the people of India. English has become a popular second language, so although many younger Indian immigrants may have some facility with English, older immigrants may not and, therefore, may need a translator for health care discussions.

Traditional Indian beliefs in health care center around what is called "ayurvedic medicine" as the means of preventing and curing illness. This methodology, originating in India thousands of years ago, views the complete human being as a combination of mind, body, senses, and soul, and looks to aid people in attaining balance between the physical, mental, and spiritual domains by suggesting specific lifestyle and nutritional guidelines, as well as herbal supplements, to assist in maintaining or restoring that balance. The Hindu concept of "karma" also plays a significant role in health and illness, as many believe that illness is caused by "karma."

Modesty is of great importance among Asian Indians, and patients usually prefer care givers of the same gender whenever possible. Direct eye contact from women to men may be avoided. Hindu married women wear a thread around their necks called *mangalsutra*, and this thread should not be removed when care is being provided.

Indian patients tend to prefer physicians who are active and appear in charge. They are more comfortable when the doctor has all the answers and most patients tend to follow the physicians medical advice without question. Health care decisions tend to be discussed by the family, with women often allowing men to play the major role in health care decision making. The elderly, as well, will tend to defer health care decisions to the family and in some situations family members may ask the physician not tell the patient the diagnosis or prognosis.

The elderly also may behave stoically when in pain, so nonverbal clues to pain are important. In addition, mental illnesses are considered a stigma, so patients often have somatic complaints when they are experiencing anxiety or depression. For this reason, the elderly are not always willing to receive counseling to deal with these types of issues.

Asian Indian American patients generally prefer to die at home. However, if institutionalization is required, one must be aware of a number of issues. For example, Hindu patients will not want to eat food containing any beef, whereas Muslim patients will not to want have anything with pork. Some patients do not like to wear hospital gowns or other clothing worn by others, even if the clothes are cleaned and sterilized. The sacred thread around the neck should not be removed or cut without the patient's permission, and as Sikh men do not cut their hair, if the hair must be cut, the reason should be carefully explained to the patient. Asian Indians who are hospitalized also tend to like visitors and expect them to stay for a long period of time.

When patients are nearing death, many of the rituals and practices are religiously based. For Hindu families, many believe that if suffering occurs prior to death, this is due to "karma." Family is often present in large numbers to be with their dying loved one. The dying person may with to be moved to the floor, to be closer to "mother earth."

After death, the family will often choose to be the ones to wash and prepare the body. Cremation is preferred over burial. Families often desire privacy after someone has passed on to allow for the specific religious rites to be performed, fol-

lowing which it is accepted practice for family members and others to openly express grief. For Hindu families, prior to cremation, a priest will offer prayers. Traditional Indian cremations take place on a wooden pyre, the body is dressed in gold-ornamented clothing, and it can take several hours for the body to burn. This is often not done in the United States, where electric cremation is the norm. Garlands of flowers, incense sticks, and purified melted butter, called *ghee*, are placed on the stretcher along with the body. Men tend to play the primary roles in funeral rites. After cremation, there is usually a mourning period of between 10 and 40 days. More detailed discussion of Hindu funeral rites can be found in the section on Hindu Americans below.

For Asian Indian Americans of other religions, the rituals of their specific faiths are generally observed.

VIETNAMESE AMERICANS

The fourth most populous group, representing 10.9% of the Asian Americans population, are the Vietnamese, with over 1.2 million people. Family loyalty is considered a premium among Vietnamese Americans, with sometimes up to four generations living under one roof to provide aid and support to one another. Due to the prolonged conflict in Vietnam in the latter part of the twentiethcentury, many immigrants suffer from varying degrees of posttraumatic stress disorder. However, due to the close-knit nature of the family unit, individuals primarily seek support for emotional distress from family, and clinicians providing such support may find it difficult to provide to patients of Vietnamese origin.

The primary religious affiliations of Vietnamese Americans are Buddhism and Roman Catholicism, with small minorities identifying with various other Far Eastern religions, Protestantism, and Islam. Ancestor worship is prominent in Vietnamese American culture, and it is not unusual for their homes to have altars dedicated to deceased relatives, with pictures, candles, incense, and religious articles and offerings on display.

The Vietnamese New Year, Tet, is an important holiday that is celebrated by most Vietnamese Americans. This usually occurs sometime between January 19 and February 20 and is considered a time of rebirth and renewal. Two other important holidays that many Vietnamese Americans continue to observe are *Thanh-Minh* and *Trung Nguyen*. *Thanh-Minh*, translated as "Day of the Dead," is celebrated in the third lunar month, and is a time when people visit the graves of their ancestors to pay their respects, clean the gravesites, offer food and flowers, and light incense sticks. It is also a day for the surviving family to gather and regroup. *Trung Nguyen*, Wandering Souls Day, occurs on the 15th day of the 7th lunar month, and is the day when souls are free to wander, and return to their homes to search for food. Vietnamese who observe this day set out large buffets to feed the wandering souls, pray for the souls, and also for their ancestors. Some of the buffets are set up outdoors to allow souls who have no family to partake as well.

Vietnamese Americans are modest and respectful. They greet with a smile and a bow. They prefer larger personal space than Western culture, and shaking hands, especially with a woman, is frowned upon unless she offers it first. Eye contact with persons considered to be of higher status, such as physicians, is avoided, and respect is shown by the slight bowing of the head or by using both hands to give something to another. Open expression of emotions is considered taboo, and indirect communication rather than confrontation is used to express disagreement.

Vietnamese believe that disease is caused by an imbalance of forces similar to the Chinese yin and yang, termed *am* and *duong*, respectively. Although many access Western medicine, they also seek Chinese herbal remedies, acupuncture, and various spiritual practices when ill. Many tend to have a fatalistic view of illness, and may view it as part of one's destiny or fate. Due to the high value placed on family, elders are cared for at home, and institutionalization is avoided.

When the end of life is approaching, most Vietnamese American families prefer that patients not be told about the terminal illness. Conversations related to decision making should be with the head of family. Patients and families also are often hesitant to ask questions openly, preferring that explanations be given in privacy. Denial or tolerance of physical pain is considered a strong character trait, so patients tend to be stoic when experiencing pain. Caregivers, therefore, should observe patient's facial expressions and body language to gain some insight as to the level of discomfort. Analgesics are often avoided due to the fear of addiction or side effects.

When death is approaching, if the patient is in a hospital or other institution, every effort is made to bring the person home. The loved one is constantly looked after by family members, and when death seems imminent, all family members are called to say their final goodbyes. Silence is often observed, and the eldest child will attempt to recall the dying person's last words of advice or counsel. It is traditional for the elder child to give the dying person another name just prior to death as well.

When a parent passes away, the children do not, traditionally, accept the idea that the person has died. They place a chopstick between the teeth of the deceased and place the body on a mat on a floor to try and bring it back to life. The eldest child then takes a shirt that the deceased had worn when alive, and waves it in the air, calling upon the soul to return to the body. Following this, the body is cleaned. Money, gold, and rice are placed in the mouth of the deceased, symbolizing that the deceased has left the world without want or hunger. The body is then wrapped in a white cloth and placed in a coffin. A prayer service is held, following which, the body is taken to the cemetery, where the funeral is held. At no time is the body left unattended by family members.

Following the funeral service, the body is lowered into the ground, incense is burned, and respects are paid to other relatives buried in the same cemetery. Three days after the funeral, incense is burned, flowers are brought, and prayers are said for the deceased. Then, once per week for 7 weeks, a memorial service is held for the deceased. Additional memorial services are held 100 days following the death, on the first anniversary of the death, and then yearly on each subsequent anniversary.

Immediate family mourns for a period of 2 years. During this time, mourners are not allowed to wear bright-colored clothing and at all memorial services, a special black or white fabric is also worn. Some have the tradition of covering their heads as well. Family members may not marry or make any significant life decisions during the 2-year period. At the end of the 2 years, one burns the fabric, signifying the end of the formal mourning period. Mourners may now marry and make other major life decisions, and the deceased is considered to be a dead ancestor, in the company of all other ancestors who have previously passed on.

KOREAN AMERICANS

Korean Americans represent the fifth highest population subgroup among Asian Americans (10.5%), with a population of over 1.2 million. Koreans share with many other Asian American peoples a strong sense of family, courtesy, and respect for the elderly. The vast majority of Korean Americans are of the Christian faith, colored with many Korean traditions. A small percentage of Koreans identify as Buddhist.

Respect is key to the Korean American. This respect may be shown by a quick "quarter-bow" while it is considered rude to direct the sole of one's shoe at another. Direct eye contact is generally avoided and body language is very important in expressing feelings and emotions. Koreans also have a sense of pride, which may result in patients or families not wanting to communicate if they feel any sense of embarrassment or shame.

The sense of family is very strong among Korean Americans. Respect for the elderly and filial piety dominate family relationships, with adult children accepting a great deal of responsibility to ensure their parents are properly cared for. Institutionalization of the elderly, therefore, is considered disrespectful and is generally frowned upon.

In addition to western medicine, Korean Americans will also rely on herbal and folk remedies, as well acupuncture, when ill. Some may also choose to utilize "spiritual healers" to drive out evil spirits that are thought to cause illness. Korean Americans, especially elderly men, will be extremely stoic when experiencing pain, although when family members are present, it is considered acceptable to be dramatic and behave in a manner suggesting that symptoms that are worse than they actually are. Pain medications are often avoided due to a fear of addiction.

When patients are nearing the end of life, decisions regarding the course of care are usually deferred to the family. A male elder, either husband, father, or eldest son, is usually the spokesman for the family. Information regarding terminal prognosis should be communicated to the family, preferably by the physician, and the family will then decide how and when the patient should be told.

When a Korean American passes away, the family may want to spend some private time with their loved one. Although Koreans may seem to cry, chant, or pray in an exaggerated way, this is considered the norm in their culture. Following death, the body is traditionally placed in a straight position, covered with a white sheet, and placed behind a partition. In front of the partition, a small table is set up with a photograph of the deceased and incense. At that point, the death is announced.

Korean funerals traditionally last for 3 days. The eldest son of the deceased assumes the role of *sangju*, ostensibly the master of ceremonies. The *sangju* will dress in a black suit and wear a hemp hat, the latter representing at time when all the clothing worn by the *sangju* was hemp. He also will wear a black ribbon on his chest or arm.

One the second day of the funeral, the *sangju* will arrange for the body to be cleaned and dressed. Although there are traditional clothes for the deceased, it is acceptable today for a suit to be worn. The body is then put into a casket, which is set behind a partition or black curtain. A table in front of the partition or curtain is set up with a picture of the deceased that has a black ribbon on it, candles, and incense. The *sangju* sits next to the table on a coarse mat (he is atoning for the sin of allowing his parent to die).

Following this, visitors are received. Mourners light a stick of incense on the table, bow at the table, and then the *sangju* and guests bow at each other. Other than a brief thank you, the *sangju* is not supposed to speak. When visitors leave, they traditionally deposit a white envelope that contains money used to help defray the cost of the funeral.

On the third day, in the morning, a short ceremony is held in the house to honor the deceased. The deceased is eulogized and incense is offered. The *sangju* and relatives then traditionally carry the casket to the burial grounds, although today they may accompany the casket using a hearse. Burial sites are traditionally on small hills, and are used for the entire extended family, often for generations. The casket is lowered and the *sangju* throws earth on the casket three times. The grave is then filled, a small mound is built on top of the grave, and the mound is then covered with grass. A small stone with the name of the deceased is buried so that the grave can be identified when the mound erodes away. A tombstone is set up in front of the grave, and a brief ceremony is held. After the burial, the *sangju* continues to wear the black ribbon for 100 days, following which a memorial service marking the formal end to funeral is held.

JAPANESE AMERICANS

Japanese Americans total approximately 1.1 million people and make up approximately 7.6%

of the Asian American population. Japanese American culture is colored by their experiences during the World War II, resulting in a high degree of assimilation in the years that followed. However, despite the desire to assimilate, many Japanese Americans have held on to a number of the traditions that they originally brought across the Pacific Ocean, although the amount of tradition followed varies by generation. For example, although many Japanese Americans adopted the Christian faith, the two primary non-Christian Japanese religions, Shintoism and Buddhism, are still deeply rooted in Japanese American cultural.

Honor and avoidance of shame dictate Japanese American behavior as it does native Japanese. Those portions of Confucian philosophy which place the highest importance on filial piety, family, and social order, also remain of paramount to Japanese Americans. Their high degree of filial piety translates into extreme devotion to parents, elders, and the extended family. This leads the elderly to the hope and expectation that, whenever possible, they will be cared for by their children at home rather than be placed in an institution.

Japanese Americans are a humble people who tend to be critical of themselves while displaying profound loyalty to family and community. Courtesy and thoughtfulness are particularly valued, and public conflict tends to be avoided. Japanese Americans, therefore, prefer indirect, rather than direct communication, when dealing with health care and other issues.

Japanese Americans who follow traditional values may be uncomfortable having direct discussions about advance care planning and end-of-life issues. When these subjects need to be broached, courteous respect is important. The male head of the household, usually the father, husband, or eldest son should be consulted on all matters, and proper deference and respect should be shown. When terminal illness strikes, some Japanese Americans have the philosophy of *Shikata ga nai*, "it cannot be helped," which allows one to stoically accept the difficult situation without imputing blame or a feeling of failure on the person or any family members. Organ donation and autopsies are generally frowned upon as there is a strong belief that a person should remain as they were at birth, and not "cut up."

A study evaluating the acculturation of Japanese Americans toward western views and comparing their views to native Japanese living in Japan was published in 2007. It showed that whether in the United States or in Japan, Japanese had negative feelings toward living in adverse health states and receiving life-sustaining treatments, which included a fear of being *meiwaku*, a physical, psychological, or financial burden on loved ones. They also shared the preference of dying *pokkuri* (popping off) before they became end stage or physically frail and preferred group-oriented decision making with family. Although both Japanese living in Japan and Japanese Americans were comfortable with advance directives, native Japanese saw written directives as intrusive. On the other hand, Japanese Americans found them to be useful as a way of reducing conflict created by a dying person's wishes and family's *kazoku nu jo*, responsibility to sustain the dying patient (Bito et al., 2007).

Japanese Americans honor their dead, and for this reason, funerals are among the most important events in the community. Although as already mentioned, many Japanese Americans have adopted the Christian faith, Buddhist customs, especially cremation, still play a major role in the funeral service. Following the deceased's passing, the body is washed by either the family or professionals on the basis of the family's preference, and gauze or cotton are placed in all body orifices. The body may be dressed in either a suit (for men) or a kimino (women and some men). Mourners will typically wear black.

Following the preparation of the body, there is a wake. The wake may be held either at the home of the deceased or at a funeral home. The body is placed in an open casket. Flowers may be reverently laid inside the coffin with the body.

In Japanense Buddhist tradition, a white kimono, leggings, sandals, paper money for the deceased to pay the toll across the "river of three hells" and a white headband with a triangle in the center are placed in the casket as well. Other burnable items the person was fond of may also be added.

Guests who come pay their respects offer *koden*, condolence money, which is traditionally contained in a thin black envelope with a white ribbon wrapped around it. Christian Japanese Americans often choose to donate this to the church as a memorial gift.

The funeral is traditionally held the day after the wake. The body is not left unattended during the night with various relatives taking turns staying up with the deceased for various periods of time. At the funeral, people may lay flowers on an altar or head table to honor the deceased. Memorial speeches are expected to be down to earth and not overloaded with theological terminology. Incense may be offered, and telegrams from friends and others are sometimes read. The eldest son or another family representative thanks all who came to pay their respects.

As already mentioned, most Japanese Americans choose cremation as the final disposition of the body. The family watches while the casket is slid into the crematorium. They are then told when to return for the remains. The family often takes a different route home to prevent the deceased's spirit from following, and food or drink may be provided for the family. In Japan, there is a custom that when family members return for the remains they pick up pieces of bone with chopsticks and place them in the urn. The urn is then wrapped in a white cloth. Some will immediately take the urn to a cemetery to be buried, whereas others will keep the urn at home until the 49th day, when there is a memorial service, following which the urn is taken for burial.

Following the cremation and initial disposition of the urn (either home or burial), there are varying customs regarding gravesite visitations and memorial services, which often continue for years after the person has passed on.

BIBLIOGRAPHY

Introduction

Alex Haley: Wikipedia, the free encyclopedia. http://en.wikipedia.org/wiki/Alex_Haley. Accessed March 2, 2009.

Berger JT: Commentary: Culture and ethnicity in clinical care. *Arch Int Med* 158:2085-2090, 1998.

Cort MA: Cultural mistrust and use of hospice care: Challenges and remedies. *J Palliat Med* 7:63-71, 2004.

Kinzbrunner BM: Jewish medical ethics and end of life care. *J Palliat Med* 7:558-573, 2004.

Krakauer EL, Crenner C, Fox K: Barriers to optimum end-of-life care for minority patients. *J Am Geriatr Soc* 50:182-190, 2002.

Melting Pot: Wikipedia, the free encyclopedia. http://en.wikipedia.org/wiki/Melting_pot. Accessed March 2, 2009.

Multiculturalism: Wikipedia, the free encyclopedia. http://en.wikipedia.org/wiki/Multiculturalism. Accessed March 2, 2009.

Smith AK, McCarthy EP, Paulk E, et al: Racial and ethnic differences in advance care planning among patients with cancer: Impact of terminal illness acknowledgement, religiousness, and treatment preferences. *J Clin Oncol* 26:4131-4137, 2008.

Welch LC, Teno JM, Mor V: End-of-life care in black and white: Race matters for the medical care of dying patients and their families. *J Am Geriatr Soc* 53:1145-1153, 2005.

African American Patients

Anderson RN, Smith BL: Deaths: Leading Causes for 2002. *National Vital Statistics Report.* Vol. 53, No. 17, Hyattsville, MD, Centers for Disease Control and Prevention. March 7, 2005.

Barrett R: Sociocultural considerations: African americans, grief, and loss. In: Doka KJ, Tucci AS, eds. *Living with Grief. Diversity and End-of-Life Care.* Washington, DC, Hospice Foundation of America, 2009, pp. 79-91.

Bullock K: Promoting advance directives among African Americans: A faith-based model. *J Palliat Med* 9(1):1983-195, 2006.

Burrs FA, Ervin MG, Harper BC: The future of hospice care for African Americans: Clinical, policy and caregiver perspectives. *Key Topics on End-of-Life Care for African Americans.* www.iceol.duke.edu/resources/lasmiles/papers. Accessed November 20, 2009.

Clayton LA, Byrd WM: *An American Health Dilemma.* New York, Routledge, 2000.

Dancy J, Davis W: Family and psycho-social dimensions of death and dying in African-Americans. www.iceol.duke.edu/resources/lastmiles/papers. Accessed November 20, 2009.

Fife R: Diversity and access to hospice care. In: Doka KJ, Tucci AS, eds. *Living with Grief. Diversity and End-of-Life Care.* Washington, DC, Hospice Foundation of America, 2009, pp. 49-62.

London G, Washington R: Spiritual care near life's end including grief and loss in the African American community. www.iceol.duke.edu/resources/lastmiles/papers. Accessed November 20, 2009.

Ludke RL, Douglas SR: Racial differences in the willingness to use hospice services. *J Palliat Med* 10(6):1329-1337, 2007.

Minkler D: U.S. minority population continues to grow. Minorities make up 34% of U.S. population in 2007. America.gov. http://www.america.gov/st/diversity-english/2008/May/20080513175840zjsredna0.1815607.html. Published May 14, 2008. Accessed January 7, 2010.

NHPCO Facts and Figures: *Hospice Care in America.* Alexandria, VA, National Hospice and Palliative Care Organization, 2009.

Payne R, Secundy M, et al: APPEAL (A Progressive Palliative Care Educational Curriculum for the Care of African Americans at Life's End). Curriculum updated 11/09.

Prograis L, Pellagrino E, eds: *African-American bioethics.* Washington, DC, Georgetown University Press, 2007.

Raghavan M, Smith A, Arnold R: African Americans and end-of-life care. *Fast Facts and Concepts #204.* EPERC. www.eperc.mcw.edu/fastFact. Accessed November 20, 2009.

Smedley B, Stith A, Nelson A, eds: *Unequal Treatment: Confronting Racial and Ethnic Disparities in Health Care.* Washington, DC, The National Academies Press, 2003.

Smith AK, McCarthy EP, Paulk E, et al: Racial and ethnic differences in advance care planning among patients with cancer: Impact of terminal illness acknowledgement, religiousness, and treatment preferences. *J Clin Oncol* 26:4131-4137, 2008.

Sullivan MA: May the circle be unbroken: The African American experience of death, dying, and spirituality. In: Parry JK, Ryan AS, eds. *A Cross-Cultural Look at Death, Dying and Religion.* Chicago, Nelson-Hall Publishers, 1995.

THINK About African Americans: *VITAS: Things hospice innovators need to know.* Miami: Vitas Innovative Hospice Care, 2008.

Torke AM, Garas NS, et al: Medical Care at the End of Life: Views of African American patients in an urban hospital. *J Palliat Med* 8(3):593-602, 2005.

Hispanic Patients

Adams CE, Horn K, Bader J: A comparison of utilization of hospice services between Hispanics and whites. *J Hosp Palliat Nurs* 7(6):328-336, 2005.

Adams CE, Horn K, Bader J: Hispanic Access to hospice services in a predominantly Hispanic community. *Am J Hosp Palliat Care* 23(1):9-16, 2006.

Clutter, AW, Nieto RD: Understanding the Hispanic Culture: Ohio State University Fact sheet HYG-5237-00.

Colon M, Lyke J: Comparison of hospice use and demographics among European Americans, African Americans, and Latinos. *Am J Hosp Palliat Care*, 20(3):182-190, 2003.

Colon M: Hospice and Latinos: A review of the Literature. *J Soc Work End Life Palliat Care* 1(2):27-43, 2005.

Gordon AK: Deterrents to access and service for blacks and Hispanics: The medicare hospice benefit, healthcare utilization, and cultural barriers. *Hosp J* 10(2):35-49, 1995.

Greiner KA, Perera S, Ahluwalia JS: Hospice usage by minorities in the last year of life: Results from the National Mortality Followback Survey. *J Am Geriat Soc* 51(7):970-978, 2003.

Hispanic: Wikipedia, the free encyclopedia. http://www.en.wikipedia.org/wiki/Hispanic. Accessed March 2, 2009.

Johnson KS, Kuchibhatala M, Sloane RJ, et al: Ethnic differences in the place of death of elderly hospice enrollees. *J Am Geriatr Soc* 53(12):2209-2215, 2005.

Letizia M, Creech S, Norton E, Shanahan M, Hedges L: Barriers to caregiver administration of pain medication in hospice care. *J Pain Symptom manage* 27(2):114-124, 2004.

Lugo L, Suro R: Pew Hispanic Center, Pew Forum on Religion and Public Life. Changing faiths: Latinos and the transformation of American religion. Washington, Pew Research Center, 2007.

Minkler D: U.S. minority population continues to grow. Minorities make up 34% of U.S. population in 2007. America.gov. http://www.america.gov/st/diversity-english/2008/May/20080513175840zjsredna0.1815607.html. Published May 14, 2008. Accessed January 7, 2010.

NHPCO Facts and Figures: *Hospice Care in America.* Alexandria, VA, National Hospice and Palliative Care Organization, 2008.

Reese D: Barriers to Culturally diverse Hospice Care: The Arkansas State Hospice and Palliative Care Association Cultural Competence Committee Needs Assessment Project, 2005. http://dailyheadlines.uark.edu/3928.htm. Accessed November 2008.

Sanjur, D: *Hispanic foodways, nutrition, and health.* Needham, MA, Allyn & Bacon, 1995.

Asian American Patients

Alagiakrishnan K, Chopra A: Health and health care of Asian Indian American elders. http://www.stanford,edu/group/ethnoger/asianindian.html. Accessed December 14, 2009.

Becker G: Dying away from home. Quandaries of migration for elders in two ethnic groups. *J Gerontol B Psychol Sci Soc Sci* 57(2):S79-S95, 2002.

Becker G, Beyenne Y, Canalita LC: Immigrating for status in late life: Effects of globalization on Filipino American veterans. *J Aging Studies* 14:273-292, 2000.

Bito S, Matsumura S, Singer MK, et al: Acculturation and end-of-life decision making: Comparison of Japanese and Japanese-American focus groups. *Bioethics* 21(5):251-262, 2007.

Clark S: Death and loss in the Philippines. http://www.indiana.edu/~famlygrf/culture/clark.html. Accessed December 11, 2009.

Fife R: Diversity and access to hospice care. In: Doka KJ, Tucci AS, eds. *Living with Grief. Diversity and End-of-Life Care.* Washington, DC, Hospice Foundation of America, 2009, pp. 49-62.

Hammond B: Japanese Buddhist Funeral Customs. http://www.tanutech.com/japan/jfunerals.html. Accessed December 15, 2009.

Ko E, Lee J: End-of-life communication: Ethnic differences between Korean American and non-Hispanic white older adults. *J Aging Health* 21:967-984, 2009.

Kwak J, Salmon JR: Attitudes and preferences of Korean-American older adults and caregivers on end-of-life care. *J Am Geriatr Soc* 55:1867-1872, 2007.

Korean Funeral Tradition: Ask a Korean! http://askakorean.blogspot.com/2008/02/dear-korean-i-just-found-out-that-my.html. Accessed December 14, 2009.

Ngan V: Funeral rites in Vietnam. http://www.vietspring.org/custom/funeral.html. Accessed December 14, 2009.

Pavri T: Asian Indian Americans. http://www.everyculture.com/multi/A-Br/Asian-Indian-Americans.html. Accessed December 11, 2009.

Population statistics and demographics: Asian-Nation: Asian American History, Demographics, and Issues. http://www.asian-nation.org/population.shtml. Accessed December 9, 2009.

Religion, spirituality, and faith: Asian-Nation: Asian American History, Demographics, and Issues. http://www.asian-nation.org/religion.shtml. Accessed December 9, 2009.

Tet Trung Nguyen (Wandering Souls Day) Vietnam: http://www.asiarooms.com/travel-guide/vietnam/vietnam-festivals-&-events/tet-trung-nguyen-(wandering-souls-day)-vietnam.html. Accessed December 15, 2009.

Thanh Minh (Day of the Dead): http://www.asiarooms.com/travel-guide/vietnam/vietnam-festivals-&-events/thanh-minh-(day-of-the-dead).html. Accessed December 15, 2009.

THINK About Asian Americans: *VITAS: Things Hospice Innovators Need to Know.* Miami, Vitas Innovative Hospice Care, 2008.

THINK About Chinese Americans: *VITAS: Things Hospice Innovators Need to Know.* Miami: Vitas Innovative Hospice Care, 2008.

THINK About Filipino Americans. *VITAS: Things Hospice Innovators Need to Know.* Miami: Vitas Innovative Hospice Care, 2008.

THINK About Japanese Americans. *VITAS: Things Hospice Innovators Need to Know.* Miami: Vitas Innovative Hospice Care, 2008.

THINK About Korean Americans. *VITAS: Things Hospice Innovators Need to Know.* Miami: Vitas Innovative Hospice Care, 2008.

THINK About Vietnamese Americans. *VITAS: Things Hospice Innovators Need to Know.* Miami: Vitas Innovative Hospice Care, 2008.

Thomas R, Wilson DM, Justice C, et al: A literature review of preferences for end-of-life care in developed countries by individuals with different cultural affiliations and ethnicity. *J Hospice Palliat Nursing* 10(3):142-161.

Vietnamese Death Traditions: http://www.ehow.com/about_5052325_vietnamese-death-traditions.html. Accessed December 14, 2009.

Wu E: Chinese funeral traditions offer link to ancestors. Dallas Morning News, June 21, 2007. http://www.dallasnews.com/sharedcontent/dws/dn/localnews/columnists/ewu/stories/DN-wu_21met.ART.West.Edition1.4435faf.html. Accessed December 10, 2009.

Yamashita Y, Young HM: Decision making at end of life among Japanese American families. *J Family Nursing* 13(2):201-225, 2007.

Yee BWK: Health and health care of Southeast Asian American Elders: Vietnamese, Cambodian, Hmong, and Laotian Elders. http://www.stanford.edu/group/ethnoger/southeastasian.html. Accessed December 8, 2009.

Yin and Yang: Wikipedia, the free encyclopedia. http://en.wikipedia.org/wiki/Yin_and_yang. Accessed December 10, 2009.

Yin and Yang: The Ki quality of food. Chinese medicine—Qi nature of foods. http://www.angelfire.com/id/croon/chinesemedicine/yangyinfoods.html. Accessed December 10, 2009.

SELF-ASSESSMENT QUESTIONS

1. All of the following barriers to hospice access are rooted in ethnic, cultural, or religious beliefs EXCEPT:

   A. The mandate to preserve life at all costs
   B. The ability to predict when someone has 6 months or less to live
   C. Mistrust of the health care system
   D. The idea that informing someone that they are terminally ill may hasten death
   E. The idea that one is never allowed to "give up"

2. All of the following statements about the cultural assessment are true EXCEPT:

   A. A cultural assessment is the part of the comprehensive assessment that elicits information about a patient's cultural, ethnic, or religious traditions.
   B. The cultural assessment may be performed separately, or have questions interspersed into other parts of the comprehensive assessment.
   C. Once the ethnic, cultural, or religious group that the patient identifies with is known, one can deduce the patient's needs.
   D. Questions in the cultural assessment may include the patient's country of birth, primary and secondary languages, and customs and rituals related to grief and mourning.
   E. It is only by performing a thorough cultural assessment that one can deliver culturally sensitive care.

3. All of the following have resulted from the African American culture of mistrust of the U.S. health care system EXCEPT:

   A. There is a high utilization of advance directives among African Americans to ensure that they receive the care they want.
   B. African American patients receive less attention by health care providers than white patients.

   C. African American patients feel they are patronized in physicians' offices.
   D. African American patients more often leave their doctors' offices unclear about their diagnosis and treatment options.
   E. Physicians are often accused of not communicating properly with African American patients.

4. All of the following are statements regarding common attitudes of African Americans toward death and dying are true EXCEPT:

   A. The deceased are treated with great reverence and respect.
   B. Death is considered as part of the continuum of life.
   C. The faith community is expected to provide comfort to families who have experienced a loss.
   D. The extended "kin network" of a person requires bereavement support following the loss of a loved one.
   E. African Americans tend to spend less discretionary income on funerals than their white counterparts.

5. True statements regarding end-of-life care decision for African American patients include all of the following EXCEPT:

   A. Many believe that choosing not to receive interventions such as CPR or a feeding tube gives the health care system a license to provide substandard care.
   B. It is important to involve spiritual counselors and "kin network" elders in advance care planning conversations.
   C. The decision to execute an advance directive can increase feelings of hopelessness in patients and families.
   D. Discussions with the patient and family about feelings of mistrust toward the health care system should be avoided.
   E. Patients and families often feel conflicted when discontinuing life-prolonging therapy as there is a perception that they are

giving up the hope that God will heal them.

6. All of the following are true statements regarding the roles of religion, the physician, and the family in shaping Hispanic cultural attitudes toward death and dying EXCEPT:

A. Irrespective of their religious faith, religion plays a significant role for Hispanic Americans when faced with end-of-life situations.

B. When making end-of-life care decisions, Hispanic Americans will more often heed the advice of their end-of-life care provider than they will the advice of their physician.

C. When there is illness in a Hispanic American family, all members of the extended family participate in the care and anticipatory grieving of the ill family member.

D. Hispanic families, in an attempt to protect the patient, often will not allow any discussion of an ill family member's terminal prognosis.

E. Although the head of the family is considered the ultimate decision maker, multiple extended family members may be actively involved in end-of-life care decision making.

7. Regarding end-of-life decision making for Hispanic Americans with respect to nutrition and hydration, each of the following statements is true EXCEPT:

A. Food is considered a powerful symbol of wellness and represents hope for improvement and cure.

B. Family members often perceive a direct correlation between nutritional support and the amount of care a loved one is receiving.

C. Allowing patients to die without food or fluid is considered to be "painful and cruel" treatment.

D. Religious beliefs may be an important factor in prompting families to request that loved ones receive artificial nutritional support or hydration.

E. Hispanic families are generally not accepting of providing small amounts of food via spoon-feeding or syringe, rather they want their loved ones to receive nutritional support via a feeding tube.

8. True statements regarding Asian Americans as a whole include all of the following EXCEPT:

A. About 45% identify themselves as Christian.

B. Most Asian American patients near the end of life are cared for in institutions.

C. Asian Americans tend to avoid discussing personal issues except with family members when seeking guidance.

D. Many Asian Americans avoid showing feelings or emotions.

E. Language barriers may be a significant challenge and require professional translators to ensure proper communication with patients.

9. Regarding caring for Asian Indian Americans, all of the following statements are true EXCEPT:

A. Modesty is of great importance and caregivers of the same gender as the patient are preferred.

B. Many Asian Indians prefer that the physician be in charge, and will usually follow the physician's advice without question.

C. Hindu women wear a thread around their necks that should be removed prior to providing care.

D. Mental illness is considered a stigma, so counseling for symptoms such as anxiety and depression is often refused.

E. The elderly may behave stoically when in pain.

10. In a 2007 study (Bito et al.) comparing the attitudes of Japanese Americans with native Japanese living in Japan, which of the following was found to be different between the two groups?

   A. Having negative feelings toward living in adverse health states and receiving life-sustaining treatments.
   B. The fear of being a physical, psychological, or financial burden on loved ones.
   C. Dying before becoming end stage or physically frail.
   D. The preference for group-oriented decision making with family.
   E. The use of advance directives as a way to reduce conflict between a dying person's wishes and the family's responsibility to sustain the dying patient.

Religious Diversity and End-of-Life Care

Barry M. Kinzbrunner, Syd Saxena, and Sara Roby

JEWISH PATIENTS

Barry M. Kinzbrunner

INTRODUCTION

Judaism is the most ancient of the monotheistic religions, tracing its origins back to the Middle East well over 3,000 years ago. The basic tenet of Jewish faith is the belief in one God, who revealed Himself to Moses and the Jewish people on Mount Sinai. Jewish traditional belief and practice is embodied in *halacha*, Jewish law, which is derived primarily from the Five Books of Moses (the first Five books of the Bible, known also to Jews as the Torah), the other books of the Bible, and an oral law, which was later written down in the ancient texts of the Mishnah and Talmud and subsequently expounded upon and codified by Jewish leaders throughout the last two millennia.

There are slightly less than 5.5 million Jews in the United States today, which represents a little over 1.5% of the total U.S. population. Approximately 10% of U.S. Jews identify themselves as Orthodox, meaning that they are observant of Jewish law and tradition and view the rabbi as the legal authority regarding Jewish law. Conservative Jews, who represent about 26% of the Jewish population, reinterpret Jewish law to fit modern society, exhibit wide variations in how they observe that reinterpreted law, and view the rabbi as an advisor rather than an authority figure. Another 35% of Jews identify with Reform Judaism, which views Jewish law as only a nonbinding guide to living a moral and ethical life. Another 9% of U.S. Jews are affiliated with several other small nontraditional denominations, and the remaining 20% are considered unaffiliated.

From the information aforementioned, it would seem that most American Jews do not follow Jewish law and tradition strictly. Yet, when the end of life approaches, Jews, as people of other faiths do, often look toward their beliefs and traditions as sources of aid and comfort during diffi-

cult times, and hence, for both the observant Jews and those who are less traditional, Jewish law and ritual can often significantly influence the wishes they or their family members are terminally ill.

JEWISH MEDICAL ETHICS AND END-OF-LIFE DECISION MAKING

Using Jewish law, the cardinal ethical principles of medical ethics have been defined from a Jewish perspective. Autonomy is voluntarily limited from the perspective that the traditional Jews choose to make decisions consistent with Jewish law. Beneficence is fully operative and encompasses both the physician's obligation to heal and the individual's obligation to seek beneficial care. Nonmaleficence, the avoidance of harm, is also incumbent on both the physician and the individual, within the constraints of an appropriate and acceptable risk/benefit analysis. Justice takes into account both the benefits to the society as well as the resources available to meet various health care needs.

Judaism believes that life is of infinite value, and yet, using these modified definitions of the ethical principles and other precepts of Jewish law, traditional Judaism recognizes terminal illness, establishing a primary definition for terminal illness as a prognosis of 1 year or less, with a second definition, "*goses,*" reserved for patients who would be described in hospice and palliative care as "actively dying." Euthanasia, assisted suicide, or any other form of intentional hastening of death is categorically forbidden. Patients who are near the end of life may refuse treatments that are deemed ineffective, futile, or will only prolong suffering, and such treatments may also be withheld. However, once treatments are started, they generally cannot be withdrawn, since withdrawal of such treatment may be seen as an active shortening of life. Food and fluid, even when provided by artificial means, are considered by all orthodox and some conservative rabbis to be basic care, and therefore, must be provided to all patients, with the only caveat being that this should be done in a way that is beneficial and not harmful. Advance directives in the form of a living will, a durable health-care power of attorney, or both, are generally permitted and organizations from all the major Jewish denominations have advance directive documents that are compatible with their understanding and interpretation of Jewish law. An important requirement for advance directives in the orthodox community, where the rabbi is the accepted authority on Jewish law, is that it is required that a rabbi knowledgeable in the area of health care decision making be included as a named surrogate in order to ensure that all such decisions are made in accordance with Jewish law.

JEWISH TRADITIONS AND RITUALS

Prayer

Jews are obligated to pray three times every day. When possible, a minimum of 10 Jewish men (or either gender in nonorthodox sects) gather together in synagogue for prayer in a group called a *minyan*, which is necessary for the recitation of certain prayers, including the mourner's *Kaddish* prayer (see Mourning and Bereavement Customs below). During weekday morning prayers, Jewish men (and some women in the Conservative movement) wear a prayer shawl, called a *tallit*, and *tefillin*, which are black leather boxes that are strapped onto the left upper arm and the forehead, which contain parchment inscribed with specific scriptural verses. The tefillin are not worn during Sabbath or holiday prayers. The afternoon prayers are held late in the day followed by evening prayers, allowing Jews who attend daily services to only come to synagogue twice a day for the three prayer services.

Sabbath and Holidays

Traditional Jews observe the Sabbath, weekly on Saturday, as a day of rest, commemorating the fact that following the six days of the creation of the world, God rested on the seventh day. During the Jewish Sabbath, which begins about one-half hour before sundown on Friday evening and ends one-half hour after sundown on Saturday night, Jews who follow the tradition are prohibited from performing many common weekday activities including using electricity, cooking, carrying in a public domain, and travelling by a motor vehicle, to name but a few. There are many rituals associated with the Sabbath, including the lighting of candles, the sanctification of the day over wine, a family meal on Friday night, a longer synagogue service with the reading of a portion from the Five Books of Moses from a handwritten parchment known as the Torah scroll, and another family meal, the Sabbath lunch.

There are also a number of Jewish holidays associated with many customs and rituals, Some of the better known Jewish holidays include Passover (during which Jews gather for a special meal called the Seder and eat unleavened bread called Matzah), Rosh Hashanah (the Jewish New Year on which a ram's horn called a Shofar is sounded), Yom Kippur (the Day of Atonement, a day of fasting and repentance), and Chanukah (the Festival of Lights during which Jews light a special candelabra for eight nights). A number of the holidays, including Passover, Rosh Hashana, and Yom Kippur have activity restrictions similar to the Jewish Sabbath.

While not all American Jews strictly observe the Sabbath or Jewish holidays in terms of ritual or activity restrictions, there are two important reasons why these special days on the Jewish calendar should become familiar to end-of-life care givers caring for Jewish patients and families. Regarding the activity restrictions on the Sabbath and major Jewish holidays, all such restrictions are set aside when someone has a life-threatening illness, even if the person is terminal and not expected to recover. Therefore, while end-of-life care providers should not meet any major challenges when caring for their patients and families on the Sabbath or a holiday, one should be aware that there will be situations where individual patients or family members who observe these restrictions may not be aware that the Sabbath and holiday prohibitions may be set aside, or may believe that the current medical situation is not severe enough to warrant violating the Sabbath or holiday. Therefore, it is important for caregivers to be aware of and sensitive to patient and family concerns when questions of Sabbath and holiday observance arise.

In regards to various rituals on the Sabbath and holidays, assisting patients in observing some of the rituals can be very meaningful when due to the nature of their illnesses, they are unable to participate in the rituals on their own. Assisting an end-of-life care patient in lighting the Chanukah menorah, arranging for a Rabbi to blow Shofar for a patient on Rosh Hashanah, or ensuring that a patient can light Shabbat candles are examples of how end-of-life caregivers can support Jewish patients and families who find these rituals important and meaningful.

Jewish Dietary Laws (Kosher)

The Jewish dietary laws (termed Kosher) are outlined in the Torah and elaborated upon by the Rabbis in the oral law. These laws are followed by orthodox Jews and to varying degrees by Jews affiliated with the conservative and reform movement. These laws include eating meat from only certain kinds of animals and birds that are slaughtered and then prepared in a specific fashion, eating only fish that have fins and scales, and not cooking or eating meat and dairy products together. Those who observe the Jewish dietary laws, keep separate dishes for meat and dairy foods as well. Caregivers need to be aware of these restrictions and make sure they do not inadvertently bring nonkosher food into a patient's home (or kosher nursing home) or use the wrong dishes if they are assisting a patient or family member at meal time. Caregivers should also be aware that even foods certified as kosher may not be considered acceptable to all Jews who state they follow the dietary laws and one should always check with the patient or family before bringing any foods into the home.

Modesty and Intergender Contact

Without delving deeply into the laws involved, suffice it to say that some orthodox Jews refrain from any physical contact with members of the opposite gender, with the exception of spouses and other immediate family members in the privacy of their own homes. While, like the laws of the Sabbath, these prohibitions are suspended when someone is ill, caregivers should be aware that some orthodox patients may be extremely uncomfortable when care, especially personal care, is provided by a member of the opposite gender. In such circumstances, it is incumbent upon the end-of-life care providers to be respectful and flexible in order to meet the needs of such patients without subjecting them to undue stress.

HOLOCAUST SURVIVORS

The specter of the systematic murder of the Jewish population of Europe by Nazi Germany during World War II, otherwise known as the Holocaust, continues to cast its shadow over the last of its survivors, who are now dying of old age. Whether Jewish holocaust survivors observe Jewish law and ritual or not, their experiences significantly color how they approach the natural end of their lives, and greatly influence their end-of-life care decisions. For example, the mandate to provide artificial nutrition and hydration (see above) is not only due to basic human needs for these patients, but for many reflects the overwhelming fear of starvation that was part and parcel of daily life under the Nazi yoke. End-of-life care providers must be aware of this and other potential challenges that Holocaust survivors face as life draws toward its close.

CARE OF THE BODY AT THE TIME OF DEATH

During the dying process, it is preferable that the patient not be left unattended. Once death occurs, it is customary for the children, close relatives, or friends who are present to close the deceased's eyes and draw a sheet over the face. The body is generally positioned so that the feet face the doorway, but is otherwise not moved. Candles are often lit, and there are various traditions as to how many and where. It is customary for friends and relatives to ask forgiveness of the deceased, and it is improper to eat or drink in the presence of the body. Cleaning and preparation of the body for internment is traditionally done by the *Chevra Kadisha*, the Jewish Burial Society, and includes the *taharah*, or ritual cleansing and the recitation of specific prayers. Therefore, if a Jewish patient is having a traditional Jewish burial, end-of-life care staff should not clean the body at the time of death, but should leave the body and allow the *Chevra Kadisha* to remove all dressings, catheters, and other medical paraphernalia.

The deceased is dressed in a simple white shroud and a male (or in some conservative and reform groups both male and female) is then wrapped in his (or her) *tallit* (prayer shawl), with one set of the corner fringes (called *tzitzit*) cut off, making it unfit to be worn. The body is then placed in a coffin made entirely of wood, which decomposes at a rate similar to the body and the cloth. It is customary to drill holes in the bottom of the casket in order to connect the body more directly with the earth to which it will be returning.

From the time of death until the funeral, the body of the deceased is never left alone, but is attended to by a watcher (*shomer* in Hebrew) who recites various Psalms until the funeral. Autopsies are generally not permitted and if they are necessary, all organs must be returned for proper burial. Embalming and cremation are generally forbidden, although currently some groups within the Reform movement permit cremation.

THE FUNERAL AND INTERNMENT OF THE BODY

Burial usually occurs within 24 hours of death. The service includes various psalms and prayers and a eulogy intended to praise the life of the deceased. Prior to the funeral, the primary mourners (see below) will perform *keriyah*, the tearing of a garment, as a demonstration of grief. (Conservative and reform Jews often choose to wear a torn black ribbon instead of tearing an article of clothing.) Following the service, the mourners accompany the deceased to the gravesite and actually participate in the burial by shoveling earth into the grave until the coffin is entirely covered. Then, following the recitation of a special Mourner's *Kaddish* prayer, the bereaved retire to the house of mourning, after being consoled by those who were present at the funeral and burial service.

THE KADDISH PRAYER

The *Kaddish* prayer is a central prayer in Jewish liturgy. It is recited in Aramaic, which was the common language of the people in ancient Israel and it can only be recited in the presence of a *minyan* (see above). The theme of the prayer is praise of God, and there is no mention of death or mourning. It is recited multiple times during a traditional Jewish prayer service, often serving to separate various parts of the daily service from one another. It is also recited following the reading of certain Jewish texts of learning, and, in the context of mourning and bereavement, is recited by someone who is in mourning.

Because of its familiarity to most Jews, the recitation of Kaddish during periods of mourning can quickly become rote and automatic for many. As that occurs, and the mind of the mourner reciting the prayer begins to wander, it allows the individual to think about and even communicate in some way with the deceased, allowing the bereaved to better cope with his loss.

MOURNING AND BEREAVEMENT CUSTOMS

There are seven relatives whose loss obligates a Jewish adult (male over the age of 13, female over the age of 12) to mourn: father, mother, sister, brother, son, daughter, and spouse. Traditional Jewish practice defines four stages of mourning:

aninus, *shiva*, *sheloshim*, and a final period that is only observed following the death of a parent, which ends 12 months after the loss.

Aninus

The first stage of mourning is called *aninus*, and it encompasses the period between the death and burial of the loved one. Despair is usually very intense (even when death is expected), yet, at the same time, the bereaved is expected to focus on ensuring that all final arrangements for the deceased have been made. In recognition of this, in addition to refraining from the social and personal activities that are traditionally forbidden during mourning (see below), the mourner is not obligated to participate in certain religious observances related to prayer.

Shiva

Shiva, traditionally lasting for 7 days (some Conservative and Reform Jews choose to only observe 3 days or 1 day), begins following the funeral. During the first three days, mourning is particularly intense, and the mourner does not traditionally respond to greetings. During the final four days, the mourner begins to emerge from the state of intense grief and is more prepared to talk about the loss.

During the *shiva* period, mourners will traditionally wear the garment or black ribbon that was torn or cut during the funeral, will sit on a low stool, and will wear slippers. Mourners are also restricted in a number of activities, including leaving the house, shaving and grooming, bathing for pleasure, working or conducting normal business activities, wearing new or freshly laundered clothes, and engaging in conjugal relations. It is traditional for friends to visit mourners during the *shiva* period to express condolences and provide emotional support. A candle is lit that will last the entire 7-day *shiva* period, and all the mirrors in the home are covered.

The traditional obligations for daily prayer that were suspended during *aninus* are resumed following the funeral, with the addition of the mourner's *Kaddish* prayer. As the mourners traditionally do not leave the house, it is common in traditional Jewish communities to conduct prayer services in house of mourning.

Sheloshim

This stage of mourning represents the 30 days following burial and includes the 7 days of *shiva*. After *shiva*, the mourner is encouraged to leave the house and begin to reintegrate into society. Certain activities, such as shaving and grooming, and attending parties and other celebratory functions with music remain prohibited under normal circumstances during the *sheloshim* period. Recitation of the *Kaddish* remains an obligation of the mourners during *sheloshim*. *Sheloshim* concludes mourning obligations for the loss of all relatives except for one's parents.

Final Mourning Period of 12 Months for One's Parent

Because of the special relationship that a child has with his or her parents, the loss of a parent is more keenly felt. Therefore, an extra period of mourning is proscribed. While business and many other activities return to normal, entertainment and amusement activities are curtailed for a period of 12 months following the funeral. Recitation of *Kaddish* during daily prayers also continues until the end of the 11th month.

Memorializing the Deceased after Formal Bereavement

While organized bereavement is discontinued after 1 year (or 30 days for other relatives), Jewish tradition continues to encourage the remembrance of those who have passed on. Toward the end of the year of mourning for a parent (or following the sheloshim for other relatives), it is not uncommon for the bereaved to gather at the gravesite of the deceased to "unveil" the headstone of the grave. This custom, called an "Unveiling," has its origins in nineteenth century American and Western Europe, includes, in addition to the "unveiling" of the headstone, the recitation of some psalms, a brief eulogy, the special Memorial prayer recited at the funeral, and the Kaddish prayer and affords the mourners another opportunity to remember the deceased.

On the yearly anniversary of the death of a loved one, or *Yahrzeit, Kaddish* is recited during prayer in remembrance of the deceased and a memorial candle is lit. Judaism also has special prayers of remembrance, the *Yizkor* service, which are recited four times a year, during the three major festivals (Passover, Shavuot, and Succot), and on Yom Kippur, to honor all those who have passed on.

Upon reflecting on the stages of mourning outlined above, one can see this as a model of healthy bereavement activities. The bereaved appropriately experience intense grieving at the time of the loss, followed by a structured decrease in the grief process, with a concomitant normalization of day-to-day activities.

MUSLIM PATIENTS

Barry M. Kinzbrunner

INTRODUCTION

Islam is the youngest of the three monotheistic religions that can trace its origin to the Middle East (the other two being Judaism and Christianity). There are between 1.6 and 1.8 billion Muslims living in the world today with a little over 7 million living in the Unites States and Canada. In Arabic, the word Islam has come to represent total submission to the will of Allah (the creator of the Universe) by conforming to His law, which was revealed to His prophet Muhammad in the Holy Book known as the *Quran*. In addition to the *Quran*, Islamic law may be derived from the *Sunnah* (the words and actions of the prophet), and the *Ijtihad* or Wisdom (which is the process of deductive logic, which gives Islamic law the dynamism to respond to the challenges of a changing world). Islamic law is also interpreted through the *Ijma*, the consensus of the Clerics, which consists of scholars charged with applying religious teachings in areas such as medicine, for example, to try and reach agreement on how to address modern advances for the wider Muslim community. The primary goal of Islamic spirituality is to please God through four steps: Faith (*Iman*: believing that Allah alone is one's Master and seeking His pleasure), Submission (*Slam*: accepting subservience to Allah), Consciousness (*Taqwa*: the readiness to undertake all that Allah has commanded), all leading to Godliness (*Ihsan*: one has attained the highest excellence in words, deeds, and thoughts).

The observance of Islam is based on the five Pillars. The first pillar is *Shahadah*, which is the expression of faith that "(t)here is no God but Allah, and Muhammad is the Messenger of Allah." Second is *Salat*, which are the mandatory daily prayers that are recited five times a day. The third pillar is *Zakat*, the giving of charity to the poor. Fourth is *Sawum*, fasting, which includes the abstinence from food, drink, and intimate relations during the daytime throughout the month of Ramadan, which is the 9th month of the Muslim lunar calendar. The fifth and final pillar is *Hajj*, which is the once in a lifetime pilgrimage to the Muslim Holy City of Mecca, required of all who are financially and physically able.

ISLAMIC MEDICAL ETHICS AND END-OF-LIFE DECISION MAKING

Islam believes in the sanctity of human life, which is derived from the *Quran*: "Whoever saves a human life saves the life of the whole mankind" (5:32). Islam also believes that one has the obligation to seek a cure when possible, but upholds the autonomous right of individuals, both male and female, to accept or refuse medical interventions when cure is not possible. The ethical principles of nonmaleficence (first do no harm) and justice are the dominant ethical values as illustrated by four major rules of Islamic medical ethics:

- Necessity overrides prohibition: items that are prohibited by Islamic law may be permissible in cases of dire medical necessity.
- Harm must be avoided at all costs.
- Accept the lesser of two harms if both cannot be avoided.
- Public interest overrides the individual interest.

Applying these principles to end-of-life decision making, it is clear that euthanasia and assisted suicide would be forbidden under Islamic law. Unless suffering from a potentially curable illness, Muslim patients may choose to accept or refuse medical interventions that are disease modifying but not curable, which would include cardiopulmonary resuscitation when a patient is suffering from a terminal illness.

Most Muslim scholars consider withholding and withdrawing of care to be morally equivalent, although some consider withholding to be ethically superior to withdrawing. Therefore, in face of terminal illness, the withholding of interventions is generally permissible, and some will even allow the withdrawal of treatment, including mechanical ventilatory support under specific circumstances. The one major exception to the permission to withhold or withdraw care relates to food and fluid, which are considered basic components of human care and, therefore, can never be withdrawn or withheld. Food and fluid should always be offered by mouth. While the prophet Muhammed discouraged forcing the sick to take food and fluids, families may desire artificial nutritional support for the patient who cannot eat or drink. Discussing the words of the prophet with the family as well as the medical issues around nutritional support and hydration near the end of life often alleviates their concerns. If a patient who is nearing death is receiving artificial nutritional support, it should not be withdrawn, but if, for example, a feeding tube is no longer functioning or comes out on its own, it does not have to be replaced.

While Islam views suffering as a way to atone for one's transgressions, the relief of suffering is considered to be very righteous. Therefore, the management of pain and other symptoms is extremely important. However, patients often have a desire to remain conscious and alert until the last moments of life in order to be able to pray and say their last words about God at the time of death. This may lead patients to refuse analgesia or only agree to reduced doses of medication because of concerns that the medication will induce an alteration in the level of consciousness. Therefore, when using opioids and other sedating medications in this population, it is important to titrate the medication carefully to avoid changes in patient sensorium and to recognize that some patients may prefer to remain alert with some degree of pain rather than have their pain completely relieved.

The Islamic faith considers the telling of lies to be a great sin. This applies in all walks of life, including health care, which means that there is an expectation that physicians will be truthful with patients regarding both diagnosis and prognosis, even when the prognosis is terminal. By informing patients and families truthfully, the physician allows the patient to have the opportunity to make peace with God, resolve personal conflicts, and make any appropriate and necessary arrangement for any personal matters. Of course, it is expected that the information be conveyed using professional communication techniques (such as those discussed in Chapter 3) that will provide the appropriate concern and sensitivity.

Muslim patients are permitted by Islamic law to have advance directives. Living will documents should include a statement that one "be permitted to die naturally with only the provision of appropriate nutrition and hydration and the administration of essential medications and the performances of any medical procedures necessary [as determined by (one's) physician] to provide (one) with comfort or to alleviate pain." In addition, the document should contain directions that the body be prepared for burial and buried according to Islamic law under the direction of family, Imam, or other qualified Muslims. Regarding durable health care power of attorney advance directives and surrogate decision making, Islamic families generally participate actively in decision making. While familial hierarchies may vary, in most situations when patients can no longer express their own wishes, parents, spouses, and elder children, in that order, are looked upon to make decisions for the patient.

ISLAMIC RITUALS AND PRACTICE

Prayer

Prayer, as one of the five pillars, is central to Islamic practice. One is required to pray five times a day (although certain prayers can be combined in a way that allows one to have three prayer sessions instead of five) during health and when ill, except when cognition is impaired. If one recovers mentally, prayers that were missed should be compensated for. One may pray alone or in a group in any clean location and sick individuals may pray while sitting or lying down. Prior to prayers, there is a ritual washing of the hands, mouth, nose, face, arms, and feet, known as the *Wadu*, which is especially important for patients who have challenges with body fluids as a result of their illnesses. For persons who cannot perform the ritual washing, there is an alternative ritual known as *Tayammum*, which involves touching clean sand with both palms and gently sweeping them over the face and the back of the hands. On Friday, which is the Muslim Sabbath, there is a special noon prayer that should be done communally in a mosque if at all possible.

In addition to the mandatory daily prayers, Muslims have a variety of prayers and rituals related to healing practices. Prayers include recitation of verses from the *Quran* and specific prophetic supplications. Many Muslims will drink Zamzam water, which can be obtained from the well in the Holy Mosque in Mecca. Others will resort to spiritual healers, amulets, and various religious symbols as well as consuming honey and black cumin (Nigella seeds), which are considered to have healing properties.

Holidays

RAMADAN Fasting, another of the five Pillars of Islam, is expressed by observant Muslims daily during the entire month of Ramadan. Muslims over the age of 12 are required to abstain from food, drink, smoking, and sexual activity from sunrise to sunset each day of the month. As the Islamic calendar is lunar, and as there is no adjustment for the difference between the lunar (354 days) and solar (365 days) calendars, the months of the Islamic calendar occur approximately 11 days earlier each year. This means that the length the daily fast during Ramadan will vary depending on the time of year when it occurs. The purpose of the fast is to help teach Muslims self-discipline, self-restraint, and generosity, as during this time Muslims are reminded of the suffering and the poor.

Elderly who are in poor health or suffer from chronic illness, people taking frequent medications, and pregnant women are among those excused from fasting. Those who cannot fast are either required to fast at another time or may give charity to the needy as a substitute. Despite these exceptions, there will be patients who desire to fast, and if they are on chronic medication (i.e., around-the-clock oral analgesia), doses might be missed without the knowledge of the interdisciplinary team. Therefore, it is important that if a Muslim patient, despite not being obligated, insists on fasting during Ramadan and is on chronic medication, that creative ways be found to alter the medication regimen (i.e., switching analgesia to once a day oral dosing, transdermal dosing, or subcutaneous infusion) to allow the patient to try and observe the fast without the added complication of missed medication leading to worsening symptoms.

On the 27th day of Ramadan, Muslims observe the *Laylat al-Qadr*, referred to as "the Night of Power" or "the Night of Destiny," which commemorates when the first verse of the *Quran* were revealed to Muhammad. The final day of Ramadan is known as *Eid-al-Fitr*, "the Festival of Fast-Breaking," which marks the end of the daily fasts.

HAJJ The fifth Pillar of Islam, *Hajj*, is the annual pilgrimage to Mecca, Saudi Arabia, which all Muslims are obligated to participate in at least once during their lifetime. The purpose of the *Hajj* is to both delete sin and improve chances for cure if one is ill, so it is not inconceivable that someone who is being cared for by a hospice may desire to perform *Hajj* before death. The yearly pilgrimage takes place from the 7th through the 13th day of Dhu al-Hijjah, the 12th month of the Islamic calendar. The last four days of the Hajj season is known as *Eid al-adha* or "the Feast of Sacrifice." Pilgrims can also go to Mecca to perform the rituals of the *Hajj* at other times of the year, and this is known as the *Omrah*, or "lesser pilgrimage."

OTHER HOLIDAYS   There are several other holidays on the Islamic calendar that bear mentioning. The first day of the first month of the Islamic calendar, Muharram, is known as *Al-Hijra*, the Islamic New Year. This marks the day that Muhammad began his migration, *Hijra* in Arabic, from Mecca to Medina in 622 CE. There are no prescribed religious rituals or observances, although some Muslims have developed the tradition of exchanging greeting cards and gifts. Most Muslims regard the day as a time for reflection on the *Hijra* and on the year to come.

The 10th day of Muharram is known as *Ashura*. This day commemorates the day, according to Muslim tradition, when *Nuh* (Noah) left the ark and the day that *Musa* (Moses) was saved from the Egyptians by Allah. Muhammad originally established this day as a fast day, but later designated Ramadan as a month of fasting and made fasting on *Ashura* voluntary, which is how this day is marked by Sunni Muslims. Shia Muslims, however, observe Ashura as a day of public grief and mourning, commemorating Hussein, son of Imam Ali and grandson of Muhammad.

The 12th day of Rabi-al-Awwal, the third month of the Muslim calendar, marks the birthday of the Prophet Muhammad. There is disagreement among Muslims whether this day should be celebrated as a holiday, as it was not observed as such during the early days of Islam. Those who think it should be observed see it as time for reading the *Quran*, and remembering the life, teachings, and the examples set by the Prophet Muhammad.

Dietary Laws

Muslims are only permitted to eat foods that are considered "*Halal*," which is an Arabic term meaning "lawful or permissible." *Halal* meat, for example, can only come from cattle and poultry that is ritually slaughtered by a Muslim, or according to some, by a Christian or a Jew as well. (For this reason, some Muslims who cannot obtain Halal meat will accept kosher meat.) Fish with scales are permitted, while fish without scales and shellfish are permitted by some and forbidden by others. Pork and all porcine products, including gelatins, are forbidden, as are animals that are killed without being ritually slaughtered.

The consumption of blood is forbidden, meaning that animals that are ritually slaughtered must have all their blood drained as part of the preparation of the meat. Muslims are permitted to receive blood transfusions and organ transplants because the blood is not being eaten or digested. Alcohol is likewise prohibited. These prohibitions extend beyond food and drink to the use of cosmetics and pharmaceuticals, except in a situation when no other option exists. Alcohol can be used for scientific, industrial, or transportation purposes.

Modesty and Intergender Contact

Modesty is important in Islam, and therefore, it is preferable that Muslim patients have caregivers of the same gender whenever possible. If a male caregiver is caring for a female patient, a female staff member should always be present. Before entering a room, one should always knock on the door and ask permission to enter in order to show a respect for the person's privacy. During an examination, exposure of body parts should be limited to the area that is being examined, and permission should be requested before exposing the specific area. It is also considered improper to talk while touching the patient. Avoidance of eye contact and handshaking between patients and caregivers of opposite genders is also common among Muslims, and non-Muslim caregivers should be sensitive to these expressions of modesty.

CARE OF THE BODY AT THE TIME OF DEATH

During the dying process, family members who are with the patient should provide comfort and remind the person of God's mercy and forgiveness. They should try to gently encourage the patient to recite the *Shahadah*, the Islamic Pillar of Faith that bears witness that "there is no God but Allah and Muhammad is His prophet." Some families also have the custom of positioning the dying patient so that s/he is facing Mecca.

After death has occurred, the loved ones who are present are encouraged to remain calm, pray for the departed, and begin preparation for the burial. While it is permitted to cry and grieve naturally, it is forbidden for those who have experienced a loss to exhibit excessive emotional reactions such as wailing or thrashing about. The eyes of the deceased should be closed, all tubes and medical paraphernalia should be removed, and the body should be covered with a clean sheet. Autopsy is forbidden except when there are legal or community health issues.

Family or other members of the community will ritually wash the body prior to burial. Clean, scented water, similar to the type used by Muslims when washing for prayer, is used. The body is then wrapped in sheets of clean white cloth.

FUNERAL AND INTERNMENT

Muslims bury their deceased as soon as possible after the death. The funeral service, known as *janazah*, is generally held outdoors, in a courtyard or public square, rather than inside a mosque. The community actively participates in the funeral service, which is similar to the structure of the daily prayers, with variations such as a lack of bowing or prostration. The prayers, for the most part, are recited silently.

The deceased is taken from the site of the funeral to the cemetery for burial. While male and female members of the community participate in the funeral service, only men generally participate in the burial. The deceased is laid in the grave, without a coffin if permissible by law, on his or her right side, facing Mecca. Islamic custom discourages the erection of tombstones or elaborate markers at the gravesite, nor does it encourage the placement of flowers or other mementos. On the day of the funeral, it is customary for the Muslim community to provide food to the family of the deceased as a sign of support and solidarity.

MOURNING AND BEREAVEMENT

Loved ones and relatives generally observe a 3-day mourning period after a loss. These days are marked by increased devotion and the avoidance of decorative clothing and jewelry. The bereaved receive visitors and condolences during this period. Widows observe an extended period of mourning, which lasts 4 months and 10 days. During this period, she is not permitted to remarry, move from her home, or wear decorative clothing or jewelry.

HINDU PATIENTS

Syd Saxena

INTRODUCTION

Hinduism is an umbrella of religious concepts and practices that has evolved on the Indian subcontinent over at least three-and-a-half millennia. Like a scientific discipline, Hinduism continuously experiments with, assimilates, and refines new ideas. Tolerance, openness, and willingness to accept diverse philosophies, deities, and symbols can be thought of as defining features of this faith. This inclusive nature and a lack of rigid institutional structures has facilitated gradual assimilation of many varied local belief systems. Thus, Hinduism has come to encompass a heterogeneous set of religious ideas, rituals, and lifestyles. As a provider of end-of-life care, one is likely to experience significant variability in the views and practices of Hindu patients, depending on education, class, and geographic background. This chapter focuses primarily on central concepts that might be useful in understanding a broad range of patients' attitudes toward death.

CONCEPTS OF DHARMA, KARMA, REINCARNATION, BRAHMAN, AND MOKSHA

Hinduism has been referred to as *Sanātana Dharma* by followers since at least the fourth century B.C. *Sanātana* may be translated as "immemorial" or "eternal". *Dharma* has multiple meanings in Sanskrit, which can include "moral order," "duty," and "right action." Therefore, the most literal translation of sanatana dharma is "eternal moral order."

Dharma is a fundamentally important concept in Hinduism. It is the concept that defines a person's unique morality, societal role, and family obligations. It can be thought of as the path of knowledge and correct action. Each individual has a unique path. For example, warriors have a path that involves killing enemies in battle, while entrepreneurs have a path which is quite different. Hinduism's emphasis on living in accordance with dharma means that anyone who is striving for spiritual knowledge and seeking the right course of ethical action is, in a broad sense, a follower of Sanātana dharma.

Karma is the Hindu concept that provides the basic framework for Hindu ethics. The word karma is often translated into English as "destiny." However, unlike the word destiny, karma does not imply absence of free will. Under the doctrine of karma, the ability to make choices remains with the individual. Karma can be thought of in a scientific sense, perhaps as we think of Newton's third law. It is a causal law that holds that all moral or immoral acts have consequences in the next life.

According to the doctrine of karma, choices made in the past have created our condition in this life. Choices made today and hereafter have a causal influence on our future lives. In short, with our actions, we either accumulate or dissipate "karmic debt." The best way to be free of karmic debt is by selfless action, or by dedicating every action as an offering to God. In addition, human beings can purify themselves of karmic debt through different *yogas* (disciplines), *kriyās* (purification processes), and *bhakti* (devotions).

Through gradual realization of the relationship between our actions and our condition, we can become enlightened and more inclined toward right choices, deeds, thoughts, and desires. After steady spiritual progress through several cycles of reincarnation, we can be absorbed into *Brahman* (the ultimate reality) and attain *Moksha* (liberation from the cycle of birth and death). The highest aim of existence is complete sublimation of the innermost self, the, *ātman* (soul), with the ultimate reality (*Brahman*).

The *Bhagavad-Gītā* is an important Hindu text. In this text, the Supreme Lord Krishna imparts wisdom to the warrior Arjuna during the time of a very difficult battle. Arjuna is pitted against his blood relatives in a profound military and spiritual struggle. He is ambivalent about his role as a warrior, and his obligation to kill enemy soldiers. Krishna reassures Arjuna that it is his duty to fight the enemy, although they are his kinsmen. Krishna states to Arjuna that though the enemies may be killed, their souls cannot be destroyed:

> Weapons do not cleave this self: fire does not burn him; waters do not make him wet; nor does the wind make him dry . . . For to the one that is born death is certain, and certain is birth for the one who has died.
>
> (Bhagavad-Gita 2.23)

Krishna also states that

> And whoever, at the time of death, gives up his body and departs, thinking of Me alone, he comes to Me; of that there is no doubt.
>
> (Bhagavad-Gita 8.5)

These passages affirm the immortality of the soul and emphasize a focus on the divine throughout the end-of-life process. They serve as comfort for the dying and form the spiritual basis for what is thought to be a good death.

THE DIETIES: BRAHMĀ, VISHNU, AND SHIVA

Hinduism is fundamentally a polytheistic religion, and it is important to recognize that the majority of Hindus choose a deity, which becomes a primary object of worship. Hindus feel a powerful, direct, personal connection with this deity and perform prayers, ceremonial worship, chanting of the deity's name, pilgrimages to sites sacred to the deity, as well as fasts on that deity's sacred days. This personal relationship is a source of profound comfort during times of distress.

The three central Hindu deities are personalized forms of Brahman (the ultimate reality). Time in the Hindu universe moves in endlessly recurring cycles, much like the motion of a wheel. The duration of the various phases of the universe's existence are calculated in units of mind-boggling astronomical duration organized around such terms as *yugas, mahāyugas, manvantaras,* and *kalpas.* The universe is seen as moving cyclically through stages of creation, sustenance, and finally, destruction. In the aftermath of destruction, creation arises once again, thus starting the process anew. This cyclical view of the universe coheres with the concept of reincarnation through the cycle of death and rebirth. Each of the three major deities represents a part of this cycle.

Brahmā is the generative spirit from which the universe arises. Brahma is traditionally depicted with four heads and four faces and four arms. With each head he continually recites one of the four Vedas (sacred texts). According to ancient Hindu texts, Brahmā is the direct offspring of Brahman (the ultimate reality) and female energy known as *Prakrti* or *Maya.* He arose from a lotus flower that grew from the navel of Vishnu. He is said to have created the human race through a set of 11 sons, who were born out of his mind rather than body. Although Brahma is one of the major gods in Hinduism, few Hindus actively worship him. In modern India, one rarely finds temples dedicated to Brahma alone. There are several thousands for both Shiva and Vishnu.

Vishnu is the harmonious, peaceful, orderly force that maintains spiritual and physical stability, thus sustaining the universe. He frequently appears on earth during times of crisis in the form of an *avatar* (incarnation). He comes to uphold dharma and restore balance to the world. Vishnu has 10 major avatars, which are described in Hindu texts called the *Purānas.* These incarnations and their Hindu names are: fish (*matsya*), tortoise (*kūrma*), boar (*varāha*), man lion (*narasimha*), dwarf (*vāmana*), axe-wielding human (*Parashurāma*), ideal person (*Rāma of the Rāmāyana*), all-attractive perfect person (*Krishna*), the enlightened (*Buddha*), and a future incarnation (*Kalkī*).

Well-known avatars of Vishnu include *Supreme Lord Krishna* who was discussed in the last section. Krishna is widely worshipped throughout India and is a source of comfort for many followers. *Rāma* is a second well-known avatar of Vishnu. His profound spiritual odyssey is the subject of the Hindu epic *Rāmāyana* (Way of Rāma). In this epic, Rāma defines the ideal roles of a good son, brother, and husband, while fighting against inherently evil demons.

Shiva is the extremely complex god of destruction. He is deeply meditative and ordinarily exists in a deep trance, but he can unleash violent, chaotic, upheaval in the universe when provoked. He is at once the "standard of invincibility, might, and terror as well as a figure of honor, delight, and brilliance." He is an ascetic who lives at the top of Mount Kalasha in the Himalayas meditating on a tiger-skin while smeared in ash, yet he is also ultimately refined. Highly mystical, he is the force that brings cycles to an end—destruction acting as a prelude to transformation, leaving pure consciousness from which the universe is reborn after destruction.

Other Gods widely worshiped by Hindus are *Devi or Shakti,* the female aspect of divinity, and

Ganesha, the elephant-headed deity associated with the removal of obstacles. It is the highly personalized worship of Gods and Goddesses that is the spiritual bread and butter of Hindus' lives. These relationships are the ultimate source of comfort for families going through grieving and the effects of loss during the end of a loved one's life.

ASHRAMA—THE FOUR STAGES OF LIFE AND THE HINDU FAMILY

Hindu thought is characterized by cycles. Cycles of birth, death, and reincarnation have been discussed, as well as cycles of creation and destruction existing within the universe. Another important concept is the Hindu life cycle. This consists of four stages or *Ashrama (āśrama)*. *Ashram* means "a place of spiritual shelter." Each stage of life is not only a sequential part of the progression from cradle to grave, but a unique time when certain aspects of spiritual development and personal growth can be cultivated. The four stages are as follows:

1. *Brahmacari-ashram (Student Life):* A stage of study with emphasis on basic learning.
2. *Grihasta-ashram (Household Life):* A stage of reproduction with emphasis on family life and work.
3. *Vanaprashta (Retired Life):* A stage of retirement from economic productivity, with emphasis on reflection and worship.
4. *Sannyasa (Renounced Life):* A stage of renunciation with emphasis on detachment from material comfort, service to mankind, and self-realization.

As originally conceived, the average human life was thought to be approximately one hundred years, with each of the four ashram periods being twenty-five years each. The ultimate goal was the ideal fulfillment of four consecutive life stages. Although to some extent, there is no longer strict adherence to the life plan as described by this doctrine, the idea of experiencing the world as an organized, sequential path of personal development

with gradual retirement and enlightenment in old age persists and remains as a powerful ideal. A life lived in this way is thought to ultimately facilitate a favorable death leading to a good reincarnation.

The life cycle is particularly important to understand in the context of untimely, premature deaths of younger individuals. As Shirley Firth has written: ". . . unfortunately, not all deaths are those of elderly people who have fulfilled their life ambitions. This situation can create problems of disclosure and withdrawal of care."

She recounts the difficulties of a Hindu family when a 3-year-old Panjabi child who suffered hypoxic brain damage after having been knocked down by a car. The family required several days to understand the concept of brain death in a child at this stage of life. Considerable time elapsed before the family was finally able to withdraw ventilatory support.

On the other hand, for more elderly patients, dwindling oral intake may be interpreted as a sign of detachment leading to spiritual purification, a defining feature of the *Sannyasa*. As Justice writes: "Not eating or drinking at the time of dying can . . . be considered an aspect of general detachment from the material world, a spiritual goal of classical Hinduism."

ANTYESHTI—FUNERAL RITES AND RITUALS: CONCEPTS OF GOOD AND BAD DEATHS

A good death occurs after the completion of the four stages of the Hindu life cycle, as described in the last section. Therefore, it comes during the period of advanced age. There is variable adherence to astrological concepts among Hindus. Theoretically, there is a proper astrological time for death for each individual.

In addition to perceptions regarding the proper timing of death, many Hindus have preferences regarding the place of death. Traditionally, the proper place of death was on the ground with the head facing north, and if possible on the banks of the Ganges River. With the advent of elevated beds in homes and hospitals, this preference has been abandoned to some extent, but it is not uncommon to hear requests from Hindu patients or family members that patients expire on the ground if possible.

Indicators of a good death are a glowing appearance with a tranquil facial expression, mouth and eyes slightly open indicating departure of the soul from the body. Sacred Ganges water, which is ordinarily kept in each household, is often placed on the lips of the corpse at or after the time of death. Bad deaths are essentially the antithesis of good deaths. They are characteristically violent, premature deaths with manifestations such as emesis, fecal or urinary incontinence, and grimacing expression visible on the face.

With the development of modern culture, a less traditional brand of Hinduism is being practiced by many devotees, especially in western countries, but also within India itself. Although this trend has flourished, the importance of ritual should not be underestimated. Ritual requirements can be powerful prescriptive forces, as illustrated in Firth's account of a Gujarati family's experience:

> An aunt was dying ... the doctors told the family, and the whole family was present at the death. But when the doctors switched off the life support machine, they wouldn't let the family give Ganges water or perform any last rites. Today, after ten years it still affects the family ... They switched off the machine, and they said they mustn't give her anything that would give her a shock and kill her straight away, that would choke her.

Several years later, this family continues to do penances because their aunt died without water, and they feel her soul is not yet free.

Good deaths require the proper funeral rites and rituals. Again, there is considerable variability in the views and practices of Hindu patients, depending on education, class, and geographic background. However, some elements of funeral rites are almost universally performed. Nearly all Hindus cremate the dead body, with the exceptions of small children and enlightened saints, whose bodies are considered pure, and are therefore buried. Cremation facilitates detachment of the departed soul from its previous body, thus al-

lowing for rapid assimilation with the oneness of God, and progression to a following incarnation.

> As a person puts on new garments, giving up old ones, the soul similarly accepts new material bodies, giving up the old and useless ones.
>
> (Bhagavad-Gita 2.22)

Again, timing is important, and funeral ceremonies should be performed as rapidly as possible—by dusk or by dawn, whichever occurs first. Generally, in India a funeral takes place within hours of death. Regulations in North American and European countries may mean that it may take much longer.

Traditionally, cremation rites are as follows: The body is washed by relatives prior to cremation. It is dressed in new clothes and finery, bedecked with flowers. Ganges water and tulasi (basil leaf) are placed in the mouth. The body is then carried by stretcher to the cremation grounds as devotional hymns are sung and the bereaved chant mantras such as "Ram Nam Satya Hai" (the name of Rama is truth). The eldest son lights the funeral pyre. At the close of the cremation, a priest or relative recites appropriate verses from scripture. There can be profound, vocal expressions of grief. Typically in India, after 3 days, the eldest son collects the ashes and places them in the Ganges. In North American or European nations, a local river of personal importance or some other location important to the family may be used, though quite a few families still ultimately return the ashes to the Ganges. Similarly, in the United States and Europe, variations on the traditional ceremony are common. For example, the body is taken by limousine to the cremation site, rather than by stretcher. The eldest son presses the incineration button rather than lighting a pyre. The basic framework, however, ordinarily remains intact.

There is a prescribed period of mourning, extending to approximately 13 days after the funeral. During this time of grief, the family is considered impure. They will not attend religious functions nor eat certain foods (e.g., sweets). It is a period for venting and demonstratively expressing grief, so that one can live unhindered by suppressed emotions thereafter. The rites are also thought to benefit the deceased by ensuring the smooth passage of the soul to a better level of existence. Most essential is the *shraddha* ceremony performed on the first anniversary of death. *Prasad,* often in the form of balls of cooked rice, are offered to God and in turn to the departed soul.

CONCLUSION

In conclusion, Hinduism is a complex, ancient belief system, which means many things to many different devotees. It is important to identify key elements of the patient's and family's belief system and attitudes surrounding death early on, striving to facilitate preferences throughout end-of-life care, death, and the rituals and the grieving process beyond. Familiarization with the broad philosophical concepts of the Hindu faith, the major Hindu deities, the Hindu life cycle, and Hindu funeral rites and rituals will serve as a solid foundation in this endeavor.

BUDDHIST PATIENTS

Sara Roby

INTRODUCTION

Buddhism is the world's fourth largest religion, with over 376 million adherents, primarily in the many nations of eastern Asia. In the United States, it represents about 0.9% of the population and is practiced by Asian immigrants and their descendants as well as a fair number of converts.

There are three major Buddhist sects, Theravada Buddhism, Mahayana Buddhism, and Tantryana Buddhism. Theravada stands for the "Way of the Elders" and this form of Buddhism is primarily practiced in nations like Sri Lanka,

Thailand, Burma, Cambodia, and Laos. It is believed to have arisen from an ancient sect known as Hinayana (Little Vehicle), and it claims to adhere to, preserve, and follow the original transmitted teachings of the Buddha (see below).

Mahayana stands for the "Big Vehicle" and this form of Buddhism is found primarily in China, Korea, and Japan. It started around the 1st century CE and broke away from Hinayana Buddhism in the fourth century CE. The Mahayana tradition developed mainly in Northern India, from which it spread into China and Tibet. Once in China, Buddhist philosophy and practice integrated Taoist and Confucian elements already present and became strongly grounded in the Chinese culture. Through China, Mahayana Buddhism also stretched to Korea, Vietnam, Cambodia, Laos, and Japan. In China, Buddhism evolved to what is known as the *Ch'an* tradition, introduced later into Korea and Japan (known there as *Zen*). Other major branches of Buddhism in Japan include Pure Land Buddhism, Nichiren, Shingon, and Tendai.

The third sect is Tantryana, also referred to as Vajrayana, which stands for the "Diamond Vehicle." It is based on both the Hinayana and Mahayana tradition and has its origins in the sixth century CE. The Tantrayana tradition of North India was introduced into Tibet around the eighth century CE. Tibet, Bhutan, and Mongolia have a virtually complete set of tantric teachings preserved. The Tibetan tradition can also be found in the Himalayan area (Northwest India), Sikkim (Northeast India), Nepal, and Mongolia (virtually identical to the Tibetan tradition). Loose ends of the Vajrayana tradition can also be found in China, Korea, and Japan.

GENERAL PRINCIPLES OF BUDDHISM

The Original Buddha

The historical Buddha (the *Awakened One*) was born Prince Siddharta Gautama, some 2,500 years ago (c. 563–483 BCE) in what is now called Lumbini in Nepal, at the foot of the Himalayas, north of the Indian subcontinent. His father was the king of the tribal clan of the Shakyas. His mother, Maya, died a week after giving birth to the child and he was raised by his loving aunt. The child's body presented marks considered special signs and as it was custom, his father consulted with a sage to decipher the meaning. The sage predicted that Siddharta Gautama would become either a great king (a "world ruler") or a great spiritual leader (a "world teacher").

While his father groomed him to be his successor, at the age of 29, as a result of what had been called the Four Passing Sights (an aged man, an ill man, a dead body taken for cremation, and a wandering holy man), he chose a spiritual path in order to find an answer to the issue of suffering. While searching for these answers during the next six years, he adopted, among other practices, asceticism, and after almost dying of starvation, he decided to abandon all these practices and to sit in meditation until he found the truth. He sat down in a place now called Bodhgaya (North India) under a Bodhi tree. Sometime later, he attained enlightenment and became known as Gautama Buddha, or simply "The Buddha," meaning "The Awakened One." He *actualised* all the potentials of a *sentient being*, liberating himself of all negative qualities. The true nature of existence and suffering (*emptiness*) through him was realized, as well as the knowledge of how to end suffering.

Seven weeks after his enlightenment, the Buddha gave his first discourse in Sarnath, near Varanasi. He taught what has become known as the *Four Noble Truths*, which constitute the core foundation of the Buddhist path. The Buddha continued to teach during his life, until he died at the age 81.

The Four Noble Truths

Regardless of the specific tradition or school one may follow within Buddhism, the *Four Noble Truths* are considered to be the central Buddhist teachings, with all teachings that have followed being derived or reflective of these profound truths.

The first of the "Noble Truths" is the *Truth of Suffering*, which as the name implies, recognizes the universality of suffering. Such suffering may take many different forms and may be encountered through our own suffering and awakening, through studying the suffering of others, or both. Our life is in the cycle of existence—*Samsara*—because of past karma, pain, and suffering caused in previous lives and by other generations. If we do not wake up to the reality of the cause of suffering and the way out of it, we will continue to enter the cycle, *Samsara*, suffering and generating suffering for others. The *Truth of Suffering* is at the heart of our existence to the point that we don't even seem to perceive it anymore or have much difficulty with it. We have learned to live with it and within it; we have excelled in creating it and multiplying it; we have found that the suffering we cause to ourselves and to others is normal and acceptable.

Second is the *Truth of the Origin of Suffering*. Buddhism views the cause of suffering as related to three basic negative emotions sometimes referred to in Buddhism as "the three poisons": anger, attachment, and ignorance. When we reflect about these negative emotions, we can see how individually, and even more importantly jointly, they underlie all of our behaviors. Suffering is never isolated, not its cause (*karma*, intentions, motivations, actions) nor its consequences. Buddhism believes in the interdependence of all: everyone and everything is linked to everything else in a never-ending circle. Ignorance blinds us from understanding the damage we cause to others by our *karma*. This karma will come back to us, sometime, somehow, somewhere; it will either affect us directly or through our descendants, family, or nation. It is a Law of the Universe.

With an understanding of suffering and what causes it, Buddhism now provides one with a way to end the suffering through the third "Noble Truth," the *Truth of the Cessation of Suffering*. Suffering can only cease when one is able to reach *Nirvana*, the ultimate state of freedom from illness, which is beyond all suffering, and outside of the cycle of existence (*Samsara*). To achieve this, one needs to end the delusions caused by three poisons mentioned above: anger, attachment, and ignorance.

To conquer the third poison, ignorance (lack of *wisdom*, conventional and ultimate wisdom), one must deeply understand the "Fourth Noble Truth," the *Truth of the Path that leads to the Cessation of Suffering*. Buddhism believes that in order to attain the highest levels of spirituality, one must train the body and mind as a single unit. As opposed to the Judeo-Christian religious tradition, where the body does not have the same value that is attributed to the *spirit*, Buddhism is essentially a nondualistic religious/spiritual proposition (body/mind as one; within/without; oneness of all things), which influences the way a Buddhist must work to understand life and existence.

The *Path that leads to the Cessation of Suffering* is also known as the *Noble Eightfold Path*. As its name already expresses, there are eight distinct domains of conduct or behavior that one must study and work to perfect and measure one's everyday life by in order to the find the path away from suffering. These behaviors are thought, speech, action, a proper livelihood that does not harm others, understanding, effort, mindfulness, and concentration. By working towards perfection in each of these areas, one can achieve a sense of balance and avoid suffering in one's life.

The Three Treasures: Buddha, Dharma, and Sangha

The Three treasures, also called the *Three Jewels*, are the symbolic spiritual space where lay and ordained Buddhist take *refuge*.

The first is *Buddha*, the Enlightened One. It refers not only to the original Buddha discussed above, but to all the Buddhas of the past, present, and future. The Buddha represents a human being who has attained the highest degree of realization; a life that has been able to see reality for what it is and has understood and directly experienced the nonduality of all things and the unity of the whole existence, visible and invisible. Buddhist vow and *take refuge in the Buddha* as a way to express the aspiration to become enlightened (not one day but everyday), help, and benefit all sentient beings through their own conduct in daily life, and live in the reality and avoid creating more delusion and karma for themselves and others. Buddha becomes the spiritual teacher and the guide, and by extension, teachers become a representation of Buddha for the disciple. For Buddhists, taking refuge in the Buddha is also an act of faith: faith that all beings are Buddha in nature and should be treated as such.

The second treasure is *Dharma*, which is a Sanskrit word meaning doctrine, law, or truth. It refers to the Buddha's Teachings, which can also be understood as the *Cosmic Law*, governing the Universe throughout the circle of time. The Buddha himself did not write anything down; his teachings came directly from the everyday experiences of the hundreds of disciples who listened and learned from and with him during his 40 years of public teaching. Following the Buddha's death, there was a gathering of his followers known as the First Buddhist Council where his disciples recited many of the Buddha's discourses from memory. This led to the institution of the first Buddhist canon, which was known as the "Three Baskets" (*Tripitaka*, in Sanskrit). The canon consists of the *Vinaya* (rules of conduct mainly for the monastic orders), the *Sutras* (discourses of the Buddha and or his immediate disciples), and the *Abhidarma* (scholastic treatises codifying and making interpretations of the Buddha's teachings). Between the years 35 and 32 BCE, it was decided to commit the oral tradition to writing. Buddhists vow *to take refuge in the Dharma* as an expression of their wish to follow and apply the teachings of Buddha in their everyday life.

The third treasure is *Sangha*, which is a Sanskrit word that refers to the community of Buddhists. It can be used to represent several levels of community: the community of all Buddhist practitioners, the community of Buddhist monks and nuns, or, in its strictest sense, the community of those who have realized emptiness. Anyone calling him or herself a Buddhist practitioner normally will be linked to a teacher and to a *sangha*, and formal ordination is not required for one to be a Buddhist or to become enlightened.

BUDDHIST ETHICS AND MORALS

Buddhists are guided by a set of Ten Precepts, which help them develop their basic attitudes toward daily life. These precepts are not viewed as proscriptive commandments imposed on one by an exterior force or superior being. Rather, they are guidelines of wisdom and common sense and are profoundly meaningful when understood as principles aiming at creating a life of compassion, harmony, and respect for all beings, based on the principles of equality (everyone and everything essentially have equal rights to live, be respected, enjoy happiness, and be free of fear and suffering) and reciprocity (we treat others with the same love, consideration, respect, and compassion, that we want to be treated with ourselves). While Buddhists do their best to adhere to these precepts as they go about their daily lives, failure to do so is seen as an opportunity for education and growth, to learn from the experience, and to try and do better the next time.

A very important aspect in one's understanding of the precepts is that one's intention is more important than the action in itself, which explains why two similar actions can have different implications and karma. While the killing of living beings, for example, is not generally permitted, killing with the intent of protecting the lives of innocent children will have a very different karma than killing for pleasure or hatred.

The first five precepts are

1. Abstain from killing living beings.
2. Abstain from taking that which is not given.
3. Abstain from sexual misconduct.
4. Abstain from false speech.
5. Abstain from distilled substances that confuse the mind (i.e., alcohol and drugs).

The precepts can also be stated in a more positive light:

1. Act with loving kindness.
2. Be open-hearted and generous.
3. Practice stillness, simplicity, and contentment.
4. Speak with truth, clarity, and peace.
5. Live with mindfulness.

They are considered training precepts and are the basic guidelines for good ethical and moral conduct. As such, they constitute the base that can then support a stable and balanced emotional, spiritual, social life, and a life of commitment and righteousness toward all beings. A Buddhist, layman, or clergy will vow to undertake the Precepts and make his/her life an expression of the Dharma (the Cosmic Law).

There are five additional precepts that a Buddhist also works toward adhering to:

6. Not talking of the faults of others.
7. Not praising oneself or slandering others.
8. Not begrudging the dharma or materials.
9. Not being angry.
10. Not slandering the Three Treasures (Buddha, Dharma, Sangha).

In addition to the Ten Precepts, there are Ten *Paramitas* (meaning gone to the other shore) or Perfections. These are a group of virtues or qualities that Buddhists follow, develop to the highest level, and incorporate into their own life experiences. They are intended to be applied toward others, as well as to the Buddhist him or herself. The Ten *Paramitas* are

1. Giving or generosity.
2. Virtue, ethics, and morality.
3. Renunciation, letting go, not grasping.
4. *Prajna* (wisdom), insight into the nature of reality.
5. Energy, vigor, vitality, diligence.
6. Patience or forbearance.
7. Truthfulness.
8. Resolution, determination, and intention.
9. Kindness, love, friendliness.
10. Equanimity.

BUDDHISM AND END-OF-LIFE CARE

Buddhist Philosophy of Life and Death

Now when the bardo of dying dawns upon me, I will abandon all grasping, yearning and attachment, Enter undistracted into a clear awareness of the teaching, And eject my consciousness into the space of unborn awareness; As I leave this compound body of flesh and blood I will know it to be a transitory illusion.

Tibetan Book of the Dead—Padmasambhava

For all Buddhist schools and its diverse sects, dying (and death) is an inextricable part of life. Life and death are not two; they are each a part of the whole, a unity, a continuous process. Life and death together are beginningless, endless, fluid, transforming itself just as water changes form without changing its nature: from solid ice to melted liquid and then to ethereal vapor, with cycle going on forever.

If from the Buddhist perspective, life is impermanent, always changing at every level; if Buddhists learn and train to see impermanence always, then they are prepared to see life and death and death and life in everything, both animated and inanimated. With proper training, a Buddhist is expected to be able to walk the path toward death with a certain amount of understanding, acceptance of the reality, and openness to deal with the fears, difficulties, and questions that come with the dying process. Clearly, no matter how well prepared one may think he or she is, when the time comes to prepare for death, sometimes months before it actually occurs, there are many uncertainties. We have very personal questions to deal with, and we have many relations with the world that will need to be faced (family, friends, animals, material things to resolve). As the dying process advances, and if we have good karma expressed through the love and support, we may find along the way, as well as the strength and courage we may awaken in order to step up to the challenges ahead; we learn to cope with the new situations at every step. This, too, is an essential part of being a Buddhist: the *here*

and now aspect of life, the focus on the present, where the past that matters is here through our karma and where one is planting, through actions, thoughts and speech, the future to come.

For a Buddhist with proper training (teacher, study, practice, and sangha), the time of death is a time to reactualize, remember, and powerfully bring forward all of what life has been about: a consistent practice of letting go, of detaching and flowing into the stream of energy "that is." Dying is dissolution of the illusory self that has taken form and shape for a brief instant in the eternity of beginningless and endless time; it is a wave returning naturally to the ocean from where it came from and becoming again a drop of water, a wave, a vapor, and again a wave in the ocean of life. Indeed beautiful, yet unsurprisingly simple and natural.

Each sect within the Buddhist tradition has its own way to express the practice and give meaning to the passage through the dying process. These may include the chanting/listening of sutras; visualizing colored lights; invoking the Buddha's name; concentrating on breathing, vocalizing a mantra, or meditating on an image (such as a mandala, an image of a teacher, or Buddha); sitting or laying down in a meditation posture; letting go of any thought, image, or existent connection; awakening through guidance specific feelings and connections to deities. For each sect, the particular practice has a powerful purpose and meaning, and follows certain rituals as in any other religion. For those whose connection with Buddhism is more emotional and spiritual than through a sustained commitment and affiliation, simplicity is usually the rule. Family, friends, or the patient can indicate what may be effective in allowing the belief to be present and honored at this time of the patient's life.

When death is very near, there is no rule. One aspires to feel within and around, pure and simple love and compassion in the midst of the reality that death imposes on all. Death can become a trap, a deadly mesh or a bumpy ride in a torrent, or it can be a smooth glide on the stream that carries one to the ocean of existence "beyond." It is said, and many times confirmed, that one dies in much the same way as one has lived: if one was unhappy during life, the dying process will likely be another obstacle. On the other hand, if one was able to transform negative experiences into positive ones, then it is likely s/he will make peace and learn what good dying may bring forward for him or herself or for others. If a person has lived a life of contentment, he or she will sooner rather than later come to terms with the inevitable. The river, the trees, the stream, the rocks, the mesh, and the open skies are all there. Each person makes choices, consciously and subconsciously, which change one's karma and, therefore, the way one leaves this visible physical existence. One may stubbornly hold on, or one may choose to let go and swim above, around, under, in-between, and through all the normal, natural, expected, and unexpected circumstances that are encountered in the way to the Ocean.

Care of the Buddhist Patient Near the End of Life

As already discussed, the Buddhist understanding of good health places an emphasis on the balanced interaction between mind and body as well between the person and the environment. Buddhists also believe that illness is inevitable during life and therefore, looking after the sick is strongly advocated. Buddhists embrace modern medicine and believe that it can be truly effective when combined with the deeper understanding of the inner issues of life that are part and parcel of Buddhist philosophy. Recitation of the precepts and virtues, for example, are believed to be endowed with healing properties. Buddhists are also open to complementary medical techniques such as acupuncture and massage.

As many Buddhists living in the United States are of Asian origin, their cultural healthcare needs may differ depending upon their nation of origin, although, in some respects, the specific behaviors seen in Asian Americans is heavily influenced by Buddhism as well. (The reader is referred to the section of Chapter 31 on Asian Americans.) For example, Buddhists in general, as well as many of the specific Asian American sub-groups, are expected to bear physical pain stoically, even if the pain is acute, so caregivers may find that patients are reluctant to take analgesics. Patients are taught to be cooperative with their caregivers, especially the physician and nurse, in order to get well. Issues related to end-of-life decision making, such as consideration for withholding or withdrawing food and fluids, should be discussed with the family.

When Buddhist patients are nearing the end of life, they generally prefer to be in a quiet place that is free of distraction. Having family or healthcare providers who visit with the patient sit in relaxed silence and provide gentle touch may be very appropriate. Patients may desire to have ritual objects surrounding them, such as pictures of their teachers, statues of the Buddha, and incense or candles. Prayers or chants, including recitation of the five precepts, by a member of the patient's spiritual community may also be desired by some. When a patient is very close to death, some Buddhist have the tradition of cleansing the patient and putting him in clean clothes in order to allow him to feel fresh and comfortable prior to passing on.

Buddhist Funeral Customs

As already mentioned, since American Buddhists come from a variety of Asian nations, and Buddhist customs have been intertwined with the customs of the specific nation (or even village within a particular country), it is very difficult to describe specific traditional Buddhist funeral customs. For many, after the patient dies, it is customary that the family clean and dress the body, as an expression of filial piety. The deceased is usually dressed in simple clothing or traditional garb, depending on local custom. The body is placed in a casket by the family, and then either placed in the appropriate room in the home where the funeral service will occur, or transported to the funeral home.

Buddhist funeral should be simple, solemn, and dignified, with money that would have been spent on more lavish arrangement being earmarked for charity for the merit of the departed. Once the casket is in its proper place, an altar is set up in front of it. With the altar is a portrait of the deceased, and offerings, including flowers, fruits, candies, and incense, are often placed on the altar. Some will also set up a Buddha image in the area of the altar.

It is not necessary for family members to dress in black (although some may choose to do so, based on local custom). Rather, clothing that is white or of a plain, somber color may be worn. During the wake, when guests come to pay their respects, they stand in front of the altar and either bow with their hands clasped together or observe a moment of silence. They may join with other mourners in chanting or if they are unable to, they should try and observe silence or only speak softly. A Buddhist monk, other officiating clergy, mourners, or lay members of the community may perform the appropriate rituals and chants, and deliver sermons in memory of the deceased.

On the morning following the wake, the deceased receives last rites, which includes various rituals and chants. The casket is then closed and transferred to the hearse so that it may be taken for cremation, which is the customary disposition of the body for the vast majority of Buddhists. During the procession to the funeral, especially if done on foot, participants should contemplate on the impermanence of life and radiate thoughts of loving kindness to the family of the deceased.

Once the body is brought to the crematorium, another ceremony with ritual chanting is performed, following which the body is cremated. Ashes are traditionally collected on the following day. Again, there are many different customs depending on the Buddhist sect and country of origin of the deceased and family. Money that was contributed by relatives and friends as a token of condolence may be used to defray funeral costs or donated to charity in the merits of the deceased. Memorial services are customarily held on the 3rd, 7th, 49th, and 100th day following the funeral. (For discussions on how Buddhist burial customs may vary among different Asian American cultures, see the section on Asian Americans in Chapter 31.)

BIBLIOGRAPHY

Jewish Patients

Babylonian Talmud Tractate. *Yoma* 85a-b.

Barile A: *Geriatric study of survivors. International Society for Yad Vashem, Martyrdom and Resistance.* March–April, 14, 2000.

David P, Pelly S, eds: *Caring for Aging Holocaust Survivors: A Practice Manual.* Toronto, Baycrest Center for Geriatric Care, 2003.

Kinzbrunner BM: Jewish medical ethics and end-of-life care. *Palliat Med* 7(4):558, 2004.

Kinzbrunner BM: Orthodox and Hasidic Perspectives. In: Doka KJ, Tucci AS, eds. *Living with Grief. Diversity and End-of-Life Care.* Washington, DC, Hospice Foundation of America, 142-150, 2009.

Koltach AJ: *The Jewish Mourner's Book of Why.* New York, Jonathan David Publishers, 1993.

Kotler-Berkowitz L, Cohen SM, Ament J, et al: *National Jewish Population Survey 2000-01. Strength, Challenge, and Diversity in the American Jewish Population.* New York, United Jewish Communities, 2004.

Lamm M: *The Jewish Way in Death and Mourning.* New York, Jonathan David Publishers, 1969.

Lamm M: Jewish perspectives on loss, grief, and end-of-life care. In: Doka KJ, Tucci AS, eds. *Living with Grief. Diversity and End-of-Life Care.* Washington, DC, Hospice Foundation of America, 2009, pp. 129-141.

Lamm M, Kinzbrunner BM: *The Jewish Hospice Manual: A Guide to Compassionate End-of-Life Care for Jewish Patients and their Families.* Miami, New York, Vitas Healthcare Corporation and National Institute for Jewish Hospice, 2003.

Rabinowicz T: *A Guide to Life. Jewish Laws and Customs of Mourning.* New Jersey, Jason Aronson Publishers, 1989.

Singer D, Grossman L, eds: *American Jewish Yearbook, 2006.* New York, American Jewish Committee. http://www.jewishvirtuallibrary.org/jsource/US-Israel/usjewpop.html. Accessed March 16, 2009.

Steinberg A: A Jewish perspective on the four principles, Chapter 7. In: Gillon R, Lloyd A, eds. *Principles of Healthcare Ethics.* Chichester, John Wiley and Sons, 1994, pp. 65-73.

Weinreb TH: Hasidic & ultra-rthodox Judaism. In: Lamm M, Kinzbrunner BM, eds. *The Jewish Hospice Manual: A Guide to Compassionate End-of-Life Care for Jewish Patients and their Families.* Miami, New York, Vitas Healthcare Corporation and National Institute for Jewish Hospice, 2003.

Muslim Patients

Al-Hijra: ReligionFacts.com. http://www.religionfacts.com/islam/holidays/hijra.htm. Accessed December 4, 2009.

American Muslim population: http://www.islamicpopulation.com/America/america_islam.html. Accessed December 2, 2009.

Asadi-Lari M, Goushegir SA, Madjd Z, Latifi NA: Spiritual care at the end of life in the Islamic context, a systematic review. *Iran J Cancer Prev* 2:63-67, 2008.

Ashura: ReligionFacts.com. http://www.religionfacts.com/islam/holidays/ashura.htm. Accessed December 4, 2009.

Athar S, Fadel HE, Ahmed WD, et al: Islamic medical ethics: the IMANA perspective. http://www.imana.org/PDF%20Files/IMANAEthicsPaperPart1.pdf. Accessed December 2, 2009.

Gatrad AR, Sheikh A: Medical ethics and Islam: Principles and practice. *Arch Dis Child* 84:72-75, 2001.

Hajj: Wikipedia, the free encyclopedia. http://en.wikipedia.org/wiki/Hajj. Accessed December 4, 2009.

Haque M, Mueenuddin H: Clinical Case: Dilemmas in end-of-life decision making for the medical tourist patient. *Virtual Mentor, Am Med Assoc J Ethics* 11(8):582-588, 2009. http://virtualmentor.ama-assn.org/2009/08/pdf/ccas2-0908.pdf. Accessed December 2, 2009.

Huda: Islamic funeral rites. Care for the dying, funeral prayers, burial, and mourning. About.com Islam. http://islam.about.com/cs/elderly/a/funerals.htm. Accessed December 3, 2009.

Huda: Milad an-Nabi—Birthday of the Prophet Muhammad. About.com Islam. http://islam.about.com/od/otherdays/a/milad.htm. Accessed December 4, 2009.

Huda: What holidays do Muslims celebrate? About.com Islam. http://islam.about.com/od/holidays/f/holidays.htm. Accessed December 3, 2009.

Islamic Dietary Laws: Wikipedia, the free encyclopedia. http://en.wikipedia.org/wiki/Islamic_dietary_laws. Accessed December 4, 2009.

Islamic New Year: Wikipedia, the free encyclopedia. http://en.wikipedia.org/wiki/Islamic_New_Year. Accessed December 4, 2009.

Muslim population worldwide. http://www.islamicpopulation.com/. Accessed December 4, 2009.

Nassar AK, Baddarni K: Islamic perspectives on life and death. Handout from Panel Presentation: 2nd International Conference on Palliative Care in Different Cultures, Eilat, Israel, Friday, March 21, 2008.

Shanawani S, Zafar S: Dying and grief in the Islamic community. In: Doka KJ, Tucci AS, eds. *Living with Grief. Diversity and End-of-Life Care.* Washington, DC, Hospice Foundation of America, 2009, pp. 151-164.

Zafir al-Shahri M, al-Khenaizan A: Palliative care for Muslim patients. *J Support Oncol* 3:432-436, 2005.

Zahedi F, Larijani B, Bazzaz JT: End-of-life ethical issues and Islamic views. *Iran J Allergy Asthma Immunol* 6(supp 5):5-15, 2007.

Hindu Patients

Firth S: *Dying, Death and Bereavement in British Hindu Community.* Leuven, Brussels, Peeters, 1997.

Firth S: End of life: A Hindu view. *Lancet* 336:682, 2005.

Friedlmeier W, Chakkarath P, Schwarz B, ed: *Culture and Human Development.* London, Psychology Press, 2005.

Justice C: *Dying the Good Death: The Pilgrimage to Die in India's Holy City.* Albany, NY, State University of New York Press, 1997.

Rama S: *Perennial Psychology of the Bhagavad Gita.* Honesdale, PA, Himalayan Institute Press, 1985.

Radhakrishnan S (translator): *Bhagvad Gita.* New York, Harper and Brothers, 1957.

Buddhist Patients

Buddhism: Religion—wiki. http://religion.wikia.com/wiki/Buddhism. Accessed December 21, 2009.

Buddhism in the United States: Wikipedia, the free encyclopedia. http://en.wikipedia.org/wiki/Buddhism_in_the_United_States. Accessed December 21, 2009.

Carrithers M: *The Buddha: A Very Short Introduction.* New York, Oxford University Press, 2001.

Coleman JW: *The New Buddhism: The Western Transformation of an Ancient Tradition.* New York, Oxford University Press, 2002.

Gethin R: *The Foundations of Buddhism*. New York, Oxford University Press, 1998.

Harris EJ: *What Buddhists Believe*. Oxford, England, Oneworld Publ., 1998.

Harvey P: *An Introduction to Buddhist Ethics: Foundations, Values and Issues*. Cambridge, Cambridge University Press, 2000.

Heine S, Charles S, Prebish, eds: *Buddhism in the Modern World: Adaptations of an Ancient Tradition*. New York, Oxford University Press, 2004.

Keown D: Buddhism: A Very Short Introduction. New York, Oxford University Press, 2000.

Keown D: *Contemporary Buddhist Ethics*. London, Curzon Press, 2000.

Lopez DS Jr., ed: *Buddhism in Practice*. Princeton, NJ, Princeton University Press, 1995.

Lopez DS, Jr., *The Story of Buddhism: A Concise Guide to Its History and Teachings*. New York, Harper, 2001.

Malaysian Buddhist Co-operative Society Berhad: A Guide to a Proper Buddhist Funeral. Buddha Dharma Education Association, Inc. http://www.buddhanet.net/pdf_file/buddhist_funeral.pdf. Accessed December 22, 2009.

Nakamura H: *Gotama Buddha: A Biography Based on the Most Reliable Texts*. Tokyo, Kosei Publ., 2001.

Powers J: *A Concise Encyclopedia of Buddhism*. Oxford, England, Oneworld Publ., 2000.

Prebish CS: *The A to Z of Buddhism*. Lanham, MD, Scarecrow Press, 2001.

Smith-Stoner M: End-of-life needs of patients who practice Tibetan Buddhism. *J Hosp Palliat Nursing* 7(4):228-233, 2005.

THINK about Buddhism: *VITAS: Things Hospice Innovators Need to Know*. Miami, Vitas Innovative Hospice Care, 2008.

SELF-ASSESSMENT QUESTIONS

1. All of the following are true regarding issues of Jewish medical ethics and end-of-life decision making, EXCEPT

    A. As life is of infinite value in Judaism, Judaism does not accept the concept of terminal illness.

    B. Providing food and fluid, even by artificial means, is considered basic care by most traditional Jews and should be provided to virtually all terminally ill patients.

    C. Euthanasia, assisted suicide, or any form of intentional hastening of death is forbidden under Jewish law.

    D. Withholding of treatment when patients are near the end of life may be permitted, while withdrawing treatment in this situation is generally forbidden.

    E. Advance directives in the orthodox Jewish community must include that a rabbi knowledgeable in healthcare matters be named as surrogate to ensure that all decisions are made according to Jewish law.

2. Each of the following statements about Jewish traditions and rituals are true, EXCEPT

    A. Jews who keep "kosher" are not allowed to eat meat and dairy foods together.

    B. During the Jewish holiday of Passover, Jews eat unleavened bread called Matzah.

    C. End-of-life caregivers are not permitted to provide care to an observant Jewish patient on the Sabbath since travelling and using electricity are not allowed.

    D. Orthodox Jewish patients may be uncomfortable if personal care is rendered by an individual of the opposite gender.

    E. On the Jewish New Year, Rosh Hashana, Jews listen to sounds that are blown on a ram's horn, called a Shofar.

3. All of the following statements regarding the care of Jewish patients at the time of death and Jewish mourning and bereavement customs are true, EXCEPT

    A. If a Jewish person is having a tradition Jewish burial, end-of-life care staff should not clean the body after the patient has passed away.

    B. Cremation is forbidden under Jewish law, although some groups in the Reform movement now permit it.

    C. During the *shiva* period, friends visit the mourners to provide comfort and support.

    D. It is permitted by Jewish law for mourners to work or conduct normal business activities during *shiva*.

    E. Jews memorialize the deceased yearly on the anniversary of the death, known as *yahrzeit*.

4. True statements concerning Islamic Medical Ethics and end-of-life decision making include all of the following, EXCEPT

    A. Euthanasia and assisted suicide are forbidden under Islamic law.

    B. While food and fluid should not be withheld orally, one is not obligated to force feed patients who cannot take food or fluid orally.

    C. Patients may desire that pain medication be withheld so they may remain alert in order to pray right before death.

    D. Items prohibited by Islamic law may not be used to treat patients, even in cases of dire medical necessity.

    E. One is not permitted to lie to a Muslim patient about his prognosis.

5. All of the following statements regarding the care of Muslim patients at the time of death and Islamic mourning and bereavement customs are true, EXCEPT

    A. When a Muslim is dying, family should be with the person to provide comfort and remind the person of God's mercy and forgiveness.

B. It is customary for Muslims to wail and thrash about excessively when a loved one passes away.

C. The funeral service is not held in a mosque, but is held in a courtyard or public square.

D. Muslims are buried without a coffin when possible, with the body laying on the right side, facing Mecca.

E. Muslim widows observe an extended mourning period of 4 months and 10 days.

6. The Hindu concept of a good death includes each of the following, EXCEPT

A. Water from the Ganges River is placed on the lips of the deceased at the time of death.

B. The head of the dying person faces north at the time of death.

C. The death occurs at the proper astrological time.

D. The body of the dying person is elevated off the ground at the time of death.

E. The deceased has a tranquil facial expression with eyes and mouth slightly open.

7. All of the following statements regarding Hindu funeral and mourning customs are true, EXCEPT

A. All Hindus, irregardless of age or social status, are cremated.

B. Funerals generally take place as soon as possible after someone passes away.

C. Three days after cremation, the eldest son collects the ashes and places them in the Ganges River or another location of importance to the family.

D. There is a 13-day period of mourning following the funeral during which family will demonstratively express grief.

E. In the western world, the eldest son will press the incinerator button at the crematorium in place of his traditional role of lighting the funeral pyre.

8. True statements regarding the Ten Precepts, which assist Buddhists in developing their basic attitudes toward daily life include all of the following, EXCEPT

A. They are not viewed as proscriptive commandments, rather, they are guidelines of wisdom and common sense.

B. Failure to adhere to the precepts is seen as an opportunity for education and growth.

C. When trying to adhere to the precepts, one's action is more important than one's intention.

D. Buddhists will vow to undertake the first five precepts on a regular basis.

E. The first five precepts are often recited by a member of the Buddhist spiritual community in the presence of one who is near death.

9. True statements concerning the care of Buddhist patients near the end of life include all of the following, EXCEPT

A. Buddhists are expected to bear pain stoically and may, therefore, be reluctant to take analgesic medications.

B. Buddhists are taught to cooperate with caregivers, especially physicians and nurse, in order to get well.

C. When nearing death, Buddhist patients desire to be in a quiet place free of distractions, with visitors or caregivers sitting in relaxed silence.

D. Buddhist patients often desire to have ritual objects surrounding them when death is near.

E. It is forbidden to change the clothes of Buddhist patients when death is near.

10. All of the following concerning Buddhist funeral customs are true, EXCEPT

A. Many Buddhist families will clean and dress the body as an expression of filial piety.

B. Buddhist funerals are traditionally simple, solemn, and dignified.

C. Guests coming to pay respects to the deceased should stand in front of the altar and either bow or observe a moment of silence.

D. The day following the wake, the body is taken to the cemetery to be buried.

E. Any money given to family as tokens of condolence may be used to defray funeral expenses or be donated to charity in memory of the deceased.

Answers to
Self-Assessment Questions

Chapter 1

1. Correct answer: D

Clinical judgment is the most important factor in determining whether a patient's prognosis is 6 months or less. The general guidelines, such as unexplained weight loss and a decrease in performance status (choice A) are useful additional factors, but are not required. Likewise, while disease specific guidelines help support the prognostic determination, patients do not need to meet all the criteria for any specific disease to determine either prognosis or diagnosis (choice B). If, based on history and clinical exam, the patient appears terminally ill, objective studies that have not already been obtained are not required (choice C). Finally, it is critically important that patients' goals are considered when determining prognosis and for appropriate end-of-life care planning (choice E).

2. Correct answer: B

The KPS does not consider the presence or absence, or the severity of patient symptoms in its evaluation (choice B). It was developed in the late 1940s as a tool to evaluate patient activity levels, as it was observed that there was correlation between patient performance and response to chemotherapy that needed to be accounted for in clinical trials (choice A). The activities the KPS considers include ambulation, self-care ability, and overall activity level. It also accounts for the extent of disease. Studies evaluating the ability of the KPS to assist in determining prognosis have demonstrated that a rapid fall of 20 to 30 units is associated with patient mortality in an average of 2 to 3 months (choice C). Additionally, patients who have a particular KPS score and have active symptoms survive for a shorter period than those whose symptoms are controlled (choice D).

3. Correct answer: C

While weight loss of 10% or more may be consistent with a prognosis of 6 months or less, the weight loss has to be unintentional and has to represent a loss of lean body mass. Although the patient in choice C has advanced congestive heart failure and may or may not have a prognosis of 6 months or less, the weight loss in this situation will not help make that determination, since it was intentional, consisted of fluid, and likely was beneficial, rather than detrimental, to the patient. On the other hand, serial functional decline evidenced in the MDS (choice A), progressive hepatomegaly in a patient with metastatic cancer (choice B), deterioration of patient's condition reported by the home health nurse (choice D), or multiple ED visits in a patient with advanced COPD (choice E) may all be indicative of deterioration in a patient's condition and help determine that a patient has a prognosis of 6 months or less.

4. Correct answer: D

The PPS assesses a patient's food and fluid intake and level of consciousness in addition to the patient activity levels that were standard in the KPS (choice D). The KPS can be used for patients with cancer as well as those with noncancer diagnoses (choice A). While a PPS score of 50 is generally viewed as associated with a prognosis of 6 months or less, a higher score does not necessarily mean that a patient does not have a less than 6 months prognosis, and may be eligible for hospice services based upon other criteria (choice B). While the PPS has been demonstrated to successfully predict patient survival at the time of admission to hospice or palliative care services, it has not been shown to be predictive of survival in the general population of patients who are chronically ill (choice C).

5. Correct answer: E

When contemplating when patients with various malignancies are approaching the end of life, there are a number of factors that must be considered. These include the natural history of the specific type of cancer (choice A), whether the patient has metastatic disease (choice B), and whether there is effective treatment available (choice C). In addition, one must be aware of the patient's goals of care, as sometimes those goals may significantly affect choices patients make regarding what types of treatments they would or would not accept, which can have an impact on prognosis (choice D).

6. Correct answer: B

While liquid morphine is often used to control symptoms of shortness of breath in patients with advanced COPD, the fact that the patient requires such therapy is not in and of itself an indicator of disease progression (choice B). (Morphine, for example, can be used to treat dyspnea secondary to pulmonary edema.) As COPD worsens, it has been shown that patients tend to require more frequent medical attention (choice A). In addition, these patients often lose significant weight because of

the increased work they have to do to breathe (choice C). Patients with advanced COPD often suffer from the comorbid condition of cor pulmonale (choice D), and are often hypoxic with oxygen saturations at or below 88% on room air (choice E).

7. Correct answer: D

As the patient has symptomatic congestive heart failure, with shortness of breath at rest and minimal exertion, he is eligible for hospice admission (choice D). While an ejection fraction of 20% is helpful additional evidence of a poor prognosis, it is not a necessary criterion in the face of clinically significant and symptomatic disease (choice A). Likewise, while a recent chest x-ray would provide additional corroborating evidence of advanced heart failure, it is not necessary or required for hospice admission (choice C). The need for maximum vasodilator therapy as a criterion is predicated on the fact that such therapy can be tolerated by the patient, and in this situation, the reason the vasodilator was reduced was because of lack of patient tolerance, a further sign of poor patient prognosis (choice B). As with all patients, the patient's autonomy is paramount, and while the physician is obligated to discuss the option of transplant with the patient, if indicated, if the patient refuses, it is not appropriate for the physician to try to force the patient to accept the procedure (choice E). It should be noted that admission to hospice would not prevent the patient from reconsidering and changing his mind at a later date.

8. Correct answer: B

The description of the patient is consistent with FAST 7 dementia, which includes the inability to ambulate without assistance and the inability to communicate. While the prognosis of patients with FAST 7 dementia without any comorbid illnesses or intercurrent illnesses may be significantly greater than 6 months (choice E), the patient as described in choice B has had two episodes of urosepsis, requiring hospitalization, and the family does not want her hospitalized again. The combination of FAST 7 dementia and the episodes of urosepsis indicate hospice eligibility. Comorbid decubitus ulcers that are associated with a high risk of mortality are stage III or IV (choice C) as is weight loss of at least 10% (choice A). While concurrent illnesses such as heart disease and diabetes can be contributory factors to a poor prognosis, in this situation, the illnesses are well controlled and not contributing to the patient's current clinical condition (choice D).

9. Correct answer: E

Hospice appropriateness is based upon patient prognosis. In ALS, rapidly progressive disease is consistent with a poor prognosis, even in the face of technological support (choice E). Although some hospice programs choose not to admit patients receiving ventilatory support (choice A), or less often, feeding tubes, other hospices are very willing and able to admit such patients. Riluzole is reported to delay the onset of ventilator dependence and extend life expectancy by only 2 months in selected patients, so its use does not change the patient's overall prognosis, and therefore, it is not necessary for the medication to be discontinued (choice B). Given the rapid progression of the patient's disease, whether or not he requires a wheelchair or is bedbound is also not relevant to hospice eligibility (choice D).

10. Correct answer: E

This patient, who appears competent and intact, refuses to be evaluated, but he clinically appears to have a life-limiting illness that is consistent with hospice eligibility, possibly either advanced cancer or advanced COPD, or, perhaps, both. As he is refusing workup or treatment, his diagnosis cannot be determined. Therefore, the diagnosis of "Debility, unspecified" or "Adult failure to thrive"

would be an appropriate option for a terminal diagnosis (choice E). Although the established criteria include a documented BMI of less than 22, in this situation, where there are well-documented signs of cachexia and significant loss of lean body mass, the patient's description, accompanied by his refusal to be weighed, should be sufficient to justify the use of the diagnosis (choice D). One cannot compel a patient to have diagnostic studies (choice A), and while a trial of antidepressants might be appropriate, as his symptoms are not likely secondary to a correctable depression, this should not be an obstacle to hospice referral either (choice B). Finally, hospice eligibility is prognosis driven (a prognosis of 6 months or less), not diagnosis driven (choice C). Diagnoses such as "Debility, unspecified" and "Adult failure to thrive" are indicated in precisely this circumstance, when a definitive terminal diagnosis is not apparent and the patient appears to have a prognosis of 6 months or less.

Chapter 2

1. Correct answer: C

Dame Cicely Saunders was a physician, a nurse, and a social worker. Although she may have had considerable experience in spiritual counseling as well, she never formally qualified as a chaplain.

2. Correct answer: D

When patients elect the MHB, they in effect exchange their standard Part A and Part B (if covered) Medicare Benefits for services under the MHB, with the exception of services for diagnoses unrelated to the terminal illness and attending physician services (choice D). To be eligible for the MHB, patients must be terminally ill, defined as a life expectancy of 6 months or less if the illness runs its normal course (choice A), and the prognosis must be certified by the Hospice Medical Director and the patient's attending physician (choice B). The benefit is divided into two 90-day periods and an unlimited number of 60-day periods, and patients can remain under the care of the hospice as long as the patient continues to have a prognosis of 6 months or less (choice D).

3. Correct answer: A

In view of the special role of the patient's attending physician, and to encourage continued attending physician involvement with the patient, reimbursement for attending physician services provided to the hospice patient are directly reimbursed to the physician under Medicare Part B (choice A). Professional services provided by hospice physicians (choice B) or consultants (choice C), although not part of the per diem hospice payment, are covered by the MHB under Medicare Part A. While chemotherapy drugs are not commonly provided by hospices due to lack of efficacy, all drugs and biologicals that are necessary for the palliation of symptoms related to the terminal illness are covered. Therefore, when a chemotherapeutic agent is being provided as part of the hospice plan care to palliate symptoms in a patient with a terminal cancer diagnosis, it is covered under the MHB (choice D). Finally, bereavement services for up to 1 year following patient death is an integral part of the MHB (choice E).

4. Correct answer: C

Both general inpatient care and continuous home care are higher levels of hospice care that have specific indications based primarily on an increase in the acute symptom management needs of the patient, which cannot be managed effectively under routine home care. Among these is uncontrolled pain that requires frequent dose adjustments and constant monitoring to achieve better control (choice C). Milder increases of pain that are amenable to less frequent adjustments in analgesia can generally be managed at a routine home care level of care (choice B). Respite inpatient care is the level of care that is most appropriate when a primary caregiver needs relief or needs to attend to their personal needs (choice A). Custodial patient needs are generally not covered beyond routine home care under the MHB, so if a patient is awaiting nursing home placement and does not have any acute medical symptoms, general inpatient care or continuous home care would not be indicated (choice D).

5. Correct answer: B

Much like the MHB, skilled care in a LTCF is a Part A Medicare benefit, and, as such, they are mutually exclusive. Therefore, as hospices are responsible for all Part A services related to a patient's terminal illness, patients cannot access both the MHB and skilled care for the same diagnosis at the same time (choice B). When a patient is a resident in a LTCF, it is considered their home and the care provided by the hospice is the same as routine home care (choice A). Room and board is not part of the MHB, so it is either paid for by the family, Medicaid (actually paid to the hospice as part of the unified rate and then "passed through" to the LTCF), or private insurance (choice C). By statute, the hospice provider is primarily responsible for the professional management of the patient living in a LTCF (choice E). To ensure that care is consistent with a palliative plan of care, the hospice and the LTCF together develop a "coordinated plan of care" to ensure that patients are properly served by both providers (choice D).

6. Correct answer: A

The hospice industry has grown significantly, with the number of patients being cared for annually more than doubling from the greater than 500,000 terminally ill patients served in 1997 to upward of 1.3 million served in 2006 (choice A). Well-documented barriers to hospice referral and hospice access include reluctance by physicians to both comfortably predict that a patient has 6 months or less to live (choice B) and to communicate this information to patients and families (choice C). The increasing availability of new and more aggressive treatment options often force patients to choose between trials of disease-modifying therapy and hospice services (choice D). Because many patients still seek hospital care at their local facility, a lack of inpatient relationships between hospices and hospitals often delays or prevents patients from receiving hospice care during or after hospitalization (choice E).

7. Correct answer: D

Nonhospice palliative care programs, much like their hospice counterparts, provide care through a team of professionals, which, at minimum generally include physicians, nurses, and social workers (choice D). Hospice care under the MHB is generally limited to patients with a prognosis of 6 months or less, while palliative care programs have the option of providing care to patients with life expectancies well beyond 6 months (choice A). Hospice care is funded primarily through the MHB, whereas there is no direct benefit defined for palliative care (choice B). Patients receiving care from a hospice must give informed consent, whereas no such consent is required to receive nonhospice palliative care services (choice C). Finally, although the MHB defines a standard array of services hospices must provide, nonhospice palliative care programs are free to determine what services they will or will not provide to the patients they care for (choice E).

8. Correct answer: B

Not only do hospital-based palliative care programs provide consultative services on medical and surgical wards, they also provide services in the ICU and other critical care areas (choice B). In fact, the ability to reduce ICU days and transition appropriate patients from critical care to palliative care is one of the major factors that are responsible for the decrease in the cost of an average inpatient day (choice A). Published studies have demonstrated that in-

patient palliative care services have improved the management of pain, dyspnea, and other common symptoms experienced by hospitalized patients with advanced life-limiting illnesses (choice C). Additional cost savings to the hospital comes from a reduction in the use of unnecessary, and often expensive, futile medical interventions (choice E). With the lack of defined reimbursement for palliative care, independent palliative care units have tended to run at a financial loss. However, the net effect on hospitals' bottom-lines appears to be positive (choice D).

9. Correct answer: C

In this study, the median time that "bridge" patients were cared for was more than twice as long (52 vs. 20 days), than those receiving traditional hospice care (choice C). However, only twice the percentage of patients (13% vs. 6%) received care for at least 6 months (choice A). In fact, the study did not examine why patients who chose the "bridge" program made the choice they did (choice D), so it is not known whether the desire to receive chemotherapy was the main reason why patients opted for the bridge program. In addition, as the study did not provide data on how many patients "crossed the bridge" to the hospice program prior to death, it is not known what percentage of patients made the transition from prehospice to hospice prior to death (choice C).

10. Correct answer: D

Attending physicians generally want to remain involved with their patients and vice versa. Therefore, the requirement by a hospice or palliative care program that their physician take over care for the attending physician would not be an important feature when looking for the best end-of-life care provider (choice D). The best end-of-life care providers are those that have evidence-based guidelines in pain and symptom management, and the outcomes data to prove it (choice A). They provide care through an interdisciplinary team of professionals trained in end-of-life care (choice B). They can manage patients wherever they need to be, whether in their own homes, LTCF facilities, or when necessary, in an inpatient setting (choice C). They also provide counseling services to family members during their loved one's illness and in the bereavement period that follows the patient's death (choice E).

Chapter 3

1. Correct answer: D

Two review articles published in 2007 (Parker et al. and Barclay et al.), examined multiple published studies on communication preferences. One of the findings was that although patients and caregivers wanted to be informed, they wanted that information presented in as positive manner as possible, and not necessarily in a frank and open way (choice D). These reviews documented that studies have shown that patients and caregivers want significant information about the illness (choice A), that their needs for information diverge over time (choice B), and that patients often do not tell their clinicians that they want to be told what is going on (choice C). Patient preferences regarding family involvement was found to vary considerably in the studies reviewed, with some showing the desire for family presence when bad news is being conveyed, some suggesting patients wanted to hear the news for themselves, and some documenting that patients did not want to hear bad news at all, but would rather have their family members be told, and they, in turn, would tell the patient whatever they thought appropriate (choice E).

2. Correct answer: C

Unfortunately, physicians are generally poorly trained to communicate bad news to patients and families (choice C), although with an increase in the available educational materials

to train practicing physicians, medical students, and residents, this is gradually changing. Physicians often do not have the time it takes to discuss bad news adequately (choice A), due to pressures in either clinic or managed care practice settings to see as many patients as possible during the day. As the messenger, physicians are often inappropriately blamed for causing the bad news that they deliver (choice B), which can be very disconcerting to one trained to help others. Furthermore, if a patient has a progressive illness despite the physician's best efforts, the physician will often experience a sense of inadequacy at having "failed" the patient (choice D). Finally, discussing bad news can often evoke significant emotions in physicians as well as in patients and families, and physicians are often very uncomfortable at having to deal with these emotions (choice E).

3. Correct answer: A

Dr. X neglected to first ask the patient whether she had any family members (choice A) that she would like to have with her when the physician gave her the news about her tests. If she did want family members present, it would have been appropriate for Dr. X to set a time later in the day to return and have the conversation when all concerned would be present. He arranged for privacy (choice B) by closing the curtain around the patient, put the patient at ease by sitting in a chair at the head of the bed to be at Mrs. Y's eye level (choice C), and held her hand (choice D) by pretending to be taking her pulse. He also did open the conversation by asking the patient her perception of the situation (choice E), which would allow him to know what the patient had been thinking or anticipating about what he had to tell her.

4. Correct answer: B

Using medical jargon and technical language to impress the patient and family will not only not give them confidence, it will likely make them more confused and frightened (choice B). Rather, medical jargon and technical terms should be avoided, in favor of terms that the patient and family can understand. When imparting knowledge, it is important to speak slowly and clearly (choice A) and to summarize and repeat information (choice D) to ensure that patients and families understand what you are saying. One should avoid giving too much information (choice C) at once to not "overload" the patient and family, reducing the chances that they are absorbing what you are telling them. One must also listen to the patient's responses (choice E) to help verify that the patient comprehends the information.

5. Correct answer: A

Telling a patient that there are no treatment options (choice A) is not only inappropriate, it is cruel and can only serve to take away hope. Furthermore, hospice as an agency provides treatment in the form of symptom-directed care, so even a hospice referral should be considered a form of treatment, rather than what you do when there is no treatment available. Setting another appointment to allow patients to ask questions (choice B) is extremely important, as patients and families often do not absorb everything they have been told, even if they think they did during the visit. Disease-directed treatment options, such as chemotherapy (choice C), are certainly part of the discussion, as are treatments focused on control of symptoms and quality of life (choice D). It is also important to make sure that patients have appropriate support at home, so confirming that the patient's daughter will be coming to take care of the patient (choice E) is very appropriate to include in the summation.

6. Correct answer: E

If a patient does not speak or understand English, a family member should NOT be used as an interpreter (choice E), as it is possible that the family member will intentionally or unintentionally filter information that he or she does not think the patient should hear. Rather, a professional interpreter should be sought. Family members can often remember things that were said, because sometimes, the patient will "tune out" once the bad news is revealed (choice A). It is important, therefore, to always ask patients if they want family members present (choice B) and even when they do not, they should be urged to bring at least one person for support (choice C). In a hospital setting, when the family is not present and the patient wants them there, the physician needs to set up a time with the patient and return to hold the discussion when the family will be at the hospital (choice D).

7. Correct answer: C

Medical decision making should NOT be based on making certain that the patient receives every treatment that is available (choice C). Rather, decisions should optimally be based on a combination of factors. Patients should be offered the best treatment options available (choice A) that are compatible with the patient's life trajectory (choice B) and in concert with the patient's wishes (choice D). Furthermore, these decisions should be based on the patient's ability to tolerate the burden of treatment (choice E).

8. Correct answer: B

If a patient has capacity, they should be included in all decisions, to the extent they choose to be involved; having these conversations does not have an adverse effect on patients (choice B). Patients with capacity should have their own stated goals and wishes respected, even if these are not the goals the family would wish for (choice A). The role of the physician in this situation is to advocate for the patient and attempt to align the family with the patient. Physicians have their own goals in these situations (choice C) and must be on guard not to put them forward too forcefully; they are the guides, not the ultimate decision makers. Goals should always be discussed in terms of what is possible and not possible to achieve (choice D). In addition, an appropriate goal is one that is beneficial for the patient (choice E).

9. Correct answer: E

Patients who advocate for themselves and are willing to confront their physicians to express their needs and wants are able to participate in effective conversations to set their own goals (choice E). These conversations do not occur, and goals are not adequately set, because of multiple barriers. Physicians create barriers by avoiding the conversation, protecting them from their own discomforts with the potential discussion (choice A). Patients are often unwilling to question a physician's recommendation if it is not what they really want in order to avoid "upsetting the physician" (choice B). Families often want patients to "fight on" even when the patient knows that he or she is not doing well, impeding the ability to have goal setting conversations (choice C). When multiple physicians are involved in a patient's care, it is often the case that no one is "in charge" and no one physician takes the responsibility of having this conversation (choice D).

10. Correct answer: D

When scheduling a goals-of-care conversation, the physician should encourage the patient to bring as many people as desired for support and to assist in the decision making (choice D). These are emotional discussions, and time should be allowed for expression of these emotions; shutting them off by stopping the conversation and rescheduling the discussion only damages the process (choice A). Although time is not limitless, a rigid time agenda does not allow for adequate decision making (choice B). Not only medical but psy-

chosocial and spiritual concerns need to be discussed (choice C), and the physician should not dominate the conversation by making recommendations that he or she encourages the patient to follow (choice E). Rather, he or she should guide the patient and family along the necessary path that will help them to make appropriate decisions for themselves.

Chapter 4

1. Correct answer: A

The attending physician (choice A) is a physician who is identified by the patient as having the most significant role in the determination of the patient's medical care. The long-term care medical director (choice B) is a physician who is responsible to oversee the medical care provided to all patients residing at all care levels in the facility. The hospice team physician (choice C) is a physician who is either employed or contracted by the hospice and responsible for providing hands-on medical care to patients cared for by the hospice. The managed care medical director (choice D) is a physician employed by a managed care organization who is responsible to oversee the medical care provided to patients on the plan. A palliative medicine consultant (choice E) is a physician who provides palliative medicine consultations to patients, generally at the request of the patient's attending physician.

2. Correct answer: D

The attending physician is NOT responsible to recertify patient prognosis if the patient has been on hospice for 90 days (choice D). The responsibility for recertification falls to the hospice medical director or hospice physician. The attending physician, however, does certify that the patient has a prognosis of 6 months or less at the time of hospice admission (choice C). The attending physician is considered a member of the hospice interdisciplinary team (choice A) and participates in the care of his or her patients to the extent desired. The attending physician usually discusses the need for end-of-life care with patients and families prior to hospice referral (choice B). In recognition of the unique relationship between the attending physician and the patient, Medicare reimburses attending physician visits under Medicare Part B (choice E).

3. Correct answer: E

While LTCF medical directors may initially identify patients who may need end-of-life care and discuss possible hospice referral with the patient and family or attending physician, it would not be appropriate for the hospice medical director to participate in this activity (choice E). It would be very appropriate, however, for the two medical directors to collaborate on a host of issues including the coordination of hospice patient care planning (choice A), education of the respective staff (choice B), development of hospice treatment guidelines that are compatible with the philosophy of the facility (choice C), and conflict resolution between the two organizations (choice D).

4. Correct answer: B

While the new CMS rules regarding hospice admission require that one of the certifying physicians document in a narrative note the reasons why the patient is eligible for hospice services, this note does not have to be written by the hospice medical director (choice B), but may be written by the certifying hospice physician (or the certifying attending physician, although the latter is highly unlikely). Supervising the hospice team physicians (choice A); providing expert consultative advice to attending physicians, hospice physicians, and hospice staff (choice C); participating in the hospice's strategic and business planning (choice D); and being involved in issues related to regu-

latory compliance and surveys (choice E) are all appropriate activities for the hospice medical director.

5. Correct answer: B

The hospice team physician's obligation to provide overall medical care to hospice patients is limited to situations in which a patient's attending physician opts not to continue to follow the patient (choice B). When the attending physician does choose to continue to follow a patient, the hospice physician's role is generally more consultative in nature and focuses primarily on the symptom management needs of the patient. The hospice physician is responsible to certify and recertify that a patient has a terminal prognosis (choice A), to participate in the interdisciplinary team meeting (choice C), to do patient visits at home (choice D), and to provide staff education and support (choice E).

6. Correct answer: D

In the hospice interdisciplinary team, the patient and family are the center of care (choice D). The team manager (choice A), primary nurse (choice B), attending physician (choice C), and hospice medical director (choice E) are all important members of the team, but all function equally with the goal of creating a plan of care that is based on the needs of and directed by the patient and family.

7. Correct answer: A

As LVNs have a limited scope of practice that prohibits them from administering medications or treatments unless supervised by the primary nurse, they cannot function in the role of the primary nurse (choice A). LVNs, however, may provide primary patient care at the bedside (choice E) and, by doing so, allow the RN primary nurse to devote more time to more complex patient needs. RNs may serve in the hospice in the roles of team manager or primary nurse (choice B). The team manager is the primary supervisor of all members of the ID team (choice C). Hospice primary nurses also function in the role of case manager (choice D), interacting with the other members of the ID team as well as the attending physician regarding patient and family needs.

8. Correct answer: C

Although it may be appropriate for a hospice chaplain to help patients ask God for forgiveness when the patient asks for this, it is inappropriate for the chaplain to assume that all patients want such help and, therefore, to provide it to all patients (choice C). Among the responsibilities of social workers is to assist patients in accessing community services (choice A), and because of these resource access responsibilities, chaplains are sometimes called upon to assist social workers in the provision of psychosocial counseling (choice B). Social workers, on the other hand, may assist chaplains in the provision of bereavement support to families after patient death (choice D). Because of the inherent challenges in working with dying patients, social workers and chaplains work together to provide staff support (choice E).

9. Correct answer: E

Because of the intimate nature of the personal care provided by CHHAs, their input at team meeting is at least as valuable as the input of the other members of the ID team, if not more so (choice E). Because of their high level of training, CHHAs may work in a patient's home independent of the supervising RN's presence (choice A) and are equipped to manage the often complicated personal hygiene needs of dying patients (choice B). The intimate nature of the care CHHAs provide often times results in their receiving the greatest thanks from family members (choice C) and in experiencing significant grief when a patient passes on, especially if they cared for the patient for a long time (choice D).

10. Correct answer: B

While as part of federal health care legislation passed in 2003, the definition of attending physician under hospice was modified to include nurse practitioners (NPs), they were prohibited from certifying a patient's prognosis (choice B) or establishing the plan of care, both of which must be done by a physician. NPs may serve as palliative care consultants (choice A), and also as part of specialty practices (for example, wound care) in hospitals and LTCFs, where they may be called upon to provide consultations to hospice or palliative care patients (choice D). Although hospices may employ NPs, they cannot bill for NP services that can either provided by an RN (choice E) or which are being provided in the role of a physician extender under the supervision of the hospice medical director (choice C).

Chapter 5

1. Correct answer: A

Unlike other health care settings where mortality is not a desired outcome, there is an expectation that patients admitted to a hospice program will die. Therefore, the use of mortality rates as a way of evaluating quality of care of an end-of-life provider has virtually no utility (choice A). However, it almost goes without saying that the adequacy of pain control (choice B) is an important measure for end-of-life providers, as pain is often a major symptom for terminally ill patients. Patients at all stages of illness are concerned with how staff communicates with them (choice C), and all providers should be monitored for the frequency of infections that occur while patients are under their care (choice E). Ultimately, all providers, including those caring for patients at the end of life, would want to know that patients, or in the case of end-of-life care providers, family members, would recommend the provider to others who need similar services (choice D).

2. Correct answer: D

Beginning in 1998, the National Hospice Work Group (NHWG) and the National Hospice and Palliative Care (NHPCO) Outcomes Taskforce developed and pilot tested several indicators of quality care at the end of life based on the end-result outcomes identified in *Pathways for Patients and Families Facing Terminal Illness*. Four measures were defined and tested, one of which was entitled "self-determined life closure." This measure evaluated the percentage of patients who had their preferences honored regarding whether or not to receive CPR and whether or not to be hospitalized while under care (choice D). Although an important preference that is included in most living will documents, artificial feeding was not one of the preferences measured by this outcome.

3. Correct answer: C

An often overlooked but essential element of symptom severity measurement in end-of-life care is the issue of the patient's (choice C) self-identified threshold for a specific symptom. Many terminally ill patients want to balance symptom relief against medication side effects that might affect their ability to interact with family or otherwise complete "unfinished business"; others may have cultural or religious reasons for rejecting medication. While professionals such as nurses (choice A), physicians (choice B), and social workers (choice E), and primary care-givers (choice D) may have input into how patients' symptoms should be managed, especially when a patient cannot self-identify an appropriate threshold, the patient should make the determination him- or herself whenever possible.

4. Correct answer: E

Typically, health-related quality-of-life measures are designed to assess the impact of illness or treatment on the patient's role and ability to function. In fact, many health-related quality-of-life instruments are constructed with the underlying assumption that functionality (choice E) and quality of life are directly proportional. Therefore, quality of life near the end of life must focus on other domains, including spiritual (choice A), psychosocial (choice B), and emotional (choice C) well-being, and the control of pain and other symptoms (choice D).

5. Correct answer: B

One of the important elements of any good quality-of-life instrument is that it is self-reported by the patient rather than observer-rated (choice B), allowing for the necessary subjectivity inherent in caring for diverse individuals. The tool should be multidimensional (choice A), evaluating all relevant spheres of personhood, including the physical, emotional, and spiritual. Both negative and positive experiences should be measured (choice C) and the scoring system should be weighted to reflect the different levels of importance patients may place on different domains being assessed (choice D). The instrument should also be easy for the patient to respond to and for staff to score (choice E), as caregivers will hesitate to utilize it if its use is perceived as burdensome.

6. Correct answer: B

Coordination of care (choice B) refers to "the processes, such as regular and parsimonious lines of communication, used to tie each provider and each episode" of care together. Continuity of care (choice A) is defined as a "thread" that connects episodes of care. Components of care (choice C) are the individual aspects of care that are coordinated together to make up an episode of care. Quality of care (choice D) can be defined as "the degree to which health care services for individuals and populations increase the likelihood of desired health outcomes and are consistent with current professional knowledge." Quality-of-life (choice E) measures are designed to assess the impact of illness or treatment on various aspects of the individual patient's role and functioning.

7. Correct answer: E

Patient/family satisfaction surveys require respondents to know what should be expected regarding services provided (choice E). However, as patients and family expectations are relatively uninformed, these surveys tend to have high scores even when the healthcare experience was less than optimal (choice B). "Patient-centered" reports allow the provider to measure how often preset standards of care are met (choice A). These reports are believed to be more accurate indicators of quality of care than patient/family satisfaction surveys (choice C). "Patient-centered" reports also allow the provider to assess the quality of a service without asking the patient/family to make a judgment about the quality of care (choice D).

8. Correct answer: B

Life review, the telling of "one's stories," and the transmission of knowledge and wisdom are tasks that provide one with a "sense of meaning about one's individual life" (choice B). Self-acknowledgment and self-forgiveness are tasks that allow one to "experience love of self" (choice A), while acceptance of dependency and decathexis are among the tasks that are associated with the "acceptance of the finality of life" (choice C). The sense of meaning about life in general is accomplished in part by achieving a sense of awe and a sense of comfort with chaos (choice D). Reconciliation, expressions of forgiveness, and leave taking are part of the work required to achieve a "sense of completion in relationships with family and friends" (choice E).

9. Correct answer: C

The MVQOLI was designed to be administered in course of routine patient visits (choice C). It is based on Byock's theoretical frame-

work of lifelong growth and development (choice E) and measures five dimensions of quality of life: symptoms, function, interpersonal relationships, emotional well-being, and transcendence (choice A). It includes a scoring protocol that "weights" each dimensional score by its importance (choice B), and may be used to inform priorities and interventions during care planning (choice D).

Chapter 6

1. Correct answer: D

Among the barriers to adequate pain management is the challenge that clinicians have in properly assessing pain (choice D). This is due to several factors including a decrease in clinical skills due to the increased reliance on technology and a lack of time to perform the comprehensive assessment required. Reluctance to report pain (choice A) is primarily a patient-related barrier, whereas a lack of knowledge regarding pain management (choice B), the fear of addiction (choice C), and the fear of premature death from opioids (choice E) are actually barriers to both patients and the clinicians who treat them.

2. Correct answer: C

The patient's description of the pain as an electric shock–like sensation coming and going in waves is most typical of neuropathic pain. Given the location and his diagnosis, the pain is most likely secondary to brachial plexopathy due to his primary lung cancer (choice C). While pain of coronary insufficiency can occur in the left arm, as a form of visceral nociceptive pain, the description is typically of a pressure-like sensation (choice A). Likewise, bone metastases in the area, as a somatic nociceptive pain, would tend to be of sharper nature (choice B). The visceral nociceptive pain of pleural disease would tend to be in the back and radiating up the shoulder rather than in the clavicle and arm (choice D). Although pain due to brain metastases is neuropathic in nature, it would be unusual to present in as localized a fashion as described (choice E).

3. Correct answer: E

Involving the patient directly in care is critical to achieving good outcomes. Therefore, although one must inform a patient about the medication he or she is to take, it is better to do so by asking whether the proposed medication makes sense and seeking the patient's agreement to take the medication, rather than just telling the patient what to do (choice E). Taking a thorough medication history including OTC medications is important to avoid such problems as acetaminophen toxicity and other potential drug–drug interactions with the medications you might be planning to prescribe (choice A). The importance of a psychosocial and spiritual history cannot be underscored enough, as the patient's perception of pain may be significantly influenced by unresolved issues in either of these areas (choice B). The history of the primary illness will help put the pain in the context of the disease process (choice C), whereas the physical examination can provide important clues as to the nature of the pain (choice D).

4. Correct answer: D

The dose-limiting property of an acetaminophen/oxycodone combination is the potential for acetaminophen toxicity with doses above 3 to 4 g/d, limiting the dosing of this combination to no more than two tablets every 4 hours (choice D). Acetaminophen does not have a ceiling effect regarding its analgesic properties (choice C). Oxycodone is an opioid that also does not have a ceiling effect (choice A), and at the doses given in the combination the risk of opioid toxicity is minimal (choice B). The combination opioid/nonopioid medications are under less regulation by the DEA than are opioids that are prescribed as stand-alone agents (choice E).

5. Correct answer: A

Mu receptors (choice A) are found at the spinal and supraspinal levels and peripherally in skin, joints, and gastrointestinal tract. Activation of the *mu* receptor produces analgesia as well as dysphoria, euphoria, respiratory depression, sedation, constipation, urinary retention, and drug dependence. Responses to activation of the *kappa* receptor (choice B) include spinal analgesia as well as sedation, dysphoria, and miosis. Although activation of the *delta* receptor (choice C) also produces analgesia, it does not appear to be clinically relevant. The *sigma* receptor (choice D), which may or may not actually be a true opioid receptor, is associated with undesirable psychotomimetic effects such as dysphoria, hallucinations, and confusion that are often seen with mixed agonist–antagonist analgesics.

6. Correct answer: B

Although morphine may be administered in a nebulized form via inhalation, this is used for the treatment of dyspnea and due to poor systemic absorption (16% bioavailability), this route of administration is not effective for the treatment of pain (choice B). All the other listed routes of administration: oral (choice A), subcutaneous (choice C), intravenous (choice D), and epidural (choice E), may be used in appropriate circumstances to achieve analgesia.

7. Correct answer: E

Morphine to methadone conversion ratios vary on the basis of the total OME a patient is taking in a 24-hour period. For the patient under discussion whose OME exceeds 1,000 mg/d, a ratio of 20:1 is appropriate (choice E). A ratio of 3:1 applies to an OME of < 100 mg/d (choice A), 5:1 applies to an OME of 101 to 300 mg/d (choice B), 10:1 to an OME of 301 to 600 mg/d (choice C), and 15:1 to an OME of 801 to 1,000 mg/d (choice D).

8. Correct answer: B

Tricyclic antidepressants (choice B) are believed to be particularly effective for dysesthetic neuropathy in which patients complain of burning, cold, or vise-like sensations. Steroids (choice A) are effective in treating neuropathic symptoms accompanied by inflammation and edema. Anticonvulsants (choice C) may be more valuable in treating episodic neuropathic pain that is lancinating or burning in nature. Local anesthetics (choice D) have shown some efficacy in the treatment of phantom pain and pain associated with diabetic neuropathy, PHN, and spinal cord injury. NMDA receptor antagonists (choice E) may be useful to treat PHN pain as well as other neuropathic conditions including postlaminectomy radicular pain.

9. Correct answer: B

The recommended dose of immediate-release opioid for breakthrough or incident pain is calculated at approximately 10% of the 24-hour total opioid dose given every 1 to 2 hours PRN. The above patient is receiving 100 mg every 12 hours, so the total 24-hour dose of opioid is 200 mg, and the correct dose for incident or breakthrough pain should be 20 mg every 1 to 2 hours as needed (choice B). A dose of 10 mg every 1 to 2 hours is adequate. Both doses of oxycodone/acetaminophen (choices C and D) provide a less than adequate amount of oxycodone (5 mg per tablet) and are not prescribed in an adequate frequency (every 4 hours as opposed to every 1–2 hours). Sustained-release oxycodone exhibits a biphasic absorption pattern, which suggests that there is an initial immediate-release of oxycodone from the tablet followed by a prolonged phase of release. However, this will only occur when the sustained-release tablet is taken, and therefore, patients still require an immediate-release medication to address incident or breakthrough pain (choice E).

10. Correct answer: C

When pain is poorly controlled, some patients, such as the one above, will resort to behaviors typically attributed to drug addicts. As the patient is behaving this way, not because of a need for mood-altering substances but for a legitimate medical reason, uncontrolled pain, this syndrome is known as pseudoaddiction (choice C). Tolerance (choice A) occurs when a patient requires an increase in opioid dose without evidence of a progressive pain stimulus due to less effectiveness of the dose of opioid that had been previously controlling the pain. Addiction (choice B) is the seeking of drugs for the purposes altering mood rather than for the treatment of pain or other legitimate medical indications. Opioid withdrawal (choice D) is the gradual decrease in opioid dose based on a decrease in the painful stimulus for which the medication was prescribed. Physical dependence (choice E) is the universal, unavoidable altered physiologic adaptation to opioid use that requires continuation of the medication in order to avoid a withdrawal reaction.

Chapter 7

1. Correct answer: C

For patients on chronic morphine who develop shortness of breath, a dosage increase of at least 25% to 50% is required in order to affect the respiratory center and reduce the breathlessness (choice C). An increase of only 10% is likely to have no significant effect on the shortness of breath (choice A), and any decrease in morphine (choices B and D) will not only not help the dyspnea, but will also likely exacerbate the patients' pain. Although morphine can occasionally cause bronchospasm due to histamine release, this usually occurs early in the course of utilizing the agent, and this patient has been on the medication chronically (choice E).

2. Correct answer: B

The timing of dyspnea may often be a clue to its etiology. When dyspnea occurs suddenly in the terminally ill, one of the causes that must be considered is pulmonary embolus (choice B). Anemia (choice A), progression of the patient's cancer (choice C), accumulation of pleural fluid (choice D), and progressive ascites (choice E) generally develop gradually, usually over several days or more.

3. Correct answer: D

Patients who are opioid naïve are sensitive to the respiratory depressant effects of morphine. Therefore, it is recommended that opioid naïve patients receive low doses of morphine, typically 2.5 to 5 mg and not 20 mg, as the starting dose (choice D). Patients who are on chronic opioids for pain management require a 25% to 50% dosage increase in order for the medication to impact dyspnea, as tolerance to respiratory depression develops with chronic opioid utilization (choice E). Morphine works by decreasing the sensitivity of the medullary respiratory center to carbon dioxide (choice A) and by reducing the carotid body's response to hypoxia (choice B). Prior to the development of diuretics, morphine was actually a treatment of choice for the management of acute pulmonary edema (choice C).

4. Correct answer: E

Nebulized morphine has been known to cause bronchospasm secondary to histamine release in the airways. Therefore, professional observation during administration of the first dose is appropriate (choice E). The starting dose of nebulized morphine is 2.5 to 10 mg (choice A), generally repeated every 4 hours as needed (choice B). Approximately one-half of studies suggest that nebulized morphine may be effective in relieving breathlessness, while the other half showed no difference between morphine and placebo (choice C). Only 16% to 19% of inhaled morphine is absorbed systemically (choice D).

5. Correct answer: A

Methylxanthines cause significant cardiac side effects and have a narrow toxic:therapeutic ratio and with the availability of safer drugs, they have fallen out of favor (choice A). Levalbuterol is not the preferred inhaled bronchodilator in end-of-life care as it has no specific benefits in this setting and it is not cost-effective when compared with albuterol (choice B). Patients with malignant pulmonary disease may benefit from inhaled short-acting bronchodilators when experiencing bronchospasm (choice C). Oral β-adrenergic agents can cause significant undesirable side effects such as anxiety, restlessness, tachycardia, insomnia, and tremors, which may adversely affect the quality of life of the patient (choice D). Inhaled ipratropium and albuterol may be used in combination, and a commercial combination inhaler is available (choice E).

6. Correct answer: C

All the choices actually are potential environmental changes that could potentially impact the patient's shortness of breath in a positive way. However, based on the information given, the only reasonable choice would be to bring in a small fan to better circulate the air (choice C). The pets (choice A), the carpet (choice B), and the goose-down pillow (choice E) have certainly been with her during a good part of her recent illness, and it is highly unlikely that she would consent to the removal of any of them, especially now that she is terminally ill. Although a quieter environment is often helpful to improve breathlessness, the patient's favorite music may itself be therapeutic. Stopping it could, in the end, have a negative effect (choice D), therefore it would also not be a reasonable option in this situation.

7. Correct answer: C

Oxygen therapy provides a psychological benefit to patients and families as it is associated with active (though not resuscitative) treatment, thus aiding in patient and family comfort (choice C). Correction of hypoxia has *not* been found to correlate with the degree of symptomatic benefit the patient experiences with oxygen therapy (choice A). It is airflow through the nasal cannula, and not improved oxygen saturation, that affects the respiratory center and reduces the sensation of breathlessness (choice D). Pulse oximetry is not required in order to provide oxygen therapy to patients on a hospice program (choice B).

8. Correct answer: B

Positioning can improve the patient's ability to cough up secretions, with optimal position for most patients being upright whenever possible (choice B). If the patient's cough were due to a left-sided effusion, then lying on his left side would be the position best suited to help control his cough (choice A). Although chest pounding can help mobilize secretions, this technique should be avoided in terminally ill patients due to the risk of possible pathologic fracture secondary to metastases or osteoporosis (choice C). When secretions are a problem, the air needs to be humidified, not dried, to help loosen and mobilize secretions (choice D).

9. Correct answer: A

Massive hemoptysis, a rare condition occurring in approximately 1% to 4% of all patients presenting with hemoptysis, is more frequently found with primary endobronchial tumors invading into a bronchial artery (choice A). Although mild to moderate hemoptysis may occur in patients with lung metastases, massive hemoptysis is rare in lung metastases because metastatic lesions remain intrapulmonary (choice B). Chronic obstructive pulmonary disease (choice C), pulmonary edema (choice D), and pulmonary embolus (choice E) are also generally associated with mild to moderate, but not massive, hemoptysis.

10. Correct answer: D

Suctioning has been noted to be ineffective and unnecessarily invasive, and should be avoided in the dying patient (choice D). Transdermal scopolamine (choice A), atropine eye drops (choice B), and sublingual hyoscyamine (choice C) have all been utilized to successfully palliate "death rattle" in terminally ill patients. Patients who receive artificial hydration or nutrition before death experience more excessive secretions than patients who are slightly dehydrated, providing them with a more comfortable, natural death. Therefore, it may be reasonable to attempt to reduce secretions by reducing the amount the patient is being fed, or discontinuing the feedings altogether in order to reduce the secretions that can result in the "death rattle" (choice E).

Chapter 8

1. Correct answer: C

The chemoreceptor trigger zone (CTZ) (choice C), located near the fourth ventricle, when exposed to various medications including opioids and chemotherapeutic agents stimulates the VC to cause nausea and vomiting. The cerebral cortex (choice A) is affected by noxious inputs from senses of taste, smell, sight, or on occasion, hearing. The vestibular apparatus (choice B) may be affected by motion, pre-existing vertigo, or advanced cerebrovascular disease with vertebrobasilar insufficiency. Vagal and sympathetic afferent nerve stimulation (choice D) may result from constipation, gastric outlet obstruction, gastroparesis, or bowel obstruction.

2. Correct answer: D

When patients have symptoms of nausea and/or vomiting, strong perfumes and after-shave lotions should be avoided (choice D). Acupressure (choice A) is a noninvasive technique that is used to treat motion sickness and has had positive effects in some patients with nausea and vomiting secondary to chemotherapy and radiation. If a patient is on emetogenic medication and it can be discontinued (choice B), it is a good idea to do so. Deep breathing and voluntary swallowing (choice C) as well as the application of cold compresses to the forehead, neck, and wrists (choice E) are other nonpharmacological methods of helping control nausea and emesis.

3. Correct answer: A

Although some in end-of-life care utilize ABHR (or a related compounded product) in gel, capsule, or suppository form as initial therapy, it is not recommended (choice A). It should only be utilized after at least two standard anti-emetic medications have been ineffective in controlling a patient's symptoms. Being a combination of four medications, its use as primary therapy would potentially expose the patient to unnecessary medication toxicity when a single medication, which would have less potential for side effects, might be just as effective. Prochlorperazine (choice B) is often used as first-line therapy and acts both at the CTZ and VC. Haloperidol (choice C), one of the components of ABHR, is sometimes used as a second-line agent and works via the cerebral cortex and CTZ. Lorazepam (choice D), another component of ABHR, primarily works at the level of the cerebral cortex. Dexamethasone (choice E) works at the level of the cerebral cortex and GI tract to reduce nausea and emesis related to increased intracranial pressure and bowel wall edema.

4. Correct answer: B

High-fiber diets (choice B) promote bowel movements due to increased bulk and fluid retention in the bowel, while low-fiber diets tend to produce constipation because of the lack of bulk and an increase in fluid reabsorption. Opioid analgesics (choice A) cause constipation by a number of mechanisms including suppression of forward peristalsis in the intestines, an increase in intestinal fluid absorption, and a reduction in intestinal se-

cretions. Spinal cord compression (choice C) may cause constipation due to lack of peristalsis leading to fecal impaction despite loss of sphincter control. Dehydration due to poor oral intake (choice D) will reduce the amount of fluid presented to the colon and also cause reabsorption of whatever fluid is presented to the colon. Hypercalcemia (choice E) causes constipation due to a combination of decreased peristalsis and dehydration.

5. Correct answer: B

When starting a patient on therapy to prevent constipation secondary to opioids, the combination of senna/docusate sodium (choice B) or a similar stool softener/laxative combination should be used. Some initially will use a stool softener alone, but there is a risk that without the laxative, the stool will not be able to be evacuated. Likewise, the laxative alone will not be effective if the patient has hard stool already present. Bisacodyl (choice C) is a laxative that is best used second line if a patient has not responded to the senna/docusate combination. Lactulose (choice D) is a hyperosmotic agent that should be used second or third line as well. Fleet enemas (choice E) should only be used if the oral agents discussed earlier do not produce the desired outcome. Methylnaltrexone (choice A) is an opioid antagonist that works peripherally and has been shown to be effective in the treatment of opioid-induced constipation. However, studies on this agent have primarily been done on patients refractory to standard therapy and its role has yet to be defined. Therefore, at present, its use should be confined to patients refractory to standard therapy.

6. Correct answer: C

Nausea and vomiting (choice C), which is primarily a central nervous system-mediated side effect of morphine, and a side effect to which patients develop tolerance, is not directly associated with opioid-induced bowel dysfunction. Symptoms that are associated with opioid-induced bowel dysfunction, include constipation (choice A), esophageal reflux (choice B) secondary to delayed gastric emptying (choice D), and abdominal cramps (choice E). Patients do not develop tolerance to symptoms of opioid-induced bowel dysfunction.

7. Correct answer: C

Aluminum-containing antacids are associated with constipation (choice C), while magnesium-containing antacids are associated with diarrhea. Overuse of laxatives (choice A) may be the most frequent cause of diarrhea in patients near the end of life. Fecal impaction (choice B) can present with diarrhea due to soft stool passing around the impaction. Antibiotics (choice D) can cause diarrhea due to changes in the flora or due to the development of pseudomembranous colitis. Radiation therapy (choice E) may cause diarrhea due to damage to the intestinal mucosa that leads to increased bowel motility and malabsorption of bile salts.

8. Correct answer: D

Rather than keeping the chin elevated and away from the chest (choice D), the chin should be kept down and toward the chest during swallowing, as this will close off the airway and decrease pressure in the throat. Providing good oral hygiene (choice E), providing food of the type and consistency the patient can swallow (choice B), and serving small meals at room temperature (choice A) are all designed to make the process of eating and swallowing easier for the patient. Keeping the head of the bed elevated both during eating and for up to 2 hours after eating (choice B) will allow gravity to assist in moving food down the esophagus and reduce aspiration risk.

9. Correct answer: B

Alcohol (choice B) causes dyspepsia by directly irritating the esophagus, rather than by reducing LES tone. The NSAIDs (choice

A), benzodiazepines (choice C), and calcium-channel blockers (choice E) all may contribute to dyspepsia by reducing LES tone, and should be discontinued, if possible, in patients with this symptom. Coffee (choice D) may also reduce LES tone and should be avoided when possible.

10. Correct answer: A

Dexamethasone (choice A), by reducing bowel wall edema, may help relieve bowel obstruction caused by tumor or adhesions. Metoclopramide (choice B), which may be helpful in treating abdominal pain due to delayed gastric emptying, may have the opposite effect if there is gastric outlet obstruction. Stool softeners may be helpful as they may allow stool to pass more freely through narrowed bowel lumen; however, stimulant laxatives such as bisacodyl (choice C) should be avoided as they may worsen the intestinal colic that accompanies bowel obstruction. Antidiarrheal agents such as loperamide (choice E), should be avoided as well, as they may make it more difficult for stool to pass through the obstructed area. Omeprazole (choice D) is a proton-pump inhibitor useful in the treatment of abdominal pain secondary to dyspepsia.

Chapter 9

1. Correct answer: C

One of the characteristics of dementia is that memory impairment exists irrespective of whether or not the patient is experiencing delirium. If the only time the patient experiences significant cognitive impairment is when delirium is present, then dementia is not the correct diagnosis (choice C). Dementia is characterized by memory impairment that includes the inability to learn new information (choice B) and/or the inability to recall previously learned information (choice D). It is also characterized by at least one additional cognitive defect that may include, among others, apraxia or aphasia (choice A). Cognitive defects associated with dementia also represent a significant decline from a patient's previous functional levels (choice E).

2. Correct answer: D

The inability to ambulate without assistance is a key characteristic of Stage 7 Alzheimer's dementia (choice D), and a key criteria that is used to determine hospice eligibility, as discussed in detail in Chapter 1. Inability to put on clothing without assistance (choice A), inability to bathe properly (choice B), urinary and/or fecal incontinence (choice C), and inability to handle the mechanics of toileting (choice E) all occur during Stage 6 dementia. Although they may be present in patients with Stage 7 disease as well, and while these functional deficits are challenging from a patient care perspective, in the absence of Stage 7 criteria as well as additional comorbid conditions and intercurrent illnesses as discussed in Chapter 1, they are generally not indicative of a terminal prognosis.

3. Correct answer: A

On the basis of the information provided, the patient, prior to his sudden change in status, has Stage 6D dementia. The sudden progression in his cognitive and functional impairment to Stage 7C would suggest the possibility that his condition may be reversible. Therefore, even though the patient has an advance directive stating that he does not want CPR or a feeding tube, the patient should not be referred to a hospice program (choice A) until it is clear that his change in condition is permanent. Common causes of reversible progression of dementia would include occult sepsis, so even in the absence of fever, cultures should be obtained and empirical antibiotics started (choice B) since in the elderly, febrile response may be blunted or delayed. All his medications should be reviewed (choice C), and agents such as hypnotics, sedatives, or an-

ticholinergic drugs that may be responsible for the change should be discontinued if possible. In order to rule out any metabolic abnormalities, serum electrolytes and a chemistry profile should be obtained (choice D). Finally, since he is now not able to eat, parenteral fluids should be provided (choice E) both to treat possible dehydration, which may be contributing to his acute change in mental status, as well as to maintain his hydration status while determining whether the change is or is not reversible.

4. Correct answer: B

Cholinesterase inhibitors have been shown to improve cognition in patients with mild to moderate Alzheimer's disease; however, they are not effective in the treatment of patients with severe dementia (choice B). Patients treated with one of these agents generally show improvement that lasts for at least 1 year (choice D), although therapy does not change the overall prognosis (choice A). Because the cholinesterase inhibitors are ineffective in patients with severe dementia, it is recommended that therapy be discontinued in institutionalized patients (choice C). Of the available agents, tacrine is generally avoided because of severe hepatoxicity (choice E).

5. Correct answer: B

Although the combination of memantine and donepezil was shown to improve cognitive impairment in patients with severe Alzheimer's disease, these patients were required to be "ambulatory or ambulatory aided" (Tariot et al., 2004) and, therefore, would not be eligible for care under the Medicare Hospice Benefit based on their stage of dementia (choice B). In a 1997 study (Sano et al.), both vitamin E (choice A) and selegiline (choice D) were shown to delay nursing home placement and death in patients with moderately advanced dementia. However, this study has never been duplicated or confirmed. Ginkgo biloba, which modestly improves cognitive function without any benefit in global functioning, increases the risk of bleeding in patients taking vitamin E and/or aspirin (choice C). Finally, regarding the cholinesterase inhibitors, there is no compelling evidence that patients may develop irreversible setbacks if these agents are discontinued and then resumed (choice E).

6. Correct answer: C

When patients with a seizure history are near the end of life and can no longer swallow, antiseizure medications should not be discontinued (choice C), but should be administered by an alternative route, in order to avoid patient and family distress if seizure activity occurs due to lack of the medication. Seizures occur as a complication in approximately 20% of patients with end-stage Alzheimer's disease (choice A) and may also be precipitated by medications including tricyclic antidepressants and phenothiazines, which are commonly used in treating end-of-life care patients (choice E). Parenteral benzodiazepines, such as lorazepam, are generally used to terminate acute seizures (choice B) and intravenous lorazepam will effectively suppress status epilepticus approximately 65% of the time (choice D).

7. Correct answer: C

Rather than suppression of NMDA receptors, the altered processing of neuronal impulses by central spinal cord neurons results in the activation of NMDA receptors (choice C), which is why methadone, which has NMDA receptor antagonist properties, is effective in the treatment of neuropathic pain. All the other choices reflect additional pathophysiological mechanisms that are believed to contribute to causing neuropathic pain.

8. Correct answer: D

Lower lumbosacral plexopathy (choice D) is characterized by pain in the buttocks, perineum, and posterolateral leg and thigh. Up-

per lumbosacral plexopathy (choice C), on the other hand, affects the low back, flank, iliac crest, or anterior thigh. Femoral entrapment neuropathy (choice A) primarily causes pain and weakness in the anteromedial thigh. Iliolingual neuropathy (choice B) causes symptoms in the inguinal region and scrotum, while obturator neuropathy (choice E) causes pain in the inguinal region and anteromedial thigh down to the knee.

9. Correct answer: A

Even though it is thought to be of central nervous system origin, phantom pain syndrome typically responds best to tricyclic antidepressants, such as nortriptyline (choice A). Dexamethasone (choice B) is a steroid, effective in the treatment of many forms of neuropathic pain that are caused by compression of nervous system structures secondary to edema. Gabapentin (choice C) is an anti-seizure medication that has become a drug of choice in the treatment of neuropathic pain for patients near the end of life. Clonidine (choice D) is an α-adrenergic agonist primarily used to treat hypertension that has efficacy in some patients with neuropathic pain. Mexiletine (choice E) is an oral antiarrhythmic agent used in the treatment of certain types of neuropathic pain.

10. Correct answer: B

Autonomic polyneuropathies (choice B) are associated with symptoms of orthostatic hypotension, cardiac arrhythmia, impotence, and/or bladder dysfunction. Diabetic peripheral neuropathy (choice A), chemotherapy-induced peripheral polyneuropathy (choice D), and paraneoplastic sensory neuropathy (choice E) all cause pain and dysesthesias in the hands and feet in the classic "stocking/glove" distribution. Guillan–Barre syndrome (choice C) is an immune-mediated demyelinating polyneuropathy causing rapidly progressive weakness in proximal and distal muscles of the extremities.

Chapter 10

1. Correct answer: B

The presence of hallucinations may be indicative of delirium, but is not present in anxiety, depression, or dementia (choice B). Labile emotional responses may be seen in patients with delirium, anxiety, and occasionally depression (choice A). A decreased level of awareness is found in both delirium and dementia (choice C), as is impairment in memory, judgment, and thinking (choice D). Speech loss is most typical of dementia (choice E).

2. Correct answer: E

Despite the reputation of delirium as being a potentially fatal disorder, studies have indicated that delirium and terminal agitation may be reversible in approximately 50% of patients without the extensive diagnostic interventions that would be incongruous with end-of-life care treatment goals (choice E). The incorrect choices only contribute to the reputation that delirium is a fatal event in patients near the end of life.

3. Correct answer: C

In this patient with a history of severe pain secondary to advanced prostate cancer, recently treated with escalating doses of morphine, it is most likely that the morphine is the cause of the delirium. Therefore, the one thing that would be least appropriate would be to continue the morphine (choice C). Rather, it would be appropriate to use the technique of opioid rotation to switch the patient to a 50% equianalgesic dose of another opioid and then titrate to effect, with the hope that pain control can be maintained and the delirium will reverse itself (choice D). Because dehydration is often a reversible primary cause of delirium and as it may also exacerbate morphine-induced delirium by causing further accumulation of toxic morphine metabolites, subcu-

taneous hydration by hypodermoclysis may be useful in this situation (choice B). Another potential cause for delirium in this patient could be hypercalcemia secondary to bone metastases from his advanced prostate cancer, so it would be reasonable to check his serum calcium level (choice E). Finally, making sure that the environment is calm, orderly, and stress free may also be of help (choice E).

4. Correct answer: B

Of the various symptoms assessed, only sedation significantly improved (83% vs. 33%, $p = 0.005$) when hydration was used as compared to placebo (choice B). Although hallucinations also were ameliorated in a higher percentage of patients (83% vs. 50%) this did not achieve statistical significance ($p = 0.208$) (choice A). There was no meaningful difference in the percentage of patients with fatigue who improved (54% vs. 62%) between the two groups (choice C). Patient perception of global well-being (choice D) and investigator perception of benefit (choice E) both favored hydration over placebo, but neither difference achieved statistical significance. This study has been expanded to include more patients and a longer follow-up period to try and better understand the role of hydration in the management of delirium and other symptoms.

5. Correct answer: A

Causes of depression near the end-of-life fall into two major categories: changes in life situations and direct or indirect effects of the terminal illness itself. There is also a third major cause, which is the exacerbation of preexisting depression (choice A), which can occur despite management of all other provocative or predisposing factors. Loss of control (choice B), loss of self-esteem (choice C), loss of independence (choice D), and alteration of the environment (choice E) are all changes in a patient's life situation that develop as a result of a terminal illness and may cause depressive symptoms or depression if not managed optimally.

6. Correct answer: A

The question "Are you depressed?" has been shown to be a reliable indicator of depression in the terminally ill when answered in the affirmative (choice A). Neurovegetative symptoms, such as altered sleep patterns (choice B) and anorexia and weight loss (choice E), are not reliable indicators of depression in the terminally ill because these symptoms are often caused by the terminal disease itself. Suicidal ideations (choice C) and a lack of interest in social interactions (choice D) may be components of normal grieving, and therefore, the clinician must explore these issues in greater depth before determining whether depression is present.

7. Correct answer: C

The psychostimulant methyphenidate (choice C) has been found to be useful in treating depression in patients near the end of life because of its rapid onset of action, with effects seen within hours of starting the agent. The TCAs amitriptyline (choice A) and desipramine (choice D) have much slower onsets of action, with amitriptyline taking up to 4–6 weeks to be effective, whereas desipramine may take approximately 2 weeks to show positive effects. The SSRI's sertraline (choice B) and escitalopram (choice E) work somewhat faster than the TCAs, with an onset of action of approximately 1 week.

8. Correct answer: E

This meta-analysis (Rief et al., 2009) evaluated 96 randomized clinical trials comparing antidepressants to placebo and found that the "placebo effect" accounted for 68% (choice E) of the improvement in symptoms in the antidepressant treated groups of patients. The fact that the "placebo effect" was seen in more than two-thirds of patients suggests that it may be

other factors, such as the time providers spend with patients, that have the greatest impact in treating depression.

9. Correct answer: D

Disorientation (choice D) is a feature of delirium that is not seen in patients with anxiety, as anxious patients do not lose awareness of self or their environment. Disorientation must be differentiated from poor concentration, which is seen in anxiety, and which may include distractibility (choice B) and an inability to focus. Other psychologic expressions of anxiety may include insomnia (choice A), irritability (choice C), and poor coping skills (choice E).

10. Correct answer: B

There is no clinical evidence base in the medical literature to support the efficacy of benzodiazepines in the treatment of anxiety (choice B). Nevertheless, they are used quite commonly in end-of-life care. As anxiety and depression coexist, antidepressants should be initiated first as benzodiazepines can worsen depression (choice A). Short-acting benzodiazepines such as midazolam have little clinical value in treating anxiety (choice D), whereas the medium-acting agent lorazepam has become the preferred agent among many (choice C) because it is shorter acting and has a better side effect profile than some of its sister medications (i.e., oxazepam), and comes in tablets and liquids, making it easier to administer. Long-acting benzodiazepines such as diazepam have accumulating active metabolites, making them less useful in the daily treatment of anxiety (choice E) as it takes many weeks to reach steady-state blood levels and toxic effects can persist long after the medication is discontinued.

Chapter 11

1. Correct answer: B

Approximately one-third of hospice patients suffer from pressure ulcers (choice B).

2. Correct answer: C

When patients who have pressure ulcers develop bacteremia, the ulcer itself is the source of the organism in half the patients (choice C).

3. Correct answer: E

This lesion would be unstageable, as the base is covered by an eschar in the wound bed preventing one from determining its true depth (choice E). Although both Stage III (choice C) and Stage IV (choice D) ulcers have full-thickness tissue loss, the lack of an eschar allows one to determine the depth of the lesion, and hence, the stage. Stage I lesions are characterized by nonblanchable redness of localized areas of skin, usually over bony prominences, with intact skin (choice A). Stage II pressure ulcers are characterized by partial-thickness loss of dermis (choice B).

4. Correct answer: B

Autolytic debridement is a technique whereby a wound is covered with a transparent film or hydrocolloid dressing, allowing macrophages and white blood cells to naturally self-digest the necrotic tissue (choice B). The topical application of enzymes to dissolve necrotic tissue is called enzymatic debridement (choice A). The removal of necrotic tissue by irrigating the wound and applying a damp to dry dressing is known as mechanical debridement (choice C), and the dissection of necrotic tissue from the wound bed with scalpel is termed surgical debridement (choice D).

5. Correct answer: B

Turning the patient is believed to be the best measure to prevent pressure ulcers (choice B). The standard is to turn patients every 2 hours, based on the observational study that patients turned on this schedule had fewer pressure ulcers than those turned less often. Although skin care is also important, the skin should be cleansed with warm water and nondrying soaps; hot water and drying soaps should be avoided (choice C). Air mattresses and other pressure-reducing surfaces may be helpful in reducing pressure ulcer risk, but none of these surfaces are a substitute for frequently turning the patient (choice A). Finally, while it is believed that nutritional support is helpful in preventing pressure ulcers, there is actually no evidence in the medical literature to support that belief. Therefore, while one can certainly try to improve the patient's nutrition orally, requesting the family to violate the patient's advance directive instructions, especially without evidence-based support, would be an inappropriate violation of patient autonomy (choice D).

6. Correct answer: A

The most appropriate intervention to treat a skin tear with moderate drainage would be a zinc oxide paste dressing, covered with a nonconforming gauze, as the zinc oxide prevents the dressing from adhering to the tear (choice A). A nonadherent gauze dressing would not be absorbent enough to be effective and the dressing may adhere to the tear (choice B). A hydrocolloid with absorbent center or foam dressing would not be the best choice as it has more absorbency than may be required (choice C). A transparent film dressing is not absorbent enough and this type of dressing may cause further trauma to the tear (choice D).

7. Correct answer: D

Using a spray air freshener may cause significant respiratory tract irritation, which could be especially problematic for this patient, who already has a severely compromised respiratory status (choice D). Saturating a cotton ball with oil of wintergreen and placing it in the patient's room (choice A), applying a charcoal pad over the dressing to absorb odor (choice B), and placing a scented dryer sheet over the air vent in the room (choice C) are all appropriate interventions that may help control the odor of a fungating skin lesion.

8. Correct answer: C

When treating pruritus, it is best to provide a topical steroid as an ointment rather than a cream, as this has the added benefit of keeping the skin moist, palliating the dryness that is often present, and avoiding the stinging sensation that sometimes accompanies application of creams (choice C). Drowsiness is a side effect of oral anti-histamines that may be exaggerated when patients are also on opioid analgesics (choice A). Because dry skin is a major cause of pruritus and often accompanies pruritus due to other causes, moisturizing the skin is an essential part of the management of pruritus (choice B). Menthol in aqueous cream applied topically can soothe the skin and act as a mild anesthetic or counter-irritant (choice D).

9. Correct answer: B

Recurrent cellulitis of the lower extremities commonly is due to streptococcal organisms associated with chronic venous stasis, or chronic lymphedema (choice B). Cellulitis due to *Staphylococcus aureus* spreads from a localized infection, such as an abscess or an infected foreign body (choice A). *Candida albicans* causes skin infections primarily in intertriginous areas of the skin where moisture accumulates (choice C). Herpes zoster causes a viral infection commonly known as shingles, which is a vesicular eruption not associated with cellulitis (choice D).

10. Correct answer: B

When treating patients for xerostomia, mouthwashes that are alcohol-based and astringent should be avoided to prevent further drying of the tissues (choice B). Sucking ice chips (choice C), chewing gum (choice A), and frequent rinsing of the mouth with tap water (choice D) are among the more common ways of treating xerostomia in patients near the end of life.

Chapter 12

1. Correct answer: D

Abnormal respiratory patterns most commonly occur during the "active" phase of dying, not during the "preactive" phase (choice D). Increased dependence on caregivers (choice A), increased sleep (choice B), a limited attention span or withdrawal from surroundings (choice C), and increased lethargy and weakness (choice E) are all characteristics of the "preactive" phase of dying, which usually begins approximately 7–14 days before death.

2. Correct answer: C

The "surge of energy" is a transient phenomenon that temporarily interrupts the dying process. However, it does not reverse the dying process and it does not indicate that the patient is likely to live for several more weeks (choice C). It occurs during the "active" phase of dying (choice A), and patients do show improvement in physical, cognitive, and functional abilities during the dying process (choice B). The "surge" may last for several hours to several days (choice D), and although death remains imminent, families often see this as a sign of hope that the patient may not be dying. Therefore, they often desire to shift goals of care to disease-directed interventions in the hope of changing the inevitable outcome (choice E).

3. Correct answer: A

When "actively" dying patients develop "disturbance" or "incident" pain, not moving them is NOT an appropriate therapeutic option (choice A). These patients may need to be moved for a variety of reasons, not the least of which is to ensure that they are kept clean and comfortable. Therefore, when these patients require significant movement or manipulation, it is recommended that they be premedicated with an appropriate dose of a short-acting analgesic approximately 30 minutes prior to the activity. Patients with "disturbance" or "incident" pain who are near death may moan, groan, or grimace when moved (choice B). The etiology of this pain has been attributed to the expected stiffness that occurs with immobility (choice C), although some have described this as an "alarm response" that occurs in patients who are sensory deprived and unaware the manipulation is coming (choice D). Families need to be taught to expect this type of response if they move the patient (choice E), and should be reassured and taught proper positioning techniques as well planning the activity in advance so the patient can be properly premedicated.

4. Correct answer: C

Although highly concentrated liquid morphine (20 mg/m) is often administered sublingually to "actively" dying patients who do not appear to be able to swallow, it does not appear to be absorbed at all through the transmucosal route (choice C). Rather it appears that the medication "trickles" down the pharynx and is absorbed conventionally through the GI tract. The reason morphine is not absorbed through the mucosa is because it is hydrophilic. Fentanyl, on the other hand, is lipophilic, allowing it to be absorbed transmucosally, making it an ideal agent for this route of administration (choice E). Unfortunately, the currently available fentanyl transmucosal products still require an intact GI tract for maximal effectiveness, as 75% of the fentanyl oralet, Actiq (choice A) and 50% of the fentanyl buccal tablet, Fentora (choice B), are absorbed through the GI mucosa, with 25% and 50% of the two products, respectively, being absorbed through the transmucosal route. Although the rectal route of analgesic administration has long been known to be effective, many caregivers prefer medication be administered via the sublingual or oral transmucosal route due to discomfort providing medication via the rectum (choice D).

5. Correct answer: D

Actively dying patients on chronic opioid therapy who develop myoclonus should NOT have all opioid analgesics discontinued as this could lead to increased pain or opioid withdrawal symptoms (choice D). Rather, if the patient's death is not imminent, rotation to an alternative opioid and/or subcutaneous hydration may be effective in treating myoclonus or any other toxic opioid complications, such as delirium. If the patient is close to death, symptomatic management with benzodiazepines for myoclonus or haloperidol for delirium (choice E) may be appropriate. Increased opioid toxicity seen in patients who are actively dying is, at least in part, secondary to the accumulation of neurotoxic opioid metabolites that cannot be properly excreted due to declining renal function (choice A). When patients are actively dying and their levels of consciousness decrease, family members are often concerned that the opioid analgesia is responsible (choice B) and often ask for the medication to be discontinued. Rather than discontinue the medication, which significantly increases the risk that the patient will either experience pain or opioid withdrawal symptoms, the dosage can be decreased up to 75% (choice C).

6. Correct answer: A

The little evidence that exists in the medical literature regarding the efficacy of oxygen in the treatment of dyspnea in actively dying patients suggests that it is most effective in hypoxemic patients, and has little effect on patients who are adequately oxygenated (choice A). A fan or cool breeze from an open window will improve the perception of breathlessness via altered stimulation of areas innervated by the trigeminal nerve (choice B). Patients who are dyspneic and on opioids for pain require a 50% increase in opioid dose to improve symptoms of breathlessness (choice C). Nebulized morphine may work via the stimulation of opioid receptors in the bronchial tree and along sensory fibers of the vagus nerve (choice D). Bronchodilators and steroids are most effectively used to treat dyspnea earlier than the actively dying phase (choice E), especially when there is airway obstruction and/or inflammation.

7. Correct answer: E

Due to the discomfort associated with suctioning, it should be avoided whenever possible and used to treat terminal congestion only when medication is ineffective or not tolerated by the patient (choice E). Terminal congestion may be defined as a collection of oscillating mucous secretion in the oropharynx and trachea during inspiration and expiration in the dying patient unable to clear secretions (choice A).

Terminal congestion is usually not perceived as uncomfortable by most patients. However, families are often troubled by the presence of the "death rattle" (choice B) as they believe the patient is uncomfortable due to the audible congestion. As patients have difficulty swallowing, liquid forms of hyoscyamine and glycopyrrolate, as well as atropine ophthalmic drops may be administered sublingually to treat terminal congestion (choice C). The anti-cholinergic agents used to treat terminal congestion may precipitate or exacerbate terminal delirium (choice D).

8. Correct answer: B

Although it has been established that dehydration may play a role in the development of terminal delirium, the question of whether all patients, especially those who are in the active phase of dying, should receive parenteral hydration has not yet been answered. Therefore, decisions regarding parenteral hydration should be made on an individual patient basis (choice B), based on each patient's clinical condition and goals of care. Confusion occurs in up to 10% of patients during the last hours of life (choice D). Nonpharmacologi-

cal interventions should include proper patient positioning and calm reassurance (choice E). Any unnecessary medications should be eliminated, and haloperidol and risperidone are the agents most commonly used to symptomatically treat delirium (choice C).

9. Correct answer: C

Nonelectrolyte containing solutions, such as D5W, are not recommended for subcutaneous infusion via hypodermoclysis (choice C) as they tend to draw fluid into the interstitial space, leading to edema and swelling, and sometime, tissue sloughing. Saline containing solutions are, therefore, recommended. 1 to 1.5 L of fluid can be safely administered to patients via hypodermoclysis (choice A) and hypodermoclysis can be safely and appropriately utilized to provide hydration to patients who desire it for cultural or religious reasons (choice D). Proctoclysis is a safe alternative to parenteral hydration (choice B), although it is, not surprisingly, used very sparingly and only when no other route of fluid administration is reasonable. Parenteral hydration continues to be requested by the families of many patients, as well as the physicians who care for them, for they believe that dying without hydration is associated with increased pain and suffering (choice E).

10. Correct answer: A

Planning funeral arrangements in advance of a patient's death has been found to be less stressful than waiting until the patient passes away, when the family is experiencing a great deal of emotional turmoil (choice A). Although it is difficult to predict exactly when someone will die, giving families a general idea when that time is coming by using time frames such as "hours versus days" or "days versus weeks," is generally acceptable (choice B). One of the more important measures that is being developed to assess quality end-of-life care is the determination of whether the patient died in the place of his or her own choosing. Therefore, it is important to reassure the family that they are doing "the right thing," when allowing the patient to die in the place chosen by the patient (choice C). When families feel guilty at wanting the death to occur to "get it over with," they need to be reassured that this is a natural feeling due to all the turmoil surrounding the event (choice D). In order to better prepare families to care for their loved ones during the last days and hours of life, families should be educated on expected symptoms during the "active"-dying process, and how to administer medication to control those symptoms (choice E).

Chapter 13

1. Correct answer: E

Based on a 2006 study (Scialla et al.), impairment in motor function was independently correlated by multivariate analysis with fatigue scores in patients with Asthenia–Fatigue syndrome (choice E). Although most patients with fatigue had serum albumin levels of less than 3.8 gm/dL (choice A), C-reactive protein levels greater than 0.5 mg/dL (choice B), hemoglobin levels below 12 gm/dL (choice C), and/or BMI less than 20 kg/m^2 (choice D), none of these were found to be independent variables by multivariate analysis.

2. Correct answer: C

Evaluation of this patient suggests that his symptoms are, at least in part, related to postural hypotension as well as dehydration, suggested by the dry mucus membranes. Therefore, the most prudent first step would be to discontinue his antihypertensive medications (choice C) and follow his blood pressures. While anemia may be associated with fatigue, the fact that this patient has pink mucus membranes and lacks conjunctival pallor does not support that his symptoms are anemia related (choice A). When diabetic patients become fatigued, it is important to maintain their current regimen. Our patient is an insulin-dependent diabetic and is in good control. There would be no reason to switch to an oral agent, and, in fact, oral hypoglycemics should be avoided in patients near the end of life with fatigue (choice B). While radiation therapy can cause fatigue, our patient completed his radiation 4 weeks ago and it was a short course to the left femur, making it most likely that any contribution to his fatigue by the radiation therapy would have nearly resolved (choice D). While methylphenidate may provide some stimulation, it is always preferable to discontinue potentially fatigue-causing medications when possible, such as the antihypertensives, as opposed to starting another medication (choice E). Furthermore, medical evidence that methylphenidate effectively treats fatigue is lacking, making its use for this symptom questionable at best.

3. Correct answer: A

Mrs. Jones' challenge is boredom during the day, which causes her to doze off, and hence, by sleeping during the day, she is unable to sleep at night. This started when her friend who was keeping her occupied by playing cards with her became ill and could no longer spend time with her. If a hospice volunteer can be found who can play cards with her as her friend did, this may resolve the patient's symptom without resorting to any additional medication (choice A). While the daytime lorazepam could be contributing to daytime drowsiness and dozing off, based on the fact that the patient believes it is the "only thing that gets me through the day," it is unlikely she will consent to discontinue the medication (choice B). If one was going to medicate her, it would most prudent to add a dose of the benzodiazepine she is already on, the lorazepam (choice C) rather than introduce another medication for sleep, such as zolpidem (choice D) or diphenhydramine (choice E). Diphenhydramine should also be avoided since it may cause increased sedation during the day, which could actually exacerbate the patient's problem.

4. Correct answer: C

There are a number of ways of causing pharyngeal stimulation that will hopefully disrupt spasms and suppress hiccups. One is placing something cold, rather than something warm (choice C), at the back of the neck. Other methods include rapid ingestion of granulated sugar (choice A), drinking from the wrong side of the cup (choice B), swallowing dry bread (choice D), or stimulating the pharynx with an oral or nasal catheter (choice E).

5. Correct answer: D

Chlorpromazine is the only pharmaceutical agent that has been approved for the treatment of hiccups (choice D). Despite this, a number of other agents have been found to be useful. Baclofen (choice A) has served as the agent of choice in hospice and palliative medicine, although it can cause increased sedation in the elderly. More recently, gabapentin (choice B) has been found to be an effective medication, and some palliative medicine experts are now suggesting it should replace baclofen as the agent of choice. Metaclopramide (choice C) may be useful in treating hiccups caused by diseases involving the upper GI tract, while prednisone (choice E) may be effective for hiccups caused by inflammatory or destructive lesions in the thorax or abdomen.

6. Correct answer: B

One of the characteristics of urinary retention due to detrussor muscle failure is decreased urgency, while urgency is typical of retention due to bladder outlet obstruction (choice B). Other characteristics of detrusor muscle failure include hesitancy (choice A), impaired bladder sensation (choice C), and long time intervals to micturition (choice D). In contrast, in addition to urgency, bladder outlet obstruction is characterized by frequency, nocturia, and a slow urinary stream.

7. Correct answer: C

Installation of formalin into the bladder has been done to treat refractory hematuria, which may cause bladder spasm, but as it is highly toxic and must be given under general or regional anesthesia, it does not have a role to play in treating patients near the end of life (choice C). Acetic acid solution (choice A) and bupivicaine (choice B) have been both found to be useful when instilled intravesically to treat bladder spasms. A case report documented the effective use of diamorphine in treating a patient with refractory bladder spasms (choice D). Chilled saline solution can be used to treat persistent hematuria, which, as already stated, can contribute to bladder spasm (choice E).

8. Correct answer: D

Drinking cranberry juice results in urine acidification, which reduces bacterial growth and the risk of bacterial infection in the bladder (choice D). Elderly debilitated patients, especially those near the end of life, often have a blunted febrile response to infection, with the result that fever is not an early sign of infection and may not occur for one or more days following infection (choice A). Many patients living in long-term care facilities develop bacterial colonization of the urinary tract without infection; therefore, without signs and symptoms of infection, antibiotics are best avoided in order to reduce the risk of the development of resistant organisms (choice B). When antibiotics are used to treat urinary tract infection, it is common to treat empirically with agents such as amoxicillin, trimethoprim/sulfamethoxizole, or ciprofloxin prior to having culture results (choice C). When the goals of care of the patient and family are to treat patient discomfort while avoiding antibiotic therapy in the face of infection, pyridium may be useful to reduce the symptoms of bladder irritation that often accompanies urinary tract infections (choice E).

9. Correct answer: B

On the basis of a retrospective analysis published in 2005, Kirkova et al. reported that when patients with advanced cancer had bilateral lower extremity edema that was asymmetrical, they had a high incidence of deep vein thrombosis as the cause (choice B). Hypoalbuminemia (choice A), congestive heart failure (choice C), plasma extravasation secondary to sensory nerve neuropeptides (choice D), and neurologic dysfunction (choice E) would be more likely to present with edema that is symmetrical as both extremities would be expected to be affected to the same degree.

10. Correct answer: A

The greatest advantage that warfarin has over LMWH in the treatment of deep vein thrombosis is that it is administered orally (choice A). LMWH, on the other hand, is given by a subcutaneous injection, and many hospice and palliative care givers believe that the burden to patients caused by needing a daily injection is very significant. Of interest is that it has been documented that patients report that treatment with warfarin has a negative impact on quality of life when compared to LMWH (choice D), especially in view of the fact that warfarin therapy requires frequent blood tests for INR monitoring (choice C), while LMWH does not. There are many drug–drug interactions associated with warfarin (choice B), including many agents used to treat other symptoms that are prevalent near the end of life, creating significant management challenges for the clinicians caring for these patients. Warfarin has been reported to cause a high incidence of bleeding complications in palliative care patients (choice E), and this has not been reported to be a major complication in patients treated with LMWH.

Chapter 14

1. Correct answer: C

In viewing the end of life as a stage of growth and development, the dying process can be a time of great achievement (choice C). Viewing death as an enemy (choice A), a sign of personal failure (choice B), a betrayal of one's body (choice D), or a shortfall in the promises of medical science (choice E) are some of the ways that death is viewed in the various established cultural and religious teachings of society.

2. Correct answer: B

Reassuring patients that they will not experience progressive symptoms near the end of life can do a lot to allay their fears about the dying process, and provides them an "opportunity" to move from fear to peace (choice B). Fearing the unknown can generate significant anxiety, and by explaining to patients and families what is going to happen, and assuring patients that they will be kept comfortable, reduces their anxiety considerably, and allows the dying process to proceed in a more peaceful fashion.

3. Correct answer: A

A critical factor in allowing someone to "die well" is one's belief about the meaning of illness in the context of his or her life. Therefore, assisting patients in working through feelings that their illness was a result of personal failure or punishment from God is an illustration of the "opportunity" to move through confusion to meaning (choice A).

4. Correct answer: E

How a patient will find hope, and in what, is entirely a unique experience. For one patient, it may mean living until they are able to take part in some significant family event. For another it may be the sense of a life well lived, a sense that they have contributed something to the world or to someone important to them.

Whatever the source, our challenge is to support patients as they reset their goals and aspirations so that they can move through despair to hope as life is drawing to a close (choice E).

5. Correct answer: C

In a perfect world, all individuals, upon death, would have full closure with all those they had connected with during their lifetime. Realistically, however, many come to this time in their life with much left undone. Often, there have been separations between family members. Many of these have gone on for years with no thought given to reconciliation until the onset of the terminal illness. Frequently, patients have been heard to say that they have forgotten what the argument was about in the first place. When a reconnection takes place, the internal conflict for the patient and family may be relieved, and the previous isolation of family members may be replaced by at least a partial restoration of the family community (choice C).

6. Correct answer: D

People in general have not prepared for the final stage of life or recognized the importance of "living until we die." Family members, trying to protect their dying loved ones, may assume that the patients are too fragile to deal with the intense emotional reactions that may result from family members' feelings and hide them. In these situations, the parties in a relationship prematurely treat each other as if the relationship were already over, and fail to see the importance of continuing to invest energy in this next, albeit probably final, stage of the relationship. Not only do patients and family members suffer premature loss in this situation, but a tremendous opportunity for final closure is often lost as well (choice D).

7. Correct answer: B

"Geotranscendence," a term originally coined by Lars Tornstam and also adopted by Joan

Erikson as an additional ninth stage in her husband Erik's eight stages of human development, is the process by which adults, as they age, developmentally turn their focus from an outward path to an inner journey as they begin to identify less with the body and more with the spirit or soul (choice B). Paul Tournier, who views life as a task to be accomplished, notes the paradox that one can never finish the task, and that the true task in the end becomes "acceptance of unfulfillment and the acceptance of the unfulfilled" (choice A). Kathleen Dowling Singh describes three stages of dying, and through this offers a theoretical structure to the nature of the profound inner changes that are taking place as the personality restructures on a deeper level in response to transpersonal forces (choice C). Victor Frankl believes that suffering is a way to discover meaning in life since when there is suffering there is an opportunity to transcend it by attaching significance to it (choice D). Finally, Erik Erickson, in his eighth and final developmental stage in life identified a psychosocial crisis of ego integrity versus despair (choice E).

8. Correct answer: A

Encouraging expressions of feelings and fears or encouraging emotional closure are ways of opening up communications between patients and families and helping to reduce the conspiracy of silence (choice A) that often interferes with patients and families relationships in the final days and weeks of life. Isolation and alienation (choice B) can be helped by general communication between patients and family members. Letting a patient know you are there and listening and communicating with family that dying people know when they are dying are ways of improving near-death awareness (choice C). Fear (choice D) may be addressed by reassuring patients that they will not be left alone and by reassuring patients that the family will be fine when they are gone. Loss (choice E) may be managed by story telling or by encouraging introspection.

9. Correct answer: E

Loss of control, loss of identity, or feeling disrespected are complaints often manifested by patients who have lost their sense of dignity or humanity (choice E). Losing the will to live and questioning the purpose of life are signs that patients have lost meaning in their lives (choice A). The need for hope (choice B) may be recognized by signs such as loss of well-being or despair. Anger at God or another spiritual source, anxiety over losing control, or feelings of guilt or shame are seen in patients who are searching for a sense of an ultimate spiritual source (choice C). The need for love and acceptance (choice D) are often characterized by feelings of alienation or isolation, fear of abandonment, or the inability to trust others.

10. Correct answer: A

Encouraging patients to discuss past accomplishments and valuing patients' accomplishments and insights are interventions that may help address patients' need for meaning (choice A). Interventions that may address the need for hope (choice B) may include helping patients identify realistic goals or discussing how it is possible to "let go of getting well" while remaining hopeful. To help patients find a sense of an ultimate spiritual source (choice C) one may discuss struggles that the patient has trying to remain in control or discuss beliefs that something beyond us give direction and meaning. Love and acceptance (choice D) may be addressed by ensuring patients that staff will be there for them and by teaching families to continue to relate to patients as intimately as possible. Lastly, allowing patients to make as many choices as possible and allowing them as much independence as possible are ways of meeting patients' needs for dignity and humanity (choice E).

Chapter 15

1. Correct answer: D

There are many components to the model of "total pain" but it is "fear of death" (choice D) that is representative of the spiritual influences on "suffering" and pain perception. Financial concerns (choice A), loss of work (choice B), and changes in social and family functioning (choice C) are all considered psychosocial influences on "suffering." The model also recognizes that there are psychosocial influences (choice E) on the perception of physical pain.

2. Correct answer: B

According to their Guidelines on Chaplaincy and Spiritual Care, Scottish National Health service's definition for spiritual and religious care states that "religious care, at its best, should always be spiritual" (choice B), whereas "spiritual care is not necessarily religious" (choice A). Clearly, spiritual care can be religious (choice C) and religious care, as already noted, should be spiritual (choice D). There are clear definitional differences between the two terms (choice E).

3. Correct answer: C

In this study, published in the *Journal of Clinical Oncology* in 2003, patients ranked "Faith in God" as the second most important factor they consider when making medical decisions, whereas physicians ranked it last (choice C). Patients and doctors agreed that the "oncologist's recommendation" was the most important factor (choice A) whereas the "family doctor's recommendation" was ranked fifth by both groups. Physicians ranked "ability to cure" second and the patients ranked it third whereas the "spouse's input" was ranked fourth by doctors and sixth by patients.

4. Correct answer: B

According to a 2005 survey, physicians were found to be more likely than the general public to cope with major problems without relying on God (choice B). In this same survey, physicians were found to be less likely than the general public to carry their religious beliefs over into other dealings in life (choice C) and were more likely than the general public to consider themselves spiritual, but not religious (choice D). Other studies have shown that family physicians are comparable to the general public regarding their religious characteristics (choice A), and they have also been found to be more religious than physicians from other specialties. In a recent study evaluating attitudes toward death and dying from traumatic injury, only 20% of trauma physicians, as opposed to 57% of the public, believe that divine intervention could save a trauma victim when the physician believed further treatment was futile (choice E).

5. Correct answer: A

A recent study of patients with probable Alzheimer's disease showed that higher levels of spirituality and participation in private religious practices slowed the rate of cognitive decline (choice A). All the other choices are true statements based on studies discussed in the chapter.

6. Correct answer: B

When taking a spiritual history, it is important to ask "open ended" questions, an example of which is: "How has your faith affected your ability to cope with your illness?" (choice B). All the other questions can be answered "yes" or "no," and if the patient answers "no," the line of questioning is often stopped cold, with no opportunity for follow-up or exploration. Avoiding questions that can be answered in the "yes/no" format is very important in order to illicit a good spiritual history.

7. Correct answer: D

There will be times when a patient will make a therapeutic choice based on religious beliefs

that will not make medical sense. In those circumstances, it is important for the physician to follow the patient's lead and to let the patient know that he or she respects his or her point of view. The physician should also attempt to work with the patient to develop a treatment plan that is mutually acceptable to both (choice D). Explaining to the patient that religion and science are not compatible will generally not influence a patient and will only serve to upset him or her (choice A). Attempting to engage the patient in a theologic discussion to get him or her to change his or her mind is likely not to be effective (choice B), nor would asking a chaplain who agrees with the physician to intervene (choice C). Even if there is disagreement between the physician and patient, having the patient seek another physician rather than trying to work toward a mutual solution will leave the patient open to feelings of abandonment (choice E).

8. Correct answer: E

Studies show that patients consider prayer to be a very important aspect of care, so when a patient requests that a physician say a prayer with him or her, it is recommended that the physician not reject the patient's request out of hand (choice E). Rather, the physician should validate the importance of prayer to the patient. Depending on the circumstances, the physician could offer passive support by politely excusing himself (choice A), stand quietly (choice B), pray quietly in a way he or she is comfortable (choice C), or fully participate (choice D).

Chapter 16

1. Correct answer: C

An assessment can best be defined as the process of collecting information from an individual about a specific situation (choice C). Choice A defines the care planning process, which comes about as a result of the information obtained during the assessment. Choice B defines the term "intervention", which are the activities delineated by the care plan. One intervention specifically relevant to psychosocial and spiritual is counseling, which is defined by choice D.

2. Correct answer: D

According to the ecosystems theory of psychosocial practice, it is the gathering of the patient's personal history (choice D), including significant moments in development, life events, family life, and the period during which the current challenges emerged, that will provide the social worker with the most significant window into the patient's psychosocial needs. History of the patient's current illness (choice A), past medical history (choice B), and current medications (choice C) are helpful adjunctive information to the social worker, but will not provide the necessary clues to fully understand the psychosocial dynamics of the situation. Obtaining a family history is important, but rather than focusing on familial medical illnesses (choice E), the focus should be on familial relationships, and if there was a death in the family, learning how the patient coped with that death is far more critical than the exact cause of the loved one's passing.

3. Correct answer: A

While social workers require a good working knowledge of a patient's physical health, they often gather much of that information by reviewing the assessment of the hospice or palliative care nurse prior to the patient encounter. In those circumstances, repeating the physical assessment would not be necessary, as it would be redundant and detract from the real goal of the visit. Therefore, it is not necessary for the social worker to confirm the information gathered by the nurse on the IDT (choice A). However, some discussion of physical issues with the patient may help the social worker establish a more comfortable relationship with the family that will allow easier

transition into discussing the more intimate psychosocial issues (choice B). In this regard, the social worker should focus on issues including understanding how well the patient and family navigate their way through the health care system (choice C), whether medication noncompliance may have a psychosocial basis (choice D), and ultimately, to be able relate physical complaints to psychosocial issues where appropriate (choice E).

4. Correct answer: E

While part of the psychosocial assessment is to evaluate the safety of the patient's neighborhood, this is considered part of the "physical environment" domain of the assessment (choice E). Membership in community or religious institutions (choice A), the role and responsibility of the primary caregiver (choice B), the level of satisfaction that the patient has with the support being provided (choice C), and whether there is any possible neglect or abuse (choice D) are all elements of the social support domain.

5. Correct answer: C

The best method for the social worker to use when assessing a patient's functionality is to ask the patient and/or caregiver to describe the course of a typical day (choice C). This will allow one to understand how the patient functions within the environment. A physical assessment will not tell one specifically how a patient can function and is outside the expertise of a social worker (choice A). Asking the patient to perform each ADL is possible but could be awkward and cumbersome if the patient has specific function deficits (choice B). Using the nurse's functional assessment may not give as true a picture of how the patient functions as the description of a typical day, as the latter factors in compensatory mechanisms that the patient may have developed that are not always detected during a more standard nursing assessment (choice D). Family members may have different perceptions regarding a patient's functionality than the reality (in part, possibly, due to denial over the patient's condition), rendering their description potentially inaccurate, as opposed to the description of the typical day, which describes the activities in a less direct and formal way (choice E).

6. Correct answer: B

It is the foundation for contracting (choice B) that "establishes a mutually agreed upon approach as to how to best meet the specific needs of the patient." Foundation for action (choice A) is the "means to guide the clinician in helping the patient through development of the individual plan of care." Foundation for personal accountability (choice C) establishes that "both the spiritual caregiver and the patient are responsible to act based on the agreed upon plan of care and can be held accountable for success or failure." Foundation for evaluation (choice D) is "established parameters that allow the spiritual care provider to reassess the patient at each visit to determine the success of various interventions." Foundation for research (choice E) is the use of "the established outcomes evaluating the success of various interventions that can be shared with others in the field."

7. Correct answer: B

The inspired assessment (choice B) can best be defined as "the innate ability of the spiritual care giver to recognize a particular situation and immediately provide the necessary spiritual or ritual care." An implicit assessment (choice A) is one in which the caregiver and patient recognize that an assessment is being performed without either acknowledging the assessment. An intuitive assessment (choice C) is one based on the "gut feeling" of the spiritual caregiver. An idiosyncratic assessment (choice D) is one in which the spiritual care provider intentionally avoids the use of formal question-ing. The explicit spiritual assessment (choice E) is one in which the spiritual care provider uses his or her skills to assess the religious and/or nonreligious spiritual needs of the patient and family.

8. Correct answer: D

Paul Pruyser (choice D) is the expert who tends to dissuade spiritual care providers from using psychological categories as he believes that spiritual care goals are different from psychological care goals. Milton Hay (choice A), an experienced hospice chaplain, developed a spiritual assessment model for use primarily by social workers, which includes the principle that psychosocial needs should be assessed because some patients do not see a distinction between spiritual and psychosocial concerns. Erin Moss (choice B), together with Keith Dobson, argue that psychology and spirituality need to be integrated when assessing end-of-life needs. George Fitchett (choice C) includes a psychosocial dimension in his 7×7 assessment model.

9. Correct answer: C

Grace or gratefulness (choice C) can be described as "kindness, generosity, and the beauty of giving and receiving." Providence (choice A) examines how a patient understands God's intentions toward him or the extent of hoping versus wishing. Faith (choice B) is defined as the affirming versus negating stance in life or the ability to commit or engage oneself. Repentance (choice D) is the "process of change from crookedness to rectitude." Communion (choice E) is the "feeling of kinship with the whole chain of being."

10. Correct answer: A

The relationship between interpersonal behavior and belief system (choice A) is included in the assessment domain of "Spiritual suffering." The perspective on the meaning of the diagnosis and prognosis (choice B) and the nature of the world view, which gives meaning to life (choice E), are both included in the "Belief system problem" domain. The level of aspiration to achieve goals (choice C) is part of the "Inner resource deficiency" domain, while the adequacy of clergy in meeting needs and requests (choice E) belongs to the "Religious need" domain.

Chapter 17

1. Correct answer: B

When working with grieving persons, it is important for caregivers to recognize that every individual has his or her own unique timetable for grief and the method for expressing that grief (choice B). Thinking that it's better not to think or talk about the pain of grief (choice A), that it takes about a year to get over a significant loss (choice C), that a mourner wants to be left alone and not talk about the loss (choice D), and that the intensity and length of one's grief reflects that person's love for the deceased (choice E) are all popular myths that are typically espoused in several western cultures.

2. Correct answer: C

Substance abuse is generally not an indication of normal grief, especially if the abuse began related to the loss. Although it may be more typical for a mourner to temporarily use alcohol or prescription medications to deal with intense grief feelings or with difficulty sleeping, when it becomes persistent and turns into substance abuse, it has escalated to a much deeper problem (choice C). Insomnia (choice A), nightmares (choice B), anger (choice D), and searching behaviors (choice E) are all considered typical grief reactions.

3. Correct answer: C

The only symptom that is typically not considered a risk factor for complicated grief is a close relationship to the deceased (choice C). Many mourners who have had a close relationship to the deceased and manage to grieve in a normal, healthy way. Someone who experiences the loss of a child (choice A) has a history of a psychiatric illness (choice B), has other significant stresses concurrent with the loss (choice D), or has had multiple recent losses (choice E) is at a much higher risk of having complicated grief. When these risk factors are noted, caregivers need to anticipate this and provide the necessary support to assist the bereaved.

4. Correct answer: A

Robert Neimeyer (choice A) comes from the "Narrative Tradition," which views the story that the mourner creates of his/her loss to be of great importance. "Reconstruct meaning" is the phrase that Neimeyer uses to describe the process by which the mourner uses narrative to help rebuild previously held assumptions and create or restore a cohesive life narrative of the deceased. The other theorists in the list have a slightly different viewpoint in how they understand grief and loss. William Worden (choice B) defines four tasks of mourning that the bereaved must complete. George Bonanno (choice C) views grieving from the point of view of the amount of resilience the bereaved possess in responding to the loss. Holly Prigerson (choice D) views grieving as a continuum and believes that complicated grief involves the persistence of certain symptoms of grief beyond a reasonable time period. Kenneth Doka (choice E) sees two distinct kinds of grieving: an intuitive response to loss and instrumental grief, which is cognitive in nature, either of which may occur independently or blended together in bereaved persons.

5. Correct answer: D

Survivors of sudden loss have a more difficult time adjusting to loss than individuals whose loved one died after a protracted illness (choice D). With sudden loss, mourners often feel they did not have a chance to say goodbye, to tie up any unfinished business, and to prepare themselves, both emotionally and financially, for the loss. On the basis of recent research, bereaved parents generally have more intense reactions than bereaved spouses (choice A), bereaved spouses generally have more intense reactions than bereaved adult children (choice B), male children generally are affected more by the loss of a parent than by the loss of a sibling (choice C), and one-third of children who lose a parent show high levels of emotional difficulty in their readjustment (choice E).

6. Correct answer: A

Searching behavior (choice A) occurs commonly in mourners experiencing normal grief. Even though it does not seem rational, it is seen as an almost subconscious attempt to reconnect with a loved one. Searching behavior is particularly common in locations where the mourner used to meet his/her loved one. When a bereaved person exhibits extreme preoccupation with the deceased (choice B), he or she significantly neglects his or her self-care (choice C), brings up themes of loss in most discussions (choice E), or is not willing to move physical possessions (choice E), the grief has clearly become more complicated and professional assistance is needed.

7. Correct answer: D

The bereaved person being discussed is having disenfranchised grief (choice D). This form of grief is characterized by the griever being deprived of validation and recognition of a loss because of constraints in openly acknowledging the loss or constraints in publicly grieving. In this situation, the bereaved was involved with a partner of the same sex who died of AIDS, and he has no one to discuss his loss with because of the unacceptable nature of his lifestyle and relationship to those he would normally seek out. Chronic grief (choice A) is defined as grief that is excessive in duration and does not reach a satisfactory conclusion. Delayed grief (choice B) occurs when the griever does not deal sufficiently with a

loss at the time when it happens. Exaggerated grief (choice C) occurs when the mourner experiences an intensification of normal grief reactions and feels overwhelmed, typically resulting in emotional distress. Masked grief (choice E) occurs when the bereaved experience symptoms and behaviors that cause difficulty in coping which they are unable to associate with the loss.

8. Correct answer: E

Mourners tend to respond favorably to social support and often seek out individuals with whom they can discuss their grief thoughts and feelings while depressed persons do not (choice E). A depressed mood (choice A), cathartic expressions (choice B), alterations in eating and sleeping patterns (choice C), and difficulty concentrating (choice D) are common to both grief and depression.

9. Correct answer: C

It would not be helpful to suggest to a mourner that they make *any* major changes or decisions soon after the loss, especially a geographic move, unless absolutely necessary (choice C). Some view such a move as an attempt to escape from the pain of grief, although it generally does not work. Validating the significance of their loss (choice A), providing education regarding the "normal" grief process (choice B), asking them about their relationship with the deceased (choice D), and suggesting they write letters to the deceased (choice E) can all be very appropriate interventions to assist the bereaved.

10. Correct answer: A

With the bereaved often experiencing prolonged and intense anxiety and/or depression, the desire to prescribe anxiolytics and antidepressants can be quite strong. It is generally agreed, however, that such medications should be prescribed as an adjunct, and not as a replacement, for other interventions (choice A). These medications should be used sparingly to avoid dependence, and there is an increased potential for suicide in bereaved individuals receiving medication (choice B). A study by Reynolds et al. on the treatment of bereavement-related major depressive episodes found that the use of the antidepressant nortriptyline was superior to placebo in achieving remission of these episodes (choice C). In fact, while antidepressants may be useful if the bereaved experience a major depressive episode, they are generally not indicated in persons with acute grief reactions (choice D).

Chapter 18

1. Correct answer: C

Although one can argue that all of these factors have some role to play in decision making when considering the appropriateness of a palliative intervention, the desires of the physician are LEAST important (choice C). There are many circumstances when a physician will recommend an intervention to a patient and the patient will not want the treatment and choose not to follow the doctor's advice (choice A). When considering whether to recommend a palliative intervention, it is also important to be confident that the intervention is likely to be effective (choice B), that it is not more toxic than can be tolerated by the patient (choice D), and that the patient will live long enough to be able to benefit from the treatment (choice E).

2. Correct answer: E

This 93-year-old woman with advanced dementia appears perfectly comfortable with no evidence of symptoms secondary to anemia, which she has likely had for some time. In any event, given her current situation, the most appropriate palliative approach to her care would be not to transfuse her since it would not improve her symptoms, and not to evaluate the anemia, since she is tolerating it well. Rather, the best approach would be to discontinue her routine blood work since there is no medical indication for drawing the hemoglobin or any

other studies at present, and also to avoid the discomfort of the venipuncture (choice E). To transfuse the patient (choice A) or start erythropoietin (choice B) might improve the results of the patient's next hemoglobin level but would not affect the patient's current clinical condition, which is one of comfort. Doing a GI work-up (choice C) or hematological work-up (choice D) would also not make any sense given the fact that she is terminally ill and not being troubled by the incidental anemia.

3. Correct answer: A

Although all the laboratory results above may be associated with altered mental status, one must always consider the potentially correctable causes and order studies in the context of the patient's illness. As hypercalcemia (choice A) is most often associated with advanced cancers, it would be the least likely abnormality responsible for this patient's altered mentation given his primary diagnosis and comorbid conditions. On the other hand, with a history of congestive heart failure on large doses of diuretics, an elevated BUN (choice B), or a low serum sodium (choice E), would not be surprising. With a history of cirrhosis and the potential of further hepatic compromise from passive congestion, a high serum ammonia would also be very possible. Finally, given that he is a long-standing diabetic patient, the possibility that he is hypoglycemic must be considered, so a low blood glucose (choice D) would also not be an unexpected finding.

4. Correct answer: B

When considering patients with end-stage diseases for surgical repair of a hip fracture, factors to consider include the patient's underlying diagnosis and comorbid illnesses, mental status, performance status, anticipated life expectancy, and prefracture ambulatory status. It is suggested that patients with a short life expectancy and who were nonambulatory prior to the fracture are least likely to benefit from surgical repair and these characteristics best fit patient B. Patient A was fully ambulatory prior to the fracture and so would likely benefit from surgery. Patient C, even though she can only walk short distances, might be able to tolerate the procedure under spinal anesthesia, and would be at increased risk of complications if she would become nonambulatory. Although some might also be concerned about doing surgery on patient D, the resultant immobilization might increase his risk of earlier mortality, so surgery should be considered for him as well.

5. Correct answer: D

In patients being considered for palliative amputation secondary to locally advanced malignancy, it has been suggested that their life expectancy be at least 3 months (choice D). It was also suggested that such patients have a performance status of greater than 50% (choice E). In a group of patient with gangrene secondary to vascular compromise who were treated without surgery, at least half the patients had significant heart disease (choice B) and almost half had a prior stroke (choice A). Patients with dry gangrene generally tolerate it well and are often more amenable to a nonsurgical approach when their overall prognosis is poor (choice C).

6. Correct answer: C

Perforation (choice C) is the most serious complication of expandable stent placement for large bowel obstruction, occurring in a little less than 4% of patients and usually requires surgical intervention. All the other complications listed do occur but are generally amenable to medical management.

7. Correct answer: B

The light source that the tumor is exposed to is contained in light-delivery catheters, not an ND-YAG laser (choice B). The patient is pretreated with a hematoporphyrin compound (choice A), which is activated and destroys the tumor tissue when exposed to the light source. PDT can be used to treat obstruction from exophytic lesions (choice C) as well as tumor ingrowth into expandable metal stents (choice D). Because the hematoporphyrin is absorbed in the skin, patients must avoid sunlight exposure and fluorescent light, as well as sources of radiant heat, for more than 1 month following treatment (choice E).

8. Correct answer: D

For this patient, sclerotherapy to prevent effusion reaccumulation is the best way to palliate his symptoms and avoid future thoracenteses. Although talc powder is very effective as a sclerotherapy agent, it requires knowledge of a special sterile technique by a pharmacist, it can cause occasional respiratory distress syndrome, and may sometimes solidify, leading to the development of residual loculated effusions (choice D). Doxycycline is a very effective sclerotherapy agent, with a reported 90% success rate for at least a 3-month duration (choice B). Its side effects include pain, fever, and cough (choice C). Bleomycin may also be used, but if patients have renal insufficiency (choice E) or are elderly, the dose needs to be adjusted. If the patient has a short life expectancy, an option to avoid sclerotherapy would be to send him home with a small, indwelling pleural catheter left in place for continued drainage (choice A).

9. Correct answer: A

This patient is suffering from malignant ascites, and while diuretics and fluid restriction are effective in controlling ascites in about 90% of patients with nonmalignant ascites, they are rarely effective in controlling ascites due to malignancy (choice A). Plasma expanders are generally not needed following paracentesis for malignant ascites (choice B). If patients require frequent abdominal taps, an implantable port-a-cath or other similar device may make frequent fluid removal easier (choice C). Sclerotherapy with doxycyline has been reported to be successful in only 30% of patients (choice D).There is evidence that insertion of peritoneovenous shunts may be beneficial in patients with malignant ascites who have a life expectancy of several months and cannot tolerate any of the other therapeutic options (choice E).

10. Correct answer: C

In a recent study regarding the treatment of patients with antibiotics in a palliative care unit, they were found to be helpful in 62% of patients. Positive outcomes were most commonly observed for infections of the urinary tract (choice C) as opposed to those with infections of the lower respiratory tract (choice B), and skin or soft tissues (choice E). Patients who were deteriorating (choice A) or in an acute phase (choice D) were also much less likely to have positive outcomes compared with those considered stable or terminal.

Chapter 19

1. Correct answer: D

In this study, which presented hypothetical case scenarios to patients with cancer, 68% (choice D) of patients said that they would opt for chemotherapy if it substantially reduced symptoms, even if there was no prolongation of life. This is in contrast to only 22% (choice A) of patients saying that they would opt for chemotherapy if the only significant outcome was a 3 month prolongation of life. This study clearly suggests that for patients with cancer, palliation of symptoms and QOL may be more important than length of life.

2. Correct answer: C

Even though a reduction in tumor mass (choice C) suggests that the chemotherapy is active, this outcome would not be included as part of a "clinical benefit response," as this is focused on outcomes that relate to patient symptoms. Decreased pain with no change in analgesic dose (choice A), improvement in

performance status (choice B) and/or weight (choice D), and a decreased analgesic dose with the same level of pain (choice E) are all considered valid outcomes that measure a "clinical benefit response."

3. Correct answer: A

In one study, "best supportive care" was defined as the best care available as judged by the attending physician, according to institutional standards (choice A). Only few "best supportive care studies" actually have attempted to control for the effects of adjunctive therapies (choice B) such as corticosteroids, which may improve symptoms on its own in some patients, or have provided detailed descriptions of patient responses to symptom management interventions (choice C). Most of these trials, by not controlling for patient/health care provider contacts in the two study arms (choice D), have failed to control for the fact that increased patient/provider contacts may have a salutary effect on symptoms. The fact that "best supportive care" as an intervention has never been standardized (choice E), places the validity of these comparative studies in question.

4. Correct answer: B

The first chemotherapy trial to utilize the "clinical benefit response" as an outcome measure involved patients with pancreatic carcinoma (choice B). Although studies with small cell (choice A) and non–small cell bronchogenic carcinoma (choice E), prostate carcinoma (choice C), and colorectal carcinoma (choice D) had occasionally utilized symptom-based or QOL-based outcomes as part of their measures, up until the description of the "clinical benefit response" in pancreatic cancer trials, the primary outcomes of chemotherapy trials focused on objective tumor response and patient survival.

5. Correct answer: E

Although there is good medical evidence that a poor performance status is associated with a lower overall response rate to chemotherapy, there is no data to support that a poor performance status is associated with a reduced likelihood of a "clinical benefit response" to palliative chemotherapy (choice E). This is because patients with a poor performance status are not included in most palliative chemotherapy studies (choice A), and one cannot extrapolate outcomes for patients with a good performance status and apply them to patients with a poor performance status. An improvement in performance status following palliative chemotherapy is considered a "clinical benefit response" (choice C). Performance status has been correlated with both degree and duration of response to radiation therapy. Patients with a poor performance status have less satisfactory pain relief (choice B) than those with a good performance status, whereas those with a good performance status have more durable pain relief (choice D) than those with a poor performance status.

6. Correct answer: C

Although all the choices are true statements regarding hypofractionation, it is the decreased risk of delayed toxicity due to short patient life expectancy (choice C) that makes hypofractionation a viable option for end-of-life care patients. In fact, it is the concern that some patients may live longer than expected and experience delayed toxicity that has been a major obstacle in getting radiation oncologists to advocate for hypofractionation in patients near the end of life. Hypofractionation does reduce the risk of acute toxicity since there are less total treatments given (choice A), and the fewer treatments result in fewer patient trips to the radiation therapy treatment center (choice B) and a more rapid onset of symptom relief (choice D).

7. Correct answer: B

Although single-fraction therapy has been recommended for patients with "poor prognostic factors" by the ACR in its recently published "Therapeutic Guidelines for the Treatment of Bone Metastases," they state that due to the risk of toxicity to adjacent structures such as the larynx, esophagus, and stomach, it should be avoided when treating vertebral metastases (choice B). Multiple studies have shown that the outcomes of single-fraction treatment is equivalent to standard multiple-fraction treatment (choice A), and in one study, toxicity was greater in the multiple-fraction arm than in the single-fraction arm (choice C). In the guidelines, one of the stated advantages of single-fraction treatment is that retreatment after a single fraction may be used to periodically reduce tumor burden (choice D). Single dose efficacy studies have shown that a single dose of 8 Gy is more effective in providing pain relief than one of 4 Gy (choice E).

8. Correct answer: C

Spinal cord compression is one of the true medical emergencies that exist in palliative care. Early recognition and treatment are crucial present as once patients become nonambulatory, which is the case in 78% of patients presenting to the radiation oncologist, the chances of recovery of function and ambulation are very small (choice C). Excruciating back pain is the most common symptom (choice A), and MRI has become an integral part of the work-up, replacing contrast myelography in most cases (choice B). Patients who are not expected to recover neurologically should still be treated with radiation therapy for pain control (choice E), and the treatment area should include at least 1 to 2 vertebrae above and below the level of the block (choice D).

9. Correct answer: E

Radiation therapy for the treatment of SVC can either be by the traditional treatment of 20 to 30 Gy in 5 to 10 fractions, or three once a week fractions of 8 Gy each, which has been shown to be equally as effective (choice E). Although SVC is considered a medical emergency, its gradual onset, in most cases, gives one some time for evaluation and treatment (choice A). Symptoms include dyspnea, hoarseness, chest pain, and syncope (choice B). Medical management consists of oxygen, diuretics, elevation of the head of the bed, and corticosteroids (choice C). Vascular stenting may be considered a viable alternative to radiation therapy in some patients (choice D).

10. Correct answer: B

Treatment of pelvic pain or bleeding secondary to recurrent gynecological or colorectal tumors can be treated with a single dose of 10 Gy to the pelvis (choice B). In fact, the dose can be repeated at monthly intervals, with a maximum of three treatments, although patients surviving more than 6 to 9 months are at high risk for severe bowel toxicity. The recent literature suggests that the placement of a self-expanding, metallic stent may be superior to EBRT in the treatment of malignant dysphagia, with a 95% success rate (choice A). Although a single 10 Gy fraction will successfully treat symptoms of pelvic disease, painful hepatomegaly should be treated with 10 fractions of 2 to 3 Gy each (choice C), and massive splenomegaly should also be treated with multiple fractions (choice D). Finally, uveal metastases should be treated in patients near the end of life, as preservation of vision can be a significant QOL issue (choice E).

Chapter 20

1. Correct answer: B

In order to be a candidate for an AICD, a patient should have an expected survival of greater than 1 year rather than less than 1 year (choice B). Other indications for AICD placement include NYHA Class II or III heart failure on optimal medical therapy (choice A), a cardiomyopathy from either ischemic or non-

ischemic heart disease with an ejection fraction of $<35\%$ (choice C), and a prior history of cardiac arrest or other hemodynamically significant ventricular arrhythmia (choice D). Additionally, in high-risk patients with a family history of sudden cardiac death, an AICD may be placed prophylactically (choice E).

2. Correct answer: D

Quality of life within 1 month of a patient being shocked by an AICD is NOT the same as for patients who have never been shocked (choice D). It is, in fact, significantly decreased, primarily due to the fact that an AICD shock is associated with significant pain and anxiety (choice C). Survival is improved in patients who had AICDs placed 30 days postmyocardial infarction and had ejection fractions below 30%, whether they had arrhythmias or not (choice A). It is also improved in patients with left ventricular dysfunction and a history of a resuscitated sudden cardiac death (choice E). Quality of life of patients with AICDs has been reported to be significantly superior to that of patients treated with amiodarone at 3 and 12 months post placement (choice B). The significance is lost at 30 months of follow-up.

3. Correct answer: E

It is not appropriate for hospices to require that patients who have an AICD have the device deactivated prior to hospice admission (choice E). In fact, it is the hospice staff who are often the first ones to broach the subject of deactivation, and often need to educate and support patients and families to help them consider the option. The deactivation process is painless to the patient (choice A). Formal deactivation requires the use of a reprogramming device that can be obtained from the manufacturer of the device (choice B). Emergency deactivation can be achieved with the use of a magnet (choice C). Patients and families should also be reassured that if the AICD has a pacemaker function, this function can be preserved when the cardioverter-defibrillator is deactivated (choice D).

4. Correct answer: A

In this 2008 study by Goldstein et al., of 15 patients with AICDs who were interviewed, it was reported that none of them were informed about the option of deactivation at the time the AICD was placed (choice A). It was also reported that none of the patients knew that deactivation was an option. When informed that it was, most patients prefer that their physician play an active role in making deactivation decisions (choice B). One patient commented that deactivation "was like an act of suicide" (choice C). Patients expressed considerable anxiety over the possibility of an AICD shock (choice D), although they all believed that the AICD device was exclusively beneficial (choice E).

5. Correct answer: D

According to a study published in 2006 (Kahn), only 2% of physicians believe that AICD deactivation is consistent with euthanasia or assisted suicide (choice D). Physicians believe that the option of AICD deactivation should be discussed as part of advance care planning (choice A); however, they rarely discuss AICD deactivation with patients (choice B). More than 50% of physicians believe that AICDs are "life sustaining" in nature (choice C) and physicians cite their own concerns about withdrawing care as a reason why they avoid discussing AICD deactivation with patients (choice E).

6. Correct answer: B

It is actually rare for deactivation of a pacemaker to result in immediate patient death (choice B) because patients are rarely 100% pacemaker dependent, and during the dying process tachycardias are the most common rhythm. However, deactivation may result in symptoms of fatigue, dizziness, or dysp-

nea (choice C) caused by the bradycardia or progressive heart failure that result from discontinuation of the device. Patients and families request pacemaker deactivation due to the mistaken belief that the pacemaker will keep the heart beating after the patient would otherwise have died, prolonging the dying process (choice A). In contrast to the 2% of physicians who believe AICD deactivation is consistent with euthanasia or assisted suicide (see question 5, above), 18.5% of the physicians surveyed in the same study (Kahn, 2006) believe the same of pacemaker deactivation (choice D). Newer pacemaker models are shielded to prevent deactivation with a magnet (choice E).

7. Correct answer: E

A patient decision to not have a pacemaker battery replaced is NOT consistent with assisted suicide (choice E). It is, in some respects, a passive form of pacemaker deactivation, and may be an appropriate decision for certain patients based on the individual patient's goals of care, current medical prognosis, ability to tolerate the procedure, and the potential risk of cardiac symptoms should the pacemaker cease to function. Pacemaker batteries generally last from 5 to 8 years (choice A), after which they require replacement, while the pacemaker leads may last for 20 years or more (choice B). Pacemaker battery replacement is a minor surgical procedure that may be performed in the outpatient setting, utilizing local anesthesia with conscious sedation (choice C). AICD battery replacement is a little more complex, as the patient has to be rendered unconscious when the defibrillator is tested so that the patient does not feel any of the pain associated with the test shock (choice D).

8. Correct answer: C

Complications of infection, bleeding, and stroke occurred in LVAD patients with twice the frequency they did in patients managed medically (choice C). LVADs were originally designed as a "bridge" to support the cardiac function until eventual cardiac transplantation, but are now used in selected patients who are not transplant candidates (choice A). In these patients, a 1-year survival is over double that of patients treated with optimal medical management (52% vs. 25%) (choice B). Patient mobility with an LVAD is limited because the power pack needs to be recharged nightly (choice D). In view of the high morbidity and mortality associated with LVADs, their role in the treatment of patients with refractory heart failure receiving hospice services is extremely limited (choice E).

9. Correct answer: E

A study evaluating the efficacy of intermittent infusion of inotropic agents in patients with refractory heart failure (Lopez-Candales et al., 2004) demonstrated that 44% of patients were able to discontinue infusions for periods ranging from 201 to 489 days (choice E). Inotropic agents may reduce hospitalization in some patients with advanced heart failure (choice A). There is an increased risk of patient mortality associated with infusion of inotropes (choice B). Intermittent infusion of inotropes improves symptoms in some patients with refractory heart failure (choice C). Intermittent infusion of inotropes may be accomplished in the home or outpatient setting (choice D).

10. Correct answer: C

Patients who have goals of care focused on symptom palliation may be appropriate to receive hospice services while awaiting transplantation (choice C). These patients usually want to be managed at home and avoid hospitalization and resuscitation, although if they can survive with palliative management until a transplant is available, they are willing to undergo the procedure. Patients who want to continue to receive care in the intensive care unit usually want all interventions, including cardiopulmonary resuscitation (CPR), to

attempt to remain alive until a transplant is available. The care these patients desire is not consistent with the palliative services hospices provide and they would not be best served receiving hospice care, rather they should continue to receive care through the acute care system (choice D). Hospices, of course, should not reject all patients awaiting transplantation, rather they should evaluate each patient's situation individually, based on the patient's goals of care (choice A). Conversely, all patients awaiting cardiac transplantation should not be admitted to hospice, because many patients need and want care that hospices are unable to provide (choice B).

Chapter 21

1. Correct answer: B

Shortness of breath is subjective and whether oxygen helps to palliate the symptoms of breathlessness is based on the whether the patient finds it helpful or not (choice B). Measurement of oxygen saturation is not an accurate gauge of whether oxygen is required or beneficial (choice A). The usefulness of oxygen therapy does not depend on administration via pressure devices (choice C), high flow rates (choice E), nor will it prevent the need to use noninvasive ventilatory devices if these are appropriate and within the patient's goals of care (choice D).

2. Correct answer: D

In the hospice setting, where the goals of the patient and family and the hospice interdisciplinary team revolve around improvement in the quality of the patient's life rather than extending the quantity of the patient's life, positive pressure ventilators are virtually never utilized (choice D) (with the one exception generally being in patients who are being admitted to hospice for the purpose of having the ventilator discontinued). Oxygen (choice A), CPAP (choice B), BiPAP (choice C), and

IPPV (choice E) are modalities that palliate symptoms in a less invasive way than mechanical ventilators and may be used when indicated and consistent with the goals of care of hospice patients.

3. Correct answer: C

BiPAP is not indicated for the relief of dyspnea secondary to physical obstruction of air flow into the trachea as may be seen in patients with head and neck cancer (choice C). BiPAP is indicated when there is hypoventilation with poor air exchange, as may be seen in such conditions as amyotrophic lateral sclerosis (choice A), muscular dystrophy (choice B), multiple sclerosis (choice D), and chest wall deformities (choice E).

4. Correct answer: B

There is no correlation between the sensation of breathlessness and oxygen saturation; a patient may sense shortness of breath with a normal saturation (choice B). Pulmonary edema can cause alveolar hypoventilation (choice A). While very unusual in a hospice setting, the use of a ventilator in a nonhospice palliative care setting can benefit patients and families by allowing them time to decide on their goals of care (choice C). Bronchodilators can be administered to patients using BiPAP (choice D). Incentive spirometry devices, while often doing no more than encouraging deep breathing, have advantages over deep-breathing exercises because the patient gains positive feedback from watching the ball rise with inspiration (choice E).

5. Correct answer: A

Given the usual advanced illness and debilitation of patients receiving hospice and palliative care, it is not appropriate to consider strenuous rehabilitation measures, such as a treadmill rehabilitation program (choice A), which would not be tolerated by the patient and which could actually cause more rapid deterioration. Incentive spirometry (choice B), chest physio-

therapy (choice C), deep-breathing exercises (choice D), and pursed-lip breathing (choice E) are all techniques that may be utilized to assist patients near the end of life, who have significant dyspnea.

6. Correct answer: D

It is generally appropriate for close family members to be with the patient during the process of discontinuing a mechanical ventilator as they can be a source of significant support for the patient (choice D). On the other hand, family members who are not supportive of this process and will be emotionally uncontrolled and disruptive should not be present (choice C). There is no reason for the facility's administrator to be present, unless he is a relative or close personal friend and has been requested to attend (choice A). If the patient is in a semi-private room, s/he must be moved to a private room for the express purpose of privacy, as having relatives of the patient in the adjoining bed, or the patient himself, present would be highly inappropriate (choice B). The facility's code team would not be required under any circumstances, as part of the premise of discontinuing the ventilator is that the patient will not be reintubated (choice E).

7. Correct answer: C

When discontinuing a mechanical ventilator in the home setting, experienced staff is crucial (choice C) and may even be more important then when this intervention is done in a facility, as the staff, who cannot call for assistance or support, needs to have the knowledge and experience to recognize and immediately deal with any problems that arise. The planning required when discontinuing a ventilator in the home is significantly greater than when the procedure is done in a facility (choice A). The electrical wiring in the house is an important issue because there have to be grounded electrical plugs for the ventilator and other medical equipment (choice B). Regardless of the location of the procedure, virtually all medications should be given intravenously (choice D). Psychosocial support is also a critical need in both the facility and the home settings (choice E).

8. Correct answer: A

The physician who writes the orders to discontinue the ventilator must have examined the patient and reviewed the records prior to giving the orders (choice A). This is an intervention that cannot be done remotely or by "standing orders." Any physician who has acquired the skills to appropriately manage patients being taken off ventilatory support can be involved in this process; specialists like pulmonologists or intensivists are not necessary (choice B). A respiratory therapist may remove the endotracheal tube; it is not required that a physician do this (choice C). The skill sets of physician and social worker are different and they serve the needs of patient and family in different ways, so both should be seen as part of the team involved in this situation. The presence of the physician does not in any way reduce the need for social workers or other disciplines to be present to support the patient and family (choice D). By the same token, while the physician should be part of the team counseling patients and families about this process, physicians should not do this independently, but should work together with the other members of the interdisciplinary team (choice E).

9. Correct answer: B

A Ramsay Score of 2 is insufficient to initiate weaning in this situation (choice B). Since respiratory distress may occur, the patient should be made unaware prior to the procedure by medicating sufficiently to induce a Ramsay Score of 5 (minimal response to stimulation) or 6 (no response to stimulation). Assuring IV access (choice A), having available sufficient quantities of opioids and benzodiazepines (choice C), having suction available in room (choice D), and assuring that all necessary clinical support staff are present (choice E) should all be done prior to any change in the ventilator settings.

10. Correct answer: C

Benzodiazepines can be effectively used to palliate respiratory distress because of their effect in relaxing and calming the patient (choice C). Since the decision should have been made that the goal of this intervention is to permanently remove ventilator support, reintubation should not be a method of palliating respiratory distress; medical management should be used (choice A). While anticholinergic medications are useful in controlling secretions, they should be administered in drop form, not via a topical patch, in order to allow tighter control over the effects and to offer a faster time to onset (choice B). Supplemental oxygen should be used postweaning as the patient's breathing may not be fully effective and this will aid in assuring comfort (choice D). The endotracheal tube should be removed to increase the patient's comfort; secretions can be managed adequately without the tube remaining in place (choice E).

Chapter 22

1. Correct answer: B

A DNR order is a physician order, which gives instructions that the patient is not to receive CPR in the event of a cardiac arrest. While the order is often the result of instructions provided by a patient through an advance directive document, the DNR order itself is NOT an advance directive (choice B). A living will is an advance directive that lists what interventions a patient does or does not desire when terminally ill or having certain irreversible medical conditions (choice A). A health care power of attorney is an advance directive through which a patient designates an individual as a surrogate who will make decisions for the patient if the patient cannot make decisions regarding care (choice C). A combined living will/health care power of attorney is an advance directive that has features of both the living will and the health care power of attorney (choice D). When a patient gives verbal instructions regarding health care choices, documented by the physician or other health care provider, this can constitute a verbal advance directive (choice E).

2. Correct answer: C

The standard for surrogate decision making is that the proxy is required to decide what the patient would want done if not incapacitated (choice C). The surrogate should not make the decision based on his or her own wishes (choice A), what the physician recommends if it is contrary to the patient's wishes (choice B), what a health care attorney would say (choice D), or consider input from multiple sources (choice E). The surrogate's obligation is to base the decision primarily on what s/he believes the patient would have chosen.

3. Correct answer: A

The Patient Self-Determination Act is a federal statute passed in November, 1990, and implemented in December 1991 that requires all Medicare and Medicaid providers to give patients the opportunity to create an advance directive (choice A). The rules defining when a living will may be applied (choice B), the requirements for appointing a durable health care power of attorney (choice C), the level of proof (verbal or written) required by a health care surrogate that the decision made is consistent with what the patient would have chosen (choice E), and the hierarchy of surrogates that may make decisions for a patient if there is no advance directive (choice D) are all governed by each individual state and differ significantly from one state to the next.

4. Correct answer: D

The key advantage to advance directives is that they allow for the respect of patient autonomy (choice D). The physician having knowledge

of patient wishes furthers the patient's autonomy being respected (choice A), by decreasing unnecessary healthcare interventions (choice C), and also decrease healthcare costs (choice E). By knowing what their loved one wants and supporting his or her autonomy, the family experiences a decrease in anxiety and guilt (choice B). But all these other advantages stem from the knowledge and respect in patient autonomy fostered by the advance directive.

5. Correct answer: A

Advance directives may be revoked by a patient at any time (choice A), and a physician should review a patient's advance directive with him or her at frequent intervals. Advance directives do not mean "don't treat" (choice B), rather they provide an individual an opportunity to let people know what treatments they want or do not want. Patients remain in control even when appointing a health care proxy, since the proxy only makes decisions when the patient is incapacitated, and the decisions the proxy makes must be consistent with what the patient would have chosen if he or she was not incapacitated (choice C). Advance directives are not only for old or sick people, but for everyone (choice D). In fact, some of the landmark cases that spurred the development of advance directives involved young people who suffered accidents that resulted in tragic outcomes requiring surrogate decisions regarding whether or not to continue certain types of supportive therapies. Legally, health care providers are compelled to honor advance directives (choice E), and in situations where a provider is unwilling to follow legal advance directive instructions, the provider should withdraw from the care of the patient and assist the patient in finding another provider who is willing to follow the advance directive instructions.

6. Correct answer: D

Research during the first decade following implementation of the PSDA showed that, unfortunately, the hoped for impact was not achieved. One major finding was that advance directives helped make end-of-life decisions in less than half of cases where a directive existed (choice D). Less than (rather than more) 50% of severely or terminally ill patients in various cited studies had advance directives in the medical record (choice A). There was no improvement in the documentation of patient preferences in the medical record of patients with advance directives (choice B) and most patients who had them did not receive any input from their physicians (choice C). As a result, care at the end of life sometimes appears to be inconsistent with the patients' preferences to forego life-sustaining treatment and patients may receive care they do not want (choice E).

7. Correct answer: C

During the physician's conversation with a patient about the creation of an advance directive, the physician should point out the pros and cons of both forms of advance directives, the living will and the durable health care power of attorney (choice C). It is better to initiate conversations about advance directives before the patient reaches a crisis situation, such as being informed that an illness is terminal (choice A). Advance directives can always be changed, and it is important for the physician to make this clear to the patient, reassure him or her that any choices that are made now can be re-examined in the future, and to revisit the advance directive choices with the patient frequently (choice B). Language in an advance directive should be very specific regarding what treatments a patient does or does not want (choice D), and one should not rely on the physician, or anyone else for that matter, to correctly interpret vague language in an advance directive document. Finally, while it is acceptable for a patient to give advance directive instructions to a physician verbally, the physician must document the conversation and the patient's choices in order for the verbal

advance directive instructions to have any true validity (choice E).

8. Correct answer: B

The outcomes for survival to discharge from the hospital following CPR for cardiac arrest are generally poor, with the best survival of 39% found in a group of cardiac patients who arrested while being cared for in the hospital (choice B). Survival to discharge following a witnessed cardiac arrest is reported at 5.2% (choice A), for the chronically ill elderly <5% (choice C), and for the ambulatory elderly at 10% (choice D). If one has a cardiac arrest and vital signs are initially present, approximately 10.2% survive to discharge (choice E).

9. Correct answer: A

Most people are poorly informed about CPR, and while most know that it includes chest compressions, a study a number of years ago showed that only approximately 36% knew that it could include placing a "tube in the windpipe" (choice A). It is well documented that the public overestimates the percentage of successful CPR outcomes (choice B). More than half of patients do not want to discuss CPR issues with their physicians (choice D), and not surprisingly, only about a quarter of people actually do have the conversation (choice E). Studies do show, however, that if patients were better informed, they would more often opt to forgo CPR during bouts of either acute or chronic illness (choice C).

10. Correct answer: E

In this patient who still wants CPR despite being terminally ill, he should continue to receive hospice care and should receive ongoing education as to why CPR will not be effective and could be potentially harmful to patients like him and their families (choice E). With this increased education, it is not uncommon that before death, patients change their minds and decide to forgo CPR. It would be inappropriate to discharge him from the hospice as he is terminally ill and needs the care, and, based on the PSDA, the patient may not be denied care based on his advance directive wishes, which in this case is to receive CPR (choice A). Telling him you will provide CPR and then not provide it by writing a DNR on his chart would be inappropriate (choice B) as it would both violate patient autonomy and entail lying to the patient. Being truthful and telling him you will not provide CPR when this is his wish remains a violation of patient autonomy (choice D). Documenting your conversation and providing CPR without any attempt at educating the patient (choice C) would also not be an appropriate action, as it has been shown that with proper education, patients often change their minds and decide to forgo CPR.

Chapter 23

1. Correct answer: D

American physicians make the distinction between the physician-assisted suicide and euthanasia (choice D), even though the majority would not participate in either (choice E). Physician-assisted suicide is not universally endorsed by national medical organizations (choice A), nor is it supported by the majority of American public (choice B). Unlike physicians, the majority of the American public does not distinguish between physician-assisted suicide and euthanasia (choice C).

2. Correct answer: A

While PAS is defined as the patient ending his own life, in the states where PAS is legal, another person may not administer the lethal medication to the patient, rather, patients must always take the medications themselves unassisted (choice A). Voluntary euthanasia means a physician and a competent patient agree to life termination (choice B), while involuntary euthanasia means that the physician acts at the request of a surrogate for

an incompetent patient (choice D). Euthanasia always implies that the physician plays an active role (choice C). However, if a physician acts alone to hasten a patient's death, without consent of the patient or her surrogate, it could be seen as murder (choice E).

3. Correct answer: E

If the negative effect occurs and there was no negligence in the performance of the act, then the physician is not considered liable for the occurrence of the negative effect (choice E), as long as the patient has knowledge that the negative effect was a possible outcome (choice C). The rule of double effect allows one to proceed with an intervention that has two possible effects, one positive and one negative, providing that the intent of the action is the positive effect (choice D), the benefit of the positive effect outweighs the burdens of the negative effect (choice A), and the negative effect is not the means to the positive effect (choice B).

4. Correct answer: E

Depression is not one of the major reasons that patients request the hastening of death, with only about 1% of patients requesting euthanasia due to this symptom (choice E). The Dutch Euthanasia Act protects practitioners if due care is taken in the performance of euthanasia and assisted suicide (choice A). The Act allows euthanasia if the patient has unbearable suffering without hope of recovery (choice B). The most common location at which the intervention of euthanasia takes place is the patient's home (choice C). With the publication of guidelines for palliative sedation in 2005, the rate of palliative sedation has increased, while the use of euthanasia has decreased (choice D).

5. Correct answer: B

The number of patients requesting prescriptions has remained relatively stable over the years (choice B), indicating that there is a defined group in the population who perceive this as an appropriate action for themselves. In fact, since the inception of the Act through 2008, less than 400 patients have actually chosen to end their own lives (choice A), which represents approximately 60% of the total number of patients who were given prescriptions by their physicians (choice C). The majority of patients requesting prescriptions had a cancer diagnosis (choice D) and the most common reason for the request was loss of autonomy (choice E).

6. Correct answer: A

While there was concern that this Act would result in a slippery slope of ever-increasing numbers of people availing themselves of the option of physician assisted death, that has not occurred (choice A). However, there has been a marked increase in the utilization of various forms of end-of-life care, resulting in better care of the dying. Knowledge and sophistication of palliative care have increased (choice B), hospice referrals in Oregon have increased (choice C), physician training in palliative care has increased (choice D), and patients and physicians communicate better regarding end-of-life choices (choice E).

7. Correct answer: E

Autonomy works both ways, and under the Oregon and Washington State acts that allow physician-assisted suicide, physicians are exempt from participation if they morally object (choice E). In fact in the entire history of the Oregon Death with Dignity Act, only 45 physicians have written the majority of the prescriptions. Nevertheless, the request for PAS under the Oregon and Washington State acts clearly derive from the principle of autonomy (choice D). Regarding the evolution of patient autonomy regarding health care decision making, the Quinlan case established the right to refuse unwanted therapies (choice A). The Cruzan case established that artificial nutrition and hydration can be refused (choice B), and the

Bouvia case (CA) established the right to control one's destiny (choice C).

8. Correct answer: D

The acceptability of a particular form of palliative sedation as legal and ethical is based on its goal and intent. Rapid sedation to suppress respiration would be consistent with the intent of shortening life, which could be considered a form of active euthanasia that is not ethically acceptable or legal in the United States (choice D). All the other forms of palliative sedation listed are legal and acceptable. Proportionate sedation has as its goal using the minimal amount of sedation needed to achieve the relief of symptoms that is acceptable to the patient (choice A). Palliative sedation to unconsciousness chooses its goal based on the fact that the continued perception of symptoms is unacceptable to the imminently dying patient (choice B). Respite sedation provides a symptomatic patient with sedation for a predetermined interval, following which the patient is brought back to consciousness (choice C). This may often break a cycle of anxiety, agitation, or insomnia, and the patient may not require further alteration of the level of consciousness afterward. Ordinary sedation is the term used to describe the intervention commonly used to relieve anxiety or depression (choice E). As a decrease in level of consciousness is not desired, if it should decrease, the sedating medication would be decreased to improve the patient's level of awareness.

9. Correct answer: C

Because of the fact that it is difficult to define or quantify, when patients request palliative sedation for existential suffering, end-of-life care providers raise significant ethical questions as to whether or not this would be an appropriate intervention (choice C). As existential suffering generally does not cause any overt physical discomfort, the option of additional psychosocial or spiritual counseling, for example, is often considered a much more appropriate intervention. Intractable pain (choice A), as well as intractable dyspnea (choice B), delirium (choice D), and nausea (choice E) may all be appropriately treated with palliative sedation when state of the art pharmacological and nonpharmacological interventions have been unsuccessful in achieving adequate symptom control.

10. Correct answer: B

Physicians often have more than one intention when an intervention is planned (choice B), so intent may not always be clearly seen. Intent allows physicians to use interventions with serious or lethal side effects as long as these were not the primary goals (choice A). It is better defined by what the clinician does, rather than by what s/he says (choice C). By focusing on intent, clinicians are able to think about the consequences of their actions before making a decision to proceed (choice D). Intent is clearly seen in actions that seem reasonable to other clinicians (choice E).

Chapter 24

1. Correct answer: D

A 2002 study in the *Journal of the American Geriatrics Society* documented that 70% of patients 80 and older would want the care they receive focused on comfort rather than life prolongation (choice D). Nevertheless, the use of life-sustaining treatments was prevalent in these patients. This study also demonstrated that the intensive care given to these patients did not affect survival, suggesting that ineffective treatments were given to patients against their stated will.

2. Correct answer: A

Beginning in 1976 with the case of Karen Ann Quinlan, the courts have affirmed the rights of individuals to refuse any unwanted intervention based on the principle of autonomy (choice A). When patients are not competent to make these decisions for themselves, a surrogate may be empowered to make these decisions on the patient's behalf. In the case of Nancy Cruzan in 1990, the US Supreme Court affirmed that feeding tubes are a medical intervention. In fact, the Cruzan case specifically stated that the administration of artificial nutrition and hydration without consent is an intrusion on personal liberty. That being said, 20 states have one or more explicit statutory provisions delineating a separate and more stringent standard for refusal of artificial nutrition and hydration. Beneficence (choice B) is the obligation to provide and receive care that is beneficial, while nonmaleficence (choice C) is the avoidance of harm. Justice (choice D) includes doing what is best for the society as a whole, which includes the allocation of resources.

3. Correct answer: C

One of the most common errors made in moral decision making is ambiguity surrounding the case. Therefore, the first thing that one should do in the decision-making process is to clarify the facts (choice C). Not only do the issues need to be clearly defined, but so does the terminology. For example, some ethicists have included spoon feeding in the definition of artificial nutrition and hydration. If this definition is to be used, all parties involved in the discussion should use the same definition so that it may then be discussed without leading to confusion or ambiguity. Identifying ethical concerns (choice A), framing the issue (choice B), and identifying and resolving conflict (choice D) are all part of Fleming's model, but they can only effectively be accomplished after the facts are clarified.

4. Correct answer: C

The salient feature of anorexia/cachexia is systemic inflammation (choice C). This mechanism for anorexia/cachexia occurs in terminal conditions as well as in progressive, potentially nonterminal conditions such as tuberculosis, malaria, and rheumatoid arthritis. Host cytokines (including interleukin 1 and 6, tumor necrosis factor, and interferon) cause wasting of peripheral tissues, which result in, among other effects, protein calorie malnutrition (choice B) and loss of fat mass (choice D), both of which give rise to unintentional weight loss (choice A).

5. Correct answer: A

REE in COPD is increased (choice A), although the reason for this is not well understood. It is not a result of inadequate intake, however, because the physiologic response to starvation is for REE to be decreased. Two main hypotheses are an increased work of breathing and a generalized hypermetabolic state similar to cardiac and cancer cachexia. Tumor necrosis factor (which inhibits lipoprotein lipase) is increased in a proportion of COPD patients.

6. Correct answer: C

Approximately 50% (choice C) of patients treated with megestrol acetate experience an increase in appetite and overall well-being, which may translate for some patients into an improvement in quality of life. In contrast, only approximately 20% of patients actually gain weight, suggesting that it is quality of life, rather than absolute weight gain, that should be the goal of therapy with megestrol acetate.

7. Correct answer: B

Although studies have shown an increase in appetite with cannabinoids, recent evidence indicates that the effects on appetite were present in placebo-treated groups as well (choice B), raising questions regarding the actual efficacy of the cannabinoids. Part of the relative ineffectiveness of these agents is thought to be due to insufficient targeting of proinflammatory cytokines. Cannabinoids have not been shown to increase muscle mass (choice A);

they can actually impair cognition (choice C) and they have a number of serious side effects, especially in the elderly (choice D).

8. Correct answer: D

Studies evaluating patient mortality following PEG tube placement have shown that up to one-half of all patients who receive a PEG tube for nutritional support succumb to their primary illness within one year of PEG placement (choice D), raising serious questions regarding the need for better patient selection. Case controlled studies have identified tube feeding as a risk factor for aspiration pneumonia (choice A). Although no prospective trials have been done, retrospective studies show only an increased risk or no benefit from tube feeding. There are no studies to date that demonstrate that wound healing improves when patients are fed via PEG tube (choice B). In addition, there are no studies that show decreased rates of infections with tube feeding (choice C). In fact, gastrostomy tubes are associated with cellulites, abscess, and diarrhea (infectious and noninfectious). There are some reports that demonstrated streptococcal bacteremia secondary to feeding tubes and evidence of bacteremia secondary to contaminated enteral solutions.

9. Correct answer: B

1999 data documented that 34% of all severely cognitively impaired nursing home residents had feeding tubes (choice B). Surveys have confirmed that physicians believe the intervention is beneficial and is the standard of care for these patients. Nursing homes receive higher reimbursements for feeding tube patients and avoid allegations of abuse and neglect for patients with severe weight loss because "everything is being done."

10. Correct answer: D

Although randomized trials have not been published to date, observational studies suggest that administration of parenteral fluids may increase blood pressure (choice D) and treat symptoms of postural hypotension in selected terminally ill cancer patients. Small amounts of parenteral fluids in selected patients may also decrease symptoms of delirium (particularly opioid induced, as renal clearance of opioid metabolites improve) (choice C), sedation (choice A), and opioid-induced myoclonus (choice B).

Chapter 25

1. Correct answer: B

Prior to the advent of antiretroviral therapy, the average survival after a first episode of PCP was approximately 10 months. Following the development of the antiretroviral agents, highly active antiretroviral therapy (HAART), and prophylactic antibiotic therapy, the average survival following the first episode of PCP is now considered indefinite (choice B). MAC (choice A), CMV (choice C), PML (choice D), and AIDS-related lymphoma (choice E) were all shown to more likely be diagnosed during the last 12 months of life (Welsh and Morse, 2002).

2. Correct answer: B

PCP occurs in approximately 80% of patients who do not receive prophylaxis. Therefore, it is reasonable, even near the end of life, to treat all patients prophylactically for PCP. CMV retinitis occurs in only approximately 25% of patients not treated prophylactically and once diagnosed, it generally responds rapidly to treatment. Therefore, primary prophylaxis to prevent CMV retinitis is generally not indicated in the palliative care setting. Regarding MAC, the toxicity of prophylaxis outweighs the potential benefits in terminally ill patients, and therefore, prophylaxis is generally not indicated.

Therefore, based on the above discussion, only PCP prophylaxis should be continued (choice B).

3. Correct answer: A

This patient should be treated for active CMV with intravenous ganciclovir (choice A). An intravitreal implant might be considered for maintenance therapy if the patient has a reasonable life expectancy, but is not indicated for primary therapy (choice B). Although cidofovir is only administered every 2 weeks (after the induction dosing of weekly for 2 weeks), which would seem to make it ideal for a hospice setting, it has significant nephrotoxicity, making it a difficult agent to use near the end of life (choice C). Foscarnet has nephrotoxicity similar to cidofovir and maintenance therapy requires daily infusions, making it even more problematic (choice D). The option not to treat is unreasonable in this situation, as the preservation of the patient's vision is a significant quality-of-life issue, and he is both active and desires to have his vision preserved (choice E).

4. Correct answer: D

AIDS-related lymphomas are generally very aggressive and they respond very poorly to antineoplastic therapy (choice D). Primary central nervous system lymphoma (PCNSL) is one type of AIDS-related lymphoma (choice C). AIDS-related Kaposi's sarcoma (KS) is a much more aggressive neoplasm than the classic form of KS (choice A) and the most common extracutaneous site of KS is the gastrointestinal tract (choice B). For both KS and AIDS-associated lymphomas, when antineoplastic therapy is not appropriate or indicated, patients should be treated symptomatically with steroids, analgesics, and other palliative measures (choice E).

5. Correct answer: C

This patient has no obvious correctable cause of fever and in view of her poor performance status, the best next step in her management would be to treat her symptomatically with steroids (choice C). Her poor performance status dictates that neither a full work-up for fever (choices D and E) nor a more limited diagnostic evaluation (choice A) would be appropriate. Additionally, given her advanced condition, treating her empirically with antibiotics without doing even a limited work-up could not be justified (choice B).

6. Correct answer: B

Dysphagia and odynophagia is usually the result of esophagitis, with Candidal infection being the most common etiology of the esophagitis (choice B). Less common causes of esophagitis include apthous ulcerations (choice A), CMV (choice C), and herpes simplex (choice D). Lesions from KS can sometimes involve the esophagus, leading to symptoms of dysphagia and odynophagia (choice E).

7. Correct answer: C

Fatigue in AIDS is associated with high levels of psychological distress (choice C). Estimates for the prevalence of fatigue in AIDS ranges from 40% to 50% (choice A), and some studies have shown a higher prevalence of fatigue in HIV-infected women compared with men (choice B). Fatigue in AIDS does correlate with advanced disease as indicated by a greater number of physical symptoms (choice D). Steroids are a mainstay of the treatment of fatigue in patients with advanced AIDS (choice E).

8. Correct answer: D

Although tricyclic antidepressants have been the traditional first-line treatment for neuropathic pain, they are of limited benefit in reducing neuropathic pain secondary to AIDS, and cause significant side effects, including somnolence and orothostatic hypotension (choice D). The prevalence of pain in advanced AIDS does range between 75% and 80% (choice A). Neuropathic pain in AIDS may be secondary to a number of drugs used to treat the AIDS virus including d4T, ddI,

and ddC (choice B), or it may be caused by HIV infection itself (choice C). Gabapentin is an anticonvulsant that is effective in the treatment of neuropathic pain (choice E).

9. Correct answer: B

AIDS Wasting syndrome includes a weight loss of at least 10%, accompanied by diarrhea, chronic weakness, and fever for at least 30 days (choice B) not attributable to another cause.

10. Correct answer: D

EF is actually very resistant to treatment and topical steroids rarely provide relief (choice D). EF lesions consist of small follicular papules and pustules (choice A), and is associated with low CD4 counts and low nadir counts (choice B). Although the etiology of EF is not clear, it is hypothesized that the rash may be secondary to hypersensitivity to the Demodex folliculorum mite (choice C). Oral metronidazole is a treatment option for EF (choice E).

Chapter 26

1. Correct answer: C

Children younger than 18 years are legally considered not competent to make decisions about their own health care, and any advance directive document created by a child younger than 18 years would not be considered legally valid (choice C). A family often views a dying child as not having had a "full and complete life" and therefore wants to do everything they can to prolong the child's life (choice A). More complex bereavement needs in pediatric hospice are the result of the overwhelming burden a parent often experiences with the loss of a child, as well the challenge of helping siblings cope with the loss of a brother or sister (choice B). Hospice admission criteria for pediatrics is much less well defined, and hospices often admit pediatric patients with prognoses much greater than the 6 months or less required in adult hospice (choice D). The developmental age of a child can significantly affect a child's understanding of life and death, and must be well understood by professional caregivers (choice E).

2. Correct answer: A

Neonates may experience increased sensitivity to pain because their inhibitory pain tracts are underdeveloped (choice A). In fact, the central nervous system of a 26-week-old fetus has the structural or neurochemical ability to experience pain (choice B) and these two facts help debunk the myth that infants do not feel pain. Children do not tolerate pain better than adults, and it has been shown that the tolerance to pain in children increases with age (choice C). Children are able to communicate appropriately about their pain within the parameters of the child's developmental age (choice D). Despite the fact that children can communicate appropriately about their pain, they often choose not to do so, sometimes due to the fear of receiving an injection (choice E).

3. Correct answer: D

A useful pneumonic to remember when assessing a child's pain is QUEST. The "S" stands for "Secure parents' involvement." It is important to include the parents in the evaluation as they know their child best and not avoid their involvement (choice D). The rest of the QUEST pneumonic, which is listed in Table 26–3, includes "Q"uestioning the child (choice A), "U"sing pain rating scales (choice B), "E"valuating behavior and physiologic changes (choice C), and "T"aking action and evaluating the results (choice E).

4. Correct answer: C

The FLACC scale looks at five different domains to assess pain: the face, the legs, activity, crying, and consolability. It then provides descriptions of observed behaviors for each area that are assigned numerical values of 0, 1, or 2, depending on the severity. In the infant being

observed, the clenched jaw (face), the constant crying (crying), and the inability to console the child (consolability) each have a value of 2 (total = 6). The tense and restless legs and continuous squirming each have a value of 1 (total = 2). The overall FLACC score for the infant, therefore, is 8 (choice C).

5. Correct answer: C

Due to a number of factors, including immature liver function, decreased renal clearance, smaller volume of distribution, and possibly increased permeability into the brain, the recommended dose of morphine in infants younger than 6 months of age should be one-fourth to one-third that of older children (choice C). The above factors combined with an infant's immature responses to hypoxia and hypercarbia significantly increase the risk of respiratory depression. Although the recommended dose of acetaminophen is the same in infants and older children, the frequency of acetaminophen administration should be decreased from every 4 hours to every 6 hours, due to a slower absorption rate and prolonged half-life in infants (choice A). Immature liver function also dictates that the medication should only be used for short period to avoid hepatotoxicity (choice B). The risk of respiratory depression as a side effect mirrors that of older children (choice D).

6. Correct answer: A

Of these agents, only chlorpromazine (choice A) can be administered to children younger than 2 years of age, although it should be avoided in infants younger than 6 months as well. Prochlorperazine (choice B), promethazine (choice C), and granisetron (choice D) are all not recommended for children younger than the age of 2.

7. Correct answer: D

There are many advantages to having a dying child cared for at home. One of these is that bereavement is less, not more, complicated for the siblings (choice D). Parents can pay more attention and provide more support to their other children (choice A), siblings can participate in the care and entertainment of their brother or sister (choice B), and the dying child will feel less isolated and have a more peaceful death (choice C).

8. Correct answer: C

It is during the ages of 6 and 12 that children begin to understand that death is permanent (choice C). Infants and toddlers younger than 3 years can only understand death as separation from parents (choice A). Between 3 and 6, children see death as the loss of a loving and protective object, but believe it to be reversible (choice B). Adolescents fully recognize death as final and irrevocable act, but often struggle with the possibility of their own death (choice D).

9. Correct answer: A

When an adult discusses death with a child, the adult should follow the child's lead regarding the timing and extent of the conversation (choice A). Communication should be brief and the conversation should be specific and literal (choice C). Expressions comparing death to a trip or a long sleep should be avoided as they can confuse the child (choice B). Nonverbal communication through such media as art and music can make the communication between adult and child easier (choice D).

10. Correct answer: C

It is important for him stay involved, and in this situation, where the physician is not experienced in the principles of hospice and palliative care, the hospice physician will provide consultative support to ensure the patient receives the best palliative care (choice C). Pediatrician involvement is important because it has been shown that maintaining the relationship between the physician and the patient and family helps ensure a smooth transition to end-of-life care (choice A). It is not reasonable nor is it good medical care to tell the pediatrician that to stay involved means he would be responsible to give all the patient's palliative care orders (choice B). Finally, for the reasons given above, it is certainly unreasonable, and against the principles of good hospice and palliative medicine, to exclude the physician from participation in the patient's care because he is inexperienced in hospice and palliative care (choice D).

Chapter 27

1. Correct answer: B

Children should only be allowed to attend funerals and memorials if they choose to (choice B). When a child chooses not to attend, it is important, though, to ascertain the reasons why the child wishes not to attend such a commemorative event. If it seems too overwhelming to them or if they are scared, the adult can describe details of the event with a child and ask again. If the child still does not wish to attend, the adult could suggest alternative commemorative activities such as planting a tree, writing a letter, etc. It is not appropriate to try and protect a child from experiencing grief (choice A), children can understand death and grief to the extent that their developmental level allows (choice C), and children are not any more resilient than adults following a loss (choice D).

2. Correct answer: B

It is thought that children do not have the mental capacity at age 4 and below to conceptualize what permanent and irreversible death might mean (choice B). They imagine that the deceased might just wake up or come back from a trip. Anxiety related to separation from a major attachment figure (choice A), irritability, protest, and crying (choice C), changes in eating and sleeping patterns (choice D), and a lack of understanding that death is something that can happen to them (choice E) are all typical grief reactions seen in infants and toddlers.

3. Correct answer: E

Whether or not children or teenagers can read does not significantly influence how they respond to grief and loss (choice E). Others can read books on grief appropriate for children to such children and they can be taught helpful truths about dying and about loss of a loved one. The developmental and chronological age of a child (choice A), the nature of the relationship with the person who died (choice B), the child's innate personality (choice C), and what they have been taught by others about death and grief (choice D) all significantly influence how children and teenagers respond to grief and loss.

4. Correct answer: D

There are times when a child becomes so preoccupied with thoughts and memories of a significant loved one that they regress to a former developmental age (one where the loved one was still alive) and begin to have difficulty functioning in one or several aspects of their life. In this case, it is often necessary to receive trained, professional help (choice D). Memory difficulties (choice A), searching behavior (choice B), difficulty concentrating (choice C), and even idealization of the deceased (choice E) are more typical grief reactions seen in children, and generally do not require professional help to resolve unless they either last an inordinately long time or significantly interfere with the child's functioning.

5. Correct answer: B

It is never healthy for any mourner, child or adult, to make a decision to "forget their loved one and move on" (choice B). Many grief experts instead say that the nature of the relationship with the loved one changes. Although the loved one is not physically there any longer, the mourner reintegrates aspects of the loved one into their lives. A return to stable eating and sleeping patterns (choice A), an increase in thinking and judgment capabilities (choice C),

and the establishment of new and healthy relationships (choice D) are all evidence that a child is adjusting to the physical loss of a loved one.

6. Correct answer: D

A teenager who is having sleep disturbances that are prolonged and include bouts of insomnia or nightmares, is suffering from a complicated grief reaction and will need professional help (choice D). Assuming mannerisms, traits or wearing clothes of the deceased (choice A), emotional regression and bed-wetting (choice B), becoming overly responsible (choice C), and needing to repeat stories of their loved one over and over again (choice E) are all considered typical teenage grief reactions and may be managed more without professional help unless they last an inordinately long time or interfere with a teenager's functioning.

7. Correct answer: D

Anger and lashing out seemingly for no reason are actually very normal grief reactions for a child (choice D). Typically, children act out their feelings and emotions through behavior. Anger is often directed at other significant adults in the child's life. A child who ruminates about how he caused the death of a loved one (choice A), extreme withdrawal, isolation, and the inability to socialize with others (choice B), pervasive fantasies that get in the way of normal functioning (choice C), and persistent assumption of the mannerisms of the deceased, including those not developmentally appropriate (choice E) are all symptoms of complicated grief and often require professional assistance by a mental health professional trained in children and grief for resolution.

8. Correct answer: A

It is generally important *not* to wait to tell a child about a dying loved one for a variety of reasons. Because of their vivid imaginations, children experience more anxiety if they suspect that something is wrong and no one is discussing it. If they are not told, they may miss important opportunities to be part of the care of their loved one, to interact in ways that may have lasting memories, etc. It is often misguided attempts by adults to protect a child that lead them to believe that they should not explain what is happening (choice A). All of the other interventions are considered very appropriate.

9. Correct answer: C

Telling a child that God wanted their loved one is wrong for several reasons. God may not have a part in the belief system of the child's family and might confuse them. It might make the child more anxious as they might believe that God might want to take them too, or take someone else that they love (choice C). The child should be assured in very specific ways how he or she will continue to be cared for (choice A), which can be aided by maintaining the child's environment and routine as much as possible (choice B). Although adults should not hide grief from children, children should be not used by adults as their sole support when grieving (choice D). It is also important for adults to respect a child who desires not to talk about his or her grief (choice E).

10. Correct answer: A

Asking the child to "calm down" may give the message that having feelings such as anger is not OK (choice A). The message should instead be that it is OK and normal to have such feelings, and that there are appropriate ways for us to express the feelings. Running or exercising (choice B) and involving the child in art work (choice C) are useful techniques to help the child channel his or her anger in a more useful direction. Asking the child about the angry feelings (choice D) or for ideas as to how he or she might respond to angry feelings (choice E), may also be very helpful.

Chapter 28

1. Correct answer: B

The process by which patients are kept in the hospital for fewer days for acute illness is a reason for the increase in emergency department (ED) visits (choice B). Patients often do not have sufficient support at home and at the first sign of anything untoward they return to the ED. Elderly patients with chronic medical problems are best evaluated by their primary physician in an outpatient setting for exacerbation of symptoms, not in the ED (choice A). Due to, among other issues, a nursing shortage, there are an insufficient number of nurses in the ED to allow for a smooth flow of patients (choice C). This creates added stress in the ED, which may be compounded if the ED is also a Level 1 trauma center (choice D). Patients who do not have medical insurance or other resources available to pay for medical care more often use the ED to receive care than those who have coverage or are able to pay for care (choice E).

2. Correct answer: C

Although dehydration is certainly one of the reasons why elderly patients may be brought to the ED for care, the most common diagnosis that prompts an elder to visit the ED is congestive heart failure (choice C). The elderly represent more than 40% of all ED visits (choice A) and more than 40% of ICU admissions from the ED (choice B). The majority of these visits occur at night or on the weekends (choice D), and most of the elderly patients seen in the ED live in long-term care facilities (choice E).

3. Correct answer: D

Elderly patients often have complicated medical problems with complex treatment regimens and variable prognoses, and are often poorly cooperative and agitated. This makes triage and management in the ED setting very challenging (choice D). The ideal ED patient is one who is easily triaged and able to be moved through the system rapidly. Such a patient would tend to have a straightforward medical problem with a defined treatment (choice A), a defined prognosis (choice B), and is relatively easy to treat and/or stabilize (choice C). Cooperation and compliance on the patient's part is also helpful in achieving effective management in the emergency setting (choice E).

4. Correct answer: E

The ED staff should be cognizant of patients who return to the ED frequently, and when such patients show signs of progressive deterioration it is very appropriate for the ED staff to discuss with the family the advisability of a hospice or palliative care referral (choice E). Advance care planning cannot be done in the hurried atmosphere of the ED (choice A), nor can counseling by staff members who may not know the patient as well as the primary physician (choice B). Care in the ED is designed to stabilize acute medical problems, and there is usually insufficient time to see to and palliate all patient needs in this service area (choice C). As an acute care service, there is no mechanism for bereavement follow-up in an ED (choice D).

5. Correct answer: E

EOL providers may provide bereavement services to family members irrespective of how short or long the patient received EOL care prior to death (choice E), even if the time is measured in minutes or hours. EOL providers may also collaborate with the ED by consulting with patients and families regarding goals of care and advance care planning conversations (choice A) and by arranging for patient transfer from the ED to an alternative setting (i.e., inpatient hospice/palliative care or home care) even if care planning is still underway (choice B). If a patient already under the care of a hospice program or other EOL

provider is brought to the ED, quick intervention by the EOL provider may prevent the patient from receiving unwanted care (choice C). EOL providers may also provide support and counseling to ED staff members (choice D).

6. Correct answer: A

Although death is an expected outcome in hospice care, it is not in the ICU (choice A). When a patient enters an ICU for care, the expectation is that there will be a positive outcome with the patient leaving the unit and the hospital. Both critical care and EOL providers care for the sickest patients in the system (choice B) and improve patient outcomes by aggressively controlling patient symptoms (choice D). Care for patients in both settings is also time intensive (choice C). When palliative care consult services are available in the ICU, there is improvement in patient and family satisfaction with the overall care provided in the critical care area (choice E).

7. Correct answer: D

A longstanding patient/physician relationship results in a decrease in medical costs because the physician knows which interventions the patient prefers. This may result in either reduction in the number of ICU days, or in many cases, avoidance of the ICU altogether (choice D). Approximately 20% of Americans die in the critical care setting (choice A) and this care consumes approximately 80% of the total costs of terminal hospital care (choice C). Most ICU deaths occur in patients older than 65 years (choice B). Increasing fragmentation of the health care system has resulted in an increase in the number of days patients spend on average in the ICU and in the cost of ICU care (choice E).

8. Correct answer: B

The "hope for the best" attitude is more common among medical practitioners and some specialists (choice B), with surgeons, being likely to continue interventions until it is clear that the patient is not going to recover. ICUs are high-tech interventional environments (choice A). Patients admitted or transferred to the ICU are assumed to have agreed to receive the type of care that is traditionally provided in this area (choice C). Medical specialists tend to be more comfortable moving away from disease-driven care when patients require chronic long-term life support, such as a tracheostomy for long-term ventilation (choice D). In surgical ICUs, EOL care decisions usually revolve around withdrawal of life sustaining measures in the last days or hours of life, when all available interventions have been exhausted (choice E).

9. Correct answer: C

Prognostic tools are derived retrospectively based on the experience of a group of patients with defined characteristics and this limits their ability to prospectively determine the prognosis of an individual patient with different clinical characteristics (choice C). On entry to the ICU, patients usually have the same goals as the clinicians caring for them, which is to improve the medical situation in order to maximize the chances of survival (choice A). Only 5% of patients in the ICU can make their own decisions (choice B). Quality of life is not one of the factors considered in tools used to prognosticate prognosis in the critical care setting (choice D). Because of the fact that prognostic tools lack the flexibility to account for individual patient characteristics that may impact individual (rather than population) outcomes, physicians are very uncomfortable with these tools (choice E).

10. Correct answer: E

As a precursor of palliative care consultations, ethics consultations, even if simply clarifying the clinical situation of the patient, have been shown to result in fewer patients proceeding with ventilator support and a greater number of patients choosing to discontinue this

intervention (choice E). Most physicians typically spend family encounter time talking rather than listening (choice A). Family meetings of any kind decrease length of stay in the ICU (choice B). Palliative care consultations have no direct effect on patient mortality (choice C), rather they effect where patients receive their care and the nature of the care they receive. Palliative care consultations have been shown to result in shorter ICU stays (choice D).

Chapter 29

1. Correct answer: B

2007 data compiled by the NHPCO showed that about 28% (choice B) of hospice patients were LTCF residents, which was a modest increase from the slightly more than 27% who were LTCF residents in 2006. It is expected that this percentage will continue to rise as the general population continues to age, and more elderly people spend their final years in a facility.

2. Correct answer: E

As both the "Skilled Nursing Facility Care Benefit" and the Medicare Hospice Benefit are Part A benefits under the Medicare program, they cannot be accessed concurrently if the skilled care is related to the terminal diagnosis (choice E) since the hospice is responsible for all care related to the terminal illness. These two benefits can theoretically be accessed concurrently if the patient's skilled care is for a need that is unrelated to the hospice terminal diagnosis, although it is often difficult to clearly determine whether the patient's two conditions are truly not related to one another. To access the "Skilled Nursing Facility Benefit," a patient must be hospitalized for 3 consecutive days within 30 days of facility admission (choice A). The skilled care the patient requires should be related to the hospitalization (choice B), can only be effectively provided in a skilled nursing facility (choice C), and, must be provided daily (choice D), with the exception of skilled rehabilitation therapy that may be delivered 5 to 6 days a week.

3. Correct answer: A

The Medicare Hospice Benefit does not cover room and board payments for patients who reside in LTCFs (choice A). Patients continue to pay for their room and board as they did before hospice enrollment, which may be privately, through long-term care insurance coverage, managed care coverage, or via Medicaid. For Medicaid patients, the room and board rate is discounted 5% and paid to the hospice under the "unified rate" program and the hospice is then responsible to pay the facility (choice C). Patients who exhibit appropriate needs can receive continuous care in the facility (choice B), and can also receive general inpatient care in the facility if the hospice and the facility have an appropriate contract in place (choice E). For the purposes of the Medicare Hospice Benefit, the LTCF is considered the patient's primary residence (choice D).

4. Correct answer: D

According to Hospice Condition of Participation (CoP) §418.112, LTCFs residents must meet the same eligibility criteria as all other hospice patients, which in the case of prognosis is 6 months or less if the illness runs its normal course (choice D). The hospice does assume responsibility for professional management of all hospice services provided to the resident in accordance with the hospice plan of care (choice B), while leaving the LTCF responsible for any non–hospice-related services required by the patient. There must be a written agreement between the hospice and the LTCF (choice A), there must be a written plan of care established by the hospice and maintained in consultation with the LTCF staff (choice E), and the hospice must orient and train the LTCF staff regarding hospice policies, procedures, and principles of hospice care and pain and symptom management (choice C).

5. Correct answer: B

Although it would be prudent for the LTCF staff to notify the hospice if a family member demands to speak to them, it is not required that this be delineated in the written agreement between the two providers (choice B). It is required to be delineated in the contract that the LTCF notify the hospice immediately if there is a significant change of any kind in the patient's condition (choice A), if a complication occurs that may require a change to the plan of care (choice C), if the patient needs transfer to a higher level of care (choice D), or if the patient passes on (choice E).

6. Correct answer: A

The hospice is responsible to provide services at the same level and extent that would have been provided had the patient been living at home. Therefore, it will not be permissible for the hospice to reduce the number of visits because the patient is residing in a LTCF facility that has its own nursing and nurses aide staff (choice A). This is also why the hospice may only use the LTCF facility nurses to assist in the administration of medications only to the same extent as the primary caregiver would have done if the patient had been living at home (choice C) and why the LTCF is responsible for the personal care and nursing needs that would have been provided by the primary caregiver at home (choice D). It is the hospice's responsibility to determine if the patient requires a change in the level of hospice care (choice B), and the written agreement must also delineate the responsibility of the hospice in providing bereavement support to LTCF staff (choice E).

7. Correct answer: C

A RAP or "Resident Assessment Protocol" is a problem-specific document that the LTCF nurse assessing a patient utilizes to further assess and care plan for the identified problem (choice C). The RAI or "Resident

Assessment Instrument" is the document used to perform the comprehensive admission assessment (choice A). The RAI includes the MDS, or "Minimum Data Set," which is a set of data obtained on patients during the comprehensive assessment (choice B) that are reported to CMS, "Center for Medicare and Medicaid Services," the government agency that oversees and administers the Medicare and Medicaid programs (choice D). An ALF, or "Adult Living Facility" is one type of LTCF (choice E).

8. Correct answer: E

As LTCF goals as defined by the RAPs are generally rehabilitative in nature and focus on improvement, and, by their nature, hospice patients are not expected to achieve improvement in many areas, goals of care for hospice patients may have to be adjusted from those typically seen in the RAPs to account for this. So, while it is important as part of a coordinated hospice/LTCF plan of care for the hospice plan to maintain as much resemblance to the RAPs as possible, it would not be appropriate to set goals for patient improvement when none is expected (choice E). On the other hand, by using the RAP problem list (choice A), using similar language (choice B), updating the care plan using the RAP process (choice C), and using similar interventions (choice D), the hospice can ensure that the LTCF staff is familiar and comfortable with the hospice plan of care, and will be able to document appropriately.

9. Correct answer: C

Studies regarding end-of-life care in LTCFs prior to the widespread incorporation of hospice services showed significant deficits in advance care planning, with one outcome being an increase in the use of feeding tubes, despite the growing body of medical evidence that artificial feedings was of limited or no benefit in many of these patients (choice C). These advance care planning deficits also resulted in lower rates of "do-not-resuscitate" orders among LTCF residents (choice E). Symptoms such as pain (choice A) and dyspnea (choice B) were documented as being poorly controlled, and family members had very low expectations regarding the quality of care they expected their loved ones to receive (choice D).

10. Correct answer: A

Studies assessing the impact of hospice services in LTCFs have shown fewer hospitalizations (choice A), as the goal is to manage the patient in place. These studies have also shown less use of feeding tubes (choice B), management of pain consistent with accepted guidelines (choice C), and a perception among family members that their loved ones care is improved following hospice admission (choice D). Also of great interest is that studies have demonstrated that the management of non-hospice patient symptoms such as pain and dyspnea have improved in facilities where hospice has a large presence (choice E).

Chapter 30

1. Correct answer: E

Geriatric patients tend to under-report pain when compared to younger patients (choice E). There are multiple reasons for this, among them the fear of loss of independence and the belief that some pain is part of the normal aging process. Geriatric patients metabolize drugs (choice A) and absorb drugs at different rates than their younger counterparts (choice B). The volume of distribution of drugs in elderly patients is different due to differences in fat content (choice C). Geriatric patients are more likely to have pain from multiple sources than younger patients (choice D).

2. Correct answer: E

Low back pain occurs in approximately 40% of the elderly, and it is the most common cause of pain in this population (choice E). Although over 75% of patients with cancer experience pain, the frequency of low back pain compared to cancer makes the former a much more common occurrence in the overall geriatric population (choice D). Chest pain (choice A), phlebitis (choice B), and constipation (choice C) may all cause pain in the elderly, but at much lower frequency than that of low back pain.

3. Correct answer: C

While some among the elderly may be stoic, this is not a trait common to the geriatric population and does not account for the fact they more commonly under-report pain than younger patients (choice C). Fear of loss of independence (choice A), the belief that pain may be a normal part of aging (choice B), the fear of being a "nuisance" (choice D), and the fear of addiction (choice E) are all reasons why the elderly under-report pain.

4. Correct answer: D

Acetaminophen should always be the first choice for mild to moderate pain due to its better tolerability in the geriatric population compared with the rest of the choices (choice D). The NSAIDs (choice A) have much too high a risk of inducing GI bleeds and renal problems to recommend them to be first-line agents. Aspirin (choice B) is relatively contraindicated (except for cardio-protectiveness) because of the high rate of GI bleeding as well as platelet inhibition. Although the Cox 2-inhibitors (choice C) may be utilized, they are never first line and some authorities suggest total avoidance of the class in this population. Propoxyphene (choice E) should never be used.

5. Correct answer: B

Meperidine is an opioid that should NEVER be used in the geriatric population (choice B). It is poorly orally bioavailable and the toxic metabolite normeperidine causes multiple side effects including dysphoria, irritability, tremors, myoclonus, seizures, as well as the possibility of encephalopathy and death. Although morphine (choice A), fentanyl (choice C), codeine (choice D), and hydrocodone (choice E) can all cause adverse side effects in the geriatric population, they are generally safe and effective when properly used.

6. Correct answer: C

Codeine (choice C) is converted to morphine, which is primarily responsible for its analgesic effects, by the cytochrome P450 enzyme CYP2D6, which is lacking in approximately 10% of the population. The other agents listed: hydrocodone (choice A), oxycodone (choice B), oxymorphone (choice D), and hydromorphone (choice E) are all primarily active and glucuronidated in the liver.

7. Correct answer: A

Fentanyl (choice A) is a lipophillic compound, making it an ideal agent to use by the transdermal route. Because of its lipophillic nature, its absorption is dependent on the degree of body fat, the hydration status of the patient, and the body temperature. Lidocaine (choice B), unlike fentanyl, is highly water soluble. It is not dependent on the factors listed and primarily works locally. Methadone (choice C) is not available in patch form. Capsaicin (choice D) provides its analgesic effects locally. Diclofenac (choice E), which was recently released in patch form, also primarily provides analgesia in the site of application and its efficacy is not dependent on the listed factors.

8. Correct answer: E

Hydromorphone (choice E) is seven times more potent in the parenteral form than parenteral morphine (choice A), making it an ideal parenteral drug when volume becomes an issue. Neither codeine (choice B) nor hydrocodone (choice C) are available in the parenteral form. Although methadone (choice D) does come in a parenteral form, due to difficulty in dosage conversions, hydromorphone should be used initially.

9. Correct answer: C

Gabapentin (choice C) is the safest and most effective of the listed agents for the treatment of neuropathic pain in the elderly. Neuropathic pain is generally less sensitive to morphine (choice A), which is why other agents, such as gabapentin, are required in addition to morphine to treat neuropathic pain. Tramadol (choice B) may be used for treatment of neuropathic pain; however, the doses needed may be excessive for the geriatric population. Amitriptyline (choice D), although an excellent choice in younger patients and a very popular drug for this purpose, is not recommended in the geriatric population due to the propensity for antihistaminic and anticholinergic side effects. Fluoxetine (choice E) and other SSRIs have only been demonstrated to have limited efficacy in the treatment of neuropathic pain.

10. Correct answer: E

Massage therapy (choice E) is the only listed therapy that has been demonstrated to release endorphines. Cold (choice A) has been shown to reduce edema, while heat (choice B) works through the mechanism of vasodilitation. The mechanism of action of TENS therapy (choice C) and vibration therapy (choice D) is via the modulation pathways.

Chapter 31

1. Correct answer: B

The difficulty that physicians may experience in being able to predict when someone has 6 months or less to live is a medical barrier to hospice access (choice B). The mandate to preserve life at all costs (choice A), mistrust of the health care system (choice C), the idea that informing someone that they are terminally ill may hasten death (choice D), and the idea that one is never allowed to "give up" (choice E) are all barriers to hospice access that are rooted in various ethnic, cultural, or religious beliefs.

2. Correct answer: C

Even though individual patients and families may identify with a specific cultural, ethnic, or religious group, the level at which they follow the traditions and practices of the group can be extremely variable. Therefore, one should never try and deduce a patient's or family's needs based on one's knowledge of the group they identify with (choice C). Rather, one must perform a thorough cultural assessment on each patient and family to be able to deliver culturally sensitive care (choice E). A cultural assessment is the part of the comprehensive assessment that elicits information about a patient's cultural, ethnic, or religious traditions (choice A). The cultural assessment may be performed separately, or have questions interspersed into other parts of the comprehensive assessment (choice B). Questions in the cultural assessment may include the patient's country of birth, primary and secondary languages, and customs and rituals related to grief and mourning (choice D).

3. Correct answer: A

Lack of trust in the health care has resulted in a low utilization of advance directives among African Americans (choice A), with one study showing that 75% of 102 patients educated about advance care planning and advance directives still refused to complete one. The culture of mistrust has also led to other significant disparities in the health care delivered to African American patients including the beliefs that they receive less attention by health care providers than white patients (choice B), they feel patronized by physicians' offices (choice C), and they more often leave their doctors' offices unclear about their diagnosis and treatment options as compared to white patients (choice D). In addition, physicians are often accused of not communicating properly with African American patients (choice E).

4. Correct answer: E

African Americans consider the funeral extremely important and have the African view that the funeral reflects the worth of the individual to the community. Therefore, they tend to spend more discretionary income on funerals than their white counterparts (choice E). African Americans tend to be accepting of death, viewing it as part of the continuum of life (choice B). They treat the deceased with great reverence and respect (choice A). There is an expectation that an individual's faith community will provide significant support and comfort to families following a loss (choice C). African Americans often have extended families called "kin networks" which may even include nonblood relatives given the title "aunt" or "uncle." These "kin networks" provide significant support when a member is terminally ill, and when the person passes on, all members of the network, whether a blood relation or not, require bereavement support (choice D).

5. Correct answer: D

When establishing a caregiving relationship with an African American patient and family, especially when advance care planning or end-of-life care decision making is involved, it has been recommended that one should directly discuss any feelings of mistrust toward the health care system with the patient and family (choice D). By doing so, it is believed that a relationship of trust between the parties can be more easily achieved. When discussing end-of-life issues with African American patients and families one should be aware that many believe that choosing not to receive interventions such as CPR or a feeding tube gives the health care system a license to provide substandard care (choice A). African American

patients and families may also feel that deciding to execute an advance directive increases feelings of hopelessness (choice C) and they may often feel conflicted when discontinuing life-prolonging therapy as there is a perception that they are giving up the hope that God will heal them (choice E). Involving spiritual counselors and "kin network" elders in these advance care planning conversations can be very important (choice B).

6. Correct answer: B

As Hispanic Americans view physicians with great respect and as major authority figures, when making end-of-life care decisions, they will more often heed the advice of their physician rather than that of their end-of-life care provider (choice B). Hispanic Americans are people of faith and, therefore, irrespective of their religious affiliation, religion plays a significant role for Hispanic Americans when faced with end-of-life situations (choice A). Family is also deeply embedded into Hispanic American culture. When there is illness in a Hispanic American family, all members of the extended family participate in the care and anticipatory grieving of the ill family member (choice C). Hispanic families, in an attempt to protect the patient, often will not allow any discussion of an ill family member's terminal prognosis (choice D). In addition, although the head of the family is considered the ultimate decision maker, multiple extended family members may be actively involved in end-of-life care decision making (choice E).

7. Correct answer: E

Although Hispanic American families believe that it is important to provide loved ones with nutritional support near the end of life, with proper education and support, many are willing to allow this to be provided noninvasively via spoon feeding or syringe, rather than resorting to a feeding tube (choice E). The importance of providing nutritional support for

Hispanic American patients near the end of life, however, cannot be emphasized enough. Food is considered a powerful symbol of wellness and represents hope for improvement and cure (choice A) and family members often perceive a direct correlation between nutritional support and the amount of care a loved one is receiving (choice B). Religious beliefs are another important factor in prompting families to request that loved ones receive artificial nutritional support or hydration (choice D). Allowing patients to die without food or fluid is considered tantamount to starving or dehydrating the patient to death, and is considered to be "painful and cruel" treatment (choice C).

8. Correct answer: B

Asian Americans have a very strong sense of family, and therefore, it is most common for patients near the end of life to be cared for by loved ones in the home, rather than in an institution (choice B). Approximately 45% of Asian Americans identify themselves as Christian (choice A), with other prominent religions among this population including Hindu (14%), Buddhist (9%), and Muslim (4%). Twenty-three percent of Asian Americans do not identify with any faith specific group. Asian Americans tend to avoid discussing personal issues except with family members when seeking guidance (choice C). They value self-control, and hence they avoid showing feelings or emotions (choice D). Language barriers, especially for more recent immigrants, may be formidable, and require professional translators to ensure that there is proper communication with patients (choice E) and that information intended for the patient is not filtered by a well-meaning family member.

9. Correct answer: C

Married Hindu women wear a thread around their necks called *mangalsutra*. This thread should *not* be removed prior to providing care (choice C). Modesty is of great importance and caregivers of the same gender as the pa-

tient are preferred (choice A). Many Asian Indians prefer that the physician be in charge, and will usually follow the physician's advice without question (choice B). The elderly may behave stoically when in pain (choice E), so verbal clues to patient discomfort are important. In addition, as mental illness is considered a stigma, counseling for symptoms such as anxiety and depression is often refused (choice D).

10. Correct answer: E

Although Japanese Americans found advance directives useful as a way of reducing conflict between a dying person's wishes and the family's responsibility to sustain the dying patient, Japanese living in Japan viewed advance directives, especially written ones, as intrusive (choice E). Whether living in the United States or in Japan, Japanese had negative feelings toward living in adverse health states and receiving life-sustaining treatments (choice A) and feared being a physical, psychological, or financial burden on loved ones (choice B). Both groups preferred group-oriented decision making with family (choice D) and preferred dying before becoming end stage or physically frail (choice C).

Chapter 32

1. Correct answer: A

Although Judaism considers life to be of infinite value, Judaism recognizes terminal illness (choice A), defined in two ways: a prognosis of one year or less and the *goses* or actively dying patient. Providing food and fluid, even by artificial means, is considered basic care by most traditional Jews and should be provided to virtually all terminally ill Jewish patients (choice B), the only exception being if a knowledgeable rabbinic authority determines that a specific patient would be harmed by providing the food or fluid. Euthanasia, assisted suicide, or any form of intentional hastening of death is forbidden under Jewish law (choice C).

Withholding of treatment when patients are near the end of life may be permitted when the treatment is deemed ineffective, futile, or prolongs suffering, while withdrawing treatment in this situation is generally forbidden (choice D). Advance directives in the orthodox Jewish community must include that a rabbi knowledgeable in healthcare matters be named as a surrogate to ensure that all decisions are made according to Jewish law (choice E).

2. Correct answer: C

While travelling and using electricity are among the activities that are not permitted on the Sabbath, the Sabbath prohibitions are suspended when someone's life is threatened, even if the person is not expected to recover. Therefore, end-of-life caregivers are absolutely permitted to provide care to an observant Jewish patient on the Sabbath (choice C). Jews who follow the Jewish dietary laws, known as "kosher" are not allowed to eat meat and dairy foods together (choice A). During the Jewish holiday of Passover, Jews eat unleavened bread called Matzah (choice B) as well as attend a special holiday meal called a Seder. As orthodox Jews generally refrain from physical contact with members of the opposite gender with the exception of their spouse and immediate family members in private, orthodox Jewish patients may be uncomfortable if personal care is rendered by an individual of the opposite gender (choice D). On the Jewish New Year, Rosh Hashana, Jews listen to sounds that are blown on a ram's horn, called a Shofar (choice E).

3. Correct answer: D

There are a number of activities that mourners are forbidden to participate in during the *shiva* period. These include leaving the house, shaving and grooming, bathing for pleasure, wearing new or freshly laundered clothes, engaging in conjugal relations, and working or conducting normal business activities (choice D). During *shiva*, it is customary for friends to visit the mourners to provide comfort and support (choice C). If a Jewish person is having a traditional Jewish burial, end-of-life care staff should not clean the body after the patient has passed away (choice A). They should leave the cleaning of the body, including the removal of any dressings, catheters, or other medical paraphernalia to the Chevra Kadisha, or Jewish burial society, who are trained in the proper preparation of the body for the funeral and burial. Cremation is forbidden under Jewish law, although some groups in the Reform movement now permit it (choice B). Jews memorialize the deceased yearly on the anniversary of the death, known as *yahrzeit* (choice E).

4. Correct answer: D

One of the four major rules of Islamic medical ethics is that necessity overrides prohibition, meaning that items prohibited by Islamic law may be used to treat patients in cases of dire medical necessity (choice D). Euthanasia and assisted suicide are forbidden under Islamic law (choice A). While food and fluid should not be withheld orally, the prophet Muhammed discouraged forcing the sick to take food and fluid. Therefore, one is not obligated to force feed patients who cannot take food or fluid orally (choice B). The treatment of pain is considered to be very righteous under Islamic law. Nevertheless, patients may desire that pain medication be reduced or withheld so they may remain alert in order to pray right before death (choice C). The Islamic faith considers the telling of lies to be a great sin. Therefore, one is not permitted to lie to a Muslim patient about his prognosis (choice E).

5. Correct answer: B

After a death, loved ones are encouraged to remain calm, pray for the departed, and begin preparation for the burial. While it is permitted to grieve naturally, excessive emotional reactions such as wailing and thrashing about are forbidden (choice B). Prior to death, family should be with the dying person to provide comfort and remind the person of God's mercy and forgiveness (choice A). The funeral service is not held in a mosque, but is held in a courtyard or public square (choice C). Muslims are buried without a coffin when possible, with the body laying on the right side, facing Mecca (choice D). Muslims observe a 3-day mourning period after the loss of a loved one. Muslim widows, however, observe an extended mourning period of 4 months and 10 days during which she is not permitted to remarry, move from her home, or wear decorative clothing or jewelry (choice E).

6. Correct answer: D

Traditionally, the proper place for a Hindu person to be in order to experience a good death is on the ground (choice D) with the head facing north (choice B), and if possible, on the banks of the Ganges River. For this reason, traditional Hindu patients and families will request that the patient be placed on the ground during the dying process. According to the Hindu faith, a good death is said to occur at the proper astrological time (choice C). The deceased will have a tranquil facial expression with the eyes and the mouth slightly open (choice E). It is traditional that water from the Ganges River be placed on the lips of the deceased at the time of death (choice A).

7. Correct answer: A

While cremation is the most common form of disposition of the remains of a Hindu person who has passed on, there are exceptions. Small children and enlightened saints have bodies that are considered pure, and, therefore, they are buried rather than cremated (choice A). Hindu funerals generally take place as soon as possible, often within hours of the death (choice B). Three days after cremation, the eldest son collects the ashes and places them in the Ganges River or another location of importance to the family (choice C). Families in North America and Europe may sometimes arrange to have ashes returned to the Ganges River. Additionally, in the western world, some Hindu traditions have had to be modified. For example, rather than lighting a funeral pyre as would be the case in India, the eldest son presses the incinerator button at the crematorium (choice E). Following the funeral, there is a 13-day period of mourning during which family will demonstratively express grief (choice D). The expression of grief allows the family to then live on, unhindered by any emotions they might have otherwise suppressed.

8. Correct answer: C

The Ten Precepts of Buddhism are a set of principles that a Buddhist chooses to live by. When one is trying to adhere to the precepts, intention is more important than the action itself (choice C). So, for example, while taking a life is a violation of one of the precepts, doing so with the intent of protecting the lives of innocent children will have a very different karma than killing for pleasure or hatred. The precepts are not viewed as proscriptive commandments, rather, they are viewed as guidelines of wisdom and common sense (choice A). Failure to adhere to the precepts is seen as an opportunity for education and growth, rather than for sanction or punishment (choice B). The first five precepts are considered of primary importance, and Buddhists will vow to undertake the first five precepts on a regular basis (choice D). In addition, the first five precepts will often be recited by a member of the Buddhist spiritual community when visiting someone who is close to death (choice E).

9. Correct answer: E

When a Buddhist patient is close to death, it is often traditional to cleanse the patient and put him in clean clothes in order to allow him to feel fresh and comfortable prior to passing (choice E). Buddhists are expected to bear pain stoically and may, therefore, be reluctant to take analgesic medications (choice A). Buddhists are taught to cooperate with caregivers, especially physicians and nurses, in order to get well (choice B). When nearing death, Buddhist patients desire to be in a quiet place free of distractions, with visitors or caregivers sitting in relaxed silence (choice C). They often desire to have ritual objects surrounding them when death is near (choice D).

10. Correct answer: D

The day following the wake, the body is taken for cremation, as this is the usual final disposition of the body chosen by the vast majority of Buddhists (choice D). At the time of death, many Buddhist families will clean and dress the body as an expression of filial piety (choice A). Buddhist funerals are traditionally simple, solemn, and dignified (choice B). Guests coming to pay respects to the deceased should stand in front of the altar and either bow or observe a moment of silence (choice C). Any money given to family as tokens of condolence may be used to defray funeral expenses or be donated to charity in memory of the deceased (choice E).

Index

Note: Page locators followed by f and t indicate figure and table respectively.